DRUG THERAPY

DECISION MAKING GUIDE

DRUG THERAPY

DECISION MAKING GUIDE

W.B. SAUNDERS COMPANY
A Division of Harcourt Brace & Company
Philadelphia London Toronto Montreal Sydney Tokyo

W.B. SAUNDERS COMPANY
A Division of Harcourt Brace & Company

The Curtis Center
Independence Square West
Philadelphia, Pennsylvania 19106

Library of Congress Cataloging-in-Publication Data

Drug Therapy Decision Making Guide / James McCormack . . . [et al.].—
1st ed.
    p.   cm.
    ISBN 0–7216–4215–2
    1. Chemotherapy—Decision making.   I. McCormack, James P.
    [DNLM: 1. Drug Therapy.   2. Decision Making.   WB 330 D7976 1995]
    RM262.D685   1996
    615.5′8—dc20
    DNLM/DLC   95-2350

DRUG THERAPY DECISION MAKING GUIDE   ISBN 0–7216–4215–2

Printed in the United States of America.

Last digit is the print number: 9   8   7   6   5   4   3

Preface

"We are overwhelmed as it is, with an infinite abundance of vaunted medicaments, and here they add another one."

Thomas Syndenham (1624–1689)

"It is an art of no little importance to administer medicines properly; but it is an art of much greater and more difficult acquisition to know when to suspend or altogether omit them."

Philippe Pinel (1745–1826)

The rational use of medications requires that treatment should optimize the benefits relative to the risks of adverse effects, their impact on quality or duration of life, and the costs incurred by the patient or third-party payer. It is becoming increasingly difficult to achieve optimal therapy for patients due to the large number of drug products available and to the rapidly growing volume of information on beneficial and adverse outcomes of treatment. It is impossible for any individual clinician to weigh the various factors involved and to reach the best single decision in each case. It is possible, however, to adopt an approach to the decision making process that will provide reasonable, if not optimal, therapy for most patients.

In writing this book, we have attempted to make explicit an approach to drug therapy that takes into account the major factors to be considered when initiating, altering, or terminating drug therapy. This approach should help the clinician to decide whether, when, and how to initiate or alter drug therapy. The method used to prepare this book was aimed at identifying the important questions that a clinician must consider when making decisions regarding drug therapy, and providing recommendations that are consistent with the information available from the literature and which other clinicians have found useful in their practices. For this purpose, the editors adopted a "template" of questions that a clinician should consider in the decision-making process. The editors then worked with a group of authors who provided their responses to these questions.

Three different templates of questions were used and incorporated into the different sections of the book: Drug Therapy for Disease States; Drug-Induced Adverse Reactions; and specific Drug Monographs. All responses were subjected to review and comment by a number of reviewers and the editors. All sections were returned to the original authors for final consideration before publication. The material in the book has been written and edited by physicians, pharmacists, and nurses and thus incorporates many useful observations from each of these disciplines.

The Drug Therapy for Disease States section is intended to assist the clinician in making decisions about when and how to use or alter drug therapy in the treatment of a particular disease and to identify an appropriate drug to prescribe. The specific drug monograph can then be consulted for more specific information regarding the best approach when using the agent. In some cases the drug will already have been chosen, and the reader will prefer to go immediately to the drug monograph. The Drug-Induced Adverse Reactions section is intended to provide specific approaches for assessing and dealing with four of the most common drug-induced reactions and the life-threatening problem of anaphylaxis.

It is anticipated that by considering the specific questions and responses listed in each chapter or monograph the reader will be encouraged to make decisions that are based on explicit factors rather than relying solely on habitual or intuitive solutions. It is in this aspect of the decision process that this book differs considerably from other books, which are usually designed to help the reader find the answer to a specific question that he or she has posed. This book is intended to achieve the former without sacrificing the practically important components of the latter. Toward this end, the second fundamental difference between this and other books of drug therapy is that we have deliberately not included certain pharmacologic/pharmacokinetic information that can readily be found elsewhere, unless explicit reference to it is important in the decision making process. When possible, we have endeavored to provide the reader with a number of particularly useful references for situations in which access to the literature is necessary. The remaining recommendations reflect the judgment and approaches of the authors, as modified by the reviewers and editors. The reader will note that we have attempted to exclude the use of terms such as "use with caution" or "monitor closely," because these terms provide no useful guidance to the clinician. Instead, if the concern is sufficiently important to mention, we have attempted to be explicit in our recommendations. We have also attempted to provide specific starting doses for drugs (rather than ranges) to indicate a clear and reasonable starting point for therapy.

We recognize that the reader may not agree with every therapeutic suggestion in this book. In addition, new evidence may become available that will alter the approach to the treatment of a specific disease state or the use of a particular drug. Nonetheless, we hope the format for decision making that is presented in this book will be helpful to the clinician in identifying the most clinically important information from the expanding medical literature and that this will lead to a more explicit and rational approach to drug therapy.

James McCormack
Glen Brown
Marc Levine
Robert Rangno
John Ruedy

Contributors

Catherine Allaire, MDCM
  Resident, Department of Obstetrics and Gynecology, University of British Columbia, Vancouver, British Columbia, Canada

Juan R. Avila, Pharm.D.
  Assistant Professor, Department of Clinical Pharmacy, Duquesne University School of Pharmacy; Psychiatric Clinical Pharmacist, St. Francis Medical Center, Pittsburgh, Pennsylvania

Terry J. Baumann, Pharm.D.
  Clinical Manager, Munson Medical Center, Traverse City, Michigan

Ann Beardsell, B.Sc.(Pharm)
  Manager, Ambulatory Pharmacy Services, St. Paul's Hospital, Vancouver, British Columbia, Canada

J. Chris Bradberry, Pharm.D.
  Professor of Pharmacy Practice and Head, Section of Pharmacy Practice, College of Pharmacy, The University of Oklahoma Health Sciences Center, Oklahoma City, Oklahoma

Glen Brown, Pharm.D.
  Satellite Manager, Pharmacy Department, St. Paul's Hospital, Vancouver, British Columbia, Canada

Bruce C. Carleton, B.Pharm., Pharm.D.
  Assistant Professor, Faculty of Pharmaceutical Sciences, University of British Columbia, Program Director, Pharmacoeconomic and Clinical Drug Research, Department of Pharmacy, British Columbia's Children's Hospital, Vancouver, British Columbia, Canada

Deborah Stier Carson, Pharm.D.
  Associate Professor, Community Pharmacy Practice and Administration, Medical University of South Carolina, Charleston, South Carolina

Frances V. H. Chow, B.Sc.(Pharm)
  Clinical Instructor, University of British Columbia, Faculty of Pharmaceutical Sciences; Clinical Pharmacist, Special Care Nursery, Royal Columbian Hospital, New Westminster, British Columbia, Canada

Robert Dombrowski, Pharm.D.
  Department of Pharmacy Services, Cleveland Veterans Administration Medical Center, Cleveland, Ohio

Jonathan A. E. Fleming, M.B., FRCP(C)
  Associate Professor, Department of Psychiatry, Faculty of Medicine, University of British Columbia; Co-Director, Sleep Disorders Program, Vancouver Hospital and Health Sciences Centre, Vancouver, British Columbia, Canada

David Forrest, M.D., FRCPC
  Fellow, Infectious Diseases and Critical Care Medicine, Clinician Investigator Program, University of British Columbia, Vancouver, British Columbia, Canada

Alfred S. Gin, Pharm.D.
Assistant Professor, Faculty of Pharmacy, University of Manitoba; Clinical Pharmacist, Infectious Diseases, Department of Pharmaceutical Services, Health Sciences Centre, Winnipeg, Manitoba, Canada

Ruby E. Grymonpre, Pharm.D.
Associate Professor, Faculty of Pharmacy, University of Manitoba, Winnipeg, Manitoba, Canada

David R. P. Guay, Pharm.D.
Associate Professor, Department of Pharmacy Practice, University of Minnesota, Minneapolis, Minnesota; Clinical Specialist, Geriatric Pharmacy Program, St. Paul-Ramsey Medical Center, St. Paul, Minnesota

Stephen F. Hamilton, Pharm.D.
Associate Professor of Pharmacy Practice and Medicine, The University of Oklahoma College of Pharmacy, Oklahoma City, Oklahoma

Stan Horton, Pharm.D.
Clinical Instructor and Postdoctoral Fellow, The University of Oklahoma Health Sciences Center, Oklahoma City, Oklahoma

Peter Jewesson, Ph.D.
Associate Professor, Faculty of Pharmaceutical Sciences, University of British Columbia, Vancouver, British Columbia, Canada

Kelly W. Jones, Pharm.D.
Assistant Professor of Family Medicine and Assistant Professor of Pharmacy, Medical University of South Carolina, Charleston, South Carolina, and University of South Carolina, Columbia, South Carolina; Director of Pharmacology Education, McLeod Regional Medical Center, Florence, South Carolina

Angela Kim-Sing, B.Sc.(Chem.), Pharm.D.
Clinical Specialist, St. Paul's Hospital, and Clinical Assistant Professor, Faculty of Pharmaceutical Sciences, University of British Columbia, Vancouver, British Columbia, Canada

Lyle K. Laird, Pharm.D.
Clinical Pharmacologist, San Antonio State Hospital; Clinical Assistant Professor, College of Pharmacy, The University of Texas at Austin and Clinical Pharmacy Programs at San Antonio, Departments of Pharmacology and Psychiatry, The University of Texas Health Science Center at San Antonio, San Antonio, Texas

Catherine Ann MacDougall, Pharm.D.
Assistant Clinical Professor, University of British Columbia; Clinical Pharmacy Specialist, Vancouver Hospital and Health Sciences Centre, Vancouver, British Columbia, Canada

Douglas L. Malyuk, B.Sc.(Pharm.), Pharm.D.
Clinical Assistant Professor, Faculty of Pharmaceutical Sciences, University of British Columbia, Vancouver, British Columbia; Assistant Director of Pharmacy Services (Clinical), Royal Columbian Hospital, New Westminster, British Columbia, Canada

Patricia Marken, Pharm.D.
Associate Professor of Pharmacy Practice and Psychiatry, Schools of Pharmacy and Medicine, University of Missouri/Kansas City; Psychopharmacy Specialist, Western Missouri Mental Health Center, Kansas City, Missouri

Leslie Mathews, B.Sc.N., R.N.
Certified Poison Information Specialist, B.C. Drug and Poison Information Centre, University of British Columbia, Vancouver, British Columbia, Canada

James McCormack, B.Sc.(Pharm), Pharm.D.
Associate Professor, Faculty of Pharmaceutical Sciences, University of British Columbia, Vancouver, British Columbia, Canada

Glenda Meneilly, B.S.P., Pharm.D.
  Assistant Professor of Clinical Pharmacy and Director, Pharm.D. Program, University of British Columbia; Clinical Pharmacist, British Columbia's Women's Hospital, Vancouver, British Columbia, Canada

Penny F. Miller, B.Sc.(Pharm.), M.A.
  Senior Instructor, Faculty of Pharmaceutical Sciences and Department of Family Practice, University of British Columbia, Vancouver, British Columbia, Canada

Julio Montaner, M.D., FRCPC, FCCP
  Associate Professor of Medicine, Department of Medicine, University of British Columbia; Director, AIDS Research and Infectious Disease Clinic, St. Paul's Hospital, Vancouver, British Columbia, Canada

Lynne Nakashima, B.Sc.(Pharm), Pharm.D.
  Clinical Assistant Professor, University of British Columbia; Coordinator, Clinical Services, British Columbia Cancer Agency, Vancouver Cancer Centre, Vancouver, British Columbia, Canada

Cindy Reesor Nimmo, M.Pharm.
  Clinical Assistant Professor, University of British Columbia, Faculty of Pharmaceutical Sciences; Clinical Pharmacy Specialist, Vancouver Hospital and Health Sciences Centre, Vancouver, British Columbia, Canada

Richard I. Ogilvie, M.D., FRCPC, FACP
  Professor of Medicine and Pharmacology, University of Toronto; Clinical Pharmacologist, The Toronto Hospital, Toronto, Ontario, Canada

Jack Onrot, B.Sc., M.D., FRCP(C)
  Clinical Associate Professor of Medicine, University of British Columbia; Consultant, Staff, St. Paul's Hospital, Vancouver, British Columbia, Canada

William A. Parker, B.Sc.(Pharm.), Pharm.D., M.B.A., FCSHP
  Instructor, School of Health Record Science, Camp Hill Medical Centre, Halifax, Nova Scotia; Pharmacist, Shoppers Drug Mart, Dartmouth, Nova Scotia, Canada

Nilufar Partovi, Pharm.D.
  Clinical Pharmacotherapeutic Specialist, Solid Organ Transplantation, Vancouver Hospital and Health Sciences Centre; Clinical Assistant Professor, Faculty of Pharmaceutical Sciences, University of British Columbia, Vancouver, British Columbia, Canada

Ian Petterson, B.Sc.(Pharm)
  Clinical Pharmacist, Pharmacy Department, Shuswap Lake General Hospital, Salmon Arm, British Columbia, Canada

Peter Phillips, M.D., FRCPC
  Clinical Associate Professor, Division of Infectious Diseases, University of British Columbia and St. Paul's Hospital, Vancouver, British Columbia, Canada

Robert Rangno, B.Sc., M.Sc., M.D., FRCP(C)
  Associate Professor, Departments of Medicine and Pharmacology, University of British Columbia; Head, Division of Clinical Pharmacology, St. Paul's Hospital, Vancouver, British Columbia, Canada

John C. Rotschafer, B.S., Pharm.D.
  Professor, College of Pharmacy, University of Minnesota, Minneapolis, Minnesota; Director, Antibiotic Pharmacokinetics Consulting Service, St. Paul Ramsey Medical Center, St. Paul, Minnesota

Robert Schellenberg, M.D.
  Professor, Department of Medicine, University of British Columbia; Active Staff, St. Paul's Hospital, Vancouver, British Columbia, Canada

Otto L. A. Schlappner, M.D., FRCP(C), FABD
  Clinical Associate Professor of Medicine and Dermatology, University of British Columbia; Active Staff, St. Paul's Hospital, Vancouver, British Columbia, Canada

Christy Silvius Scott, Pharm.D.
Assistant Professor, Division of Pharmacy Practice, School of Pharmacy, The University of North Carolina; Clinical Pharmacy Specialist, North Carolina Children's Hospital, Chapel Hill, North Carolina

Karen F. Shalansky, Pharm.D.
Clinical Assistant Professor, University of British Columbia, Faculty of Pharmaceutical Sciences; Clinical Pharmacy Specialist, Vancouver Hospital and Health Sciences Centre, Vancouver, British Columbia, Canada

Stephen Shalansky, Pharm.D.
Clinical Pharmacist, Pharmacy Department, Lions Gate Hospital, North Vancouver, British Columbia, Canada

Steven W. Stanislav, Pharm.D.
Clinical Assistant Professor, College of Pharmacy, The University of Texas at Austin; Clinical Pharmacologist, The Healthcare Rehabilitation Center and Austin State Hospital, Austin, Texas

Jerry W. Taylor, Pharm.D., B.C.P.S.
Clinical Pharmacy Specialist, St. Joseph Hospital and Health Center, Bryan, Texas

Udho Thadani, M.B.B.S., MRCP, FRCP(C), FACC
Professor of Medicine, Vice Chief of Cardiology, and Director of Clinical Research, Cardiology Section, University of Oklahoma Health Sciences Center, Oklahoma City, Oklahoma

James E. Tisdale, B.Sc.(Pharm), Pharm.D.
Assistant Professor, College of Pharmacy and Allied Health Professions, Wayne State University; Coordinator, Education and Training, Department of Pharmacy Services, Henry Ford Hospital, Detroit, Michigan

Kyle Vance-Bryan, Pharm.D.
Assistant Professor of Pharmacy, College of Pharmacy, University of Minnesota, Minneapolis; Critical Care Specialist, Section of Clinical Pharmacology, St. Paul-Ramsey Medical Center, St. Paul, Minnesota

Julia Vertrees, Pharm.D.
Clinical Pharmacologist, San Antonio State Hospital; Clinical Assistant Professor, College of Pharmacy, The University of Texas at Austin and Clinical Pharmacy Programs at San Antonio, Department of Pharmacology, The University of Texas Health Science Center at San Antonio, San Antonio, Texas

C. Wayne Weart, Pharm.D.
Professor of Community Pharmacy Practice and Administration and Associate Professor of Family Medicine, Medical University of South Carolina, Charleston, South Carolina

J. Scott Whittaker, B.Sc., M.D.
Clinical Assistant Professor, University of British Columbia; Active Staff, St. Paul's Hospital, Vancouver, British Columbia, Canada

Eric M. Yoshida, M.D., FRCPC
Gastroenterology Fellow, Department of Medicine, University of British Columbia, Vancouver, British Columbia, Canada

Rick Zabinski, Pharm.D.
Manager, Medical Education, Miles Inc., West Haven, Connecticut

George G. Zhanel, Pharm.D., Ph.D.
Associate Professor and Head, Division of Clinical Sciences, Faculty of Pharmacy, and Assistant Professor, Department of Medical Microbiology, Section of Infectious Diseases, Faculty of Medicine, University of Manitoba; Coordinator of Antibiotic Research Program, Section of Infection Control, Department of Medicine, Health Sciences Centre, Winnipeg, Manitoba, Canada

Reviewers

How to Use This Book

This book is divided into two sections. Section I provides suggestions for the use of drugs in the treatment of more than 50 different disease states. This section is divided alphabetically into nine different areas: cardiovascular, endocrinology, gastrointestinal, infectious diseases/AIDS-related illness; neurology, obstetrics/gynecology, psychiatry, respiratory, and rheumatology. Each area is divided into topics on drug therapy for common disease states or conditions that are found in these areas. The last chapter in this section provides suggestions for the treatment of five specific drug-induced adverse reactions. Section II provides information on more than 300 commonly used drugs. Drugs within this section are listed alphabetically by generic name.

All chapters or monographs in each section are written in a similar format to allow the reader to become familiar with the location of specific information. The following formats are used within each chapter or monograph.

Section I, Chapters 1 to 10 (Drug Therapy for Disease States)

What Are My Goals of Treatment?
What Evidence Is Available to Support Drug Therapy?
When Should I Consider Drug Therapy?
What Drug Should I Use as Initial Treatment?
What Dosage Should I Use?
How Long Should I Treat with My Initial Regimen?
What Efficacy Parameters Should I Follow, and How Frequently Do I Have to Assess My Patient?
Should I Add Another Drug or Substitute Therapy if My Initial Drug Therapy Fails?
How Long Should I Continue Drug Therapy?

Section I, Chapter 11 (Drug-Induced Adverse Reactions)

My Patient Has Developed an Adverse Reaction; How Do I Determine if This Is Drug Induced?
What Drugs Are Most Likely to Cause This Adverse Reaction?
What Are the Characteristics of This Adverse Reaction?
How Do I Treat This Adverse Reaction?
How Quickly Should My Patient Respond, and What Should I Monitor with Regard to Efficacy of My Treatment?
Do I Have to Stop the Administration of the Drug That Is Causing This Adverse Reaction?
How Long Should I Treat This Adverse Reaction?

Section II (Drug Monographs)

When Should I Use This Drug?
When Should I Not Use This Drug?
What Contraindications Are There to the Use of This Drug?
What Drug Interactions Are Clinically Important?
What Route and Dosage Should I Use?
What Should I Monitor with Regard to Efficacy and Toxicity?
How Long Do I Treat Patients with This Drug?
How Do I Decrease or Stop the Administration of This Drug?
What Should I Tell My Patient About This Drug?
Therapeutic Tips for the Use of This Drug

Contents

I Drug Therapy for Disease States

1 CARDIOVASCULAR DISEASES 2

DRUG THERAPY FOR HYPERTENSION, 2
James McCormack and Robert Rangno

DRUG THERAPY FOR CONGESTIVE HEART FAILURE, 9
Jack Onrot

DRUG THERAPY FOR ISCHEMIC HEART DISEASE (ANGINAL SYNDROMES AND MYOCARDIAL INFARCTION), 13
Stephen F. Hamilton, Stan Horton, and Udho Thadani

DRUG THERAPY FOR CARDIAC ARRHYTHMIAS, 22
James E. Tisdale

DRUG THERAPY FOR RAYNAUD'S SYNDROME, 30
Richard I. Ogilvie

DRUG THERAPY FOR INTERMITTENT CLAUDICATION, 31
Richard I. Ogilvie

DRUG THERAPY FOR PULMONARY EMBOLISM OR DEEP VEIN THROMBOSIS, 32
Douglas L. Malyuk

DRUG THERAPY FOR HYPERLIPIDEMIAS, 34
Stephen Shalansky and Robert Dombrowski

DRUG THERAPY FOR ISCHEMIC CEREBROVASCULAR DISEASE, 37
J. Chris Bradberry

2 ENDOCRINOLOGICAL DISORDERS 41

DRUG THERAPY FOR DIABETES MELLITUS, 41
Christy Silvius Scott

DRUG THERAPY FOR HYPOTHYROIDISM, 49
Ruby E. Grymonpre

3 GASTROINTESTINAL DISEASES 50

DRUG THERAPY FOR GASTROESOPHAGEAL REFLUX, 50
James McCormack and Glen Brown

DRUG THERAPY FOR PEPTIC ULCER DISEASE AND STRESS ULCERS, 51
James McCormack and Glen Brown

DRUG THERAPY FOR INFLAMMATORY BOWEL DISEASE, 56
J. Scott Whittaker

DRUG THERAPY FOR CONSTIPATION, 60
Leslie Mathews

DRUG THERAPY FOR NAUSEA AND VOMITING, 64
Lynne Nakashima

4 INFECTIOUS DISEASES 69

DRUG THERAPY FOR URINARY TRACT INFECTION, 69
George G. Zhanel

DRUG THERAPY FOR PNEUMONIA, 74
James McCormack

DRUG THERAPY FOR INTRAABDOMINAL INFECTIONS, 78
David R. P. Guay

DRUG THERAPY FOR INFECTIVE ENDOCARDITIS, 80
John C. Rotschafer

DRUG THERAPY FOR MENINGITIS, 83
James McCormack

DRUG THERAPY FOR SEXUALLY TRANSMITTED DISEASES, 85
Catherine Allaire and James McCormack

DRUG THERAPY FOR SOFT TISSUE INFECTIONS, 91
Catherine Ann MacDougall and James McCormack

DRUG THERAPY FOR OSTEOMYELITIS, 94
Catherine Ann MacDougall and James McCormack

DRUG THERAPY FOR THE PREVENTION OF POSTOPERATIVE INFECTIONS, 96
David Forrest

DRUG THERAPY FOR COUGHS AND THE COMMON COLD, 98
Penny F. Miller

5   AIDS-RELATED ILLNESS 100
DRUG THERAPY FOR HUMAN IMMUNODEFICIENCY VIRUS INFECTION, 100
Julio Montaner and Peter Phillips

DRUG THERAPY FOR *PNEUMOCYSTIS CARINII* PNEUMONIA, 102
Julio Montaner and Peter Phillips

DRUG THERAPY FOR HIV-RELATED CANDIDIASIS, 103
Peter Phillips

DRUG THERAPY FOR AIDS-RELATED CYTOMEGALOVIRUS DISEASE, 105
Peter Phillips

DRUG THERAPY FOR CEREBRAL TOXOPLASMOSIS IN PATIENTS WITH AIDS, 106
Peter Phillips

DRUG THERAPY FOR CRYPTOCOCCAL MENINGITIS IN PATIENTS WITH AIDS, 107
Peter Phillips

DRUG THERAPY FOR AIDS-RELATED *MYCOBACTERIUM AVIUM* INFECTION, 108
Peter Phillips

DRUG THERAPY FOR HIV-RELATED HERPES SIMPLEX VIRUS (HSV) INFECTION, 110
Peter Phillips

DRUG THERAPY FOR HIV-RELATED VARICELLA-ZOSTER VIRUS INFECTIONS, 111
Peter Phillips

6   NEUROLOGICAL DISEASES 113
DRUG THERAPY FOR EPILEPSY, 113
William A. Parker

DRUG THERAPY FOR PARKINSON'S DISEASE, 117
Ruby E. Grymonpre

DRUG THERAPY FOR PAIN, 119
Terry J. Baumann

DRUG THERAPY FOR MIGRAINE HEADACHE, 124
Jerry W. Taylor

7   OBSTETRICAL AND GYNECOLOGICAL CONDITIONS 128
DRUG THERAPY FOR BIRTH CONTROL, 128
Deborah Stier Carson

DRUG THERAPY FOR LABOR INDUCTION, 132
Glenda Meneilly

DRUG THERAPY FOR LABOR INHIBITION, 134
Glenda Meneilly

8 PSYCHIATRIC DISORDERS 136

DRUG THERAPY FOR DEPRESSION, 136
Lyle K. Laird and Julia Vertres

DRUG THERAPY FOR PSYCHOSIS, 139
Juan R. Avila and Patricia Marken

DRUG THERAPY FOR ANXIETY DISORDERS, 143
Steven W. Stanislav and Patricia Marken

DRUG THERAPY FOR BIPOLAR DISORDERS, 147
Steven W. Stanislav and Patricia Marken

DRUG THERAPY FOR INSOMNIA, 150
Jonathan A. E. Fleming

9 RESPIRATORY DISEASES 154

DRUG THERAPY FOR ASTHMA AND CHRONIC OBSTRUCTIVE PULMONARY DISEASE, 154
Karen F. Shalansky and Cindy Reesor Nimmo

10 RHEUMATIC DISEASES 158

DRUG THERAPY FOR RHEUMATOID ARTHRITIS AND OSTEOARTHRITIS, 158
Kelly W. Jones

DRUG THERAPY FOR OSTEOPOROSIS, 163
Deborah Stier Carson

DRUG THERAPY FOR GOUT, 166
C. Wayne Weart

11 DRUG-INDUCED ADVERSE REACTIONS 168

DRUG-INDUCED SKIN RASH, 168
Otto L. A. Schlappner

DRUG-INDUCED ANAPHYLAXIS, 171
Robert Schellenberg

DRUG-INDUCED DIARRHEA, 172
James McCormack

DRUG-INDUCED CONSTIPATION, 174
Leslie Mathews

DRUG-INDUCED NAUSEA AND VOMITING, 176
Lynne Nakashima

II Drug Monographs

ACEBUTOLOL, 181
Robert Rangno and James McCormack

ACETAMINOPHEN, 181
Terry J. Baumann and Jerry W. Taylor

ACETOHEXAMIDE, 182
Christy Silvius Scott

ACYCLOVIR, 182
Ann Beardsell

ADENOSINE, 184
James E. Tisdale

ALLOPURINOL, 185
C. Wayne Weart

ALPRAZOLAM, 186
Steven W. Stanislav and Patricia Marken

AMANTADINE, 187
Ruby E. Grymonpre

AMIKACIN, 189
David R. P. Guay and Ann Beardsell

AMILORIDE, 190
Ian Petterson

AMINOPHYLLINE, 191
Karen F. Shalansky and Cindy Reeser Nimmo

AMIODARONE, 192
James E. Tisdale

AMITRIPTYLINE, 194
Lyle K. Laird and Julia Vertrees

AMOXAPINE, 195
Lyle K. Laird and Julia Vertrees

AMOXICILLIN, 195
John C. Rotschafer and Kyle Vance-Bryan

AMOXICILLIN-CLAVULANATE, 196
John C. Rotschafer, Kyle Vance-Bryan,
and Rick Zabinski

AMPHOTERICIN B, 197
Peter Jewesson

AMPICILLIN, 199
John C. Rotschafer, Kyle Vance-Bryan,
and Rick Zabinski

AMPICILLIN-SULBACTAM, 200
John C. Rotschafer, Kyle Vance-Bryan,
and Rick Zabinski

ANTACIDS, 200
James McCormack

ASPIRIN, 202
Kelly W. Jones, Terry J. Baumann,
and Jerry W. Taylor

ASTEMIZOLE, 205
Penny F. Miller

ATENOLOL, 206
Robert Rangno and James McCormack

AZATHIOPRINE, 207
Kelly W. Jones and J. Scott Whittaker

AZTREONAM, 208
James McCormack

BACAMPICILLIN, 209
John C. Rotschafer, Kyle Vance-Bryan,
and Rick Zabinski

BECLOMETHASONE DIPROPIONATE, 209
Karen F. Shalansky and Cindy Reeser Nimmo

BENAZEPRIL, 211
Jack Onrot and James McCormack

BENDROFLUMETHIAZIDE
(BENDROFLUAZIDE), 211
Ian Petterson

BENZTROPINE, 212
Ruby E. Grymonpre

BETAXOLOL, 213
Robert Rangno and James McCormack

BIPERIDEN, 213
Ruby E. Grymonpre

BISACODYL, 213
Leslie Mathews

BITOLTEROL, 215
Karen F. Shalansky and Cindy Reesor Nimmo

BRETYLIUM TOSYLATE, 215
James E. Tisdale

BROMOCRIPTINE, 216
Ruby E. Grymonpre

BUDESONIDE, 217
Karen F. Shalansky and Cindy Reesor Nimmo

BULK-FORMING LAXATIVES, 218
Leslie Mathews

BUMETANIDE, 221
Ian Petterson

BUPRENORPHINE, 221
Terry J. Baumann

BUPROPION, 222
Lyle K. Laird and Julia Vertrees

BUSPIRONE, 223
Steven W. Stanislav and Patricia Marken

BUTORPHANOL, 225
Terry J. Baumann

CALCITONIN, 225
Deborah Stier Carson

CALCIUM, 226
Eric M. Yoshida and Angela Kim-Sing

CAPTOPRIL, 228
Jack Onrot and James McCormack

CARBAMAZEPINE, 232
William A. Parker, Steven W. Stanislav,
and Patricia Marken

CARTEOLOL, 235
Robert Rangno and James McCormack

CASCARA, 235
Leslie Mathews

CASTOR OIL, 236
Leslie Mathews

CEFACLOR, 236
Bruce C. Carleton

CEFAMANDOLE, 236
Bruce C. Carleton

CEFAZOLIN, 236
Bruce C. Carleton

CEFIXIME, 238
Bruce C. Carleton

CEFONICID, 239
Bruce C. Carleton

CEFOPERAZONE, 239
Bruce C. Carleton

CEFORANIDE, 239
Bruce C. Carleton

CEFOTAXIME, 239
Bruce C. Carleton

CEFOTETAN, 240
Bruce C. Carleton

CEFOXITIN, 241
Bruce C. Carleton

CEFTAZIDIME, 242
Bruce C. Carleton

CEFTIZOXIME, 243
Bruce C. Carleton

CEFTRIAXONE, 244
Bruce C. Carleton

CEFUROXIME, CEFUROXIME AXETIL, 245
Bruce C. Carleton

CEPHALEXIN, 246
Bruce C. Carleton

CEPHRADINE, 247
Bruce C. Carleton

CHLORAL HYDRATE, 247
Jonathan A. E. Fleming

CHLORAMPHENICOL, 247
George G. Zhanel and Alfred S. Gin

CHLORDIAZEPOXIDE, 248
Steven W. Stanislav and Patricia Marken

CHLORPROMAZINE, 248
Juan R. Avila and Patricia Marken

CHLORPROPAMIDE, 251
Christy Silvius Scott

CHLORTHALIDONE, 252
Ian Petterson

CHLORPHENIRAMINE, 253
Penny F. Miller

CHOLESTYRAMINE, 255
Stephen Shalansky and Robert Dombrowski

CHOLINE MAGNESIUM TRISALICYLATE, 256
Kelly W. Jones

CIMETIDINE, 257
James McCormack and Glen Brown

CIPROFLOXACIN, 259
Peter Jewesson

CLINDAMYCIN, 261
David R. P. Guay and Ann Beardsell

CLOFAZIMINE, 263
Ann Beardsell

CLOFIBRATE, 264
Stephen Shalansky and Robert Dombrowski

CLOMIPRAMINE, 264
Lyle K. Laird and Julia Vertrees

CLONAZEPAM, 265
Steven W. Stanislav, Patricia Marken,
and William A. Parker

CLOTRIMAZOLE, 267
Peter Jewesson

CLOXACILLIN, 268
John C. Rotschafer, Kyle Vance-Bryan,
and Rick Zabinski

CODEINE, 269
Terry J. Baumann

COLCHICINE, 269
C. Wayne Weart

COLESTIPOL, 271
Stephen Shalansky and Robert Dombrowski

CROMOLYN, 272
Karen F. Shalansky and Cindy Reesor Nimmo

CYCLOPHOSPHAMIDE, 273
Kelly W. Jones

CYCLOSPORINE, 274
Nilufar Partovi

CYPROHEPTADINE, 277
Jerry W. Taylor

DANTHRON, 277
Leslie Mathews

DAPSONE, 278
Ann Beardsell

DESIPRAMINE, 279
Lyle K. Laird and Julia Vertrees

DEXAMETHASONE, 280
Karen F. Shalansky and Cindy Reesor Nimmo

DEXTROMETHORPHAN, 280
Penny F. Miller

DIAZEPAM, 281
Steven W. Stanislav and Patricia Marken

DICLOFENAC, 283
Kelly W. Jones

DICLOXACILLIN, 283
John C. Rotschafer, Kyle Vance-Bryan,
and Rick Zabinski

DIFLUNISAL, 283
Kelly W. Jones

DIGOXIN, 284
Jack Onrot

DIHYDROERGOTAMINE, 286
Jerry W. Taylor

DILTIAZEM, 287
Stephen F. Hamilton, Stan Horton,
and Udho Thadani

DIMENHYDRINATE, 290
Lynne Nakashima

DIPHENHYDRAMINE, 291
Penny F. Miller

DIPYRIDAMOLE, 292
J. Chris Bradberry

DISOPYRAMIDE, 293
James E. Tisdale

DOCUSATE, 294
Leslie Mathews

DOMPERIDONE, 295
Lynne Nakashima

DOXEPIN, 295
Lyle K. Laird and Julia Vertrees

DOXYCYCLINE, 297
Alfred S. Gin and George G. Zhanel

DRONABINOL, 298
Lynne Nakashima

DROPERIDOL, 298
Lynne Nakashima

DYPHYLLINE, 299
Karen F. Shalansky and Cindy Reesor Nimmo

ENALAPRIL, 299
Jack Onrot and James McCormack

EPHEDRINE, 300
Karen F. Shalansky and Cindy Reesor Nimmo

EPINEPHRINE, 300
Karen F. Shalansky and Cindy Reesor Nimmo

ERGOTAMINE TARTRATE, 301
Jerry W. Taylor

ERYTHROMYCIN, 303
Alfred S. Gin and George G. Zhanel

ESMOLOL, 305
Robert Rangno and James McCormack

ESTROGENS, 306
Deborah Stier Carson

ETHAMBUTOL, 308
Ann Beardsell

ETHOSUXIMIDE, 309
William A. Parker

ETODOLAC, 311
Kelly W. Jones

FAMOTIDINE, 311
James McCormack and Glen Brown

FENOFIBRATE, 312
Stephen Shalansky and Robert Dombrowski

FENOPROFEN, 313
Kelly W. Jones

FENOTEROL, 313
Karen F. Shalansky and Cindy Reesor Nimmo

FENTANYL, 313
Terry J. Baumann

FLECAINIDE, 314
James E. Tisdale

FLUCLOXACILLIN, 316
John C. Rotschafer, Kyle Vance-Bryan,
and Rick Zabinski

FLUCONAZOLE, 316
Peter Jewesson

FLUCYTOSINE (5-FC,5-fluorocytosine), 317
Peter Jewesson

FLUNISOLIDE, 319
Karen F. Shalansky and Cindy Reesor Nimmo

FLUOXETINE, 319
Lyle K. Laird and Julia Vertrees

FLUPHENAZINE, 320
Juan R. Avila and Patricia Marken

FLURBIPROFEN, 321
Kelly W. Jones

FOLIC ACID, 322
Eric M. Yoshida and Angela Kim-Sing

FOSINOPRIL, 323
Jack Onrot and James McCormack

FUROSEMIDE, 324
Ian Petterson

GANCICLOVIR, 326
Ann Beardsell

GEMFIBROZIL, 328
Stephen Shalansky and Robert Dombrowski

GENTAMICIN, 329
David R. P. Guay

GLICLAZIDE, 333
Christy Silvius Scott

GLIPIZIDE, 333
Christy Silvius Scott

GLYBURIDE (GLIBENCLAMIDE), 334
Christy Silvius Scott

GLYCERIN, 335
Leslie Mathews

GOLD COMPLEXES, 335
Kelly W. Jones

GUAIFENESIN, 337
Penny F. Miller

HALOPERIDOL, 338
Juan R. Avila and Patricia Marken

HEPARIN, 339
Frances V. H. Chow

HYDROCHLOROTHIAZIDE, 341
Ian Petterson

HYDROCORTISONE SODIUM SUCCINATE, 345
Karen F. Shalansky and Cindy Reesor Nimmo

HYDROMORPHONE, 345
Terry J. Baumann

HYDROXYCHLOROQUINE, 347
Kelly W. Jones

IBUPROFEN, 348
Kelly W. Jones, Terry J. Baumann,
and Jerry W. Taylor

IMIPENEM-CILASTATIN, 350
James McCormack

IMIPRAMINE, 351
Lyle K. Laird and Julia Vertrees

INDAPAMIDE, 355
Ian Petterson

INDOMETHACIN, 355
C. Wayne Weart

INSULIN, 356
Christy Silvius Scott

IPRATROPIUM, 362
Karen F. Shalansky and Cindy Reesor Nimmo

IRON, 363
Eric M. Yoshida and Angela Kim-Sing

ISOCARBOXAZID, 365
Lyle K. Laird and Julia Vertrees

ISOMETHEPTENE MUCATE, 365
Jerry W. Taylor

ISONIAZID, 365
Ann Beardsell

ISOPROTERENOL, 367
Karen F. Shalansky and Cindy Reesor Nimmo

KETOCONAZOLE, 367
Peter Jewesson

KETOPROFEN, 368
Kelly W. Jones

KETOROLAC, 369
Kelly W. Jones

KETOTIFEN, 370
Karen F. Shalansky and Cindy Reesor Nimmo

LABETALOL, 371
Robert Rangno and James McCormack

LACTULOSE, 372
Leslie Mathews

LEVODOPA-BENSERAZIDE, 373
Ruby E. Grymonpre

LEVODOPA-CARBIDOPA, 374
Ruby E. Grymonpre

LEVORPHANOL, 376
Terry J. Baumann

LEVOTHYROXINE, 376
Ruby E. Grymonpre

LIDOCAINE, 377
James E. Tisdale

LISINOPRIL, 379
Jack Onrot and James McCormack

LITHIUM, 380
Steven W. Stanislav and Patricia Marken

LORATADINE, 381
Penny F. Miller

LORAZEPAM, 382
Steven W. Stanislav, Patricia Marken,
William A. Parker, and Jonathan A. E. Fleming

LOVASTATIN, 385
Stephen Shalansky and Robert Dombrowski

LOXAPINE, 387
Juan R. Avila and Patricia Marken

MAGNESIUM, 388
Leslie Mathews, James McCormack,
and Glenda Meneilly

MAPROTILINE, 390
Lyle K. Laird and Julia Vertrees

MECLIZINE, 390
Lynne Nakashima

MECLOFENAMATE, 391
Kelly W. Jones

MEFENAMIC ACID, 391
Kelly W. Jones

MEPERIDINE, 391
Terry J. Baumann

MESALAMINE (5-AMINOSALICYLIC ACID), 392
J. Scott Whittaker

METFORMIN, 394
Christy Silvius Scott

METHADONE, 395
Terry J. Baumann

METHOTREXATE, 396
Kelly W. Jones

METHYLPREDNISOLONE, 398
Karen F. Shalansky and Cindy Reesor Nimmo

METHYSERGIDE, 399
Jerry W. Taylor

METOCLOPRAMIDE, 400
Lynne Nakashima

METOLAZONE, 402
Ian Petterson

METOPROLOL, 402
Robert Rangno and James McCormack

METRONIDAZOLE, 403
David R. P. Guay

MEXILETINE, 405
James E. Tisdale

MICONAZOLE, 406
Peter Jewesson

MINERAL OIL, 408
Leslie Mathews

MINOCYCLINE, 408
Alfred S. Gin and George G. Zhanel

MISOPROSTOL, 408
James McCormack and Glen Brown

MORICIZINE, 409
James E. Tisdale

MORPHINE, 410
Terry J. Baumann

MULTIVITAMIN PREPARATIONS, 413
Angela Kim-Sing and Eric Yoshida

NABILONE, 414
Lynne Nakashima

NABUMETONE, 415
Kelly W. Jones

NADOLOL, 416
Robert Rangno and James McCormack

NAFCILLIN, 420
John C. Rotschafer, Kyle Vance-Bryan,
and Rick Zabinski

NALBUPHINE, 421
Terry J. Baumann

NALIDIXIC ACID, 421
Peter Jewesson

NALOXONE, 422
Terry J. Baumann

NAPROXEN, 422
Kelly W. Jones

NETILMICIN, 423
David R. P. Guay

NIACIN, 423
Stephen Shalansky and Robert Dombrowski

NIFEDIPINE, 424
Stephen F. Hamilton, Stan Horton,
and Udho Thadani

NITROFURANTOIN, 426
George G. Zhanel

NITROGLYCERIN, 427
Stephen F. Hamilton, Stan Horton,
and Udho Thadani

NIZATIDINE, 431
James McCormack and Glen Brown

NORFLOXACIN, 431
Peter Jewesson

NORTRIPTYLINE, 432
Lyle K. Laird and Julia Vertrees

NYSTATIN, 433
Peter Jewesson

OMEPRAZOLE, 434
James McCormack and Glen Brown

ONDANSETRON, 435
Lynne Nakashima

ORCIPRENALINE, METAPROTERENOL, 436
Karen F. Shalansky and Cindy Reesor Nimmo

ORPHENADRINE, 436
Ruby E. Grymonpre

OXACILLIN, 436
John C. Rotschafer, Kyle Vance-Bryan,
and Rick Zabinski

OXAPROZIN, 436
Kelly W. Jones

OXAZEPAM, 437
Steven W. Stanislav, Patricia Marken,
and Jonathan A. E. Fleming

OXTRIPHYLLINE, 437
Karen F. Shalansky and Cindy Reesor Nimmo

OXYCODONE, 438
Terry J. Baumann

OXYTOCIN, 438
Glenda Meneilly

PARALDEHYDE, 440
Jonathan A. E. Fleming

PENBUTOLOL, 440
Robert Rangno and James McCormack

PENICILLAMINE, 440
Kelly W. Jones

PENICILLIN, 442
John C. Rotschafer, Kyle Vance-Bryan,
and Rick Zabinski

PENTAMIDINE, 445
Ann Beardsell

PENTAZOCINE, 447
Terry J. Baumann

PENTOBARBITAL, 447
Jonathan A. E. Fleming

PENTOXIFYLLINE, 447
Richard I. Ogilvie

PERPHENAZINE, 448
Lynne Nakashima

PHENELZINE, 448
Lyle K. Laird and Julia Vertrees

PHENOBARBITAL, 451
William A. Parker and Jonathan A. E. Fleming

PHENOLPHTHALEIN, 453
Leslie Mathews

PHENYLBUTAZONE, 453
Kelly W. Jones

PHENYLPROPANOLAMINE, 453
Penny F. Miller

PHENYTOIN, 454
William A. Parker

PHOSPHORUS, 458
Angela Kim-Sing and Eric Yoshida

PIMOZIDE, 459
Juan R. Avila and Patricia Marken

PINDOLOL, 459
Robert Rangno and James McCormack

PIPERACILLIN, 460
John C. Rotschafer, Kyle Vance-Bryan,
and Rick Zabinski

PIRENZPINE, 461
James McCormack and Glen Brown

PIROXICAM, 461
Kelly W. Jones

POLYETHYLENE GLYCOL-ELECTROLYTE
SOLUTION, 461
Leslie Mathews

POTASSIUM, 463
Eric Yoshida and Angela Kim-Sing

PRAVASTATIN, 465
Stephen Shalansky and Robert Dombrowski

PREDNISONE, 465
Karen F. Shalansky, Cindy Reesor Nimmo,
and J. Scott Whittaker

PRIMIDONE, 469
William A. Parker

PROBENECID, 469
C. Wayne Weart

PROBUCOL, 471
Stephen Shalansky and Robert Dombrowski

PROCAINAMIDE, 472
James E. Tisdale

PROCATEROL, 474
Karen F. Shalansky and Cindy Reesor Nimmo

PROCHLORPERAZINE, 474
Lynne Nakashima

PROCYCLIDINE, 476
Ruby E. Grymonpre

PROGESTINS, 476
Deborah Stier Carson

PROMETHAZINE, 477
Lynne Nakashima

PROPAFENONE, 478
James E. Tisdale

PROPOXYPHENE, 479
Terry J. Baumann

PROPRANOLOL, 480
Robert Rangno and James McCormack

PROTRIPTYLINE, 481
Lyle K. Laird and Julia Vertrees

PSEUDOEPHEDRINE, 481
Penny F. Miller

PYRAZINAMIDE, 483
Ann Beardsell

QUINAPRIL, 483
Jack Onrot and James McCormack

QUINIDINE, 484
James E. Tisdale

RAMIPRIL, 486
Jack Onrot and James McCormack

RANITIDINE, 487
James McCormack and Glen Brown

RIFAMPIN (RIFAMPICIN), 488
Ann Beardsell

RITODRINE, 489
Glenda Meneilly

SALBUTAMOL, ALBUTEROL (IN USA), 491
Karen F. Shalansky and Cindy Reesor Nimmo

SALMETEROL, 493
Karen F. Shalansky and Cindy Reesor Nimmo

SALSALATE, 493
Kelly W. Jones

SCOPOLAMINE, 494
Lynne Nakashima

SECOBARBITAL, 495
Jonathan A. E. Fleming

SELEGILINE, 495
Ruby E. Grymonpre

SENNA, 496
Leslie Mathews

SIMVASTATIN, 497
Stephen Shalansky and Robert Dombrowski

SODIUM PHOSPHATE, 497
Leslie Mathews

SOTALOL, 499
James E. Tisdale

SPIRONOLACTONE, 500
Ian Petterson

STREPTOKINASE, 502
Stephen F. Hamilton, Stan Horton,
and Udho Thadani

SUCRALFATE, 503
James McCormack and Glen Brown

SULFINPYRAZONE, 504
C. Wayne Weart

SULFASALAZINE (5-AMINOSALICYLIC ACID
BOUND TO SULFAPYRIDINE), 506
J. Scott Whittaker and Richard I. Ogilvie

SULINDAC, 508
Kelly W. Jones

SUMATRIPTAN, 509
Jerry W. Taylor

TEMAZEPAM, 509
Jonathan A. E. Fleming

TENOXICAM, 510
Kelly W. Jones

TERBUTALINE, 511
Karen F. Shalansky and Cindy Reesor Nimmo

TERFENADINE, 512
Penny F. Miller

TETRACYCLINE, 513
Alfred S. Gin and George G. Zhanel

THEOPHYLLINE, 514
Karen F. Shalansky and Cindy Reesor Nimmo

THIETHYLPERAZINE, 517
Lynne Nakashima

THIORIDAZINE, 517
Juan R. Avila and Patricia Marken

THIOTHIXENE, 518
Juan R. Avila and Patricia Marken

TICARCILLIN, 519
John C. Rotschafer, Kyle Vance-Bryan,
and Rick Zabinski

TICARCILLIN-CLAVULANATE, 519
John C. Rotschafer, Kyle Vance-Bryan,
and Rick Zabinski

TICLOPIDINE, 520
J. Chris Bradberry

TIMOLOL, 521
Robert Rangno and James McCormack

TISSUE PLASMINOGEN ACTIVATOR
(ALTEPLASE), 521
Stephen F. Hamilton, Stan Horton,
and Udho Thadani

TOBRAMYCIN, 522
David R. P. Guay

TOCAINIDE, 522
James E. Tisdale

TOLAZAMIDE, 524
Christy Silvius Scott

TOLBUTAMIDE, 524
Christy Silvius Scott

TOLMETIN, 527
Kelly W. Jones

TRANYLCYPROMINE, 528
Lyle K. Laird and Julia Vertrees

TRAZODONE, 528
Lyle K. Laird, Julia Vertrees, and
Jonathan A. E. Fleming

TRIAMCINOLONE ACETONIDE, 529
Karen F. Shalansky and Cindy Reesor Nimmo

TRIAMTERENE, 529
Ian Petterson

TRIAZOLAM, 529
Jonathan A. E. Fleming

TRIHEXYPHENIDYL, 531
Ruby E. Grymonpre

TRIMETHOPRIM-SULFAMETHOXAZOLE
(TMP/SMX, CO-TRIMOXAZOLE), 531
George G. Zhanel and Ann Beardsell

TRIMIPRAMINE, 533
Lyle K. Laird and Julia Vertrees

VALPROIC ACID, 533
Lyle K. Laird and Julia Vertrees

VANCOMYCIN, 536
George G. Zhanel

VERAPAMIL, 538
Stephen F. Hamilton, Stan Horton,
and Udho Thadani

VITAMIN B12 (Cobalamin), 541
Eric Yoshida and Angela Kim-Sing

VITAMIN K (Phytonadione), 542
Eric Yoshida and Angela Kim-Sing

WARFARIN, 543
Frances V. H. Chow

ZIDOVUDINE (AZT), 545
Ann Beardsell

ZOLPIDEM, 548
Jonathan A. E. Fleming

ZOPICLONE, 548
Jonathan A. E. Fleming

I

Drug Therapy for
Disease States

1 | CARDIOVASCULAR DISEASES

DRUG THERAPY FOR HYPERTENSION

James McCormack and Robert Rangno

▶ *What Are My Goals of Treatment?*

Acute (crisis) hypertension

to reduce blood pressure rapidly when elevations are associated with immediate life-threatening hypertensive situations (e.g., malignant hypertension, dissecting aneurysm, eclampsia, pheochromocytoma, and cocaine abuse)

Chronic (noncrisis) hypertension

to reduce the amplifier effect of hypertension on atherogenesis which in turn reduces the long-term risk of fatal and nonfatal target organ damage (e.g., strokes, myocardial infarction [MI], and heart and renal failure)

to reduce blood pressure safely to a proven acceptable range and to avoid hypotension, which may also provoke stroke, MI, or renal failure (JAMA 1991;165:489–495)

to avoid all adverse drug effects, because hypertension is usually asymptomatic and adverse effects decrease the patient's compliance and hence the drug's effectiveness

to choose the least expensive drug that has been shown to improve outcome, not just lower blood pressure, and thus to optimize long-term cost-effectiveness

to appreciate that many patients achieve an optimum reduction of blood pressure with a drug dosage that is $1/4$–$1/2$ of the normal recommended dosage

to consider future gradual antihypertensive drug dosage reduction and possible discontinuation of therapy to reevaluate diagnosis, nondrug therapy, optimum class of drug, and dosage

▶ *What Evidence Is Available to Support Drug Therapy for Hypertension?*

Malignant hypertension (retinal hemorrhage, papilledema, or encephalopathy) and hypertensive crisis (e.g., pulmonary edema, dissecting aneurysm, and eclampsia)

- prior to the use of drug therapy, observers reported near 100% 1 year mortality (Br J Med 1959;2:969–980)
- overzealous rate of blood pressure reduction, however, can result in complications of fatal and nonfatal reduction in target organ perfusion of brain, heart, and kidneys (Acta Med Scand 1980;207:253–257)

Moderate to severe hypertension (diastolic pressure greater than 106 and less than 115 mmHg)

- Veterans Administration Cooperative Study proved that hydrochlorothiazide, reserpine, and hydralazine substantially decreased the occurrence of fatal and nonfatal stroke, MI, heart failure, and renal failure (JAMA 1967;202:1028–1034)

Mild hypertension (diastolic pressure between 90 and 105 mmHg)

- diuretic and beta-adrenergic blocking agent (beta-blocker) therapy produce a relative reduction in the frequency of fatal and nonfatal strokes of 40% or an absolute reduction from 1.9% to 1% during 4–5 years of treatment (Hypertension 1989;13[suppl I]:I-36–I-44)
- evidence also suggests that renal failure, left ventricular hypertrophy, and congestive heart failure (CHF) are diminished
- reduction in coronary heart disease (CHD) by treating mild hypertension has been disappointingly smaller in middle-aged patients (Am Heart J 1987;4:1018–1023) but more impressive in the elderly

Hypertension in the elderly

- series of studies in elderly patients with mild hypertension have shown, especially with the use of low-dose diuretics, a reduction in the incidence of fatal and nonfatal cerebrovascular, coronary events and heart failure (Br Med J 1992;304:412–416)
- treatment of isolated systolic hypertension in the elderly with diuretic plus or minus beta-blocker reduced stroke, MI, and mortality (JAMA 1991;265:3255–3264)

▶ *When Should I Consider Drug Therapy?*

Acute (crisis) hypertension

Acute target organ damage is present (with or without symptoms)

- if encephalopathy, pulmonary edema, papilledema or hemorrhage, dissecting aneurysm, caused by malignant hypertension, eclampsia, or pheochromocytoma is present, irrespective of the diastolic pressure value, blood pressure should be lowered aggressively, within 30 minutes to 2 hours
- avoid hypotension (i.e., lower blood pressure to a diastolic value of approximately 110 mmHg within the first 1–2 hours)

Chronic (noncrisis) hypertension

Diastolic pressure repeatedly exceeds 115 mmHg in a patient with no target organ damage (with or without symptoms)

- even diastolic pressures up to 140 mmHg in the absence of target organ damage do not require emergency reduction
- rapid reduction has been shown to increase the risk of cerebrovascular and coronary hypoperfusion (Br Med J 1975;4:739, Ann Intern Med 1976;84:696–699)
- blood pressure in these patients should be lowered with drugs, starting immediately but being accomplished gradually (over days)

Diastolic pressure repeatedly exceeds 100 mmHg but is less than 115 mmHg after 3–6 months of appropriate nonpharmacological measures

- even in patients without risk factors, blood pressure

should be lowered slowly (over weeks) with drugs (Hypertension 1986;8:444–467)

Diastolic pressure is repeatedly between 95 and 100 mmHg after 3–6 months of appropriate nonpharmacological measures

- in patients with other cardiovascular risk factors, blood pressure should be lowered slowly (over weeks) with drugs

Isolated systolic pressure is repeatedly greater than 160 mmHg (diastolic pressure < 90 mmHg) after 3–6 months of appropriate nonpharmacological measures

- blood pressure should be lowered with drugs in a patient with other cardiovacular risk factors

Elderly (older than 65 years)

- indications and goals are different in the elderly with regard to the level at which treatment is initiated and the magnitude of the reduction (Can Med Assoc J 1986; 135:741–745)
- in general, treatment thresholds are 5–10 mmHg higher
- there is no evidence of a benefit from pharmacological therapy in patients older than 80 years; however, judicious use of nonpharmacological therapy is suggested

▶ *What Drug Should I Use for Initial Treatment?*

Acute (crisis) hypertension

In these patients, typically the choice of drug has been based on a predictable route of administration (IV) and titratability; however, oral routes can be used in cases of crisis hypertension (Br J Clin Pharmacol 1986; 21:377–383) and in patients in whom IV access is not possible or feasible • The IV route should be used in patients with hypertensive heart failure and/or encephalopathy, as the response is predictable and easily titratable

NITROPRUSSIDE

- has instant onset and reversibility and no central nervous system (CNS) effects
- requires an infusion pump and constant monitoring

DIAZOXIDE

- rapid onset, sustained effect, and no CNS effects
- preferable over nitroprusside when infusion pumps are not available and/or continuous pressure monitoring is not possible

LABETALOL

- has rapid onset with sustained effect; causes no rebound tachycardia and no CNS effects
- in hypertension-tachycardia syndrome following severe injury to the head or the chest, labetalol may be preferable to nitroprusside because, in contrast to nitroprusside, it results in a decrease in cerebral blood flow (Crit Care Med 1988;16:1159–1160, Crit Care Med 1988; 16:765–768) and this may limit cerebral bleeding

ORAL ATENOLOL OR NADOLOL, NIFEDIPINE, CAPTOPRIL

- all of these agents have been shown to be effective (Lancet 1985;2:34–35, Br J Clin Pharmacol 1986;21:377–383) in the treatment of acute (crisis) hypertension and should not be considered suboptimum therapy
- these agents are also useful for the initial treatment of patients with no target organ damage who have diastolic pressures that repeatedly exceed 115 mmHg

- the onset of action of angiotensin converting enzyme (ACE) inhibitors other than captopril is likely too slow for them to be used in this condition
- although nifedipine is the most commonly used agent, there is no evidence that it is any more effective than the other agents
- the choice among these oral agents should be based on cost and the ultimate usefulness of the drug for long-term control (see below)
- many of these patients require more than one drug for adequate long-term control
- doses at the higher end of the dosing range should be given initially
- although diuretics have not been studied in the treatment of acute (crisis) hypertension, if a diuretic is considered for long-term therapy, start administration of a diuretic along with one of the above agents

Chronic (noncrisis) hypertension

Initial drug choice depends on the presence or absence of other concomitant disease states, side effects, and cost

- there are no clinically useful indicators (e.g., age, race, or renin status) for deciding which drug will work
- primarily, consider drugs that have been proved to reduce mortality and morbidity (diuretics and beta-blockers) because an equivalent reduction in blood pressure by two different drugs does not necessarily confer an equal reduction in target organ damage (Br Med J 1992; 304: 405–412)
- useful to select drugs that may also treat another disease state, if present
- equal (60–80%) chance of any patient responding to any particular drug group
- the best approach is sequential monotherapy by initially choosing the most appropriate single representative of a drug class and trying it

Patients with no concomitant disease
HYDROCHLOROTHIAZIDE, CHLORTHALIDONE

- are as effective as any of the other antihypertensive agents in lowering blood pressure; allow once a day dosing; have few adverse effects with low dosage; have proven effectiveness in reducing mortality and morbidity secondary to strokes, MI (JAMA 1991;265:3255–3264), and heart and renal failure; and are inexpensive
- have additive hypotensive effects with most other antihypertensives and are especially useful in combination with beta-blockers and ACE inhibitors (Arch Intern Med 1990;150:1175–1183)
- drugs of choice in elderly patients with either diastolic or isolated systolic hypertension because of unquestionable effectiveness (JAMA 1991;265:3255–3264); and diuretics produce a reduction in the number of hip fractures in men and women because they cause reduced osteoporosis (Br Med J 1990;301:1303–1305)
- the choice between hydrochlorothiazide and chlorthalidone should be based on cost

NADOLOL, ATENOLOL

- if hydrochlorothiazide or chlorthalidone is not effective or tolerated, most beta-blockers allow once a day dosing, adverse effects are low with low doses, they have proven efficacy in influencing mortality and morbidity, and they are usually less expensive than other agents
- nadolol, a nonselective beta-blocker with low lipid solubility should be tried initially, as it has proven effective-

ness and has many advantages over propranolol (nadolol can be given once a day and has more consistent absorption characteristics than does propranolol)

- the beta$_2$-blockade of nadolol may offer a distinct advantage by blockade of epinephrine (beta$_2$)–induced arrhythmia and hypokalemia
- other once-daily beta-blockers (e.g., atenolol and acebutolol) may be used instead of nadolol if they are less expensive than nadolol (no generic is available for acebutolol) or if there is a problem with cold extremities, which may be worsened by beta$_2$-antagonism
- there is no evidence that beta-blockers such as atenolol and nadolol result in a lower quality of life than do other agents such as the ACE inhibitors and calcium channel blockers (Circulation 1991;84[suppl VI]:VI-108–VI-118)
- beta-blockers, along with ACE inhibitors and calcium channel blockers, reduce microalbuminuria in patients with essential hypertension (Hypertension 1993;21:810–815), and no antihypertensive class is unique in its ability to slow the progression of diabetic renal disease (South Med J 1994;84:1043–1053)

ANGIOTENSIN CONVERTING ENZYME INHIBITORS, CALCIUM CHANNEL BLOCKERS, ALPHA-ANTAGONISTS

- one of these agents should be chosen if the above agents are ineffective, not tolerated, or contraindicated
- there are no data proving that these agents decrease mortality or morbidity associated with hypertension
- decision among these agents should be based on convenience (once a day dosing) and cost, as all these agents are equally effective at lowering blood pressure

Patients with concomitant disease states
Ischemic heart disease
NADOLOL, ATENOLOL

- these are effective drugs for ischemic heart disease, are usually less expensive than calcium channel blockers, and can be given once daily

DILTIAZEM, NIFEDIPINE, VERAPAMIL

- if beta-blockers are not effective or tolerated, calcium channel blockers are also effective in patients with ischemic heart disease
- all calcium channel blockers are equally effective; however, diltiazem is usually the best tolerated calcium channel blocker and should be chosen over other agents unless there are significant price differences

Previous myocardial infarction
NADOLOL, ATENOLOL, METOPROLOL, PROPRANOLOL

- both selective and nonselective agents have been shown to reduce morbidity and mortality, although the absolute reduction in mortality is greater when nonselective agents are used (Lancet 1986;2:57–66, N Engl J Med 1981;304:801–807, Prog Cardiovasc Dis 1985;27:335–371)
- most beta-blockers with intrinsic sympathomimetic activity, except acebutolol (Am J Cardiol 1990;66:24C–31C), have been shown not to have an effect on mortality after an MI (Am J Cardiol 1990;66:9C–20C, Prog Cardiovasc Dis 1985;27:335–371)
- nadolol and atenolol have advantages over the other agents with proven effectiveness in that they can be dosed once daily and have low lipid solubility
- only timolol, propranolol, metoprolol, and acebutolol

have been shown to have significant long-term effect on mortality, and some clinicians suggest that only those beta-blockers with proven long-term postinfarction effects should be used for prophylaxis (Circulation 1991;84[suppl VI]:VI-101–VI-107)
- the data for empirical use of calcium antagonists after MI have consistently been negative, and they should not be used after MI unless the patient is unresponsive to beta-blocker therapy

CAPTOPRIL, ENALAPRIL, LISINOPRIL, BENAZEPRIL, FOSINOPRIL, RAMIPRIL, QUINAPRIL

- ACE inhibitors are useful in patients who have had an MI and have left ventricular dysfunction, as increased length of survival has been shown (N Engl J Med 1992;327:669–677)

Congestive heart failure
HYDROCHLOROTHIAZIDE, CHLORTHALIDONE

- effective for both hypertension and mild CHF and less expensive than ACE inhibitors

CAPTOPRIL, ENALAPRIL, LISINOPRIL, BENAZEPRIL, FOSINOPRIL, RAMIPRIL, QUINAPRIL

- all ACE inhibitors are likely equally effective, and the decision about which agent to use should be based on convenience (all but captopril can be given once daily) and cost

NADOLOL, ATENOLOL, ACEBUTOLOL

- beta-blockers have traditionally not been used in patients with CHF but old and newer data (Am J Med 1992;92:527–538) show that, when they are introduced slowly, they often improve (not worsen) CHF, whereas calcium channel blockers, especially verapamil and diltiazem usually worsen CHF (Circulation 1990;82:2254–2257)

Chronic obstructive pulmonary disease and asthma
HYDROCHLOROTHIAZIDE, CHLORTHALIDONE

- useful because no effect on pulmonary function and less expensive than other agents

CAPTOPRIL, ENALAPRIL, LISINOPRIL, BENAZEPRIL, FOSINOPRIL, RAMIPRIL, QUINAPRIL

- ACE inhibitors have no effect on asthma but are more expensive than diuretics

DILTIAZEM, NIFEDIPINE, VERAPAMIL

- calcium channel blockers have no effect on pulmonary function, but use only if ACE inhibitors are not effective or tolerated, as calcium blockers are usually more expensive

ATENOLOL

- even beta$_1$-selective agents are contraindicated, as they can cause bronchoconstriction and worsening of asthma
- low doses of beta$_1$-selective agents may be tried as a last choice in chronic obstructive pulmonary disease (COPD) but not in asthma

Non–insulin-dependent diabetes
NADOLOL, ATENOLOL, HYDROCHLOROTHIAZIDE, CHLORTHALIDONE

- adverse effects on blood glucose level may largely be avoided with smaller yet still effective doses of these agents

- long-term treatment with diuretics rarely, if ever, cause diabetes (Drugs Ther Perspectives 1993;1[9]:13–14)
- data suggest that, with long-term use, diuretics, beta-blockers, and ACE inhibitors all prevent the onset of microalbuminuria in patients with non–insulin-dependent diabetes and do not worsen glycemic control (Hypertension 1993;21:786–794)
- these agents need not be avoided in patients with non–insulin-dependent diabetes

CAPTOPRIL, ENALAPRIL, LISINOPRIL, BENAZEPRIL, FOSINOPRIL, RAMIPRIL, QUINAPRIL

- no effect on diabetes and may improve insulin sensitivity

DILTIAZEM, NIFEDIPINE, VERAPAMIL

- no effect on diabetes, but use only if ACE inhibitors are not effective or tolerated, as calcium channel blockers are usually more expensive

Insulin-dependent diabetes
HYDROCHLOROTHIAZIDE, CHLORTHALIDONE

- when used in low doses, there is little if any effect in the insulin-dependent diabetic, and these agents are effective and inexpensive

ANGIOTENSIN CONVERTING ENZYME INHIBITOR, CLONIDINE, METHYLDOPA, CALCIUM CHANNEL BLOCKER, PRAZOSIN

- can be considered if hydrochlorothiazide is not effective or tolerated because these agents have little effect on blood glucose levels

NADOLOL, ATENOLOL

- may be used in low dose if there are no other useful alternatives
- nonselective beta-blockers can mask the symptoms associated with hypoglycemia (except sweating, which is enhanced) and may inhibit glycogenolysis which may cause prolonged hypoglycemia in the event of excessive insulin administration
- beta-blockers, along with ACE inhibitors and calcium channel blockers, reduce microalbuminuria in patients with essential hypertension (Hypertension 1993;21:810–815) and no antihypertensive class is unique in its ability to slow the progression of diabetic renal disease (South Med J 1994;84:1043–1053)

Mild hyperlipidemia (i.e., that which does not require drug therapy)
HYDROCHLOROTHIAZIDE, CHLORTHALIDONE

- the lipid changes are usually slight, are short lived, and are of no proven consequence, and diuretics are less expensive than other agents
- despite the potential of small changes in lipids, complications secondary to atherosclerosis are decreased, not increased, with these agents (e.g., reduction in the occurrence of MIs in elderly patients receiving these agents) (Br Med J 1992;304:412–416)

NADOLOL, ATENOLOL

- if thiazide diuretics are not effective, beta-blockers can be used because the lipid changes are usually slight, are short lived, and are of no proven consequence
- reversal of atherosclerosis has been shown to occur even when serum lipid levels increase (J Hypertens 1991;9[suppl]:S21–S25)

Moderate to severe hyperlidemia (i.e., that which requires drug therapy)
ANGIOTENSIN CONVERTING ENZYME INHIBITORS

- no effect on lipids but more expensive than hydrochlorothiazide

CALCIUM CHANNEL BLOCKERS

- no effect on lipids, but use only if ACE inhibitors are not effective or tolerated, as calcium channel blockers are usually more expensive

HYDRALAZINE, PRAZOSIN

- actually decrease lipid levels but there is no proven clinical benefit of this small lipid decrease

Atrial fibrillation
NADOLOL, ATENOLOL

- beta-blockers are useful if the heart rate is not controlled with digoxin and/or is excessively rapid during exercise
- are less expensive than verapamil and can be used once daily
- more data on newer beta-blockers (N Engl J Med 1992;326:1264–1271)

VERAPAMIL

- use in patients who do not respond to digoxin and beta-blockers as long as the patient does not have poor left ventricular function

Ventricular arrhythmias
NADOLOL, ATENOLOL

- for symptomatic benign ventricular arrhythmias (that are nonsustained, are hemodynamically stable, and are not associated with structural heart disease), beta-blockers are preferable to other antiarrhythmic agents because of the benign nature of these arrhythmias and because of the relatively low incidence of adverse effects of beta-blockers compared with other antiarrhythmic drugs (Drugs 1974;7:118–129)

Migraine
NADOLOL, ATENOLOL

- propranolol, atenolol, metoprolol, and nadolol are all effective for migraine prophylaxis
- timolol and acebutolol are somewhat effective, and pindolol and oxprenolol are ineffective
- nadolol should be tried initially, as it has proven effectiveness, has the advantage over propranolol of being given once a day, and has more consistent absorption characteristics
- agents such as acebutolol and atenolol can be used if they are less expensive than nadolol

Gout
- usually avoid diuretics, as these agents increase serum uric acid levels and may precipitate a gouty attack

Symptomatic prostatic hyperplasia
PRAZOSIN, TERAZOSIN

- may decrease urethral spasm

Menopausal symptoms
CLONIDINE

- clonidine, in addition to having an antihypertensive effect, also reduces menopausal symptoms

- may be useful in patients who have contraindications or intolerance to hormone replacement

Pregnancy

BETA-BLOCKERS, METHYLDOPA, HYDRALAZINE

- are safe and effective

▶ *What Dosage Should I Use?*

Acute (crisis) hypertension

NITROPRUSSIDE

- 10 μg/min IV increasing by 10 μg/min at 10 minute intervals until blood pressure is controlled or a maximum of 100 μg/min is reached

DIAZOXIDE

- 50 mg IV bolus at 10 minute intervals until blood pressure is controlled

LABETALOL

- when used intravenously in hypertensive emergencies, administration by infusion provides a smoother, less precipitous fall in blood pressure compared with that achieved with intermittent bolus injections (Br J Clin Pharmacol 1982;13[suppl 1]:97s–99s)
- start with 20 mg/h and double the dosage every 30 minutes until a satisfactory response is obtained or a maximum dose rate of 160 mg/h is reached
- in hypertension complicating acute MI, start the infusion at 15 mg/h and increase gradually to a maximum of 120 mg/h, depending on blood pressure response

ORAL BETA-BLOCKERS, CALCIUM CHANNEL BLOCKERS, ANGIOTENSIN CONVERTING ENZYME INHIBITORS

- doses at the higher end of the dosing range should be given initially to allow for rapid (over 1–2 hours) reduction in blood pressure

ATENOLOL

- 100 mg PO daily

NADOLOL

- 80 mg PO daily

NIFEDIPINE

- 10 mg PO (5 mg in patients such as the elderly in whom cerebral hypoperfusion is a potential hazard), and repeat every 6 hours as needed
- do not use the sublingual route, as nifedipine is not absorbed by the oral mucosa; however, biting the capsule and swallowing the contents increases the rate of absorption by about 5–10 minutes (Am J Med 1986;81[suppl 6A]:2–5)

CAPTOPRIL

- 25 mg PO and repeat Q6H PRN

Chronic (noncrisis) hypertension

Start with a low dosage and increase slowly (increase dosages every 2–4 weeks) • Effective dosages are often lower than those recommended in most texts

HYDROCHLOROTHIAZIDE, CHLORTHALIDONE

- start with 12.5 mg PO daily
- some clinicians advocate the use of 6.25 mg as a starting dose, but the difficulty in attaining this dose makes it impractical

- dosage may be increased every 4 weeks if the current dosage is not adequately controlling blood pressure
- dosage should rarely exceed 25 mg and never exceed 50 mg daily, as there is no greater hypotensive effect with higher dosage and an increased incidence of adverse reactions occurs

NADOLOL

- 20 mg PO daily
- increase the dosage every 4 weeks by 20 mg PO daily until an effect is seen
- dosage increases up to 80 mg PO daily may be necessary in some patients, but no benefit is likely to result from further increases

ATENOLOL

- 25 mg PO daily
- increase the dosage every 4 weeks by 25 mg PO daily until an effect is seen
- dosage increases up to 100 mg PO daily may be necessary in some patients, but no benefit is likely to result from further increases

CAPTOPRIL

- 6.25 mg PO BID
- increase the dosage by 12.5 mg PO daily every 4 weeks until adequate blood pressure is achieved or a maximum daily dosage of 150 mg is reached
- twice-daily dosing is usually necessary for captopril

ENALAPRIL

- 2.5 mg PO daily
- increase the dosage by 2.5 mg PO daily every 4 weeks until adequate blood pressure is achieved or a daily dosage of 20 mg is reached (dosages as high as 40 mg PO daily have been used)
- twice-daily dosing with this agent is not necessary unless side effects preclude once-daily dosing

LISINOPRIL

- 2.5 mg PO daily
- increase the dosage by 2.5 mg PO daily every 4 weeks until adequate blood pressure is achieved or a daily dosage of 20 mg is reached
- limited value in exceeding a total daily dosage of 20 mg (dosages as high as 80 mg PO daily have been used)

DILTIAZEM

- 60 mg of diltiazem SR (a twice-daily product) PO BID increasing the dosage every 4 weeks by 60 mg/d until an effect is seen or a maximum dosage of 300 mg/d is reached
- 180 mg of diltiazem CD (a once-daily product) PO daily, increasing the dosage every 4 weeks by 60 mg/d until an effect is seen or a maximum dosage of 300 mg/d is reached
- sustained-release preparations are recommended, as they are more convenient and usually not much different in price from the regular-release products (unless generic regular release is available)
- the regular-release form is started at 30 mg PO Q6H, increasing the dosage every 4 weeks by 30 mg PO Q6H until an effect is seen or a maximum dosage of 360 mg/d is reached

VERAPAMIL

- 120 mg of verapamil SR (a once-daily product sometimes given twice daily when dosages exceed 240 mg/d) PO daily increasing the dosage every 4 weeks by 120 mg/d

until an effect is seen or a maximum dosage of 480 mg/d is reached
- sustained-release preparations are recommended, as they are more convenient and usually not much different in price from the regular-release products (unless generic regular release is available)
- the regular-release form is started at 80 mg PO Q8H, increasing the dosage every 4 weeks by 80 mg PO Q6H until an effect is seen or a maximum dosage of 360 mg/d is reached

NIFEDIPINE

- 30 mg of nifedipine XL PO daily, increasing the dosage every 4 weeks by 30 mg/d until an effect is seen or a maximum dosage of 90 mg/d is reached
- 10 mg of nifedipine PA PO BID, increasing the dosage every 4 weeks by 20 mg/d until an effect is seen or a maximum dosage of 80 mg/d is reached
- sustained-released preparations are recommended, as they are more convenient and usually not much different in price from the regular-release products (unless generic regular release is available)
- the regular-release form is started at 10 mg PO TID, increasing the dosage every 4 weeks by 10 mg PO TID until an effect is seen or maximum dosage of 90 mg/d is reached

See Drug Monographs for Further Dosing Schedules

▶ How Long Should I Treat with My Initial Regimen?

Acute (crisis) hypertension

- until diastolic pressure is sustained between 100 and 110 mmHg for most patients
- for patients with dissecting aneurysms, drug therapy should be given until the systolic pressure is 110 mmHg or less
- start long-term drug therapy as soon as possible

Chronic (noncrisis) hypertension

- patients with blood pressures greater than 115 mmHg or patients with symptoms should be evaluated again within 48 hours to ensure that at least a 5–10 mmHg drop in blood pressure has occurred
- for patients with blood pressures less than 115 mmHg, assess the effect of each dose increment and reevaluate drug therapy every 2–4 weeks, depending on what is convenient for the patient and the clinician

▶ What Efficacy Parameters Should I Follow and How Frequently Do I Have to Assess My Patient?

Acute (crisis) hypertension
Blood pressure
- preferably measure intraarterial blood pressure; however, if this is not available, perform indirect (cuff) measurements every 5 minutes until the desired blood pressure is reached and then every hour, ensuring that the diastolic pressure does not go below 100 mmHg during the first 1–2 days due to the concern of hypoperfusion
- the ideal rate of blood pressure reduction in this condition is unknown; however, the goal should be to lower pressures to the desired range within 30 minutes to 2 hours (i.e., to approximately 180/110 mm/kg initially)

Electrocardiographic measurements
- continuous electrocardiographic (EKG) monitoring is

recommended until a stable blood pressure reduction has been achieved and sustained
- this is done to look for evidence of coronary ischemia, and if this occurs, treat as for angina (also consider that blood pressure may have been lowered too far)

Chronic (noncrisis) hypertension
Blood pressure
- patients with blood pressures greater than 115 mmHg or patients with symptoms should be evaluated again within 48 hours to ensure that at least a 5–10 mmHg drop in blood pressure has occurred
- for patients with blood pressures less than 115 mmHg, follow-up blood pressure determinations should be done within a couple of weeks
- at each visit, do two blood pressure measurements, supine or sitting, after the patient has been resting without conversation for 5–10 minutes
- continue to do this every 4 weeks to assess the effect of each new drug or dosage until control is achieved
- for most patients with mild hypertension, blood pressure measurements 2–4 times per year are sufficient after blood pressure is controlled

Evidence of end-organ damage
- if blood pressure is well controlled and no other disease states (e.g., diabetes) exist, measure baseline serum creatinine, blood glucose, and serum cholesterol levels and perform urinalysis and repeat every 5 years
- repeat every year if other disease states are present

Left ventricular hypertrophy
- when diagnosed by EKG or echocardiogram, left ventricular hypertrophy is a major risk factor for sudden death or MI
- left ventricular hypertrophy can be reversed by most old and new antihypertensive drugs, but the ultimate benefit is unknown; therefore, routine evaluation is not recommended unless there is evidence of valve disease

▶ Should I Add Another Drug or Substitute Therapy If My Initial Drug Therapy Fails?

Acute (crisis) hypertension
- labetalol is often a rational addition (with vasodilators) to avoid or reverse reflex tachycardia and to decrease shear force

Chronic (noncrisis) hypertension
If no effect seen with the initial dosage after 4–8 weeks
- increase the dosage of the drug, and reassess after 4–8 weeks
- if there is still no response, stop administration of the drug and start a low dosage of a drug from a different class

If a clinically important drop in blood pressure is achieved (although not to the desired level) with the first drug, with no adverse effects
- continue the first drug and add a second drug (in low dosage) and titrate upward as with the first drug

If a clinically important drop in blood pressure is achieved with the first drug but adverse effects are present
- adverse effects are usually extensions of known pharmacological effects and indicate excessive dosage and/or unique sensitivity
- if they are intolerable, discontinue the drug
- if the adverse effect is tolerable and the patient has had

a satisfactory blood pressure response, the dosage of the drug should be decreased

- if the adverse effect continues despite dosage reductions, discontinue the drug and replace with a different drug class
- if the adverse effect is biochemical, it usually resolves with dosage reduction and should not prompt discontinuation of drug therapy unless adverse effects become clinically important

If little or no response occurs with the first drug despite increasing dosages

- first drug should be discontinued, and administration of another drug from a different class should be started

▶ *How Long Should I Continue Drug Therapy?*

Acute (crisis) hypertension

- drug discontinuation is not advised in patients with severe to malignant hypertension or target organ damage (e.g., MI, CHF, stroke, or renal failure); however, continual reassessment allows the hypertension to be treated with the least number of drugs at the lowest dosage that reduces the incidence of adverse effects, reduces the frequency of drug administration, and is more cost-effective

Chronic (noncrisis) hypertension

Stepped-down therapy, in general, should be considered in patients whose blood pressures during the previous few visits have been well controlled

- approximately 50% of patients with well-controlled blood pressures successfully undergo either a reduction in dosage or number of drugs and remain normotensive for a time, but unfortunately, this time period varies from patient to patient and consistent reevaluation is necessary
- this return to normal blood pressure levels may be explained by a reversal of cardiac and vascular changes that may occur after prolonged treatment with drug therapy and may be a means of "setting back the clock" of primary hypertension evolution or may reflect an incorrect initial diagnosis
- as with every treatment, not every patient's blood pressure successfully responds to drug discontinuation or drug dosage reduction
- patients most likely to have a successful reduction or discontinuation of therapy may be predicted by a low pretreatment blood pressure (mild hypertension, diastolic pressure < 100 mmHg), no evidence of target organ damage, requirement for only monotherapy for blood pressure control, and achievement of weight loss, salt restriction, increased exercise, and decreased alcohol intake
- reassessment allows a reevaluation of the efficacy of nondrug measures in the treatment of hypertension, such as reduction of weight and salt and alcohol intake

Approach to drug reevaluation

- very gradual dosage and drug discontinuation, along with a precise discussion of why drug reduction is being done and what the goals of therapy are, avoids most of the patient's psychological dependence
- in patients with blood pressure controlled with single-drug therapy, the dosage should be reduced by 50%, with reassessment of blood pressure at 2 weeks
- if the patient is still normotensive, reduce the dosage by another 50% (i.e., to 25% of the initial dose) and recheck the blood pressure in another 2 weeks
- if the blood pressure is still well controlled, discontinue the drug and recheck the blood pressure in 2 weeks

- so-called rebound hypertension does not occur if the dosage is gradually tapered with dosage reductions of no more than 50% at 2–4 week intervals
- the final dose before full drug discontinuation should be less than $1/4$ of the dose of the initial therapy
- in patients receiving multiple-drug therapy, first reduce the most expensive agent and/or the drug most likely to cause adverse effects
- occasionally, during hypertensive withdrawal, a previously masked symptom may emerge (e.g., angina or migraine when a beta-blocker is stopped), and reinstitution of the drug may be necessary
- after drug therapy has stopped, patients should have their blood pressure checked every month for 6 months and then every 3–4 months
- drug therapy, at a low dose with a single inexpensive drug, should be reinstituted if the patient becomes hypertensive again

Useful References

Recommendations of the Canadian Consensus Conference on non-pharmacological approaches to the management of high blood pressure. Can Med Assoc J 1990;142:1397–1409

Canadian Hypertension Society Consensus Conference on the pharmacological treatment of hypertension. Can Med Assoc J 1989;140:1141–1146

Brunner HR, Ménard J, Waeber B, et al. Treating the individual hypertensive patient: Considerations on dose, sequential monotherapy and drug combinations. J Hypertens 1990;8:3–11

Fletcher AE, Franks PJ, Bulpitt CJ. The effect of withdrawing antihypertensive therapy: A review. J Hypertens 1988;6:431–436

Joint National Committee on Detection, Evaluation, and Treatment of High Blood Pressure. The Fifth Report of the Joint National Committee on Detection, Evaluation, and Treatment of High Blood Pressure (JNC V). Arch Intern Med 1993;153:154–183

DRUG THERAPY FOR CONGESTIVE HEART FAILURE

Jack Onrot

▶ *What Are My Goals of Treatment?*

to improve exercise tolerance and quality of life
to prolong survival
to improve hemodynamics

▶ *What Evidence Is Available to Support Drug Therapy for Congestive Heart Failure?*

Symptomatic relief, improved exercise tolerance, and enhanced quality of life

- diuretics, ACE inhibitors (Am Heart J 1985;110:439–447), and digoxin (Am J Cardiol 1988;61:371–375) improve symptoms

Prolonged survival

- ACE inhibitors (N Engl J Med 1987;316:1429–1435) and hydralazine with isosorbide (N Engl J Med 1986;314: 1547–1562) have been shown to prolong survival
- ACE inhibitors are superior to hydralazine and isosorbide (N Engl J Med 1991;325:303–310)

Improved hemodynamics

- diuretics (Am J Cardiol 1979;43:86–90), ACE inhibitors (Am Heart J 1985;110:439–447), digoxin (J Am Coll Cardiol 1989;13:134–142), and nitrates all reduce preload
- ACE inhibitors (Am Heart J 1985;110:439–447) and digoxin (JAMA 1988;259:539–544) improve cardiac output

▶ When Should I Consider Drug Therapy?

Congestive heart failure

- in all patients after symptomatic heart failure is documented and acute reversible precipitating factors are ruled out
- symptoms warranting therapy include shortness of breath, decreased exercise tolerance, orthopnea, and nocturnal polyuria
- in patients with acute CHF, drug therapy should be started immediately on presentation

▶ What Drug Should I Use for Initial Treatment?

Congestive heart failure

Acute pulmonary edema

OXYGEN

- supplemental oxygen should be administered to maximize arterial oxygenation

MORPHINE

- morphine is effective in reducing preload and reducing dyspnea

FUROSEMIDE

- furosemide mobilizes interstitial lung fluid and promotes a rapid diuresis

NITROGLYCERIN

- short-acting nitrates (e.g., sublingual nitroglycerin) may be useful in reducing preload in patients slow to respond to diuretic therapy
- nitroglycerin should be administered if furosemide does not reduce symptoms within 30 minutes (of the first IV dose)
- there is a danger of decreasing preload, which leads to decreased cardiac output

CAPTOPRIL

- captopril is not commonly used initially to treat acute pulmonary edema
- captopril is used after diuresis has been initiated with furosemide (should not be used initially during times of rapid diuresis)
- used initially in small doses, and titrated to response
- concern exists with the use of ACE inhibitors in the context of rapid diuresis, as they may cause a clinically important drop in blood pressure and an increase in serum creatinine levels
- captopril is preferred in the acute setting because it has a faster onset (30 minutes) and peak activity (60–90 minutes) than other ACE inhibitors; this allows easier titration, and if side effects occur, they are less prolonged
- after the patient has been stabilized, the ACE inhibitors for long-term therapy should be chosen on the basis of cost and frequency of administration

DIGOXIN

- may be useful in the acute setting, especially if ventricular rate control in atrial fibrillation is needed

DOBUTAMINE

- parenteral inotropes should be added only if systemic perfusion is impaired and tissue perfusion is compromised (cardiogenic shock)

- dobutamine is usually preferred over dopamine because it has a more direct effect (it does not work via cardiac norepinephrine release)
- parental inotropes should be used only in the intensive care setting with continual hemodynamic monitoring

DOPAMINE

- dopamine should be chosen over dobutamine if the patient is hypotensive, because in high doses, dopamine not only increases cardiac output but also increases blood pressure
- in low doses, dopamine is also useful in patients with decreased renal blood flow, as it increases renal blood flow

NITROPRUSSIDE

- useful if the patient has severe hypertension and heart failure, as it has balanced arterial and venous effects

Mild to moderate chronic congestive heart failure

FUROSEMIDE

- oral furosemide should be the initial drug therapy selected, on the basis of consistent beneficial effects and synergistic effects seen with subsequent additional therapy
- furosemide should be chosen over thiazide diuretics because it is more effective, has a faster onset, provides more diuresis, and causes less metabolic changes than do thiazides when used in equivalent natriuretic doses
- ACE inhibitors, in the absence of furosemide, may be ineffective (Lancet 1987;2:709–711)

HYDROCHLOROTHIAZIDE

- useful when mild CHF coexists with hypertension
- the diuretic effect (versus the antihypertensive effect) of hydrochlorothiazide is not always maintained for an extended period

CAPTOPRIL, ENALAPRIL, LISINOPRIL, BENAZEPRIL, FOSINOPRIL, RAMIPRIL, QUINAPRIL

- all ACE inhibitors are likely equally effective; however, captopril and enalapril have been the ACE inhibitors shown to provide survival benefit (N Engl J Med 1987;316:1429–1435, N Engl J Med 1991;325:293–302, N Engl J Med 1991;325:303–310)
- decision about which agent to use should be based on dosing frequency (all but captopril can be given once daily) and cost
- these agents are best used in conjunction with furosemide (Ann Intern Med 1984;100:777–782)
- no evidence exists to support the use of ACE inhibitors alone in heart failure
- also useful in maintaining normokalemia in patients receiving diuretics, as they indirectly reduce aldosterone secretion
- ACE inhibitors in patients with CHF and hypertension are useful because ACE inhibitors prolong survival and because they treat both disease states
- also useful in patients who have had an MI and have left ventricular dysfunction, as increased length of survival has been shown (N Engl J Med 1992;327:669–677)
- in general, unless there is a contraindication, patients with symptomatic CHF should receive an ACE inhibitor

DIGOXIN

- most patients with severe heart failure need a loop diuretic, ACE inhibitor, and digoxin (JAMA 1988;259: 539–544)

- triple therapy is warranted for patients who fail to respond to a loop diuretic plus ACE inhibitors
- because digoxin works by improving contractility, it is useful only in patients with decreased systolic left ventricular function and heart failure (many patients with CHF have normal systolic left ventricular function but diastolic dysfunction [impedance to filling] because of thickened left ventricular myocardium; this is the situation in hypertensive cardiomyopathy or early hypertensive cardiomyopathy)
- in hypertensive patients with CHF, assessment of left ventricular function (echocardiography or multigated angiography) is recommended to determine the feasibility of digoxin therapy (i.e., do not use if solely diastolic dysfunction)
- digoxin should be used in all patients with concomitant atrial fibrillation and may be especially beneficial in patients with an S_3 heart sound (Drugs 1986;32:538–568)

METOLAZONE

- useful in diuretic-resistant states (i.e., patients who do not respond to two consecutive doublings of their previously stable furosemide dosage)
- even in low doses, when metolazone is combined with furosemide, a dramatic diuresis may occur
- be aware of hypokalemia, hypomagnesemia, hypotension, and prerenal failure with rapid diuresis

SPIRONOLACTONE

- used only in addition to other diuretics
- useful if hypokalemia persists despite the use of ACE inhibitors
- spironolactone is preferable to the other potassium-sparing diuretics, as it has the most diuretic effect
- beware of hyperkalemia when spironolactone is combined with ACE inhibitor

NITRATES, HYDRALAZINE

- may prolong survival but should be used only in patients intolerant to ACE inhibitors (N Engl J Med 1986;314: 1574–1552)

BETA-BLOCKERS AND CALCIUM CHANNEL BLOCKERS

- can be a useful adjunct to other agents in patients who have heart failure due to underlying hypertensive heart disease (i.e., echocardiogram shows left ventricular hypertrophy with normal systolic function but abnormal diastolic filling–diastolic dysfunction)
- patients with diastolic dysfunction respond to agents such as beta-blockers and calcium channel blockers, which relax the heart in diastole
- decision between these agents should be on the basis of concomitant disease states (see chapter on hypertension)
- the clinician should be aware that these drugs can worsen heart failure in some patients with systolic dysfunction

▶ *What Dosage Should I Use?*

Congestive heart failure
Acute pulmonary edema
OXYGEN

- high flow initially

MORPHINE

- 1–5 mg IV depending on patient's size

FUROSEMIDE

- 20 mg IV if the patient is furosemide naive, and if no response occurs in 30 minutes, double the dose (40 mg IV), and if there is still no response after another 30 minutes, give 80 mg IV
- if the patient is already receiving furosemide, begin with an IV dose equal to the previous PO maintenance dosage and then double every 30 minutes until a response is seen
- after symptoms begin to resolve and edema begins to clear, therapy can be switched to the oral route

NITROGLYCERIN

- 0.4 mg (0.3 mg in Canada owing to different available dosage forms) placed under the tongue or one spray on the tongue every 3 minutes until symptoms improve or systolic blood pressure is less than 90 mmHg

CAPTOPRIL

- 6.25 mg PO as a single dose, and assess the blood pressure every 15–30 minutes for 1¹/₂ hours
- if the patient does not become hypotensive with this dose, it is unlikely that he or she will become hypotensive with further doses (Eur Heart J 1992;13:1521–1527)
- if the patient tolerates the 6.25 mg dose, give 6.25 mg PO BID
- double dosage every 2–3 days until CHF is controlled or the patient experiences orthostatic hypotension (the usual maintenance dosage is 75–150 mg daily)
- maintain systolic blood pressure at greater than 90 mmHg
- optimum dosage is difficult to determine, but attempt to avoid hypotensive symptoms and drops in blood pressure on standing, maintain normokalemia, and minimize adverse effects

DIGOXIN

- digoxin is rarely given as an IV loading dose for the treatment of heart failure (except for patients with acute pulmonary edema) and is used more frequently for rate control in atrial fibrillation
- 0.013 mg/kg (Ann Intern Med 1968;69:703–717) rounded to the closest 0.25 mg dose is the initial loading dose over the first 24 hours
- if the total loading dose is 0.75 mg or greater, administer an initial dose of 0.5 mg IV
- if the total loading dose is less than 0.75 mg, administer an initial dose of 0.25 mg IV
- remainder of calculated loading dose should be administered orally or IV (if patient cannot tolerate oral medications) in 0.25 mg increments every 6 hours
- follow loading dose with a maintenance dosage of 0.25 mg PO daily in young patients or 0.125 mg PO daily in patients older than 65 years of age or patients with renal dysfunction
- titration of dose upward beyond the above doses is not useful except to control rate in atrial fibrillation

Chronic congestive heart failure
FUROSEMIDE

- 20 mg PO daily
- double the dosage every 3–4 days until desired clinical response attained
- too low a dosage is characterized by worsening symp-

toms, high jugular venous pressure, edema, crackles, S_3 heart sound, and weight gain
- too high a dosage is indicated by a lowish jugular venous pressure, rising urea/creatinine ratio, weight loss, and orthostatic hypotension
- divide the dose if the patient has paroxysmal nocturnal dyspnea (give dose before dinner, not at bedtime)

HYDROCHLOROTHIAZIDE

- 25 mg PO daily if being used as sole diuretic therapy
- dosage may be increased after 2 weeks to 50 mg PO daily if the current dosage is not adequately controlling the edema
- adverse metabolic effects at dosages greater than 50 mg limit effectiveness; however, doses up to 100 mg PO daily can be tried in patients unresponsive to 50 mg PO daily
- in cardiac failure, thiazides are effective in potentiating the action of loop diuretics (furosemide), especially in resistant heart failure
- in patients already receiving furosemide, start with low doses (12.5 mg daily) and be aware of possible profound volume depletion and electrolyte disturbances with standard doses (Ann Intern Med 1991;114:886–894)

CAPTOPRIL

- 6.25 mg PO BID
- rapidity of dosage escalation depends on the severity of symptoms
- dosage may be increased daily if necessary
- no value in exceeding a total daily dose of 150 mg
- frequent small Q6H doses may be required if the hypotensive effects of large doses prevent twice-daily administration (BID dosing, however, is usually appropriate)

ENALAPRIL

- 2.5 mg PO daily
- rapidity of dosage escalation depends on the severity of symptoms
- in general, increase dosages weekly; however, dosages may be increased daily
- no value in exceeding a total daily dose of 40 mg

LISINOPRIL

- 2.5 mg PO daily
- rapidity of dosage escalation depends on the severity of symptoms
- in general, increase dosages weekly; however, dosages may be increased daily
- no value in exceeding a total daily dose of 40 mg

DIGOXIN

- 0.25 mg PO daily in young patients
- 0.125 mg PO daily in patients older than 60 years of age
- titration of dose upward is not useful except to control rate in atrial fibrillation

METOLAZONE

- 2.5 mg PO daily as sole diuretic
- 1.25 mg PO daily if added to furosemide for diuretic synergy because of concerns of overdiuresis, electrolyte depletion, and prerenal insufficiency
- double the dosage every 3–4 days, based on response, up to a maximum of 20 mg PO daily

SPIRONOLACTONE

- 50 mg PO daily

- double the dosage weekly, based on response, up to a maximum of 400 mg PO daily

NITRATES, HYDRALAZINE

- begin with hydralazine 25 mg PO BID and nitroglycerin (equivalent to isosorbide dinitrate 20 mg PO QID)

▶ *How Long Should I Treat with My Initial Regimen?*

Congestive heart failure

Acute pulmonary edema

- continue furosemide, adding captopril and increasing dosages daily until symptoms resolve
- if desired effect is not obtained then add digoxin
- a second diuretic is sometimes needed for synergy
- most patients with moderate to severe CHF should begin ACE inhibitors regardless of symptoms because of survival benefits
- many patients will require digoxin for symptom control
- reserve parenteral inotropes for cardiogenic shock

Chronic congestive heart failure

- continue furosemide, titrating to volume and clinical status

▶ *What Efficacy Parameters Should I Follow and How Frequently Do I Have to Assess My Patient?*

Congestive heart failure

Acute pulmonary edema

Pulmonary signs and symptoms

- for a parenteral furosemide dose, relief of dyspnea may occur within 5 minutes, the onset of diuresis occurs in 15–30 minutes (peak, approximately 1 hour) and the duration of effect is 3–4 hours
- for an oral dose, the onset of diuresis is 30–60 minutes (peak, 1–2 hours) and the duration of effect is 4–6 hours
- patients should initially be assessed after each dose of furosemide
- do arterial blood gas determinations initially and repeat hourly if indicated
- look for relief of dyspnea, orthopnea, paroxysmal nocturnal dyspnea, and distribution of crackles
- after the patient is stable, monitor the patient daily while receiving IV furosemide
- in general, follow the parameters that were abnormal initially

Other signs and symptoms

- assess jugular venous pressure, peripheral edema, weight, and liver size after each dose of furosemide
- jugular venous pressure should be normal to slightly increased (be aware that right-sided filling pressures do not always accurately reflect left-sided pressure)
- after acute symptoms have improved, assess the patient at least twice daily for the next 48 hours
- assess weight daily while in hospital

Urea, creatinine, and sodium levels

- may improve if cardiac output is improved, and in patients who are hyponatremic, the serum sodium level may normalize
- in overdiuresis, the level of urea increases out of proportion to the creatinine level increase
- monitor daily in patients with acute disease who are undergoing rapid diuresis
- in patients with severe chronic CHF, accept modest urea

and creatinine level increases above baseline values if this is needed to maintain optimum symptom control

Chronic congestive heart failure

Signs and symptoms

- decreased dyspnea, orthopnea, paroxysmal nocturnal dyspnea, fatigue, ankle swelling, fine crackles on chest auscultation, body weight, liver size, and presence or absence of S_3 heart sound
- jugular venous pressure should be normal to slightly increased
- after the patient is discharged, assess within a week of discharge
- after the patient is stabilized, decrease the frequency of monitoring
- for patients with mild symptoms, assess weekly until symptoms are controlled

▶ Should I Add Another Drug or Substitute Therapy If My Initial Drug Therapy Fails?

Congestive heart failure

Acute pulmonary edema, chronic congestive heart failure

- further therapy should be added, not substituted, especially for loop diuretics because other drugs work best in conjunction with diuretics (Ann Intern Med 1984; 100:777–782)

▶ How Long Should I Continue Drug Therapy?

Congestive heart failure

Acute pulmonary edema, chronic congestive heart failure

- seek the lowest dosage of furosemide compatible with maximum symptom relief
- if nitrates have been used, their administration should be discontinued and the patient assessed for the need for long-term diuretic and vasodilator therapy
- usually need less diuretic when the patient is stable and free from acute precipitants that may have brought the patient to medical attention (therefore, a trial of a decreased dosage of the diuretic is warranted after the patient has been stabilized for 2–3 months; however, one can rarely withdraw diuretics completely)
- because of a demonstrated survival benefit, patients with severe disease who are receiving ACE inhibitors should not have drugs discontinued unless adverse effects occur

Useful References

Guyatt GH. The treatment of heart failure. A methodological review of the literature. Drugs 1986;32:538–568
Parmley WW. Pathophysiology and current therapy of congestive heart failure. J Am Coll Cardiol 1989;13:771–785

DRUG THERAPY FOR ISCHEMIC HEART DISEASE (ANGINAL SYNDROMES AND MYOCARDIAL INFARCTION)

Stephen F. Hamilton, Stan Horton, and Udho Thadani

▶ What Are My Goals of Treatment?

Anginal syndromes

to decrease the frequency and severity of angina
to decrease myocardial oxygen demand and ischemia and to increase exercise tolerance

to increase blood flow to the ischemic area
to halt the progression of coronary artery disease
to prevent progression to acute MI
to prolong life and improve the quality of life

Myocardial infarction

to minimize the loss of myocardium and the subsequent risk of CHF
to prolong life and improve the quality of life
to prevent ischemia-induced arrhythmia

▶ What Evidence Is Available to Support Drug Therapy for Ischemic Heart Disease?

Anginal syndromes

Decreasing symptoms of angina

- nitrates such as isosorbide dinitrate (Am J Cardiol 1984;53:700–705, Postgrad Med 1992;91:307–318), isosorbide-5-mononitrate (Circulation 1991;84[suppl II]: II730), buccal nitroglycerin (Am Heart J 1983;105:848–854), and nitroglycerin in unstable angina (Am J Cardiol 1983;51:694–698, Circulation 1987;76[suppl IV]:128) have been shown to reduce anginal symptoms
- beta-blockers and calcium channel blockers are also effective in reducing symptoms of chronic angina and/or decreasing myocardial oxygen demand (Cardiol Clin 1991;9:73–87, Cardiovasc Drugs Ther 1987;1:411–430)
- when calcium channel blockers are directly compared for therapy of angina they all seem equally effective (Cardiovasc Drugs Ther 1987;1:411–430)
- for variant angina, first-generation calcium channel blockers have all been shown to decrease symptoms and to decrease nitroglycerin consumption at an acceptable level of adverse effects in short- and long-term studies (Am Heart J 1983;106:1341–1347)

Increasing exercise tolerance

- objective evidence of increasing treadmill walking time and decreasing determinants of myocardial oxygen demand has been documented with the nitrates, beta-blockers, and calcium antagonists
- no form of nitrates provides continuous prophylaxis; however, intermittent therapy with prolonged nitrate-free intervals increases treadmill walking time but may leave the patient unprotected during the nitrate-free period (Postgrad Med 1992;91:307–318)
- beta-blockers also increase exercise tolerance (Am J Med 1980;68:243–250)
- improvement in total exercise time and reduction of significant ST segment depression have been shown with diltiazem (Am J Cardiol 1982;49:573–577), verapamil (Am J Med Sci 1966;251:552–562), nifedipine (Am J Cardiol 1979;44:811–816), and nicardipine (Br J Clin Pharmacol 1985;20:195S–205S, Br J Clin Pharmacol 1985;20:187S–194S)

Decreasing ischemia

- little data suggest that nitrates can reduce ST segment abnormalities (Am J Cardiol 1985;56:322–326) or improve resting left ventricular function during continuous or frequent daily therapy (Circulation 1974;50:108–113, Circulation 1975;51:140–145, Am J Cardiol 1986;58:38B–42B)
- intermittent therapy with topical nitrates has been shown to reduce ambulatory myocardial ischemia (Am J Cardiol 1991;68:857–862)
- for silent myocardial ischemia, the number of episodes of ST segment deviations have been decreased by beta-blockers (Am J Cardiol 1988;61:18B–21B), verapamil

(Am J Cardiol 1982;49:125–132), diltiazem (G Ital Cardiol 1985;15:1085–1089), nifedipine (Am J Cardiol 1980;45:825–830), and nicardipine (Am J Cardiol 1985;56:232–236) in patients with severe angina during daily activity and/or with significant pain at rest

Prevention of progression to acute myocardial infarction

- both aspirin and heparin have been shown to decrease the progression from unstable angina to MI (N Engl J Med 1985;313:1369–1375, N Engl J Med 1983;309:396–403, N Engl J Med 1988;319:1105–1111)
- beta-blockers have been used for acute intervention in unstable angina and fewer patients went on to develop MI with atenolol (Lancet 1986;2:57–69), propranolol (Clin Pharmacol Ther 1975;17:232, Br Med J 1975;1:117–119), and metoprolol (N Engl J Med 1983;308:614–618, Br Heart J 1986;56:400–413), and a metaanalysis led to the same conclusion (Circulation 1983;67[suppl I]:I32–I41)
- overall, there are few data to support the routine use of calcium antagonists for primary or secondary intervention in MI

Prolongation of life

- aspirin was the first drug shown to decrease mortality in unstable angina (N Engl J Med 1983;309:396–403), and its beneficial effects have been confirmed in subsequent studies (N Engl J Med 1985;313:1369–1375, N Engl J Med 1988;319:1105–1111)
- heparin has been found equally effective as aspirin in decreasing mortality in one study of unstable angina (N Engl J Med 1988;319:1105–1111)
- thrombolytics have not decreased mortality of unstable angina, and therefore risks outweight benefits (Clin Cardiol 1990;13:679–686)

Myocardial infarction

Minimization of loss of myocardium

- early treatment with IV nitroglycerin in patients with acute MI prevents infarct expansion (ventricular remodeling) measured at 6 weeks after infarction (Circulation 1987;76[suppl IV]:IV128)
- the extent of left ventricular asynergy and the evidence of infarction expansion were reduced by the combination of coronary reperfusion (mechanical or pharmacological) and IV nitroglycerin administration in patients with acute MI (J Am Coll Cardiol 1988;11[Suppl A]:90A)
- short-term administration of IV nitroglycerin to patients with acute MI resulted in improvement of electrocardiographical evidence of myocardial ischemia, regardless of the level of left ventricular function (Br Heart J 1976;38:612–621)

Prolongation of life

- early treatment (within 10 hours of symptoms' onset) of patients with acute MI with 48 hours of IV nitroglycerin resulted in a trend toward decreases in 3 month mortality, in-hospital death, infarct extension, and new onset of CHF in a small (n = 104) study, but the results did not reach statistical significance (Circulation 1983;68:576–588)
- a metaanalysis of 7 studies (n > 1000) revealed a reduction in mortality (14%) for the group receiving IV nitroglycerin versus 21% for the control patients (Circulation 1985;72[Suppl III]:III-24)
- the use of beta-blockers in the postinfarct period has conclusively resulted in a reduction in mortality, reinfarction, and sudden cardiac death: alprenolol (Lancet 1974;2:1157–1172, Lancet 1979;2:865–867), metoprolol (Am J Cardiol 1984;53[suppl]:1D–50D), timolol (Br

Med J 1982;284:155–160), and propranolol (Circulation 1985; 72:449–455, Am Heart J 1979;97:797–807)
- pooled data (Prog Cardiovasc Dis 1985;27:335–371) suggest that beta-blockers with intrinsic sympathomimetic activity (ISA) are less effective than those without ISA
- conflicting data exist for acebutolol (Am J Cardiol 1990;66:24C–31C) but the beta-blockers with ISA are of no advantage
- verapamil (Am J Cardiol 1990;66:779–785) has not been shown to decrease mortality but does decrease the combined end points of death and adverse cardiovascular events in patients with MI without CHF
- a review of two verapamil studies (Danish Verapamil Infarction Trials I and II) concluded that verapamil decreases mortality after MI (these patients did not receive beta-blockers) (Am J Cardiol 1990;66:331–401, Am J Cardiol 1990;66:855–856)
- the overall benefit of verapamil on reducing reinfarction and mortality in patients after MI is weak (Am J Cardiol 1991;67:1295–1367)
- diltiazem (N Engl J Med 1986;315:423–429, N Engl J Med 1988;319:385–392) did not alter the mortality of MI in 14 day or 25 month follow-up, but did reduce the frequency of reinfarction in patients with non–Q wave MI at 14 days in patients without evidence of pulmonary congestion on chest X-rays and/or ejection fractions greater than 40%
- all thrombolytic agents have been effective in myocardial salvage and impressive in decreasing mortality (by 25–40%) from acute MI: streptokinase (Lancet 1986; 1:397–401, Lancet 1988;2:349–360), tissue plasminogen activator (Lancet 1988;2:525–533), anistreplase plasminogen streptokinase activator complex (Lancet 1990; 335:427–431) and a recent comparative trial: Global Utilization of Streptokinase and Tisysue Plasminogen Activator for Occluded Coronary Arteries (GUSTO) (N Engl J Med 1993;329:673–682)
- when aspirin or heparin is used concomitantly, mortality may be decreased (by 40-50%)

▶ When Should I Consider Drug Therapy?

Suspected angina

- all patients with suspected angina should receive drug therapy in an attempt to decrease the frequency and severity of angina and thereby improve the quality of life

Chronic stable angina

- all patients with suspected or proven chronic stable angina should receive drug therapy in an attempt to decrease symptoms after an evaluation to rule out other causes of their symptoms
- maintenance therapy should be considered for patients who are psychologically troubled by recurrent angina or who have angina pain more than 2–3 times a week

Unstable angina

- all patients with suspected or proven unstable angina should receive drug therapy in an attempt to relieve symptoms and prevent MI

Acute myocardial infarction

- all appropriate patients with a suspected or proven MI should receive thrombolytic therapy
- appropriate patients are those without contraindications to thrombolytic therapy with pain for 12 hours or less and ST segment elevation in two contiguous leads
- much research is underway, and similar patients older than 75 years seem to benefit as much or more than younger patients do, but the frequency of major and fatal bleeding complications is higher

- absolute contraindications to thrombolytic therapy are active internal bleeding, suspected aortic dissection, diabetic hemorrhagic retinopathy, any other ophthalmic hemorrhages, history of cerebrovascular accident known to be hemorrhagic, recent head trauma, known intracranial neoplasm, pregnancy, blood pressure greater than 200/120 mmHg, and history of allergic reactions to any thrombolytic agent
- relative contraindications (if evidence of an MI is strong enough, thrombolytic therapy should still be used) to thrombolytic therapy are history of severe hypertension, history of cerebrovascular accident, significant liver dysfunction, active peptic ulcer, patients taking oral anticoagulants, surgery or trauma from 2 weeks to 6 months previously (trauma or surgery within less than 2 weeks is an absolute contraindication), and traumatic cardiopulmonary recuscitation
- when patients present with a convincing history of an acute MI within 12 hours of symptoms and have uninterpretable ST segments (e.g., bundle branch block), the patient should be treated with thrombolytic therapy unless contraindications are present
- all postinfarction patients should be considered candidates for prophylactic therapy in an attempt to reduce mortality and sudden cardiac death

▶ *What Drug Should I Use for Initial Treatment?*

Suspected angina
SUBLINGUAL NITROGLYCERIN

- any patient with suspected anginal symptoms should have sublingual nitroglycerin available and be instructed in its use
- sublingual nitroglycerin is rapid acting, effective, convenient for the patient to use and carry around, and inexpensive
- sublingual nitroglycerin is also useful as prevention before planned exercise that may bring on symptoms
- nitroglycerin tablets and nitroglycerin spray are equally effective
- nitroglycerin spray is more expensive per dose than the tablets; however, if nitroglycerin is used only infrequently, it may be more cost-effective because nitroglycerin tablets are outdated after 6 months, while the spray is good for 3 years

Chronic stable angina
ASPIRIN

- all patients with proven chronic stable angina (men and women) should be treated with daily aspirin, as aspirin has been shown to decrease mortality from MIs and other thromboembolic events (Cardiology 1990;77[suppl 2]:99–109, Lancet 1988;2:349–360, Ann Pharmacother 1992;26:1530–1533)

SUBLINGUAL NITROGLYCERIN

- all patients with chronic stable angina should have sublingual nitroglycerin available and be instructed in its use (see above)

Initial drug choice for long-term treatment depends on the presence or absence of other concomitant disease states, side effects, and cost

Patients with no concomitant disease
NADOLOL, ATENOLOL

- beta-blockers should be the first-choice therapy, in conjunction with PRN sublingual nitroglycerin, because they are inexpensive, are effective, can be given once per day, and decrease the chance of an arrhythmia, reinfarction, and sudden cardiac death after MI
- even in patients with mixed angina (angina at exercise and rest) in whom coronary vasospasm may play a role in the cause of the pain, beta-blockers are as effective as calcium channel blockers (Br Heart J 1987;57:505–511)
- calcium channel blockers are expensive and usually must be given more than once daily
- nadolol, a nonselective beta-blocker with low lipid solubility should be tried initially, as it has proven effectiveness and has many advantages over propranolol (can be given once a day and has more consistent absorption characteristics)
- the beta$_2$-blockade of nadolol may offer a distinct advantage by blockade of epinephrine (beta$_2$)–induced arrhythmia and hypokalemia
- other once-daily beta-blockers (e.g., atenolol and acebutolol) may be used instead of nadolol if they are less expensive than nadolol (no generic is available for acebutolol) or if the patient has a problem with cold extremities, which may be worsened by beta$_2$-antagonism

ISOSORBIDE-5-MONONITRATE, ISOSORBIDE DINITRATE

- oral nitrates have a long history of efficacy and safety, low cost, and lack of serious side effects and should be used in patients in whom beta-blockers are ineffective or not tolerated (Postgrad Med 1992;91:307–318)
- development of tolerance during long-term therapy with nitrates, however, is a major limitation
- isosorbide-5-mononitrate (not available in Canada) has dependable bioavailability because it does not require conversion from dinitrate to mononitrate and has proven efficacy in dosages that tend to circumvent tolerance
- isosorbide dinitrate has been widely studied, but there are inadequate data proving that tolerance is circumvented after the second and third dose of the day during 3 times daily therapy (Am J Cardiol 1992;70:43B–53B)
- halitosis (bad breath), flushing, and drug rash have not been reported with isosorbide mononitrate, as they have been with isosorbide dinitrate
- nitroglycerin tablets and capsules are popular products; however, the evidence of their efficacy and dosing regimens are extrapolated from studies with poor controls or presumed from knowledge of other nitrate products (their use is not recommended)

TRANSDERMAL NITROGLYCERIN

- nitroglycerin patches are more expensive than generic oral isosorbide dinitrate and should be used only if the patient cannot tolerate oral medications or does not like taking pills
- nitroglycerin patches must be removed for 10–12 h/d to avoid the development of tolerance (Postgrad Med 1992;91:307–318) and dose titration is essential
- nitroglycerin ointment is inconvenient and messy, and its only advantage over oral nitrates is that the effect can be stopped relatively quickly by wiping it off

DILTIAZEM, NIFEDIPINE, VERAPAMIL

- useful additions if beta-blockers and nitrates are not effective
- all calcium channel blockers are equally effective; however, diltiazem is usually the best tolerated calcium channel blocker and should be chosen over other agents unless there are significant price differences

- in Printzmetal's angina, an uncommon condition, calcium channel blockers are more effective than beta-blockers

Patients with concomitant disease states

Hypertension

NADOLOL, ATENOLOL

- beta-blockers are chosen over nitrates to treat both the hypertension and angina with a single agent, and beta-blockers are less expensive than calcium antagonists
- see above for which beta-blocker to choose

DILTIAZEM, NIFEDIPINE, VERAPAMIL

- if patients are unable to take beta-blockers, calcium antagonists are excellent alternatives
- see above for which calcium channel blocker to choose

ISOSORBIDE-5-MONONITRATE, ISOSORBIDE DINITRATE, TRANSDERMAL NITROGLYCERIN

- if anginal symptoms are poorly controlled with a beta-blocker or a calcium channel blocker regimenn, the addition of a nitrate is recommended because of the long-term experience with the combination of nitrates and a beta-blocker and expense considerations
- the consideration for the additions of the second or third agent for control of angina is similar in these patients to the case with chronic stable angina after hypertension is controlled

Congestive heart failure or impaired left ventricular function (ejection fraction < 40%)

ISOSORBIDE-5-MONONITRATE, ISOSORBIDE DINITRATE, TRANSDERMAL NITROGLYCERIN

- nitrates are effective and inexpensive and are the agents of first choice, as they do not depress left ventricular function
- nitrates may be used in these patients even when mitral regurgitation is present
- beta-blockers are not generally used in patients with CHF; however, when introduced slowly, they can improve, not worsen, CHF
- verapamil and diltiazem can both depress left ventricular function and should not be used in patients with CHF
- nifedipine may be useful if reduction in afterload exceeds the negative inotropic effect
- calcium antagonists have the potential to depress left ventricular function and have exacerbated symptoms of CHF in some patients with ejection fractions less than 30%

Postmyocardial infarction

NADOLOL, ATENOLOL, PROPRANOLOL, METOPROLOL

- patients should be treated empirically with beta-blockers after an MI (Am J Cardiol 1990;66:3C–8C) because there are convincing data that reinfarction, sudden cardiac death, and overall mortality are reduced
- only timolol, propranolol, metoprolol, and acebutolol have been shown to have significant long-term effects on mortality, and some clinicans suggest that only those beta-blockers with proven long-term postinfarction effects should be used for prophylaxis (Circulation 1991;84[suppl VI]:VI-101–VI-107)
- both selective and nonselective agents have been shown to reduce morbidity and mortality, although the absolute reduction in mortality is greater when nonselective agents are used (Lancet 1986;2:57–66, N Engl J Med 1981;304:801–807, Prog Cardiovasc Dis 1985;27:335–371)
- most beta-blockers with intrinsic sympathomimetic activity, except acebutolol (Am J Cardiol 1990;66:24C–31C) have been shown not to have an effect on mortality after an MI (Am J Cardiol 1990;66:9C–20C, Prog Cardiovasc Dis 1985;27:355–371)
- nadolol and atenolol have advantages over metoprolol and propranolol in that they can be dosed once daily and have low lipid solubility; however, no studies have shown long-term effects on mortality with these agents
- data for both propranolol (Circulation 1982;66[Suppl II]:II-328) and metoprolol (Circulation 1982;66[Suppl II]:II-144) are consistent with the hypothesis that beta-blockers decrease ventricular ectopy after MI
- the data for empirical use of calcium antagonists after MI have been consistently negative, and these agents should not be used unless the patient has angina that is not reponsive to beta-blocker therapy

Arrhythmias

NADOLOL, ATENOLOL

- recurrent supraventricular tachycardia or paroxysmal atrial fibrillation in patients with angina can be controlled with antianginals having atrioventricular (AV) nodal blocking properties
- a beta-blocker is a good first choice because beta-blockers block AV nodal conduction and have proven long-term benefit in patients with angina
- the use of beta-blockers to prevent ventricular ectopy is controversial
- the Cardiac Arrhythmia Suppression Trial (CAST) study suggests that it is best to avoid treatment of ventricular ectopy with type IC antiarrhythmic agents without electrophysiological or rigorous exercise and ambulatory Holter monitoring data, and this is probably also true for type IA antiarrhythmics (N Engl J Med 1991;324:781–788)
- empirical use of amiodarone or sotalol has been shown to reduce sudden cardiac deaths in patients with documented ventricular tachycardia after a myocardial infarction (Am J Cardiol 1993;72:62F–69F)

VERAPAMIL

- verapamil should be chosen, as it decreases AV nodal conduction more than the other calcium channel blockers and should be used if the patient is unable to tolerate a beta-blocker

ISOSORBIDE-5-MONONITRATE, ISOSORBIDE DINITRATE, TRANSDERMAL NITROGLYCERIN

- should be used in patients with greater than first-degree AV block, as beta-blockers, verapamil, and diltiazem are relatively contraindicated

Chronic obstructive pulmonary disease and asthma

ISOSORBIDE-5-MONONITRATE, ISOSORBIDE DINITRATE, TRANSDERMAL NITROGLYCERIN

- nitrate therapy is the first choice for patients with angina and concomitant COPD or asthma because nitrates are effective in treating angina and have no effect on pulmonary disease
- calcium antagonists are a good second choice in patients with COPD or asthma
- beta-blockers are best avoided in COPD or asthma; however, low doses of beta$_1$-selective agents may be tried as a last choice in COPD (but not asthma)

Diabetes mellitus

ISOSORBIDE-5-MONONITRATE, ISOSORBIDE DINITRATE, TRANSDERMAL NITROGLYCERIN

- nitrate therapy is the best first-choice therapy for patients with angina and diabetes mellitus; however, diabetics tend to be prone to postural hypotension, and patients should be made aware of this potential
- beta-blockers can mask the symptoms associated with hypoglycemia (except sweating) and may inhibit glycogenolysis, prolonging hypoglycemia in the event of excessive insulin administration
- these problems are much less likely in patients not taking insulin (i.e., patients with non–insulin-dependent diabetes mellitus)
- beta$_1$-selective blocking agents can be used in low doses for diabetic patients taking oral hypoglycemics

DILTIAZEM

- diltiazem may be used, but nifedipine should be avoided, as it may cause severe hypotension in diabetic patients with autonomic insufficiency

Intermittent claudication

- nitrates, beta-blockers, and calcium channel blockers can be used safely in the presence of intermittent claudication, provided that there is no evidence of resting leg ischemia, in which case beta-blockers should be avoided (Arch Intern Med 1991;151:1705–1707)
- decision among these agents should be as above for patients with no concomitant disease

Raynaud's phenomenon

NIFEDIPINE

- patients with both Raynaud's phenomenon and angina can have both conditions effectively treated with nifedipine (Lancet 1982;2:1299–1301)
- nifedipine has proven efficacy in Raynaud's phenomenon, and is the most studied calcium channel blocker for this disease
- diltiazem and nicardipine have been shown to be effective for Raynaud's phenomenon but have not been as extensively studied (Hypertension 1991;17:593–602)
- beta-blockers are best avoided in Raynaud's phenomenon because they may exaggerate the normal fall in digital arterial pressure in response to cooling (Br J Clin Pharmacol 1982;13[suppl 2]:317S–320S) and there are some reports of digital gangrene (Br Med J 1979;1:721–722, Br Med J 1979;1:955, Lancet 1978;1:1216)

ISOSORBIDE-5-MONONITRATE, ISOSORBIDE DINITRATE, TRANSDERMAL NITROGLYCERIN

- an excellent second choice for angina complicated by Raynaud's phenomenon, as they have a vasodilatory effect

Migraine

NADOLOL, ATENOLOL

- beta-blockers can decrease the incidence of migraine headaches and are preferred for first-line therapy in these patients with angina
- see above for which beta-blocker to choose

VERAPAMIL

- is also effective in migraine headaches
- potent vasodilators such as nitrate and nifedipine may worsen a migraine headache and should be avoided

Hyperthyroidism

NADOLOL, ATENOLOL

- beta-blockers have been shown to be effective in controlling anxiety, tachycardia, palpitations, and tremors in hyperthyroidism and are agents of first choice (Drugs 1984;27:425–446)
- see above for which beta-blocker to choose

Unstable angina

SUBLINGUAL NITROGLYCERIN

- sublingual nitroglycerin can be safely given if systolic blood pressure is at least 90 mmHg, and doses can be repeated every 3–5 minutes
- multiple doses may be required and can be given as long as systolic blood pressure is at or above 90 mmHg

MORPHINE

- provides analgesic effect and reduces myocardial oxygen demand by reducing ventricular preload but blocks the patient's perception of pain, which is an important indication of ischemia

ASPIRIN

- all patients with strongly suspected or proven unstable angina should receive an oral aspirin tablet (N Engl J Med 1988;319:1105–1111), as it has been shown to decrease mortality in unstable angina (N Engl J Med 1983; 309:396–403) and its beneficial effects have been confirmed in subsequent studies (N Engl J Med 1985;313: 1369–1375, N Engl J Med 1988;319:1105–1111)
- aspirin has been shown to decrease the progression of unstable angina to MI (N Engl J Med 1985;313:1369–1375, N Engl J Med 1983;309:396–403, N Engl J Med 1988; 319:1105–1111)

HEPARIN

- all patients with chest pain at rest (symptomatic proven unstable angina) should receive IV heparin to prevent thrombus formation (Clin Cardiol 1990;13:679–686, N Engl J Med 1988;319:1105–1111)
- warfarin is not usually added initially because of the possibility of the patient's undergoing coronary artery surgery or angioplasty

INTRAVENOUS NITROGLYCERIN

- all patients who remain symptomatic after sublingual nitroglycerin administration or have recurrent pain should receive IV nitroglycerin for 48 hours (Clin Cardiol 1990;13:679–686), and the dose should be titrated to appropriate reductions in blood pressure
- it is thought that IV dosing with titration upward overcomes the problem of nitrate tolerance

ISOSORBIDE-5-MONONITRATE, ISOSORBIDE DINITRATE, TRANSDERMAL NITROGLYCERIN

- switch to a nonparenteral form of nitrate preparation after the patient is stabilized (usually after 48 hours of IV therapy or 24 hours of freedom from pain)
- decision between oral route and transdermal route should be based on the patient's preference and cost
- transdermal patch may be more convenient initially for the nursing staff (once-daily application)

NADOLOL, ATENOLOL, METOPROLOL, PROPRANOLOL

- patients with symptomatic, unstable angina who are

treated as above and do not respond should receive IV atenolol (or IV metoprolol in Canada) (Clin Cardiol 1990;13:679–686) unless their heart rate is less than 60 bpm, systolic blood pressure is less than 100 mmHg, or there are contraindications to the use of beta-blockers

- although parenteral therapy is usually recommended, oral administration can also be used with the realization that absorption of the agent takes about 30 minutes (some clinicians recommend the IV route for the first dose possibly to reduce the size of a potential or occurring infarction)
- the decision between IV atenolol and metoprolol should be based on cost
- after the initial parenteral dose, oral therapy with a beta-blocker (nadolol or atenolol) should be started
- patients with symptomatic unstable angina who are treated as above, including IV beta-blockers, and who do not respond should be invasively evaluated (cardiac catheterization) for use of intracoronary thrombolytic therapy or mechanical revascularization.

Acute myocardial infarction

- all patients should be treated empirically with beta-blockers (unless there are contraindications to beta-blockers) after an MI (Am J Cardiol 1990;66:3C–8C) because there are convincing data that they reduce the frequency of reinfarction, sudden cardiac death and overall mortality after MI

As above for unstable angina, plus
STREPTOKINASE

- streptokinase is the drug of first choice because of equivalent efficacy to tissue plasminogen activator in reducing mortality, and it is less expensive
- all appropriate patients with a suspected or proven MI should receive thrombolytic therapy
- appropriate patients are those without contraindications to thrombolytic therapy with pain lasting 12 hours or less and ST segment elevation in two contiguous leads
- when patients have a convincing history of an acute MI within 12 hours of symptoms and have uninterpretable ST segments (e.g., bundle branch block), the patient should be treated with thrombolytic therapy unless contraindications are present

TISSUE PLASMINOGEN ACTIVATOR (ALTEPLASE)

- drug of choice if patients have received streptokinase, have been given anisoylated plasminogen streptokinase activator complex, or have been treated for a streptococcal infection within the previous year because these patients have streptococcal antibodies, which neutralize the streptokinase and could cause severe allergic reactions
- may be better in hypotensive patients, as streptokinase causes a higher incidence of hypotension than does tissue plasminogen activator, although thrombolytic-induced hypotension is uniformly transient and easily managed with IV fluid administration (Pharmacotherapy 1992; 12:440–444)

ASPIRIN

- aspirin therapy should be given early to all patients
- routine use of heparin rather than aspirin to reduce mortality or reinfarction after streptokinase cannot be recommended at this time (Chest 1992;102:456S–481S, Lancet 1988;2:349–360)
- aspirin can be used in patients who require long-term

warfarin administration, as evidenced by a pilot study of ischemic heart disease (Eur Heart J 1988;836–843) and mechanical heart valves (Can J Cardiol 1991;7[suppl A]:95A)

- aspirin should be continued in all patients indefinitely unless a contraindication exists

HEPARIN

- all patients with an MI should receive heparin to prevent thromboembolism, further coronary artery thrombosis, mural thrombus, and systemic embolism (Chest 1992; 102[suppl]:456S–481S)
- heparin therapy should be instituted, even in patients who do not receive thrombolytic therapy
- heparin should be used to prevent coronary reocclusion with tissue plasminogen activator and should be started concomitantly with tissue plasminogen activator to help decrease the risk of reocclusion
- the American College of Chest Physicians offers a grade C (their weakest) recommendation for the use of heparin after thrombolysis with streptokinase, which has not been strengthened by the results of the GUSTO trial (N Engl J Med 1993;329:673–682)
- heparin therapy should be used for high-risk patients to prevent deep vein thrombosis
- high-risk patients are those older than 70 years old with a history of previous MI, large anterior MI, heart failure, or shock
- a preventive subcutaneous regimen should be considered in patients who are immobilized for longer than 3 days, are obese, or have signs of chronic venous insufficiency

WARFARIN

- for many patients, the risks of standard warfarin therapy are high and prolonged anticoagulation after an MI is not warranted until definitive data are available from ongoing trials
- consider warfarin in patients with a prior embolus, left ventricular thrombus, large anterior infarcts, atrial fibrillation, or left ventricular aneurysm or patients who have or develop left ventricular dysfunction (failure), who do not have contraindications to anticoagulation, and who are willing to undergo regular medical and laboratory follow-up
- start warfarin administration after arterial punctures are no longer required

COLACE

- stool softeners are routinely given to prevent straining and vagally mediated heart block

LIDOCAINE

- cardioversion should be used to treat ventricular fibrillation and unstable symptomatic ventricular tachycardia; however, the routine prophylactic use of lidocaine for the prevention of ventricular fibrillation or in the presence of frequent premature ventricular contractions is not recommended
- lidocaine has been shown to reduce the incidence of primary ventricular fibrillation following acute MI, but has not been shown to influence mortality positively, and evidence suggests that routine prophylaxis may increase mortality
- the American Heart Association and the American College of Cardiology recommend the prophylactic administration of lidocaine to patients with suspected acute MI

who experience frequent (>6/min) ventricular premature beats (VPBs), closely coupled (R-on-T) VPBs, multiform VPBs or VPBs that occur in short bursts of three or more in succession (N Engl J Med 1974;291:1324–1326; Arch Intern Med 1989;149:2694–2698; Circulation 1990; 82:664–707)

- if the patient is receiving an IV beta-blocker, there is likely little reason to add lidocaine
- ventricular arrhythmias appearing 48 hours or longer after an acute MI are associated with an increased risk of sudden cardiac death and should be aggressively investigated and not treated empirically, as empirical therapy with class IC and possibly IA antiarrhythmic agents is associated with increased mortality (N Engl J Med 1991;324:781)

PROCAINAMIDE

- procainamide should be given to patients in whom lidocaine fails to control ventricular arrhythmias

BRETYLIUM TOSYLATE

- can be used in patients who fail to respond to lidocaine or procainamide

MAGNESIUM

- there is evidence from a single trial and a metaanalysis that magnesium may reduce mortality (Am J Cardiol 1991;68:87D–100D, Circulation 1992;86:774–779)

▶ What Dosage Should I Use?

Suspected angina

SUBLINGUAL NITROGLYCERIN

- 0.4 mg (0.3 mg in Canada owing to different dosage forms) placed under the tongue at the onset of symptoms or for prophylaxis before planned exercise
- for the lingual spray, spray on the tongue at the onset of symptoms or as prevention before planned exercise
- patients should discontinue the activity that produced the symptoms and be seated
- this dose should be repeated at 3–5 minute intervals, and if the symptoms are not relieved within 3 doses (15 minutes), the patient should seek emergency medical assistance

Chronic stable angina

ASPIRIN

- 325 mg of enteric-coated aspirin PO daily

SUBLINGUAL NITROGLYCERIN

- as above

NADOLOL

- 40 mg PO daily is given for the initial treatment of angina
- increases in the dosage by 40 mg daily can be made every 3 days until symptoms are controlled or a maximum dosage of 240 mg PO daily is reached
- can also be titrated until exercise-induced heart rate is decreased by 15%

ATENOLOL

- 50 mg PO daily is given for the initial treatment of angina
- increases by 50 mg daily can be made every 3 days until symptoms are controlled or a maximum dosage of 200 mg PO daily is reached

- can also be titrated until exercise-induced heart rate is decreased by 15%

ISOSORBIDE-5-MONONITRATE (QUICK-RELEASE PRODUCT)

- 20 mg PO at 8 AM and 3 PM is effective and avoids tolerance for the regular-release tablets (Ann Intern Med 1994;120:353–359)
- increase the dosage to 40 mg PO with the same dosage schedule after 1 week of therapy if symptoms are not controlled

ISOSORBIDE DINITRATE (QUICK-RELEASE PRODUCT)

- 30 mg PO at 7 AM and 12 noon avoids tolerance for the subsequent 7 AM dose, but the 12 noon dose may not be as effective

TRANSDERMAL NITROGLYCERIN

- 0.4 mg/h for 12–14 h/d applied to provide coverage during the time of maximum symptoms
- dosage titration is essential, and the dosage can be increased every 2–3 days until symptoms are controlled or a maximum of 2 mg/h has been given
- the large doses cover a large surface area and are unacceptable to many patients (J Am Coll Cardiol 1989; 13:786–795)

DILTIAZEM

- 60 mg of diltiazem SR (a twice-daily product) PO BID, increasing the dosage by 60 mg/d at weekly intervals until symptoms are controlled or a maximum dosage of 300 mg/d is reached
- 180 mg of diltiazem CD (a once-daily product) PO daily, increasing the dosage by 60 mg/d at weekly intervals until symptoms are controlled or a maximum dosage of 300 mg/d is reached
- sustained-release preparations are recommended, as they are more convenient and usually not much different in price from the regular-release products (unless a generic regular release is available)
- the regular-release form is started at 30 mg PO Q6H, increasing the dosage weekly by 30 mg PO Q6H until symptoms are controlled or a maximum dosage of 360 mg/d is reached

VERAPAMIL

- 120 mg of verapamil SR PO daily (a once-daily product sometimes given twice daily when dosages exceed 240 mg/d), increasing the dosage weekly by 120 mg daily until symptoms are controlled or a maximum dosage of 480 mg PO daily is reached
- sustained-release preparations are recommended, as they are more convenient and usually not much different in price from the regular release products (unless a generic regular release is available)
- regular-release form is started at 80 mg PO Q8H, increasing the dosage weekly by 80 mg daily until symptoms are controlled or a maximum dosage of 360 mg/d is reached

NIFEDIPINE

- 30 mg of nifedipine XL PO daily, increasing the dosage weekly by 30 mg daily until symptoms are controlled or a maximum dosage of 90 mg PO daily is reached
- 10 mg of nifedipine PA PO BID (only available in Canada), increasing the dosage weekly by 20 mg daily until symp-

toms are controlled or a maximum dosage of 80 mg PO daily is reached
- sustained-release preparations are recommended, as they are more convenient and usually not much different in price from the regular-release products (unless a generic regular release is available)
- the regular-release form is started at 10 mg PO TID and increased weekly by 10 mg PO TID until a maximum dosage of 90 mg/d is reached

Unstable angina

SUBLINGUAL NITROGLYCERIN

- given as above if systolic blood pressure is at least 90 mm Hg, and repeated every 5 minutes

MORPHINE

- 2 mg IV every 5 minutes PRN for relief of chest pain but should be reserved for those patients who fail to respond to nitroglycerin because morphine clouds the perception of pain
- adjust the dosage on the basis of the response to each dose and titrate to achieve pain control and to maintain an adequate level of sedation and respiratory rate
- although peak respiratory depression occurs at 10 minutes after the dose, if the patient is still in pain 5 minutes after the dose of morphine, it is highly unlikely that respiratory depression at 10 minutes will occur, and the patient should be given morphine every 5 minutes until relief of pain
- IM injections should be avoided because they can raise creatine kinase values, and serious IM bleeding can occur in anticoagulated patients

ASPIRIN

- 325 mg PO at suspicion of unstable angina diagnosis
- if enteric-coated tablets are used, tablets should be chewed

HEPARIN

- 100 units/kg (either 5000 units, 7500 units, or 10,000 units) IV bolus followed by a continuous infusion of 1250 units/h for 48–72 hours (N Engl J Med 1988;319:1105–1111)
- measure partial thromboplastin time (PTT) 6 hours after the initiation of infusion and 6 hours after every dosage change
- adjust the dosage to prolong activated PTT to 2–2$\frac{1}{2}$ times normal values (normal = 25–35 seconds)

INTRAVENOUS NITROGLYCERIN

- start with a constant infusion of 10 μg/min
- increase the infusion rate by 10 μg/min (by 25 μg/min when the dosage has reached 50 μg/min) every 5–10 minutes until the signs and symptoms of ischemia are absent or the mean arterial blood pressure is decreased by 10% in previously normotensive patients (30% in previously hypertensive patients), keeping systolic blood pressure at or above 90 mm Hg (Am J Cardiol 1989;64:581–587)
- if the increase in heart rate is more than the decrease in systolic blood pressure, there is a detrimental effect on the double product (heart rate multiplied by systolic blood pressure, which is a bedside estimate of myocardial oxygen demand and should decrease with effective therapy) and the dosage should be decreased
- there is no absolute maximum dose; however, dosages of 200 μg/min or higher may be required, provided that hypotension is avoided

- if invasive monitoring is available, a decrease in the pulmonary capillary wedge pressure of 10–30% is a reasonable goal
- when discontinuing IV nitroglycerin, the dosage should be titrated downward while another nitroglycerin dosage form (oral or topical) is being titrated upward (e.g., apply a nitrate patch and 15 minutes later start decreasing nitroglycerin infusion by 10 μg/min every 5 minutes until the infusion is stopped or symptoms recur); if symptoms recur, add another patch and continue to decrease the infusion

ISOSORBIDE-5-MONONITRATE, ISOSORBIDE DINITRATE, TRANSDERMAL NITROGLYCERIN

- as above

ATENOLOL

- 5 mg IV over 5 minutes and follow with another 5 mg IV 10 minutes later unless heart rate is <60 beats/min or systolic blood pressure is <100 mmHg
- patients who tolerate the IV doses should receive 50 mg orally 2 hours after the last IV dose and again in 12 hours
- a dosage of 100 mg orally PO daily is continued until the patient is discharged unless side effects or contraindications occur

METOPROLOL

- 5 mg IV every 2 minutes until heart rate is <60 beats/min or systolic blood pressure is <100 mmHg or a maximum of 3 doses
- follow parenteral therapy with an oral beta-blocker as above under atenolol (if metoprolol is chosen, start with 50 mg PO BID, increasing up to 100 mg PO BID after 3–4 days)

PROPRANOLOL

- 1 mg IV over 2 minutes and follow with another 1 mg IV 2–3 minutes later unless heart rate is <60 beats/min or systolic blood pressure is less than 100 mmHg
- follow parenteral therapy with an oral beta-blocker as above under atenolol (if propranolol is chosen, start with 40 mg PO Q8H and increase the dose every 2–3 days until 60 mg PO TID is reached)

Acute myocardial infarction

As above for unstable angina, plus

STREPTOKINASE

- 1.5 million units IV over 1 hour (Lancet 1987;2:871–874, Lancet 1988;2:349–360)

TISSUE PLASMINOGEN ACTIVATOR

- 15 mg IV bolus followed by 0.75 mg/kg (not to exceed 50 mg) over 30 minutes; then 0.5 mg/kg (up to 35 mg) over the next 60 minutes (N Engl J Med 1993;329:673–682)

ASPIRIN

- 325 mg PO at diagnosis
- if enteric-coated tablets are used, tablets should be chewed

HEPARIN

- as above

WARFARIN

- 10 mg PO daily and titrated to an international normalized ratio (INR) of 2–3

COLACE

- 100 mg PO BID

LIDOCAINE

- 1.5 mg/kg IV (usually 100 mg) over 1–2 minutes as an initial loading dose
- 5–10 minutes later, administer a second loading dose of 0.75 mg/kg IV (usually 50 mg) over 1–2 minutes
- maximum loading dose is 3 mg/kg (JAMA 1992; 268:2199–2241)
- if arrhythmia suppression occurs, follow the loading dose with a maintenance dose
- breakthrough ventricular arrhythmias are managed by giving additional boluses of 0.5 mg/kg and increasing the maintenance infusion by 1 mg/min up to 4 mg/min
- maintenance dosage of 3 mg/min in patients younger than 65 years without acute MI, CHF, or chronic liver disease
- 2 mg/min in patients older than 65 years of age, those with acute MI, and those receiving concomitant beta-adrenergic receptor blocking agent therapy
- 1.5 mg/min in patients with chronic liver disease or both acute MI and CHF
- 1 mg/min in patients with CHF and those older than 65 years of age with chronic liver disease

PROCAINAMIDE

- 17 mg/kg IV (12 mg/kg in patients with CHF or renal failure) administered at a rate of 20 mg/min (Eur J Clin Pharmacol 1978;13:303–308)
- a maintenance infusion of 2.8 mg/kg/h (1.9 mg/kg/h in patients with moderate CHF; 1 mg/kg/h in patients with severe CHF or renal failure) should follow the loading dose

BRETYLIUM TOSYLATE

- for hemodynamically unstable ventricular tachycardia or ventricular fibrillation, the initial loading dose should be 5 mg/kg administered undiluted by rapid IV injection
- if no response occurs in 3–5 minutes for ventricular fibrillation or 5–15 minutes for ventricular tachycardia, administer 10 mg/kg undiluted by rapid IV injection
- if no response occurs in several minutes, administer an additional dose of 10 mg/kg undiluted by rapid IV injection

▶ How Long Should I Treat with My Initial Regimen?

Suspected angina

- initial treatment with sublingual nitroglycerin should continue as long as patients are suspected or known to have angina
- patients should be evaluated within 4 weeks with some provocative test such as a symptom-limited exercise treadmill test or an exercise or pharmacological stress test with thallium perfusion imaging
- maintenance therapy should be considered for patients who are psychologically troubled by recurrent angina or who have angina pains more than 2–3 times a week

Chronic stable angina

- initial treatment with the first-line drug of choice should be continued until the patient's condition deteriorates or the patient undergoes a revascularization procedure
- if the patient's condition deteriorates at any time, continue to increase the dosage of the first agent until toxicity develops or the maximum dosage is achieved

- if the patient's condition deteriorates, a second-line agent should be added if not contraindicated
- if optimal therapy with 2 drugs is unable to control symptoms, a third drug can be used unless contraindicated

Unstable angina, acute myocardial infarction

- treat until stabilized
- the patient should stabilize within 24 to 48 hours, and if not, should be evaluated for revascularization procedures
- continue heparin administration for 3–4 days or until the patient is stable
- when the patient is free from ventricular arrhythmias for 12–24 hours, the antiarrhythmic drug can be discontinued

▶ What Efficacy Parameters Should I Follow and How Frequently Do I Have to Assess My Patient?

Suspected angina

- relief of chest pain should be evaluated for efficacy of sublingual nitroglycerin at 5 minute intervals, and if the symptoms are not relieved within 3 doses (15 minutes), the patient should seek emergency medical assistance

Chronic stable angina

- relief of chest pain and decreased frequency of chest pain
- reduction in the use of nitroglycerin tablets
- resolution of ST segment depression or reduction in the amount of total daily ischemia on Holter monitoring should be achieved for silent ischemia
- patient should be evaluated every time the dosage of an antianginal drug needs to be increased
- patients should be reevaluated with treadmill exercise tests when symptoms change or at least every 3 years

Unstable angina

- relief of chest pain and decreased frequency of chest pain
- frequency of assessment depends on the frequency of chest pain
- serial creatine kinase determinations and EKGs in first 24 hours are used to rule out an MI
- reduced frequency of original complaints (e.g., shortness of breath)
- ST-T wave abnormalities should resolve and not reoccur

Acute myocardial infarction

- relief of chest pain and decreased frequency of chest pain
- frequency of assessment depends on the frequency of chest pain and complications of MI (cardiogenic shock, arrhythmias, septal rupture)

▶ Should I Add Another Drug or Substitute Therapy If My Initial Drug Therapy Fails?

Anginal symptoms

- add chronic maintenance drugs as you would for chronic stable angina

Chronic stable angina, unstable angina

- increase the dosage of first drug until efficacy is seen or the maximum dosage is achieved
- if no effect has been seen with the first drug stop it and start administration of a second-line drug
- if some effect has been seen with maximum dosages of the first drug, add a second-line drug
- if optimal therapy with two drugs is unable to control symptoms, the third-line agent should be added unless contraindicated
- combination therapy with nitrates and a beta-blocker has been shown to be superior to a beta-blocker alone in a

study of acute disease (J Am Coll Cardiol 1985; 6:1395–1401), and the major benefits of each offset the major side effects of the other

- calcium antagonists may be added when optimal two drug therapy (nitrates and beta-blockers) are not adequate for symptom control (Am Heart J 1989;118:1093–1097) or if the patient is unable to tolerate a beta-blocker
- triple-drug therapy (maximum therapy) is not necessarily optimum and should be reserved for those patients still symptomatic while receiving double-drug (nitrates and beta-blockers) therapy (J Am Coll Cardiol 1984;3: 1051–1057)
- combined therapy can decrease perfusion pressure, resulting in decreased exercise time compared with that documented on optimal single or double (nitrate and beta-blocker) drug therapy
- bepridil has been shown to be effective in increasing treadmill walking time and reducing the frequency of anginal episodes (Circulation 1985;71:98–103) and may be of particular value in angina refractory to optimal double- or triple-drug therapy
- angiography should be used to assess risks and benefits of revascularization procedures for patients who do not respond adequately

Acute myocardial infarction

- patients with persistent ischemia or hemodynamic compromise should undergo coronary angiography

▶ How Long Should I Continue Drug Therapy?

Anginal symptoms

- therapy is lifelong

Chronic stable angina

- maintenance drug therapy should likely be continued indefinitely; however, changes in the patient's lifestyle and the natural history of the disease will suggest reevaluation for the lowest effective dosage, replacement with a better or less expensive agent, dosage decrease, or even drug discontinuation

Unstable angina

- maintenance drug therapy should likely be continued indefinitely

Acute myocardial infarction

- continue warfarin for 3 months after MI and continue aspirin indefinitely
- treat with prophylactic therapy lifelong if tolerated
- beta-blocker therapy has been shown to reduce mortality for at least 6 years after MI; therefore, beta-blockers are continued as long as the patient tolerates the therapy

Useful References

Pepine CJ. Is silent ischemia a treatable risk factor in patients with angina pectoris? Circulation 1990;82:135–142

von Dohlen TW, Rogers WB, Frank MJ. Pathophysiology and management of unstable angina. Clin Cardiol 1989;12:363–369

Thadani U, Hamilton SF, Olson E, et al. Transdermal nitroglycerin patches in angina pectoris: Dose, titration, duration of effect, and rapid tolerance. Ann Intern Med 1986;105:485–492

Engles McAnally L, Corn CR, Hamilton SF. Aspirin for the prevention of vascular death in women. Ann Pharmacother 1992;26:1530–1533

Gunnar RM, Passamani ER, Bourdillon PD, et al. Guidelines for the early management of patients with acute myocardiual infarction. Report of the American College of Cardiology/American Heart Association Task Force on Assessment of Diagnostic and Therapeutic Cardiovascular Procedures (Subcommittee to Develop Guidelines for the Early Management of Patients with Acute Myocardial Infarction). J Am Coll Cardiol 1990;2:249–292

Yusuf S, Petor L, Lewis J, et al. Beta-blockade during and after myocardial infarction: An overview of the randomized trials. Prog Cardiovasc Dis 1985;27:335–371

Chadda K, Goldstein, Byington R, Curb JD. Effect of propranolol after acute myocardial infarction in patients with congestive heart failure. Circulation 1986;3:503–510

Muller DWM, Topol EJ. Selection of patients with acute myocardial infarction for thrombolytic therapy. Ann Intern Med 1990;113:949–960

DRUG THERAPY FOR CARDIAC ARRHYTHMIAS

James E. Tisdale

▶ What Are My Goals of Treatment?

Atrial fibrillation or flutter

to control ventricular rate in patients with acute, chronic, or paroxysmal atrial fibrillation or flutter

to restore sinus rhythm in patients experiencing an acute episode of paroxysmal atrial fibrillation or flutter

to prevent or reduce the frequency of recurrent episodes of paroxysmal atrial fibrillation or flutter

to reduce the risk of systemic embolization and stroke

Atrioventricular (AV) nodal reentrant tachycardia (the most common form of paroxysmal supraventricular tachycardia)

to terminate the tachycardia and to restore sinus rhythm

to maintain sinus rhythm or to reduce the frequency of episodes of AV nodal reentrant tachycardia

Ventricular arrhythmias

to terminate symptomatic ventricular arrhythmias

to prevent subsequent episodes of symptomatic ventricular arrhythmias

to prevent sudden cardiac death in patients with potentially lethal ventricular arrhythmias in survivors of out-of-hospital sudden cardiac death

▶ What Evidence Is Available to Support Drug Therapy for Cardiac Arrhythmias?

Atrial fibrillation or flutter

- treatment has been shown to control ventricular rate, resulting in improvement in blood pressure and enhanced cardiac output in some patients
- in addition, treatment may result in alleviation and/or prevention of symptoms and an enhanced sense of well-being (Drugs 1990;40:841–853)
- anticoagulation has been demonstrated to reduce the risk of embolization and stroke in both rheumatic and non-rheumatic atrial fibrillation (N Engl J Med 1990;323: 1505–1511; N Engl J Med 1990;322:863–868)

Atrioventricular nodal reentrant tachycardia

- termination of an acute episode of paroxysmal supraventricular tachycardia results in alleviation of symptoms associated with the tachycardia
- pharmacological therapy has been shown to reduce the frequency of episodes of symptomatic paroxysmal supraventricular tachycardia (Am J Cardiol 1988;62:56D–61D; Ann Intern Med 1991;114:189–194)

Ventricular arrhythmias

- treatment of acute episodes of symptomatic ventricular arrhythmias may result in the restoration of sinus rhythm and alleviation of symptoms (Circulation 1963;28: 486–491; Lancet 1990;336:670–673)

- no data support the treatment of asymptomatic ventricular arrhythmias, and treatment with certain drugs may be harmful in specific patient populations (Am J Cardiol 1990;66:423–428; N Engl J Med 1989;321:406–412)
- identification and prescription of an antiarrhythmic drug that has been shown to render previously inducible sustained ventricular tachycardia noninducible or that results in favorable modification (decreased rate, shortened duration, and/or reduction of associated symptoms) of an arrhythmia that remains inducible in the electrophysiology laboratory is associated with significantly reduced mortality compared with that for patients for whom an effective drug could not be identified during electrophysiologic testing (J Am Coll Cardiol 1987;10:83–89)
- in survivors of out-of-hospital cardiac arrest, identification and prescription of a drug that renders previously inducible ventricular tachycardia noninducible or that favorably modifies the arrhythmia in the electrophysiology laboratory significantly reduces the chance of recurrence of cardiac arrest (N Engl J Med 1988;318:19–24)

▶ When Should I Consider Drug Therapy?

Atrial fibrillation or flutter
Control of ventricular rate
- attempt to control ventricular rate in all patients with atrial fibrillation or flutter, unless it is transient, is asymptomatic, and/or is due to a correctable underlying cause or intrinsic AV nodal disease prevents the ventricular rate from becoming excessive
- drugs for control of ventricular rate should be administered prior to attempting pharmacological conversion
- unless patients are hemodynamically unstable, rate control is always attempted prior to electrical or pharmacological conversion because quinidine, procainamide, and disopyramide have some anticholinergic activity and therefore may theoretically accelerate conduction through the AV node

Conversion to sinus rhythm
- there is little evidence that drugs for control of ventricular rate are effective for converting patients to normal sinus rhythm
- drugs that may be given intravenously for rate control are not significantly better than placebo for the restoration of normal sinus rhythm (N Engl J Med 1992;326:1264–1271)
- conversion to sinus rhythm should not be attempted in patients with chronic atrial fibrillation (duration >1 year) or in patients with left atrial size greater than 45 mm (as determined by echocardiography), as it is usually unsuccessful (Ann Intern Med 1966;65:216–224; Circulation 1976;53:273–279)
- an attempt should be made to convert all patients with relatively new onset (>1 week and <12 months) asymptomatic or mildly symptomatic atrial fibrillation or flutter with left atrial size less than 45 mm or with acute paroxysmal atrial fibrillation or flutter to normal sinus rhythm when control of ventricular response has been achieved (Ann Intern Med 1966;65:216–224; Clin Pharm 1983;2:312–320)
- patients with acute hemodynamically unstable atrial fibrillation or flutter (hypotension, angina, heart failure) should undergo electrical cardioversion because the delay in conversion with drug therapy may be detrimental (Am Heart J 1986;111:1150–1161)
- hemodynamically stable patients should have either electrical or pharmacological cardioversion, and at present, there are no studies that compare these methods (N Engl J Med 1992;326:1264–1271)
- on the basis of noncomparative trials, electrical cardioversion appears to be more successful than pharmacological conversion
- electrical cardioversion is always preferred in hemodynamically unstable patients
- IV pharmacological cardioversion may be preferable if hospitalized patients have acute atrial fibrillation and when general anesthesia is either undesirable or unavailable
- in most other situations, electrical cardioversion may be preferable because the administration of oral antiarrhythmic agents is associated with a relatively high incidence of adverse effects (N Engl J Med 1992;326:1264–1271)
- electrical cardioversion should not be attempted in patients with digitalis toxicity, as they may be at increased risk of developing ventricular arrhythmias

Maintenance of sinus rhythm
- only patients with frequent and/or symptomatic attacks of paroxysmal atrial fibrillation or flutter should receive long-term therapy to maintain sinus rhythm

Anticoagulation
- patients with paroxysmal or nonvalvular chronic atrial fibrillation should receive anticoagulation if other factors such as hypertension, coronary artery disease, or CHF are present (Arch Intern Med 1990;150:1598–1603)
- all other patients with atrial fibrillation should have anticoagulation with warfarin to minimize the chance of systemic embolization from a cardiac source (Am J Cardiol 1990;65:24C–28C; N Engl J Med 1990;323:1505–1511, Am J Cardiol 1990;65:24C–28C, N Engl J Med 1992;326:1264–1271) if patients do not have contraindications to anticoagulation

Atrioventricular nodal reentrant tachycardia
Acute episode
- patients with an acute episode of symptomatic, hemodynamically stable AV nodal reentrant tachycardia that does not respond to carotid sinus massage or the Valsalva maneuver (Am Heart J 1986;111:1150–1161) should receive pharmacological therapy
- patients who are hemodynamically unstable and/or are experiencing severe symptoms should undergo electrical cardioversion (Am Heart J 1986;111:1150–1161)

Long-term therapy
- patients with frequent or severely symptomatic episodes of AV nodal reentrant tachycardia (Clin Pharm 1983;2:312–320) or patients with symptomatic AV nodal reentrant tachycardia associated with ventricular preexcitation syndromes, such as the Wolff-Parkinson-White syndrome (Cardiovasc Med 1984;9:873–891), should be seen by a cardiac electrophysiologist, and an attempt to electrically ablate the pathway should be made to avoid long-term pharmacological therapy
- if electrical therapy fails or is not desired by the patient, pharmacological therapy should be considered

Ventricular arrhythmias
- all patients with ventricular tachycardia who are hemodynamically unstable and/or are experiencing severe symptoms (syncope, angina, shortness of breath, heart failure) (JAMA 1992;268:2199–2241)
- patients with ventricular fibrillation require immediate asynchronous defibrillation (JAMA 1992;268:2199–2241)

- patients with symptomatic ventricular ectopic activity, symptomatic nonsustained (>3 beats but <30 seconds in duration and spontaneously terminating) or symptomatic sustained (>30 seconds in duration) ventricular tachycardia require treatment
- patients with frequent complex ventricular activity that is asymptomatic do not require therapy
- patients who have been resuscitated from an episode of documented ventricular fibrillation require acute drug therapy until potential causes of the arrhythmia are identified and corrected, if possible, and if no identifiable causes are found, long-term therapy may be required (Circulation 1989;80:1925–1939)
- survivors of an out-of-hospital episode of sudden cardiac death not associated with acute MI may require long-term drug therapy as guided by electrophysiological studies (Circulation 1989;80:1925–1939)

▶ *What Drug Should I Use for Initial Treatment?*

Atrial fibrillation or flutter

Control of ventricular rate

DIGOXIN

- considered the drug of choice for most patients for control of ventricular rate, because CHF is often present in patients with atrial fibrillation or flutter (Drugs 1990;40:841–853; Clin Pharm 1983;2:312–320), and verapamil can worsen CHF
- digoxin has been shown to achieve reductions in resting heart rate during chronic atrial fibrillation or flutter; however, digoxin may have relatively little effect on heart rate during exercise in these patients (Ann Intern Med 1991;114:573–575; Drugs 1986;31:185–197)
- digoxin should not be administered to patients with atrial fibrillation who are known to have Wolff-Parkinson-White syndrome or other syndromes characterized by ventricular preexcitation, as it may paradoxically increase the ventricular rate (Circulation 1977;56:260–267)
- digoxin may be ineffective in patients with paroxysmal atrial fibrillation (sinus rhythm punctuated by attacks of fibrillation) (N Engl J Med 1992;326:1264–1271) and less effective in rate control for patients with high catecholamine level states (e.g., following coronary artery bypass)
- although there is some evidence that digoxin may not be effective in paroxysmal atrial fibrillation, it is still considered the drug of choice by some clinicians (especially because many of these patients have heart failure)

NADOLOL, ATENOLOL, METOPROLOL, PROPRANOLOL, ESMOLOL

- useful if rate is not controlled with digoxin and/or is excessively rapid during exercise
- may have a faster onset than digoxin
- less expensive than verapamil and can be used once daily
- more data on newer beta-blockers (N Engl J Med 1992;326:1264–1271)
- nadolol is a nonselective beta-blocking, lipid-insoluble, once-daily agent
- atenolol can be used if it is less expensive or if there is a problem that may be worsened by beta$_2$-antagonism (e.g., cold extremities), but not in the presence of asthma, because any beta-blockers are potentially dangerous in such patients and their use must be discouraged
- nadolol and atenolol have the advantage over metoprolol and propranolol in that they can be dosed once daily and

have low lipid solubility; however, no studies have shown long-term effects on mortality after MI with these agents
- atenolol (in USA), metoprolol, propranolol, and esmolol are available as parenteral agents
- in patients with a history of MI, some clinicians suggest that only those beta-blockers with proven long-term post-infarction effects be used for prophylaxis (Circulation 1991;84[suppl VI]:VI-101–VI-107)
- only timolol, propranolol, metoprolol, and acebutolol have been shown to have significant long-term effects on postinfarction mortality
- parenteral esmolol (a short-acting beta-blocker) can be used instead of the other beta-blockers in patients with poor ventricular dysfunction because it has a short half-life and its effects disappear quickly

VERAPAMIL

- use in patients who do not respond to digoxin and beta-blockers as long as patient does not have poor left ventricular function
- verapamil should also be used after digoxin and beta-blockers to control ventricular rate in patients with paroxysmal atrial fibrillation or flutter, even though digoxin may not be sufficiently effective in these patients (Br Heart J 1990;63:225–227)
- verapamil may be more effective than digoxin in controlling ventricular rate in atrial fibrillation or flutter associated with increases in circulating catecholamines (anxiety, exercise)

DILTIAZEM

- intravenous diltiazem is an alternative to parenteral verapamil if the negative inotropic effects of verapamil would be detrimental to the patient (likely neither verapamil nor diltiazem should be used on a long-term basis if the patient has left ventricular dysfunction)

Conversion to sinus rhythm

QUINIDINE

- quinidine should be considered the drug of choice because it is the agent for which the most efficacy data exist and because many patients have CHF (N Engl J Med 1992;326:1264–1271)
- however, concern about possible adverse effects of quinidine therapy on mortality is provoking reevaluation of its use in atrial fibrillation or flutter (Circulation 1990;82:1106–1116)

FLECAINIDE

- flecainide should be considered in patients intolerant to quinidine who have no history of ischemic heart disease or left ventricular dysfunction (Am J Cardiol 1986;58:496–498)

PROCAINAMIDE

- procainamide should be considered for patients intolerant to quinidine who have ischemic heart disease or left ventricular dysfunction
- IV procainamide should be administered to patients with atrial fibrillation or flutter who are known to have ventricular preexcitation such as Wolff-Parkinson-White syndrome because procainamide blocks conduction in the accessory pathway and, unlike digoxin or verapamil, may not increase ventricular rate in this situation (Cardiol Clin 1990;8:503–521)
- IV procainamide is the drug of choice if rapid conversion is required (and electrical cardioversion cannot be per-

formed) because quinidine should not be given intravenously, as it causes hypotension

Maintenance of sinus rhythm

QUINIDINE

- metaanalysis of several studies suggests that, although quinidine is significantly more effective than placebo at maintaining sinus rhythm in patients with atrial fibrillation or flutter, it may increase mortality
- until these findings are confirmed in a prospective trial, and until the effects on mortality of other antiarrhythmic drugs used for this indication are evaluated, quinidine should remain the drug of first choice for the maintenance of sinus rhythm (Circulation 1990;82:1106–1116, Medical Lett Drugs Ther 1991;33:55–60)
- quinidine therapy may be preferable to therapy with procainamide, as more data supporting the efficacy of quinidine exist (Am Heart J 1986;111:1150–1161)

Anticoagulation

WARFARIN

- short-term anticoagulation with warfarin 3 weeks prior to attempting conversion (electrically or pharmacologically) to sinus rhythm should be considered for patients with atrial fibrillation/flutter of duration longer than 2 days (Chest 1992;102[suppl]:426S–433S) and should be continued until normal sinus rhythm has been maintained for 4 weeks
- at this time, evidence supporting the efficacy of warfarin for the prevention of stroke in atrial fibrillation is stronger than that for aspirin (Circulation 1991;84:527–539, Chest 1992;104:426S–433S)

HEPARIN

- for emergency cardioversion (patients with angina or hemodynamic complications), start heparin administration immediately (if patient has been in atrial fibrillation for longer than 2 days)

Atrioventricular nodal reentrant tachycardia

Acute episodes

ADENOSINE

- is considered the drug of choice for the acute termination of AV nodal reentrant tachycardia because of its shorter half-life and significantly lower incidence of hypotension compared with verapamil (Ann Intern Med 1991;114:513–515, JAMA 1992;268:2199–2241)

VERAPAMIL

- is considered the drug of choice when adenosine does not work or when the arrhythmia returns following adenosine treatment (JAMA 1992;268:2199–2241)
- verapamil should not be used for the treatment of a wide QRS tachycardia unless it is known to be supraventricular in origin; administration of verapamil in patients with ventricular tachycardia may result in acceleration of the tachycardia and severe hemodynamic deterioration (Am J Cardiol 1987;59:1107–1110)

ESMOLOL

- if adenosine and verapamil are ineffective or contraindicated, esmolol may be used (except in patients with severe left ventricular dysfunction or contraindications to beta-blockade)

DIGOXIN

- digoxin should be used in patients in whom adenosine,

verapamil, and esmolol are ineffective or contraindications to these agents exist

Long-term therapy

DIGOXIN

- there are no studies comparing the efficacy of agents for prevention of AV nodal reentrant tachycardia, but most sources consider digoxin to be the drug of choice (Arch Intern Med 1987;147:1706–1716)
- therapy may be selected empirically for patients with AV nodal reentrant tachycardia that is not life-threatening and not associated with serious symptoms
- few data exist comparing the efficacy of drugs for the suppression of recurrent episodes of AV nodal reentrant tachycardia
- because response to IV verapamil does not accurately predict long-term response to oral verapamil (Circulation 1980;62:996–1010) and because many of these patients have concomitant left ventricular dysfunction, digoxin is a reasonable choice as a first-line agent

VERAPAMIL

- can be used when digoxin is ineffective

NADOLOL, ATENOLOL, METOPROLOL, PROPRANOLOL

- see above under atrial fibrillation or flutter

Electrophysiological testing

- for patients with recurrent AV nodal reentrant tachycardia that is potentially life-threatening or is associated with serious symptoms (hemodynamic instability, syncope), and in those with Wolff-Parkinson-White syndrome with the potential for rapid atrial fibrillation, selection of appropriate long-term oral drug therapy should be guided by invasive electrophysiological testing

Ventricular arrhythmias

Treatment of acute symptomatic ventricular arrhythmias

LIDOCAINE

- lidocaine is considered the drug of choice, as it is effective and is associated with a lower incidence of hypotension than IV procainamide (Lancet 1990;336:670–673, Circulation 1963;28:486–491, JAMA 1992;268:2199–2241)

PROCAINAMIDE

- used in patients unresponsive to lidocaine (JAMA 1992;268:2199–2241)

BRETYLIUM

- used in patients unresponsive to lidocaine or procainamide (JAMA 1992;268:2199–2241)

Long-term therapy for ventricular arrhythmias

NADOLOL, ATENOLOL, METOPROLOL

- for symptomatic benign ventricular arrhythmias (that are nonsustained, are hemodynamically stable, and are not associated with structural heart disease), beta-blockers are preferable to other antiarrhythmic agents because of the benign nature of these arrhythmias, and because of the relatively low incidence of adverse effects of beta-blockers compared with those of other antiarrhythmic drugs (Drugs 1974;7:118–129)
- for symptomatic premature ventricular depolarizations or nonsustained ventricular tachycardia after acute MI, beta-blockers are preferable to other antiarrhythmic

agents because they have been shown to suppress arrhythmias and to reduce mortality in patients who have survived acute MI (JAMA 1982;247:1707–1724; N Engl J Med 1983;308:614–618)

- nadolol and atenolol have advantages over metoprolol and propranolol in that they can be dosed once daily and have low lipid solubility; however, no studies have shown long-term effects with these agents on mortality after MI
- in patients with a history of MI, some clinicians suggest that only those beta-blockers with proven long-term postinfarction effects should be used for prophylaxis (Circulation 1991;84[suppl VI]:VI-101–VI-107)
- only timolol, propranolol, metoprolol, and acebutolol have been shown to have significant long-term effects on postinfarction mortality
- sotalol can be used in patients with refractory ventricular tachycardia (sotalol has not been shown to reduce mortality after MI and causes torsades de pointes in 2–8% of patients) (N Engl J Med 1994;331:33–38)

Therapy determined by serial drug testing during electrophysiological studies

- patients with symptomatic ventricular arrhythmias (that are nonsustained, are usually hemodynamically stable, and are associated with structural heart disease and a moderate to high risk of sudden cardiac death) should be referred to an electrophysiologist for an assessment of the severity of arrhythmias and selection of appropriate therapy
- during serial drug testing in the electrophysiology laboratory, class IA drugs should be tested initially (usually procainamide or quinidine); if ventricular arrhythmias remain inducible, class IB agents (usually mexiletine) should be tested; if ventricular arrhythmias remain inducible, but a partial response is observed with the class IA drug or mexiletine, a combination of the class IA drug and mexiletine should be tested; if ventricular arrhythmias remain inducible, testing of sotalol should be considered; if arrhythmias remain inducible, amiodarone should be tested; if arrhythmias remain inducible on amiodarone, the drug may be prescribed anyway, or nonpharmacological management should be considered, depending on physician and patient preference (Am J Cardiol 1988;62:39H–45H, Clin Pharm 1991;10:195–205)
- patients with sustained ventricular tachycardia or survivors of ventricular fibrillation or out-of-hospital sudden cardiac death should not be treated empirically but should be referred for invasive electrophysiological studies (Clin Pharm 1991;10:195–205)

▶ What Dosage Should I Use?

Atrial fibrillation or flutter

Control of ventricular rate

DIGOXIN

- 0.013 mg/kg of ideal body weight (Ann Intern Med 1968;69:703–117) for the loading dose
- if the total loading dose is to be greater than 0.75 mg, administer an initial dose of 0.5 mg
- if the total loading dose is to be less than 0.75 mg, administer an initial dose of 0.25 mg
- remainder of calculated total dose administered in 0.25 mg increments every 3–4 hours
- complete load should be given even if ventricular rate control is achieved with the first or second dose

- 0.25 mg PO daily as maintenance dosage
- 0.125 mg daily in patients with renal impairment or who are receiving drugs that may interact with digoxin to cause elevation in serum digoxin concentration

NADOLOL

- if the patient is not symptomatic and rapid rate control is desired, start with 20 mg PO daily and increase every 2–3 days by 20 mg PO daily until the heart rate is controlled or a maximum dosage of 160 mg/d is reached
- not available as a parenteral agent

ATENOLOL

- 5 mg IV over 5 minutes and if tolerated (systolic BP >100 mmHg, heart rate >60 bpm) give second dose of 5 mg IV 10 minutes later (IV atenolol is not available in Canada)
- do not push IV dose until a response is seen, as betablockers do not always work and can precipitate asystole
- parenteral route is used if the patient is symptomatic and the goal is to control the ventricular rate rapidly
- if the patient is not symptomatic and rapid rate control is desired, start with 25 mg PO daily and increase every 2–3 days by 25 mg PO daily until the heart rate is controlled or a maximum dosage of 200 mg/d is reached

METOPROLOL

- 5 mg IV every 5 minutes until the heart rate is less than 100 bpm, symptoms are alleviated or 15 mg is reached
- do not push IV dose until a response is seen, as betablockers do not always work and can precipitate asystole
- if the patient is not symptomatic and rapid rate control is desired start with 25 mg PO daily and increase every 2–3 days by 25 mg PO daily until the heart rate is controlled or a maximum dosage of 200 mg/d is reached

PROPRANOLOL

- 1 mg IV every 2 minutes until the heart rate is less than 130 bpm (or 100 bpm if angina or CHF is present) or 0.1 mg/kg (7–10 mg) is reached

ESMOLOL

- 500 μg/kg IV over 1 minute as a loading dose followed by 50 μg/kg/min as the initial maintenance infusion
- if inadequate response after 4 minutes, repeat loading dose of 500 μg/kg over 1 minute and increase maintenance infusion rate to 100 μg/kg/min
- if inadequate response after 4 minutes, repeat loading dose of 500 μg/kg/min over 1 minute and increase maintenance infusion rate to 150 μg/kg/min
- if inadequate response after 4 minutes, repeat loading dose of 500 μg/kg/min and increase maintenance infusion rate to the maximum recommended rate of 200 μg/kg/min (Am Heart J 1986;111:42–48)
- as desired heart rate is approached, the incremental dosage for maintenance may be reduced from 50 to 25 μg/kg/min while the interval titration steps are increased from 4 to 10 minutes (Drugs 1987;33:392–412)

VERAPAMIL

- 2.5 mg IV over 2–3 minutes
- if arrhythmia persists, additional doses of 2.5 mg every 5 minutes should be administered to a maximum of 10 mg or development of hypotension
- pretreatment with calcium chloride 1 g IV over 10 minutes may prevent many of the hypotensive effects of verapamil without antagonizing the negative dromotropic effects (Am J Cardiol 1991;67:300–304)

DILTIAZEM

- 20 mg IV over 2 minutes and if heart rate goal not achieved, give 25 mg IV 15 minutes later
- give 10 mg/h IV continuous infusion; if heart rate goal not achieved increase to 15 mg/h

Conversion to sinus rhythm and maintenance of sinus rhythm

QUINIDINE

- 200 mg of quinidine sulfate PO Q2H until conversion or a maximum dose of 1200 mg PO in 12 hours is reached (Am J Cardiol 1986;58:496–498)
- follow the loading dose with a longer-acting agent such as 324 mg PO TID of quinidine gluconate or 500 mg PO BID of quinidine bisulfate (not available in USA)
- the bisulfate products allow twice-daily administration (versus every 6 hours for the sulfate)
- parenteral quinidine is usually avoided owing to problems with hypotension

FLECAINIDE

- 100 mg PO Q12H
- titrate the dose upward in increments of 50 mg PO Q12H every 4 days to a maximum of 300 mg PO Q12H

PROCAINAMIDE

- 17 mg/kg IV (usually 1 g) administered at a rate of 20 mg/min (Eur J Clin Pharmacol 1978;13:303–308)
- a maintenance infusion of 2.8 mg/kg/h should follow the loading dose
- after a patient has been stabilized on IV procainamide (conversion to sinus rhythm), the total daily dose of oral procainamide should approximate the total daily IV dose, divided every 4 hours if a conventional-release preparation is used and every 6 hours if a sustained-release preparation is used (most clinicians use the sustained-release preparation)
- when oral procainamide therapy is desired for a patient not receiving IV procainamide therapy, an initial daily dose of 50 mg/kg PO divided every 4 hours (conventional-release preparations) or every 6 hours (sustained-release preparations) is recommended (most clinicians use the sustained-release preparation, as there is likely no clinical difference and it allows a more convenient dosing schedule) (JAMA 1971;215:1454–1460)

WARFARIN

- 10 mg PO daily for 3 days, and titrate to achieve an INR of 2–3 (prothrombin time 1.3–1.5 times control values) (N Engl J Med 1990;323:1505–1511)
- titrate to achieve an INR of 2.5–3.5 for patients with mechanical prosthetic valves (Chest 1992;102[suppl]: 445S–455S)

Atrioventricular nodal reentrant tachycardia
Acute episodes

ADENOSINE

- 6 mg IV over 1–2 seconds
- if no response within 2 minutes, give another 12 mg IV over 1–2 seconds, and an additional dose of 12 mg may be administered over 1–2 seconds if necessary 1–2 minutes later (Drugs 1991;41:596–624)

VERAPAMIL

- see above under atrial fibrillation or flutter

ESMOLOL

- see above under atrial fibrillation or flutter

DIGOXIN

- see above under atrial fibrillation or flutter

Long-term therapy
DIGOXIN

- 0.25 mg PO daily
- 0.125 mg daily in patients with renal impairment or who are receiving drugs that may interact with digoxin to cause elevation in serum digoxin concentration

BETA-BLOCKERS

- see above under atrial fibrillation or flutter

Ventricular arrhythmias
LIDOCAINE

- 1.5 mg/kg IV (usually 100 mg) over 1–2 minutes as an initial loading dose
- 5–10 minutes later, administer a second loading dose of 0.75 mg/kg IV over 1–2 minutes
- maximum loading dose is 3 mg/kg (JAMA 1992;268: 2199–2241)
- maintenance dosage of 3 mg/min in patients younger than 65 years without acute MI, CHF, or chronic liver disease
- 2 mg/min in patients older than 65 years of age, those with acute MI, and those receiving concomitant beta-adrenergic receptor blocking agent therapy
- 1.5 mg/min in patients with chronic liver disease or both acute MI and CHF
- 1 mg/min in patients with CHF and those older than 65 years of age with chronic liver disease

PROCAINAMIDE

- as above for atrial fibrillation

BRETYLIUM

- 5 mg/kg IV over 8–10 minutes
- if ventricular tachycardia persists administer second dose of 5 mg/kg IV over 8–10 minutes
- maintenance dose of 2 mg/min (1 mg/min in patients with renal impairment)

NADOLOL

- 80 mg PO daily (40 mg PO daily in patients with low blood pressure, heart rate <60 bpm, or concomitant therapy with agents that depress function of the sinoatrial [SA] or AV nodes) and increase every 2–3 days until beta-blockade is achieved (resting heart rate and heart rate during exercise is suppressed) or a dosage of 160 mg PO daily is reached

ATENOLOL

- 50 mg PO daily (25 mg PO daily in patients with low blood pressure, heart rate < 60 bpm, or concomitant therapy with agents that depress function of the SA or AV nodes) and increase every 2–3 days until beta-blockade is achieved (resting heart rate and heart rate during exercise is suppressed) or a dosage of 100 mg PO daily is reached

METOPROLOL

- 50 mg PO BID (25 mg PO BID in patients with low blood pressure, heart rate < 60 bpm, or concomitant therapy with agents that depress function of the SA or AV nodes) and increase every 2–3 days until beta-blockade is achieved (resting heart rate and heart rate during exercise is suppressed) or a dosage of 100 mg PO BID is reached

▶ **How Long Should I Treat With My Initial Regimen?**

Atrial fibrillation or flutter

Control of ventricular rate

- the ventricular rate should decrease during the 6–8 hour period of the loading dose of digoxin
- therapy should be continued until precipitating factors have been reversed (if they can be identified and are reversible)
- if the rate is not controlled with digoxin, nadolol or verapamil should replace digoxin if the patient can tolerate these agents

Conversion to sinus rhythm

- quinidine therapy should promote cardioversion within 8–24 hours
- if conversion to normal sinus rhythm is not achieved within 24 hours, continue oral quinidine until electrical conversion can be performed (some clinicians believe that quinidine may facilitate electrical conversion but there is little evidence of this)
- if electrical conversion is not an option, switch to another agent

Atrioventricular nodal reentrant tachycardia

Acute episodes

- adenosine should terminate the arrhythmia within 5 minutes
- verapamil should terminate the arrhythmia within 15–20 minutes
- if the arrhythmia persists despite maximum dosages, confirmation of the diagnosis is required
- treatment should be discontinued on restoration of sinus rhythm

Long-term therapy

- the frequency of episodes of paroxysmal supraventricular tachycardia should be reduced within several days to weeks of drug initiation
- if the frequency has not decreased, use of an alternative agent should be considered

Ventricular arrhythmias

Treatment of acute symptomatic ventricular arrhythmias

- treatment should be continued until the underlying cause of arrhythmia is corrected or until the patient is evaluated for oral antiarrhythmic therapy
- if the patient is referred for electrophysiological testing, antiarrhythmic medications should be discontinued at least 5 half-lives prior to the study while the patient is in a monitored environment

▶ **What Efficacy Parameters Should I Follow and How Frequently Do I Have to Assess My Patient?**

Atrial fibrillation or flutter

Control of ventricular rate

Electrocardiogram

- during acute loading, the patient's EKG should be monitored continuously until loading of digoxin is complete

Vital signs

- every 15 minutes until stable, then every 4 hours for 24 hours
- resting apical ventricular rate of 60–80 bpm is a reason-

able target, although 90–100 bpm or decrease of 20% may be acceptable if the patient is asymptomatic at this heart rate
- presence or absence of symptoms related to arrhythmia (palpitations, shortness of breath, dizziness, angina)

Serum digoxin concentrations

- need not be determined unless signs or symptoms of digoxin toxicity are suspected
- if the ventricular rate is within the desired range and there is no evidence of digoxin toxicity, the digoxin dosage should be considered appropriate

Conversion to normal sinus rhythm

Electrocardiogram

- monitor continuously for 24–48 hours for confirmation of cardioversion and for recurrence of arrhythmias

Vital signs

- monitor heart rate and blood pressure

Maintenance of sinus rhythm

Electrocardiogram

- QRS duration and QT intervals should be monitored in patients receiving quinidine or procainamide within 1 week of each dosage increase
- increases in the duration of the QRS complex or QT interval of greater than 25% suggests that further dosage increases should be avoided to prevent induction of ventricular arrhythmias

Serum quinidine or procainamide concentrations

- measurements are not necessary unless noncompliance or toxicity is suspected because clinical monitoring is more relevant for efficacy than is a serum concentration
- titrate the dosage to efficacy or toxicity

Prothrombin time

- if the patient is receiving warfarin, titrate to achieve an INR of 2–3 (prothrombin time 1.3–1.5 times control values) (N Engl J Med 1990;323:1505–1511)
- titrate to achieve an INR of 2.5–3.5 in patients with prosthetic valves

Atrioventricular nodal reentrant tachycardia

Acute episodes

Electrocardiogram

- the EKG should be monitored continuously until the arrhythmia has stopped

Vital signs

- should be assessed every 5 minutes during drug administration
- presence or absence of symptoms related to arrhythmia (palpitations, shortness of breath, dizziness, angina)

Long-term therapy

- frequency or duration of episodes (may be evaluated by ambulatory or transtelephonic EKG or by the patient's reports of symptom frequency)
- patients should be assessed every few weeks during the first few months of therapy and every few months thereafter

Ventricular arrhythmias

Acute symptomatic ventricular arrhythmias

Vital signs

- heart rate, blood pressure, respiratory rate
- should be assessed continuously until arrhythmia is under control

- presence or absence of symptoms related to arrhythmia (palpitations, shortness of breath, dizziness, angina, syncope)

Electrocardiogram

- frequency of ventricular ectopic activity and rate and duration of episodes of ventricular tachycardia
- should be assessed continuously until arrhythmia is under control

Serum lidocaine concentrations

- if the patient's ventricular arrhythmia is under control and no toxicities are present, the lidocaine dosage should be considered appropriate and no measurement of concentration is required
- if signs or symptoms of lidocaine toxicity are present, or if an inadequate response is achieved with the current dosage, a serum lidocaine concentration should be obtained
- if arrhythmia recurs, obtain a serum concentration and increase the dosage by 0.5–1 mg/min pending the results of concentration determination (if the concentration is between 2 and 6 mg/L change to a different drug)

Long-term therapy

- patient should be evaluated every few weeks during the first few months of therapy and every few months thereafter, depending on the frequency of symptomatic episodes
- any episodes of symptomatic ventricular arrhythmia should be reported to the physician

▶ *Should I Add Another Drug or Substitute Therapy If My Initial Drug Therapy Fails?*

Atrial fibrillation or flutter

Control of ventricular rate

- if acute control of ventricular rate is not achieved following a complete loading dose of IV digoxin, start verapamil administration
- like digoxin, verapamil should not be administered to patients with atrial fibrillation known to have a ventricular preexcitation syndrome such as Wolff-Parkinson-White syndrome
- if oral digoxin therapy is not successful in controlling ventricular rate during chronic or paroxysmal atrial fibrillation, verapamil 80 mg PO Q8H may be initiated in patients without left ventricular systolic dysfunction
- the dosage may be gradually titrated upward to a maximum daily dose of 360 mg according to heart rate response during the rhythm

Conversion to sinus rhythm

- if oral quinidine therapy is not successful in restoring or maintaining sinus rhythm or reducing the frequency of attacks of paroxysmal atrial fibrillation or flutter, a number of alternative therapies may be considered
- in patients with no history of MI and without left ventricular dysfunction, flecainide 100 mg PO Q12H may be initiated
- titrate the dosage upward in increments of 50 mg Q12H every 4 days to a maximum of 300 mg Q12H
- dosage increases should be based on clinical response (termination of atrial fibrillation or flutter or reduction in the frequency of symptomatic episodes) (N Engl J Med 1989;321:406–412, Am J Cardiol 1991;67:713–717)
- in patients with a past history of MI or with mild or moderate left ventricular dysfunction, sustained-release procainamide 50 mg/kg PO daily, divided Q6H may be initiated
- the dosage may be titrated upward in increments of

250 mg PO Q6H according to response (termination of atrial fibrillation or flutter or reduction in the frequency of symptomatic episodes)
- maximum effective dosages vary, but patients usually do not require more than 1.5 g PO Q6H

Atrioventricular nodal reentrant tachycardia

Acute episodes

- if adenosine is ineffective in terminating an episode of AV nodal reentrant tachycardia, verapamil may be used
- if full doses of adenosine are ineffective in terminating the arrhythmia, the origin of the tachycardia should be reconsidered
- esmolol may be used in patients without asthma or severe left ventricular dysfunction
- in patients with asthma or severe left ventricular dysfunction, IV digoxin may be used as the second line of therapy
- if adenosine is unavailable, IV procainamide may be used in patients who are known to have an extranodal accessory pathway (such as in Wolff-Parkinson-White syndrome)
- procainamide should be administered in single doses of 100 mg every 5 minutes at a rate of 20 mg/min until the tachycardia is terminated or until a dose of 17 mg/kg has been infused (12 mg/kg in patients with renal failure) (Ann Intern Med 1973;78:183–193; Eur J Clin Pharmacol 1978;13:303–308)

Long-term therapy

Therapy selected empirically

- if digoxin is ineffective alone, a beta-blocker may be added
- if the patient is asthmatic, has severe left ventricular dysfunction, or fails to respond to the combination of digoxin and a beta-blocker, a number of options exist
- in patients with a history of MI or mild to moderate left ventricular dysfunction, quinidine gluconate 324 mg PO TID or quinidine bisulfate 500 mg PO BID (not available in USA) may be prescribed
- in patients with no history of MI or left ventricular dysfunction, flecainide 100 mg PO Q12H may be used
- in patients with a history of MI but no history of left ventricular dysfunction, verapamil may be used

Therapy guided by electrophysiological testing

- choice of drugs in patients refractory to initial therapy should continue to be guided by electrophysiological testing

Ventricular arrhythmias

Acute episodes

- if acute control of symptomatic ventricular arrhythmias cannot be achieved with lidocaine, procainamide may be administered at 17 mg/kg of ideal body weight (IBW) (12 mg/kg in the presence of severe renal impairment) administered intravenously over 1 hour, followed by a maintenance infusion of 2.8 mg/kg/h
- if more rapid arrhythmia control is necessary, the loading dose may be administered at a rate no faster than 50 mg/min (J Am Coll Cardiol 1991;17:1581–1586)
- if neither is effective use bretylium
- if none of these drugs is effective, cardioversion should be used

Long-term therapy

- if therapy with beta-receptor blocking agents fails in patients with symptomatic benign arrhythmias, quinidine gluconate 324 mg PO TID or quinidine bisulfate 500 mg PO BID (not available in USA) may be substituted

- in this situation, however, consultation with an electrophysiologist for assessment and selection of therapy is appropriate
- if therapy is being guided by electrophysiological testing, therapy should continue to be guided by electrophysiological studies in patients refractory to initial therapy

► How Long Should I Continue Drug Therapy?

Atrial fibrillation or flutter
- patients with acute atrial fibrillation or flutter for which an underlying cause can be identified require rate control therapy until the underlying cause can be corrected
- patients with chronic or paroxysmal atrial fibrillation or flutter require rate control therapy indefinitely
- patients with paroxysmal atrial fibrillation or flutter require therapy for the maintenance of sinus rhythm indefinitely
- patients with rheumatic or nonrheumatic chronic atrial fibrillation or flutter and those with rheumatic paroxysmal atrial fibrillation or flutter require anticoagulation indefinitely

Atrioventricular nodal reentrant tachycardia
Acute episodes
- therapy should be continued until arrhythmia is terminated

Long-term therapy
- unless nonpharmacological arrhythmia cure (such as radiofrequency ablation or surgery) is attempted and achieved, therapy is required indefinitely

Ventricular arrhythmias
Acute episodes
- treatment should continue until the underlying cause of the arrhythmia is corrected
- if no correctable cause exists, therapy should continue until the patient can be evaluated for oral therapy
- if the patient is to undergo electrophysiological testing, antiarrhythmic drugs should be discontinued at least 5 half-lives prior to the baseline study, if the patient can tolerate discontinuation of therapy

Long-term therapy
- therapy may be required indefinitely if contributing factors cannot be reversed

Useful References

Pritchett ELC. Management of atrial fibrillation. N Engl J Med 1992; 326:1264–1271

Mannino MM, Mehta D, Gomes JA. Current treatment options for paroxysmal supraventricular tachycardia (editorial). Am Heart J 1994;127: 475–480

Emergency Cardiac Care Committee and Subcommittees, American Heart Association. Adult advanced cardiac life support. JAMA 1992; 268:2199–2241

Tisdale JE, Webb CR. Are antiarrhythmic drugs obsolete? Clin Pharm 1992; 11:714–726

DRUG THERAPY FOR RAYNAUD'S SYNDROME

Richard I. Ogilvie

► What Are My Goals of Treatment?
to reduce the frequency, severity, or duration of attacks

► What Evidence Is Available to Support Drug Therapy for Raynaud's Syndrome?

Frequency and severity of attacks
- the frequency and severity of attacks is reduced by 25% with calcium channel blockers (nifedipine) compared with placebo (Drugs 1989;37:700–712)
- 60–70% of patients experience clinical improvement with nifedipine

► When Should I Consider Drug Therapy?

Immediate treatment, long-term prevention
- only after secondary causes have been ruled out, such as power tool use, drugs (bleomycin, cisplatin, cyclosporine, beta-blockers, antimigraine drugs, oral contraceptives), neurovascular compression (carpal tunnel syndrome, thoracic outlet), occlusive arterial disease, hematological disorders, and connective tissue diseases (symptoms may precede diagnosis by 3–16 years)
- after nondrug preventive measures have failed, such as cessation of smoking and avoidance of precipitating factors (e.g., reducing exposure to cold and avoiding vibrating tools)

► What Drug Should I Use for Initial Treatment?

Immediate treatment or prophylaxis, long-term prevention
NIFEDIPINE
- proven efficacy and is the most studied calcium channel blocker
- diltiazem and nicardipine have been shown to be effective but have not been as extensively studied (Hypertension 1991;17:593–602)
- nisoldipine is probably less effective than nifedipine (Eur J Clin Pharmacol 1987;33:27–30)
- verapamil does not appear to be effective (J Clin Pharmacol 1982;22:74–76)
- ketanserin (not available) has been shown to decrease the frequency but not the severity of attacks (J Cardiovasc Pharmacol 1984;6:975–976)
- reserpine has been suggested, but no trials have evaluated efficacy with this drug

► What Dosage Should I Use?

Immediate treatment or prophylaxis
NIFEDIPINE
- 10 mg PO just prior to cold exposure or at the onset of an attack
- do not use sublingual route, as nifedipine is not absorbed by the oral mucosa; however, biting the capsule and swallowing the contents increases the rate of absorption

Long-term prevention
NIFEDIPINE
- 10 mg PO Q8H
- nifedipine (Adalat PA—Canada only) mg PO Q12H or nifedipine (Procardia XL, Adalat XL) 30 mg PO daily may decrease the incidence of adverse effects associated with nifedipine use but is more expensive (Hypertension 1991;17:593–602)

► How Long Should I Treat with My Initial Regimen?

Immediate treatment or prophylaxis
- effect is usually obtained with first dose

Long-term prevention

- limit use to period of cold exposure or emotional stress, which triggers attacks

▶ *What Efficacy Parameters Should I Follow and How Frequently Do I Have to Assess My Patient?*

Immediate treatment or prophylaxis

- reduction in severity and duration of attack

Long-term prevention

- subjective improvement seen as a reduction in the frequency, severity, or duration of attacks best determined by diary records

▶ *Should I Add Another Drug or Substitute Therapy If My Initial Drug Therapy Fails?*

Immediate treatment or prophylaxis, long-term prevention

- if nifedipine is not effective, it is unlikely that other calcium channel blockers will work
- other classes of drugs (e.g., reserpine) have limited utility but can be tried
- if nifedipine is effective but not tolerated, diltiazem at 30 mg PO Q8H may be effective with fewer adverse effects

▶ *How Long Should I Continue Drug Therapy?*

Immediate treatment or prophylaxis

- repeated doses every 8 hours may be required if precipitating factors continue

Long-term prevention

- treatment with nifedipine can be continued as long as symptoms recur during drug-free periods

Useful References

Crisanti JM. Raynaud's phenomenon. Am Family Physician 1990;41: 134–142

Roath S. Management of Raynaud's phenomenon: Focus on new treatments. Drugs 1989;37:700–712.

Cardelli MB, Kleinsmith DM. Raynaud's phenomenon and disease. Med Clin North Am 1989;73:1127–1141

Coffman JD. Raynaud's phenomenon: An update. Hypertension 1991;17: 593–602

DRUG THERAPY FOR INTERMITTENT CLAUDICATION

Richard I. Ogilvie

▶ *What Are My Goals of Treatment?*

to improve mobility and quality of life
to increase walking distance and time to claudication to a clinically important degree
to increase capacity for regular dynamic leg exercise

▶ *What Evidence Is Available to Support Drug Therapy for Intermittent Claudication?*

Increase in walking distance

- 50% increase in pain-free walking distance in patients with moderately severe claudication treated with pentoxifylline (Ann Intern Med 1990;113:135–146)

- statistically demonstrable improvement following drug therapy may not always be clinically important and is unpredictable (Ann Intern Med 1990;113:135–146)

Increased resting and hyperemic calf blood flow

- blood flow increases in patients with peripheral artery disease treated with pentoxifylline (Drugs 1987;34:50–97)

▶ *When Should I Consider Drug Therapy?*

Intermittent claudication

- only after nondrug measures have been shown to be ineffective, such as cessation of cigarette smoking and regular performance of dynamic leg exercise (30 minutes each day)
- cessation of smoking and regular dynamic leg exercise for a 3 month period may be of more benefit than drug therapy (Ann Intern Med 1990;113:135–146)
- after control of diabetes mellitus, angina pectoris, congestive heart failure, and hyperlipidemia, drug therapy should be implemented
- patients with symptoms of moderate severity for longer than 1 year may have a better drug response (Am J Surg 1990;160:266–270)

▶ *What Drug Should I Use for Initial Treatment?*

Intermittent claudication

PENTOXIFYLLINE

- no other drugs, including vasodilators, have demonstrable efficacy (Ann Intern Med 1990;113:135–146)

▶ *What Dosage Should I Use?*

Intermittent claudication

PENTOXIFYLLINE

- 400 mg PO TID with meals

▶ *How Long Should I Treat With My Initial Regimen?*

Intermittent claudication

- improvement may be seen after 2–4 weeks
- if an improvement of at least 25–50% is not seen after 8 weeks, drug therapy should be discontinued

▶ *What Efficacy Parameters Should I Follow and How Frequently Do I Have to Assess My Patient?*

Intermittent claudication

- assess efficacy at 4 week intervals
- subjective improvemnt in pain-free walking distance
- objective improvement in pain-free treadmill walking distance
- an improvement by 80–100 m for everyday walking should be expected (Circulation 1989;80:1549–1556)

▶ *Should I Add Another Drug or Substitute Therapy If My Initial Drug Therapy Fails?*

Intermittent claudication

- no other drugs, including vasodilators, have demonstrable efficacy and therefore are not recommended

▶ *How Long Should I Continue Drug Therapy?*

Intermittent claudication

- if improvement is noted at 8 weeks, continue for 6 months followed by a 2 month drug-free period for reassessment

- reassessment is needed as patient may improve on drug therapy, which increases the ability to exercise and may decrease the need for the drug

Useful References

Ward A, Clissold SP. Pentoxifylline. Drugs 1987;34:50–97

Radack K. Conservative management of intermittent claudication. Ann Intern Med 1990;113:135–146

Lindgärde F, Jelnes R, Bjorkman H, et al. Conservative drug treatment in patients with moderately severe chronic occlusive peripheral arterial disease. Circulation 1989;80:1549–1556

AbuRahma AF, Woodruff BA. Effects and limitations of pentoxifylline therapy in various stages of peripheral vascular disease of the lower extremity. Am J Surg 1990;160:266–270

DRUG THERAPY FOR PULMONARY EMBOLISM OR DEEP VEIN THROMBOSIS

Douglas L. Malyuk

▶ What Are My Goals of Treatment?

to prevent recurrence and extension of thrombi and emboli

to promote thromboembolic resolution and speed resolution of symptoms (pain and inflammation)

to decrease mortality from thromboemboli (Harrison's Principles of Internal Medicine 1990:1090–1096)

to reduce the risk and severity of postphlebotic syndrome

▶ What Evidence Is Available to Support Drug Therapy for Pulmonary Embolism or Deep Vein Thrombosis?

Mortality

- mortality in untreated pulmonary embolism ranges from 25–42% (Chest 1992;102:408S–425S, Pharmacotherapy: A Pathophysiologic Approach 1989:324–345)
- survival rates as high as 92% when treated adequately have been reported (Pharmacotherapy: A Pathophysiologic Approach 1989:324–345)

Severity of postphlebotic syndrome

- fibrinolytic therapy has been shown to reduce severity (Chest 1992;102:408S–425S)

Recurrence prevention

- recurrent deep vein thrombosis (DVT) occurs in 29–47% of patients if adequate anticoagulation with either heparin or anticoagulants is not continued after initial heparin therapy (N Engl J Med 1991;324:1565–1574)
- recurrence can be reduced to less than 5% if adequate anticoagulation is maintained (Chest 1992;102:408S–425S, N Engl J Med 1991;324:1565–1574)

▶ When Should I Consider Drug Therapy?

Deep vein thrombosis or pulmonary embolism

- drug therapy should be started immediately in patients with suspected or diagnosed DVT or pulmonary embolism

Venous thromboembolism prevention

Bedridden patients with one or more of the following risk factors should receive prophylaxis

- advanced age (older than 40 years)
- prolonged immobility or paralysis
- prior venous thromboembolism
- cancer
- surgical operations (particularly those involving the lower extremities or pelvis)
- obesity
- varicose veins
- CHF
- oral contraceptive use
- patients with known hypercoagulable states

Drug therapy is not required for low-risk general surgery patients without any of the above risk factors

▶ What Drug Should I Use for Initial Treatment?

Deep vein thrombosis or pulmonary embolism

HEPARIN

- heparin acts immediately to inhibit cascade and speeds resolution of symptoms
- if the patient is pregnant, use only heparin until postpartum then institute warfarin administration
- heparin is the anticoagulant of choice in pregnancy because it does not cross the placenta (N Engl J Med 1991;324:1565–1574, Chest 1992;102:385S–390S)

WARFARIN

- allows for oral anticoagulation; however, it takes 3–5 days to become effective and must be overlapped with heparin administration

Venous thromboembolism prevention

HEPARIN

- low-dose heparin is effective, safe, and requires little if any monitoring
- patients who have hip fractures or multiple trauma as well as those undergoing neurosurgical procedures or knee or hip replacement surgery should not receive low-dose heparin for DVT prophylaxis (Chest 1992;102:391S–407S)

WARFARIN

- for all patients who are undergoing elective hip surgery or have fractured hips, as warfarin has been shown to be more effective than low-dose heparin (Chest 1992;102:391S–407S)

▶ What Dosage Should I Use?

Deep vein thrombosis or pulmonary embolism

HEPARIN

- 100 units/kg (either 5000 units, 7500 units, or 10,000 units) IV bolus followed by a continuous infusion of 1250 units/h
- measure PTT 6 hours after initiation of infusion and 6 hours after every dosage change
- adjust the dosage to prolong PTT to 1½–2 times normal value (normal = 25–35 seconds) (Table 1–1)

WARFARIN

- 10 mg PO daily starting at the same time as heparin administration
- adjust the dosage to achieve an INR of 2–3 (a PT ratio of 1.3–1.5 times control values)
- during the first 2–3 days of therapy, desirable increase in PT is only 1–2 s/d and changes greater than this suggest that the dosage may be too high
- if PT increases are greater than 1–2 s/d, reduce the daily dosage by 50%

Table 1–1 • Heparin Dosage Adjustment Guidelines

PTT Results	Dosage Adjustment	Time of Repeated PTT
<50	give 5000 unit bolus and increase infusion by 100 units/h	Repeat in 6 hours
50–59	increase infusion by 100 units/h	Repeat in 6 hours
60–85	no change	Repeat next morning
86–95	decrease infusion by 100 units/h	Repeat next morning
96–120	stop infusion for 30 minutes and decrease infusion by 100 units/h	Repeat in 6 hours
>120	stop infusion for 60 minutes and decrease infusion rate by 200 units/h	Repeat in 6 hours

- in general, titrate the daily dosage by 0.5–2 mg on the basis of PT results
- changes in the dosage after the initiation of therapy should not occur more frequently than every 4–5 days because of warfarin's long half-life

Venous thromboembolism prevention

HEPARIN

- 5000 units SC 2 hours prior to surgery and 5000 units SC Q8H

WARFARIN

- 5 mg PO daily starting 3–4 days prior to surgery
- PT should be approximately 2 seconds over baseline levels prior to surgery
- continue warfarin after surgery keeping an INR of 2–3 (a PT ratio of 1.3–1.5 times control values)

▶ *How Long Should I Treat with My Initial Regimen?*

Deep vein thrombosis or pulmonary embolism

- heparin should be given for a minimum of 5 days but should not be discontinued before warfarin therapy has yielded an INR of 2–3 (a PT ratio of 1.5–2 times control values) (Chest 1992;102:408S–425S, N Engl J Med 1991;324:1565–1574)
- in pregnancy heparin should be given in full IV dosages for 7–10 days followed by subcutaneous injections given every 12 hours to prolong 6 hour postinjection PTT to a PTT 1.5–2 times control values until delivery (warfarin can then be started post-partum) (Chest 1992;102:385S–390S)

Venous thromboembolism prevention

- should be continued until patient is ambulatory (i.e., no longer confined to bed)

▶ *What Efficacy Parameters Should I Follow and How Frequently Do I Have to Assess My Patient?*

Deep vein thrombosis or pulmonary embolism

Venous thrombosis

Limb circumference, swelling, tenderness, perfusion
- assess patient daily

PTT and INR
- measure PTT every 6 hours until heparin achieves the desired PTT, then monitor daily

- measure INR daily until stable, then weekly for 2 weeks, then every 2–3 weeks

Pulmonary embolism

Apprehension, cough, pleuritic chest pain, hemoptysis
- assess patient daily

PTT and INR
- measure PTT every 6 hours until heparin achieves the desired PTT, then monitor daily
- measure INR daily until stable, then weekly for 2 weeks, then every 2–3 weeks

Venous thromboembolism prevention

Clinical signs
- monitor daily for signs of venous thromboembolism, such as changes in limb circumference, swelling, tenderness, and perfusion

PTT
- most patients do not require PTT measurements when receiving low-dose heparin
- if patients are malnourished, have prior coagulation problems, or are receiving broad-spectrum antibiotics, do baseline coagulation studies (PTT) and repeat in 3 days to evaluate the effect of heparin
- if baseline PTT is already elevated, do not start heparin administration until PTT is normalized

▶ *Should I Add Another Drug or Substitute Therapy If My Initial Drug Therapy Fails?*

Deep vein thrombosis or pulmonary embolism

- thrombolytic therapy with streptokinase should be considered in the initial treatment of patients with life-threatening acute massive embolism who are hemodynamically unstable if there are no contraindications to treatment (Chest 1992;102:408S–425S)
- administration of heparin should be stopped and streptokinase should be started after a PTT or thrombin time is 1½ times control values or less
- heparin administration should be restarted when the streptokinase is stopped and the PTT or thrombin time is 1½ times control values or less

▶ *How Long Should I Continue Drug Therapy?*

Deep vein thrombosis or pulmonary embolism

- heparin should be given for a minimum of 5 days but should be continued until warfarin therapy has yielded an INR of 2–3 (a PT ratio of 1.3–1.5 times control values) (Chest 1992;102:408S–425S, N Engl J Med 1991;324:1565–1574)
- warfarin should be continued for 3 months for the first episode, for 1 year for the second episode, and indefinitely for more than 2 episodes

Venous thromboembolism prevention

- should be continued until patient is ambulatory (i.e., no longer confined to bed)
- patients with recurrent venous thrombosis or a continuing risk factor such as antithrombin III deficiency, protein C or S deficiency, or malignancy should be treated indefinitely (Chest 1992;102:391S–407S)

Useful References

Hyers TM, Hull RD, Weg JG. Antithrombotic therapy for venous thromboembolic disease. Chest 1992;102:408S–425S.

Hirsch J. Heparin. N Engl J Med 1991;324:1565–1574.

Rodvold KA, Quandt CM, Friedenberg WR. Thromboembolic disorders. In: Dipiro JT, Talbert RL, Hayes PE, et al, eds. Pharmacotherapy: A pathophysiologic approach. New York: Elsevier, 1988:324–345.

Moser KM. Pulmonary thromboembolism. In: Wilson JD, Braunwald E, Isselbacher KJ, et al, eds. Harrison's Principles of Internal Medicine, 12th ed. New York: McGraw-Hill, 1990:1090–1096.

Ginsberg JS, Hirsh J. Use of anticoagulants during pregnancy. Chest 1989;95:156S–160S.

Clagett GP, Anderson FA Jr, Levine MN, et al. Prevention of venous thromboembolism. Chest 1992;102(suppl 4):391S–470S.

DRUG THERAPY FOR HYPERLIPIDEMIAS

Stephen Shalansky and Robert Dombrowski

▶ What Are My Goals of Treatment?

to prevent progression of coronary atherosclerosis
to lower cholesterol with a minimum of adverse drug effects
to promote regression of atherosclerosis
to choose a regimen affordable to the patient
to involve the patient in the decision-making process
to prevent morbidity or mortality associated with CHD

▶ What Evidence Is Available to Support Drug Therapy for Hyperlipidemias?

Coronary heart disease in patients with increased cholesterol levels

- in normotensive nonsmoking men, death from CHD was 1.6/1000 if serum cholesterol levels were less than 182 mg/dL (4.7 mmol/L) and was 6.4/1000 if the serum cholesterol level was greater than 245 mg/dL (6.3 mmol/L) (Arch Intern Med 1988;148:36–69)
- in hypertensive men who smoked, death from CHD was 6.3/1000 with a serum cholesterol level less than 182 mg/dL compared with 21.4/1000 with a serum cholesterol level greater than 245 mg/dL (Arch Intern Med 1988;148:36–69)

Coronary heart disease reduction in patients treated for hypercholesterolemia

CHOLESTYRAMINE

- patients treated for an average of 7.4 years with dietary therapy and cholestyramine had a 19% reduction in risk of definite CHD and/or definite nonfatal MI, with events occurring in 155/1906 in the group treated with cholestyramine and in 187/1900 in the placebo group (JAMA 1984;251:351–364)
- overall mortality was not changed

GEMFIBROZIL

- patients receiving 600 mg twice daily of gemfibrozil for 5 years had a 34% reduction (1.4% absolute reduction) in the incidence of CHD (defined as MI or cardiac death) compared with the placebo group (56/2051 in the gemfibrozil group versus 84/2030 in the placebo group) (N Engl J Med 1987;317:1237–1245)
- overall mortality was unchanged (placebo group, 42/2030; gemfibrozil group, 45/2051)

NIACIN

- patients receiving niacin and dietary therapy for 6 years during a study were followed 9 years later and had an overall lower mortality rate (52%) when compared with the placebo–dietary group (58%) (J Am Coll Cardiol 1986;6:1245–1255)

SIMVASTATIN

- patients with angina pectoris or previous myocardial infarction and a serum cholesterol of 5.5–8.0 mmol/L on a lipid lowering diet were treated with either simvastatin or placebo
- over 5.4 years 11.5% of the patients in the placebo group and 8.2% of patients in the simvastatin group died (Lancet 1994;344:1383–1389)

Atherosclerosis regression

- in 80 men given colestipol and niacin for 2 years versus 82 men given placebo, atherosclerotic plaquing, demonstrated by angiogram, was stable in 36 patients and reversed in 13 patients in the treatment group compared with 30 and 2 patients, respectively, in the placebo group (JAMA 1987;257:3233–3240)
- patients with familial hypercholesterolemia have shown regression of coronary atherosclerosis while receiving colestipol, niacin, or lovastatin (JAMA 1990;264:3007–3012)

Coronary heart disease in patients with increased triglyceride levels

- hypertriglyceridemia as a risk factor for the development of CHD remains uncertain and is currently not treated (Arterioscler Thromb 1991;11:2–15)

Coronary heart disease reduction in patients treated for hypertriglyceridemia

- no studies of treatment directly aimed at patients with increased triglyceride levels are presently available (Br Med J 1992;304:394–396)

Ability to lower lipid levels

- individual patient responses are variable; however, the percentages in Table 1–2 represent a range

▶ When Should I Consider Drug Therapy?

Hypercholesterolemia

- the decision to use drug therapy should be based on at least two cholesterol/triglyceride levels, presence or absence of coronary heart disease or other atherosclerotic disease (cerebrovascular or occlusive peripheral vascular disease), and CHD risk factors (male ≥ 45, female ≥ 55 or premature menopause without estrogen replacement therapy, family history of premature coronary heart disease, current cigarette smoking, diabetes mellitus, hypertension, HDL cholesterol < 35 mg/dL [0.9 mmol/L])
- an HDL level of >60 mg/dL (1.6 mmol/L) is considered a negative risk factor
- the patient should always be involved in the decision and should be told of the absolute benefits and risks of therapy

Patients without coronary heart disease or atherosclerotic disease and with fewer than two risk factors

Young adult men (<35 years of age)

- drug therapy in this group should be considered only when LDL cholesterol is >220 mg/dL (5.7 mmoles/L) despite a 6 month trial of intensive dietary therapy (JAMA 1993;269:3015–3023)

Males ≥ 35 years of age

- recommend drug therapy if LDL is >190 mg/dL

Table 1–2 • **Lipid-lowering effect**

	Total Cholesterol	LDL Cholesterol	HDL Cholesterol	Triglycerides
cholestyramine or colestipol	decreased by 15–30%	decreased by 15–35%	increased by 10–38%	increased by 5–40%
niacin	decreased by 10–30%	decreased by 15–30%	increased by 5–30%	decreased by 10–30%
fibric acid derivatives	decreased by 2–10%	decreased by 5–18%	increased by 5–25%	decreased by 10–50%
HMG-CoA reductase inhibitors	decreased by 24–35%	decreased by 25–45%	increased by 8–23%	decreased by 8–25%

(4.9 mmoles/L) or total cholesterol is >260 mg/dL (6.7 mmol/L) after a 6 month trial of intensive dietary therapy and exercise

Premenopausal women
- drug therapy in this group should be considered only when LDL cholesterol is >220 mg/dL (5.7 mmol/L) despite a 6 month trial of intensive dietary therapy and exercise (JAMA 1993;269:3015–3023)
- because of the low risk of coronary heart disease in this patient population, drug therapy is often delayed until after the menopause

Postmenopausal women
- drug therapy in this group should be considered only when LDL cholesterol is >220 mg/dL (5.7 mmol/L) despite a 6 month trial of intensive dietary therapy (JAMA 1993;269:3015–3023)
- clinicians should be aware that the relationship between coronary heart disease and cholesterol levels is less consistent in women over the age of 65 than that seen in other groups (JAMA 1994;272:1335–1340)

Patients >65 years of age
- moderate dietary therapy and exercise cannot be discouraged in this patient population; however, no data support or refute drug therapy in this patient population
- despite this lack of evidence, some clinicians suggest that elderly patients who are not of advanced physiological or chronological age and who do not suffer from severe life-limiting illnesses (congestive heart failure, dementia, cancer) should receive drug therapy in a similar fashion to middle-aged patients
- patients of advanced physiological or chronological age or those with severe life-limiting illness should not receive drug therapy or aggressive non-drug therapy (JAMA 1993;269:3015–3023)

Patients without coronary heart disease or atherosclerotic disease but with two or more risk factors
- recommend drug therapy if LDL is >160 mg/dL (4.1 mmol/L) or total cholesterol is still >240 mg/dL (6.2 mmol/L) after a 6 month trial of intensive dietary therapy

Patients with definite coronary heart disease (prior MI or angina) or atherosclerotic disease
- start drug therapy if LDL is still >130 mg/dL (3.4 mmol/L) or total cholesterol is still >200 mg/dL (5.2 mmol/L) after a 6 month trial of intensive dietary therapy

Hypertriglyceridemia
- consider drug therapy only in patients with symptomatic (pancreatitis, xanthomas) hypertriglyceridemia as there is no evidence yet to support the treatment or screening of patients with asymptomatic elevated triglycerides (BMJ 1992;304:394–396)

Mixed hyperlipidemia (hypercholesterolemia and hypertriglyceridemia)
- treat as above for hypercholesterolemia

▶ *What Drug Should I Use for Initial Treatment?*

Hypercholesterolemia

HMG-CoA REDUCTASE INHIBITORS (LOVASTATIN, PRAVASTATIN, SIMVASTATIN, FLUVASTATIN)
- HMG-CoA reductase inhibitors are recommended as first line agents because they have proven efficacy in the reduction of cardiovascular mortality and morbidity (Lancet 1994;344:1383–1389) and they are better tolerated than niacin or the bile acid sequestrants
- choose the least expensive of either lovastatin, pravastatin, simvastatin, or fluvastatin, as these agents are likely equally effective and equally well tolerated

BILE ACID SEQUESTRANTS (CHOLESTYRAMINE, COLESTIPOL)
- bile acid sequestrants are recommended (assuming they are tolerated) if HMG-CoA reductase inhibitors are ineffective or not tolerated, as bile acid sequestrants have proven efficacy and safety in the reduction of cardiovascular disease and cardiovascular mortality
- choose the least expensive of either cholestyramine (4 g dose) or colestipol (5 g dose) as these agents are equally effective and equally tolerated

NIACIN
- should be considered first line therapy for patients in whom cost is a limiting factor as niacin is less expensive than HMG-CoA reductase inhibitors and bile acid sequestrants
- while niacin does lead to a reduction in cholesterol, there is more evidence for a positive effect on cardiovascular disease, especially in primary prevention, with the HMG-CoA reductase inhibitors and bile acid sequestrants
- also chosen in patients when HMG-CoA reductase inhibitors or bile acid sequestrants are ineffective or not well tolerated
- side effects such as fllushing, gastrointestinal discomfort, hyperglycemia, liver toxicity, and hyperuricemia may limit its use

FIBRIC ACID DERIVATIVES (GEMFIBROZIL, FENOFIBRATE)
- fibric acid derivatives generally decrease LDL cholesterol less than bile acid sequestrants, niacin, or HMG CoA reductase inhibitors and in some cases may increase LDL cholesterol
- should be considered only if all other agents have failed
- this is true despite the results of the Helsinki trial showing gemfibrozil to be safe and effective in treating hyperlipidemias (N Engl J Med 1987;317:1237–1245)
- there is an apparent inconsistency in gemfibrozil's effects, which may be related to triglyceride levels
- the Helsinki trial results showed that gemfibrozil can actually increase LDL cholesterol in patients with very elevated triglyceride levels (>500 mg/dL [>5.6 mmol/L]),

while decreasing LDL in patients with normal or moderately elevated triglyceride levels

- unless there is significant cost advantage, gemfibrozil should be used over fenofibrate as there are no long-term studies evaluating fenofibrate's effect on cardiovascular morbidity and mortality

Hypertriglyceridemia

FIBRIC ACID DERIVATIVES (GEMFIBROZIL, FENOFIBRATE)

- these agents are recommended because gemfibrozil has proven efficacy in reducing the incidence of cardiovascular disease and has its main effect on triglycerides
- unless there is significant cost advantage, gemfibrozil should be used over fenofibrate as there are no long-term studies evaluating fenofibrate's effect on cardiovascular morbidity and mortality

NIACIN

- not as effective in reducing triglycerides as fibric acid derivatives but is much less expensive and should be considered if fibric acid derivatives are not effective or tolerated

Mixed hyperlipidemias (hypercholesterolemia and hypertriglyceridemia)

NIACIN

- niacin is recommended (if it is tolerated) because it has proven efficacy in the reduction of cardiovascular disease, lowers triglycerides, raises HDL, lowers LDL, and is the least expensive agent

HMG-CoA REDUCTASE INHIBITORS

- choose for patients who cannot take or tolerate niacin
- choose the least expensive of either lovastatin, pravastatin, simvastatin, or fluvastatin as these agents are equally effective and equally well tolerated

FIBRIC ACID DERIVATIVES

- fibric acid derivatives have only a small effect on cholesterol and should be used only if niacin and HMG-CoA reductase inhibitors are ineffective or triglycerides are over 500 mg/dL (5.6 mmol/L)

BILE ACID SEQUESTRANTS

- bile acid sequestrants raise triglycerides and are therefore not particularly useful
- may be used in combination with gemfibrozil or niacin, particularly in patients who develop myositis on the combination of gemfibrozil and lovastatin

▶ *What Dosage Should I Use?*

Hypercholesterolemia, hypertriglyceridemia, mixed hyperlipidemias

LOVASTATIN

- 10 mg PO daily with the evening meal
- double the dosage if an adequate response has not been seen within 4 weeks

PRAVASTATIN

- 10 mg PO daily at bedtime
- double the dosage if an adequate response has not been seen within 4 weeks

SIMVASTATIN

- 10 mg PO daily

- double the dosage if an adequate response has not been seen within 4 weeks

FLUVASTATIN

- 20 mg PO daily
- double the dosage if an adequate response has not been seen within 4 weeks

CHOLESTYRAMINE, COLESTIPOL

- 2 g (1/2 packet) of cholestyramine PO daily initially and titrate up every 2–3 days by 2 g PO daily until 4 g PO BID is reached, as this may increase tolerability
- give BID dosing with breakfast and the evening meal to increase tolerability
- increase the dosage to 12 g PO daily (4 g PO in the morning and 8 g with the evening meal) if inadequate response occurs in 4 weeks
- continue to increase the dosage by 4 g (1 scoop) per week up to a maximum dosage of 24 g/d (12 g in the morning and 12 g with the evening meal); however, be aware that most patients do not tolerate dosages greater than 16 g/d
- 2 g of cholestyramine equals 2.5 g of colestipol

NIACIN

- 100 mg PO TID with meals, and increase the dosage every 2–3 days by 100 mg/dose over 2 weeks until a dosage of 500 mg PO TID is reached
- usually, at least 500 mg PO TID must be given to see an effect on lipids
- increase the dosage of niacin up to 4 g/d if inadequate response occurs in 4 weeks

GEMFIBROZIL

- 600 mg PO BID

FENOFIBRATE

- 100 mg PO TID with meals

▶ *How Long Should I Treat with My Initial Regimen?*

Hypercholesterolemia, hypertriglyceridemia, mixed hyperlipidemias

- continue therapy, if tolerated, for 3 months before deciding whether to add or substitute therapy

▶ *What Efficacy Parameters Should I Follow and How Frequently Do I Have to Assess My Patient?*

Hypercholesterolemia, hypertriglyceridemia, mixed hyperlipidemias

Total cholesterol and fractionated lipid profile

- initially measure baseline lipid values (cholesterol levels, fractionated lipid profile) when deciding on initiating drug therapy for hyperlipidemias
- in patients with no coronary heart disease or atherosclerotic disease and with fewer than 2 CHD risk factors, lower total cholesterol levels below 240 mg/dL (6.2 mmol/L) and LDL cholesterol levels below 160 mg/dL (4.1 mmol/L)
- in patients with no coronary heart disease or atherosclerotic disease and with 2 or more CHD risk factors, lower total cholesterol levels below 200 mg/dL (5.2 mmol/L) and LDL cholesterol levels below 130 mg/dL (3.4 mmol/L)
- for patients with coronary heart disease or atherosclerotic

disease lower LDL cholesterol to below 100 mg/dL (2.6 mmol/L)

- complete lipid profiles should be measured at 1 and 3 months
- if goals are achieved then, check annually

Evidence of coronary heart disease

- MI, angina, coronary bypass grafting

Risk factors

- reduce risk factors such as obesity and smoking
- control risk factors such as diabetes and hypertension

▶ *Should I Add Another Drug or Substitute Therapy If My Initial Drug Therapy Fails?*

Hypercholesterolemia, hypertriglyceridemia, mixed hyperlipidemias

If at 3 months the drug is tolerated and there has been at least a 15% decrease in lipids but not to the desired level

- continue the first drug and add second-line agent
- if adding another drug, monitor as if initiating therapy

If the drug is not tolerated or there is less than a 15% decrease in total cholesterol levels

- stop the first drug and start administration of second-line drug
- if changing drugs, monitor as if initiating therapy

▶ *How Long Should I Continue Drug Therapy?*

Hypercholesterolemia, hypertriglyceridemia, mixed hyperlipidemias

- while drug therapy can be continued for many years and possibly a lifetime, one should consider reducing or stopping drug therapy if the desired LDL cholesterol level is maintained for 2 years (continue dietary therapy) to reestablish the diagnosis and to check the efficacy of nondrug measures
- measure total cholesterol levels 4 to 6 weeks after stopping drugs and at 3 months; if elevated, restart therapy

Useful References

Expert Panel on Detection, Evaluation, and Treatment of High Blood Cholesterol in Adults. Summary of the second report of the National Cholesterol Education Program (NCEP) expert panel on detection, evaluation, and treatment of high blood cholesterol in adults. JAMA 1993; 269:3015–3023

Carter BL, Bakht FR. Therapy for hypercholesterolemia. Prim Care September 1990;17(3):479–493

Wones RG. Screening, diagnosis, and treatment of hypercholesterolemia. Prim Care January 1990;16(1):479–497

Kafonek SD, Kwiterovich PO. Treatment of hypercholesterolemia in the elderly. Ann Intern Med 1990;112:723–725

Labreche DG. Reassessment of the value of lowering serum cholesterol. Clin Pharm 1988;7:592–603

DRUG THERAPY FOR ISCHEMIC CEREBROVASCULAR DISEASE

J. Chris Bradberry

▶ *What Are My Goals of Treatment?*

Transient ischemic attacks

to reduce and/or eliminate transient ischemic attacks (TIAs) and to prevent stroke

to treat risk factors for stroke, which include control of hypertension, hyperlipidemia, obesity, tobacco use, diabetes, and other risk factors (Stroke 1984;15:1105, Neurol Clin 1983;1:317, JAMA 1982;247:633–638)

to identify patients with greater than 70% carotid stenosis ipsilateral to hemispheric or ocular symptoms related to ischemia who are best managed by endarterectomy

Progressing stroke

to stop and/or reverse the stroke syndrome

Completed stroke

to prevent additional stroke

Prevention of cardiogenic cerebral embolism

to prevent stroke

▶ *What Evidence Is Available to Support Drug Therapy for Ischemic Cerebrovascular Disease?*

Transient ischemic attacks

- TIAs precede 20% of strokes
- both aspirin and ticlopidine reduce the risk of stroke or death over 3–5 years (by approximately 20% relative reduction and 5% absolute reduction) in patients with TIAs or strokes (Lancet 1991;338:1345–1349, Br Med J 1988;296:320–331)
- secondary prevention of TIAs with drug therapy is well documented (Med J Aust 1991;154:477–480, Br Med J 1988;296:320–321)
- ticlopidine reduces the stroke rate in patients with TIAs marginally better than aspirin does (N Engl J Med 1989;321:501–507)

Progressing stroke

- no clear evidence of benefit from drug intervention with antiplatelet agents
- anticoagulants have been used in ischemic stroke if hemorrhage has been ruled out

Completed Stroke

- ticlopidine treatment produces a 30% risk reduction in stroke, MI, and vascular death compared with placebo (Lancet 1989;2:1215–1220)
- no evidence of aspirin benefit for stroke survivors with serious neurological deficit

Prevention of cardiogenic cerebral embolism

- cardiogenic embolism is the major cause of cerebral embolism (Chest 1986;89[suppl 2]:82S) and accounts for up to 23% of all ischemic strokes (Chest 1986;89[suppl 2]:82S)
- warfarin decreases the incidence of TIAs and strokes in patients with nonvalvular atrial fibrillation (Lancet 1989;1:175–179)

▶ *When Should I Consider Drug Therapy?*

Transient ischemic attacks

- as soon as possible after diagnosis of TIAs
- TIAs are diagnosed by a history of brief ischemic neurological deficits
- clinical symptoms depend on the vascular territory involved (carotid or vertebrovasilar)

Progressing stroke

- anticoagulation is controversial, and the use of heparin is anecdotal
- anticoagulation should be used only in cases of progressing stroke in which hemorrhage has been ruled out by computed tomographic (CT) scan and there are major

progressing neurological deficits; otherwise, do not anti-coagulate

Completed stroke

- anticoagulation is recommended only for the prevention of recurrent cardioembolic stroke
- antiplatelet therapy should be used in patients if there is potential for a good quality of life and no major neurological damage has occurred after a stroke
- although not clear, anecdotal evidence suggests that antiplatelet agents be started within hours if possible

Prevention of cardiogenic cerebral embolism

Atrial fibrillation

- achieve long-term anticoagulation for patients with chronic rheumatic or nonrheumatic atrial fibrillation (Am J Cardiol 1990;65:24C–28C; N Engl J Med 1990;323:1505–1511), rheumatic paroxysmal atrial fibrillation (Am J Cardiol 1990;65:24C–28C), and nonvalvular chronic atrial fibrillation if cardiac disease such as hypertension, coronary artery disease, or CHF is present (Arch Intern Med 1990;150:1598–1603)
- all other patients with atrial fibrillation should be anticoagulated to minimize the chance of systemic embolization from a cardiac source (Am J Cardiol 1990;65:24C–28C; N Engl J Med 1990;323:1505–1511, Am J Cardiol 1990; 65:24C–28C, N Engl J Med 1992;326:1264–1271) if no contraindication to anticoagulation is present
- short-term anticoagulation prior to attempting to convert (electrically or pharmacologically) to sinus rhythm should be considered for patients who have been in atrial fibrillation or flutter for longer than 2 days (Chest 1992; 102[suppl]:426S–433S)
- long-term therapy with warfarin has been shown to be significantly more effective than aspirin for the prevention of stroke in atrial fibrillation (Lancet 1989;1:175–179, N Engl J Med 1990;323:1505–1511; N Engl J Med 1990; 322:863–868)

Heart valves

- all patients with mechanical prosthetic or bioprosthetic cardiac valves should receive some sort of anticoagulant or antiplatelet therapy (Chest 1989;95:107S–117S)

Myocardial infarction

- all patients with an MI should receive some type of anticoagulant or antiplatelet agent to decrease the incidence of systemic thromboembolism (see below for choice of agent)

▶ What Drug Should I Use for Initial Treatment?

Transient ischemic attacks

ASPIRIN

- agent of choice because of its antiplatelet activity, low cost, and efficacy (Pharmacotherapy: A Pathophysiologic Approach 1993;336–356)
- although ticlopidine was shown to be slightly more effective than aspirin (13% incidence of stroke for aspirin versus 10% for ticlopidine), ticlopidine had a higher incidence of adverse effects (diarrhea, rash, and severe neutropenia) (N Engl J Med 1989;321:501–507)
- ticlopidine is far more expensive and less convenient to take than aspirin

TICLOPIDINE

- use if aspirin is contraindicated or is ineffective in reducing attacks

Progressing stroke

HEPARIN PLUS WARFARIN

- anticoagulation for this condition is controversial, and the use of heparin is anecdotal
- anticoagulation should be used only in cases of progressing stroke if hemorrhage has been ruled out by CT scan and there are major progressing neurological deficits; otherwise, do not anticoagulate
- begin as soon as hemorrhagic stroke is ruled out (Chest 1986;89[suppl 2]:82S, Stroke 1989;20:1407)
- aspirin has no proven role
- studies with tissue plasminogen activator are presently ongoing

Completed stroke

ASPIRIN

- drug of choice for male patients following a completed stroke
- aspirin is effective, well tolerated, and inexpensive

TICLOPIDINE

- there is a suggestion that ticlopidine is slightly more effective in female patients (Neurology 1992;42:111–115)
- some clinicians suggest that ticlopidine should be used in patients with significant neurological deficit

Prevention of cardiogenic cerebral embolism

Atrial fibrillation

WARFARIN

- warfarin should be used if no contraindications exist
- in patients to undergo cardioversion, warfarin should be started 3 weeks prior to cardioversion
- for emergency cardioversion (patients with angina or hemodynamic complications), start warfarin administration immediately
- warfarin is more effective than aspirin for the prevention of stroke in atrial fibrillation (Lancet 1989;1:175–179, N Engl J Med 1990;323:1505–1511; N Engl J Med 1990; 322:863–868)
- initial treatment with heparin is not needed

ASPIRIN

- use if warfarin is contraindicated

Heart valves

Mechanical prosthetic valves

HEPARIN WITH WARFARIN

- warfarin is needed for long-term anticoagulation
- heparin need only be used if the patient cannot take warfarin

ASPIRIN

- use if warfarin is contraindicated, and use in additon to warfarin if patient has systemic embolism while receiving adequate warfarin therapy (Chest 1992;102[suppl]: 445S–455S)

DIPYRIDAMOLE

- although some studies have shown no benefit, this agent should be used if patient has systemic embolism and warfarin and aspirin are not allowed

Bioprosthetic mitral valves

WARFARIN

- warfarin is needed as long-term anticoagulation

- heparin need only be used if the patient cannot take warfarin

ASPIRIN

- chosen over warfarin because risk of embolization is low in these patients

Myocardial infarction

ASPIRIN

- aspirin therapy should be given early to all patients
- routine use of heparin rather than aspirin following streptokinase cannot be recommended to reduce mortality or reinfarction at this time (Chest 1992;102:456S–481S, Lancet 1988;2:349–360)
- aspirin can be used in patients who will require long-term warfarin administration, as evidenced by a pilot study of ischemic heart disease (Eur Heart J 1988;9:836–843) and mechanical heart valves (Can J Cardiol 1991;7[suppl A]:95A)
- aspirin administration should be continued in all patients indefinitely unless a contraindication exists

HEPARIN

- all patients with an MI should receive heparin to prevent thromboembolism, further coronary artery thrombosis, mural thrombus, and systemic embolism (Chest 1992; 102[suppl]:456S–481S)
- heparin therapy should be instituted even in patients who do not receive thrombolytic therapy
- heparin should be used to prevent coronary reocclusion with tissue plasminogen activator and should be started concomitantly with tissue plasminogen activator to help decrease the risk of reocclusion
- the American College of Chest Physicians offers a grade C (their weakest) recommendation for the use of heparin after thrombolysis with streptokinase, which has not been strengthened by the results of the GUSTO trial (N Engl J Med 1993;329:673–682)
- heparin therapy should be used for high-risk patients to prevent DVT
- high-risk patients are those older than 70 years, with a history of previous MI, large anterior MI, heart failure, or shock
- a preventive subcutaneous regimen should be considered in patients who are immobilized for longer than 3 days, are obese, or have signs of chronic venous insufficiency

WARFARIN

- for many patients, the risks of standard warfarin therapy are high and prolonged anticoagulation after an MI is not warranted until definitive data are available from ongoing trials
- consider warfarin in patients with a prior embolus, left ventricular thrombus, large anterior infarct, atrial fibrillation, or left ventricular aneurysm or patients who have or develop left ventricular dysfunction (failure); who do not have contraindications to anticoagulation; and who are willing to undergo regular medical and laboratory follow-up
- start warfarin after arterial punctures are no longer required

▶ *What Dosage Should I Use?*

Transient ischemic attacks

ASPIRIN

- 325 mg (enteric coated) PO daily (Br Med J 1988; 296:316–320)

- although low-dose aspirin (30–75 mg PO daily) has been shown to be effective (N Engl J Med 1991;325:1261–1266, Lancet 1991;338:1345–1349), these dosage forms are sometimes difficult to find and may be more expensive than the 325 mg dose
- if 325 mg is not well tolerated, use the lower-dose version, or give 325 mg PO every other day

TICLOPIDINE

- 250 mg PO BID (N Engl J Med 1989;321:501–507)

Progressing stroke

HEPARIN

- 100 units/kg (either 5000 units, 7500 units, or 10,000 units) IV bolus followed by a continuous infusion of 1250 units/h started after hemorrhagic stroke has been ruled out
- adjust the dosage to prolong PTT $1\frac{1}{2}$–2 times normal values (normal = 25–35 seconds)

WARFARIN

- 10 mg PO daily titrated to an INR of 2–3

Completed stroke

ASPIRIN, TICLOPIDINE

- as above for TIAs

Prevention of cardiogenic cerebral embolism

Atrial fibrillation, heart valves, myocardial infarction

HEPARIN

- 100 units/kg (either 5000 units, 7500 units, or 10,000 units) IV bolus followed by a continuous infusion of 1250 units/h
- adjust the dosage to prolong PTT $1\frac{1}{2}$–2 times normal values (normal = 25–35 seconds)

WARFARIN

- 10 mg PO daily titrated to an INR of 2.5–3.5 for patients with mechanical prosthetic valves and 2–3 for those with bioprosthetic valves (Chest 1992; 102[suppl]:445S–455S), MI, or atrial fibrillation

DIPYRIDAMOLE

- 100 mg PO Q6H (Chest 1992;102[suppl]:445S–455S)

ASPIRIN

- 325 mg PO daily

▶ *How Long Should I Treat with My Initial Regimen?*

Transient ischemic attacks

- if patient has more than one TIA while receiving drug therapy, that therapy should be stopped and the alternative therapy tried

Progressing stroke

- continue anticoagulation until either the patient's condition has stabilized or roughly 3–5 days
- if the stroke has not stabilized after 48 hours of therapy, stop anticoagulation and be sure worsening of the clinical condition is not due to hemorrhagic stroke or another medical condition

Completed stroke

- indefinitely

Prevention of cardiogenic cerebral embolism

Atrial fibrillation, heart valves

- heparin should be given for a minimum of 5 days but

should not be discontinued before warfarin therapy has yielded a therapeutic INR (Chest 1989;95:37S–51S, N Engl J Med 1991;324:1565–1574)
- warfarin should be continued as long as risk of embolism persists

Myocardial infarction
- continue heparin administration for 3–4 days or until patient is stable

▶ What Efficacy Parameters Should I Follow and How Frequently Do I Have to Assess My Patient?

Transient ischemic attacks
Occurrence of transient ischemic attacks
- assess the patient monthly initially, and tell the patient to contact you if any future TIAs occur (loss of vision in one eye, dizziness, weakness on one side, numbness in face, arm, or leg)
- if no TIAs occur during the first 3 months, assess every 6 months thereafter

Progressing stroke
Stroke stabilization
- assess whether the stroke is stabilizing or not

PTT and INR
- measure PTT every 6 hours until it is in the target range, then monitor daily
- measure INR daily until INR stable, then weekly for 2 weeks, then every 2–3 weeks (Chest 1989;95:37S–51S)

Completed stroke
- no efficacy parameters other than future strokes

Prevention of cardiogenic cerebral embolism
Evidence of cerebral embolism
- TIAs or strokes

PTT and INR
- measure PTT every 6 hours until it is in the target range, then monitor daily
- measure INR daily until INR stable, then weekly for 2 weeks, then every 2–3 weeks (Chest 1989;95:37S–51S)

▶ Should I Add Another Drug or Substitute Therapy If My Initial Drug Therapy Fails?

Transient ischemic attacks
- if neither aspirin nor ticlopidine is effective, consider low-dose warfarin (INR of 2–3)
- anticoagulation with heparin or warfarin in TIAs produces no change in mortality but some reduction in the rate of TIA recurrence, as has been shown in some studies

Progressing stroke
- if the stroke has not stabilized after 48 hours of therapy, stop anticoagulation and be sure worsening of the clinical condition is not due to hemorrhagic stroke or another medical condition

Completed stroke
- substitute aspirin for ticlopidine or vice versa

Prevention of cardiogenic cerebral embolism
- not clear what should be done (Chest 1992;102[suppl]: 529S–537S)

▶ How Long Should I Continue Drug Therapy?

Transient ischemic attacks
- continue therapy indefinitely

Progressing stroke
- continue anticoagulation until either the patient's condition has stabilized or a maximum of 2 weeks has elapsed
- if the stroke has not stabilized after 48 hours of therapy, stop anticoagulation and be sure worsening of the clinical condition is not due to hemorrhagic stroke or another medical condition

Completed stroke
- evidence of benefit exists for up to 2–3 years, and therapy should likely be continued indefinitely

Prevention of cardiogenic cerebral embolism
Atrial fibrillation
- continue anticoagulation for 4 weeks after successful cardioversion
- maintain long-term anticoagulation for patients with chronic rheumatic or nonrheumatic atrial fibrillation (Am J Cardiol 1990;65:24C–28C, N Engl J Med 1990;323: 1505–1511), rheumatic paroxysmal atrial fibrillation (Am J Cardiol 1990;65:24C–28C), and nonvalvular chronic atrial fibrillation if cardiac disease such as hypertension, coronary artery disease, or CHF is present (Arch Intern Med 1990;150:1598–1603)

Heart valves
Mechanical prosthetic valves
- mechanical valves necessitate anticoagulation indefinitely (J Am Coll Cardiol 1986;8:41B)

Bioprosthetic mitral valves
- bioprosthetic mitral valves necessitate warfarin for 3 months followed by low-dose aspirin indefinitely; however, warfarin should be continued indefinitely in patients with a history of systemic embolism

Bioprosthetic aortic valves
- continue aspirin indefinitely

Myocardial infarction
- continue warfarin for 3 months after MI and continue aspirin indefinitely

Useful References

1990 Heart and Stroke Facts. Dallas, TX: American Heart Association, 1989

Easton JD, Hart RG, Sherman DG, et al. Diagnosis and management of ischemic stroke. Part 1. Threatened stroke and its management. Curr Probl Cardiol 1983;8:1–80

Dyken ML, Wolf PA, Barnett HJM, et al. Risk factors in stroke—A statement for physicians by the Subcommittee on Risk Factors and Stroke of the Stroke Council. Stroke 1984;15:1105–1111

Wolf PA, Kannel WB, Verter J. Current status of risk factors for stroke. Neurol Clin 1983;1:317–343

Hypertension Detection and Follow-up Program Cooperative Group. Five year findings of the Hypertension Detection and Follow-up Program. III. Reduction in stroke incidence among persons with high blood pressure. JAMA 1982;247:633–638

Bradberry JC. Stroke. In: Dipiro, J, Talbert RL, Hayes PE, et al, eds. Pharmacotherapy: A Pathophysiologic Approach. New York: Elsevier, 1993:336–356

UK-TIA Study Group. United Kingdom transient ischaemic attack (UK-TIA) aspirin trial: Interim results. Br Med J 1988;296:316–320

Hass WK, Easton D, Adams HP, et al. A randomized trial comparing ticlopidine hydrochloride with aspirin for prevention of stroke in high-risk patients. N Engl J Med 1989;321:501–507

Sherman DG, Dyken ML, Fisher M, et al. Cerebral embolism. Chest 1986;89(suppl 2):82S–98S

Cerebral Embolism Task Force. Cardiogenic brain embolism. The second report of the Cerebral Embolism Task Force. Arch Neurol 1989; 46:727–743

Chesebro JH, Adams PC, Fuster V, et al. Antithrombotic therapy in patients with valvular heart disease and prosthetic heart valves. J Am Coll Cardiol 1986;8:41B–46B

Stroke 1989. Recommendations on stroke prevention, diagnosis, and therapy. Report of the WHO Task Force on stroke and other cerebrovascular disorders. Stroke 1989;20:1407–1431

MacMahon S, Sharpe N. Long-term antiplatelet therapy for the prevention of vascular disease. Med J Aust 1991;154:477–480

Antiplatelet Trialists Collaboration. Secondary prevention of vascular disease by prolonged antiplatelet treatment. Br Med J 1988;296:320–321

Third ACCP Consensus Conference on Antithrombotic Therapy. Chest 1992;102(suppl):529S–537S

2 | ENDOCRINOLOGICAL DISORDERS

DRUG THERAPY FOR DIABETES MELLITUS

Christy Silvius Scott

▶ What Are My Goals of Treatment?

(Can Med Assoc J 1992;147:697–712, N Engl J Med 1989; 321:1231–1240)

to relieve the symptoms of diabetes (polyuria, polydipsia, polyphagia, fatigue, and blurred vision)

to avoid hypoglycemia

to prevent diabetic ketoacidosis

to improve the patients' quality of life

to promote normal growth and development in children and adolescents

to prevent and treat long-term complications (retinopathy, neuropathy, nephropathy, atherosclerotic heart disease, peripheral vascular disease, and recurrent infections)

▶ What Evidence Is Available to Support Drug Therapy for Diabetes Mellitus?

Effect on symptoms

Insulin-dependent diabetes mellitus

- without exogenous insulin, patients die of ketoacidosis

Non–insulin-dependent diabetes mellitus

- patients are at risk for nonketotic hyperglycemic hyperosmolar coma without treatment (Diabetic Med 1988;5: 275–281)

Mortality and morbidity

- studies suggest that patients with marked hyperglycemia are at an increased risk for the development of microvascular disease (Lancet 1976;2:1009–1012, Lancet 1980; 2:1050–1052, Diabetes Care 1990;13:1011–1019)
- studies of animal models suggest that improved blood glucose level control decreases the progress of retinopathy, nephropathy, and neuropathy (Diabetes 1977;26: 760–769, Diabetes 1980;29:509–515, Diabetes Care 1990; 13:1011–1019)

- limited prospective studies in patients with insulin-dependent diabetes mellitus (IDDM) suggest that improved glycemic control might prevent deterioration of microvascular complications in some patients (Lancet 1983;1:204–208, Lancet 1986;2:1300–1304, Diabetes Care 1990;13:1011–1019)
- Diabetes Control and Complications Trial (DCCT) was a multicenter prospective trial that showed that in patients treated for a mean of 6.5 years with intensive insulin therapy there was a delay in the onset and a slowing of the progression of diabetic nephropathy, retinopathy, and neuropathy (N Engl J Med 1993;329:977–986)

▶ When Should I Consider Drug Therapy?

Definition of diabetes in nonpregnant adults

(Diabetes 1979;28:1039–1057, Can Med Assoc J 1992;147: 697–712)

- random plasma glucose level greater than 200 mg/dL (11.1 mmol/L) with symptoms of diabetes such as polydipsia, polyuria, polyphagia, weight loss, fatigue, and blurred vision
- fasting plasma glucose level greater than 140 mg/dL (7.8 mmol/L) on at least 2 occasions
- if diabetes is suspected, but plasma glucose level is less than 140 mg/dL (7.8 mmol/L), administer 75 g of oral glucose; plasma glucose levels of >200 mg/dL (11.1 mmol/L) at the 2-hour sample and at least 1 other sample between 0 and 2 hours (1/2, 1, or 1 1/2 hours) is diagnostic of diabetes
- impaired glucose tolerance is not an indication for glucose-lowering therapy
- deciding whether the patient has IDDM or non–insulin-dependent diabetes mellitus (NIDDM) may sometimes be difficult, but treatment should begin after the diagnosis is made

Insulin-dependent diabetes mellitus

- treat all patients immediately to treat or prevent ketoacidosis

Non–insulin-dependent diabetes mellitus

(Can Med Assoc J 1992;147:697–712, Physician's Guide to Non–Insulin-Dependent (Type II) Diabetes: Diagnosis and Treatment, 1988:48)

Severe, symptomatic hyperglycemia, particularly if patients are nonobese (fasting plasma glucose level > 200 mg/dL [11.1 mmol/L])

- all patients require drug therapy to be initiated from the outset along with a diet and exercise program

Moderate hyperglycemia (fasting plasma glucose level between 140 and 199 mg/dL [7.8–11 mmol/L]) without significant symptoms

- initially, prescribe a program of diet and exercise designed to achieve ideal body weight (IBW)
- if the maximum effects of diet and exercise fail to achieve adequate glycemic control after 2–3 months, initiate drug therapy

Mild hyperglycemia (fasting plasma glucose level between 115 and 139 mg/dL [6.4–7.7 mmol/L])

- should be managed with dietary therapy and exercise at least initially, for up to 6 months
- if dietary therapy and exercise fail to control blood glucose, then initiate drug therapy

▶ *What Drug Should I Use for Initial Treatment?*

Insulin-dependent diabetes mellitus

INSULIN

- insulin must be used for initial and long-term management of all patients to prevent diabetic ketoacidosis and to achieve metabolic target levels (Diabetes Care 1991;14 [suppl 2]:30–33)

Available products

HUMAN, BEEF, PORK, BEEF-PORK INSULINS

- most clinicians recommend initiating treatment with human insulin to minimize the potential for immunological complications, which may result from use of the more antigenic beef-pork mixed species insulins; however, the evidence to support this practice is not conclusive (Diabetes Care 1989;12:641–648)
- there is no clinical difference between biosynthetic and semisynthetic human insulins (Diabetes Care 1989;12: 641–648)
- patients who require insulin on only an intermittent or short-term basis (e.g., with total parenteral nutrition supplementation or after surgery in patients with NIDDM) or who have gestational diabetes should use human insulin to decrease the possibility of present or future immunological complications
- patients who have disease that is stabilized with beef-pork insulins (less expensive than human insulins) and who are experiencing no adverse effects do not need to be switched to human insulin
- there appears to be an increased risk of severe hypoglycemia when patients are transferred from animal source insulins to human insulins (Br Med J 1991;303:617–621)
- there are several different formulations of insulin, and they vary with respect to time to peak effect and duration of effect

Short acting

(onset, 1/2–1 hour; peak, 2–4 hours; duration, 5–7 hours)

INSULIN INJECTION (REGULAR INSULIN, CRYSTALLINE ZINC INSULIN)—AVAILABLE AS HUMAN OR ANIMAL SPECIES INSULIN

- preferred subcutaneous rapid-acting insulin and the only agent that can be used intravenously

PROMPT INSULIN ZINC SUSPENSION (SEMILENTE)

- should not be used instead of regular insulin because its onset of action is less prompt and its duration is more prolonged

Intermediate acting

(onset 1–3 hours; peak, 6–12 hours; duration, approximately 24 hours)

ISOPHANE INSULIN SUSPENSION (NPH) AND INSULIN ZINC SUSPENSION (LENTE)—AVAILABLE AS HUMAN OR ANIMAL SPECIES INSULIN

- are widely used and can be considered interchangeable
- NPH may be mixed with regular insulin in the same syringe; Lente may not, as the extra zinc binds with the regular insulin, changing it to intermediate acting
- human Lente insulin may have a slightly longer duration of action than does human NPH insulin

Long acting

(onset 6 hours; peak, 18–24 hours [10–14 hours for human]; duration, 36 hours [16–18 hours for human])

EXTENDED INSULIN ZINC SUSPENSION (ULTRALENTE) (AVAILABLE AS HUMAN OR BEEF INSULIN)

- is the preferred type in this class

PROTAMINE ZINC INSULIN

- no longer available

Premixed fixed ratios of Regular and NPH insulin (USA: 70/30, 50/50; Canada: 90/10, 85/15, 80/20, 70/30, 50/50)

- are generally recommended for convenience in selected patients whose diabetes has previously been stabilized with mixed-dose regimens and should not be used for initiating insulin therapy

Non–insulin-dependent diabetes mellitus

- Patients who are older than 40 years and obese, have a fasting plasma glucose level less than 180 mg/dL (10 mmol/L), and have had diabetes for less than 5 years are more likely to have satisfactory results from the use of oral hypoglycemics (N Engl J Med 1989;321: 1231–1245, Can Med Assoc J 1991;145:1571–1581)

Nonobese (within 120% of IBW) and young (<40 years old) patients willing to inject insulin and self-monitor blood glucose levels and those patients with severe, symptomatic hyperglycemia

INSULIN

- these patients are generally started on insulin, especially if they are symptomatic and have urinary ketones, because they rarely respond to oral agents (Can Med Assoc J 1991;145:1571–1581, Diabetes Care 1990;13:1240–1262)

Obese (>120% of IBW) and/or older (>40 years old) patients with moderate hyperglycemia and without significant symptoms

Oral hypoglycemic agents

- because obese diabetic patients are in a state of insulin resistance, large doses of insulin may be required and euglycemia may be difficult to achieve (N Engl J Med 1989;321:1231–1245)
- insulin may also be lipogenic and may promote further weight gain; therefore, oral hypoglycemics are the preferred agent (Diabetes Care 1990;13:1240–1262)

- on average, oral agents decrease blood glucose concentrations by 50–70 mg/dL (3–4 mmol/L)
- incidence of hypoglycemia, the most troubling side effect of these agents, is connected to the duration of action and the potency of the medications (Drugs 1981;22:211–245, 295–320)
- patient risk factors for severe hypoglycemia include age older than 60 years, renal insufficiency (secondary to decreased clearance and accumulation of active metabolites), alcoholism, poor dietary habits, and concomitant medication administration (N Engl J Med 1989; 321: 1231–1245, Horm Metab Res 1985;17[suppl 150]: 111–115, Endocrinol Metab Clin North Am 1989;18: 163–183, Diabetes Care 1989;12:203–208)
- although there are no studies demonstrating the greater effectiveness of second- over first-generation sulfonylureas (Diabetes Care 1992;15:737–754), most studies suggest that the maximum doses of chlorpropamide, glyburide, and glipizide are equally efficacious and appear superior to those of tolazamide, acetohexamide, and tolbutamide (N Engl J Med 1989;321:1231–1245)
- sulfonylureas are contraindicated in patients who have sulfa allergies or who are pregnant or nursing

TOLBUTAMIDE

- shortest duration of action (6–10 hours) and least potent agent; therefore, administered 2–3 times a day
- probably associated with the fewest serious adverse effects (Drugs 1981;22:211–245, N Engl J Med 1989;321: 1231–1245)
- is less expensive than glyburide, gliclazide, and glipizide but has the disadvantage of having to be dosed 2–3 times daily
- useful for patients who have developed severe hypoglycemia while receiving the other agents despite dosage reductions, patients at high risk for hypoglycemia (N Engl J Med 1989;321:1231–1245) and patients who cannot afford more expensive agents
- metabolized to inactive compounds and, therefore, may safely be used in patients with renal insufficiency

GLYBURIDE (GLIBENCLAMIDE)

- duration of action is 18–24 hours and, therefore, may be dosed 1–2 times per day
- glyburide is as effective as other oral hypoglycemics and can be given less frequently than tolbutamide
- highest incidence of hypoglycemia occurs with glyburide and chlorpropamide (5 times more common than with tolbutamide, 2 times more frequent than with glipizide and gliclazide) (Diabetes Care 1989;12:203–208, Drugs 1981;22:211–245, N Engl J Med 1989;321:1231–1245); hospitalizations due to hypoglycemia occur most frequently with glyburide (Br Med J 1988;296:949–950, Diabetes Res Clin Pract 1991;14:139–148)
- almost all severe cases of hypoglycemia have involved patients older than 70 years (Comprehensive Therapy 1979;5:21–29, Diabetes Care 1992;15:737–754)
- because of the increased incidence of hypoglycemia with glyburide, the cost advantage of glyburide may be offset
- increased incidence of hypoglycemia may be due to a greater magnitude and duration of suppression of hepatic glucose production compared with that achieved with glipizide (Diabetes Care 1992;15:737–754)
- metabolized to active metabolite 4–hydroxyglyburide, which is retained in renal insufficiency (Drugs 1981; 22:211–245, 295–320)

- avoid in patients with renal insufficiency
- is a reasonable starting medication for younger patients with good renal function who desire less frequent dosing schedules

GLIPIZIDE (USA ONLY)

- similar potency and duration of action to those of glyburide
- more expensive than glyburide
- causes a lower incidence (approximately 50% less) of hypoglycemia in comparison with glyburide (Drugs 1981; 22:211–245)
- metabolized to inactive compounds
- therefore, reserve for patients with renal insufficiency who desire once-daily dosing and are willing to pay more for the convenience
- tolbutamide is probably a better choice for patients older than 60 years owing to decreased potency and duration of action (Drug Ther Bull 1987;25:13–16)

GLICLAZIDE (CANADA ONLY)

- similar potency and duration of action to those of glyburide
- less than 20% is metabolized to active metabolites; however, they may be retained in renal failure (Can Med Assoc J 1992;124:1571–1581, Clin Pharmacokinet 1981; 6:215–241)
- also reduces platelet adhesiveness and impairs aggregation, enhances fibrinolytic activity, possesses antithrombotic activity, and is a free radical scavenger; however, the extent to which these effects alter the microvascular long-term complications in patients with diabetes is unknown (Metabolism 1992;41:33–39, 40–45, JAMA 1991; 90[suppl 6A]:50S–54S)
- cost is higher than with glyburide or tolbutamide
- the future role of gliclazide depends on its ability to decrease the long-term microvascular complications of diabetes; presently its role is unclear

CHLORPROPAMIDE

- chlorpropamide causes a relatively high incidence of hypoglycemia, which may be prolonged for several days after discontinuation; a disulfiram-type reaction with alcohol; and syndrome of inappropriate secretion of antidiuretic hormone (SIADH), which can produce profound hyponatremia; therefore, it is rarely used (N Engl J Med 1989;321:1321–1345, Drugs 1981;22: 211–245)
- is the only truly once a day oral hypoglycemic agent and should be used only in patients who require twice-daily dosing with glyburide, glipizide, or gliclazide (e.g., when higher dosages of these agents are used and twice-daily dosing is required)
- 20% is eliminated unchanged by the kidneys and, therefore, this drug should not be used in the elderly or patients with renal insufficiency (N Engl J Med 1989;321:1231–1245, Drugs 1981;22:211–245)

METFORMIN (CANADA ONLY)

- metformin differs from sulfonylureas because, by itself, it does not produce hypoglycemia or promote weight gain (Diabetes Care 1992;15:755–772)
- if patients are obese (>120–160% of IBW), metformin as sole therapy may be tried initially, as it can decrease insulin resistance without increasing hyperinsulinemia in these patients, which is often the reason for their glucose intolerance (Diabetes Care 1992;15:755–772)

- blood glucose concentrations usually decrease by more than 36 mg/dL (2 mmol/L) (Diabetes Care 1992;15: 755–772)
- metformin is also commonly used in combination with other oral hypoglycemics if the patient has failed to respond to therapy with maximum doses of sulfonylureas
- metformin should not be used in patients with renal, hepatic, or cardiac insufficiency or with hypoxia because of the concern for the development of lactic acidosis (Diabetes Care 1992;15:755–772)
- metformin has been shown to decrease risk factors for cardiovascular disease (N Engl J Med 1989;321: 1321–1345, Diabetes Care 1993;16:621–629)

ACETOHEXAMIDE, TOLAZAMIDE (USA ONLY)

- offer no advantages over other available agents and have active metabolites that are retained in renal failure

▶ ## What Dosage Should I Use?

Insulin-dependent diabetes mellitus

Insulin

(doses in parentheses are for a 60 kg patient)

- 0.5 unit/kg/day (30 units)
- insulin can be initiated in either a BID (before breakfast and dinner) or TID regimen (before breakfast and dinner and at bedtime)

BID regimen

- more convenient than the TID regimen; however, the patient must eat a bedtime snack before retiring to avoid hypoglycemic reaction in early morning (2–4 AM)
- suggested starting regimen: give $^2/_3$ of the total daily dose (20 units) before breakfast, with $^2/_3$ of the morning dose (14 units) given as an intermediate-acting insulin and $^1/_3$ (6 units) given as regular insulin; give $^1/_3$ of the total daily dose (10 units), before dinner with $^1/_2$ (5 units) given as an intermediate-acting insulin and $^1/_2$ (5 units) given as a short-acting insulin
- short-acting insulins provide coverage for breakfast and dinner; intermediate-acting insulins provide coverage for lunch and bedtime snack and supply basal amounts throughout the day
- evening dose of intermediate-acting insulin may have to be given at bedtime (TID regimen) rather than before dinner in patients who experience 3 AM hypoglycemia followed by fasting 7 AM hyperglycemia owing to a peak effect of insulin occurring during early morning hours followed by counterregulatory hormones causing increased glucose production and hyperglycemia. (Diabetes Mellitus, Theory and Practice 1990:526–546, Diabetes Care 1988;37:1608)
- insufficient duration of action of the intermediate-acting insulin administered before dinner may also cause 7 AM fasting hyperglycemia; administering the NPH at bedtime may be required

TID regimen

- allows more flexibility than the BID regimen and can be more readily adjusted (time and amount)
- give a mixed dose (as above for the BID regimen)—$^2/_3$ of the total daily dose (20 units) before breakfast, with $^2/_3$ of the morning dose (14 units) given as an intermediate-acting insulin and $^1/_3$ (6 units) given as a short-acting insulin, and split the dinner dose by giving $^1/_6$ of the daily dose (5 units) of short-acting insulin before dinner and $^1/_6$ of the daily dose (5 units) of intermediate-acting insulin at bedtime

Further insulin dosage adjustments should be based on blood glucose measurements

- gradually increase or decrease the daily dosage by 1–2 units/d as needed to achieve desired glycemic control
- early (3–6 months, up to 2 years) in the course of insulin-dependent diabetes mellitus (IDDM), during a period of relative remission ("honeymoon period"), insulin requirements may fall to as low as 0.2 unit/kg/d; insulin therapy must not be interrupted despite low requirements because of the concern for future immunological reactions (Diabetes Care 1987;10:164)
- aggressive therapy (intensive insulin therapy with three or more insulin doses per day based on frequent blood glucose levels) is recommended for most young, otherwise healthy patients to normalize blood glucose levels and thereby potentially to minimize the incidence and severity of long-term complications (N Engl J Med 1993; 329:977–986)
- consider a less aggressive approach for elderly patients in whom long-term complications are absent and/or unlikely to develop during their expected lifetime (Diabetes Care 1990;13:1011–1019, Clin Diabetes 1985;3: 73–90)
- do not attempt to achieve a degree of blood glucose control tighter than that which can be attained safely without frequent and/or severe hypoglycemic episodes
- accept higher plasma glucose values in patients who are predisposed to hypoglycemia, unaware of the signs and symptoms, and/or likely unable to recover
- dosage adjustments should not be made more frequently than every 3 days (so that a pattern may be established)
- in general, dosage changes of greater than 10% should not be done except in the acute care setting

Non–insulin-dependent diabetes mellitus

INSULIN

- 0.2–0.5 unit/kg (actual body weight) of intermediate-acting insulin (NPH or Lente) given once daily before breakfast is the most common starting dose (usually approximately 20 units as a starting dose) (Diabetes Care 1990;13:1240–1262, Can Med Assoc J 1991;145: 1571–1581)
- alternatively, long-acting beef or mixed beef-pork Ultralente may be given once daily in the evening to supply 24 hour basal insulin levels (long-acting human Ultralente insulin is usually given twice daily) (Diabetes Care 1990;13:1240–1262)
- if the patient is in the hospital and has urinary ketones, 4–6 units of regular insulin every 6 hours should be administered until ketosis is resolved (Diabetes Care 1990; 13:1240–1262)
- for patients in the hospital, dosages may be increased by 20–40% daily, with close monitoring, to pursue more efficient and cost-effective therapy (Diabetes Care 1990; 13:1240–1262
- for outpatients, dosage increases of 2–5 units/d may be made every 3 days (Can Med Assoc J 1991;145:1571–1581)
- if the NPH dose in the morning reaches 60–80 units without achieving a desirable 7 AM fasting blood glucose level, a second dose of NPH should be added at bedtime (Diabetes Care 1990;13:1240–1262) so that 50–70% of the daily dose is administered before breakfast and 30–50% of the daily dose is administered before dinner (Can Med Assoc J 1991;145:1571–1581)

- owing to inherent insulin resistance, daily doses may exceed 1 unit/kg in order to achieve euglycemic control (Can Med Assoc J 1991;145:1571–1581)
- after euglycemia is achieved, dosage decreases may be necessary because insulin sensitivity improves with control of blood glucose levels (Can Med Assoc J 1991;145:1571–1581, Diabetes Care 1990;13:1240–1262)

TOLBUTAMIDE

- 250 mg PO BID administered 30 minutes before meals
- increase the dosage weekly by 250 mg increments until glycemic control or a maximum daily dose of 3000 mg is reached
- daily doses greater than 1500 mg should be divided TID
- average daily dose is 1500 mg (N Engl J Med 1989; 321:1231–1245)

GLYBURIDE

- 2.5 mg PO daily
- timing of the dose in relation to meals appears to be irrelevant with long-term therapy (Diabetes Care 1990; 13[suppl 3]:26–31)
- increase the dosage weekly by 2.5 mg increments until glycemic control or a maximum daily dose of 20 mg is reached
- average daily dose is 7.5 mg (N Engl J Med 1989; 321:1231–1245)
- daily doses greater than 10 mg should be divided BID because patients requiring high doses likely require a split dose to ensure adequate effective concentrations throughout the day

GLIPIZIDE (USA ONLY)

- 5 mg PO daily
- food delays the absorption of glipizide; however, with long-term therapy, this delay is not clinically important and administration before meals is not necessary (Diabetes Care 1990;13[suppl 3]:26–31)
- increase the dosage weekly by 2.5 mg increments until glycemic control or a maximum daily dose of 40 mg is reached
- average daily dose is 10 mg (N Engl J Med 1989;321: 1231–1245)
- daily doses greater than 15 mg PO should be divided BID because patients requiring high doses likely require a split dose to ensure adequate effective concentrations throughout the day

GLICLAZIDE (CANADA ONLY)

- 40 mg PO daily
- timing of the dose in relation to meals appears to be irrelevant with long-term therapy (Eur J Clin Pharmacol 1990;38:465–467)
- increase the dosage weekly by 40 mg increments until glycemic control or a maximum daily dose of 320 mg is reached
- daily doses greater than 160 mg should be divided BID because patients requiring high doses likely require a split dose to ensure adequate effective concentrations throughout the day

CHLORPROPAMIDE

- 100 mg PO daily
- increase the dosage every 2 weeks by 100 mg increments until glycemic control or a maximum daily dose of 500 mg is reached

- the average daily dose is 250 mg (N Engl J Med 1989; 321:1231–1245)
- all doses should be given once daily

METFORMIN (CANADA ONLY)

- 500 mg PO BID given with meals to prevent or decrease gastrointestinal upset (Diabetes Care 1992;15: 755–772)
- increase the dosage weekly by 500 mg increments until glycemic control or a maximum daily dose of 3000 mg is reached
- average daily doses are 1500–1700 mg (Diabetes Care 1992;15:755–772)
- dosages of 3 g daily (1 g TID) are not usually tolerated (Diabetes Care 1992;15:755–772)

▶ *How Long Should I Treat with My Initial Regimen?*

Insulin-dependent diabetes mellitus

INSULIN

- continue with initial insulin treatment regimens as long as adequate control is maintained
- if patients initially receiving beef-pork insulins experience any immunological reactions, switch to human insulin

Non–insulin-dependent diabetes mellitus

INSULIN

- if insulin requirements are 20 units/d or less, a trial with a sulfonylurea alone is warranted (Diabetes Care 1990; 13:1240–1262)
- definite indications for insulin withdrawal are sustained excellent control and suspected hypoglycemia (Br Med J 1981;283:1386–1388, Diabetes Care 1990;13:1240–1262)

TOLBUTAMIDE, GLYBURIDE, GLIPIZIDE, GLICLAZIDE, CHLORPROPAMIDE, METFORMIN

- continue therapy until adequate control is achieved or the maximum daily dosage is reached (N Engl J Med 1989;321:1231–1245)
- approximately ⅓ of all patients with NIDDM receiving sulfonylureas fail to respond to therapy, most often owing to dietary noncompliance (N Engl J Med 1989;321: 1231–1245)
- if only a partial response has been seen with maximum dosages of the first agent, add metformin if available (Can Med Assoc J 1992;147:697–712, N Engl J Med 1989; 321:1231–1245)
- some patients who do not respond to tolbutamide, acetohexamide, or tolazamide may respond to glyburide, glipizide, or chlorpropamide (N Engl J Med 1989;321: 1231–1245)
- patients who do not respond to glyburide, glipizide, or chlorpropamide do not usually respond to a different sulfonylurea (N Engl J Med 1989;321:1231–1245)
- patients who do not respond to oral agents should be treated with insulin (Diabetes Care 1990;13:1240–1262, Can Med Assoc J 1992;147:697–712)
- if the obese patient is receiving insulin and the disease is well controlled, tapering and withdrawal of insulin administration should be considered (the obesity may partly be due to insulin therapy) (Diabetes Care 1990;13: 1240–1262)
- according to several studies, many patients receiving insulin (especially those who are obese) could be managed without it (Diabetes Care 1990;13:1240–1262)

▶ What Efficacy Parameters Should I Follow and How Frequently Do I Have to Assess My Patient?

- frequency of assessment in an individual patient depends on the type, severity, and complications of diabetes; the difficulty experienced in controlling blood glucose levels; changes in therapy; and other medical conditions (Diabetes Care 1993;16[suppl 2]:4–13)
- all patients should be referred to a diabetes education center after diagnosis and periodically attend refresher courses (Diabetes Care 1993;16[suppl 2]:4–13)

Insulin-dependent and non–insulin-dependent diabetes mellitus

(Diabetes Care 1993;16[suppl 2]:4–13)

- daily contact may be required during the initiation of insulin therapy or after any major change in the insulin regimen and should continue until satisfactory control is achieved, the risk of hypoglycemia is low, and the patient demonstrates competence in following therapy
- after a major change in insulin therapy, contact with the patient should be made within at least 1 week
- weekly contact may be required during the initiation of dietary therapy or a regimen of oral medications until acceptable glucose level control and competence in following therapy is achieved
- after a major change in oral therapy, contact with the patient should occur within 1 month
- in general, regular office visits are scheduled every 3 months for patients receiving insulin and every 6 months for other patients
- children and adolescents should be managed in consultation with persons who have expertise in treating diabetes in this age group

Patients who are injecting insulin

(Diabetes Care 1993;16[suppl 2]:4–13)

- all insulin-treated patients and those with poorly controlled NIDDM should be taught self-monitoring of blood glucose levels
- in patients with IDDM receiving intensive therapy (3–4 injections a day) and requiring insulin dosage on the basis of the interpretation of blood glucose testing results, testing should initially be done as frequently as 4–8 times daily (before and 2 hours after meals, at bedtime, and between 2 and 4 AM)
- this intensive schedule need not be followed every day during stable periods and can be adjusted (e.g., only 3 d/wk) or can be staggered (e.g., before breakfast and lunch 1 day and before dinner and at bedtime on the following day)
- patients receiving minimum insulin therapy may be required to test blood glucose levels only once or twice daily (e.g., before breakfast and/or supper) and, during stable periods, only 3–7 times per week (Can Med Assoc J 1992;147:697–712)
- frequency and scheduling of blood glucose testing must be individualized according to the type of diabetes, the goals of and the agents used for treatment, the extent of blood glucose fluctuation, and the patient's willingness to self-monitor
- every 4–6 months, a blood glucose level obtained by the patient should be compared simultaneously with a laboratory-measured blood glucose level to verify patient self-monitoring technique (Can Med Assoc J 1992;147:697–712)

Self-monitoring of preprandial blood glucose levels

(N Engl J Med 1989;321:1231–1245, Can Med Assoc J 1992;147:697–712)

- 80–120 mg/dL (4.4–6.7 mmol/L) is considered good or optimum control
- 120–140 mg/dL (6.7–7.8 mmol/L) is considered acceptable control
- 140–180 mg/dL (7.8–10 mmol/L) is considered fair control
- greater than 180 mg/dL (>10 mmol/L) is considered poor control
- patients should strive for levels in the optimum range; for elderly patients, fair control is acceptable
- all patients must be carefully taught by a qualified trainer how to use the individual testing devices to try to minimize errors (Diabetes Care 1993;16:60–65)
- in the elderly, it may be best to avoid devices that necessitate wiping blood from sticks or pressing buttons to start the timer (Br Med J 1992;305:1171–1172)

Urine glucose levels

(Diabetes Care 1993;16[suppl 2]:39)

- patients should monitor blood glucose, not urine glucose, levels
- normal renal threshold for glucose is 180 mg/dL (10 mmol/L)
- renal threshold may be increased in patients with diabetes of long duration or may be decreased in children and pregnant women
- urine glucose concentration may affect the results
- reflects only an average level of blood glucose since last voiding
- hypoglycemia cannot be detected
- color tests used for urine testing are not very accurate

Patients with non–insulin-dependent diabetes mellitus who are not injecting insulin

- although this schedule is controversial, patients should self-monitor blood glucose levels at least before breakfast (fasting) and dinner (Can Med Assoc J 1992;147:697–712, Diabetes Care 1993;16:60–64)
- some studies suggest that self-monitoring of glucose levels in patients with NIDDM is not helpful in the overall treatment of the disease (Br Med J 1992;305:1194–1196, Br Med J 1992;305:1171–1172, Am J Med 1986;81:830–835, Diabetes Care 1990;13:1044–1050)
- if the patient is not willing to self-monitor blood glucose levels, urine glucose testing should be used (Physician's Guide to Non-Insulin-Dependent (Type II) Diabetes: Diagnosis and Treatment, 1988)
- frequency and scheduling of self-tests must be individualized to the goals of and the agents used for treatment, the extent of blood glucose fluctuation, and the patient's willingness to self-monitor

Glycosylated hemoglobin

(N Engl J Med 1989;321:1231–1245, Can Med Assoc J 1992;147:697–712)

- glycosylated hemoglobin (e.g., HbA_{1c}) is expressed as a percentage of total hemoglobin
- hemoglobin is slowly and irreversibly glycosylated throughout the life of the red blood cell; the amount that is glycosylated depends on blood glucose concentrations
- because the life of a red blood cell is approximately 120 days, measuring HbA_{1c} values more frequently than 4 times per year is not beneficial
- best index of glycemic control because it reflects the mean blood glucose values over the preceding 6–10 weeks

- HbA$_{1c}$ values <6% suggest hypoglycemia; ask about symptoms
- HbA$_{1c}$ values should be determined in all diabetics at least every 6 months, but preferably every 3 months in insulin-treated patients and non–insulin-treated patients with poor glycemic control
- HbA$_{1c}$ values <6% suggest hypoglycemia; ask about symptoms
- HbA$_{1c}$ values of 6–8% suggest good glucose control
- HbA$_{1c}$ values of 8–11% suggest fair glucose control
- HbA$_{1c}$ values of 11–13% suggest poor glucose control
- upper limit of normal varies from laboratory to laboratory: in general, an HbA$_{1c}$ level within 1% of the upper limit reflects good control; within 1–3%, acceptable control; and greater than 3% above normal, poor control
- the goal of therapy is to have HbA$_{1c}$ values suggesting good control

Urinary ketones

(Diabetes Care 1993;16[suppl 2]:4–13)

- indicative of impending ketoacidosis
- patient with IDDM should test urine for ketones when periods of stress or acute illness are experienced and when blood glucose levels consistently exceed 240 mg/dL (13.4 mmol/L) or symptoms of diabetic ketoacidosis (nausea, vomiting, abdominal pain) are present
- if ketones are present, medical advice should be sought

Eye examination

(Diabetes Care 1993;16[suppl 2]:16–18, Can Med Assoc J 1992;147:697–712)

- retinal examination by an ophthalmologist should be performed at least once annually in all patients with a 5 year history of IDDM
- patients with NIDDM should have a complete eye examination at the time of diagnosis and then yearly
- pregnant women with preexisting diabetes should have a complete eye examination during the first trimester and be followed closely throughout the remaining months

Lipid profile

(Diabetes Care 1993;16[suppl 2]:4–13, 106–112, Can Med Assoc J 1992;147:697–712)

- in adults, monitor fasting serum triglyceride and total high-density lipoprotein and calculated low-density lipoprotein cholesterol levels once yearly
- if abnormalities exist, complete the above testing every 4 months
- in children, complete testing as for adults at the time of diagnosis; if any abnormality exists, complete testing annually; if no abnormality exists, complete testing every 2 years
- high triglyceride and low-density lipoprotein cholesterol levels may be associated with poor glycemic control
- dyslipidemia should first be treated by weight reduction (if necessary), decreased saturated fat and cholesterol intake, and increased exercise
- if response is not adequate with nonpharmacological treatment in 4 months, then drug therapy to lower lipid levels should be considered

Blood pressure

(Diabetes Care 1993;16[suppl 2]:4–13)

- measure blood pressure at regular office visits
- the results do not affect diabetic therapy but may suggest the need for further diet consultation or antihypertensive drug therapy

- because hypertension contributes to the risk and progression of diabetic complications, increased blood pressure should be treated aggressively

Renal profile

(Diabetes Care 1993;16[suppl 2]:4–13, Can Med Assoc J 1992;147:697–712)

- at diagnosis and once yearly, a routine urinalysis and serum creatinine level should be completed
- in patients past puberty or younger patients with a 5 year history of diabetes, total urinary protein excretion should be determined yearly (if possible, by a microalbuminuria method)
- if abnormalities are present, the above testing should be done during all regular office visits
- if declining renal function or persistent proteinuria is confirmed, the patient should be referred to a nephrologist specializing in diabetic renal disease

Neurological profile

(Diabetes Care 1993;16[suppl 2]:4–13, Can Med Assoc J 1992;147:697–712)

- sensory, motor, and autonomic nervous systems may be affected by diabetes
- a complete neurological examination should be completed at the time of diagnosis and at least annually

Foot care

(Diabetes Care 1993;16[suppl 2]:4–13, Can Med Assoc J 1992;147:697–712)

- a complete foot and leg examination should be completed at the time of diagnosis and at regular office visits
- patients should routinely inspect their feet for any abnormality each evening

Symptoms

- reduction in symptoms such as polyuria, polydipsia, yeast and urinary tract infections

▶ *Should I Add Another Drug or Substitute Therapy If My Initial Drug Therapy Fails?*

Insulin-dependent diabetes mellitus

(Applied Therapeutics 1993;72-1–72-51)

- insulin is the only medication that is useful for controlling blood glucose in IDDM
- dosage adjustments may be necessary; however, they should be done only after 3 days if eating and blood glucose patterns are unchanged
- usually, for every 50 mg/dL (2.5 mmol/L) that blood glucose levels differ from the established goal, adjust the insulin dosage by 1–2 units
- if prebreakfast blood glucose level is high or low, increase or decrease, respectively, predinner or bedtime intermediate or long-acting insulin administration
- if prelunch glucose level is high or low, increase or decrease, respectively, prebreakfast regular insulin administration
- if predinner glucose level is high or low, increase or decrease, respectively, prebreakfast intermediate-acting insulin or prelunch regular insulin administration
- if bedtime glucose level is high or low, increase or decrease, respectively, predinner regular insulin administration
- if 3 AM glucose level is high or low, increase or decrease, respectively, predinner intermediate-acting insulin or give intermediate-acting insulin at bedtime instead

Non–insulin-dependent diabetes mellitus

- primary failure (occurs in approximately 30% of patients) with oral hypoglycemic agents is thought to be due to poor patient selection, dietary therapy failure, and/or severely impaired pancreatic function (N Engl J Med 1989;321:1231–1245)
- secondary failure (5–10% of patients each year who once were controlled no longer respond) with oral hypoglycemic agents is thought to be due to poor patient selection, failure with dietary therapy, drug interactions, or ongoing diminishing pancreatic function (N Engl J Med 1989; 321:1231–1245)

INSULIN

- if premeal blood glucose levels are excessive, intensify the insulin regimen by adding premeal injections of regular insulin twice daily before breakfast and dinner (Diabetes Care 1990;13:1011–1020)
- at this stage, oral therapy is not beneficial because beta cell function is probably inadequate (Diabetes Care 1990;13:1011–1020) and these patients should be treated as patients with IDDM

ORAL HYPOGLYCEMIC AGENTS

Switching to or adding another oral hypoglycemic agent

- if adequate control is not achieved with chlorpropamide, gliclazide, glipizide, or glyburide, the patient is unlikely to benefit by changing to another sulfonylurea (N Engl J Med 1989;321:1231–1245)
- approximately 50% of patients who have failed treatment with a sulfonylurea respond to metformin (N Engl J Med 1989;321:1231–1245)
- there is no indication for the simultaneous use of two sulfonylureas (N Engl J Med 1989;321:1231–1245)
- when sulfonylurea therapy is insufficient (blood glucose level has lowered, but not reached the set goal), the addition of metformin, if available, is an alternative to the initiation of insulin therapy (Can Med Assoc J 1992;147:1231–1245)
- by adding metformin therapy, blood glucose levels usually decrease by an additional 25–35 mg/dL (1.5–2 mmol/L) (Diabetes Care 1990;13:1011–1020)
- if the patient's blood glucose level is 180–230 mg/dL (10–13 mmol/L) while receiving maximum doses of a sulfonylurea, metformin should be added (Diabetes Care 1990;13:1240–1262)
- if the patient's blood glucose level is greater than 230 mg/dL (13 mmol/L) while receiving maximum doses of a sulfonylurea, the therapy should be switched to insulin (Diabetes Care 1990;13:1240–1262)

Switching to insulin or combining insulin with sulfonylurea therapy

- where metformin is not available, insulin therapy must be initiated in patients whose control is unsatisfactory with a sulfonylurea
- with failure to respond to a sulfonylurea, switching to insulin therapy alone is preferable to adding insulin therapy, although somewhat controversial (Can Med Assoc J 1992;147:697–712, Diabetes Care 1990;13:1011–1020, 1240–1262, N Engl J Med 1989;321:1231–1245)
- in obese patients, if insulin administration has been instituted and glycemic control is not attained with insulin doses greater than 100 units/d, a sulfonylurea may be added to therapy (Diabetes Care 1990;13:1240–1262, Diabetes Care 1992;15:953–959)
- the addition of insulin to oral therapy may cause a drop in blood glucose level by approximately 40–50 mg/dL (2.2–2.8 mmol/L) or control may be the same; insulin doses may need to be adjusted accordingly; however, this benefit may be only temporary (Diabetes Care 1990;13:1240–1262)

▶ How Long Should I Continue Drug Therapy?

Insulin-dependent diabetes mellitus

- patients require insulin treatment continuously for the rest of their lives
- early in the course of IDDM, during a period of relative remission (honeymoon period), insulin requirements may fall to as low as 0.2 unit/kg/d; insulin therapy must not be interrupted, despite low requirements, because of the concern for future immunological reaction (Diabetes Care 1987;10:164)

Non–insulin-dependent diabetes mellitus

INSULIN

- each patient should be viewed as a candidate for insulin withdrawal
- if insulin requirements are 20 units/d or less, a trial with a sulfonylurea alone is warranted (Diabetes Care 1990;13:1240–1262)
- definite indications for insulin withdrawal are sustained excellent control and suspected or repeated hypoglycemia (Br Med J 1981;283:1386–1388, Diabetes Care 1990;13:1240–1262)

ORAL HYPOGLYCEMIC AGENTS

- patients responding satisfactorily to sulfonylurea treatment should have a 6 month trial of dosage reduction to determine whether a lower dosage is acceptable (N Engl J Med 1989;321:1231–1245)
- decrease the dosage by the same increments used to increase the dosage every 2 weeks (see above discussion of dosage)
- patients with good glycemic control with modest dosages of an oral agent may maintain satisfactory control after withdrawal of the drug (N Engl J Med 1989;321: 1231–1245)
- patients need to have the importance of diet and exercise reemphasized so that a trial without oral therapy can occur
- obese patients who require less than 40 units/d of insulin should be given a trial of an oral hypoglycemic agent alone (Diabetes Care 1990;13:1240–1262)

Useful References

American Diabetes Association. Clinical practice recommendations, 1992–93. Diabetes Care 1993;16(suppl 2):1–118

Bailey CJ. Biguanides and NIDDM. Diabetes Care 1992;15:755–772

Expert Committee of the Canadian Diabetes Advisory Board. Clinical practice guidelines for treatment of diabetes mellitus. Can Med Assoc J 1992;147:697–712

Gerich JE. Oral hypoglycemic agents. N Engl J Med 1989;321:1231–1245

Genuth S. Insulin use in NIDDM. Diabetes Care 1990;13:1240–1262

Groop LC. Sulfonylureas in NIDDM. Diabetes Care 1992;15:737–754

Koda-Kimble MA. Diabetes mellitus. In: Koda-Kimble MA, Young LY, eds: Applied Therapeutics, The clinical use of drugs, 3rd ed. Vancouver, WA: Applied Therapeutics, Inc, 1992

Physician's Guide to Insulin-Dependent (Type I) Diabetes: Diagnosis and Treatment. New York: American Diabetes Association, 1988

Physician's Guide to Non–Insulin-Dependent (Type II) Diabetes: Diagnosis and Treatment. New York: American Diabetes Association, 1988

Rodger W. Non–insulin-dependent (type II) diabetes mellitus. Can Med Assoc J 1991;145:1571–1581

Turner RC, Hohman RR. Insulin use in NIDDM. Rationale based on pathophysiology of disease. Diabetes Care 1990;13:1011–1020

DRUG THERAPY FOR HYPOTHYROIDISM

Ruby Grymonpre

▶ What Are My Goals of Treatment?

to restore patients to the euthyroid state

to provide symptomatic relief of the signs and symptoms of hypothyroidism (cool and dry skin, lethargy, cold intolerance, constipation, weight gain, slowed reflexes, edema, brittle hair and nails, coarse voice, and so on)

to normalize serum thyroxine (T_4) and thyrotropin (thyroid-stimulating hormone [TSH]) concentrations (JAMA 1990;263:1529–1532)

▶ What Evidence Is Available to Support Drug Therapy for Hypothyroidism?

Control signs and symptoms

- levothyroxine prevents the wide variety of symptomatic and metabolic disturbances associated with insufficient thyroid production

▶ When Should I Consider Drug Therapy?

Hypothyroidism

In patients with signs and symptoms of hypothyroidism and TSH level greater than 15 mU/L and T_4 level below normal values

- signs and symptoms of hypothyroidism can be treated effectively with thyroid hormone replacement

In patients with mild or no symptoms of hypothyroidism and moderately elevated TSH level (6–15 mU/L) and T_4 within normal limits

- approximately 80% of patients in this category ultimately experience overt hypothyroidism, and early rather than late treatment in this group with subclinical disease is appropriate (South Med J 1989;82:681–685)

TSH levels within normal limits (0.5–6 mU/L) and T_4 level low or low normal

- thyroid hormone replacement is not required

▶ What Drug Should I Use for Initial Treatment?

Hypothyroidism

LEVOTHYROXINE

- levothyroxine (T_4) has a number of advantages over other thyroid hormone preparations (e.g., desiccated thyroid hormone)
- these advantages include uniform potency, relatively low cost, and lack of foreign protein antigenicity (Aust Pharmacist 1990;9:196–200)
- it has been suggested that triiodothyronine (T_3) is safer than levothyroxine because T_3 is more potent and has a shorter half-life (2–3 days) and serum levels fall more rapidly on drug discontinuation; however, advantages with T_3 are offset by difficulties in dosage regulation, which can result in more frequent cardiovascular problems and symptoms of hyperthyroidism

▶ What Dosage Should I Use?

Hypothyroidism

LEVOTHYROXINE

- 0.1 mg PO daily for young, otherwise healthy patients (Thyroid Function and Disease 1990:274–291)
- 0.05 mg PO daily for patients older than 45 years of age with no cardiac disease
- 0.025 mg PO daily for elderly patients and patients with cardiac disease or long-standing hypothyroidism
- therapy that is initiated too aggressively may lead to thyroid hormone toxicity, including chest pain, increased pulse rate, palpitation, excessive sweating, headache, heat intolerance, and nervousness

▶ How Long Should I Treat with My Initial Regimen?

Hypothyroidism

- increase the dosage by 0.025 mg increments every 4 weeks until TSH levels are within normal limits
- some patients (elderly, those with cardiac disease) are able to tolerate a maximum daily dose of only 0.05–0.075 mg of levothyroxine
- the half-life of levothyroxine is approximately 7 days, and therefore, TSH measurements and subsequent dosage adjustments should be made no more frequently than every 4 weeks

▶ What Efficacy Parameters Should I Follow and How Frequently Do I Have to Assess My Patient?

Hypothyroidism

Thyrotropin and thyroxine levels

- optimal thyroid hormone replacement is achieved when TSH and T_4 levels are normal
- measure TSH and T_4 every 4 weeks until these values are within normal limits
- TSH level should not be suppressed to undetectable levels, as this increases the risk of physiological abnormalities affecting cardiac, renal, hepatic, and bone tissue (Mayo Clin Proc 1988;63:1223–1229)
- during long-term replacement therapy, T_4 level is not a reliable monitoring variable because it is often above normal values
- as long as the TSH level is within normal limits, ignore an increased T_4 level
- after an optimum levothyroxine dosage has been established, evaluate TSH levels annually
- in patients known to be compliant, TSH can be monitored every 4–5 years to ensure that levothyroxine requirements are not decreasing with age

Free thyroxine index

- use of free thyroxine index is redundant and an excessive use of laboratory resources

Triiodothyronine levels

- T_3 is often within normal limits in early or mild hypothyroidism and, for diagnostic purposes, is an insensitive indicator of hypothyroidism (Can Med Assoc J 1981; 124:1181–1183)
- is usually not readily available

Thyrotropin-releasing hormone

- TSH response to thyrotropin releasing hormone has been used to fine-tune the optimum levothyroxine dosage; however, this is not clinically practical

Signs and symptoms of hypothyroidism

- assess symptoms every 4 weeks until the dosage is stabilized
- some reversal of hypothyroid symptoms such as reduced skin temperature and physical activity changes occur

within 2–3 weeks of therapy; however, maximum effects are not noticed until 4–6 weeks, and certain symptoms (e.g., anemia, hair or skin changes) need several months of replacement therapy for reversal

▶ *Should I Add Another Drug or Substitute Therapy If My Initial Drug Therapy Fails?*

Hypothyroidism

- thyroid hormone replacement is the only therapy available for hypothyroidism

▶ *How Long Should I Continue Drug Therapy?*

Hypothyroidism

- therapy with levothyroxine is usually lifelong
- transient forms of hypothyroidism (subacute thyroiditis, postpartum thyroiditis) do not usually necessitate lifelong thyroid replacement therapy

Useful References

Brown CA, Hennessey JV. Clinical significance of mildly elevated thyrotropin levels with normal thyroxine levels. South Med J 1989;82:681–685

Hamburger JI, Kaplan MM. Hypothyroidism: Don't treat patients who don't have it. Postgrad Med 1989;86:67–74

Northcutt RC, Stiel JN, Hollifield JW, et al. The influence of cholestyramine on thyroxine absorption. JAMA 1969;208:1857–1861

Oppenheimer JH, Volpe R. Measurement of thyroid function. In: Burrow GN, Oppenheimer JH, Volpe R, eds. Thyroid Function and Disease. Philadelphia: WB Saunders, 1990

Ross DS. Subclinical hyperthyroidism: Possible danger of overzealous thyroxine replacement therapy. Mayo Clin Proc 1988;63:1223–1229

Rubinoff H, Fireman BH. Testing for recovery of thyroid function after withdrawal of long-term suppression therapy. J Clin Epidemiol 1989;42:417–420

Surks MI, Chopra IJ, Mariash CN, et al. American Thyroid Association guidelines for the use of laboratory tests in thyroid disease. JAMA 1990;263:1529–1532

Thyroxine replacement therapy—too much of a good thing? Lancet 1990; 336:1352–1353

Volpe R. Hypothyroidism. In: Burrow GN, Oppenheimer JH, Volpe R, eds. Thyroid Function and Disease. Philadelphia, WB Saunders, 1990

Wong MM, Volpe R. What is the best test for monitoring levothyroxine therapy? Can Med Assoc J 1981;124:1181–1183

3

GASTROINTESTINAL DISEASES

DRUG THERAPY FOR GASTROESOPHAGEAL REFLUX

James McCormack and Glen Brown

▶ *What Are My Goals of Treatment?*

to ameliorate signs and symptoms, especially heartburn, because complications can occur with even mild symptoms

to prevent irritation of the distal esophagus, which could produce strictures or perforations

▶ *What Evidence Is Available to Support Drug Therapy for Gastroesophageal Reflux?*

Ameliorate symptoms

- efficacy depends on the initial severity of disease
- 40–60% of patients had symptomatic improvement while receiving H_2 antagonists compared with 10–35% of patients receiving placebo (Am J Gastroenterol 1989;84: 245–248)
- 60–90% of patients show endoscopic improvement (Am J Gastroenterol 1989;84:245–248)

Prevent long-term complications

- approximately 50% of patients exhibit long-term improvement with ongoing drug therapy (Arch Intern Med 1987;147:1701–1702)

▶ *When Should I Consider Drug Therapy?*

Reflux esophagitis

- drug therapy should be considered in all patients with symptoms of reflux (substernal sensation of warmth or

burning, regurgitation, or dysphagia) who do not respond to nondrug measures such as avoidance of foods that reduce lower esophageal sphincter pressure or worsen symptoms, avoidance of lying down directly after meals, ingestion of smaller meals, elevation of the head of the bed by 4–6 inches, smoking cessation, and loss of weight

▶ *What Drug Should I Use for Initial Treatment?*

Reflux esophagitis

Mild to moderate disease

CIMETIDINE

- all H_2 antagonists have equivalent efficacy
- cimetidine is the least expensive of all the H_2 antagonists

RANITIDINE, FAMOTIDINE, NIZATIDINE

- if patients are receiving drugs that have the potential to interact with cimetidine, choose either ranitidine, famotidine, or nizatidine, whichever is the least expensive

OMEPRAZOLE

- high costs and unknown long-term effects of omeprazole relegate it to the treatment of patients with severe, refractory reflux esophagitis

ANTACIDS

- should be concurrently prescribed on an as needed basis for symptom relief, but only if the patient describes symptomatic relief after antacid administration

Severe disease

OMEPRAZOLE

- is more effective than H_2 antagonists and promotility

agents in the treatment of severe or erosive esophagitis and is considered the drug of choice

▶ What Dosage Should I Use?

Reflux esophagitis

CIMETIDINE

- 400 mg PO BID
- 400 mg PO HS if the patient has only nighttime symptoms

RANITIDINE

- 150 mg PO BID
- 150 mg PO HS if the patient has only nighttime symptoms

FAMOTIDINE

- 20 mg PO BID
- 20 mg PO HS if the patient has only nighttime symptoms

NIZATIDINE

- 150 mg PO BID
- 150 mg PO HS if the patient has only nighttime symptoms

ANTACIDS

- usual dose is 30 mL of the regular-strength antacids or 15 mL of the double- or extra-strength antacids as needed for symptoms up to 6 times per day
- usual tablet dose is 2 tablets of regular-strength antacids or 1 tablet of the double- or extra-strength antacids as needed for symptoms up to 6 times per day
- see drug monograph on antacids for more dosing information

OMEPRAZOLE

- start with 20 mg PO daily for mild to moderate disease
- start with 40 mg PO daily for severe disease

▶ How Long Should I Treat with My Initial Regimen?

Reflux esophagitis

Mild to moderate disease

- initial treatment should be 4 weeks in duration, and if no relief occurs, double the dosage of the H_2 antagonist and continue therapy for a total of 8 weeks
- approximately 50% of patients have complete relief with H_2 antagonist therapy
- after symptoms are controlled, cut back the dosage by 50% every few weeks to identify the lowest effective dose

Severe disease

- give omeprazole for 4 weeks, if no response occurs, continue for another 4 weeks
- if still no response occurs, increase the dosage to 60 mg PO daily
- after symptoms are controlled, cut back the dosage by 50% every few weeks to identify the lowest effective dosage (some patients will be controlled with 20 mg PO every 2 days)

▶ What Efficacy Parameters Should I Follow and How Frequently Do I Have to Assess My Patient?

Reflux esophagitis

Signs and symptoms

- decrease in symptoms, including heartburn, pain on swallowing, and sour or bitter taste in mouth
- aim is to be virtually symptom free
- initially assess the patient every month and then every

3–6 months after symptoms are under control to encourage lifestyle changes (losing weight, and so on)

▶ Should I Add Another Drug or Substitute Therapy If My Initial Drug Therapy Fails?

Reflux esophagitis

Mild to moderate disease

- if the patient remains symptomatic after 8 weeks of H_2 antagonist therapy, the patient should have endoscopy to confirm the diagnosis and to assess the severity of irritation
- stop the H_2 antagonist and start omeprazole 40 mg PO daily for 4 weeks; if no response occurs, continue for another 4 weeks
- if still no response occurs, increase the dosage to 60 mg PO daily
- in patients who do not respond to omeprazole, add a promotility agent
- although metoclopramide is the least expensive of the promotility agents, it is associated with a large number of central nervous system adverse effects such as sedation and has the potential to cause movement disorders
- domperidone (10 mg PO QID) is less expensive than cisapride and should be tried initially for this reason

Severe disease

- in patients who do not respond to omeprazole 60 mg PO daily, add domperidone 10 mg PO QID

▶ How Long Should I Continue Drug Therapy?

Reflux esophagitis

Mild to moderate disease

- approximately 80% of patients experience relapse within a year after discontinuation of immediate treatment
- patients with frequent relapse should be considered for long-term prophylaxis
- prophylaxis usually necessitates dosages equivalent to treatment; however, after symptoms are controlled, cut back the dosage by 50% every few weeks to identify the lowest effective dosage

Severe disease

- continued treatment with a successful drug regimen is recommended
- risks of long-term omeprazole therapy are not yet completely characterized; however, patients with severe disease in which omeprazole has been effective should have therapy continued indefinitely

Useful References

Pope CE. Acid reflux disorders. N Engl J Med 1994;331:656–660
Sontag SJ. Medical management of reflux esophagitis. Role of antacids and acid inhibition. Med Clin North Am 1990;19:683–712
Tytgat GNJ. Drug therapy of reflux oesophagitis: An update. Scand J Gastroenterol 1989;24(suppl 168):38–49

DRUG THERAPY FOR PEPTIC ULCER DISEASE AND STRESS ULCERS

James McCormack and Glen Brown

▶ What Are My Goals of Treatment?

to ameliorate symptoms of peptic ulcer disease

to promote ulcer healing

to prevent complications of peptic ulcer disease (hemorrhage or perforation)

to prevent recurrences of peptic ulcer disease

to prevent complications of stress ulcers

▶ *What Evidence Is Available to Support Drug Therapy for Peptic Ulcer Disease or Stress Ulcers?*

Ulcer pain

- treatment decreases the incidence of intractable pain or worsening of symptoms (Gastroenterology 1986;90: 478–481)

Rate of ulcer healing

- antacids, H_2 antagonist, sucralfate, and misoprostol have all been shown to be superior to placebo in the degree of ulcer healing, with ulcer healing of 40% with placebo and 70–80% with drug therapy after 8 weeks of therapy (Gastroenterology 1986;90:478–481)
- omeprazole appears to heal a greater percentage of ulcers (85–95%) than do H_2 antagonists when these agents are given for similar duration of treatment (N Engl J Med 1989;320:69–75)

Incidence of complications from peptic ulcer disease

- no evidence is available that drug therapy decreases the incidence of gastrointestinal hemorrhage and perforation in patients without evidence of previous complications (Gastroenterology 1986;90:478–481)
- for patients with a healed duodenal ulcer after severe hemorrhage, maintenance therapy with an H_2 antagonist decreases the incidence of recurrent hemorrhage (N Engl J Med 1994;330:382–386)

Rate of ulcer recurrences

- frequency of ulcer recurrences is decreased when long-term maintenance therapy with antacids, H_2 antagonists, sucralfate, misoprostol, and omeprazole is used (Am J Gastroenterol 1988;83:607–617, Digestion 1990;47[suppl 1]:64–68)
- frequency of ulcer recurrences during a 12 month period is decreased when H_2 antagonists are given with a 12 day course of metronidazole and amoxicillin (85% recurrence in the group given ranitidine alone versus 8% in the group receiving ranitidine combined with metronidazole and amoxicillin) (N Engl J Med 1993;328:308–312)
- frequency of ulcer recurrences is also decreased when omeprazole is combined with amoxicillin (Am J Gastroenterol 1993;88:481–483)
- a 1 week course of triple therapy (bismuth, metronidazole, and tetracycline) has been shown to eradicate *Helicobacter pylori* (Lancet 1994;343:508–510)

Surgery, incidence of rebleeding, deaths

- metaanalysis suggests that early parenteral use of H_2 antagonists versus placebo reduces the chance of surgery (18.8% with drug versus 20.6% with placebo), the incidence of persistent or recurrent bleeding (10.2% versus 12.9%), and deaths (5.1% versus 7.2%) in patients with acute upper gastrointestinal hemorrhage (N Engl J Med 1985;313:660–666)
- however, two double-blind trials of high-dose IV omeprazole or high-dose IV famotidine versus placebo (use of oral agents starting approximately 72 hours after hospital admission) failed to demonstrate any difference in either morbidity or mortality in patients with acute upper gastro-

intestinal hemorrhage (Br Med J 1992;304:143–147, Lancet 1992;340:1058–1062)

Stress ulcer occurrence

- incidence of overt bleeding is reduced (Ann Intern Med 1987;106:562–567)

▶ *When Should I Consider Drug Therapy?*

Dyspepsia

- any patient not responding to PRN antacid therapy over 1–2 weeks should receive a 2 week trial in an attempt to control symptoms

Duodenal or gastric ulcer

Suspected or endoscopically proven duodenal or gastric ulcer, suspected or endoscopically proven duodenal or gastric ulcer due to nonsteroidal antiinflammatory drugs (NSAIDs)

- use drug therapy in all patients with a suspected or proven ulcer, because drug therapy increases the rate of healing and decreases ulcer pain

Prevention of peptic ulcer disease recurrence

- since 20–40% of patients will not have a recurrence, antibiotic therapy can be delayed until after the first relapse (Can Med Assoc J 1994;150:189–198)
- antibiotic therapy should be given to patients presenting with, or with a history of, severe complications (bleeding, perforation)

Prevention of NSAID-induced ulcers

- consider prophylactic therapy in patients receiving NSAIDs who are older than 60 years of age, have a past history of peptic ulcer, are also receiving corticosteroids or anticoagulants, or are poor surgical risks if ulcer complications occur (Mayo Clin Proc 1992;67:354–364)

Acute upper gastrointestinal hemorrhage

- while early parenteral treatment does not affect morbidity and mortality, all patients with acute upper gastrointestinal hemorrhage should receive an agent to promote healing of the ulcer

Stress ulcer prophylaxis

- for patients with extensive burns, central nervous system injury, prolonged hypotension, sepsis, uncorrectable coagulopathy, and acute respiratory failure (undergoing ventilation) or hepatic failure (Am J Gastroenterol 1990; 85:95–96)
- stress ulcer prophylaxis is not needed if the patient is not at risk for gastrointestinal hypoperfusion or is receiving feeding by gastric administration

Zollinger-Ellison symdrome

- when symptomatic with either ulcer pain, complications, or diarrhea

▶ *What Drug Should I Use for Initial Treatment?*

Dyspepsia, duodenal or gastric ulcer

Suspected or endoscopically proven gastric or duodenal ulcer

ANTACIDS

- should be concurrently prescribed on a PRN basis for symptom relief, but only if the patient describes symptomatic relief after antacid administration

CIMETIDINE

- drug of choice for initial treatment of peptic ulcer disease because it has few adverse effects, can be given once daily, and is less expensive than other treatment modalities such as other H_2 antagonists, sucralfate, and omeprazole
- all H_2 antagonists have equivalent efficacy and toxicity (N Engl J Med 1990;323:1749–1755)

RANITIDINE, FAMOTIDINE, NIZATIDINE

- if the patient is receiving drugs that have the potential to interact with cimetidine, choose either ranitidine, famotidine, or nizatidine, whichever is the least expensive

OMEPRAZOLE

- high costs and unknown long-term effects of omeprazole relegate it to a second-line regimen at present because most patients respond to other less expensive agents
- use in patients who have not responded to a 12 week course of H_2 antagonists

SUCRALFATE

- use if H_2 antagonists or omeprazole cannot be used because of intolerance or documented drug interactions
- sucralfate needs to be given twice daily and is more expensive than cimetidine

MISOPROSTOL

- not recommended, as it is no more effective than H_2 antagonists, but is more expensive than cimetidine; is usually dosed 4 times per day compared with once to twice a day with other agents; and produces a high incidence of diarrhea

ANTIBIOTICS

- use of antibiotics to eradicate *Helicobacter pylori*, a potential cause of peptic ulcer disease, is recommended for all patients with documented *H. pylori* infection
- several regimens with different combinations of antibiotics for varying durations have been used (Am J Gastroenterol 1992;87:1716–1727) (see below under prevention of peptic ulcer recurrence)

Suspected or endoscopically proven gastric or duodenal ulcer due to NSAIDs
(if NSAID administration can be stopped)

CIMETIDINE

- H_2 antagonists appear to be effective, cause a lower incidence of adverse effects than does misoprostol, and are convenient to take

RANITIDINE, FAMOTIDINE, NIZATIDINE

- use if the patient is receiving drugs that have the potential to interact with cimetidine
- choose either ranitidine, famotidine, or nizatidine, whichever is the least expensive

OMEPRAZOLE

- may be more effective than H_2 antagonists but at present should be used only in patients who do not respond to H_2 antagonists

Prevention of peptic ulcer disease recurrence
CIMETIDINE

- all H_2 antagonists have equivalent efficacy and toxicity

in prophylactic dosages, and cimetidine is the least expensive (N Engl J Med 1990;323:1749–1755)

RANITIDINE, FAMOTIDINE, NIZATIDINE

- if there is concern with cimetidine drug interactions, use one of the other H_2 antagonists, whichever is the least expensive

SUCRALFATE

- use sucralfate if the patient is unable to tolerate H_2 antagonists

ANTIBIOTICS

- if patients have *H. pylori*–associated chronic peptic ulcer disease, a course of antibiotics should be offered as an option over surgery or long-term drug therapy
- several regimens have been shown to be effective, and the decision among these regimens should be based on convenience, toxicity, and cost
- H_2 antagonist for 6–10 weeks plus metronidazole and amoxicillin for 12 days (N Engl J Med 1993;328:308–312)
- bismuth compound (colloidal bismuth subcitrate not available in North America but bismuth subsalicylate is available) plus metronidazole and tetracycline for 2 weeks (useful if the patient is penicillin allergic)
- omeprazole plus amoxicillin for 2 weeks (Am J Gastroenterol 1993;88:491–495)
- 1 week with triple therapy (bismuth, metronidazole, and tetracycline) has also been shown to eradicate *H. pylori* (Lancet 1994;343:508–510)

Prevention of NSAID-induced ulcers
MISOPROSTOL

- misoprostol has been shown to be effective in preventing endoscopically proven NSAID-induced ulceration (Lancet 1988;2:1277–1280), and other agents have generally been no better than placebo (Mayo Clin Proc 1992;67:354–364)
- at present, there is no published evidence that misoprostol prevents ulcer complications and death (Am J Gastroenterol 1991;86:264–266)
- for all patients receiving NSAIDs, ensure they are on the lowest effective dose and/or that acetaminophen in appropriate doses (up to 1 g PO QID) is ineffective

CIMETIDINE

- H_2 antagonists appear to reduce the incidence of duodenal ulcers but not gastric ulcers and should be chosen in patients who cannot tolerate misoprostol

Acute upper gastrointestinal hemorrhage

- although many clinicians recommend a parenteral acid-suppressing agent (H_2 antagonists or omeprazole), evidence suggests that these agents are no more effective than placebo in the first 48–72 hours in preventing complications such as rebleeding, the need for surgery, and death (BMJ 1992;304:143–147, Lancet 1992;340:1058–1062)
- all patients should receive an oral agent to help to heal the ulcer, and the decision as to which agent to use should be as above under duodenal or gastric ulcer

Stress ulcer prophylaxis
SUCRALFATE

- is preferred agent if oral or nasogastric administration is possible because it is less expensive than parenteral H_2 antagonists, likely does not increase the chance of nosocomial pneumonia, and does not require pH measurement of gastric contents (Lancet 1989;2:1255–1256)

CIMETIDINE, RANITIDINE, FAMOTIDINE

- if oral administration is not possible, use the least expensive parenteral H_2 antagonist (consider cost and frequency of administration)

Zollinger-Ellison syndrome
OMEPRAZOLE

- drug of choice because it is more effective than other agents, requires the patient to take fewer pills (than with H_2 antagonists), and is usually less expensive in comparable doses needed to treat this disease (N Engl J Med 1990;323:1749–1755)

▶ *What Dosage Should I Use?*

Dyspepsia, duodenal or gastric ulcer
Suspected or endoscopically proven gastric or duodenal ulcer
ANTACIDS

- total daily dosage equivalent to 180 mEq of acid-neutralizing capacity, administered PO QID is enough to treat an ulcer (Scand J Gastroenterol 1986;21:385–391)
- can be ordered on a PRN basis for symptomatic relief (in addition to regular doses of antacid or other drugs used to treat ulcers)
- see drug monograph on antacid for more information on dosing

CIMETIDINE

- 800 mg PO HS
- 400 mg PO BID if the patient has frequent daytime ulcer pain

RANITIDINE

- 300 mg PO HS
- 150 mg PO BID if the patient has frequent daytime ulcer pain

FAMOTIDINE

- 40 mg PO HS
- 20 mg PO BID if the patient has frequent daytime ulcer pain

NIZATIDINE

- 300 mg PO HS
- 150 mg PO BID if the patient has frequent daytime ulcer pain

OMEPRAZOLE

- 20 mg PO daily

SUCRALFATE

- 2 g PO BID

Prevention of peptic ulcer disease recurrence
CIMETIDINE

- 400 mg PO HS

RANITIDINE

- 150 mg PO HS

FAMOTIDINE

- 20 mg PO HS

NIZATIDINE

- 150 mg PO HS

SUCRALFATE

- 1 g PO BID

ANTIBIOTICS

- treatment dose of an H_2 antagonist (see above) plus 750 mg of amoxicillin PO TID and metronidazole 500 mg PO TID
- 2 Pepto-Bismol tablets (524 mg of bismuth subsalicylate) PO QID plus metronidazole 500 mg PO QID and tetracycline 500 mg PO QID
- omeprazole 20 mg PO BID plus amoxicillin 500 mg PO QID

Prevention of NSAID-induced ulcers
MISOPROSTOL

- 100 μg PO QID

Stress ulcer prophylaxis
SUCRALFATE

- 1 g PO or via nasogastric tube QID

CIMETIDINE

- 300 mg IV Q6H titrated to keep gastric pH greater than 4 at all times
- infusion of drug is not clinically superior (although it does produce better pH control) to intermittent therapy and should be used only if more practical or economical than intermittent injections
- analysis of aspirates of gastric fluid should be done Q4H and the dosage increased in 150 mg increments to maintain gastric pH of greater than 4 at all times

RANITIDINE

- 50 mg IV Q8H titrated to keep gastric pH greater than 4 at all times
- analysis of aspirates of gastric fluid should be done Q4H and the dosage increased in 25 mg increments to maintain gastric pH greater than 4 at all times

FAMOTIDINE

- 20 mg IV Q12H titrated to keep gastric pH greater than 4 at all times
- analysis of aspirates of gastric fluid should be done Q4H and the dosage increased in 10 mg increments to maintain gastric pH greater than 4 at all times

Zollinger-Ellison syndrome
OMEPRAZOLE

- 40 mg PO daily
- increase the dosage every 3–4 weeks on the basis of symptoms
- dosages as high as 120 mg PO Q8H, titrated on the basis of basal acid output, have been used

▶ *How Long Should I Treat with My Initial Regimen?*

Dyspepsia

- treat for 2 weeks, and stop drug therapy if the patient becomes symptom free

Duodenal or gastric ulcer
Suspected or proven gastric or duodenal ulcer

- initial treatment should be 6 weeks in duration

- patient should be assessed after 1 week for relief of symptoms
- if there is no relief after 1 week, endoscopy or reendoscopy is recommended
- if there is relief of symptoms, continue therapy for a total of 6 weeks

Suspected or endoscopically or barium study–proven gastric or duodenal ulcer due to NSAIDs

- 8 weeks for duodenal ulcers, 12 weeks for gastric ulcers (Gastroenterology 1989;96:662–674)

Prevention of peptic ulcer disease recurrence

- if prophylaxis with acid-suppressing therapy is indicated, a minimum of 2 years of therapy is recommended

Prevention of NSAID-induced ulcers

- for the duration of NSAID use

Acute upper gastrointestinal hemorrhage

- as above under duodenal or gastric ulcer

Stress ulcer prophylaxis

- until the patient is out of the intensive care unit or is being gastrically fed

Zollinger-Ellison syndrome

- treatment is indefinite

▶ *What Efficacy Parameters Should I Follow and How Frequently Do I Have to Assess My Patient?*

Dyspepsia, duodenal or gastric ulcer

Signs and symptoms

- patient should be assessed after 1 week for relief of symptoms
- pain (dull ache, burning, gnawing) in abdomen, an exaggerated hunger sensation, and a sensation of fullness may be described by the patient as symptoms of peptic ulcer disease
- successful therapy should be confirmed through the absence of occult blood in stool

Endoscopy

- if no relief after 1 week, endoscopy or reendoscopy is recommended
- for duodenal ulcers, reendoscopy is not needed unless symptoms persist
- for gastric ulcers, reendoscopy is recommended to ensure that complete healing has occurred because loss of symptoms is well described in malignant ulcers.

Prevention of peptic ulcer disease recurrence

- recurrence of symptoms

Prevention of NSAID-induced ulcers

- signs and symptoms of peptic ulcer disease

Stress ulcer prophylaxis

Absence of visual blood in gastric aspirates

- assess every 4 hours
- if the aspirate contains blood, the need for endoscopy should be evaluated

Gastric pH

- assess every 4 hours (if the patient is receiving H_2 antagonist) and titrate to a gastric pH greater than 4 at all times

Hemoglobin

- measure daily, as changes in hemoglobin concentration may indicate possible hemorrhage

Zollinger-Ellison syndrome

- check symptoms such as gastrointestinal pain and diarrhea

▶ *Should I Add Another Drug or Substitute Therapy If My Initial Drug Therapy Fails?*

Dyspepsia

- if no improvement in symptoms following 2 weeks of therapy, the patient should undergo endoscopy to confirm diagnosis

Duodenal or gastric ulcer

- if symptoms remain after 6 weeks of initial therapy, the patient should undergo endoscopy to confirm the diagnosis and rule out gastrointestinal malignancy
- if the diagnosis is confirmed, treat for another 6 weeks
- if symptoms still persist or the ulcer is not healed, start administration of omeprazole 20 mg PO daily
- do not combine agents, as there is no evidence that combinations of any two of the above agents result in a higher cure rate than does a single agent used alone (Lancet 1988;1:1383–1385, N Engl J Med 1991;325:1017–1025, Am J Gastroenterol 1993;88:675–679)

Prevention of peptic ulcer disease recurrence

- combination therapy has not been effective
- if the patient experiences an ulcer while receiving maintenance therapy, treat as an ulcer and then continue with maintenance therapy
- if patients have *H. pylori*–associated chronic peptic ulcer disease, a course of antibiotics should be offered as an option over surgery or long-term drug therapy

Prevention of NSAID-induced ulcers

- if bleeding occurs while on misoprostol, omeprazole 20 mg PO daily should be used

Stress ulcer prophylaxis

- if the patient bleeds while taking one agent, switch to another agent for a full course of therapy

Zollinger-Ellison syndrome

- dosages as high as 120 mg PO Q8H of omeprazole, titrated on the basis of basal acid output, have been used

▶ *How Long Should I Continue Drug Therapy?*

Dyspepsia

- if symptoms are controlled, non-drug measures and PRN antacids can be continued indefinitely

Duodenal or gastric ulcer

- initial H_2 antagonist therapy should be continued for 6 weeks
- if not cured after 6 weeks, continue therapy for another 6 weeks
- if subsequent omeprazole therapy is required, a 4 week trial is warranted

Prevention of peptic ulcer disease recurrence

- indefinitely; however, consideration should be given to a trial without drug for patients who have remained symptom free for longer than 2 years
- if the peptic ulcer disease was associated with complications (e.g., bleeding and perforation), consideration should be given to the ability of the patient to cope with further complications when deciding on the duration of therapy

- if peptic ulcer disease recurs, endoscopy and sampling for *H. pylori* should be completed, and if the culture is positive, antibiotic therapy should be instituted
- treatment dose of an H$_2$ antagonist (see above) for 6 weeks plus amoxicillin 750 mg PO TID and metronidazole 500 mg PO TID for 12 days
- 2 Pepto-Bismol tablets (524 mg of bismuth subsalicylate) PO QID plus metronidazole 500 mg PO QID and tetracycline 500 mg PO QID each taken for 14 days
- omeprazole 20 mg PO BID plus amoxicillin 500 mg PO QID; both for 2 weeks
- if patient cannot tolerate 2 weeks of therapy, 1 week of therapy may be sufficient to eradicate *H. pylori* (Lancet 1994;343:508–510)

Prevention of NSAID-induced ulcers

- for the duration of the NSAID therapy

Stress ulcer prophylaxis

- until the patient no longer exhibits risk factors or is being gastrically fed
- in general, if a patient is no longer in an intensive care unit or burn ward and does not have sepsis or central nervous system injury, prophylaxis can be stopped

Zollinger-Ellison syndrome

- treatment is lifelong

Useful References

Freston JW. Overview of medical therapy of peptic ulcer disease. Med Clin North Am 1990;19:121–140

Veldhyzen van Zan SJ, Sherman PM. Indications for treatment of *Helicobacter pylori* infection: A systematic overview. Can Med Assoc J 1994;150(2):189–197

DRUG THERAPY FOR INFLAMMATORY BOWEL DISEASE

J. Scott Whittaker

▶ What Are My Goals of Treatment?

Ulcerative proctitis or colitis

to ameliorate completely the symptoms, which may include rectal bleeding, diarrhea, urgency, tenesmus, and abdominal cramps
to return the colonic or rectal mucosa to normal
to prevent recurrences

Crohn's disease

to reduce or, if possible, eliminate symptoms of the disease, which include abdominal pain, diarrhea, fever, and perianal problems
endoscopic or radiologic improvement is not currently a primary goal of treatment because there is no good correlation of results of these investigations and the clinical state of the patient
to prevent recurrences

▶ What Evidence Is Available to Support Drug Therapy for Inflammatory Bowel Disease?

Ulcerative proctitis or colitis

- corticosteroids and mesalamine (5-aminosalicylic acid [5-ASA])–containing regimens have been shown to improve the rate of remission and to provide symptomatic relief (Gut 1960;1:217–222)
- frequency of recurrences of ulcerative colitis is reduced by 60% when oral 5-ASA therapy, in the form of sulfasalazine, is given (Lancet 1965;1:185–188)

Crohn's disease

- corticosteroids and 5-ASA–containing regimens have improved the rate of remission (Gastroenterology 1979; 77:847–869)
- frequency of recurrences of Crohn's disease may be reduced by the use of oral 5-ASA therapy, but this has not been well established (Aliment Pharmacol Ther 1990;4: 55–64)

▶ When Should I Consider Drug Therapy?

Ulcerative proctitis

- if symptoms consist of only rectal bleeding, no therapy is required in patients younger than 40 years
- in the older patient, ongoing rectal bleeding may interfere with the recognition of the development of a neoplasm
- incidence of colorectal carcinoma is not increased in patients with ulcerative proctitis
- if the patient is bothered by the presence of rectal bleeding or the symptoms of proctitis (urgency and/or tenesmus)

Ulcerative colitis

- whenever symptoms occur, including rectal bleeding, diarrhea, and abdominal pain
- for maintenance of remission after treatment of an acute exacerbation

Crohn's disease

- whenever symptoms affect the quality of life of the patient

▶ What Drug Should I Use for Initial Treatment?

Ulcerative proctitis

TOPICAL 5-ASA SUPPOSITORIES

- effective and less toxic than corticosteroids
- topical administration is at least as effective as oral administration and has the potential for fewer systemic effects (N Engl J Med 1980;303:1499–1502)

HYDROCORTISONE SUPPOSITORY

- use if the patient has had failure or intolerance to 5-ASA

HYDROCORTISONE RECTAL FOAM (CORTIFOAM), PRAMOXINE RECTAL FOAM (PROCTOFOAM)

- if suppositories are ineffective, use hydrocortisone foam

PREDNISONE

- if topical therapy is ineffective, give a 4 week course of prednisone

Ulcerative colitis

Mild to moderate disease

TOPICAL 5-ASA ENEMAS

- a trial of topical 5-ASA enemas should be given to patients with mild to moderate disease limited to the rectosigmoid, as topical therapy has fewer adverse effects than does oral therapy and provides quick relief of symptoms
- topical 5-ASA enemas should also be used in patients in combination with oral 5-ASA when minor but annoying distal symptoms persist after instituting oral therapy for 3–4 weeks

BETAMETHASONE ENEMA

- may be used in the same manner as 5-ASA enemas, but they are probably less effective than topical 5-ASA (Lancet 1981;2:270–271) and should therefore be used only when the 5-ASA enemas have failed
- if a 2 week course of the 5-ASA enemas fails, try a 2 week trial of a betamethasone enema

HYDROCORTISONE ENEMA

- hydrocortisone enemas can be used but most clinicians use betamethasone enemas because the glucocorticoid effects are greater with hydrocortisone

ORAL 5-ASA

- in disease limited to the rectosigmoid, if urgency and tenemus limit the retention time for enemas and thus the effectiveness of these agents, oral 5-ASA should be used
- if complete relief of symptoms occurs with oral therapy, no enema therapy need be given
- if there are some residual mild distal symptoms (some urgency, bleeding, mucus), a nightly 5-ASA enema should be used in conjunction with oral 5-ASA
- in patients with mild to moderate disease not limited to the rectosigmoid, oral 5-ASA should be used as first-line therapy
- all patients with established ulcerative colitis should be offered maintenance therapy with some 5-ASA agent

Oral 5-ASA products

SULFASALAZINE (5-ASA BOUND TO SULFAPYRIDINE)

- sulfasalazine is much less expensive than the new 5-ASA medications, and when sulfasalazine is well tolerated by the patient, this drug is a good choice in ulcerative colitis
- there are rare but serious side effects with sulfasalazine, which has led some gastroenterologists to use the newer non–sulfa-containing 5-ASA preparations, but there is no evidence that these new preparations are more effective than sulfasalazine, and they cost considerably more
- sulfasalazine needs bacterial action to split; therefore, it is useful only in colonic inflammatory disease
- if the patient develops gastrointestinal intolerance to sulfasalazine, try the enteric-coated product

ASACOL (USA OR CANADA)

- 5-ASA (mesalamine) completely enveloped by a resin, Eudragit-S, which delivers 5-ASA to the colon
- use instead of sulfasalazine in patients who are allergic to sulfa or intolerant of sulfasalazine
- dosage of non–sulfa-containing 5-ASA products can be increased up to 4–6 g/d of 5-ASA, which is usually higher than dosages achievable with sulfasalazine
- chosen over Mesasal or Salofalk or Rowasa, as Asacol allows better delivery to the distal colon
- Pentasa releases 5-ASA throughout the small bowel but has also been effective in ulcerative colitis

MESASAL OR SALOFALK (CANADA), ROWASA (USA)

- 5-ASA (mesalamine) completely enveloped by a resin, Eudragit-L, which delivers some 5-ASA to the colon and some to the small bowel
- use only if above 5-ASA products are not tolerated or effective
- because some 5-ASA is released in the small bowel, less 5-ASA is reaching the colon, and more 5-ASA is excreted

in the urine, which theoretically might increase the risk of the rare renal toxicity that has been described with the use of 5-ASA preparations (Gut 1990;31:1271–1276)

DIPENTUM (USA OR CANADA)

- 2 5-ASA (olsalazine) molecules bound together
- use only when other 5-ASA products are not tolerated because this product causes the highest incidence of diarrhea (Gastroenterology 1986;90:1024–1030)
- patient is usually given a trial of corticosteroids before switching to this agent

Severe disease or failure of topical and oral 5-ASA therapy

PREDNISONE

- oral prednisone is effective, but because of long-term adverse effects, it should be used only in patients who fail to respond to other therapy, unless the disease is severe
- use if disease is severe (>6 bloody bowel movements per day) with systemic signs and symptoms (fever, weight loss)
- there is no therapeutic gain to adding 5-ASA compounds to prednisone during initial therapy

HYDROCORTISONE

- IV hydrocortisone should be used only in patients who have failed to respond to oral prednisone or patients ill enough to require hospitalization

Crohn's disease

- treatment of Crohn's disease depends on the location of the disease to some extent and on the severity of symptoms
- approximately 55% of all patients with Crohn's disease have ileocolitis, with the colitis being predominantly right sided
- a further 30% have only terminal ileal involvement, and therefore therapies should take into account that 85% of all patients have terminal ileal involvement (albeit possibly asymptomatic)

Colitis

TOPICAL 5-ASA OR CORTICOSTEROIDS

- topical 5-ASA or corticosteroids have a limited role in Crohn's disease because the majority of patients do not have left-sided colitis as their major problem
- in patients in whom the left side of the colon is the predominant site, topical therapy can be considered similar to the case with ulcerative colitis (see above)

ORAL 5-ASA

- oral sulfasalazine is effective for Crohn's disease involving the colon (Gastroenterology 1979;77:847–869) and is used as first-line therapy in Crohn's colitis except in severe disease, when corticosteroids are preferred
- the efficacy of the new 5-ASA agents in the treatment of Crohn's colitis is similar to that of oral sulfasalazine

PREDNISONE

- although the efficacy of steroids in Crohn's colitis has not been well demonstrated to be superior to that of sulfasalazine, studies show that patients with Crohn's disease (all patients) tend to respond more quickly and better with steroids
- many gastroenterologists prefer to use prednisone in severely ill patients with Crohn's colitis

- prednisone is effective and should be used in patients with severe disease
- because of long-term adverse effects, it should be used only in patients with mild disease who fail to respond to other therapies

HYDROCORTISONE

- IV hydrocortisone should be used only in patients who have failed to respond to oral prednisone or patients ill enough to require hospitalization

METRONIDAZOLE

- widely used in the perianal disease, which may accompany Crohn's disease, although the reports of its efficacy are anecdotal
- as effective as sulfasalazine in 1 study (Gastroenterology 1982;83:550–562), but generally it is used only when the other short-term agents such as 5-ASA and steroids have failed, because efficacy is not definitively demonstrated and long-term toxicities (neuropathies) are common

Ileitis and ileocolitis

Oral 5-ASA

PENTASA (USA OR CANADA)

- 5-ASA (mesalamine) coated with a semipermeable ethylcellulose membrane, which releases 5-ASA throughout the small bowel
- preferred product for widespread disease, as 5-ASA is released throughout the small bowel
- sulfasalazine, Dipentum, and Asacol release 5-ASA in only small amounts in the small bowel and hence are not recommended when ileal disease is prominent

MESASAL OR SALOFALK (CANADA), ROWASA (USA)

- use instead of Pentasa if colonic involvement is known to be more significant (based on X-ray studies or colonoscopy)
- the decision between these agents should be based on cost

PREDNISONE

- mild and moderate Crohn's disease are also often treated with prednisone when the disease involves the small intestine and until other medications are shown to be effective in small intestinal disease, steroids are the drug of first choice
- severe Crohn's disease, regardless of the site of disease, should be treated with corticosteroids
- in severe cases of Crohn's disease, abscess formation and perforation are possible complications, and there is always the concern that systemic corticosteroids may mask these inflammatory conditions
- the clinician should always be cognizant that florid symptoms and signs may be absent when high-dose corticosteroids are used
- there is no therapeutic gain to adding 5-ASA compounds to prednisone during initial therapy, except in the first 6 weeks (Ann Intern Med 1991;114:445–450)

HYDROCORTISONE

- for severe cases requiring hospitalization and parenteral therapy

AZATHIOPRINE,
MERCAPTOPURINE (6-MERCAPTOPURINE)

- chronic, unresponsive Crohn's disease has been success-

fully treated with azathioprine and its active metabolite 6-mercaptopurine
- it is essential to recognize that these medications take months for onset of effect, and hence these medications have no role in acute, severe disease
- initial reports showed no efficacy of azathioprine, but these studies were criticized because only a 17 week treatment period was used (Gastroenterology 1979;77: 847–869, Gastroenterology 1981;80:193–196)
- later studies used a 1 or 2 year treatment period, and the drugs were effective (N Engl J Med 1980;302:981–987)
- these antimetabolites are most often used in concert with other medications, particularly steroids, and may have some steroid-sparing effect
- in general, these drugs are used as a last resort, owing to the known side effects, especially pancreatitis, leukopenia, and the potential long-term oncogenic effects

▶ *What Dosage Should I Use?*

Ulcerative proctitis

TOPICAL 5-ASA SUPPOSITORIES

- 500 mg rectally daily at bedtime
- 500 mg rectally BID (in the morning and at bedtime) should be used if single-dose therapy is ineffective after 1 week

HYDROCORTISONE SUPPOSITORY

- 40 mg rectally BID (in the morning and at bedtime)

HYDROCORTISONE RECTAL FOAM

- 100 mg rectally BID (in the morning and at bedtime)

PREDNISONE

- 30 mg PO daily for 1 week, reduce to 20 mg PO daily for 1 week, reduce to 10 mg PO daily for 1 week, then reduce to 5 mg PO daily for 1 week, then stop

Ulcerative colitis

TOPICAL 5-ASA ENEMAS

- 4 g enema daily at bedtime and retain for as long as possible (minimum, 1 hour)
- 4 g BID (in the morning and at bedtime) should be used if single-dose therapy is ineffective after 1 week

BETAMETHASONE ENEMA

- 5 mg in 60 mL daily at bedtime

HYDROCORTISONE ENEMA

- 100 mg enema in 60 mL daily at bedtime

Oral 5-ASA products

SULFASALAZINE

- 1 g PO BID and increase every 4 days by 1 g/d until 4 g/d is reached (in 4 divided doses) or the patient develops intolerable side effects
- dosage greater than 4 g/d is usually not well tolerated; however, a dosage up to 6 g may be used if the patient can tolerate it
- 1 g PO BID as a maintenance dose after remission has been induced
- use enteric-coated product if gastrointestinal symptoms are a problem

ASACOL

- 1200 mg PO QID for flare-ups
- 400 mg PO TID for maintenance

MESASAL OR SALOFALK, ROWASA

- 1000 mg PO QID for flare-ups
- 500 mg PO TID for maintenance

DIPENTUM

- 1000 mg PO BID for flare-ups and after 4 days increase to 1000 mg TID to decrease the chance of diarrhea with this product
- 500 mg PO BID for maintenance

PREDNISONE

- 40 mg PO daily for 1–2 weeks, depending on response
- decrease the dosage to 30 mg PO daily for 1 week, then reduce daily dosage by 5 mg every week
- BID dosing may be used in patients with nocturnal gastrointestinal symptoms

HYDROCORTISONE

- 100 mg IV Q8H for a 5 day course in patients with severe cases or patients who do not respond to prednisone

Crohn's disease

TOPICAL 5-ASA, TOPICAL CORTICOSTEROIDS, PREDNISONE, HYDROCORTISONE

- as above

ORAL 5-ASA

- as above for ulcerative colitis, except that maintenance therapy is not used, because the efficacy of maintenance therapy is not established
- treat for 10–14 days after relief of symptoms (usual course of therapy is 6–8 weeks)

PENTASA

- 1000 mg PO QID for flare-ups

METRONIDAZOLE

- 250 mg PO QID
- 500 mg PO TID for severe perineal disease

AZATHIOPRINE, 6-MERCAPTOPURINE

- start at 50 mg PO daily
- increase to 75 or even 100 mg/d (or 2 mg/kg) if the initial dosage is not effective after 3 months

▶ *How Long Should I Treat with My Initial Regimen?*

Ulcerative proctitis

Acute symptoms

TOPICAL 5-ASA THERAPY

- if initial therapy is not having any effect on symptoms in 7–10 days, the dosage should be increased for another week, and if still not successful, switch to a 2 week trial of topical corticosteroid therapy

ORAL 5-ASA

- should be used for up to 6 weeks; if the patient's condition deteriorates or the treatment fails, use corticosteroids

Ulcerative colitis

PREDNISONE

- for lesser forms of colitis, prednisone may be used in doses of 20 mg or higher for 6 weeks, and if there is no effect and if 5-ASA preparations have not worked, a 5

day course of IV hydrocortisone in the hospital should be considered

HYDROCORTISONE

- for toxic megacolon, IV hydrocortisone is used for 48 hours, and if there is no change in the patient's condition, subtotal colectomy is advised
- for severe colitis, IV hydrocortisone is used for up to 14 days, and if there is no improvement, subtotal colectomy is advised

Crohn's disease

Acute symptoms

TOPICAL THERAPY

- use for 7 days, and if no change in symptoms occurs, use oral corticosteroids

ORAL 5-ASA

- symptoms may persist for 2–3 weeks before improvement is seen
- 5-ASA is used for 6 weeks in high doses (or 10–14 days after relief of symptoms) and then stopped
- complete relief of symptoms may not occur, and then a decision regarding continuing with a small dose of corticosteroid, 5-ASA, azathioprine, or 6-mercaptopurine has to be made

PREDNISONE

- prednisone for acute disease is used for about 2 weeks and then tapered over about 6 weeks

METRONIDAZOLE

- 8 weeks
- for perianal disease, much longer therapy may be needed, as drainage increases and many of the perianal symptoms quickly return when metronidazole administration is stopped

▶ *What Efficacy Parameters Should I Follow and How Frequently Do I Have to Assess My Patient?*

Ulcerative proctitis or colitis

- in general, patients should be seen within 2 weeks of starting therapy, particularly if steroids are being employed, because tapering of steroids should begin no later than 2 weeks after starting therapy
- for toxic megacolon, patients should be evaluated several times a day while in the hospital

Signs and symptoms

- diarrhea, urgency, tenesmus, blood per rectum, abdominal pain, fever, and weight status should improve
- symptoms begin to improve with steroids (topical or oral) within a week, but with 5-ASA, this may take a few days longer

Laboratory parameters

- indicators of inflammation (increased white blood cell count, including left shift) and of blood loss from ulceration (decreased hemoglobin concentration) should improve in 1 week
- in severely ill hospitalized patients, these counts are done daily
- in less ill outpatients, these are repeated after a week

X-rays

- for toxic megacolon, X-rays (3 views of the abdomen) should be taken daily to assess colonic distention

• if there is no improvement after 48 hours or if complications (e.g., perforation) have occurred, the patient should undergo subtotal colectomy

Crohn's disease

• treat for 1–2 weeks and reassess the patient

Signs and symptoms

• diarrhea, abdominal pain, fever, abdominal distention, and tenderness, size of mass (if present), appetite
• these symptoms may persist for 2–3 weeks before improvement is seen, and complete reflief of symptoms may not occur

Laboratory parameters

• indicators of inflammation (increased white blood cell count, including left shift) and of blood loss from ulceration (decreased hemoglobin concentration) should improve in 1 week
• in severely ill hospitalized patients, these counts are done daily
• in less ill outpatients, these are repeated after a week

▶ *Should I Add Another Drug or Substitute Therapy If My Initial Drug Therapy Fails?*

Ulcerative proctitis

• if patient has had failure of treatment with or intolerance to topical 5-ASA, switch to topical hydrocortisone enema
• if topical therapy is ineffective, give a 4 week course of prednisone if the patient understands and agrees regarding the risks and benefit of this therapy

Ulcerative colitis

• if there has not been some improvement after 10–14 days, the initial dosage of the drug used should be increased or another form of therapy should be used
• usually, this means switching to steroids from other therapies, or being admitted for IV hydrocortisone administration and possibly nutritional therapy such as total parenteral nutrition or an elemental diet (although nutrition plays no role in disease modification, just supportive therapy)

Crohn's disease

• there is no evidence of increased efficacy in combining 5-ASA and steroids; however, in patients with distal Crohn's disease who are unable to retain enemas, initial therapy with prednisone leading to some improvement may allow the patient to take topical therapy and reduce the time of prednisone administration
• sometimes, only a week to 10 days of prednisone administration is needed and the disease can then be treated with 5-ASA
• chronic, unresponsive Crohn's disease has been successfully treated with azathioprine and its active metabolite 6-mercaptopurine (N Engl J Med 1980;302:981–987, Scand J Gastroenterol 1985;20:1197–1203)
• it is essential to recognize that azathioprine and 6-mercaptopurine take months for onset of effect, and hence, these medications have no role in acute, severe disease
• in general, these drugs are used as a last resort, owing to the known side effects, especially pancreatitis, leukopenia, and the potential long-term oncogenic effects
• if the measures fail, and especially if the patient is doing poorly while receiving high-dose prednisone in the acute phase, admission to the hospital for nutritional support such as total parenteral nutrition and enteral feeding is advised

▶ *How Long Should I Continue Drug Therapy?*

Ulcerative proctitis

Maintenance therapy

• not recommended
• with frequent flares 5-ASA suppositories (250 mg) can be used every other night at bedtime

Ulcerative colitis

Maintenance therapy for remission in ulcerative colitis

• 5-ASA for maintenance is used indefinitely
• for maintenance therapy of ulcerative colitis, the drug is continued indefinitely, as relapses occur in only 20% of the patients receiving the drug versus 73% of patients receiving no therapy (Lancet 1965;2:185–188)
• some patients who have had infrequent flares (e.g., every few years) with no maintenance treatment (patients who have undiagnosed disease or who refused maintenance) can just use drug therapy for treatment of flares of the disease

Crohn's disease

• partial remissions are common, and frequently patients receive therapy for many months, usually at ever-decreasing dosages
• for the patient with Crohn's disease in remission, the drug may be stopped abruptly 10–14 days after the patient is symptom free

---

DRUG THERAPY FOR CONSTIPATION

Leslie Mathews

▶ *What Are My Goals of Treatment?*

to establish regular, comfortable stooling that empties the rectum, using the least number of drugs in the lowest dosages for the shortest duration of time

to establish the normal frequency of stools; most adults and children (99%) have 3 or more bowel movements per week (Hosp Pract 1990;25:89–100)

to address effectively other risk factors: low-residue diet, deficient fluid intake, lack of regular physical exercise, poor bowel habits, use of constipating medications, and laxative abuse, and to treat any underlying predisposing conditions

to prevent or reverse the sequelae (fecal impaction, intestinal obstruction, and so on) associated with constipation

to prevent or minimize the adverse effects associated with laxative use

to prevent laxative dependence

to relieve the discomfort associated with constipation

▶ *What Evidence Is Available to Support Drug Therapy for Constipation?*

• it is estimated that 900 people die annually in the USA from diseases associated with or related to constipation (Dis Colon Rectum 1989;32:1–8)
• constipation can cause other complications (e.g., fecal impaction, intestinal obstruction or perforation, fecal and urinary incontinence, megacolon, stercoraceous ulceration, urinary tract infections, gastrointestinal bleeding, anorexia, generalized weakness, and mental disturbances (Gastroenterol Clin North Am 1990;9:405–418)

- straining to defecate causes changes in intrathoracic pressure, leading to a reduction in coronary, cerebral, and peripheral circulation (Clin Geriatr Med 1988;4:571–588)
- other potential problems with straining: development of hernias, worsening of symptoms of gastroesophageal reflux (Clin Geriatr Med 1988;4:571–588), transient ischemic attacks, and syncope in elderly patients with cerebrovascular disease or deficient baroreceptor reflexes (Gastroenterol Clin North Am 1990;9:405–418)

▶ *When Should I Consider Drug Therapy?*

Fecal impaction

- all patients with fecal impaction should be treated immediately (within hours)

Acute constipation

- treat all patients constipated as a result of acute illness, surgery, perianal disease, severe abdominal or perineal muscle weakness, drug therapy, irritable bowel syndrome, uncomplicated diverticular disease, neurological deficits, severe debilitation, and immobility
- treat within hours to days

Chronic constipation

- after 2–4 weeks of appropriate nonpharmacological measures (J Gerontol Nursing 1990;16:4–11)
- after weeks of a dietary trial of increased fiber for recurrent constipation or after regular laxative use (Am J Gastroenterol 1985;80:303–309)

Bowel preparation

- in patients who are to undergo colonoscopy, barium enema, or elective colorectal surgery

▶ *What Drug Should I Use for Initial Treatment?*

Initial drug choice depends on the type and severity of constipation, the effect desired, and the underlying pathophysiological conditions

Fecal impaction

SODIUM PHOSPHATE (FLEET) ENEMA

- drug of choice for severe impaction after or instead of manual disimpaction
- convenient and easier to administer than many enemas because it is premixed, the nozzle is prelubricated, it uses a low volume, and it uses less nursing time than other enemas

MAGNESIUM CITRATE, SULFATE, OR HYDROXIDE; SENNA; CASCARA; BISACODYL; LACTULOSE; BALANCED ELECTROLYTE SOLUTION (POLYETHYLENE GLYCOL–ELECTROLYTE SOLUTION [PEG-ES])

- after impaction is cleared with enemas, give one of the above agents to empty the colon completely
- decision among these agents should be based on side effects, cost, and the duration of therapy that will be necessary
- oral osmotic agents (magnesium) and the oral stimulant laxatives are usually well tolerated and are less expensive than lactulose
- magnesium citrate is preferable to magnesium sulfate because it is likely better tolerated by the patient (magnesium sulfate has an intensely bitter taste) and is less likely to produce fluid and electrolyte imbalance

OTHER LAXATIVE THERAPY (SENNA, CASCARA, BISACODYL, LACTULOSE, BULK-FORMING LAXATIVES)

- likely required after the colon has been emptied to prevent further impactions
- decision among these agents is based on reason for constipation, side effects, the duration of therapy, and cost (see below under acute and chronic constipation)

Acute constipation

Rapid response not desired

BULK-FORMING LAXATIVES

- effective within 2–3 days, well tolerated, and safe in long-term use in conjunction with increased dietary fiber
- choice of product (dietary fiber, commercial powders, crystals, tablets) depends on the patient's acceptance of texture and taste (tasteless, minty, orange flavored, and so on) and excipients (low sodium, sugar free), and cost
- these agents do not work as rapidly as the stimulant laxatives or lactulose

Rapid response desired

BISACODYL, SENNA, CASCARA

- effective within 6–24 hours
- all stimulant laxatives are equally effective and are less expensive than lactulose
- although some authors have advocated the use of senna instead of other stimulants, claiming that it is the mildest and that standardized senna is the most physiological of all the nonfiber laxatives (Pharmacology 1988;36[suppl 1]:230–236), there are no good studies to confirm or deny these claims
- should be used only short term, as other agents are safer and more effective for long-term treatment
- decision about which stimulant laxative to use should be based on availability and cost

MAGNESIUM CITRATE, SULFATE, OR HYDROXIDE

- useful for short-term use
- are equally effective, and have similar adverse effects, when compared with stimulant laxatives
- choice between these agents and stimulant laxatives should be based on availability, cost, and patient preference
- magnesium hydroxide preferred over magnesium citrate or sulfate due to milder action (less cathartic)

LACTULOSE

- if stimulant laxatives or magnesium is ineffective or not tolerated, oral lactulose can be tried, as it is effective and most patients prefer this over an enema or a suppository
- more expensive than stimulant laxatives or magnesium hydroxide but can be used long term

Constipation associated with hard, dry stools or conditions in which straining should be avoided

(e.g., anorectal disorders, hernias, recovery from myocardial infarction, and cerebrovascular accident)

BULK-FORMING LAXATIVES

- used to maintain soft, bulky stools that are easily passed (Dis Colon Rectum 1987;30:780–781)
- increased bulk does not necessarily mean increased straining
- are effective and can be used regularly

LACTULOSE

- if bulk-forming laxatives are contraindicated, ineffective, or not tolerated
- softens stool by retaining water in the lumen of the bowel
- chosen over magnesium hydroxide, as these patients likely require long-term therapy (longer than 1 week) and magnesium should be given for only occasional or short-term use

Constipation related to pregnancy, uncomplicated diverticular disease, irritable bowel syndrome, and low-residue diet

BULK-FORMING LAXATIVES

- effective (variably and initially may not be) and safe in long-term use in conjunction with increased dietary fiber
- increase bulk of stool, decrease colonic transit time, and increase frequency of stools
- decision about which bulk-forming laxative to use should be based on availability, cost, and patient preference

Chronic constipation
Ambulatory or elderly patients
BULK-FORMING LAXATIVES

- useful in patients who are elderly or when constipation is related to a low-residue diet, pregnancy, acute or chronic illness, and constipating medications
- effective and safe in long-term use in conjunction with increased dietary fiber
- many patients respond well, requiring no alternative drug therapy (Br Med J 1990; 300:1063–1065)

LACTULOSE

- if bulk-forming laxatives contraindicated, ineffective, or not tolerated
- softens stools by retaining water in the lumen of the bowel
- chosen over magnesium hydroxide, stimulant laxatives, and docusate, as these agents should not be used long term

DOCUSATE

- suitable for short-term use only (7 days)
- clinical and laboratory evidence suggests that docusate can be hepatotoxic and may increase absorption of the hepatobiliary toxins (Med Clin North Am 1989;73: 1502–1509)
- is effective in producing soft stools, which are easy to pass without a great increase in bulk
- use for hard, dry stools only if lactulose is ineffective or not tolerated

Constipation in bedbound patients, neurogenic constipation, and constipation in debilitated or terminally ill patients

LACTULOSE

- should be used because it softens stool, prevents impaction, and is likely a better choice over bulk-forming laxatives
- these patients may also require regular stimulation of the rectal mucosa with suppositories or enemas

Atonic or severe idiopathic constipation
GLYCERIN SUPPOSITORY

- glycerin is necessary in those conditions in which the rectum is filled but the defecation reflex is not triggered,

or intestinal transit time is severely delayed, because it stimulates the rectal mucosa
- glycerin is sometimes referred to as a stimulant laxative but is generally classified as an osmotic laxative
- is less likely to produce anorectal irritation and is less expensive than bisacodyl suppository

Bowel preparation
BALANCED ELECTROLYTE SOLUTION (PEG-ES)

- drug of choice for bowel preparation for colonoscopy, barium enema study, and elective colorectal surgery because is as effective as or better than standard hydration, cathartic, and enema regimens and causes the best and most complete evacuation of the gastrointestinal tract (Gastroenterology 1983;84:1512–1516)
- patients prefer PEG-ES over enema or cathartic preparation because it is more convenient (5 hours versus 3 days), is more rapidly active, and causes less discomfort (Clin Pharm 1985;4:414–424)

SODIUM PHOSPHATE (FLEET) ENEMA

- if patient cannot use oral PEG-ES
- may need to use in conjunction with oral bisacodyl

▶ What Dosage Should I Use?
Fecal impaction
SODIUM PHOSPHATE (FLEET) ENEMA

- one 120 mL enema per rectum daily
- repeat once if ineffective (e.g., not retained until abdominal cramping felt or little or no stool evacuated)

MAGNESIUM CITRATE, SULFATE OR HYDROXIDE

- minimum effective dose is 80 mEq of magnesium PO daily
- increase the dosage as needed after 24 hours by 40 mEq to a maximum of 240 mEq PO daily
- 100 mL of magnesium citrate contains approximately 80 mEq of magnesium ion
- 10 g of magnesium sulfate contains approximately 80 mEq of magnesium ion (dilute in 250 mL of water)
- 1 g of magnesium hydroxide contains approximately 35 mEq of magnesium ion (30 mL of milk of magnesia contains approximately 80 mEq of magnesium ion)

BALANCED ELECTROLYTE SOLUTION (PEG-ES)

- 2 L given orally or via nasogastric tube
- give another 2 L the following day if the first 2 L is not effective (Age Ageing 1986;15:182–184)

OTHER LAXATIVE THERAPY

- see below

Acute constipation
BULK-FORMING LAXATIVES

- dosage varies with type of bulk-forming laxative and product format (see drug monograph on bulk-forming laxatives)
- psyllium hydrophilic powder
- usual dosage for constipation is 1 teaspoon or package 1–3 times per day PO mixed in 250 mL of fluid
- optimum dosage for irritable bowel syndrome is 20 g/day (Gut 1987;28:150–155)
- other types of bulk-forming laxatives include methylcellulose, grain and fruit fibers, sterculia gum, malt soup extract, and calcium polycarbophil

- other preparations are also available, which may be more acceptable to the patient and therefore increase compliance (e.g., psyllium is available as a tablet, wafer, or crystal format)

BISACODYL

- 5 mg PO daily
- increase the dosage as needed after 24 hours by 5 mg to a maximum of 15 mg PO daily

SENNA

- 15 mg PO daily
- increase the dosage as needed after 24 hours by 7.5 mg to a maximum of 60 mg PO daily

CASCARA

- aromatic fluid extract 5 mL PO daily
- others: fluid extract 1.5 mL, bark 1 g, extract 0.4 mL daily

MAGNESIUM CITRATE, SULFATE, OR HYDROXIDE

- as above

LACTULOSE

- give 15 mL PO BID (can be given as a single dose but may cause more nausea and vomiting) and increase the dosage after 24–48 hours, if no response, to a total daily maximum of 60 mL
- higher dosages are less likely to be tolerated and are more likely to produce fluid and electrolyte problems

Chronic constipation

BULK-FORMING LAXATIVES

- as above

LACTULOSE

- as above

DOCUSATE

- there is little therapeutic difference among the different docusate salts
- 100 mg PO BID of docusate sodium or potassium (or 240 mg PO daily of docusate calcium)
- assess effectiveness after 3 days and increase as needed to a maximum of 500 mg PO daily of docusate sodium or 300 mg PO daily of docusate potassium

GLYCERIN SUPPOSITORY

- 3 g suppository rectally administered 30 minutes after a meal to take full advantage of gastrocolic reflex

Bowel Preparation

BALANCED ELECTROLYTE SOLUTION (PEG-ES)

- 4 L (1 gallon) orally over 3 hours (240 mL every 10–15 minutes) given 4–5 hours before colonoscopy
- give the night before surgery or barium enema study
- can be given by nasogastric tube (20–30 mL/min)

SODIUM PHOSPHATE (FLEET) ENEMA

- one 120 mL enema given at least 2 hours before procedure

▶ *How Long Should I Treat with My Initial Regimen?*

Fecal impaction

SODIUM PHOSPHATE (FLEET) ENEMA

- watery evacuation within 5–30 minutes, depending on retention time

MAGNESIUM HYDROXIDE, CITRATE, OR SULFATE

- magnesium hydroxide used as a laxative produces one or more bowel movements within 6–12 hours magnesium citrate or magnesium sulfate used as a cathartic produces watery stools within 1–3 hours

BALANCED ELECTROLYTE SOLUTION (PEG-ES)

- produces liquid stool within 30–60 minutes

Acute constipation

BULK-FORMING LAXATIVES

- produces soft, formed stool within 1–5 days

STIMULANT LAXATIVES

- soft or semiliquid stool occurs within 6–24 hours after administration of oral preparations and within 15–60 minutes after rectal suppository administration

MAGNESIUM HYDROXIDE

- magnesium hydroxide produces one or more bowel movements within 6–12 hours

LACTULOSE

- should produce a soft or semifluid stool in 6–24 hours, with full effects within 48 hours

Chronic constipation

BULK-FORMING LAXATIVES

- produces soft, formed stool within 1–5 days

LACTULOSE

- should produce a soft or semifluid stool in 6–24 hours, with full effects within 48 hours

DOCUSATE

- produces soft stool within 1–3 days

GLYCERIN SUPPOSITORY

- should see effect within 15–60 minutes

Bowel preparation

BALANCED ELECTROLYTE SOLUTION (PEG-ES)

- give over 3 hours, 4–5 hours before colonoscopy
- give the night before surgery or barium enema study

SODIUM PHOSPHATE (FLEET) ENEMA

- watery evacuation within 5–30 minutes, depending on retention time

▶ *What Efficacy Parameters Should I Follow and How Frequently Do I Have to Assess My Patient?*

Fecal impaction, acute constipation, chronic constipation, bowel preparation

Frequency of bowel movements

- for chronic constipation, compare with what is usual for each individual
- this can normally vary from 3 times a day to once a week
- assess the patients on a daily basis
- for time course of effect, see above

Consistency of stool

- goal is soft, well-formed stools that are relatively bulky

▶ Should I Add Another Drug or Substitute Therapy If My Initial Drug Therapy Fails?

Fecal impaction

- if sodium phosphate enema is unsuccessful, consider manual disimpaction after stool softening with a docusate or mineral oil enema (if stool is hard or dry)
- depending on results; follow with balanced electrolyte solution

Acute constipation

- if bulk-forming laxatives are ineffective after 3 days, use magnesium hydroxide PO or a stimulant laxative
- glycerin suppositories and/or enema solutions (tap water, sodium phosphate [Fleet], saline) may be necessary as a single dose when constipation is resistant to oral laxatives

Chronic constipation

- if bulk-forming laxatives are ineffective, add lactulose
- if glycerin is ineffective, a bisacodyl suppository every second day may be necessary

Bowel preparation

- if balanced electrolyte solution fails, use sodium phosphate enema or oral bisacodyl plus bisacodyl suppository or enema

▶ How Long Should I Continue Drug Therapy?

Fecal impaction

- continue until impaction is cleared
- prevent further impaction with drug therapy until predisposing factors are eliminated (e.g., immobility, low-residue diet, anorectal injury)

Acute constipation

- avoid use for longer than 7 days
- if needed for longer than this, consider increasing the bulk in the patient's diet and/or using bulk-forming laxatives

Chronic constipation

- bulk-forming laxatives can be continued indefinitely, if needed
- with others, best to limit use to 7 days whenever possible
- drug trials have shown that approximately 50% of patients who use laxatives regularly redevelop normal bowel habits if laxative administration is stopped (Postgrad Med 1983;74:143–149)

Bowel preparation

- continue until rectal return is clear (usually requires 4 L over 3 hours)

Useful References

Tedesco FJ. Laxative use in constipation. Am J Gastroenterol 1985; 80:303–309
Rousseau P. Treatment of constipation in the elderly. Postgrad Med 1988; 83:339–349

DRUG THERAPY FOR NAUSEA AND VOMITING

Lynne Nakashima

▶ What Are My Goals of Treatment?

to prevent or relieve the distressing symptoms associated with nausea and vomiting of any cause

to prevent or reduce the inexorable nausea and vomiting associated with chemotherapy and thus allow completion of effective chemotherapy programs

to prevent life-threatening complications such as electrolyte imbalances, dehydration, and malnutrition

▶ What Evidence Is Available to Support Drug Therapy for Nausea and Vomiting?

Motion sickness

- prophylactic treatment with scopolamine, promethazine, or dimenhydrinate is effective in 90% of patients susceptible to motion sickness (Drugs 1979;17:471–479)

Postoperative nausea and vomiting

- incidence of nausea and vomiting associated with anesthesia is about 30%, and prophylaxis or treatment can often be useful (Can Anaesth Soc J 1984;31:407–415)
- postoperative nausea and vomiting necessitates treatment in only about 5% of postoperative patients (Can Anaesth Soc J 1986;33:22–31)

Nausea and vomiting associated with chemotherapy

- prophylactic treatment for patients treated with antineoplastic agents is imperative, as nausea and vomiting can curtail effective chemotherapy (Pharmacotherapy 1990; 10:129–145)
- prophylaxis and treatment of chemotherapy-induced nausea and vomiting may eliminate symptoms in up to 82% of patients (Am J Hosp Pharm 1988;45:1322–1328)

Pregnancy

- routine drug therapy for prophylaxis or treatment is not recommended unless severe hyperemesis gravidarum is present
- nausea and vomiting is usually self-limited and intermittent (Drugs 1992;43:443–463)

▶ When Should I Consider Drug Therapy?

Prophylaxis

Motion sickness

- in patients with a previous history of nausea and vomiting associated with motion sickness during travel

Postoperative nausea and vomiting

- routine prophylaxis after surgery is discouraged (Drugs 1981;22:246–253) because nausea and vomiting necessitating treatment is seen in only about 5% of postoperative patients (Can Anaesth Soc J 1986;33:22–31) and some drugs used for the treatment of postoperative nausea and vomiting can cause hypotension and movement disorders
- patients at high risk for aspiration (e.g., patients who have their jaws occluded by wires after oral surgery or patients with a history of moderate to severe postoperative vomiting) should receive prophylactic therapy

Chemotherapy-induced nausea and vomiting

- prophylactic therapy should be used if chemotherapy has either a high or a moderate emetogenic potential
- for drugs with low emetogenic potential, prophylactic therapy should be used in patients who experienced nausea or vomiting on a previous course of these drugs
- high emetogenic potential drugs: cisplatin, cyclophosphamide, dacarbazine, dactinomycin, mechlorethamine, and streptozocin (Recent Results Cancer Res 1991;121:68–85)
- moderate emetogenic potential drugs: carmustine, cytarabine, daunorubicin, doxorubicin, lomustine, procarbazine, and carboplatin

- low emetogenic potential drugs: fluorouracil (5-fluoro-uracil), bleomycin, chlorambucil, etoposide, hydroxy-urea, methotrexate, mitomycin C, vinblastine, vincris-tine, and vindesine
- it is important to prevent anticipatory nausea and vom-iting because nausea and vomiting usually worsens with each cycle and up to 30% of patients refuse further treat-ment related to intolerable nausea and vomiting (J Clin Oncol 1989;7:1142–1149)

Migraine

- if nausea and vomiting is routinely associated with mi-graine headaches on the basis of the patient's history

Treatment

Pregnancy

- routine treatment of pregnancy-induced nausea and vom-iting is not suggested (owing to the potential for terato-genic effects associated with drug therapy) unless pro-tracted vomiting (hyperemesis gravidarum) occurs or if nondrug measures such as ingesting crackers and tea before morning rising, taking small, light, appetizing meals, and keeping head movement to a minimum have failed (Drugs 1992;43:443–463)

Postoperative nausea and vomiting

- for patients with prolonged nausea (longer than 30 min-utes) or repeated episodes of vomiting unrelieved by de-creasing vestibular stimulation (head movement)
- therapy is not recommended for patients who experience transient nausea and vomiting as a result of excessive fluid intake or vestibular stimulation

Gastric stasis

- characterized by intractable nausea and vomiting (espe-cially shortly after eating) (Ann Intern Med 1984;101: 211–218), bloating, and early satiety
- treatment should be tried after diagnostic studies have ruled out other underlying disease states and other causes of nausea and vomiting (Am J Gastroenterol 1985;80: 210–218)

Intractable nausea and vomiting

- when nondrug measures have failed such as having no oral intake (for a short period) or oral intake guided by the patient with small, frequent amounts of any noncar-bonated liquid and keeping movement to a minimum by resting in bed or a chair to avoid vestibular stimulation

▶ *What Drug Should I Use for Initial Treatment?*

Initial antiemetic choice, dosage, and route of adminis-tration depends on the underlying cause of nausea and vomiting • For treatment of nausea and vomiting, the decision should initially be based on potential adverse effects, as no one agent has proved more effective than any other agent

Prophylaxis

Motion sickness

DIMENHYDRINATE

- for mild to moderate travel by road (e.g., automobile), air, or sea, especially if sedation is desired
- decision between dimenhydrinate and promethazine should be based on cost

PROMETHAZINE

- as above

TRANSDERMAL SCOPOLAMINE

- for rough seas and extended journeys (Pharmacotherapy 1982;2:29–31)
- more convenient than promethazine or dimenhydrinate, as it can be applied every 3 days
- causes less sedation than does promethazine or dimenhy-drinate, but causes a high incidence of anticholinergic effects
- confusion and psychosis in the elderly have been reported
- urinary retention in elderly men is a problem with this agent
- also effective after nausea has started (Drugs 1992; 43:443–463)

MECLIZINE

- almost as convenient as scopolamine, as it can be given once daily and is less expensive than scopolamine

Postoperative nausea and vomiting

DROPERIDOL

- considered antiemetic of choice to control postoperative vomiting prophylactically owing to its effectiveness and long duration of action (Can Anaesth Soc J 1979;26: 125–127, Drugs 1992;43:443–463, Anesth Analg 1974;53: 361–364, Anesth Analg 1977;56:674–677)
- only drug that appears truly to prevent nausea and vom-iting; however, it produces dysphoria in some patients, delays awakening, and prolongs time to discharge from the postanesthetic care unit
- in general, prophylactic antinauseants are not recom-mended

Chemotherapy-induced nausea and vomiting

- choice of drug depends on the emetogenic potential of the drug administered
- in combination chemotherapy, antiemetic therapy should be based on the drug with the highest emetogenic poten-tial in the combination

High emetogenic potential

ONDANSETRON

- although ondansetron is expensive, it is chosen in this case, as it is the most effective agent available for pre-venting nausea and vomiting in patients receiving highly emetogenic therapy
- expense of ondansetron must be compared with the cost of preparing the parenteral 3 or 4 agent regimens and the cost of rescue medications (Eur J Cancer 1993; 29A(3):303–306)
- ondansetron is well tolerated by most patients

DEXAMETHASONE

- add to ondansetron, as it is a useful concomitant anti-emetic, plus it occasionally makes patients feel better
- ondansetron in combination with dexamethasone, is more effective than ondansetron alone (J Clin Oncol 1991;9: 675–678)
- corticosteroids, in most trials, confer a positive benefit when added to antiemetic therapy (Recent Results Cancer Res 1991;121:91–100)
- although most studies have used dexamethasone, other corticosteroids are likely also useful

PROCHLORPERAZINE, PERPHENAZINE, THIETHYLPERAZINE

- these agents are added for breakthrough nausea and vom-iting experienced with prophylactic regimens

- these agents are likely equally effective, and the decision among them should be based on cost and availability

METOCLOPRAMIDE, DIPHENHYDRAMINE, DEXAMETHASONE, AND LORAZEPAM

- useful combination when ondansetron cannot be used
- lorazepam is added for its amnestic properties

Moderate or low emetogenic potential

PROCHLORPERAZINE, PERPHENAZINE, THIETHYLPERAZINE

- these agents are likely equally effective, and the decision among them should be based on cost and availability
- the phenothiazines are widely used but are not superior to metoclopramide in terms of effectiveness or adverse effects
- the phenothiazines are available in a variety of dosage forms (injection, oral, rectal) which can be an advantage in terms of ease of administration
- thiethylperazine cannot be given intravenously
- there is no rectal formulation of perphenazine
- these agents are less expensive than metoclopramide

METOCLOPRAMIDE

- useful if one of the above agents cannot be used or is ineffective
- dystonic reactions, tetanus, restlessness, facial spasms, involuntary movement, torticollis, and muscular twitching occur in about 3% of patients (Pharmacotherapy 1990;10:129–145)
- patients younger than age 30 years have a higher incidence of acute extrapyramidal effects (Br Med J 1985;291:930–932)

DEXAMETHASONE

- add to either prochlorperazine or metoclopramide, as it is a useful concomitant-antiemetic, plus it occasionally makes patients feel better

Migraine

METOCLOPRAMIDE

- if the patient is experiencing nausea or vomiting with the headache, use metoclopramide
- metoclopramide enhances subsequent analgesic absorption, as well as providing an antimigraine effect

DOMPERIDONE

- domperidone is associated with fewer extrapyramidal reactions than is metoclopramide; however, it has not been directly compared with metoclopramide (Drugs 1992;43: 443–463)
- although it is likely useful in this setting, domperidone has not been evaluated in patients with migraine, and unlike metoclopramide, it cannot be given parenterally

Treatment

Pregnancy

PYRIDOXINE

- drug therapy should be used only after all other measures (dietary modifications, and so on) are unsuccessful
- although pyridoxine's usefulness has not been confirmed in clinical trials, it is the least likely agent to be toxic (Drugs 1992;43:443–463)

MECLIZINE

- use if pyridoxine is unsuccessful

PROMETHAZINE, PROCHLORPERAZINE, METOCLOPRAMIDE

- all have been tried
- there is no evidence available to support the use of one agent over another
- there is also not enough information available to say that any one of these agents is completely safe

Postoperative nausea and vomiting

PROCHLORPERAZINE, PERPHENAZINE, THIETHYLPERAZINE

- these agents are likely equally effective, and the decision among them should be based on cost and availability
- these agents likely cause less sedation than does dimenhydrinate
- thiethylperazine cannot be given intravenously
- there is no rectal formulation of perphenazine

PROMETHAZINE

- should be chosen for patients undergoing ear surgery owing to its anticholinergic and antihistaminic activity (Can Anaesth Soc J 1984;31:407–415)

METOCLOPRAMIDE

- useful if above agents cannot be used or are ineffective

DIMENHYDRINATE

- if sedation is desired, choose dimenhydrinate instead of the above agents

HALOPERIDOL

- likely causes less sedation and less orthostatic hypotension than do the above agents but causes a greater incidence of acute extrapyramidal or dystonic reactions
- is more expensive than prochlorperazine, perphenazine, or thiethylperazine

Gastric stasis

DOMPERIDONE

- increases sphincter tone and improves gastric emptying
- if oral route is available, choose domperidone over metoclopramide, as it produces fewer adverse effects

CISAPRIDE

- cisapride is expensive, and although it does improve gastric emptying, it does not have any antiemetic activity

METOCLOPRAMIDE

- also increases lower esophageal sphincter tone and improves gastric emptying
- metoclopramide should be chosen only if an IV route is required

Intractable nausea and vomiting

DIMENHYDRINATE, PROCHLORPERAZINE, PERPHENAZINE, THIETHYLPERAZINE

- these agents are likely equally effective, and the decision among them should be based on cost and availability

▶ What Dosage Should I Use?

All antiemetic drugs and dosages are adjusted according to the patient's tolerance and the efficacy

• A parenteral or rectal route of administration should be used if the oral route is not tolerated

Prophylaxis
Motion sickness

DIMENHYDRINATE

• 50 mg PO Q12H starting 1–2 hours prior to departure

PROMETHAZINE

• 25 mg PO Q12H starting 1–2 hours prior to departure

TRANSDERMAL SCOPOLAMINE

• apply a 1.5 mg patch to skin at least 4 hours prior to departure
• replace every 72 hours (Pharmacotherapy 1982;2:29–31)

MECLIZINE

• 50 mg PO daily starting 1–2 hours before leaving
• some clinicians suggest starting administration of this agent the day before leaving because it may have a long onset of action

Postoperative nausea and vomiting

DROPERIDOL

• 0.0175 mg/kg IV, as a single dose at the end of surgery

Chemotherapy-induced nausea and vomiting
High emetogenic potential

ONDANSETRON

• 8 mg (0.15 mg/kg) PO 30 minutes prior to chemotherapy (give intravenously at same dose if the patient is already vomiting)
• use PO dosing before chemotherapy unless the patient has preexisting nausea and vomiting because the oral dose is half the cost of IV therapy and is just as effective
• follow the prechemotherapy dose with 8 mg PO Q8H, starting 4 hours after chemotherapy

DEXAMETHASONE

• 10 mg PO 30 minutes prior to chemotherapy (give intravenously at same dose if the patient is already vomiting)
• follow the prechemotherapy dose with 4 mg PO Q8H, starting 4 hours after chemotherapy

PROCHLORPERAZINE

• 10 mg IV, IM, PO, or PR Q3H PRN for breakthrough nausea and vomiting

PERPHENAZINE

• 5 mg IV or IM Q3H PRN for breakthrough nausea and vomiting

THIETHYLPERAZINE

• 10 mg IM, PO, or PR (PR and IM not available in Canada) Q3H PRN for breakthrough nausea and vomiting

METOCLOPRAMIDE

• 1 mg/kg IV or PO 30 minutes prior to chemotherapy, then 1 mg/kg IV or PO Q3H for 3 doses
• replace parenteral metoclopramide (if patient can tolerate oral therapy) with 10 mg PO Q6H, starting 6 hours after the last 1 mg/kg dose (maximum daily dose 12 mg/kg)
• if emesis is uncontrolled and adverse effects are not present, increase the dosage by 20 mg increments to a maxi-

mum of 3 mg/kg until optimum effect is obtained (Am J Hosp Pharm 1988;45:1322–1328)

DIPHENHYDRAMINE

• 50 mg IV (usually mixed with metoclopramide) 30 minutes prior to chemotherapy and with each 1 mg/kg dose of metoclopramide
• after the 1 mg/kg dose of metoclopramide has been given, replace the parenteral diphenhydramine with 25 mg PO Q6H

LORAZEPAM

• 1 mg IV or sublingually 30 minutes prior to chemotherapy
• continue lorazepam Q12H for the duration of chemotherapy

Moderate or low emetogenic potential

PROCHLORPERAZINE

• 10 mg PO 30 minutes prior to chemotherapy (give intravenously at same dose if the patient is already vomiting)
• follow with 10 mg PO Q6H for 24 hours and then 10 mg PO PRN for 3–4 days

PERPHENAZINE

• 8 mg PO 30 minutes prior to chemotherapy
• follow with 8 mg PO Q6H for 24 hours and then 8 mg PO PRN for 3–4 days

THIETHYLPERAZINE

• 10 mg PO 30 minutes prior to chemotherapy (give IM at same dose if the patient is already vomiting)
• follow with 10 mg PO Q6H for 24 hours and then 10 mg PO PRN for 3–4 days

METOCLOPRAMIDE

• 20 mg PO 30 minutes prior to chemotherapy (give intravenously at same dose if the patient is already vomiting)
• follow with 20 mg PO Q6H for 24 hours and then 20 mg PO PRN for 3–4 days

DEXAMETHASONE

• 10 mg PO 30 minutes prior to chemotherapy (give intravenously at same dose if the patient is already vomiting)
• follow with 4 mg PO Q8H for 24 hours

Migraine

METOCLOPRAMIDE

• 10 mg PO TID
• 10 mg IV Q8H if the patient is vomiting

DOMPERIDONE

• 10 mg PO TID

Treatment
Pregnancy

PYRIDOXINE

• 50 mg PO Q12H PRN
• increase to 100 mg PO BID if nausea and vomiting persists
• 50 mg IV Q6H has been used in hospitalized patients (Drugs 1992;43:443–463)

MECLIZINE

• 50 mg PO daily PRN

PROMETHAZINE

• 25 mg PO Q12H PRN

PROCHLORPERAZINE

- 12.5 mg IM Q4H PRN

METOCLOPRAMIDE

- 10 mg IM Q4H PRN

Postoperative nausea and vomiting

PROCHLORPERAZINE

- 10 mg IV or IM Q3H PRN for breakthrough nausea and vomiting
- 10 mg PO Q3H PRN may be used if patient can tolerate sips of fluid
- can also be used rectally 25 mg Q6H (only 10 mg suppository available in Canada)

PERPHENAZINE

- 5 mg IV or IM Q3H PRN for breakthrough nausea and vomiting
- 8 mg PO Q3H PRN may be used if patient can tolerate sips of fluid

THIETHYLPERAZINE

- 10 mg IM Q3H PRN for breakthrough nausea and vomiting
- 10 mg PO Q3H PRN may be used if the patient can tolerate sips of fluid

PROMETHAZINE

- 25 mg IV or IM Q3H PRN for breakthrough nausea and vomiting
- 25 mg PO Q3H PRN may be used if the patient can tolerate sips of fluid

METOCLOPRAMIDE

- 10 mg IV or IM Q3H PRN for breakthrough nausea and vomiting
- 10 mg PO Q3H PRN may be used if the patient can tolerate sips of fluid

DIMENHYDRINATE

- 50 mg IV or IM Q3H PRN for breakthrough nausea and vomiting
- 50 mg PO Q3H PRN may be used if the patient can tolerate sips of fluid

HALOPERIDOL

- 0.5 mg IM Q8H PRN for breakthrough nausea and vomiting

Gastric stasis

DOMPERIDONE

- 10 mg PO 30 minutes before meals and at bedtime

METOCLOPRAMIDE

- 10 mg PO 30 minutes before meals and at bedtime

Intractable nausea and vomiting

DIMENHYDRINATE, PROCHLORPERAZINE, PERPHENAZINE, THIETHYLPERAZINE

- as above under treatment of postoperative nausea and vomiting

▶ *How Long Should I Treat with My Initial Drug Therapy?*

Prophylaxis

Motion sickness

- for the duration of the trip

Postoperative nausea and vomiting

- use a single dose of droperidol

Chemotherapy-induced nausea and vomiting

High, moderate emetogenic potential or low emetogenic potential

- all prophylactic agents are given round-the-clock for the first 24 hours, and then the patient is reassessed
- if the patient has exhibited little if any nausea and vomiting, switch to oral PRN medications
- if the patient has had episodes of nausea and/or vomiting in the previous 24 hours, continue agents on a regularly dosed basis for another 24 hours and then reassess the patient

Migraine

- if 2 doses of metoclopramide do not provide relief, switch to an alternative agent

Treatment

Pregnancy

- reassess the effect of each dose of medication
- if no effect occurs after a couple of doses, switch to a different agent

Postoperative nausea and vomiting

- try 1–2 doses, and if no effect is seen, try a different agent

Gastric stasis

- try for a few days, and if no effect is seen, try a different agent

General

- if nausea and vomiting is not controlled within the first 12–24 hours, the patient should be reassessed and an alternative agent should be used

▶ *What Efficacy Parameters Should I Follow and How Frequently Do I Have to Assess My Patient?*

Frequency of assessment depends on the severity and frequency of nausea and vomiting

Number and severity of vomiting episodes

- determine the time of day, the force, description of vomitus, and associated symptoms

Fluid balance

(only needed if vomiting occurs for a prolonged period)

- assess jugular venous pressure and orthostatic changes in blood pressure and heart rate; any decrease in upright diastolic pressure plus a rise in heart rate of 20 bpm or greater is abnormal
- oliguria
- weight
- rising values of hematocrit and creatinine, urea, sodium, and bicarbonate levels plus decreasing potassium and chloride levels are an indication of dehydration

▶ *Should I Add Another Drug or Substitute Therapy If My Initial Drug Therapy Fails?*

Motion sickness, postoperative nausea and vomiting, migraine, pregnancy, gastric stasis, intractable nausea and vomiting

- if the first drug is ineffective, discontinue the first drug and begin administration of a drug from a different class of antiemetics

Chemotherapy-induced nausea and vomiting

High emetogenic potential

- if patient vomits while taking ondansetron and dexamethasone, switch to the parenteral route

Moderate emetogenic potential

- if the initial drugs fail to prevent or treat nausea or vomiting after 24 hours, stop these agents and start ondansetron plus dexamethasone regimen

Low emetogenic potential

- If the initial drug did not work, switch to one of the alternative agents
- base choice on costs and potential adverse effects
- if none of these agents work, add dexamethasone (Hosp Pharm 1988;45:1322–1328)

▶ *How Long Should I Continue Drug Therapy?*

Prophylaxis

Motion sickness

- for the duration of the trip

Postoperative nausea and vomiting

- 1 dose only

Chemotherapy-induced nausea and vomiting

- treat patients for 24 hours after chemotherapy, then re-evaluate the patient
- for cisplatin-induced nausea and vomiting, delayed symptoms may occur up to 1 week after the last dose of chemotherapy and treatment should last for up to 1 week after chemotherapy

- if there is previous experience with the drug, base duration of use on how the patient responded the first time (e.g., if the drug was used for 24 hours and the patient went home and experienced substantial nausea and vomiting, give as a regular dose for a longer period of time)

Migraine

- for 2–3 days

Treatment

Pregnancy

- treatment should continue until symptoms resolve

Postoperative nausea and vomiting

- if regular prophylactic therapy is required, treat for 24 hours
- use PRN antiemetics for 2–3 days after surgery

Gastric stasis

- treatment should continue until underlying pathophysiology is resolved or until symptoms resolve

Intractable nausea and vomiting

- therapy should be continued on a PRN basis until vomiting is controlled and the underlying pathophysiological changes are treated

Useful References

Barbezat GO. The vomiting patient: A rational approach. Drugs 1981; 22:246–253.

Eburn E. Choosing the right anti-emetic. Nurs Times 1989;85(24):36–38

Hanson JS, McCallum RW. The diagnosis and management of nausea and vomiting: a review. Am J Gastroenterol 1985; 80(3):210–218.

Malagelada JR, Camilleri M. Unexplained vomiting: A diagnostic challenge. Ann Intern Med 1984;101:211–218.

Mitchelson F. Pharmacological agents affecting emesis. A review part I. Drugs 1992;43:295–315

Mitchelson F. Pharmacological agents affecting emesis. A review part II. Drugs 1992;43:443–463

Palazzo MGA. Anaesthesia and emesis II: Prevention and management. Can Anaesth Soc J 1984;31:407–415.

Van der Vliet W. Controlling chemotherapy induced emesis. Pharm Pract September 1991:21–29

Wood CD. Antimotion sickness and antiemetic drugs. Drugs 1979; 17:471–479.

4

INFECTIOUS DISEASES

DRUG THERAPY FOR URINARY TRACT INFECTION

George G. Zhanel

▶ *What Are My Goals of Treatment?*

to ameliorate the signs and symptoms of upper and lower urinary tract infections

to prevent sepsis and death

to prevent reinfection

to preserve renal function

▶ *What Evidence Is Available to Support Drug Therapy for Urinary Tract Infections?*

Ameliorates signs and symptoms

- signs and symptoms of acute lower urinary tract infection (frequency; urgency; dysuria, with or without turbid, smelly urine; and fever) or acute upper urinary tract infection (fever, chills, and flank pain, with or without lower

Table 4–1 • Antibiotic Susceptibility Chart

	Streptococcus pneumoniae/ S. viridans/S. faecalis (Enterococcus faecalis)	Staphylococcus aureus or S. epidermidis Non–Penicillinase Producing/ Penicillinase Producing/ Methicillin Resistant	Escherichia coli or Proteus mirabilis	Klebsiella pneumoniae	Haemophilus influenzae (Ampicillin Sensitive/ Ampicillin Resistant)	Neisseria gonorrhoeae (Non–Penicillinase Producing/ Penicillinase Producing)/ Neisseria meningitidis	Pseudomonas aeruginosa or Acinetobacter calcoaceticus	Anaerobes Above the Diaphragm (Anaerobic Cocci)	Anaerobes Below the Diaphragm (Bacteroides fragilis)
penicillin V or G	yes/yes/var	yes/no/no	no	no	no/no	yes/no/yes	no	yes	no
amoxicillin, ampicillin, pivampicillin	yes/yes/var	yes/no/no	yes	no	yes/no	yes/no/yes	no	yes	no
amoxicillin-clavulanate	yes/yes/yes	yes/yes/no	yes	yes	yes/yes	yes/yes/yes	no	yes	yes
cloxacillin, nafcillin	yes/yes/yes	yes/yes/no	no	no	no/no	no/no/no	no	yes	no
piperacillin	yes/yes/yes	yes/no/no	yes	yes	yes/var	yes/no/no	yes	yes	yes
ticarcillin-clavulanate	yes/yes/no	yes/yes/no	yes	yes	yes/yes	yes/yes/yes	yes	yes	yes
cefazolin, cephalexin	yes/yes/no	yes/yes/no	yes	yes	no/no	no/no/no	no	yes	no
cefuroxime, cefuroxime axetil, cefaclor	yes/yes/no	yes/yes/no	yes	yes	yes/yes	yes/yes/yes	no	yes	no
cefoxitin, cefotetan, ceftizoxime	yes/yes/no	yes/yes/no	yes	yes	yes/yes	yes/yes/no	no	yes	yes
ceftriaxone, cefotaxime	yes/yes/no	yes/yes/no	yes	yes	yes/yes	yes/yes/yes	no	yes	no
cefixime	yes/yes/no	no/no/no	yes	yes	yes/yes	yes/yes/yes	no	yes	no
ceftazidime	yes/yes/no	no/no/no	yes	yes	yes/yes	yes/var/no	yes	yes	no
aztreonam	no/no/no	no/no/no	yes	yes	yes/yes	yes/yes/no	no	no	no
imipenem	yes/yes/yes	yes/yes/no	yes	yes	yes/yes	yes/yes/yes	yes	yes	yes
amikacin, tobramycin, gentamicin, netilmicin	synergy with penicillins and vancomycin	synergy with penicillins and vancomycin	yes	yes	yes/yes	no/no/no	yes (tobramycin more active)	no	no
chloramphenicol	yes/yes/no	yes/yes/var	yes	yes	yes/yes	yes/no/yes	no	yes	yes
ciprofloxacin, norfloxacin	no/no/yes	yes/yes/no	yes	yes	yes/yes	yes/yes/yes	yes	no	no
clindamycin	yes/yes/no	yes/yes/no	no	no	no/no	no/no/no	no	yes	yes
trimethoprim-sulfamethoxazole	yes/yes/yes	yes/yes/var	yes	yes	yes/yes	no/no/yes	no	var	no
erythromycin	yes/yes/no	yes/yes/no	no	no	yes/var	yes/no/no	no	yes	no
metronidazole	no/no/no	no/no/no	no	no	no/no	no/no/no	no	no	yes
tetracycline, doxycycline	yes/yes/no	no/no/no	var	no	yes/yes	var/var/yes	no	yes	yes (doxycycline) var (tetracycline)
vancomycin	yes/yes/yes	yes/yes/yes	no	no	no/no	no/no/no	no	yes	no

yes = clinically useful; no = not clinically useful; var = variable depends on local sensitivities.

tract symptoms) are alleviated with appropriate antimicrobial therapy

Prevents sepsis and death

- occasionally, gram-negative sepsis and death complicate urinary tract infection, and this can be prevented with appropriate antimicrobial therapy (Urol Clin North Am 1986;13:627–635)

Prevents reinfection

- although many patients have a reinfection, antibiotics reduce the relapse rate in selected populations (Arch Intern Med 1990;150:1389–1396)

Preserves renal function

- antibiotics have reduced the development of pyelonephritis in selected populations (pregnant women, preschoolers) with bacteriuria (Arch Intern Med 1990;150:1389–1396)

▶ When Should I Consider Drug Therapy?

Upper urinary tract infection (pyelonephritis)

- treat all patients when an upper urinary tract infection is suspected on the basis of clinical symptoms such as flank pain, fever, dysuria, frequency, and urgency
- confirmation can be made by the presence of more than 10^2 colony-forming units (CFU) per milliliter of 1 species on a clean-catch midstream urine specimen and/or pyuria defined as more than 5–10 white blood cells per $400\times$ field on the spun sediment

Lower urinary tract infection (cystitis)

- patients with dysuria, frequency, urgency, and pyuria and more than 10^2 CFU/mL of 1 species should be treated

Asymptomatic bacteriuria

- defined as an absence of symptoms and 2 separate clean-catch voided urine specimens, with both yielding positive cultures ($\geq 10^5$ CFU/mL) of the same organism
- should be treated in neonates, preschool-aged children, pregnant women, men younger than 60 years of age, and patients with abnormal obstructed urinary tracts and in patients after genitourinary manipulation or instrumentation (Arch Intern Med 1990;50:1389–1396)

Catheter-related infection

- treat bacteriuria only if the patient is symptomatic
- catheter must be removed if infection is to be completely eradicated

Recurrent lower urinary tract infection

- low-dose long-term prophylaxis should be used in women who experience more than 3 symptomatic recurrences a year (considered a reinfection with the same or a different organism)

Acute bacterial prostatitis

- treat patients with symptoms of fever, lower back and perineal pain, discomfort on voiding, and tender, swollen prostate on palpation, and the presence of pyuria and bacteriuria
- in patients with apparent acute bacterial prostatitis, prostatic massage should not be done because of the risk of precipitating bacteremia

Chronic bacterial prostatitis

- treat patients who have some disruption of urine, urgency, and some discomfort
- differentiate between chronic bacterial prostatitis and nonbacterial prostatitis by using a Meares-Stamey procedure (a collection of serial aliquots of urine before and after prostatic massage)

▶ What Drug Should I Use for Initial Treatment?

Upper urinary tract infection (pyelonephritis)

Patients who are severely ill

AMPICILLIN WITH GENTAMICIN

- patients with high fever, chills, nausea or vomiting, and hypotension are at risk for sepsis and require treatment with parenteral antibiotics
- ampicillin and gentamicin have activity against organisms that commonly cause urinary tract infection. *Escherichia coli*, *Proteus* sp., *Klebsiella-Enterobacter* sp., *Pseudomonas aeruginosa*, and *Enterococcus*

CEFTRIAXONE, CEFOTAXIME

- use in patients with a contraindication to aminoglycoside therapy (poor renal function)

CEFTAZIDIME PLUS TOBRAMYCIN

- use in patients with hospital-acquired infection in which *Pseudomonas* or other resistant organisms may be present
- if patient has renal dysfunction, use ceftazidime as sole therapy

CIPROFLOXACIN

- use parenteral ciprofloxacin if the patient is beta-lactam allergic
- oral ciprofloxacin is useful as step-down therapy (for aminoglycoside or cefotaxime, ceftriaxone, or ceftazidime) after the patient has improved

Patients who are mildly to moderately ill

TRIMETHOPRIM-SULFAMETHOXAZOLE

- patients who are reliable and compliant may be treated orally (Am J Med 1988;85:793–798)
- trimethoprim-sulfamethoxazole is as effective as other agents if organisms are sensitive, provides convenient twice-daily dosing, and is less expensive than the newer agents

CIPROFLOXACIN

- use ciprofloxacin if the patient is allergic to trimethoprim-sulfamethoxazole
- ciprofloxacin should be chosen over norfloxacin for systemic infections (pyelonephritis)

Lower urinary tract infection (cystitis), asymptomatic bacteriuria, and catheterrelated infection

TRIMETHOPRIM-SULFAMETHOXAZOLE

- is as effective as other agents (may be better than amoxicillin) if organisms are sensitive, provides convenient twice-daily dosing, and is less expensive than newer agents

AMOXICILLIN

- if the patient is allergic to trimethoprim-sulfamethoxazole

CIPROFLOXACIN

- if the patient is allergic to both trimethoprim-sulfamethoxazole and beta-lactams

- norfloxacin should be chosen over ciprofloxacin if it is less expensive or if patient is receiving concurrent theophylline or warfarin owing to a possible interaction between theophylline or warfarin and ciprofloxacin

Recurrent lower urinary tract infection

TRIMETHOPRIM-SULFAMETHOXAZOLE

- inexpensive and effective prophylaxis

NITROFURANTOIN

- if the patient is allergic to trimethoprim-sulfamethoxazole

Acute or chronic bacterial prostatitis
Patients who are severely ill
AMPICILLIN WITH GENTAMICIN

- ampicillin and gentamicin have activity against organisms that commonly cause prostatitis

CIPROFLOXACIN

- use parenteral ciprofloxacin if the patient is beta-lactam allergic

Patients who are mildly to moderately ill
TRIMETHOPRIM-SULFAMETHOXAZOLE

- patients who are reliable and compliant may be treated orally (Am J Med 1988;85:793–798)
- trimethoprim-sulfamethoxazole penetrates the prostate well, provides convenient twice-daily dosing, and is less expensive than the newer agents

CIPROFLOXACIN

- use if the patient is allergic to trimethoprim-sulfamethoxazole, as ciprofloxacin has good activity against common infecting organisms and good penetration into the prostate tissue
- demonstrates a broader spectrum than does erythromycin or tetracycline and demonstrates better penetration into the prostate than do amoxicillin and cephalosporins

▶ *What Dosage Should I Use?*

Upper urinary tract infection (pyelonephritis)
Patients who are severely ill
AMPICILLIN

- 1 g IV Q6H

GENTAMICIN

- 2 mg/kg IV Q8H

CEFTRIAXONE

- 1 g IV Q24H

CEFOTAXIME

- 1 g IV Q8H

CEFTAZIDIME

- 1 g IV Q8H

TOBRAMYCIN

- 2 mg/kg IV Q8H

CIPROFLOXACIN

- 200 mg IV Q12H

Patients who are mildly to moderately ill
TRIMETHOPRIM-SULFAMETHOXAZOLE

- 160 mg/800 mg (1 double-strength tablet) PO BID

CIPROFLOXACIN

- 500 mg PO BID

Lower urinary tract infection (cystitis), asymptomatic bacteriuria, and catheterrelated infection

TRIMETHOPRIM-SULFAMETHOXAZOLE

- 160 mg/800 mg PO BID

AMOXICILLIN

- 500 mg PO Q8H

CIPROFLOXACIN

- 250 mg PO BID

NORFLOXACIN

- 400 mg PO BID

Recurrent lower urinary tract infection
TRIMETHOPRIM-SULFAMETHOXAZOLE

- 40 mg/200 mg PO HS or after intercourse in women whose infections occur in association with sexual activity
- alternative regimen, in the compliant patient, is treatment initiated by the patient at the first signs of a urinary tract infection (dosages as above for lower urinary tract infection)

NITROFURANTOIN

- 50 mg PO HS or after intercourse in women whose infections occur in association with sexual activity

Acute or chronic bacterial prostatitis
Patients who are severely ill
AMPICILLIN

- 2 g IV Q6H

GENTAMICIN

- 2 mg/kg IV Q8H

CIPROFLOXACIN

- 200 mg IV Q12H

Patients who are mildly to moderately ill
TRIMETHOPRIM-SULFAMETHOXAZOLE

- 160 mg/800 mg PO BID

CIPROFLOXACIN

- 500 mg PO BID

▶ *How Long Should I Treat with My Initial Regimen?*

Upper urinary tract infection (pyelonephritis)
Patients who are severely ill

- initially, treat for 48–72 hours in the hospital, and base further therapy on an assessment of the patient
- when chills, nausea, and vomiting abate; blood pressure normalizes; and the patient has been afebrile for at least 48 hours, change to trimethoprim-sulfamethoxazole 160 mg/800 mg PO BID (if the patient is allergic, use amoxicillin 500 mg PO TID), assuming the organisms are sensitive

Patients who are mildly to moderately ill

- initially, treat for 48–72 hours at home and instruct the patient to telephone if there is no improvement

Lower urinary tract infection (cystitis)

- 72 hours; the patient should be instructed to telephone or return to the clinic if there is no response after this time
- single-dose therapy is also effective (DICP 1988;22: 21–24); however, with 3 day therapy, patients take antibiotics for the duration of their symptoms and have a slightly lower relapse rate

Asymptomatic bacteriuria

- treat for 3 days, 7 days if the patient is pregnant
- in women after short-term catheterization and without abnormalities of the urinary tract, a single dose of trimethoprim-sulfamethoxazole 160 mg/800 mg PO is adequate (Ann Intern Med 1991;114:713–719)

Catheter-related infection

- treat for 5 days (Geriatrics 1988;43(8):43–48)

Recurrent lower urinary tract infection

- use prophylaxis for 6 months, then discontinue and reassess

Acute or chronic bacterial prostatitis

- for acute prostatitis, treat for a total of 30 days (Med Clin North Am 1991;75:405–424)
- for chronic prostatitis, treat for a total of 6 weeks
- symptoms usually resolve over 7 days, but a prolonged treatment course is mandatory for eradication

▶ What Efficacy Parameters Should I Follow and How Frequently Do I Have to Assess My Patient?

Upper urinary tract infection (pyelonephritis)

Patients who are severely ill

Signs and symptoms

- temperature, chills, dysuria, and blood pressure should be assessed Q6H for 3 days
- incidence of nausea and vomiting should be assessed Q12H for 3 days

Microbiological findings

- urine and blood samples for culture and sensitivity testing should be taken prior to starting antibiotics
- a repeat culture should be obtained a few days after therapy is completed to ensure eradication of the organism

Patients who are mildly to moderately ill

Signs and symptoms

- measure temperature and evaluate symptoms (dysuria) 48–72 hours after the start of therapy

Microbiological findings

- urine and blood samples for cultures and sensitivity testing should be taken prior to starting antibiotics

Lower urinary tract infection (cystitis)

Signs and symptoms

- urgency, frequency, and dysuria should disappear after 24–48 hours if appropriate therapy has been instituted

Microbiological findings

- for initial or infrequent lower urinary tract infections, cultures are not needed as long as treatment is successful
- if symptoms persist after the initial antibiotic treatment course, urine cultures should be obtained to verify the sensitivity of offending organism to the antibiotic
- follow-up urine cultures are mandatory within 1–2 weeks

of completion of therapy in children, pregnant women, patients with recurrent symptomatic upper urinary tract infection, and patients at high risk for renal damage, even if they are asymptomatic (Ann Intern Med 1989;111: 906–917)
- repeated cultures are not required in nonpregnant women who remain asymptomatic

Asymptomatic bacteriuria

- repeat cultures 7 days after treatment

Catheter-related bacteriuruia

- cultures are not needed

Recurrent lower urinary tract infection

- frequency of recurrent urinary tract infections

Acute or chronic bacterial prostatitis

Signs and symptoms

- should resolve over several days and should be assessed weekly

Microbiological findings

- sensitivity of bacteria to the antibiotic should be confirmed on urine culture

▶ Should I Add Another Drug or Substitute Therapy If My Initial Drug Therapy Fails?

Upper urinary tract infection (pyelonephritis)

- if signs or symptoms do not abate in 48–72 hours, therapy should be changed on the basis of antibiotic susceptibility test results

Lower urinary tract infection (cystitis)

- if signs or symptoms (dysuria, frequency, and urgency, with or without fever) do not abate in 48–72 hours, therapy should be changed on the basis of antibiotic susceptibility test results

Asymptomatic bacteriuria

- if initial therapy fails, further therapy should be based on antibiotic susceptibility test results

Catheter-related infection

- if sign or symptoms have not abated after a second 5 day course of antibiotics

Recurrent lower urinary tract infection

- if initial therapy fails, further therapy should be based on antibiotic susceptibility test results

Acute bacterial prostatitis

- if signs or symptoms do not abate within 7 days, therapy should be changed on the basis of antibiotic susceptibility test results

Chronic bacterial prostatitis

- if signs or symptoms have not abated within 14 days, therapy should be changed on the basis of culture and sensitivity testing data (even with correct treatment, not all symptoms may go away)

▶ How Long Should I Continue Drug Therapy?

Upper urinary tract infection (pyelonephritis)

- 14 days total (IV and PO) (Ann Intern Med 1987; 106:341–345)

Lower urinary tract infection (cystitis)

3 days

- single-dose therapy is also effective (DICP 1988;

22:21–24); however, with 3 day therapy, patients take antibiotics for the duration of their symptoms and have a slightly lower relapse rate

- use for women and children with uncomplicated urinary tract infection

7–10 days

- use a longer treatment for men (Ann Intern Med 1989;15:138–150); patients with complicated urinary tract infection, low socioeconomic status (more likely to have "silent" renal infection), urological abnormalities, and renal disease or kidney stones; diabetics or patients receiving immunosuppressive agents; and patients with a history of urinary tract infection caused by resistant organisms

If patients experience relapse

- patients require assessment for the reason for relapse (e.g., renal involvement, structural abnormalities, and chronic bacterial prostatitis)
- if the patient experiences relapse after a 3 day or 7–10 day course, treat for 2 weeks
- if the patient experiences relapse after 2 weeks, treat for 6 weeks
- if the patient experiences relapse after 6 weeks, treat for 6 months

Asymptomatic bacteriuria

- 3 days

Catheter-related bacteriuria

- 5 days

Recurrent lower urinary tract infection

- for 6 months, then stop drug administration and reassess

Acute bacterial prostatitis

- 30 days (Med Clin North Am 1991;75:405–424)

Chronic bacterial prostatitis

- 6 weeks with initial therapy
- if relapse occurs, treat for 3 months
- if relapse occurs again, treat for 6 months
- if the patient subsequently experiences relapse, chronic suppressive therapy with ciprofloxacin 250 mg PO daily is indicated

Useful References

Johnson JR, Stamm WE. Urinary tract infection in women: Diagnosis and treatment. Ann Intern Med 1989;111:906–917
Lipsky BA. Urinary tract infections in men. Epidemiology, pathophysiology, diagnosis and treatment. Ann Intern Med 1989;110:138–150
Meares EM. Prostatitis. Med Clin North Am 1991;75:405–424
Safrin S, Siegel D, Black D. Pyelonephritis in adult women: Inpatient versus outpatient therapy. Am J Med 1988;85:793–798
Seuker WO, Stahelin HB. Practical management of catheter-associated UTIs. Geriatrics 1988;43(8):43–48
Zhanel GG, Ronald AR. Single-dose versus traditional therapy for uncomplicated UTI. DICP 1988;22:21–24
Zhanel GG, Harding GKM, Guay DRP. Asymptomatic bacteriuria. Which patients should be treated? Arch Intern Med 1990:150:1389–1396
Zhanel GG, Harding GKM, Nicolle LE. Asymptomatic bacteriuria in patients with diabetes mellitus. Rev Infect Dis 1991;13:150–154

DRUG THERAPY FOR PNEUMONIA

James McCormack

▶ What Are My Goals of Treatment?

to ameliorate signs and symptoms (fever, shortness of breath, cough, and chest pain)

to prevent sepsis and death
to prevent complications such as empyema, abscess, bronchiectasis, and purulent pericarditis

▶ What Evidence Is Available to Support Drug Therapy for Pneumonia?

Mortality is associated with pneumonia

- 10% of patients admitted to a hospital with pneumonia die (Am J Med 1990;89:713–721)
- mortality increases to 40% in the elderly (Geriatrics 1990;45:49–55)

Antibiotic treatment improves outcome

- signs and symptoms of pneumonia are alleviated with appropriate antimicrobial therapy

▶ When Should I Consider Drug Therapy?

Pneumonia

- antibiotics should be given to patients presenting with a cough, dyspnea, increased sputum production, or pleuritic chest pain when associated with a radiological diagnosis of pneumonia
- although a high fever may be seen in patients presenting with pneumonia, many patients, especially the elderly, may have only a low-grade fever
- elevated white blood cell count is usually seen; however, in the elderly, immunocompromised patients, and patients with viral pneumonia, the white blood cell count may be normal or low
- prior to initiation of antibiotic therapy, a Gram stain and culture of the sputum and 2 blood cultures should be done
- a Gram stain should be considered useful for diagnosis only if polymorphonuclear neutrophils (PMNs) are abundant (>25/high-power field) and no or few (<10/high-power field) epithelial cells are seen

▶ What Drug Should I Use for Initial Treatment?

Community-acquired pneumonia

Mildly to moderately ill patients with no underlying disease states

Gram stain is not possible or unobtainable or Gram stain shows no organisms

ERYTHROMYCIN

- erythromycin is the drug of choice, as it covers the main organisms responsible for pneumonia in this patient population (*Streptococcus pneumoniae* and *Mycoplasma pneumoniae*), whereas penicillin does not cover mycoplasma
- should also be used in patients who do not present with abrupt onset of fever, chills, and pleuritic pain, which are classic signs and symptoms of bacterial pneumonia, as these patients may have atypical pneumonia (*M. pneumoniae*, *Legionella pneumophila*, or *Chlamydia pneumoniae*) (Clin Chest Med 1987;8:441–453)

AMOXICILLIN

- useful in patients with a history of intolerance to erythromycin
- amoxicillin covers most common pathogens, with the exception of *Mycoplasma*, *Legionella*, and *Chlamydia*

Gram stain shows gram-positive diplococci (Streptococcus pneumoniae)

PENICILLIN

- penicillin is the drug of choice in patients with pneumococcal pneumonia, as it is effective, well tolerated, and inexpensive

TRIMETHOPRIM-SULFAMETHOXAZOLE

- if the patient is penicillin allergic, trimethoprim-sulfamethoxazole has good activity against *Pneumococcus* and is better tolerated than erythromycin

ERYTHROMYCIN

- if the patient is allergic to penicillins and sulfa drugs

Gram stain shows gram-negative coccobacilli (Haemophilus influenzae)

CEFUROXIME AXETIL OR AMOXICILLIN-CLAVULANATE

- in many areas, the rate of ampicillin-resistant *H. influenzae* is too high to warrant the empirical use of amoxicillin in patients with a potentially life-threatening infection (pneumonia)
- even in areas with a low incidence, agents with activity against ampicillin-resistant *H. influenzae* should be used until culture and sensitivity testing results are available
- these agents also have good activity against other gram-negative organisms that may be present (e.g., *Klebsiella*)
- the decision between cefuroxime axetil and amoxicillin-clavulanate should be based on cost

TRIMETHOPRIM-SULFAMETHOXAZOLE

- if the patient is penicillin allergic, trimethoprim-sulfamethoxazole may be used as it has good activity against ampicillin-resistant *H. influenzae*
- trimethoprim-sulfamethoxazole is very inexpensive and could be chosen over cefuroxime axetil and amoxicillin-clavulanate for patients who cannot afford these agents

Mildly to moderately ill patients with underlying disease states such as alcoholism and chronic obstructive pulmonary disease (these patients have a high incidence of infections caused by gram-negative organisms)

Gram stain is not possible or unobtainable or Gram stain shows either gram-negative coccobacilli or no organisms

CEFUROXIME

- is the drug of choice, as cefuroxime has good activity against *S. pneumoniae*, ampicillin-resistant *H. influenzae*, and *Klebsiella* and is well tolerated and inexpensive when compared with other parenteral antibiotics with similar spectrum of activity

TRIMETHOPRIM-SULFAMETHOXAZOLE

- should be used if patients are truly allergic to penicillins, as it has good activity against ampicillin-resistant *H. influenzae*, *S. pneumoniae*, and *Klebsiella*

ERYTHROMYCIN WITH CIPROFLOXACIN

- should be used if the patient is allergic to both penicillins and sulfa drugs

Gram stain shows gram-positive diplococci (Streptococcus pneumoniae)

PENICILLIN

- parenteral penicillin is the drug of choice in patients with pneumococcal pneumonia, as it is effective, well tolerated, and inexpensive

TRIMETHOPRIM-SULFAMETHOXAZOLE

- if the patient is penicillin allergic, trimethoprim-sulfamethoxazole has good activity against pneumococcus and is better tolerated than erythromycin

ERYTHROMYCIN

- if the patient is allergic to both penicillin and trimethoprim-sulfamethoxazole

Gram stain shows gram-positive cocci in clusters (Staphylococcus aureus)

NAFCILLIN, CLOXACILLIN

- drugs of choice for sensitive gram-positive staphylococcal organisms, as cloxacillin and nafcillin are less expensive than vancomycin
- these agents also have good activity against *S. pneumoniae*

VANCOMYCIN

- drug of choice if patients are allergic to penicillin and/or resistant gram-positive organisms are suspected

Gram stain shows gram-negative rods

CEFUROXIME

- for cases of community-acquired pneumonia, cefuroxime covers most potential pathogens including *S. pneumoniae*, *H. influenzae*, *Klebsiella pneumoniae*, and oral anaerobes and can be used until specific organisms have been identified

TRIMETHOPRIM-SULFAMETHOXAZOLE

- if the patient is penicillin allergic, trimethoprim-sulfamethoxazole has good activity against many gram-negative organisms and has good coverage against pneumococcus

Severely ill patients

ERYTHROMYCIN PLUS CEFTRIAXONE

- useful in severely ill patient with a community-acquired pneumonia, as this combination covers most organisms and further therapy can be determined on the basis of culture and sensitivity testing results
- if gram-negative organisms are seen on Gram stain add gentamicin to ensure adequate coverage until culture and sensitivity testing results are available

Hospital-acquired pneumonia

CEFTAZIDIME

- use if the patient is ventilated and gram-negative organisms have been seen on a Gram stain
- ceftazidime should be chosen initially because it has good activity against *P. aeruginosa* and can be used until organisms have been identified
- acts against streptococcus, but has poor activity against staphylococci
- empirical therapy is very dependent on the individual institution's normal flora

TOBRAMYCIN

- tobramycin should be added to the above regimens if the patient is severely ill to ensure adequate coverage of *P. aeruginosa*

ERYTHROMYCIN

- should be added to ceftazidime until a causative organism has been identified on either culture or a good Gram stain to allow coverage of *Mycoplasma* and *Legionella* (especially if *Legionella* is common in a particular hospital or institution)

- if *Legionella* is not suspected, only add erythromycin if the patient is not responding to the above therapy

Patients with proven atypical pneumonias (*Mycoplasma, Legionella*)

ERYTHROMYCIN

- drug of choice for these infections if tolerated
- in patients who are severely ill, rifampin should be added

TETRACYCLINE, DOXYCYCLINE

- useful in patients who cannot tolerate erythromycin
- both drugs equally effective
- doxycycline has the advantages of less frequent dosing (BID for doxycycline versus QID for tetracycline) and may be taken with food
- use tetracycline in patients who cannot afford doxycycline

TRIMETHOPRIM-SULFAMETHOXAZOLE

- can be used for *Legionella* pneumonia if erythromycin or tetracycline cannot be used or tolerated

Aspiration or lung abscess

Aspiration need not be treated if the patient is not ill or there are no spreading infiltrates, as aspiration is often sterile (just observe the patient) • For aspiration, do a Gram stain, and if no organisms are seen, no antibiotics are required

PENICILLIN

- drug of choice if the pneumonia is community acquired and/or gram-positive organisms are seen on Gram stain, as it provides good coverage against gram-positive organisms and anaerobes typically found in the lung
- penicillin is also less expensive and better tolerated than clindamycin

CLINDAMYCIN

- if the patient is allergic to penicillin

CEFUROXIME

- if the patient is mildly to moderately ill and gram-negative organisms are seen on Gram stain

CLINDAMYCIN PLUS CEFOTAXIME OR CEFTRIAXONE

- if pneumonia is hospital acquired or the patient is very ill and/or if gram-negative organisms are seen on Gram stain

CLINDAMYCIN PLUS CIPROFLOXACIN

- if pneumonia is hospital acquired and the patient is penicillin allergic

▶ What Dosage Should I Use?

Community-acquired pneumonia

Mildly to moderately ill patients with no underlying disease states

ERYTHROMYCIN

- 500 mg PO QID with food or milk
- 500 mg IV Q6H if the patient needs hospitalization

AMOXICILLIN

- 500 mg PO TID
- ampicillin 500 mg IV Q6H if the patient needs hospitalization

PENICILLIN

- 500 mg–600 mg (depending on available dosage form)
- 600,000 IV Q6H if the patient needs hospitalization

TRIMETHOPRIM-SULFAMETHOXAZOLE

- 160 mg/800 mg PO BID

CEFUROXIME AXETIL

- 500 mg PO BID
- cefuroxime 750 mg IV Q8H if the patient needs hospitalization

AMOXICILLIN-CLAVULANATE

- 500 mg PO TID

Mildly to moderately ill patients with underlying disease state such as alcoholism and chronic obstructive pulmonary disease

AMPICILLIN

- 1 g IV Q6H

CEFUROXIME

- 750 mg IV Q8H

CIPROFLOXACIN

- 500 mg PO Q12H or 200 mg IV Q12H if parenteral therapy is required

PENICILLIN

- 2 million units IV Q6H

TRIMETHOPRIM-SULFAMETHOXAZOLE

- 160 mg/800 mg IV Q8H

ERYTHROMYCIN

- 500 mg IV Q6H and 1 g IV Q6H if *Legionella* is suspected

NAFCILLIN, CLOXACILLIN

- 1 g IV Q6H

VANCOMYCIN

- 15 mg/kg IV Q12H

Severely ill patients

ERYTHROMYCIN

- 1 g IV Q6H

CEFTRIAXONE

- 2 g IV Q24H

GENTAMICIN

- 2 mg/kg IV Q8H

Hospital-acquired pneumonia

CEFTAZIDIME

- 1 g IV Q8H
- 2 g IV Q8H if severe

TOBRAMYCIN

- 2 mg/kg IV Q8H

ERYTHROMYCIN

- 1 g IV Q6H

Patients with proven atypical pneumonias (*Mycoplasma, Legionella*)

ERYTHROMYCIN

- 500 mg PO QID if the patient is moderately ill (1 g PO QID if *Legionella* is suspected)
- 500 mg IV Q6H if the patient is severely ill (1 g IV Q6H if *Legionella* is suspected)

TETRACYCLINE

- 500 mg PO QID if the patient is moderately ill
- 500 mg IV Q6H if the patient is severely ill

DOXYCYCLINE

- 100 mg PO BID if the patient is moderately ill
- 100 mg IV Q12H if the patient is severely ill

TRIMETHOPRIM-SULFAMETHOXAZOLE

- 160 mg/800 mg PO BID if the patient is moderately ill
- 160 mg/800 mg IV Q8H if the patient is severely ill

Aspiration or lung abscess

PENICILLIN

- 2 million units IV Q4H

CLINDAMYCIN

- 600 mg IV Q8H
- 900 mg IV Q8H if the condition is severe

CEFUROXIME

- 750 mg IV Q8H

CEFOTAXIME

- 1 g IV Q8H
- 2 g IV Q8H if the condition is severe

CEFTRIAXONE

- 1 g IV Q24H
- 2 g IV Q24H if the condition is severe

CIPROFLOXACIN

- 500 mg PO Q12H or 200 mg IV Q12H if parenteral therapy is required

▶ How Long Should I Treat with My Initial Regimen?

Pneumonia

- initially, treat for 48–72 hours, and base further therapy on the assessment of clinical improvement and culture and sensitivity testing results

▶ What Efficacy Parameters Should I Follow and How Frequently Do I Have to Assess My Patient?

Pneumonia

Signs and symptoms

- evaluate signs and symptoms such as cough, dyspnea, and temperature daily if parenteral therapy is required or follow up at 48–72 hours after the start of therapy if oral antibiotics are being used
- for severely ill patients, monitor cough, dyspnea, temperature, and blood pressure Q6H for 3 days

Microbiological findings

- sputum and blood samples for Gram stain, cultures, and sensitivity testing should be obtained before starting antibiotic administration
- culture results are much more reliable if they are consistent with Gram stain findings and if the associated Gram stain was of good quality
- Gram stain results can be found out immediately and can guide empirical antibiotic treatment
- identification of the organism can be made within 24–36 hours, and sensitivities should be known within 48–60 hours
- repeat cultures only if patient does not respond or symptoms return

Chest X-ray

- initial chest X-ray aids in diagnosis
- focal findings suggest a bacterial infection
- diffuse infiltrates suggest infection with a virus or *Mycoplasma*
- repeat X-ray only if patient does not respond or symptoms return

White blood cell count

- initial white blood cell count helps in diagnosis

Immunoglobulin assay for *Mycoplasma*

- if *Mycoplasma* is suspected, order immunoglobulin assay
- cold agglutinins are often absent in mild *Mycoplasma* infections

Arterial blood gas values

- assess in the severely ill patient, and repeat on the basis of results

▶ Should I Add Another Drug or Substitute Therapy If My Initial Drug Therapy Fails?

Pneumonia

Patients who fail to respond after 24–48 hours of antibiotic therapy

- further antibiotic treatment should be based on culture and sensitivity testing results
- if antibiotic therapy is appropriate (on the basis of culture and sensitivity testing), continue therapy, as some cases of pneumonia may take 4–5 days to respond
- in patients who remain sick despite negative Gram stain and cultures, add erythromycin 500 mg PO QID to cover *Mycoplasma* and *Legionella*
- also need to consider rare pathogens such as fungi and tuberculosis and the need for invasive diagnostic techniques

▶ How Long Should I Continue Drug Therapy?

Pneumonia

- if the patient responds rapidly, a 10 day course of therapy is sufficient
- oral antibiotics should be considered after the patient has clinically improved and has been afebrile for 48 hours
- if the patient responds slowly or has a pneumonia caused by gram-negative organisms, *Mycoplasma,* or *Legionella,* a 14 day course of therapy should be given (Clin Chest Med 1991;12:237–242, Ann Intern Med 1987; 106:341–345)
- a pneumonia caused by *Legionella* may require 3 weeks of treatment if patient responds slowly

Useful References

Pomilla PV, Brown RB. Outpatient treatment of community acquired pneumonia. Arch Intern Med 1994;154:1793–1802
Rodnick JE, Gude JK. Diagnosis and antibiotic treatment of community acquired pneumonia. West J Med 1991 154:405–409

DRUG THERAPY FOR INTRAABDOMINAL INFECTIONS

David R. P. Guay

▶ What Are My Goals of Treatment?

to prevent systemic infectious complications, including multiple organ system failure

to minimize local spread of the infection

to amalgamate drug therapy effectively with nondrug therapeutic measures (abscess drainage via percutaneous or laparotomy approach, surgical repair of perforated bowel and injured organs), as adequate drainage or debridement is of paramount importance

▶ What Evidence Is Available to Support Drug Therapy for Intraabdominal Infections?

To prevent systemic infectious complications

- reduces the chance of clinical sepsis, multiple organ system failure, and death

To minimize local spread of infection

- early therapy for primary (spontaneous) and secondary bacterial peritonitis and cholecystitis or cholangitis reduces mortality rate and systemic infectious complications, including empyema and pericholecystic abscess formation (Emerg Med Clin North Am 1989;7:611–629, Hepatology 1983;3:545–549)

▶ When Should I Consider Drug Therapy?

Intraabdominal infections

Spontaneous bacterial peritonitis (in cirrhotic patients)

- treat patients with fever, abdominal tenderness (may be absent), leukocytosis, and hypoactive bowel sounds
- diagnosis is confirmed with a peritoneal puncture showing more than 500 white blood cells per milliliter or more than 200 PMN/mL of ascitic fluid with a pH of 7.35
- always do a Gram stain on spun fluid to help with the antibiotic choice

Secondary bacterial peritonitis

- treat patients with diffuse abdominal tenderness, fever, reduced bowel sounds, and leukocytosis

Abdominal trauma

- treat any patient with a penetrating abdominal wound

Gangrenous or perforated appendix

- treat any patient with fever, leukocytosis, and diffuse abdominal pain

Cholecystitis or cholangitis

- treat any patient with fever, right upper quadrant abdominal pain, leukocytosis and ultrasonographic evidence of gallstones, thickened gallbladder wall or dilated gallbladder or bile ducts, or biochemical evidence of cholestasis (e.g., increased alkaline phosphatase or gammaglutamyl transferase levels or conjugated hyperbilirubinemia)

▶ What Drug Should I Use for Initial Treatment?

Intraabdominal infections

Spontaneous bacterial peritonitis (in cirrhotic patients)

AMPICILLIN PLUS CEFOTAXIME OR CEFTRIAXONE

- covers enterococci, Enterobacteriaceae, and aerobic streptococci
- decision between cefotaxime and ceftriaxone is based on cost
- ampicillin plus an aminoglycoside may be used; however, some studies suggest an increased incidence of nephrotoxicity in cirrhotic patients receiving aminoglycosides, but this is not yet clearly delineated (Gastroenterology 1982;82:97–105, Hepatology 1985;5:457–462)

VANCOMYCIN PLUS CIPROFLOXACIN

- if the patient is penicillin allergic

Secondary bacterial peritonitis, abdominal trauma, gangrenous or perforated appendix, and cholecystitis or cholangitis

METRONIDAZOLE PLUS GENTAMICIN

- provides excellent coverage against anaerobes and gram-negative organisms and is usually less expensive than cefoxitin, cefotetan, or ceftizoxime or clindamycin plus gentamicin

CEFOXITIN, CEFOTETAN, CEFTIZOXIME

- if the risk of renal impairment from aminoglycoside is high (in cases of elderly patients, preexisting renal failure, otic or vestibular dysfunction, and previous aminoglycoside treatment), one of these agents should be chosen
- decision among these agents should be based on cost and the frequency of dosing

CLINDAMYCIN PLUS GENTAMICIN

- although this regimen is as effective as metronidazole and gentamicin, clindamycin is usually more expensive than metronidazole and clindamycin causes diarrhea and occasionally pseudomembranous colitis

AMPICILLIN

- Add to the above regimens for enterococcal coverage if enterococcus is the predominant organism seen on culture

IMIPENEM/CILASTATIN

- use if the patient has had multiple surgical procedures during the present hospital admission because such patients are at higher risk for infection with hospital-acquired pathogens
- use in combination with gentamicin in life-threatening infections

PIPERACILLIN

- likely as effective as cefoxitin, cefotetan, or ceftizoxime but must be dosed more frequently (Q4H), which makes it inconvenient to use
- provides adequate coverage against enterococcus, which, if needed, provides a useful advantage over cefoxitin, ceftizoxime, or cefotetan
- also covers *P. aeruginosa;* however, this pathogen is not usually seen in bowel flora

▶ What Dosage Should I Use?

Intraabdominal infections

AMPICILLIN

- 1 g IV Q6H
- 2 g IV Q6H if the condition is severe

CEFOTAXIME

- 1 g IV Q8H
- 2 g IV Q8H if the condition is severe

CEFTRIAXONE

- 1 g IV Q24H
- 2 g IV Q24 if the condition is severe

VANCOMYCIN

- 1 g IV Q12H

CIPROFLOXACIN

- 200 mg IV Q12H
- 400 mg IV Q8H if the condition is severe

GENTAMICIN

- 1.5 mg/kg Q8H
- 2 mg/kg Q8H if the condition is severe

METRONIDAZOLE

- 500 mg IV Q8H

CLINDAMYCIN

- 600 mg IV Q8H
- 900 mg IV Q8H if the condition is severe

CEFOXITIN

- 1 g IV Q6H
- 2 g IV Q6H if the condition is severe

CEFOTETAN

- 1 g IV Q12H
- 2 g IV Q12H if the condition is severe

CEFTIZOXIME

- 1 g IV Q8H
- 2 g IV Q8H if the condition is severe

IMIPENEM/CILASTATIN

- 0.5 g IV Q6H
- 1 g IV Q6H if the condition is severe

PIPERACILLIN

- 2 g IV Q4H
- 3 g IV Q4H if the condition is severe

▶ How Long Should I Treat with My Initial Regimen?

Intraabdominal infections

- initially, treat for 48–72 hours, and base further therapy on the assessment of clinical improvement and culture and sensitivity testing results

▶ What Efficacy Parameters Should I Follow and How Frequently Do I Have to Assess My Patient?

Intraabdominal infections

Clinical response

- diminution of abdominal pain, reduction in fever and abdominal tenderness, lack of purulent discharge, and return of bowel sounds.
- initially, the patient should be assessed twice daily
- after the patient is stabilized, daily examination should guide evaluation of the patient's status

White blood cell count

- initial white blood cell count helps in diagnosis

Microbiological findings

- tailor empirical therapy to culture and sensitivity testing results
- repeated cultures are necessary only if the clinical response is inadequate or suppurative complications occur

Ascitic fluid

- in spontaneous bacterial peritonitis (ascites), follow the patient clinically and repeat the peritoneal puncture only if treatment failure is suspected

▶ Should I Add Another Drug or Substitute Therapy If My Initial Drug Therapy Fails?

Intraabdominal infections

Spontaneous bacterial peritonitis

- subsequent therapy should be based on culture and sensitivity testing results of initial or repeated paracentesis specimens

Secondary bacterial peritonitis

- if initial therapy fails, a laparotomy or a paracentesis should be conducted to obtain fluid for culture and sensitivity testing
- changes in therapy are guided by culture and sensitivity testing results

Abdominal trauma

- if initial therapy fails to resolve symptoms, a swab of the abdominal wound and paracentesis (under ultrasonographic guidance) or laparotomy to obtain specimens for culture and sensitivity testing should be done and further therapy should be based on the results of this testing

Gangrenous or perforated appendix

- add coverage for enterococcus (ampicillin), and perform a radiological test to determine the absence of abscess formation

Cholecystitis or cholangitis

- a radiological test should be conducted to confirm the diagnosis
- if the diagnosis is verified, surgical treatment should be performed rather than altering drug therapy

▶ How Long Should I Continue Drug Therapy?

Intraabdominal infections

Oral antibiotics should be considered after the patient has clinically improved and has been afebrile for 48 hours.

Spontaneous bacterial peritonitis, secondary bacterial peritonitis, abdominal trauma, gangrenous or perforated appendix, and cholecystitis or cholangitis

- treatment should continue for a minimum of 10 days; however, extend therapy if the patient has not been asymptomatic for longer than 72 hours

Useful References

Hackford AW. Intra-abdominal sepsis: A medical-surgical dilemma. Clin Ther 1990;12(suppl B):43–53

Levison ME, Bush LM. Peritonitis and other intra-abdominal infections. In: Mandell GL, Douglas RG Jr, Bennett JE, eds. Principles and Practice of Infectious Diseases, 3rd ed. New York: Churchill Livingstone, 1990: 636–670

Macho JR, Meyer AA. Management of sepsis following injury. Crit Care Clin 1986;2:869–876

Tam J, Guglielmo BI. Microbiology and antibiotics in infectious abdominal emergencies. Emerg Med Clin North Am 1989;7:611–629

DRUG THERAPY FOR INFECTIVE ENDOCARDITIS

John C. Rotschafer

▶ What Are My Goals of Treatment?

to eradicate the infection and to sterilize the infected site

to prevent or limit heart valve damage

to prevent the development or worsening of congestive heart failure and conduction defects

to prevent embolic sequelae of infectious endocarditis

to prevent endocarditis by using appropriate prophylaxis

▶ What Evidence Is Available to Support Drug Therapy for Endocarditis?

Mortality

- in the preantibiotic era, infective endocarditis was a universally fatal disease
- even with aggressive antibiotic therapy, surgery, and cardiac valve replacement, infective endocarditis still has a 10–80% mortality, depending on the underlying pathogen (Principles and Practice of Infectious Diseases 1990: 670–706, Rev Infect Dis 1987;9:891–907, JAMA 1989; 261:1471–1477)

Prophylaxis

- precise risk of endovascular infection associated with particular cardiac defects is not known, and randomized, controlled clinical trials involving the broad scope of patients thought to be affected have not been undertaken to determine the risks and benefits of prophylaxis
- 1 study in patients with prosthetic cardiac valves was successful in demonstrating the efficacy of prophylaxis (Z Kardiol 1986;75:8–11)
- it has been estimated that, even if prophylaxis is completely effective, fewer than 10% of cases of endocarditis can be prevented (Ann Intern Med 1991;114:803–804), and it is generally accepted that antibiotic prophylaxis for bacterial endocarditis is primarily indicated for moderate- to high-risk patients

▶ When Should I Consider Drug Therapy?

Suspected or proven infective endocarditis

If the patient is not acutely ill and not in congestive heart failure

- wait for culture results before starting specific antibiotic administration, except for patients with classic signs of endocarditis (Osler's nodes, splinter hemorrhages, and Janeway's lesions) to prevent the chance of ongoing valvular damage or septic emboli

If the patient is acutely ill or has cardiac or neurological complications

- antibiotic therapy should be started immediately after culture specimens have been obtained

Bacterial endocarditis prophylaxis

- prophylaxis should be used in patients with cardiac conditions known to place patients at risk (mitral valve prolapse with regurgitation, an indwelling nonnative cardiac valve, a previous history of endocarditis, a history of congential heart malformations, surgically constructed systemic-pulmonary shunts, and cardiomyopathy) who are undergoing certain dental, medical, or surgical procedures known to place the patient at risk for bacterial endocarditis (Circulation 1991; 83:1174–1178)
- dental or surgical procedures known to place these patients at risk for bacterial endocarditis include tonsillectomy and/or adenoidectomy, rigid (not flexible) bronchoscopy, esophageal dilatation or sclerotherapy, professional cleaning of teeth or any dental procedure likely to induce gingival bleeding, surgical procedures of respiratory or intestinal mucosa, gallbladder surgery, vaginal hysterectomy, vaginal delivery in which there is evidence of infection, procedures to incise and drain infected areas of the body, prostatic surgery, cystoscopy, and urethral dilatation or catheterization when a urinary tract infection is present

▶ What Drugs Should I Use for Initial Treatment?

Suspected or proven infective endocarditis

If the patient is not acutely ill and not in congestive heart failure

Therapy after culture and sensitivity testing results are known

(JAMA 1989;261:1471–1477)

PENICILLIN G

- for penicillin-sensitive streptococci (minimum inhibitory concentration [MIC] < 0.1 mg/L) if the patient is 65 years or older or has renal or auditory impairment and no prosthetic valve

PENICILLIN G AND GENTAMICIN

- for penicillin-sensitive streptococci (MIC < 0.1 mg/L) if the patient is younger than 65 years and has no renal or auditory impairment
- for intermediately sensitive streptococci (MIC 0.1–1.0 mg/L)
- for penicillin-sensitive enterococci
- for penicillin-sensitive diphtheroids (JK diphtheroids, a frequent cause of endocarditis, are often penicillin-resistant and need vancomycin)
- for culture-negative cases

CLOXACILLIN OR NAFCILLIN

- for penicillin-resistant *S. aureus*
- addition of gentamicin has reduced the time of bacteremia but not morbidity (Ann Intern Med 1988;109:619–624)
- there are no trials to show that cefazolin is as good as cloxacillin or nafcillin, and cefazolin may penetrate vegetations less well

VANCOMYCIN

- for penicillin-resistant diphtheroids
- for penicillin-sensitive streptococci (MIC < 0.1 mg/L) and a history of an immediate-type hypersensitivity reaction to penicillin
- for methicillin-resistant *S. aureus* with a native valve
- for *S. aureus* and a history of an immediate-type hypersensitivity reaction to penicillin

VANCOMYCIN AND GENTAMICIN

- for methicillin-resistant *S. aureus* with a prosthetic valve

- for penicillinase-producing enterococcus
- if the patient has a history of an immediate-type hypersensitivity reaction to penicillin and has penicillin-sensitive streptococci (MIC < 0.1 mg/L) or if the patient is younger than 65 years and has no renal or auditory impairment
- penicillin-resistant streptococci (MIC ≥ 2.0 mg/L)
- gentamicin-sensitive diphtheroids
- culture-negative endocarditis if the patient has a history of an immediate-type hypersensitivity reaction to penicillin

VANCOMYCIN AND RIFAMPIN AND GENTAMICIN

- for methicillin-resistant *S. aureus* or *S. epidermidis* if the patient does not respond to vancomycin and gentamicin
- if staphylococcus is resistant to gentamicin, use another aminoglycoside, and if it is resistant to all aminoglycosides, omit aminoglycosides

CEFTRIAXONE

- for sensitive gram-negative organisms
- because therapy is for 4–6 weeks, ceftriaxone is recommended because of the ease of administration (once daily) versus that of cefotaxime (3 times daily)

CEFTAZIDIME AND TOBRAMYCIN

- if *P. aeruginosa* is present

METRONIDAZOLE

- for anaerobes such as *Bacteroides fragilis;* however, this is rare

AMPHOTERICIN AND FLUCYTOSINE

- for fungal endocarditis
- always needs surgery

If the patient is acutely ill or has cardiovascular or neurological complications

- antibiotics should be started immediately after cultures have been drawn

Native valve endocarditis

PENICILLIN G AND GENTAMICIN

- if the patient is 65 years or older or has auditory or renal dysfunction, just use penicillin
- if the patient is allergic to penicillin, substitute vancomycin for penicillin G; however, skin testing and potential desensitization should be considered, as the patient needs to be treated for an extended period and penicillin is less toxic and less expensive than vancomycin

New valvular insufficiency or suspected intravenous drug abuser

VANCOMYCIN AND GENTAMICIN

- vancomycin should be used until culture and sensitivity testing results are known because of the potential for methicillin-resistant staphylococcal organisms
- also useful if the patient is penicillin allergic
- substitute cloxacillin or nafcillin or penicillin for vancomycin after sensitivities are known if the organism is sensitive to one of these agents

Prosthetic valve endocarditis

VANCOMYCIN AND GENTAMICIN

- as above

Bacterial endocarditis prophylaxis

Dental, oral, or respiratory tract procedures

Patients able to tolerate oral medications

- amoxicillin

Patients able to tolerate oral medications but allergic to penicillins

- erythromycin

Patients unable to tolerate oral medications

- ampicillin

Patients unable to tolerate oral medications and allergic to penicillins

- vancomycin

Genitourinary or gastrointestinal procedures

Patients not allergic to penicillins

- ampicillin and gentamicin

Patients allergic to penicillins

- vancomycin and gentamicin

▶ What Dosage Should I Use?

Suspected or proven infective endocarditis

For all patients, whether acutely ill or not

PENICILLIN G

- 4 million units IV Q4H (5 million units IV Q4H for intermediately sensitive streptococci)

CLOXACILLIN OR NAFCILLIN

- 2 g IV Q4H

GENTAMICIN, TOBRAMYCIN

- 1 mg/kg IV Q8H
- low doses required because only using with beta-lactams or vancomycin for synergy against enterococci or staphylococci
- low doses should also be used because an aminoglycoside may be needed for up to 2–4 weeks, and it is best to use a low dose to minimize toxicity

VANCOMYCIN

- 15 mg/kg IV Q12H

RIFAMPIN

- 600 mg PO Q24H

CEFTRIAXONE

- 2 g IV Q24H

CEFTAZIDIME

- 2 g IV Q8H

METRONIDAZOLE

- 500 mg IV Q8H

AMPHOTERICIN

- common maintenance dosage is 0.6 mg/kg/d
- maximum daily dosage of 1 mg/kg in severe infections (as tolerated by the patient)

FLUCYTOSINE

- 37.5 mg/kg PO Q6H (rounded to nearest 500 mg)

Bacterial endocarditis prophylaxis

Dental, oral, or respiratory tract procedures

Patients able to tolerate oral medications

AMOXICILLIN

- 3 g PO 1 hour before the procedure and 1.5 g PO 6 hours after the first dose

Patients able to tolerate oral medications but allergic to penicillins

ERYTHROMYCIN

- 1000 mg PO 2 hours before the procedure and 500 mg PO 6 hours after the first dose

Patients unable to tolerate oral medications

AMPICILLIN

- 2 g IV or IM 30 minutes before the procedure or at induction of anesthesia and 1 g IV or IM 6 hours after the first dose

Patients unable to tolerate oral medications and allergic to penicillins

VANCOMYCIN

- 1 g IV 1 hour prior to the procedure

Genitourinary or gastrointestinal procedures

Patients not allergic to penicillins

AMPICILLIN

- 2 g IV or IM 30 minutes before the procedure or at induction of anesthesia and amoxicillin 1.5 g 6 hours after the first dose (ampicillin 2 g IV can be used if the patient is not able to take amoxicillin by mouth)

GENTAMICIN

- 1.5 mg/kg (maximum 80 mg) IV or IM 30 minutes before the procedure

Patients allergic to penicillins

VANCOMYCIN

- 1 g IV 1 hour prior to the procedure

GENTAMICIN

- 1.5 mg/kg (maximum 80 mg) IV 1 hour prior to the procedure

▶ *How Long Should I Treat with My Initial Regimen?*

Suspected or proven infective endocarditis

- may take 5–7 days to see a decrease in fever and sterile blood cultures
- precise identification of the causative organism may permit changes in antibiotic choice

▶ *What Efficacy Parameters Should I Follow and How Frequently Do I Have to Assess My Patient?*

Suspected or proven infective endocarditis

Blood cultures

- always obtain 3 blood cultures prior to antibiotic therapy
- identity of the bacterial pathogens and results of antibiotic susceptibility studies should be available within 72 hours
- in a patient who becomes afebrile, further cultures during therapy need not be obtained because, even in patients who respond to therapy, blood cultures can remain positive for at least 5–7 days after the initiation of antibiotic administration
- if the patient remains febrile after 4 days, repeat cultures if the organism remains unknown
- after the completion of antibiotic therapy, 1 set of blood cultures should be obtained 1 month after therapy to document blood sterility

Temperature

- measure temperature Q6H; however, remember that patients may remain febrile with positive blood cultures throughout the first week of therapy

Heart murmur

- change could indicate valvular damage

Signs of congestive heart failure

- should be checked on a daily basis

Neurological status

- examination should be performed on a daily basis

Blood pressure

- widening pulse pressure suggests valvular insufficiency

Serum bactericidal titers

- not needed if infection is caused by sensitive streptococci
- should be obtained if organisms are resistant or tolerant to one of the drugs being used, or if the patient is having a poor clinical response
- serum bactericidal titers should be greater than 1:8 at the time of the peak antibiotic concentration (Am J Med 1975;58:209–215, N Engl J Med 1985;312:968–974, Am J Med 1985;78:262–269, Am J Med 1982;73:260–267)
- if they are not, increase the dosage if the dosage can safely be increased; if not, change the drug

Echocardiogram

- not a useful outcome measure, unless it is indicated by factors suggesting valve damage and the need for surgery such as a change in murmurs or cardiac failure
- most useful for identifying native valve endocarditis and is of limited value in prosthetic heart valve endocarditis (Principles and Practice of Infectious Diseases 1990: 670–706) because of echo distortion
- echocardiography can detect valve vegetations of greater than 2 mm
- sensitivity of the procedure has varied from less than 50% to greater than 90% and false-positive studies are rare, but a normal echocardiogram does not rule out infective endocarditis; however, an esophageal echocardiogram is of greater sensitivity and specificity
- new diagnostic criteria have been proposed and suggest using transesophageal echo as part of the diagnostic criteria and to identify when surgery is necessary (Infect Dis Clin North Am 1993;7:1–8)

Bacterial endocarditis prophylaxis

- no efficacy variables to follow other than the absence of signs and symptoms of endocarditis

▶ *Should I Add Another Drug or Substitute Therapy If My Initial Drug Therapy Fails?*

Suspected or proven infective endocarditis

Addition of other antibiotics

- addition of adjunctive antibiotics should be considered on a case by case basis
- patients with lack of response to appropriate antibiotic therapy and/or with worsening signs of congestive heart failure should be evaluated for possible surgery and/or valve replacement

RIFAMPIN

- add rifampin if the patient has an intracellular (PMN) staphylococcal infection, a prosthetic valve is present, staphylococcal tolerance (minimum bactericidal concentration [MBC]/MIC ratio > 32) is suspected, or the patient is rapidly deteriorating; however, there is little evidence that this helps (A Textbook for the Clinical Application of Therapeutic Drug Monitoring 1986:353–363, Ann Intern Med 1991;115:674–680)

- serum inhibitory and bactericidal titers should be done while the patient remains on single antibiotic therapy, and these tests are repeated after the rifampin is added and has reached steady state levels
- rifampin use should be questioned if a 2-fold or greater improvement in serum bactericidal titer is not seen (A Textbook for the Clinical Application of Therapeutic Drug Monitoring 1986:353–363)
- potential for adverse drug reactions to rifampin should be factored into the decision to use this drug

▶ *How Long Should I Continue Drug Therapy?*

Suspected or proven infective endocarditis

PENICILLIN G

- 4 weeks for penicillin-sensitive streptococci (MIC < 0.1 mg/L) if the patient is 65 years or older or has renal or auditory impairment and no prosthetic valve

PENICILLIN G AND GENTAMICIN

- 2 weeks (gentamicin for 2 weeks) for penicillin-sensitive streptococci (MIC < 0.1 mg/L) if the patient is younger than 65 years and has no renal or auditory impairment
- 4 weeks (6 weeks if there is a prosthetic valve, symptoms for longer than 3 months, or negative culture) plus gentamicin for 2 weeks for penicillin-sensitive streptococci (MIC < 0.1 mg/L)
- 4 weeks for both drugs for intermediately sensitive streptococci (MIC 0.1–1.0 mg/L), enterococci, and penicillin-sensitive diphtheroids

CLOXACILLIN OR NAFCILLIN

- 4 weeks for penicillin-resistant *S. aureus*
- some clinicians suggest that the duration of therapy for right-sided *S. aureus* endocarditis be 4 weeks and that left-sided *S. aureus* endocarditis be treated for 4–6 weeks, depending on the clinical response (Infect Dis Clin North Am 1993;7:53–68)

VANCOMYCIN

- 4 weeks for methicillin-resistant *S. aureus* with native valve, penicillin-sensitive streptococci (MIC < 0.1 mg/L) and a history of an immediate-type hypersensitivity reaction to penicillin, and *S. aureus* and a history of an immediate-type hypersensitivity reaction to penicillin
- some clinicians suggest that the duration of therapy for right-sided *S. aureus* endocarditis be 4 weeks and that left-sided *S. aureus* endocarditis be treated for 4–6 weeks, depending on the clinical response (Infect Dis Clin North Am 1993;7:53–68)
- 6 weeks for penicillin-resistant diphtheroids

VANCOMYCIN AND GENTAMICIN

- 4 weeks for both drugs for penicillinase-producing enterococcus, intermediately or penicillin-resistant streptococci (MIC ≥ 0.1 mg/L), enterococci, penicillin-sensitive diphtheroids, or negative cultures in patients with a history of an immediate-type hypersensitivity to penicillin
- 4 weeks for vancomycin (2 weeks for gentamicin) for penicillin-sensitive streptococci (MIC < 0.1 mg/L) if the patient is younger than 65 years and has no renal or auditory impairment

- 6 weeks (gentamicin for 2 weeks) for methicillin-resistant *S. aureus* if there is a prosthetic valve

VANCOMYCIN, RIFAMPIN, AND GENTAMICIN

- 6 weeks (gentamicin for 2 weeks) for methicillin-resistant *S. aureus* or *S. epidermidis* if the patient does not respond to vancomycin and gentamicin

CETAZIDIME OR CEFTRIAXONE AND GENTAMICIN OR TOBRAMYCIN

- 6 weeks total therapy for gram-negative organisms
- if *P. aeruginosa* is the causative organism, continue therapy with the aminoglycoside for the full 6 weeks unless toxicity occurs
- for other gram-negative organisms, the aminoglycoside may be stopped after 2 weeks
- once the bacterial load is decreased and the patient has clinically improved, for patients in whom the organism is sensitive, guinolones may be used to facilitate outpatient therapy

METRONIDAZOLE

- 6 weeks for anaerobes such as *B. fragilis*

AMPHOTERICIN AND FLUCYTOSINE

- 6–8 weeks for fungi

Useful References

Bisno AL, Dismukes WE, Durack DT, et al. Antimicrobial treatment of infective endocarditis due to viridans streptococci, enterococci, and staphylococci. JAMA 1989;261:1471–1477

Dajani AS, Bisno AL, Chung KJ. et al. Prevention of bacterial endocarditis. JAMA 1990;264:2919–2922

Korzeniowski O, Sande MA. Combination antimicrobial therapy for *Staphylococcus aureus* endocarditis in patients addicted to parenteral drugs and in nonaddicts. Ann Intern Med 1982;97:496–503

Levine DP. Slow response to vancomycin or vancomycin plus rifampin in methicillin-resistant *Staphylococcus aureus* endocarditis. Ann Intern Med 1991;115:674–680

Rotschafer JC. Vancomycin. In: Taylor WJ, Caviness MHD, eds. A Textbook for the Clinical Application of Therapeutic Drug Monitoring. Irving, TX: Abbott Laboratories, 1986:353–363

Scheld WM, Sande MA. Endocarditis and intravascular infection. In: Mandell GI, Douglas RG Jr, Bennett JE, eds. Principles and Practice of Infectious Diseases, 3rd ed. New York: Churchill Livinstone, 1990: 670–706

Wilson WR, Steckleberg JM, eds. Infective endocarditis. Infect Dis Clin North Am 1993;7:1–170

DRUG THERAPY FOR MENINGITIS

James McCormack

▶ *What Are My Goals of Treatment?*

to ameliorate signs and symptoms
to start antibiotic administration rapidly to prevent the development of seizures, deafness, focal neurological sequelae, coma, and death

▶ *What Evidence Is Available to Support Drug Therapy for Meningitis?*

Mortality is associated with meningitis

- mortality from meningitis is high: *S. pneumoniae* (26%), *Neisseria meningitidis* (10%), and *H. influenzae* (6%) (JAMA 1985;253:1749–1754)

Antibiotic treatment improves outcome

- signs and symptoms of meningitis are alleviated with appropriate antimicrobial therapy, and complications are reduced

Sepsis and death are prevented

- cure rates of up to 95% are seen when third-generation cephalosporins are used to treat gram-negative meningitis (Am J Med 1981;71:693–703)

▶ *When Should I Consider Drug Therapy?*

Meningitis

- antibiotics should be given to all patients presenting with a fever, headache, meningism (nuchal rigidity, Brudzinski's sign, or Kernig's sign), and signs of cerebral dysfunction with cerebrospinal fluid (CSF) showing elevated opening pressure (usually >300 mmH$_2$O), elevated white blood cell count (>100/mm^3), increased protein levels (>50 mg/dL), and decreased glucose level (<40 mg/dL)
- in the elderly, fever and altered mental status are the main symptoms of meningitis, although patients can have signs of meningeal irritation (Geriatrics 1990;45:63–75)
- empirical antibiotic administration should be started as soon as possible after a Gram stain of the CSF is obtained
- if there is a clinical suspicion of bacterial meningitis and there is any delay in doing a lumbar puncture (even 30–60 minutes), the first dose of an antibiotic should not be withheld (the first dose has little effect on the evaluation of the CSF)
- in stable patients with a CSF examination that shows no organisms, normal protein and glucose levels, and only a slightly elevated white blood cell count, antibiotics can likely be withheld and a second examination of the CSF can be done in 6–12 hours (if a repeated CSF examination shows increased white blood cell count or decreasing glucose level or the clinical status of the patient worsens, empirical antibiotic therapy should be started)
- Gram stain of the CSF can identify the organism in 50–90% of cases
- cultures should be done and are positive in 80% of patients
- blood cultures should also be obtained

▶ *What Drug Should I Use for Initial Treatment?*

Meningitis

Gram stain results are not yet available or Gram stain shows no organisms

AMPICILLIN PLUS CEFOTAXIME OR CEFTRIAXONE

- ampicillin covers *S. pneumoniae* and *N. meningitidis*, *Listeria monocytogenes*, and ampicillin-sensitive *H. influenzae*, which are the most common organisms in the adult patient population
- use in conjunction with cefotaxime or ceftriaxone, especially in adults 50 years or older or patients with a history of head injury, concurrent sinusitis, otitis media, pneumonia or epiglottitis, diabetes, alcoholism, or hypogammaglobulinemia to cover ampicillin-resistant *H. influenzae* and other gram-negative organisms that may be present (Infect Dis Clin North Am 1990;4:645–659)
- decision between cefotaxime and ceftriaxone should be based on cost and the frequency of administration

CHLORAMPHENICOL

- drug of choice in patients truly allergic to penicillins and cephalosporins, as it covers most of the potential causative organisms

VANCOMYCIN

- use in patients with suspected shunt infections to cover either *S. aureus* or *S. epidermidis* until culture and sensitivity testing results are known

VANCOMYCIN PLUS CEFTAZIDIME

- use in patients who are severely ill with suspected shunt infections to cover *S. aureus*, *S. epidermidis*, and gram-negative organisms (*Pseudomonas* possible) until culture and sensitivity testing results are known

Gram stain shows gram-positive diplococci (*Streptococcus pneumoniae*) or gram-negative diplococci (*Neisseria meningitidis*)

PENICILLIN

- penicillin is the drug of choice in patients with pneumococcal or meningococcal meningitis, as it is effective, well tolerated, and inexpensive

CHLORAMPHENICOL

- if the patient is truly allergic to penicillins and cephalosporins, chloramphenicol has good activity against pneumococcus and has good penetration into the CSF

Gram stain shows gram-negative organisms

CEFOTAXIME, CEFTRIAXONE

- good CSF penetration and good activity against most potential gram-negative organisms
- decision between these agents should be based on cost

CEFTAZIDIME PLUS TOBRAMYCIN

- if *P. aeruginosa* is suspected or proven, this combination should be used because cefotaxime does not have good activity against *P. aeruginosa*

CHLORAMPHENICOL

- choose as empirical therapy if the patient is truly allergic to penicillins or cephalosporins
- patient should then be desensitized to penicillins so that a third-generation cephalosporin may be used, as chloramphenicol is often not very active against some gram-negative organisms

Gram stain shows gram-positive cocci in clusters (*Staphylococcus aureus* or *S. epidermidis*)

VANCOMYCIN

- although cloxacillin or nafcillin can be effective, these agents should not be used until sensitivities have been determined

Gram stain shows gram-positive rods

AMPICILLIN

- active against *L. monocytogenes*

TRIMETHOPRIM-SULFAMETHOXAZOLE

- if the patient is penicillin allergic

Further antibiotic treatment should be based on culture and sensitivity testing results

▶ *What Dosage Should I Use?*

Meningitis

AMPICILLIN

- 2 g IV Q4H

CEFOTAXIME

- 2 g IV Q8H

CEFTRIAXONE

- 2 g IV as a first dose, then 1 g IV Q12H until the patient is stable, then switch the dosage to 2 g IV Q24H

CHLORAMPHENICOL

- 2 g IV Q6H

VANCOMYCIN

- 20 mg/kg IV Q12H

PENICILLIN

- 4 million units IV Q4H

TRIMETHOPRIM-SULFAMETHOXAZOLE

- 10 mg/kg (trimethoprim component) daily IV divided Q8H

CEFTAZIDIME

- 2 g IV Q8H

TOBRAMYCIN

- 2 mg/kg IV Q8H

▶ *How Long Should I Treat with My Initial Regimen?*

Meningitis

- initially, treat for 48–72 hours, and base further therapy on the assessment of clinical improvement and culture and sensitivity testing results

▶ *What Efficacy Parameters Should I Follow and How Frequently Do I Have to Assess My Patient?*

Meningitis

Signs and symptoms

- fever, headache, meningism (nuchal rigidity, Brudzinski's sign, or Kernig's sign), and signs of cerebral dysfunction Q4H for 3 days then daily
- vital signs Q4H, as sepsis is common
- Glasgow Coma Scale in severely ill patients

Microbiological findings

- CSF and blood samples (2 sets) for Gram stain, cultures, and sensitivity testing should be taken prior to starting antibiotic therapy
- Gram stain results can be found out immediately and can guide empirical antibiotic treatment
- identification of the organism can be made within 24–36 hours, and sensitivities should be known within 48–60 hours
- repeat cultures only if no response or relapse of symptoms occurs
- a second tube should be taken to allow for latex agglutination tests for antigens to common meningeal pathogens (*H. influenzae*, pneumococcus, *E. coli*, *N. meningitidis*, and group B streptococcus) if the Gram stain has not been helpful

Cerebrospinal fluid examination

- measure white blood cell count, protein and glucose levels in the CSF
- total and differential white blood cell counts are important to distinguish between bacterial and other potential causes of meningitis

- in bacterial meningitis, the CSF white blood cell count is usually greater than 1000/mm³ and if PMNs are greater than 90%, viral meningitis is unlikely
- in bacterial meningitis, the CSF protein level is usually elevated, but it is not greatly elevated in patients with viral meningitis
- in bacterial meningitis, the CSF glucose level is usually low (<50 mg/dL or 50–60% of a simultaneous blood glucose value), whereas in viral meningitis, it is usually normal

▶ *Should I Add Another Drug or Substitute Therapy If My Initial Drug Therapy Fails?*

Meningitis

Further antibiotic treatment should be based on culture and sensitivity testing results

Gram-positive meningitis

- if patients fail to respond to initial antibiotic therapy, add rifampin

Gram-negative meningitis

- if patients fail to respond, give intrathecal or intraventricular aminoglycosides

▶ *How Long Should I Continue Drug Therapy?*

Meningitis

- 7 days for patients who respond quickly if meningitis is caused by *S. pneumoniae;* however, treat for 10 days if the patient responds slowly
- 10 days for patients who respond quickly if meningitis is caused by *N. meningitidis* or *H. influenzae;* however, treat for 14 days if the patient responds slowly
- 10 days for shunt infections caused by *S. aureus* or *S. epidermidis* (Infect Dis Clin North Am 1990;4:677–791)
- 21 days if meningitis is caused by gram-negative organisms (stop aminoglycoside administration after 10 days because of increased risk of toxicity)

Useful References

Mattison HR, Roberts NJ. Central nervous system infections. In: Reese RE, Betts RF, eds. A Practical Approach to Infectious Diseases. Boston: Little, Brown, 1991:108–145

Roos KL. Meningitis as it presents in the elderly: Diagnosis and care. Geriatrics 1990;45:63–75

Scheld WM, Wispelwey B, eds. Meningitis. Infect Dis Clin North Am 1990

Tunkel AR, Wispelwey B, Scheld WM. Bacterial meningitis: Recent advances in pathophysiology and treatment. Ann Intern Med 1990; 112:610–623

DRUG THERAPY FOR SEXUALLY TRANSMITTED DISEASES

Catherine Allaire and James McCormack

▶ *What Are My Goals of Treatment?*

Urethritis or cervicitis

to ameliorate signs and symptoms such as irritation in the distal urethra, urethral discharge, and vaginal discharge

to prevent complications (e.g., sterility and disseminated infection) of untreated disease

Vaginitis

to ameliorate signs and symptoms such as vaginal discharge, pruritus, unpleasant odor, and external dysuria or pain on intercourse

Pelvic inflammatory disease

to ameliorate signs and symptoms such as lower abdominal pain, abnormal vaginal bleeding or discharge, dyspareunia, cervical motion tenderness, adnexal tenderness or mass, fever, and purulent cervical discharge

to prevent abscess formation, sepsis, and death

to prevent tubal damage (infertility and ectopic pregnancies)

to prevent chronic pelvic pain syndromes

Genital ulcers

to ameliorate signs and symptoms

to decrease recurrences

to prevent late complications of untreated syphilis if ulcer caused by *Treponema pallidum*

▶ What Evidence Is Available to Support Drug Therapy for Sexually Transmitted Diseases?

Urethritis or cervicitis

- *Chlamydia* infection and gonorrhea are eradicated with appropriate treatment
- pelvic inflammatory disease (PID) cases have declined in jurisdictions with aggressive treatment strategies aimed at these conditions

Vaginitis

- symptoms are alleviated with appropriate treatment

Pelvic inflammatory disease

- antibiotic therapy is associated with a clinical cure rate of 90–100% (Rev Infect Dis 1990;12:S656–664)
- antibiotics decrease the frequency of persistent masses and ruptured abscesses (Fertil Steril 1965;16:125)
- aggressive antibiotic treatment combined with early surgical intervention has significantly decreased mortality from ruptured tuboovarian abscesses, which is the most serious complication of PID
- early diagnosis and effective treatment can decrease long-term sequelae of PID (Contraception 1987;36:111–128)

Genital ulcers

- primary syphilis and chancroid are curable with appropriate treatment
- primary herpes may be ameliorated and recurrences reduced

▶ When Should I Consider Drug Therapy?

Urethritis

- urethritis is suspected in a male patient who reports irritation in the distal urethra and urethral discharge
- infection can be confirmed when 4 PMNs or more per high-power field are seen on microbiological examination of discharge
- if a smear shows less than 4 PMNs per high-power field, treatment may be withheld pending results of gonorrhea culture and *Chlamydia* testing
- if no urethral discharge is present, delay treatment until microbiological results are known unless the patient is at high risk or unlikely to return for follow-up
- if women have these symptoms and if no organism is found (uretheral syndrome), consider a sexually transmitted disease and evaluate as below for cervicitis

Cervicitis

- for all patients with vaginal discharge, lower abdominal discomfort, deep dyspareunia, and/or abnormal vaginal bleeding
- cervicitis is best diagnosed by the presence of yellow mucopurulent discharge on a swab taken from the endocervix
- smear may help by showing the presence of *Neisseria gonorrhoeae,* but the PMN count, in contrast to that from the urethra, is of poor predictive value
- treatment should be offered to those with the above clinical diagnosis or to those with *Chlamydia trachomatis* or *N. gonorrhoeae* isolated from the cervix

Vaginitis

- all patients with mild to moderate erythema and vaginal discharge, pruritus, unpleasant odor, external dysuria, or pain on intercourse should be evaluated as follows:
- speculum examination with visual inspection of vaginal discharge and cervix and *Chlamydia* test and gonorrhea culture from the cervix
- slide for bacterial vaginosis (Gram stain)
- slide for trichomonas (wet mount)
- slide for yeast (Gram stain or potassium hydroxide)
- vaginal pH (pH of <4.5 usually excludes a diagnosis of bacterial vaginosis)
- whiff test (smell vaginal secretions for amine odor after the application of potassium hydroxide) is useful for diagnosis of bacterial vaginosis
- detection of yeasts in the absence of symptoms does not necessitate treatment
- asymptomatic patients with bacterial vaginosis undergoing an endometrial biopsy, hysteroscopy, hysterosalpingogram, or intrauterine device insertion should receive treatment before these procedures to decrease the risk of infection

Pelvic inflammatory disease

- antibiotic treatment should be given to all patients clinically suspected of having PID on the basis of having lower abdominal pain, cervical motion tenderness, and one of these findings: temperature >38°C, leukocytosis >10,500 WBC/mm^3, culdocentesis yielding peritoneal fluid containing WBCs or bacteria, inflammatory mass on pelvic exam or ultrasound, elevated ESR, cervical Gram stain revealing gram-negative diplococci, or positive *Chlamydia* test
- clinical diagnosis is only approximately 65% accurate (Am J Obstet Gynecol 1969;105:1088–1098) when laparoscopy is used for verification
- most importantly, a low threshold for treatment is wise, as minimally symptomatic infection may cause extensive tubal disease

Genital ulcers

- all patients with ulcers or vesicles (painful or painless)
- type of treatment should be based on clinical suspicion and the type of lesion

▶ What Drug Should I Use for Initial Treatment?

Sexual contacts of patients with pelvic inflammatory disease, syphilis, *Trichomonas* infection, and any form of urethritis or cervicitis should be treated in the same way as the index case

Urethritis

Urethral discharge shows 4 PMNs or more per high-power field and no diplococci (Chlamydia)

DOXYCYCLINE

- doxycycline is active against *C. trachomatis* and can be given twice daily, and food does not affect the absorption

TETRACYCLINE

- tetracycline may be used if the patient cannot afford doxycycline

ERYTHROMYCIN

- if the patient cannot take tetracyclines, erythromycin has activity against *C. trachomatis*
- erythromycin is the drug of choice if the patient is pregnant

AZITHROMYCIN

- single dose of this agent has been shown to be as effective as a 7 day course of doxycycline (Am J Med 1991;91[suppl 3A]:19S–22S) and may be useful in the noncompliant patient; it is much more expensive than a 7 day course of doxycycline
- does not appear to be effective for gonorrhea

Urethral discharge shows 4 PMNs or more per high-power field and gram-negative intracellular diplococci (gonorrhea) or no results are available

CEFIXIME WITH TETRACYCLINE OR DOXYCYCLINE

- cefixime covers *N. gonorrhoeae* and is a single-dose oral treatment that is as effective as, and less expensive than, ceftriaxone
- tetracycline or doxycycline should be added because coexisting *C. trachomatis* is often present

CEFTRIAXONE WITH TETRACYCLINE OR DOXYCYCLINE

- ceftriaxone should be used instead of cefixime in cases of epididymitis owing to a lack of experience with cefixime in this condition

CIPROFLOXACIN WITH TETRACYCLINE OR DOXYCYCLINE

- if the patient is penicillin allergic
- single dose of ciprofloxacin is effective for *N. gonorrhoeae* and the tetracycline will cover for *C. trachomatis*

Cervicitis

- because a cervical stain is only 50% positive for gonorrhea, all cervicitis should be treated as above for urethritis, including treatment for *Chlamydia,* because of frequent concomitant infection

Vaginitis

Endocervical discharge

- if patient has an endocervical discharge, treat as above for urethritis or cervicitis

Gram stain of vaginal swab shows gram-positive and/or gram-negative coccobacilli, vaginal pH is 5–6, and whiff test result is positive (bacterial vaginosis)

METRONIDAZOLE

- is effective for treatment of bacterial vaginosis, as it covers *Gardnerella vaginalis, Mycoplasma hominis,* and other typical organisms
- it is less expensive than clindamycin
- metronidazole should be avoided in pregnancy; however, in patients with severe symptoms, a single 2 g dose can be used after the first trimester

CLINDAMYCIN

- if patients cannot take metronidazole

Wet mount (saline) shows the presence of motile trichomonads

METRONIDAZOLE

- only effective treatment of trichomonas infection
- treatment of the partner is also required to prevent reinfection

Wet mount (potassium hydroxide) shows the presence of mycelia (yeasts)

TOPICAL MICONAZOLE, CLOTRIMAZOLE, OR TERCONAZOLE

- these agents are more effective than nystatin (Obstet Gynecol 1976;48:491–494) and can be given as a short course of therapy
- all these agents appear to be equally effective in a 3 day regimen, and the decision among these agents should be based on cost

FLUCONAZOLE

- is an effective single-dose oral agent, and should be used if the patient fails to respond to topical therapy
- ketoconazole is also effective but necessitates a 3 day course

Pelvic inflammatory disease

Inpatient treatment

- inpatient treatment is advisable for all first episodes of acute PID in women of childbearing age
- current recommendations for hospitalization are uncertain diagnosis, inability to rule out surgical emergencies such as appendicitis and ectopic pregnancy, suspected pelvic abscess, pregnancy, prepubertal child or adolescent, severe illness precluding outpatient treatment, failure to respond to outpatient therapy, inability to arrange outpatient follow-up within 72 hours, immunocompromised patient, intrauterine device user, temperature greater than 38°C (100.4°F), and upper peritoneal signs
- no single agent has been proved as efficacious as combination therapy (JAMA 1991;266:2605–2611)

CEFOXITIN, CEFTIZOXIME, OR CEFOTETAN WITH DOXYCYCLINE OR TETRACYCLINE

- covers organisms implicated in PID, namely *C. trachomatis, N. gonorrhoeae,* aerobes (*E. coli,* streptococci), and anaerobes (*Bacteroides* sp.)
- proven efficacy and lower toxicity than clindamycin and gentamicin make this combination first choice in mildly to moderately ill hospitalized patients
- selection of cephalosporin depends on cost
- doxycycline has the advantages over tetracycline of less frequent dosing (BID for doxycycline versus QID for tetracycline), can be used in patients with decreased renal function, and may be taken with food

CLINDAMYCIN WITH GENTAMICIN

- regimen of choice if the patient is penicillin allergic or if the patient cannot tolerate or take doxycycline (e.g., pregnant patients)
- better anaerobic (especially against *Bacteroides*) and gram-positive aerobic coverage make it first-line therapy for patient with sepsis or evidence of tuboovarian abscess (Rev Infect Dis 1983;5[suppl]:876–884)

- patient not responding to cefoxitin and doxycycline might respond to this alternative combination (Am J Obstet Gynecol 1988;158:734)
- clindamycin is also clinically effective against *C. trachomatis* (Ann Intern Med 1986;104:187–193)

Outpatient therapy

CEFTRIAXONE WITH DOXYCYCLINE OR TETRACYCLINE

- broad-spectrum coverage for common etiological agents of PID, especially penicillinase-producing *N. gonorrhoeae*
- inadequate anaerobic coverage; therefore, not used for inpatient therapy

CEFTRIAXONE WITH ERYTHROMYCIN

- if the patient cannot tolerate or take doxycycline (e.g., pregnant patient)

CEFOXITIN WITH PROBENECID AND DOXYCYCLINE OR TETRACYCLINE

- also used if less expensive than the above combination

CIPROFLOXACIN WITH DOXYCYCLINE

- if the patient is penicillin allergic

METRONIDAZOLE

- usually not required for outpatient treatment, but can be added to the above regimens in cases in which anaerobes are strongly suspected

Genital ulcers

Clinical suspicion and lesions suggest syphilis

(usually painless lesions with raised border and indurated base), dark-field microscopy shows corkscrew spirochetes, or direct fluorescent antibody test shows spirochetes

PENICILLIN G

- drug of choice for syphilis and less expensive than ceftriaxone or doxycycline

DOXYCYCLINE OR TETRACYCLINE

- if the patient is penicillin allergic

Clinical suspicion and lesions suggest herpes

(usually painful, grouped vesicles or ulcers), and dark-field microscopy does not show corkscrew spirochetes

ACYCLOVIR

- only presently available agent effective for the treatment of genital herpes
- oral acyclovir shortens duration of pain, healing, and viral shedding (N Engl J Med 1983;308:916–921) in first infections
- acyclovir may be used for recurrent infections, but it is not as effective as for initial infections
- topical acyclovir is not effective (Med Lett 1991;33:119–124)
- acyclovir also decreases the rate of recurrence when taken prophylactically and should be tried in patients with poor immune status, severe recurrent episodes, or more than 6 episodes per year

Clinical suspicion and lesions suggest chancroid

(usually superficial, shallow lesions with a ragged edge), and dark-field microscopy does not show corkscrew spirochetes (obtain smear for *Haemophilus ducreyi*)

CEFTRIAXONE

- effective, better tolerated, and more convenient than erythromycin
- treatment of the partner is required

ERYTHROMYCIN

- if the patient is penicillin allergic and can be used if the patient is pregnant

▶ *What Dosage Should I Use?*

Urethritis or cervicitis

DOXYCYCLINE

- 100 mg PO BID

TETRACYCLINE

- 500 mg PO QID

ERYTHROMYCIN

- 500 mg PO QID

AZITHROMYCIN

- 1 g as a single dose

CEFIXIME

- 400 mg PO as a single dose

CEFTRIAXONE

- 250 mg IM as a single dose

CIPROFLOXACIN

- 500 mg PO as a single dose

Vaginitis

- use doses as above if treating a patient with an endocervical discharge

METRONIDAZOLE

- 500 mg PO BID for bacterial vaginosis
- 2 g PO as a single dose for trichomoniasis

CLINDAMYCIN

- 300 mg PO BID

MICONAZOLE

- 200 mg vaginal suppository nightly for 3 nights

CLOTRIMAZOLE

- two 100 mg vaginal suppositories nightly for 3 nights

TERCONAZOLE

- 80 mg vaginal suppository nightly for 3 nights

FLUCONAZOLE

- 150 mg PO as a single dose

Pelvic inflammatory disease

Inpatient therapy

CEFOXITIN

- 1 g IV Q6H
- 2 g IV Q6H if the disease is severe

CEFOTETAN

- 1 g IV Q12H
- 2 g IV Q12H if the disease is severe

CEFTIZOXIME

- 1 g IV Q8H
- 2 g IV Q8H if the disease is severe

DOXYCYCLINE

- 100 mg IV Q12H
- 100 mg PO Q12H if the patient can tolerate oral medications

TETRACYCLINE

- 500 mg IV Q6H
- 500 mg PO Q6H if the patient can tolerate oral medications

CLINDAMYCIN

- 600 mg IV Q8H
- 900 mg IV Q8H if the disease is severe

GENTAMICIN

- 1.5 mg/kg IV Q8H

Outpatient therapy

CEFTRIAXONE

- 250 mg IM as a single dose

DOXYCYCLINE

- 100 mg PO BID

TETRACYCLINE

- 500 mg PO Q6H

CIPROFLOXACIN

- 500 mg PO BID

ERYTHROMYCIN

- 500 mg PO QID

CEFOXITIN

- 2 g IV as a single dose

PROBENECID

- 1 g PO as a single dose

METRONIDAZOLE

- 500 mg PO Q8H

Genital ulcers

PENICILLIN G

- 2.4 million units of benzathine penicillin G IM as a single dose for early syphilis (shorter than 1 year in duration)
- 2.4 million units of benzathine penicillin G IM weekly for 3 weeks for late syphilis (longer than 1 year in duration)
- 2 million units of aqueous penicillin G IV Q4H for 10 days followed by 2.4 million units of benzathine penicillin G weekly for 3 weeks for neurosyphilis

DOXYCYCLINE OR TETRACYCLINE

- as above

ACYCLOVIR

- 400 mg PO TID for first episode and recurrent infections
- 5 mg/kg IV Q8H or 400 mg PO 5 times daily (if the patient can take oral medication) for immunocompromised patients
- for prophylaxis, start with 200 mg PO BID, and if not

effective, increase the dosage to as much as 400 mg PO 5 times daily

CEFTRIAXONE

- 250 mg IM as a single dose

ERYTHROMYCIN

- 500 mg PO Q6H

▶ *How Long Should I Treat With My Initial Regimen?*

Urethritis or cervicitis

- doxycycline, tetracycline, and erythromycin should initially be continued for 7 days
- ceftriaxone and ciprofloxacin are single-dose therapy

Vaginitis

- as above for urethritis if endocervical discharge is present
- 7 days for bacterial vaginosis
- single dose for trichomoniasis
- 3 days for yeast infections

Pelvic inflammatory disease

Inpatient therapy

- evaluate for clinical improvement 24–48 hours after the initiation of inpatient therapy

Outpatient therapy

- evaluate for clinical improvement 48–72 hours after the initiation of outpatient therapy

Genital ulcers

Syphilis

- single dose for early syphilis
- weekly penicillin for 3 weeks for late syphilis
- 14 days for doxycycline (4 weeks if late syphilis)
- 10 days of aqueous penicillin plus 3 weeks of benzathine penicillin for neurosyphilis

Herpes

- treat initial infection for 7 days (10 days if lesions heal slowly)
- treat recurrent episodes for 5 days
- for prophylaxis, stop treatment after 6–9 months to determine if the frequency or severity is sufficient to warrant prevention (Antimicrob Agents Chemother 1987;31: 361–367)
- in immunocompromised patients, prophylactic treatment should likely continue indefinitely

Chancroid

- ceftriaxone as a single dose
- erythromycin for 7 days

▶ *What Efficacy Parameters Should I Follow and How Frequently Do I Have to Assess My Patient?*

Urethritis, cervicitis, and vaginitis

Signs and symptoms

- significant improvement in signs and symptoms (pain, tenderness, discharge, and erythema) should occur within 48–72 hours of starting therapy

Microbiological findings

- repeated testing is not required in patients whose initial test results were negative and is not cost effective in other patients

Pelvic inflammatory disease
Signs and symptoms

- significant improvement in pain, tenderness, fever, and leukocytosis should occur within 48–72 hours after starting therapy
- patients should also be reevaluated at the end of treatment and several weeks later for tenderness, masses, and vaginal discharge
- repeated cultures are not useful unless *C. trachomatis* is identified initially (identify asymptomatic carriers)

Genital ulcers

- healing of ulcers and decrease in pain
- for syphilis, VDRL test should be done every 3 months for a year, and if they show a 4-fold rise, the patient should be retreated

▶ Should I Add Another Drug or Substitute Therapy If My Initial Drug Therapy Fails?

Urethritis or cervicitis

- recurrent nongonococcal urethritis or cervicitis (in the absence of new sexual contacts) can be treated with erythromycin 500 mg PO QID for 14 days

Vaginitis

- for trichomoniasis, a full course of metronidazole (500 mg PO BID for 10 days) should be used
- for bacterial vaginosis, switch to clindamycin
- for yeast infections, a second course of topical therapy should be tried, and if this is not effective, fluconazole should be tried
- for patients with recurrent yeast vaginitis, clotrimazole 100 mg intravaginally for 5 days with menses can be tried (fluconazole 100 mg PO weekly can be used in patients unwilling or unable to use topical therapy)

Pelvic inflammatory disease
Inpatient therapy

- if no clinical improvement is noted or symptoms and signs worsen, suspect a tuboovarian abscess or other pelvic pathology (appendicitis, ectopic pregnancy, endometriosis, and ovarian torsion)
- ultrasound or computed tomographic (CT) scan and/or laparoscopy is indicated to clarify the diagnosis
- if the patient has PID confirmed by laparoscopy and is unimproved after therapy with cefoxitin and doxycycline, a trial of clindamycin and gentamicin is indicated
- if a tuboovarian abscess is diagnosed and the patient is clinically stable and unresponsive to cefoxitin and doxycycline, a trial of clindamycin and gentamicin is indicated
- if a patient with tuboovarian abscess does not improve clinically after 48–72 hours of clindamycin and gentamicin therapy, surgical intervention is indicated
- ruptured tuboovarian abscess (acute peritonitis, septic shock) is a surgical emergency, but concurrent antibiotic coverage with clindamycin and gentamicin improves the outcome

Outpatient therapy

- if the patient shows only minimal or no clinical improvement after 72 hours of therapy, admit the patient to the hospital for inpatient therapy

Genital ulcers
Syphilis

- if rapid plasma reagin or VDRL titer increases 4-fold or

more with follow-up after treatment, therapy should be repeated

Herpes

- no other effective drugs are yet available (foscarnet may be used to treat acyclovir-resistant herpes in the compromised host)

Chancroid

- switch to an alternative agent, or base further treatment on sensitivities

▶ How Long Should I Continue Drug Therapy?

Urethritis or cervicitis

- doxycycline, tetracycline, and erythromycin should be continued for 7 days
- ceftriaxone, cefixime, and ciprofloxacin are single-dose therapies

Vaginitis

- as above for urethritis if endocervical discharge is present
- 7 days for bacterial vaginosis
- single dose for trichomoniasis
- for yeast infections, a 3 day topical course is usually effective

Pelvic inflammatory disease
Inpatient therapy

- continue the initial regimen until 48 hours after clinical improvement
- after discharge from the hospital, continue doxycycline 100 mg PO BID or clindamycin 450 mg PO TID for a total of 10–14 days, depending on which regimen was used in the hospital (both regimens provide adequate coverage against *C. trachomatis*)

Outpatient therapy

- continue oral antibiotics for 10–14 days, depending on how quickly the patient responded

Genital ulcers
Syphilis

- single dose of benzathine penicillin for early syphilis
- weekly penicillin for 3 weeks for late syphilis
- 14 days for doxycycline
- 10 days of aqueous penicillin plus 3 weeks of benzathine penicillin for neurosyphilis

Herpes

- 7 days for acyclovir for the initial infection
- for prophylaxis, stop treatment after 6–9 months to determine if the frequency or severity is sufficient to warrant prevention (Antimicrob Agents Chemother 1987;31: 361–367)
- in immunocompromised patients, prophylactic treatment should likely continue indefinitely

Chancroid

- ceftriaxone as a single dose
- erythromycin for 7 days

Useful References

Drugs for sexually transmitted diseases. Med Lett 1994;36:1–6
McCormack WM. Pelvic inflammatory disease. N Engl J Med 1994; 330:115–119
Sweet RL, Gibbs RS. Infectious Diseases of the Female Genital Tract, 2nd ed. Baltimore: Williams & Wilkins, 1990

DRUG THERAPY FOR SOFT TISSUE INFECTIONS

Catherine Ann MacDougall and James McCormack

▶ What Are My Goals of Treatment?

to ameliorate signs and symptoms
to prevent sepsis and death
to prevent complications such as tissue necrosis, ulceration, abscesses, bullae, local extension of infection, neurological lesions, contiguous focus osteomyelitis, bone destruction, loss of limb, lymphangitis, and thrombophlebitis

▶ What Evidence Is Available to Support Drug Therapy for Soft Tissue Infections?

Cellulitis, Animal Bites, Human Bites

Antibiotic treatment improves outcome

- signs and symptoms of infection (local tenderness, pain, erythema, swelling, ulceration, necrosis, and wound drainage) are alleviated with appropriate antimicrobial therapy (Emerg Med Clin North Am 1992;10:753–765, Emerg Med Clin North Am 1992;10:719–736, J Fam Pract 1989;28:713–718)
- signs and symptoms of systemic infection (malaise, fever, chills, and hypotension) are alleviated with appropriate antimicrobial therapy

Erysipelas

- erysipelas will respond quickly to antibiotics with activity against group H streptococci (Andrew's Diseases of the Skin, 1990:277–278)

▶ When Should I Consider Drug Therapy?

Cellulitis

- treat all patients, even without a definite lesion, when cellulitis is suspected (local tenderness, pain, swelling, warmth, and erythema) secondary to trauma or an underlying skin lesion
- malaise, fever, and chills may also be present in patients with cellulitis
- patients with mild cellulitis (no evidence of systemic infection) do not require antibiotics and can be treated with local wound care (cleaning or irrigation of the site with soap and water)
- acute traumatic wounds do not require routine antibiotic therapy unless there is evidence of an infection or the patient is immunocompromised, as prophylactic antibiotic therapy does not appear to decrease the chance of infection (Emerg Med Clin North Am 1992;10:753–765)
- a course of antibiotic therapy should be given to patients with an acute traumatic wound only if they are found to be immunocompromised (patients with diabetes mellitus, peripheral vascular disease, acquired immunodeficiency syndrome [AIDS], long-term steroid use, and leukopenia)
- do not treat patients presenting with *Pseudomonas* folliculitis or "hot tub folliculitis" (papules, pustules, or nodules) who give a history of being in a whirlpool, hot tub, or swimming pool and have a rash in the bathing suit area

Animal bites

- need for antibiotics for dog bites is controversial and should be guided by wound characteristics

- antibiotics should be used if the wound involves the hand, is near joints or involves deep punctures, if irrigation of the lacerations is difficult, if the patient is immunocompromised (i.e., with diabetes, after splenectomy), or if the wound is not well perfused (Postgrad Med 1992:92(July):134,136,139–144,146,149, Emerg Med Clin North Am 1992;10:719–736)
- all cat bites should likely be treated, as there is a 50% incidence of infection after cat bites (Clin Infect Dis 1992;14:633–640)

Human bites

- if the bite does not involve the hand and the patient has been seen within approximately 12 hours of the injury, treatment can consist of simple irrigation (Ann Intern Med 1988;17:1317–1327)
- if the hand has been bitten, the patient has not been seen within 12 hours of the injury, or the patient is immunocompromised, antibiotics should be used

Erysipelas

- treat all patients when erysipelas is suspected
- erysipelas is distinguished from typical cellulitis in that the lesions are warm, shiny, red, and swollen and have a definite margin
- lesions are commonly found on the face or legs

▶ What Drug Should I Use for Initial Treatment?

Cellulitis

CLOXACILLIN OR NAFCILLIN

- drugs of choice if staphylococcal and streptococcal organisms are suspected or proved, or if there are no clues as to what organisms are present
- these drugs have good activity against staphylococcal and streptococcal organisms and they are less expensive than agents such as dicloxacillin and flucloxacillin
- cloxacillin as sole therapy is also useful for patients with soft tissue infections resulting from IV drug abuse because gram-negative organisms are rarely causative (Can J Infect Control 1993;8:7–9)
- some clinicians suggest adding penicillin to cloxacillin or nafcillin in moderately to severely ill patients; however, this is likely not needed if high-dose cloxacillin or nafcillin (2 g IV Q6H) is used
- dicloxacillin produces slightly higher total serum concentrations than does cloxacillin; however, it is more highly protein bound than cloxacillin, and thus, at similar dosages, dicloxacillin produces slightly lower free serum concentrations (Br Med J 1970;4:455–460)
- flucloxacillin (not available in USA) produces similar total serum concentrations to dicloxacillin but is less protein bound and produces higher free concentrations than does either cloxacillin or dicloxacillin
- the small differences in pharmacokinetics between these drugs have never been shown to affect clinical outcome

PENICILLIN

- drug of choice if only streptococcal organisms are suspected (if the cellulitis is well demarcated and there are no pockets of pus or evidence of vein thrombosis) or proved because penicillin has good activity against group A beta-hemolytic streptococcus
- penicillin is effective, well tolerated, less expensive than cloxacillin or clindamycin, and is usually better tolerated than erythromycin

CEFAZOLIN, CEPHALEXIN

- can be used in place of cloxacillin or nafcillin if they are less expensive
- cefazolin and cephalexin have good activity against staphylococcal and streptococcal organisms

ERYTHROMYCIN

- erythromycin has activity against staphylococcal and streptococcal organisms and is less expensive than oral clindamycin
- useful in mildly to moderately ill patients with a documented history of penicillin allergy in whom oral therapy can be used (if the patient is severely ill, clindamycin should be chosen over erythromycin, as it has better activity against gram-positive organisms than does erythromycin)

CLINDAMYCIN

- if the patient is moderately to severely ill with a documented history of penicillin allergy, as clindamycin has better activity against gram-positive organisms than does erythromycin
- if parenteral therapy is required, clindamycin is less expensive than either parenteral erythromycin or vancomycin
- also useful when both gram-positive and anaerobic organisms are suspected (devitalized tissue, necrosis, foul smelling tissue, crepitus, and intraabdominal surgery wound infection)

CLOXACILLIN OR NAFCILLIN WITH METRONIDAZOLE

- same spectrum as clindamycin and can be used if the combination is less expensive than clindamycin

VANCOMYCIN

- if methicillin-resistant staphylococci are suspected or proven

High-risk patients

CLOXACILLIN OR NAFCILLIN WITH GENTAMICIN

- for high-risk patients (patients undergoing hemodialysis and patients with underlying debilitating diseases) and/or patients in whom both gram-positive and gram-negative organisms are suspected or proven pathogens
- cloxacillin or nafcillin with gentamicin provides activity against the common organisms causing cellulitis in these patients (*S. aureus* [penicillin resistant], *E. coli,* and *K. pneumoniae*)
- aminoglycosides, when used for a short period of time (5–7 days) are effective, safe, and inexpensive

CLOXACILLIN OR NAFCILLIN WITH CIPROFLOXACIN

- as above under cloxacillin or nafcillin with gentamicin in those patients in whom aminoglycosides are contraindicated

CLINDAMYCIN WITH GENTAMICIN

- for high-risk patients if an abscess is present or for patients in whom anaerobic and gram-negative organisms are suspected (devitalized, necrotic, foul-smelling tissue or abdominal surgery wound)

CEFOXITIN, CEFOTETAN, CEFTIZOXIME, PIPERACILLIN

- for high-risk patients when aminoglycosides are contraindicated
- decision among these agents should be based on cost

CLINDAMYCIN WITH CIPROFLOXACIN

- in high-risk patients when aminoglycosides are contraindicated and the patient has an allergy to penicillins

Animal bites

CLOXACILLIN WITH PENICILLIN

- combination provides coverage for the predominant organisms in dog and cat bites (alpha-hemolytic streptococci, *S. aureus, Pasteurella multocida,* and anaerobic bacteria, particularly *Bacteroides* species and *Fusobacterium* species) (J Fam Pract 1989;28:713–718)

AMOXICILLIN-CLAVULANATE

- can be used, as it covers most of the potential organisms; however, it is usually more expensive than cloxacillin with penicillin and has not been demonstrated to be superior to this combination

DOXYCYCLINE

- useful if the patient is penicillin allergic
- although clindamycin or erythromycin may be useful, they have limited activity against *P. multocida*

Human bites

CLOXACILLIN WITH PENICILLIN

- this combination provides coverage for the predominant organisms in human bites (alpha-hemolytic streptococci, *S. aureus, Eikenella corrodens, Corynebacterium* spp. and *Bacteroides* spp.) (J Fam Pract 1989;28:713–718)
- therapy should not be simply a penicillinase-resistant penicillin (cloxacillin) or a first-generation cephalosporin (cephalexin) alone because *E. corrodens* is commonly resistant to these antibiotics

AMOXICILLIN-CLAVULANATE

- can be used, as it covers most of the potential organisms; however, it is usually more expensive than cloxacillin with penicillin and has not been demonstrated superior to this combination
- if the anaerobic flora of the patient's community is frequently resistant to penicillin, amoxicillin-clavulanate should be considered the drug of choice

DOXYCYCLINE

- useful if the patient is penicillin allergic
- although clindamycin or erythromycin may be useful, they have limited activity against *E. corrodens*

Erysipelas

PENICILLIN

- penicillin has activity against the organism that causes erysipelas (group A streptococci)

ERYTHROMYCIN

- if there is a documented history of penicillin allergy, erythromycin is effective for the treatment of erysipelas

CLINDAMYCIN

- if parenteral therapy is required for a penicillin-allergic patient

▶ *What Dosage Should I Use?*

Cellulitis, animal bites, human bites, and erysipelas
Mild to moderate conditions (oral therapy required)

CLOXACILLIN

- 500 mg PO Q6H

PENICILLIN V

- 250–300 mg (depending on available dosage forms) PO Q6H

CEPHALEXIN

- 500 mg PO Q6H

ERYTHROMYCIN

- 500 mg PO Q6H

CLINDAMYCIN

- 300 mg PO Q6H

METRONIDAZOLE

- 500 mg PO Q8H

AMOXICILLIN-CLAVULANATE

- 500 mg PO Q8H

DOXYCYCLINE

- 100 mg PO Q12H

Moderate to severe conditions (parenteral therapy required)

CLOXACILLIN OR NAFCILLIN

- 1 g IV Q6H if the condition is moderate
- 2 g IV Q6H if the condition is severe

PENICILLIN G

- 1 million units IV Q6H if the condition is moderate
- 2 million units IV Q6H if the condition is severe

CEFAZOLIN

- 1 g IV Q8H if the condition is moderate
- 2 g IV Q8H if the condition is severe

VANCOMYCIN

- 15 mg/kg IV Q12H

GENTAMICIN

- 2.0 mg/kg IV Q8H

CLINDAMYCIN

- 600 mg IV Q8H if the condition is moderate
- 900 mg IV Q8H if the condition is severe

METRONIDAZOLE

- 500 mg IV Q8H

CEFOXITIN

- 1 g IV Q6H if the condition is moderate
- 2 g IV Q6H if the condition is severe

CEFOTETAN

- 1 g IV Q12H if the condition is moderate
- 2 g IV Q12H if the condition is severe

CEFTIZOXIME

- 1 g IV Q8H if the condition is moderate
- 2 g IV Q8H if the condition is severe

PIPERACILLIN

- 1 g IV Q6H if the condition is moderate
- 2 g IV Q4H if the condition is severe

CIPROFLOXACIN

- 500 mg PO Q12H or 200 mg IV Q12H if parenteral is therapy required for moderate infections
- 750 mg PO Q12H or 400 mg IV Q12H if parenteral therapy is required for severe infections

▶ *How Long Should I Treat with My Initial Regimen?*

Cellulitis, animal bites, human bites, and erysipelas

- initially, treat for 48–72 hours, and base further therapy on the assessment of clinical improvement and culture and sensitivity testing results (if obtained)
- duration of parenteral antibiotic therapy prior to switching to oral therapy depends on the patient's clinical response and the likelihood of recurrence

▶ *What Efficacy Parameters Should I Follow and How Frequently Do I Have to Assess My Patient?*

Cellulitis, animal bites, human bites, and erysipelas
Signs and symptoms

- local tenderness, pain, erythema, swelling, ulceration, necrosis, wound drainage, malaise, fever, and chills
- assess the patient daily

Microbiological findings

- in otherwise healthy individuals, identification of the causative organism in cases of cellulitis is unnecessary
- appropriate empirical treatment is effective in the vast majority of patients, and an attempt to isolate the organism is often fruitless (Arch Intern Med 1990;150: 1907–1912)
- although organisms are often not cultured, attempts at identification of the organism (a needle aspiration or punch biopsy at the leading edge of the cellulitis) is recommended if initial treatment fails or if the patient is immunocompromised, has potential joint or tendon damage, or has a life-threatening infection necessitating hospitalization
- if a culture of the site is done, specimens for blood cultures should also be obtained
- anaerobic cultures need be performed only when anaerobes are suspected (the wound contains necrotic tissue, is foul smelling, or crepitance is present)
- Gram stain results can be found out immediately and guide empirical antibiotic treatment
- identification of the organism can be made within 24–36 hours, and sensitivities should be known within 48–60 hours

▶ *Should I Add Another Drug or Substitute Therapy If My Initial Drug Therapy Fails?*

Cellulitis, animal bites, human bites, and erysipelas
Patients who fail to respond after 48–72 hours of antibiotic therapy

- further antibiotic treatment should be based on culture and sensitivity testing results
- surgical consultation may be required

How Long Should I Continue Drug Therapy?

Cellulitis, animal bites, human bites, and erysipelas

- usual duration is 10 days, or 4–5 days after the patient has become afebrile and has clinically improved
- if using parenteral treatment, consider switching to oral therapy after the patient has become afebrile and has been clinically improved for 1–2 days

Useful References

Goldstein EJ. Bite wounds and infection. Clin Infect Dis 1992;14:633–640

Lindsey D. Soft tissue infections. Emerg Med Clin North Am 1992; 10:737–751

Powers RD. Soft tissue infections in the emergency department: The case for the use of ''simple'' antibiotics. South Med J 1991;84:1313–1315

DRUG THERAPY FOR OSTEOMYELITIS

Catherine Ann MacDougall and James McCormack

What Are My Goals of Treatment?

to ameliorate signs and symptoms

to prevent sepsis and death

to prevent complications such as tissue necrosis, bone destruction, loss of limb, abscesses, local extension of infection, neurological lesions, amyloidosis (rare), and epidermoid carcinoma (rare)

What Evidence Is Available to Support Drug Therapy for Osteomyelitis?

Morbidity is associated with osteomyelitis

- appropriate treatment can prevent loss of limb in diabetic patients with osteomyelitis of the foot (Am J Med 1987; 83:653–660)

Antibiotic treatment improves outcome

- signs and symptoms of acute osteomyelitis (fever, chills, night sweats, malaise, anorexia, weight loss, pain, limitation of motion, swelling, redness, warmth, and tenderness over the area of involved bone) are alleviated with appropriate antimicrobial therapy
- signs and symptoms of chronic osteomyelitis such as drainage from wounds and sinus tracts can often be alleviated with appropriate antimicrobial therapy

When Should I Consider Drug Therapy?

Acute osteomyelitis (hematogenous or contiguous)

- treat all patients when osteomyelitis is suspected on the basis of clinical symptoms such as pain, limitation of motion, swelling, redness, warmth, tenderness over the area of involved bone, fever, chills, night sweats, malaise, anorexia, weight loss, and positive blood cultures
- treat patients as soon as possible after presentation and diagnosis of osteomyelitis
- prior to the initiation of antibiotic therapy, a Gram stain and culture of the blood should be done

Chronic osteomyelitis

- most cases of adult osteomyelitis are subacute or chronic (Drugs 1993;45:29–43)
- treat all patients presenting with fever, regional soft tissue swelling, tenderness, erythema, warmth, drainage from wounds or sinus tracts, and limitation of motion of an affected area that has occurred within 1–2 months of a predisposing situation such as trauma, bacteremia, surgery, soft tissue infection, diabetes mellitus, and peripheral vascular disease
- radiological evidence of osteomyelitis (cortical bone erosion) is also useful for diagnosis
- for most cases of chronic osteomyelitis, it is not urgent to start antibiotic therapy immediately
- start antibiotic treatment after the results of cultures (blood and bone) and sensitivities are determined (Hosp Formul 1993;28:63–85)

What Drug Should I Use for Initial Treatment?

Most cases of osteomyelitis necessitate local debridement surgery in addition to antibiotic therapy (Ann Intern Med 1991;114:986–987) • For cases of osteomyelitis associated with a prosthetic device, removal of the device along with antibiotic therapy is almost always required • Below are guidelines for empirical therapy; however, antibiotic therapy in most cases can and should be guided by culture and sensitivity testing results

Acute or chronic osteomyelitis

CLOXACILLIN, NAFCILLIN

- cloxacillin and nafcillin have good activity against the most common organisms causing osteomyelitis (staphylococci)
- less expensive and less toxic than clindamycin (which can cause diarrhea and/or C. difficile infection) but has to be given more frequently than clindamycin (Q4H versus Q8H)

CLINDAMYCIN

- drug of choice if there is documented history of penicillin allergy
- also useful when both gram-positive and anaerobic organisms are suspected
- is less expensive than vancomycin plus has activity against anaerobes

CLOXACILLIN OR NAFCILLIN WITH METRONIDAZOLE

- has the same spectrum of activity as clindamycin and can be used if this combination is less expensive than clindamycin

High-risk patients

CLOXACILLIN OR NAFCILLIN WITH GENTAMICIN

- for high-risk patients (IV drug abusers, patients undergoing hemodialysis, and patients with underlying debilitating diseases)
- cloxacillin or nafcillin with gentamicin provides activity against the common organisms causing osteomyelitis in these patients (S. aureus, E. coli, K. pneumoniae, and H. influenzae)
- if anaerobes are suspected, add metronidazole or use clindamycin with gentamicin (the decision between these regimens should be based on cost and potential toxicities)

CLINDAMYCIN WITH GENTAMICIN

- useful combination in patients who have a history of penicillin allergy and who are at high risk; patients with peripheral vascular disease (diabetes); or patients with osteomyelitis if the skull, the facial bones, the mandible, the sacrum (especially with decubitus ulcers), the hand

(after human bite), or the pelvis (after intraabdominal infections) is involved
- clindamycin with gentamicin has activity against the common organisms causing osteomyelitis in these patients (*S. aureus, E. coli, K. pneumoniae, H. influenzae,* and anaerobes)

CLINDAMYCIN WITH CEFTRIAXONE OR CEFOTAXIME

- in above patients in whom aminoglycosides are contraindicated

CLINDAMYCIN WITH CIPROFLOXACIN

- in above patients when aminoglycosides are contraindicated and the patient is allergic to penicillins

VANCOMYCIN

- as empirical therapy until sensitivities are known in patients with osteomyelitis if prosthetic joints are involved
- vancomycin has activity against the common organisms causing osteomyelitis in patients with prosthetic joints (*S. aureus* and *S. epidermidis*) (Infect Dis Clin North Am 1989;3:329–338)
- if organisms are not methicillin resistant, switch to cloxacillin or nafcillin after sensitivities are known

▶ *What Dosage Should I Use?*

Acute or chronic osteomyelitis

At this time, oral therapy cannot be recommended for the *initial* treatment of osteomyelitis, and further conclusive studies are needed (Drugs 1993;45:29–43)

CLOXACILLIN, NAFCILLIN

- 2 g IV Q4H

CLINDAMYCIN

- 600 mg IV Q8H

METRONIDAZOLE

- 500 mg IV Q8H

GENTAMICIN

- 1.5 mg/kg IV Q8H

CEFTRIAXONE

- 2 g IV Q24H

CEFOTAXIME

- 2 g IV Q8H

CIPROFLOXACIN

- 400 mg IV Q12H

VANCOMYCIN

- 15 mg/kg IV Q12H

▶ *How Long Should I Treat with My Initial Regimen?*

Acute osteomyelitis

- initially, treat for 48–72 hours, and base further therapy on the assessment of clinical improvement (may not be seen this early) and culture and sensitivity testing results

Chronic osteomyelitis

- if debridement surgery and empirical antibiotic therapy are required immediately, initially give antibiotics for

48–72 hours, and base further therapy on the assessment of clinical improvement and culture and sensitivity testing results

▶ *What Efficacy Parameters Should I Follow and How Frequently Do I Have to Assess My Patient?*

Acute or chronic osteomyelitis

Signs and symptoms
- initially assess signs and symptoms daily (pain, limitation of motion, swelling, redness, warmth, tenderness over the area of involved bone, fever, chills, night sweats, malaise, anorexia, and drainage from wounds and sinus tracts)

Microbiological findings
- in most patients with osteomyelitis, especially when associated with peripheral vascular disease, or in patients with chronic osteomyelitis, needle aspiration or bone biopsy should be done prior to the initiation of empirical antibiotic therapy to allow for confirmation of the pathogen and tailoring of therapy
- identification of the organism can be made within 24–36 hours, and sensitivities should be known within 48–60 hours

Serum bactericidal titers
- some clinicians recommend that serum bactericidal titers be followed to assess the adequacy of treatment, evaluate compliance, and ensure that adequate concentrations are obtained when oral therapy is used (Drugs 1993;45:29–43)
- varying recommendations for specific titers are available—trough titers greater than or equal to 1:8 (J Infect Dis 1987;155:968–972) or 1:2 (Drugs 1993;45:29–43)
- if titers are below the desired level, it is likely best to increase the dosage only if a patient is not responding well (on the basis of clinical and laboratory measures); this is especially true if the antibiotics the patient is receiving have some dose-related toxicities (e.g., aminoglycosides) (Drugs 1993;45:29–43)

▶ *Should I Add Another Drug or Substitute Therapy If My Initial Drug Therapy Fails?*

Acute or chronic osteomyelitis

- further antibiotic treatment should be based on culture and sensitivity testing results

▶ *How Long Should I Continue Drug Therapy?*

Acute or chronic osteomyelitis

- treat patients with at least 4 weeks of parenteral antibiotics after debridement surgery (the duration of therapy is based on the patient's clinical response)
- if an amputation is done proximal to the site of the infection, only prophylactic antibiotics are required (Hosp Formul 1993;28:63–85)
- if the bone is removed and there is still evidence of soft tissue infection, the patient should receive a 2 week course of antibiotics
- for patients with a prosthetic device, treat for 4–6 weeks with parenteral antibiotics followed by 3–6 months of oral antibiotics
- treat patients with peripheral vascular disease with at least 4 weeks of parenteral antibiotics and follow with oral antibiotics until there is no evidence of inflammation (on the basis of clinical or radiological evidence) (Am J Med 1987;83:653–660)

- duration of parenteral antibiotic therapy prior to switching to oral therapy depends on the patient's clinical response
- in patients receiving aminoglycosides as part of their parenteral regimen, consideration should be given to switching to either cefotaxime, ceftriaxone, or a quinolone after 10–14 days of aminoglycoside therapy to decrease the chance of serious ototoxicity
- use of oral antibiotics should follow parenteral therapy only when the pathogen is known and the patient can be relied on to be compliant with the oral antibiotic regimen
- oral antibiotics commonly used are cloxacillin 1 g PO Q6H, ciprofloxacin 750 mg PO BID, and clindamycin 300 mg PO Q6H

Useful References

Dirschl DR, Almekinders LC. Osteomyelitis—Common causes and treatment recommendations. Drugs 1993;45:29–43

Mandell GL, Douglas RG Jr, Bennett JE, eds. Principles and Practice of Infectious Diseases, 3rd ed. New York: Churchill Livingstone, 1990

Reese RE, Betts RF, eds. A Practical Approach to Infectious Diseases, 3rd ed. Toronto: Little, Brown, 1991

Vibhagool A, Calhoun J, Mader J, et al. Therapy of bone and joint infection. Hosp Formul 1993;28:63–85

DRUG THERAPY FOR THE PREVENTION OF POSTOPERATIVE INFECTIONS

David Forrest

▶ What Are My Goals of Treatment?

to prevent infection when normally sterile tissues (including blood) are likely to be contaminated with bacterial pathogens, both endogenous and exogenous

to reduce morbidity and mortality associated with wound infection after surgery

▶ What Evidence Is Available to Support the Use of Prophylactic Antibiotics?

Decreased incidence of postoperative infection

- early experiments in animal models (Ann Surg 1946; 124:268–276, Surgery 1961;50:161–168), as well as numerous clinical studies, demonstrated the efficacy of perioperative antibiotic administration in reducing the incidence of postoperative infections, particularly wound infections (Principles and Practice of Infectious Diseases 1990:2245–2257)

Reduction in perioperative morbidity

- decrease in postoperative infections is associated with a concomitant reduction in perioperative morbidity and a decrease in the length of the postoperative hospital stay (Arch Surg 1993;128:79–88)

Reduction in perioperative mortality

- reduction in mortality has been shown (N Engl J Med 1986;315:1129–1138)

Cost-effectiveness

- although prophylactic antibiotic administration represents a substantial proportion of hospital budgets, there is good evidence that appropriate use of prophylactic antibiotics is cost-effective (N Engl J Med 1986;315: 1129–1138, J Antimicrob Chemother 1984;14[suppl 13]: 33–37, Ann Surg 1977;185:264–268)

▶ When Should I Consider Drug Therapy?

Antibiotic prophylaxis is not indicated for every surgical procedure • Prophylactic antibiotics should not be used indiscriminately because of the risk for selection and superinfection with antibiotic-resistant organisms, the development of antibiotic-induced pseudomembranous colitis, idiosyncratic adverse drug reactions, and cost • Antibiotic prophylaxis is distinct from treatment of established clinical infection

Clean procedures

- if there is no entry into the respiratory, gastrointestinal, or genitourinary tracts and no major breaks in surgical technique, the incidence of postoperative infection is approximately 5% and antibiotic prophylaxis is *not* routinely indicated
- prophylactic antibiotics are indicated for clean surgical procedures that involve implantation of prosthetic material or in patients who are significantly immunocompromised

Surgical prophylaxis

Neurosurgery

- recommended for CSF shunt procedures in institutions with high infection rates and for high-risk craniotomies

Head and neck surgery

- recommended for procedures involving an incision through the oral cavity or pharynx

Cardiac surgery

- recommended for median sternotomy, coronary artery bypass grafting, and valve surgery

Noncardiac thoracic surgery

- recommended for lobectomy, pneumonectomy, and pacemaker insertion
- no proven benefit in cases of thoracic surgery associated with trauma unless there is esophageal perforation

Peripheral vascular surgery

- recommended for all prosthetic grafts, including abdominal aortic and lower extremity vascular surgery
- no proven benefit in surgery on the carotid arteries and upper extremities

Gastroduodenal surgery

- recommended only when there is a high risk of postoperative infection such as in the presence of diseases or drugs that alter upper gastrointestinal motility or gastric pH or in the presence of bleeding, obstruction, malignancy, or morbid obesity
- gastric bypass

Biliary tract surgery

- recommended only if there is high risk of postoperative infection (risk factors such as age older than 70 years, previous biliary surgery, evidence of obstruction of the biliary tract, acute cholecystitis, and endoscopic or percutaneous instrumentation)

Colorectal surgery

- recommended in all elective and emergency colorectal surgery

Appendectomy

- recommended for all patients

Surgery for abdominal trauma

- recommended for blunt abdominal trauma necessitating laparotomy or penetrating abdominal injury

- antibiotics should be considered therapeutic and not prophylactic in situations in which perforation of a viscus is encountered

Gynecological surgery
- recommended for hysterectomy (abdominal or vaginal)
- recommended for second-trimester instillation abortion and first-trimester induced abortion with a history of previous PID
- prophylactic antibiotics are not indicated for routine dilatation and curettage

Obstetrical surgery (cesarean section)
- recommended only if there is high risk of postoperative infection such as with duration of labor longer than 6 hours with rupture of membranes, premature rupture of membranes, multiple vaginal examinations, and poor socioeconomic status

Urological surgery
- bacteriuria (whether believed to be indicative of infection or not) should be treated with a therapeutic preoperative course of antibiotics, with the specific antibiotics being based on appropriate culture and sensitivity testing results
- if therapy cannot be completed preoperatively, the course should be given through the operative period

Orthopedic surgery
- recommended for arthroplasty (including joint replacement)
- recommended for open reduction of a fracture or lower extremity amputation as these are considered contaminated procedures

▶ *What Drug Should I Use for Initial Treatment?*

Parenteral antibiotic prophylaxis should generally be administered at or shortly before the start of the procedure • Induction of anesthesia is a convenient time for the initiation of such prophylaxis (Principles and Practice of Infectious Diseases 1990:2245–2257)

Surgical prophylaxis

Non–penicillin-allergic patients

Neurosurgery
- vancomycin and gentamicin

Head and neck surgery
- clindamycin and gentamicin

Cardiac surgery
- cefuroxime (J Thorac Cardiovasc Surg 1992;104:590–599)
- in institutions in which there is a high incidence of infection with coagulase-negative *Staphylococcus* species or methicillin-resistant *Staphylococcus* species, use vancomycin

Noncardiac thoracic surgery, peripheral vascular surgery, gastroduodenal surgery, biliary tract surgery, and orthopedic surgery
- cefazolin
- in institutions in which there is a high incidence of infection with coagulase-negative *Staphylococcus* species or methicillin-resistant *Staphylococcus* species, use vancomycin for noncardiac thoracic surgery, peripheral vascular surgery, and orthopedic surgery

Appendectomy, surgery for abdominal trauma, emergency colorectal surgery, and lower extremity amputation
- cefoxitin, ceftizoxime, or cefotetan
- whichever of these agents is least expensive

Colorectal surgery
- mechanical bowel preparation is essential but is not sufficient alone to prevent postoperative infection
- neomycin plus erythromycin on the day prior to surgery and cefoxitin, ceftizoxime, or cefotetan immediately perioperatively

Gynecological surgery
- cefazolin for hysterectomy
- penicillin G for induced abortion in the first trimester in patients with a history of PID

Obstetrical surgery
- cefazolin for cesarean section (after clamping the umbilical cord) or second-trimester instillation abortion

Penicillin-allergic patients

Neurosurgery
- vancomycin and gentamicin

Head and neck surgery
- clindamycin and gentamicin

Cardiac, noncardiac thoracic, peripheral vascular, and orthopedic surgery
- vancomycin

Gastroduodenal, biliary tract, and emergency colorectal surgery; appendectomy; surgery for abdominal trauma; and lower extremity amputation
- clindamycin and gentamicin

Colorectal surgery
- neomycin plus erythromycin on the day prior to surgery and clindamycin or gentamicin immediately perioperatively

Gynecological surgery
- doxycycline for hysterectomy
- metronidazole for second-trimester instillation abortion
- doxycycline should be used for induced abortion in the first trimester in patients with a history of PID

Obstetrical surgery
- clindamycin and gentamicin for cesarean section (after clamping the umbilical cord)

▶ *What Dosage Should I Use?*

Surgical prophylaxis

Antibiotics administered as a single dose (except as indicated) • Repeated doses of penicillin, cefazolin, cefoxitin, cefuroxime, and clindamycin are recommended if surgery is longer than 4 hours (all other agents have a sufficiently long half-life or have a postantibiotic effect which allows for a single dose to be used, as for gentamicin)

CEFAZOLIN
- 1 g IV (2 g in knee arthroplasty if a tourniquet is used)

CEFOXITIN, CEFTIZOXIME, CEFOTETAN
- 2 g IV

CEFUROXIME (FOR CARDIAC SURGERY)
- 1.5 g IV Q12H for 48 hours or until all drainage tubes have been removed (Clin Pharm 1992;11:483–513)

VANCOMYCIN

- 15 mg/kg IV (administer Q12H for 48 hours or until all drainage tubes have been removed for cardiac surgery)

GENTAMICIN

- 2 mg/kg IV

NEOMYCIN, ERYTHROMYCIN

- 1 g PO of each at 1 PM, 3 PM, and 11 PM on the day prior to surgery

CLINDAMYCIN

- 600 mg IV

METRONIDAZOLE

- 500 mg IV

DOXYCYCLINE

- 200 mg IV

PENICILLIN G

- 2 million units IV

▶ *How Long Should I Treat with My Initial Regimen?*

Surgical prophylaxis

Single dose

- in general, only a single preoperative dose of parenteral antibiotic is indicated
- there is no clear evidence that postoperative administration of antibiotics (in addition to appropriately administered preoperative and intraoperative antibiotics) is associated with a reduction in postoperative infection rate
- evidence indicates that multiple doses of antibiotics are no more effective than single doses and may select out more resistant bacteria (Ann Intern Med 1972;76: 843–894, Br Med J 1977;1:1254–1256, Br J Surg 1980; 67:90–92)
- for cardiac surgery, a 48 hour course is suggested; however, there are reports that a single dose may be effective (J Thorac Cardiovasc Surg 1992;104:590–599)
- see above for indications for a repeated dose during surgery

▶ *What Efficacy Parameters Should I Follow and How Frequently Do I Have to Assess My Patient?*

Surgical prophylaxis

Postoperative infection

- evidence of postoperative infection such as fever, wound erythema, tenderness, discharge, and healing delays

▶ *Should I Add Another Drug or Substitute Therapy If My Initial Drug Therapy Fails?*

Surgical prophylaxis

If postoperative infection occurs

- if any postoperative infection occurs, treat with a full course of antibiotics against the causative organisms

▶ *How Long Should I Continue Drug Therapy?*

Surgical prophylaxis

- in general, only a single preoperative dose of parenteral antibiotic is indicated

Useful References

Antimicrobial prophylaxis in surgery. Med Lett 1989;31:105–108

Bergquist EJ, Murphey SA. Prophylactic antibiotics for surgery. Med Clin North Am 1987;71:357–368

Kaiser AB. Postoperative infections and antimicrobial prophylaxis. In: Mandell GL, Douglas RG Jr, Bennett JE, eds. Principles and Practice of Infectious Diseases, 3rd ed. New York: Churchill Livingstone, 1990: 2245–2257

Page CP, Bohnen JM, Fletcher JR, et al. Antimicrobial prophylaxis for surgical wounds. Arch Surg 1993;128:79–88

Van Scoy RE. Prophylactic use of antimicrobial agents in adult patients. Mayo Clin Proc 1987;62:1137–1141

DRUG THERAPY FOR COUGHS AND THE COMMON COLD

Penny F. Miller

▶ *What Are My Goals of Treatment?*

to relieve symptoms of the common cold such as sneezing, increased nasal secretions and congestion, coughing, and aches and pains that are most disturbing to the patient

to use the least number of drugs in the lowest effective dosages while keeping adverse effects at the absolute minimum

▶ *What Evidence Is Available to Support Drug Therapy for Coughs and the Common Cold?*

Coughs

- dextromethorphan and codeine have both been shown to be effective in suppressing coughs (Eur J Clin Pharmacol 1979;16:393–397)
- ability of guaifenesin to increase sputum production and decrease sputum viscosity, thereby facilitating expectoration, has been demonstrated in chronic coughing associated with chronic obstructive pulmonary disease, and consequently it is considered safe and effective as an expectorant for the common cold (Health Protection Branch. Second Report of the Expert Advisory Committee on Nonprescription Cough and Cold Remedies. Health and Welfare Canada, 1989:1–50)

Relief or decreased severity of common cold symptoms

- symptoms of the common cold such as runny nose, congestion, sneezing, and cough are relieved but drugs do not shorten the course of the condition or abort the cold (Health Protection Branch. First Report of the Expert Advisory Committee on Nonprescription Cough and Cold Remedies. Health and Welfare Canada, 1988:1–51) or eradicate the more than 200 viruses responsible for the common cold

Decreased lost time

- lost time from school or work is likely to be reduced by the reduction of cold symptoms, although there is no supportive evidence

Reduction of bacterial infection

- reduction of secondary bacterial infections such as otitis media and sinusitis is not proved

▶ *When Should I Consider Drug Therapy?*

Coughs

- when symptoms of a productive or nonproductive cough

interfere with daily activities or disturb sleep (coughs associated with uncomplicated colds are not usually productive)

Common cold

- drugs decrease the severity of symptoms and should be considered at any time during the presence of symptoms, especially when they interfere with daily activities or worsen other preexisting medical conditions (coughing with stress incontinence, a productive cough with chronic obstructive pulmonary disease, nasal congestion when traveling by air, and so on)

▶ *What Drug Should I Use for Initial Treatment?*

Coughs

Nonproductive cough

DEXTROMETHORPHAN

- has proven efficacy equal to that of codeine (J Int Med Res 1983;11:92–100)
- causes less sedation, constipation, histamine release, and abuse potential than does codeine

Productive cough

GUAIFENESIN

- some evidence of efficacy as an expectorant (Federal Register 1989;54(38):8507) and negligible side effects

Common cold (drug choice depends on the presence of specific symptoms)

Sneezing and/or runny nose

CHLORPHENIRAMINE

- antihistamines have proven efficacy for symptoms such as runny nose and sneezing
- chlorpheniramine has widespread use, has a relatively low incidence of sedation (20–35% compared with 10% with placebo) (N Engl J Med 1991;325:860–869) and anticholinergic side effects, works rapidly, and is less expensive than the newer antihistamines (Health Protection Branch. First Report of the Expert Advisory Committee on Nonprescription Cough and Cold Remedies. Health and Welfare Canada, 1988:1–51)
- antihistamines do not appear to reduce congestion
- agents such as diphenhydramine and promethazine, although effective, are not usually recommended, as they may produce excessive drowsiness
- some of the newer second-generation antihistamines (astemizole) have a slower onset of action and do not have the anticholinergic effects likely required to have an effect on the symptoms of sneezing and runny nose

Nasal congestion

XYLOMETAZOLINE (TOPICAL)

- has proven efficacy, a long duration of action (8–12 hours), and less rebound congestion and lacks a stinging sensation on application that occurs with some other topical decongestants (Self Medication. Reference for Health Professionals, CPhA 1992)
- topical decongestants should be used when a fast and intense decongestant effect is desired for a few days or intermittently or when sympathetic side effects must be avoided
- oral decongestants are preferred if prolonged therapy (i.e., longer than 3–7 days) is required and sympathetic

side effects can be well tolerated or if rebound congestion has already occurred with topical use

PSEUDOEPHEDRINE (ORAL)

- has proven efficacy, a low vasopressor effect, and low abuse potential; is available as single-entity oral preparations; and is inexpensive
- phenylpropanolamine, although also effective and safe when given in recommended doses (Health Protection Branch. Third Report of the Expert Advisory Committee on Nonprescription Cough and Cold Remedies. Health and Welfare Canada, 1989:1–32), is only available in combination products in Canada, and abuse has been reported

Aches and Pains

ACETAMINOPHEN

- has analgesic efficacy equivalent to that of aspirin but does not have an antiplatelet effect and causes less gastrointestinal upset
- acetaminophen is also not associated with Reye's syndrome in children

Fever

- fever is not associated with the common cold so analgesic or antipyretic agents are included for their pain-relieving properties only

Combination products

- single-entity products are preferred; however, if two or more symptoms are bothersome and treatment is desired, any combination of the above is considered acceptable (Health Protection Branch. First Report of the Expert Advisory Committee on Nonprescription Cough and Cold Remedies. Health and Welfare Canada, 1988:1–51)

▶ *What Dosage Should I Use?*

Coughs

DEXTROMETHORPHAN

- 15 mg PO Q4H PRN for symptoms up to a maximum dosage of 120 mg PO daily

GUAIFENESIN

- 200 mg PO Q6H PRN for symptoms to a maximum dosage of 2400 mg PO daily

Common cold

CHLORPHENIRAMINE

- 4 mg PO Q6H PRN for symptoms up to a maximum dosage of 24 mg PO daily

XYLOMETAZOLINE (TOPICAL)

- 0.1%—2–3 drops or sprays in each nostril Q8H PRN for symptoms

PSEUDOEPHEDRINE

- 60 mg PO Q6H PRN for symptoms to a maximum dosage of 240 mg PO daily

ACETAMINOPHEN

- 325 mg PO Q4H PRN for symptoms up to a maximum dosage of 650 mg PO Q4H PRN for symptoms

▶ *How Long Should I Treat with My Initial Regimen?*

Coughs and common cold

- antihistamines should reduce runny nose and sneezing within 2–3 hours

- with topical decongestants, the effect should be seen within 5–10 minutes
- with oral decongestants and oral cough suppressants, the effect should be seen within 30–60 minutes

▶ *What Efficacy Parameters Should I Follow and How Frequently Do I Have to Assess My Patient?*

Coughs and common cold

- follow the frequency and severity of symptoms such as sneezing and/or runny nose, nasal congestion, cough, and aches and pains
- monitor for relief or a reasonable degree of reduction (50–60%) of these symptoms

▶ *Should I Add Another Drug or Substitute Therapy If My Initial Drug Therapy Fails?*

Coughs

Nonproductive cough

- increase dextromethorphan to maximum dosage of 120 mg PO daily
- if this is not effective, codeine (10 mg PO Q4H) may be tried as an alternative agent; however, there is no evidence that codeine is any more effective than dextromethorphan

Productive cough

- increase guaifenesin to a maximum dosage of 2400 mg PO daily
- there are no other expectorants that have demonstrated efficacy
- increase fluid intake (6–8 cups of water a day) and humidify air

Common cold

Sneezing and/or runny nose

- if sedation is a problem, but the antihistamine is effective, reduce the dosage by 50%

- if an antihistamine is not effective, use oral pseudoephedrine
- if congestion is severe, add pseudoephedrine to chlorpheniramine

Nasal congestion

- if initial topical therapy fails, try oral pseudoephedrine
- if initial oral therapy fails, try topical xylometazoline
- if CNS stimulation with oral pseudoephedrine is a problem, switch to topical xylometazoline

Aches and pains

- if not relieved at maximum dosage of 650 mg PO Q4H of acetaminophen, the diagnosis should be reconsidered

▶ *How Long Should I Continue Drug Therapy?*

Coughs

- some coughs may persist longer than a week, and these should be evaluated

Common cold

- because the common cold is a self-limiting condition lasting no longer than 5–7 days, treatment should not extend beyond this time
- topical decongestants should be limited to 3 days of continuous use to prevent rebound congestion; however, xylometazoline may be used for up to 7 days if needed
- if symptoms continue beyond this time, reevaluate the diagnosis

Useful References

Health Protection Branch. First Report of the Expert Advisory Committee on Nonprescription Cough and Cold Remedies. Health and Welfare Canada, 1988:1–51.

Health Protection Branch. Second Report of the Expert Advisory Committee on Nonprescription Cough and Cold Remedies. Health and Welfare Canada, 1989:1–50.

Health Protection Branch. Third Report of the Expert Advisory Committee on Nonprescription Cough and Cold Remedies. Health and Welfare Canada, 1989:1–32.

5

AIDS-RELATED ILLNESS

DRUG THERAPY FOR HUMAN IMMUNODEFICIENCY VIRUS INFECTION

Julio Montaner and Peter Phillips

▶ *What Are My Goals of Treatment?*

to prolong life
to prolong the disease-free interval
to enhance the quality of life

▶ *What Evidence Is Available to Support Drug Therapy for HIV Disease?*

Survival

- zidovudine (AZT) prolongs life in patients with acquired immunodeficiency syndrome (AIDS) or AIDS-related complex (N Engl J Med 1987;317:185–191, N Engl J Med 1992;326:437–443)
- it has become apparent that the overall effect on survival is not different if AZT alone is used early or late in the course of the disease (Lancet 1993;341:889); however,

this issue is less relevant since dideoxyinosine (ddI) and dideoxycytidine (ddC) have become available

Disease-free interval

- AZT prolongs the disease-free interval in patients with CD4 counts less than 500/mm^3 (regardless of their clinical status) (N Engl J Med 1987;317:185–191)

Effect on surrogate markers

- AZT and ddI have a beneficial short-term effect on surrogate markers of human immunodeficiency virus (HIV) disease such as increasing CD4 counts and decreasing levels of p24 antigen
- simultaneous combination of AZT and ddI or ddC may provide greater and more persistent beneficial effects on surrogate markers of HIV disease than does monotherapy

▶ When Should I Consider Drug Therapy?

Human immunodeficiency virus infection

Asymptomatic patients

- if the CD4 count is consistently less than 500/mm^3 (N Engl J Med 1990;322:941–949)

Patients with AIDS-related complex or AIDS

- regardless of CD4 count (N Engl J Med 1987;317:185–191)

Patients with HIV-related thrombocytopenia

- regardless of CD4 count (J AIDS 1990;3:565–570)

▶ What Drug Should I Use for Initial Treatment?

Human immunodeficiency virus infection

ZIDOVUDINE (AZT)

- initial drug of choice

DIDEOXYINOSINE (ddI)

- ddI should be used in patients who have progressed despite zidovudine administration or who are intolerant of zidovudine

DIDEOXYCYTIDINE (ddC)

- not recommended for use as single therapy

STAVUDINE (D4T)

- recently approved by FDA for individuals who fail or cannot tolerate any of the above

▶ What Dosage Should I Use?

Human immunodeficiency virus infection

ZIDOVUDINE (AZT)

- 200 mg PO TID, although some clinicians recommend 100 mg PO Q4H while the patient is awake (dosage regimen likely does not matter as long as the patient receives 500–600 mg PO daily)
- 400 mg PO TID if central nervous system involvement by HIV is apparent (rarely justified)
- 100 mg PO QID if there is evidence of bone marrow dysfunction or hepatic diseases
- 100 mg PO QID is the lowest dosage at which a clinical benefit has been demonstrated (Br Med J 1992;304:13–17)
- beneficial effect on surrogate markers has been demonstrated with dosages of AZT as low as 300 mg/d; however,

the clinical impact of this dosage of AZT has not yet been demonstrated

DIDEOXYINOSINE (ddI)

- for a patient weighing 35–49 kg, give 150 mg PO BID; 50–74 kg, give 200 mg PO BID; and 75 kg or greater, 300 mg PO BID (the last dose is rarely recommended)

DIDEOXYCYTIDINE (ddC)

- 0.75 mg PO TID in simultaneous combination with AZT

▶ How Long Should I Treat with My Initial Regimen?

Human immunodeficiency virus infection

- if the patient is stable, consider adding ddI or changing to ddI (if the patient is intolerant of AZT) after 4–6 months of therapy with AZT, because this delays disease progression and decline in CD4 count

▶ What Efficacy Parameters Should I Follow and How Frequently Do I Have to Assess My Patient?

Human immunodeficiency virus infection

Clinical progression

- patients with low CD4 counts but no other symptoms of HIV infection generally do not notice any difference with AZT administration, except that their disease does not progress and infections do not develop as soon as expected without AZT
- patients with some consitutional symptoms (fever, night sweats, and weight loss) generally notice an improvement within 2–8 weeks
- many patients respond with a transient increase in CD4 counts
- patients with HIV-related dementia may show some improvement in cognitive function
- patients with HIV-related thrombocytopenia may show higher platelet counts for some time
- for the first 6 weeks of therapy, patients should be monitored every 1–2 weeks
- if stable, patients can be monitored every 4–8 weeks

CD4 counts

- every 3–6 months if initially greater than 300/mm^3 to guide the introduction of *Pneumocystis carinii* pneumonia (PCP) prophylaxis, and every 3 months if less than 300/mm^3 to guide the use of alternative therapy

▶ Should I Add Another Drug or Substitute Therapy If My Initial Drug Therapy Fails?

Human immunodeficiency virus infection

- if disease progression occurs despite AZT administration, ddI should be added to therapy or used as monotherapy if the patient is intolerant of zidovudine
- patients who experience intolerance of AZT should be given ddI, as the spectrum of adverse effects of ddI (see above for dosage) is significantly different from that of AZT
- ddC can be used in combination with AZT

▶ How Long Should I Continue Drug Therapy?

Human immunodeficiency virus infection

- antiretroviral agents do not prevent the ultimate development of disease, rather delay it

- antiretroviral therapy should be continued for life, even in the face of clinical progression of HIV disease, as long as the patient tolerates the drug

DRUG THERAPY FOR *PNEUMOCYSTIS CARINII* PNEUMONIA

Julio Montaner and Peter Phillips

▶ What Are My Goals of Treatment?

to reduce mortality
to prevent respiratory failure
to ameliorate the symptoms of PCP
to prevent or postpone the development of PCP

▶ What Evidence Is Available to Support Drug Therapy for AIDS-Related PCP?

Treatment of the acute episode

- antimicrobial therapy reduces the mortality of AIDS-related PCP (N Engl J Med 1990;323:769–775, Ann Intern Med 1991;114:948–953)
- adjunctive corticosteroid therapy further reduces mortality and accelerates the defervescence of AIDS-related PCP (Ann Intern Med 1990;113:15–20, N Engl J Med 1990;323:1500–1504, Tubercle and Lung Disease 1993; 74:173–177)

Prophylaxis

- prevents 85% or more of PCP relapses over 6 months (Ann Intern Med 1991;114:948–953)

▶ When Should I Consider Drug Therapy?

Treat as soon as possible

- PCP is extremely frequent among patients with advanced HIV disease who have a CD4 count of $200/mm^3$ or less
- presence of a dry cough, dyspnea, fever, a clear chest on examination, and a recent elevation of serum lactic dehydrogenase (LDH) levels are all useful supporting evidence of a diagnosis of PCP
- diagnostic confirmation necessitates obtaining tracheo-bronchial secretions, usually through sputum induction or bronchoscopic bronchoalveolar lavage
- many times, this cannot be achieved on an emergency basis, and therefore, treatment can be started prior to diagnosis
- unfortunately PCP's differential diagnosis is extensive and includes other readily treatable conditions, such as bacterial pneumonia and tuberculosis, that can seriously deteriorate if an empirical course of anti-PCP medications is undertaken; therefore, etiological confirmation of the diagnosis is highly desirable

Prophylaxis

- any HIV-infected individual who has had a previous episode of PCP or who has a CD4 count less than $200/mm^3$ should receive PCP prophylaxis
- PCP prophylaxis is also recommended if there is evidence of recurrent oral candidiasis, if the CD4 fraction is less than 15%, if there is a diagnosis of AIDS, or if there are unexplained constitutional symptoms such as persistent weight loss and fever

▶ What Drug Should I Use for Initial Treatment?

Treatment

TRIMETHOPRIM-DAPSONE

- preferred regimen for mild to moderately severe PCP that can be treated on an outpatient basis with an oral regimen, as it is effective and inexpensive

TRIMETHOPRIM-SULFAMETHOXAZOLE

- is preferred if there is known dapsone intolerance, or if the initial hemoglobin level is below 110 g/L, because dapsone is known to produce methemoglobinemia and hemolytic anemia in a dose-related fashion
- if concomitant bacterial infection is present or suspected, trimethoprim-sulfamethoxazole is also preferred because of its inherent antimicrobial activity
- trimethoprim in combination with either sulfamethoxazole or dapsone is preferred over pentamidine because of the cost of pentamidine

ATOVAQUONE

- less efficacy than trimethoprim-sulfamethoxazole but better tolerated
- reserved for mild to moderate PCP in patients who are intolerant of trimethoprim-sulfamethoxazole who can take oral medications

PENTAMIDINE

- is reserved for patients with a well-documented history of sulfa intolerance who require IV therapy (e.g., severe PCP) or who cannot tolerate oral medications
- aerosol pentamidine should not be used for the treatment of PCP because it has poor distribution to the areas of the lungs that are more heavily affected

PREDNISONE

- should be added to the initial treatment in patients with moderate to severe respiratory distress defined by an arterial oxygen pressure of less than 75 mmHg while the patient is breathing room air
- even patients with milder PCP are likely to benefit

Prophylaxis

TRIMETHOPRIM-SULFAMETHOXAZOLE

- most effective regimen
- more convenient and less expensive than aerosol pentamidine
- trimethoprim-sulfamethoxazole has a rather high incidence (50%) of adverse drug reactions (rash, nausea, fever, and neutropenia), particularly among HIV-infected individuals

DAPSONE

- intermittent dapsone administration should be used if trimethoprim-sulfamethoxazole cannot be tolerated
- do not take dapsone simultaneously with ddI (separate administration by several hours) because the ddI buffer may decrease the bioavailability of dapsone

AEROSOL PENTAMIDINE

- reasonable option for patients intolerant of sulfa drugs or those who have evidence of bone marrow dysfunction
- long-term use appears to increase the risk of pneumothorax

- avoid aerosolized pentamidine in patients with severe or poorly controlled asthma because it precipitates bronchospasm

▶ What Dosage Should I Use?

Treatment

TRIMETHOPRIM

- 20 mg/kg PO daily divided QID or 200 mg PO QID

DAPSONE

- 100 mg PO daily

SULFAMETHOXAZOLE

- 100 mg/kg PO daily divided QID
- when using trimethoprim-sulfamethoxazole, this equals approximately 2 double-strength tablets QID

ATOVAQUONE

- 750 mg PO TID

PENTAMIDINE

- 4 mg/kg IV daily

PREDNISONE

- 40 mg PO BID for 1 week, followed by 40 mg PO daily for 1 week, and then followed by 20 mg PO daily for 1 week

Prophylaxis

TRIMETHOPRIM-SULFAMETHOXAZOLE

- 1 double-strength tablet PO daily

DAPSONE

- 100 mg PO 3 times weekly

AEROSOL PENTAMIDINE

- 60 mg every 2–3 days for 5 doses followed by 60 mg every 2 weeks via ultrasonic nebulizer (FISONeb) or 300 mg every month via continuous, flow-driven nebulizer (Respigar II), whichever is available
- routine premedication with salbutamol is recommended to decrease the risk of bronchospasm

▶ How Long Should I Treat with My Initial Regimen?

Treatment

- 14 days of therapy is usually adequate
- 21 days if the patient responds slowly

Prophylaxis

- continue for life

▶ What Efficacy Parameters Should I Follow and How Frequently Do I Have to Assess My Patient?

Treatment

- response to treatment should be monitored using clinical variables such as respiratory rate, fever, heart rate, as well as pulse oximetry in moderate to severe cases
- patients treated with dapsone have at least some degree of hemolytic anemia, which is associated with an increase in serum lactic dehydrogenase (LDH) levels that should not be misinterpreted as worsening of the PCP

- monitor the patient once or twice weekly as an outpatient if milder disease is present
- daily or more frequent inpatient monitoring if moderate to severe disease is present

Prophylaxis

- before starting PCP prophylaxis, a chest x-ray should be obtained to ensure that there is no active pulmonary disease (in particular, subclinical pulmonary tuberculosis should be ruled out if aerosol pentamidine will be used)
- simple spirometry is also advisable to rule out asthma in patients who will be treated with aerosolized pentamidine
- no specific ongoing monitoring is required
- PCP can occur despite adequate prophylaxis, and its presentation may be unusual

▶ Should I Add Another Drug or Substitute Therapy If My Initial Drug Therapy Fails?

Treatment

- patients should generally improve within 3–5 days of initiating antimicrobial therapy
- deterioration occurring within the first 3–5 days of treatment indicates the need for a thorough reassessment of the case to rule out other concomitant or complicating conditions (e.g., pulmonary embolism, pneumothorax, and bacterial or viral infection)
- if deterioration occurs in a patient not previously receiving corticosteroids, prednisone should be added to the regimen
- lack of improvement after 5–7 days of appropriate treatment justifies a change to an alternative antimicrobial agent
- combination of the above-mentioned regimens is not recommended, as this does not enhance therapeutic efficacy and it certainly potentiates toxicity
- clindamycin-primaquine is a promising combination currently under investigation

▶ How Long Should I Continue Drug Therapy?

Treatment

- 14 days of therapy is usually adequate
- if the patient is clinically improving and afebrile after 5–7 days of therapy, the IV pentamidine may be switched to a combination of oral dapsone (100 mg PO daily) and trimethoprim (200 mg PO QID) for the remainder of the 14 days, which enables the patient to be treated at home
- 21 days, if the patient responds slowly
- after the initial treatment is completed, patients should be prescribed PCP prophylaxis for life

Prophylaxis

- for life

DRUG THERAPY FOR HIV-RELATED CANDIDIASIS

Peter Phillips

▶ What Are My Goals of Treatment?

to control symptoms such as local pain, altered taste and dysphagia, and visible oral white lesions

▶ *What Evidence Is Available to Support Drug Therapy for HIV-Related Candidiasis?*

Control of symptoms

- treatment eradicates the lesions, controls the symptoms (Rev Infect Dis 1990;12[suppl 3]:334–337, Postgrad Med 1988;84:193–205), and facilitates nutrition, particularly if there is esophageal involvement

▶ *When Should I Consider Drug Therapy?*

Oropharyngeal candidiasis

- usually a presumptive diagnosis based on signs and symptoms
- diagnosis confirmed by Gram stain or potassium hydroxide smear
- mouth culture is not required

Esophageal candidiasis

- this is the most likely diagnosis in any patient with HIV or AIDS (who is not already receiving antifungal therapy) presenting with dysphagia or odynophagia
- rapid symptomatic response shortly after initiating specific therapy obviates the need for endoscopy in these patients (Am J Gastroenterol 1989;84:143–146); however, if symptoms persist, endoscopy should be performed to rule out other potentially treatable pathogens such as herpes simplex virus (HSV) and cytomegalovirus (CMV)

▶ *What Drug Should I Use for Initial Treatment?*

Oropharyngeal candidiasis

CLOTRIMAZOLE

- topical agents should initially be used because they are associated with less toxicity and less potential for drug interactions
- unfortunately, compliance with these regimens may be poor, and this often mandates a change to systemic antifungal therapy such as ketoconazole, fluconazole, or itraconazole (see below under esophageal candidiasis)
- clotrimazole is preferred as the initial treatment of oropharyngeal candidiasis, as it may be better tolerated than nystatin; however, clotrimazole is more expensive than nystatin

NYSTATIN

- equally effective as clotrimazole but may be less well tolerated

Esophageal candidiasis

KETOCONAZOLE

- ketoconazole is the preferred agent for the initial treatment of esophageal candidiasis, as it is less expensive than fluconazole
- not tolerated as well and somewhat less effective than fluconazole (Ann Intern Med 1992;117:655)

ITRACONAZOLE

- itraconazole and ketoconazole both given as 200 mg PO daily resulted in similar response rates for both esophageal and oropharyngeal candidiasis (ICAAC 1992, abstract 1117, p 297)

FLUCONAZOLE

- use if there is failure to achieve some symptomatic improvement after 5–7 days with ketoconazole or initially if a drug interaction may be more likely to result in failed

therapy with ketoconazole or itraconazole (e.g., rifampin, H_2 blockers, and omeprazole)

▶ *What Dosage Should I Use?*

Oropharyngeal candidiasis

CLOTRIMAZOLE

- 1 troche (10 mg) 5 times a day
- 1 vaginal suppository (100 mg) dissolved slowly in the mouth TID if troches are not available (Dig Dis Sci 1991;36:279–281) and increase to 5 times a day if TID dosing is not effective

NYSTATIN

- 1 vaginal tablet (100,000 units) dissolved slowly in the mouth TID (up to 5 a day depending on response)
- suspension is generally less effective owing to decreased contact time but can be used at 500,000 units in a swish and swallow route QID
- choice of the above depends on the patient's preference

KETOCONAZOLE

- 200 mg PO daily

ITRACONAZOLE

- start with 100 mg PO BID for 3 days, then give 100 mg PO daily
- if no response within a week, increase the dose to 200 mg PO daily

FLUCONAZOLE

- start with 100 mg PO daily for 1 day, then give 50 mg PO daily
- if no response within a week, increase the dose to 100 mg PO daily
- 150 mg PO as a single dose has been effective

Esophageal candidiasis

KETOCONAZOLE

- 200 mg PO daily (200 mg PO BID if disease is moderate to severe)

ITRACONAZOLE

- 200 mg PO daily

FLUCONAZOLE

- 200 mg PO followed by 100 mg PO daily

▶ *How Long Should I Treat with My Initial Regimen?*

Oropharyngeal candidiasis

- 1 week and at least 2 days after the symptoms have resolved
- patient should respond within a few days to a week
- single-dose fluconazole may be used

Esophageal candidiasis

- treat for at least 2–3 weeks and 1 week after the resolution of symptoms

▶ *What Efficacy Parameters Should I Follow and How Frequently Do I Have to Assess My Patient?*

Oropharyngeal candidiasis

- reduction in pain and disappearance of lesions
- assess symptoms once or twice weekly, but no specific

monitoring is required unless the condition does not improve

Esophageal candidiasis

- relief of dysphagia and odynophagia
- assess symptoms daily for inpatients or weekly for outpatients
- endoscopy is not required unless symptoms persist

▶ *Should I Add Another Drug or Substitute Therapy If My Initial Drug Therapy Fails?*

Oropharyngeal candidiasis

- the response rate to topical therapy usually decreases with repeated episodes, as often evidenced by an increased amount of time needed to achieve symptomatic relief with each new episode as well as a shortening of the symptom-free interval between episodes and, in this case, it is useful to change to systemic antifungal therapy
- systemic therapy should be recommended if persistent symptoms are severe enough to warrant the increased expense and potential adverse effects or drug interactions of the systemic agents
- combination of topical and systemic therapy is not recommended, as it usually does not increase efficacy
- preliminary studies indicate that itraconazole solution (200 mg PO daily) may be effective in fluconazole-resistant mucosal candidiasis (IXth International Conference AIDS 1993:abstract PO–B09–1394:368)
- patients who do not respond to itraconazole solution should be considered for treatment with amphotericin B

Esophageal candidiasis

- failure to achieve some symptomatic improvement after 5–7 days of therapy warrants consideration of a change to fluconazole if the diagnosis was confirmed by endoscopy
- endoscopic diagnosis should be considered in patients who do not respond to fluconazole
- see under oropharyngeal candidiasis for treatment of fluconazole-resistant mucosal candidiasis

▶ *How Long Should I Continue Drug Therapy?*

Oropharyngeal candidiasis, esophageal candidiasis

- relapses occur frequently, and it has not been determined which of the following approaches is most effective: repeated courses of antifungal agents for symptomatic recurrences, intermittent topical or systemic antifungal therapy, or indefinite daily maintenance antifungal therapy (topical or systemic)
- if patients notice that episodes occur frequently (e.g., monthly), intermittent treatment with fluconazole 150 mg PO once weekly should be considered (J Infect Dis 1990;21:55–60)
- if this fails to control the recurrences, continuous therapy should be considered

---

DRUG THERAPY FOR AIDS-RELATED CYTOMEGALOVIRUS DISEASE

Peter Phillips

▶ *What Are My Goals of Treatment?*

to arrest the progression of disease in the involved eye (or eyes) and to preserve vision and prevent blindness in patients with CMV chorioretinitis

to control symptoms in patients with gastrointestinal infection

to reduce morbidity and mortality related to other sites of CMV visceral infection (e.g., lung, brain, and hepatobiliary system)

▶ *What Evidence Is Available to Support Drug Therapy for CMV Disease?*

Vision

- untreated CMV chorioretinitis leads to blindness and can be successfully delayed or averted with the use of ganciclovir (Ann Intern Med 1991;115:665–673, N Engl J Med 1992;326:213–220)

Gastrointestinal symptoms

- gastrointestinal infection by CMV can produce a variety of syndromes; among the most common are esophagitis and colitis, which can be very symptomatic
- clinical responses may be achieved with ganciclovir therapy (Ann Intern Med 1992;116:63–77)
- randomized placebo-controlled trial showed some evidence of benefit in ganciclovir-treated patients (J Infect Dis 1993;167:278–282)

Other sites of infection

- there are no controlled studies to indicate the efficacy of ganciclovir or foscarnet for AIDS-related CMV disease in other organs

▶ *When Should I Consider Drug Therapy?*

Chorioretinitis

- chorioretinitis should be treated promptly after the detection of characteristic retinal lesions

Gastrointestinal disease

- pathological confirmation (typical intranuclear inclusions in cytomegalic cells with or without positive culture or antigen detection in tissue by immunohistochemistry) should be obtained before initiating treatment

▶ *What Drugs Should I Use for Initial Treatment?*

Chorioretinitis, gastrointestinal disease

GANCICLOVIR

- foscarnet and ganciclovir have been equally effective for delaying the progression of retinitis (N Engl J Med 1992;326:213–220)
- some improvement in median survival time has been seen with foscarnet (12 months) compared with ganciclovir (8 months), although this finding has yet to be confirmed in other studies (N Engl J Med 1992;326:213–220)
- foscarnet is somewhat more toxic, inconvenient regarding administration (infusion pump), and more expensive than ganciclovir

FOSCARNET

- foscarnet therapy may be associated with clinical response in patients failing to respond to ganciclovir therapy

▶ *What Dosage Should I Use?*

Chorioretinitis

GANCICLOVIR

- 5 mg/kg IV Q12H for 14 days (21 days if patient responds slowly) followed by a maintenance dosage of 5 mg/kg IV daily, or 6 mg/kg IV daily for 5 d/wk in patients not willing to do 7 d/wk maintenance

FOSCARNET

- 60 mg/kg IV over 1 hour Q8H for 14 days (21 days if patient responds slowly) followed by a maintenance dosage of 120 mg/kg IV daily (over 2 hours) administered via pump to avoid inadvertent rapid infusion (use 90 mg/kg IV daily if the patient is fluid overloaded or at risk for toxicity)
- alternative induction dosage is 100 mg/kg IV Q12H for 14–21 days (VIth International Conference AIDS 1990: abstract ThB434)
- foscarnet doses greater than 60 mg/kg are given over 2 hours with 500–1000 mL of normal saline to reduce the risk of nephrotoxicity

Gastrointestinal disease

GANCICLOVIR

- 5 mg/kg IV Q12H for 14–21 days
- role of maintenance therapy is unclear in gastrointestinal disease
- some clinicians reserve maintenance therapy for patients having frequent recurrences

FOSCARNET

- 60 mg/kg IV Q8H for 14–21 days

▶ *How Long Should I Treat with My Initial Regimen?*

Chorioretinitis

- treat for at least 2–3 weeks before switching to another agent
- chorioretinitis usually necessitates lifelong maintenance therapy

Gastrointestinal disease

- 14–21 days
- response should be seen in 7–10 days

▶ *What Efficacy Parameters Should I Follow and How Frequently Do I Have to Assess My Patient?*

Chorioretinitis

- ophthalmological assessment for evidence of progression
- patients should be assessed every 1–2 weeks until retinitis is inactive and then monthly by an experienced ophthalmologist

Gastrointestinal disease

- relief of diarrhea, abdominal discomfort, and fever
- assess clinical changes in symptoms daily initially and then 2–3 times a week

▶ *Should I Add Another Drug or Substitute Therapy If My Initial Drug Therapy Fails?*

Chorioretinitis, gastrointestinal disease

- if there is no clinical response to treatment (e.g., continued progression of retinitis and persistent gastrointestinal symptoms) after 2–3 weeks, consider changing ganciclovir to foscarnet or vice versa

▶ *How Long Should I Continue Drug Therapy?*

Chorioretinitis

- if the patient becomes blind in 1 eye but the other eye is not affected, either continue maintenance therapy to try to prevent retinitis in the remaining eye or consider stopping and providing close follow-up of the remaining eye
- if a decision is made to stop maintenance therapy, reinduction and maintenance can be restarted if the second eye becomes involved

Gastrointestinal disease

- some authorities (Ann Intern Med 1992;116:63–77) recommend maintenance therapy; however, some clinicians reserve maintenance therapy for patients with frequent recurrences

---

DRUG THERAPY FOR CEREBRAL TOXOPLASMOSIS IN PATIENTS WITH AIDS

Peter Phillips

▶ *What Are My Goals of Treatment?*

to prevent progression of the disease
to improve symptoms such as headaches, motor-sensory deficits, and seizures
to reduce the size of the lesions as visualized by computed tomographic (CT) scan

▶ *What Evidence Is Available to Support Drug Therapy for Cerebral Toxoplasmosis in Patients with AIDS?*

Response rate

- with appropriate therapy, a 65–90% response rate measured as relief of symptoms and improvement in CT scan can be expected in patients with AIDS-related cerebral toxoplasmosis (Ann Neurol 1986;19:224–238, Am J Med 1988;84:94–100, Am J Med 1989;86:521–527)

Relapse prevention

- without lifelong suppressive therapy, relapse is predictable (Am J Med 1988;84:94–100)

▶ *When Should I Consider Drug Therapy?*

Toxoplasmosis

- when a known HIV-infected individual has neurological symptoms and a CT scan of the head demonstrates compatible lesions
- in these cases, pathological confirmation of the cause is not required (Am J Med 1989;86:521–527)
- atypical lesions or the suspicion of a cause other than toxoplasmosis (e.g., lack of response to standard treatment), particularly if serum serological study is negative for toxoplasmosis, may necessitate brain biopsy for confirmation of diagnosis

▶ *What Drugs Should I Use for Initial Treatment?*

Toxoplasmosis

SULFADIAZINE AND PYRIMETHAMINE

- less expensive than clindamycin and pyrimethamine (Ann Intern Med 1992;116:33–43)

CLINDAMYCIN AND PYRIMETHAMINE

- if the patient is sulfa allergic

FOLINIC ACID

- should be added to either regimen to decrease the frequency of drug-induced hematological toxicity

CORTICOSTEROIDS

- steroids should be reserved for patients with life-threatening cerebral edema related to mass lesions
- steroids may be associated with improvement in central nervous system lymphoma and therefore confuse the results of empirical therapy for toxoplasmosis

▶ *What Dosage Should I Use?*

Toxoplasmosis

SULFADIAZINE

- 4–8 g/d (100 mg/kg/d) PO in 4 divided doses

PYRIMETHAMINE

- 100 mg PO BID for 1 day followed by 75 mg PO daily

CLINDAMYCIN

- 900 mg IV Q6H for 3 weeks until marked clinical improvement occurs
- if no clinical improvement occurs, increase the dose to 1200 mg IV Q6H
- once marked clinical improvement has occurred, give 300 mg PO QID for 3 more weeks (Ann Intern Med 1992; 116:33–43)

FOLINIC ACID

- 10 mg PO daily

▶ *How Long Should I Treat with My Initial Regimen?*

Toxoplasmosis

- treat for 6 weeks, at which time there has usually been marked clinical improvement
- lesions that fail to respond to antitoxoplasmosis therapy within 7–14 days should be considered for diagnostic stereotactic brain biopsy, unless the patient's general medical condition and short-term prognosis are poor (Neurosurgery 1992;30:186–190)
- major symptomatic improvement can be expected to occur within 7–14 days of the initiation of therapy

▶ *What Efficacy Parameters Should I Follow and How Frequently Do I Have to Assess My Patient?*

Toxoplasmosis

- assess daily for clinical improvement in headaches, fever, and neurological signs

Computed tomographic scan

- improvement of lesions on the CT scan of the head can be expected to occur after 2–4 weeks of therapy
- a repeated CT scan should be done 2–3 weeks after starting treatment

▶ *Should I Add Another Drug or Substitute Therapy If My Initial Drug Therapy Fails?*

Toxoplasmosis

- continue pyrimethamine but switch sulfadiazine to clindamycin or vice versa
- regimen of clarithromycin plus pyrimethamine has been associated with favorable results (Interscience Conference on Antimicrobial Agents and Chemotherapy 1990:abstract 1158, p. 279)

new agent, atovaquone, is currently available for patients who fail to respond to or cannot tolerate conventional therapy (VIIth International Conference AIDS 1991:abstract W.B. 31, Vol 2, p. 30)

▶ *How Long Should I Continue Drug Therapy?*

Toxoplasmosis

- maintenance therapy should be continued lifelong (sulfadiazine 500 mg PO QID and pyrimethamine 50 mg PO daily and folinic acid 5 mg PO daily, which can be increased to 20 mg PO daily if hematological toxicity persists)
- without maintenance treatment, relapse is the rule, even after normalization of the CT scan (Am J Med 1989; 86:521–527)

DRUG THERAPY FOR CRYPTOCOCCAL MENINGITIS IN PATIENTS WITH AIDS

Peter Phillips

▶ *What Are My Goals of Treatment?*

to provide symptomatic relief of headache, photophobia, fever, and decreased level of consciousness
to sterilize the cerebrospinal fluid
to decrease mortality
to reduce progression of the disease

▶ *What Evidence Is Available to Support Drug Therapy for Cryptococcal Meningitis in Patients with AIDS?*

Mortality

- untreated cryptococcal meningitis is universally fatal
- before the AIDS era, a 65% cure rate was reported using standard doses of amphotericin B
- in the context of AIDS, cryptococcal meningitis is probably incurable with the currently available regimens; however, it is temporarily suppressed by amphotericin B with resolution of symptoms
- 30–50% 1 year relapse rate occurs in patients not receiving lifelong suppressive therapy versus rare relapses occurring with lifelong fluconazole suppression (N Engl J Med 1992;326:793–798)

▶ *When Should I Consider Drug Therapy?*

Cryptococcal meningitis

- treatment should be initiated immediately after diagnosis, which is made by demonstrating the fungus in the cerebrospinal fluid using India ink smear, cryptococcal antigen, or culture
- cerebrospinal fluid variables in patients with cryptococcal meningitis in the context of AIDS are often normal or minimally abnormal (often few or no cells and glucose and protein may be normal)

▶ *What Drugs Should I Use for Initial Treatment?*

Cryptococcal meningitis

AMPHOTERICIN B PLUS FLUCYTOSINE

- combination has been shown to be the treatment of choice in non-AIDS patients (N Engl J Med 1979;301:126), but

it is unclear whether it is more effective than amphotericin alone in AIDS patients (Ann Intern Med 1990;113: 183–187, N Engl J Med 1992:326:83–89)
- add flucytosine unless there are significant cytopenias or renal impairment

FLUCONAZOLE

- fluconazole is considered to be less effective than amphotericin B as initial therapy but might be considered in selected cases if there is mild disease without poor prognostic factors (e.g., abnormal mental status, or both cryptococcal antigen titer > 1:1024 and cerebrospinal fluid white blood cell count < 20/mm^3 [N Engl J Med 1992;326:83–89])
- use if the patient develops severe intolerance of amphotericin

ITRACONAZOLE

- use if the patient refuses to take amphotericin and/or is refractory to or intolerant of fluconazole
- less effective than amphotericin B (AIDS 1992;6:185–190)

▶ *What Dosage Should I Use?*

Cryptococcal meningitis

AMPHOTERICIN B

- administer 0.7 mg/kg IV daily until there is marked improvement (usually 2–3 weeks), and then complete a 10 week course of fluconazole 400 mg PO daily (N Engl J Med 1992;327:565–566)

FLUCYTOSINE

- 25 mg/kg PO Q6H

FLUCONAZOLE

- 400 mg PO daily

ITRACONAZOLE

- 200 mg PO BID

▶ *How Long Should I Treat with My Initial Regimen?*

Cryptococcal meningitis

- for 10 weeks, and expect clinical response in 1–2 weeks for most patients

▶ *What Efficacy Parameters Should I Follow and How Frequently Do I Have to Assess My Patient?*

Cryptococcal meningitis

- relief of headache, neurological signs, and fever
- assess daily until clinical response occurs, then 1–2 times a week until the patient has completed 10 weeks of treatment
- periodic lumbar punctures to check for reduction in CSF cryptococcal antigen titer and sterilization of CSF may not be necessary in patients who are doing well clinically
- if initial lumbar puncture indicates elevated opening pressure or clinical course suggests development of raised intracranial pressure, repeated lumbar punctures may be required (+/− repeat CT head scans)
- optimal management of elevated intracranial pressure has not been determined in this situation

▶ *Should I Add Another Drug or Substitute Therapy If My Initial Drug Therapy Fails?*

Cryptococcal meningitis

- intrathecal amphotericin B is not indicated because of significant risks of complications and uncertain additional benefit
- in patients failing to respond to amphotericin B, consider increasing the amphotericin dosage to 1 mg/kg/d and adding flucytosine while ruling out complications such as raised intracranial pressure with or without hydrocephalus

▶ *How Long Should I Continue Drug Therapy?*

Cryptococcal meningitis

- lifelong suppressive therapy should be undertaken
- fluconazole 200 mg PO daily is clearly the preferred approach (N Engl J Med 1992;326:793–798, N Engl J Med 1991;324:580–584) despite its cost and potential drug interactions, because it has greater efficacy, convenience (once-daily oral dosing), and tolerance compared with amphotericin
- the relapse rate with maintenance therapy is 6% with fluconazole and 24% with itraconazole

---

DRUG THERAPY FOR AIDS-RELATED *MYCOBACTERIUM AVIUM* INFECTION

Peter Phillips

▶ *What Are My Goals of Treatment?*

to control constitutional symptoms (fever, chills, night sweats, malaise, and fatigue) and, in some patients, gastrointestinal symptoms (abdominal pain and diarrhea), and thereby to improve the patient's quality of life

to prolong life

▶ *What Evidence Is Available to Support Drug Therapy for AIDS-Related* Mycobacterium avium *Infection?*

Improvement in symptoms with multiple-drug regimens

- constitutional complaints (fevers, chills, and malaise) are more responsive to therapy than are weight loss, diarrhea, and anemia (N Engl J Med 1991;324:1332–1338)
- 1 randomized placebo-controlled trial in HIV-infected patients has been reported, in which microbiological efficacy was demonstrated (J Infect Dis 1993;168:112–119)

Prolonged survival

- evidence suggests that survival is prolonged in patients receiving multiple-drug regimens compared with the case for untreated patients (J Infect Dis 1991;164:994–998)
- no randomized comparative trial, but some reports have questioned the survival benefit with current regimens for the treatment of *M. avium* infection in AIDS patients (AIDS 1991;5:1036–1038)
- preliminary results indicate that rifabutin prophylaxis in advanced HIV disease provides some protection against the development of *M. avium* bacteremia

Prophylaxis of *Mycobacterium avium* infection

- *M. avium* mycobacteremia is approximately twice as frequent with placebo compared with rifabutin 300 mg PO daily (VIII International Conference AIDS 1992:abstract WeB 1055)
- clarithromycin also is effective prophylaxis and may be associated with a survival benefit (ICAAC, Abstract A/ 2 October 1994)

▶ When Should I Consider Drug Therapy?

Treatment

- any patient with documented invasive or disseminated infection with *M. avium*
- disseminated disease is most often diagnosed by mycobacterial blood culture, which may take up to 6 weeks before becoming positive
- less often, the diagnosis is made by smear, histological study, and/or culture of bone marrow, lymph node, or occasionally liver biopsy specimen (N Engl J Med 1991;324:1332–1338)
- most patients are symptomatic, but occasionally symptoms have largely resolved by the time a microbiological diagnosis is made
- it is currently unclear whether such asymptomatic patients with documented disseminated disease should be treated differently from those who remain symptomatic
- patients who have *M. avium* recovered from the respiratory or gastrointestinal tracts may be colonized but do not necessarily have invasive or disseminated infection
- colonization may not necessarily give way to disseminated infection, even if it is untreated (J Infect Dis 1991;163:1326–1335); appropriate management of colonized patients has not been defined

Prophylaxis

- patients with an absolute CD4 count of less than 100/mm^3 should be offered prophylaxis

▶ What Drug Should I Use for Initial Treatment?

Treatment

- several multiple-drug regimens have been reported to be associated with clinical improvement, but optimal therapy has not been identified by way of randomized comparative trials to date
- at least 2 drugs in combination, including a macrolide (clarithromycin or azithromycin) plus ethambutol with or without a rifamycin (e.g., rifampin or rifabutin), ciprofloxacin, or clofazimine (Clin Infect Dis 193;17:7–20)

CIPROFLOXACIN, CLOFAZIMINE, RIFAMPIN, AND ETHAMBUTOL

- an alternative regimen (N Engl J Med 1991;324: 1332–1338)

Prophylaxis

RIFABUTIN

- drug of choice

CLARITHROMYCIN

- for patients who cannot tolerate rifabutin

▶ What Dosage Should I Use?

When starting multiple-drug regimens for *M. avium* infection, it may be useful to introduce the drugs sequentially over the first 1–2 weeks, so that there may be greater opportunity for identifying which drugs may be responsible for specific adverse effects

Treatment

ETHAMBUTOL

- 15 mg/kg PO daily

CIPROFLOXACIN

- 750 mg PO BID

CLOFAZIMINE

- 100 mg PO daily

RIFAMPIN

- 600 mg PO daily (or 10 mg/kg if body weight < 50 kg)

CLARITHROMYCIN

- 500 mg PO BID

AZITHROMYCIN

- 600–1200 mg PO daily

Prophylaxis

RIFABUTIN

- 150 mg PO BID

CLARITHROMYCIN

- 500 mg PO BID

▶ How Long Should I Treat with My Initial Regimen?

Treatment?

- oral medications are continued indefinitely
- addition or substitution of other antimycobacterial drugs should be considered in patients who experience adverse effects or remain symptomatic after the first few weeks of treatment

▶ What Efficacy Parameters Should I Follow and How Frequently Do I Have to Assess My Patient?

Treatment

Signs and symptoms

- fevers, chills, night sweats, malaise, fatigue, weight loss, abdominal pain, and diarrhea
- there are usually few or no physical signs to follow other than body weight and possibly the presence of a lesion in patients with localized disease (e.g., regional lymphadenopathy)
- patients should also be advised to report new or worsening diarrhea while taking such regimens, because *Clostridium difficile* colitis is a possible complication
- patients should be assessed every 1–2 weeks during the first 1–2 months of treatment but more often for severe cases

Laboratory variables

Complete blood count

- monthly or more frequently if there is severe disease, to detect progressive anemia and cytopenias due to bone marrow involvement, which may persist despite treatment

Blood cultures

- to document reduction or clearance of mycobacteremia, particularly in patients who have persistent symptoms

Prophylaxis

- Prior to initiating rifabutin, a mycobacterial culture should be performed to exclude unrecognized MAC infection, in addition to a chest x-ray and sputum specimen to exclude active pulmonary tuberculosis
- investigate for *M. avium* infection (mycobacterial blood culture) if patient develops suggestive findings (unexplained fevers, or hematocrit <30% or serum albumin <3.0 g/dL) in association with ≤50 CD4 cells/mm^3 (Clin Infect Dis 1994;19:668–674)

▶ Should I Add Another Drug or Substitute Therapy If My Initial Drug Therapy Fails?

Treatment

- drugs associated with the greatest potential cost, toxicity, and inconvenience should be the first to be removed from the multiple-drug regimen if substitution is being considered
- although there are no clear guidelines, patients initially treated with ciprofloxacin, clofazamine, rifampin, and ethambutol (N Engl J Med. 1991;324:1332–1338) may have clarithromycin substituted for rifampin, as rifampin seems more likely to be associated with adverse effects
- clarithromycin 500 mg PO BID may be added to the regimen in patients who remain symptomatic after the first few weeks of treatment (Am Rev Respir Dis 1991;144:564–569) if it is not included in the initial regimen
- use of other antimycobacterial drugs such as ethionamide and cycloserine is discouraged because of the associated toxicities (N Engl J Med 1991;324:1332–1338)
- amikacin has not yet been shown to provide additional benefit in multidrug regimens (Clin Infect Dis 1993; 17:7–20) and is associated with considerable inconvenience (IV route of administration) and potential toxicity
- antiinflammatory drugs may be considered for patients with marked constitutional complaints (especially high fevers) unresponsive to antimycobacterial therapy, when other causes of fever have been excluded

Prophylaxis

- if the patient develops adverse effects of rifabutin (e.g., uveitis, arthritis, pseudojaundice) then consider clarithromycin 500 mg PO BID for prophylaxis (Interscience Conference on Antimicrobial Agents and Chemotherapy 1994, abstract A/2)

▶ How Long Should I Continue Drug Therapy?

Treatment

- lifelong, although clinical trials have not addressed this question
- number of patients, even after 1 year or longer of treatment, can develop recurrent symptoms and mycobacteremia when antimycobacterial medication administration is stopped

Prophylaxis

- lifelong

DRUG THERAPY FOR HIV-RELATED HERPES SIMPLEX VIRUS (HSV) INFECTION

Peter Phillips

▶ What Are My Goals of Treatment?

to shorten the duration and reduce the severity of HSV primary infection at mucocutaneous sites

to reduce the number of recurrences of mucocutaneous infection with chronic suppressive therapy

to reduce the morbidity and mortality associated with visceral HSV infection

▶ What Evidence Is Available to Support Drug Therapy for HIV-Related HSV Infection?

Shortened duration of disease

- both primary and secondary infections with HSV at ano-genital and perioral as well as other mucocutaneous sites may be effectively treated with oral or IV acyclovir (N Engl J Med 1983;308:916–921, Am J Med 1988;85: 301–306)

Prevention of recurrences

- the frequency of recurrences is reduced with acyclovir (J Am Acad Dermatol 1988;18:186)

Visceral infection

- morbidity and mortality are reduced with acyclovir treatment of visceral HSV infection (e.g., encephalitis and hepatitis) (N Engl J Med 1986;314:144–149)

▶ When Should I Consider Drug Therapy?

Active infection

- all patients with suspected (pending the results of viral studies) and proven primary HSV infection at mucocutaneous or deep visceral sites should be treated
- patients who are receiving either ganciclovir or foscarnet for induction or maintenance treatment of CMV disease usually do not require acyclovir because both of these CMV antiviral agents have activity against HSV

Suppression

- long-term suppression should be considered in patients with frequent recurrent episodes of mucocutaneous infection

▶ What Drug Should I Use for Initial Treatment?

Active infection, suppression

ACYCLOVIR

- acyclovir is the drug of choice for HSV infections, as it is better tolerated than ganciclovir and foscarnet and is more effective than vidarabine
- acyclovir is also available as an oral medication, whereas the others are not

▶ What Dosage Should I Use?

Active infection

ACYCLOVIR

Mild infections

- 200 mg PO 5 times daily (some clinicians recommend 400 mg PO TID) for active HSV infection at mucocutaneous sites
- give 400 mg PO 5 times daily if there is inadequate response to the lower dosage

Severe episodes

- 5 mg/kg IV Q8H
- 10 mg/kg IV Q8H for patients with deep visceral HSV infections (e.g., encephalitis and hepatitis)

Suppression

ACYCLOVIR

- start with 400 mg PO BID, and if not effective, increase the dosage to as much as 400 mg PO 5 times daily (Ann Intern Med 1993;118:268–272)

▶ *How Long Should I Treat with My Initial Regimen?*

Active infection

ACYCLOVIR

Mild infections
- 10 days

Severe episodes
- continue parenteral therapy until there has been a clinical response, at which time treatment may be changed to oral acyclovir, and complete a 10 day course
- for visceral infection, treatment should be completed parenterally

Suppression

ACYCLOVIR

- indefinitely

▶ *What Efficacy Parameters Should I Follow and How Frequently Do I Have to Assess My Patient?*

Active infection

Mild infections • clinical resolution
- for mucocutaneous disease, lesions should be followed clinically for evidence of healing (crusting and then reepithelialization)
- reevaluate at 7–10 days to ensure that clinical resolution has occurred
- follow-up viral cultures are unnecessary, except in patients who have persistent mucocutaneous lesions caused by HSV despite appropriate treatment with acyclovir, and in such patients, the possibility of acyclovir-resistant HSV should be excluded

Severe episodes • clinical resolution
- daily clinical evaluation is required
- depending on clinical response, deep visceral infection may necessitate monitoring appropriate for the site of involvement (e.g., serial CT head scans, electroencephalograms, liver enzymes, and chest x-rays)

Suppression

- periodic evaluation every few months; recurrent lesions unresponsive to high-dose acyclovir suggest possible acyclovir-resistant strains

▶ *Should I Add Another Drug or Substitute Therapy If My Initial Drug Therapy Fails?*

Active infection

Mild infections
- if oral acyclovir proves ineffective for mucocutaneous disease, treatment should be changed to IV acyclovir at a dosage of 5 mg/kg IV Q8H

Severe episodes
- if acyclovir-resistant HSV is strongly suspected (preferably documented), treatment of mucocutaneous disease should be foscarnet 40 mg/kg IV Q8H (N Engl J Med 1991;325:551–555, Am J Med 1992;90:30s–35s) (each dose is infused with an infusion pump or other accurate flow regulators to avoid inadvertent rapid IV administration)
- hydration with IV saline (500–1000 mL before each induction or maintenance dose of foscarnet) is recommended to reduce the frequency of nephrotoxicity (Ann Intern Med 1990;113:332)

- duration of foscarnet therapy in acyclovir-resistant HSV must be individualized according to the clinical response
- when lesions have healed, which often takes 2 weeks or longer of treatment, foscarnet therapy can be stopped and high-dose oral acyclovir administration may be started, because some residual HSV in nerve roots may remain sensitive to acyclovir (however, patients often require long-term IV foscarnet suppressive therapy)

Suppression

- although many first recurrences of acyclovir-resistant HSV infection are sensitive to acyclovir, second recurrences are acyclovir resistant (N Engl J Med 1991; 352:551–555)
- documented acyclovir-resistant strains should be treated with foscarnet 90 mg/kg once dialy for 5–7 d/wk as needed (N Engl J Med 1989;320:297–300)

▶ *How Long Should I Continue Drug Therapy?*

Active infection

Mild infections
- 10 days

Severe episodes
- continue parenteral therapy until there has been a clinical response, at which time treatment may be changed to oral acyclovir, and complete a 10 day course
- for acyclovir-resistant HSV infection continue foscarnet until clinical resolution (usually 2–3 weeks or longer)

Suppression

- indefinitely

DRUG THERAPY FOR HIV-RELATED VARICELLA-ZOSTER VIRUS INFECTIONS

Peter Phillips

▶ *What Are My Goals of Treatment?*

to shorten the duration of illness and to reduce the time to crusting and healing of skin lesions for both herpes zoster (shingles) and varicella (chickenpox)
to reduce the morbidity and mortality associated with deep visceral infection with varicella-zoster virus (VZV)

▶ *What Evidence Is Available to Support Drug Therapy for HIV-Related VZV Infections?*

Shortened duration

- efficacy of drug therapy in VZV infections has been established in other immunocompromised patient populations (N Engl J Med 1986;314:208–212)
- duration of illness and the time to crusting and healing of lesions in patients with dermatomal infections (herpes zoster) and disseminated infection (varicella) may be reduced with IV or oral acyclovir treatment (AIDS 1988;2 [suppl 1]:5191–5193, Ann Ophthalmol 1988;20:480–482)

Decreased progression

- reduction of the rate of progression from localized to disseminated herpes zoster has been accomplished with

the use of IV acyclovir in other immunocompromised patient populations, but this has not been studied in AIDS patients
- postherpetic neuralgia is not prevented or reduced in severity by steroid treatment

▶ When Should I Consider Drug Therapy?

Suspected or proven herpes zoster (shingles)
- treat suspected or proven infections

Suspected or proven varicella (chickenpox)
- diagnosis may be confirmed by antigen detection and immunofluorescent stains of material obtained from lesions and by viral culture
- treat all cases in HIV-infected patients

Chronic varicella syndrome
- occasional patients may experience a chronic varicella syndrome (J Am Acad Dermatol 1988;18:584–585) and require long-term oral acyclovir to try to reduce the number of skin lesions

▶ What Drugs Should I Use for Initial Treatment?

Suspected or proven herpes zoster (shingles), suspected or proven varicella (chickenpox), chronic varicella syndrome

ACYCLOVIR
- drug of choice, as it is more effective and less toxic than vidarabine for VZV infection (N Engl J Med 1986; 314:208–212)
- acyclovir is better tolerated than ganciclovir, foscarnet, and vidarabine

▶ What Dosage Should I Use?

Suspected or proven herpes zoster (shingles)

ACYCLOVIR
- 800 mg PO 5 times daily
- 10 mg/kg IV Q8H for severe episodes and those with ophthalmic involvement
- if no response, increase dose to 12 mg/kg IV Q8H

Suspected or proven varicella (chickenpox)

ACYCLOVIR
- 10 mg/kg IV Q8H
- if no response, increase dose to 12 mg/kg IV Q8H

Chronic varicella syndrome

ACYCLOVIR
- 10 mg/kg IV Q8H for 7–10 days followed by long-term treatment
- if no response, increase dose to 12 mg/kg IV Q8H

▶ How Long Should I Treat with My Initial Regimen?

Suspected or proven herpes zoster (shingles)
- 7–10 days

Suspected or proven varicella (chickenpox)
- until there is no further development of new lesions and old lesions are crusting, which usually involves at least 7 days of IV treatment

Chronic varicella syndrome
- probably indefinite suppressive therapy

▶ What Efficacy Parameters Should I Follow and How Frequently Do I Have to Assess My Patient?

Suspected or proven herpes zoster (shingles)
Clinical variables
- development of new lesions as well as the healing (crusting and reepithelialization) of existing lesions
- follow-up once or twice weekly for mild to moderate episodes and more frequently for severe or ophthalmic involvement
- patients should be observed for evidence of secondary bacterial infections occurring at the site of herpes zoster skin lesions

Suspected or proven varicella (chickenpox)
Clinical variables
- development of new lesions, as well as the healing (crusting and reepithelialization) of existing lesions, and fever
- follow-up should be daily initially
Laboratory variables
- chest X-ray and oxygen saturation in cases of varicella pneumonia
- liver enzyme levels if associated hepatitis occurs

Chronic varicella syndrome
- assess the development of new lesions

▶ Should I Add Another Drug or Substitute Therapy If My Initial Drug Therapy Fails?

Suspected or proven herpes zoster (shingles), suspected or proven varicella (chickenpox)
- if there is no response to oral acyclovir, switch to IV acyclovir for herpes zoster
- if there is still no response after approximately 1–2 weeks, investigational antiviral therapy for herpes zoster may be considered if available (e.g., BV-ara-U [Bristol Myers-Squibb])
- vidarabine has been effective in the management of herpes zoster (N Engl J Med 1982;307:971–975) in other patient populations but may be associated with greater toxicity

Chronic varicella syndrome
- if this remains unresponsive to high-dose oral or IV acyclovir, consider acyclovir-resistant varicella and treat with foscarnet 40 mg/kg IV Q8H for 2–4 weeks (Ann Intern Med 1990;112:187–191)
- if 40 mg/kg IV Q8H is ineffective, consider increasing dose to 60 mg/kg IV Q8H

▶ How Long Should I Continue Drug Therapy?

Suspected or proven herpes zoster (shingles), suspected or proven varicella (chickenpox)
- both herpes zoster and varicella can usually be treated with a 7–10 day course of acyclovir

Chronic varicella syndrome
- indefinitely
- acyclovir-resistant VZV infection has been reported in AIDS patients, particularly in association with long-term use of acyclovir (Ann Intern Med 1990;112:187–191)
- foscarnet is the drug of choice for acyclovir-resistant VZV infection (Ann Intern Med 1991;115:19–21)

6 | NEUROLOGICAL DISEASES

DRUG THERAPY FOR EPILEPSY

William A. Parker

▶ What Are My Goals of Treatment?

to reduce seizure frequency and severity (complete seizure control may not always be possible) with an acceptable incidence of side effects

to educate the patient regarding epilepsy, the types of seizures that may be experienced, and the importance of lifestyle changes and compliance with drug therapy in the control of seizures

▶ What Evidence Is Available to Support Drug Therapy for Epilepsy?

Seizure control

- approximately 80% of all epileptic patients experience control of their disease or show a significant reduction in severity of seizures with appropriate anticonvulsant therapy (Antiepileptic Drugs 1972;87–101, A Textbook of Epilepsy 1988;421–483)
- efficacy varies according to the age at onset, the seizure type and severity, and the serum anticonvulsant level (Prognosis of Patients with Epilepsy 1968, Epilepsia 1973;14:93)
- reduces the chance of trauma arising from seizures (head-banging, falling, and experiencing prolonged anoxia with status epilepticus and/or aspiration and its complications)

▶ When Should I Consider Drug Therapy?

Generalized seizures (no primary focus), partial seizures (with or without secondarily generalized tonic-clonic seizures)

- it is not necessary to start drug therapy for the first seizure unless there is a lesion found on computed tomographic scan or an epileptic focus seen on electroencephalogram (EEG)
- start drug therapy when there is a history of recurrent seizures (more than one) that cannot be explained by drug or alcohol abuse, cardiac arrhythmias, metabolic disorder, or other nonepileptiform cause
- patient's particular seizure type must be identified first on the basis of a description of the seizure by an observer; the history of any recentor past head trauma; drug history and drug or alcohol abuse; and detailed neurological examination, complete blood count, serum electrolyte determination, liver function tests, urinalysis, VDRL test, skull X-rays, and computed tomographic scan

Status epilepticus

- when status epilepticus is present (repetitive seizure activity in which the patient does not regain consciousness between seizures or there is a continuous, single seizure episode lasting 30 minutes or longer, with or without

alteration of consciousness), immediate treatment is required

Alcohol withdrawal (treatment and prevention of seizures)

- all patients with the potential for alcohol withdrawal syndrome should receive prophylactic drug therapy to help prevent signs and symptoms of alcohol withdrawal and to prevent further potential alcohol withdrawal seizures
- all alcohol withdrawal seizures should be treated because they can be life-threatening

▶ What Drug Should I Use for Initial Treatment?

Rational drug selection is based on the seizure type, and initial treatment should be with one drug, as monotherapy permits easier titration and assessment of the drug's effect or toxicity

Generalized seizures (no primary focus)
Tonic-clonic seizures

VALPROIC ACID

- is effective and is better tolerated than phenytoin or carbamazepine
- phenytoin and carbamazepine cause a greater incidence of central nervous system adverse effects
- also useful if the patient has generalized tonic-clonic and absence seizures, as valproic acid works on both seizure types

CARBAMAZEPINE

- many clinicians prefer carbamazepine over phenytoin as initial therapy owing to fewer adverse effects, easier dose titration, and fewer cosmetic side effects than with phenytoin
- carbamazepine is more expensive than phenytoin and must be dosed twice a day, compared with once-daily dosing for phenytoin

PHENYTOIN

- phenytoin is the drug of choice if an agent must be given parenterally
- phenytoin causes more cosmetic side effects than does carbamazepine (hirsutism, coarsening of facial features, and gingival hyperplasia) and may cause a greater incidence of adverse cognitive effects than does carbamazepine
- phenytoin has the advantages of being given once a day and being inexpensive

PHENOBARBITAL

- use only if valproic acid, phenytoin, or carbamazepine is not effective
- phenobarbital is effective but has a greater potential for causing sedation or behavioral disturbances than do the other agents

Absence seizures
ETHOSUXIMIDE

- as effective as valproic acid
- ethosuximide is preferred because of the risk of serious hepatotoxicity and pancreatitis with valproic acid, although risk of valproic acid hepatotoxicity is much lower in adults than in children

VALPROIC ACID

- can be used if there is a contraindication to the use of ethosuximide or ethosuximide is ineffective
- drug of choice if multiple seizures are present because ethosuximide is effective only for absence seizures

CLOBAZAM (CANADA ONLY), CLONAZEPAM, NITRAZEPAM

- these agents are effective alternative drugs in treating patients who do not tolerate or respond to first-line drugs
- they are second-line drugs owing to central nervous system and behavioral side effects and the potential for loss of efficacy after several months
- many clinicians prefer clobazam to clonazepam because it has fewer psychomotor side effects

Myoclonic seizures (including juvenile myoclonic epilepsy)
VALPROIC ACID

- drug of choice, as it is the most effective agent for juvenile myoclonic epilepsy

CLOBAZAM (CANADA ONLY), CLONAZEPAM, NITRAZEPAM

- see above under absence seizures

Partial seizures (with or without secondarily generalized tonic-clonic seizures)
CARBAMAZEPINE, PHENYTOIN

- phenytoin and carbamazepine are equally effective, and the decision between these agents is as above under generalized seizures
- phenytoin is the drug of choice if parenteral therapy is required

VALPROIC ACID

- not as effective as carbamazepine and phenytoin, but is an alternative in patients who do not respond to or cannot tolerate phenytoin or carbamazepine (N Engl J Med 1992;327:765–771)

PHENOBARBITAL, CLOBAZAM

- use only if the above agents are ineffective

Status epilepticus
LORAZEPAM

- is the first choice for many clinicians, as it distributes out of the central nervous system more slowly and may work longer than diazepam (even though it has a shorter half-life than does diazepam), but the clinical significance of this is not known (Pharmacotherapy: A Pathophysiologic Approach 1992:864–878)

DIAZEPAM

- as effective as and less expensive than lorazepam
- when given intravenously, diazepam causes more irritation than does lorazepam and is absorbed erratically when given intramuscularly

PHENYTOIN

- should be started as soon as possible after the initial dose of the benzodiazepine
- may not be needed after a history has been determined, but it is best to load the patient with phenytoin initially and then to decide in 12–24 hours whether the patient requires maintenance phenytoin therapy

PHENOBARBITAL

- use if the patient is still having seizures 1 hour after a phenytoin load (usually given while preparing the patient to be moved to the intensive care unit)

Alcohol withdrawal (treatment and prevention of seizures)
DIAZEPAM

- both diazepam and lorazepam are effective for preventing alcohol withdrawal seizures
- diazepam has a longer duration of action than does lorazepam and other benzodiazepines, which may be useful when stopping diazepam administration (self-titrating)
- some clinicians prefer lorazepam over diazepam, because if an IM agent is required (in addition to an oral agent for backup), IM lorazepam is absorbed more rapidly and completely than IM diazepam

LORAZEPAM

- as for status epilepticus, many clinicians prefer lorazepam for the treatment (i.e., not prevention) of seizures secondary to alcohol withdrawal

PHENYTOIN

- not effective for the prevention of alcohol withdrawal seizures (Ann Emerg Med 1991;20:520–522, Am J Med 1989;87:645–648)
- if there is a question about the coexistence of epilepsy, a phenytoin loading dose is administered and maintenance therapy is begun
- after the patient is stabilized, obtain the history and stop phenytoin administration if epilepsy is ruled out

▶ *What Dosage Should I Use?*

When there is little urgency for completely protecting the patient from recurrent seizures, minimize side effects by gradually increasing the drug dosage to the full initial dose (see below) • Further dosages must be slowly and carefully adjusted according to individual requirements and clinical response, rather than relying solely on serum drug concentrations

Generalized seizures (no primary focus), partial seizures (with or without secondarily generalized tonic-clonic seizures), alcohol withdrawal (treatment and prevention of seizures), status epilepticus
VALPROIC ACID

- 15 mg/kg/d as a starting dose
- if immediate response not needed, it is best to start administration at 500 mg PO HS and increase by 500 mg daily every 5–7 days to minimize gastrointestinal side effects
- final total daily dose depends on the frequency of seizures and the patient's ability to tolerate the drug
- patients with primary generalized seizures require 1500–2000 mg PO daily divided BID to TID depending on tolerance

- patients with juvenile myoclonic epilepsy generally require lower dosages
- patients previously receiving valproic acid can initially be given divalproex (enteric coated) at the same daily dosage
- divalproex is often the agent used in a BID regimen to reduce the incidence of gastrointestinal upset

ETHOSUXIMIDE

- loading dose is not appropriate
- initial dose is 250 mg BID
- data suggest that patients can successfully be managed on once-daily therapy, but gastrointestinal distress appears to be dose related and most patients better tolerate a BID regimen
- maintenance dosage is 20 mg/kg/d; achieve by increasing the daily dosage by 250 mg every 5 days until seizure control is achieved or side effects become intolerable

PHENYTOIN

Orally with no loading dose

- 300 mg PO daily HS
- 400 mg PO daily HS if the patient weighs more than 70 kg
- to reduce initial gastrointestinal or central nervous system side effects, start slowly; give 100 mg PO daily HS for 3 days, then 200 mg PO daily HS for 3 days, and then 300 mg PO daily HS (400 mg for patients weighing > 70 kg)
- once-daily dosing is appropriate if capsules are used (sustained release)
- if tablets or suspension is used, the daily dose must be split and given BID
- in patients who clear the drug rapidly, have side effects, or tend to forget some doses, phenytoin should be given in 2 divided doses

Oral loading dose

- oral loading dose should be used in patients when rapid (within 8–12 hours) attainment of effective serum concentrations is needed (for a patient who has had several recent seizures)
- without a loading dose, steady state serum concentrations may not be achieved for a couple of weeks
- 15 mg/kg (usually 1 g given PO as 400 mg, 300 mg, and 300 mg administered at 3 hour intervals)
- initiate maintenance dosage the following day

Intravenous (if the oral route is not available or for status epilepticus)

- 15 mg/kg IV given no faster than 50 mg/min
- start the maintenance dosage the following day
- if only the parenteral route is available, give 100 mg IV TID or 200 mg IV Q12H as the maintenance dosage

CARBAMAZEPINE

- 200 mg PO BID, if an immediate response is needed
- if an immediate response is not needed, give 100 mg PO daily for 3 days; increase to 100 mg PO BID for 3 days, and then 100 mg PO every morning and 200 mg PO every evening for 3 days; and then increase to 200 mg PO BID, as this regimen should decrease the initial gastrointestinal upset and dizziness seen with this agent
- avoid single doses greater than 400 mg to minimize gastrointestinal upset

LORAZEPAM

- administer 2 mg IV over 30–60 seconds, and if seizures are not controlled and no cardiorespiratory depression occurs, give another 2 mg in 2–5 minutes

- further 2 mg IV can be given 10–20 minutes later if tonic-clonic seizures continue (this rarely happens) while phenytoin is being administered
- to prevent alcohol withdrawal seizures, give 2 mg PO TID for 2 days, 2 mg PO BID for 2 days, and 2 mg PO daily for 1 day and then stop

DIAZEPAM

- administer 5 mg IV over 30–60 seconds, and if seizures are not controlled and no cardiorespiratory depression occurs, give another 5 mg in 2–5 minutes
- a further 10 mg IV can be given 10–20 minutes later if tonic-clonic seizures continue
- to prevent alcohol withdrawal seizures, give 10 mg PO Q1H until the patient is sedated and then given 10 mg PO TID for 2–3 days

PHENOBARBITAL

- 30 mg PO TID, increasing by 60 mg/d every 5 days until seizure control is achieved, side effects become intolerable, or a maximum dosage of 250 mg PO daily is reached
- maintenance dosage can be consolidated into a single nightly dose because of the drug's long half-life
- takes 2–3 weeks to reach steady state concentration
- for status epilepticus, give 250 mg IV at a maximum rate of 60 mg/min and repeat in 30 minutes if seizures are not controlled to a maximum dose of 20 mg/kg
- maximum drug effect may not be seen for up to 30 minutes, so give the drug time to work before reinjecting to avoid overdose

CLOBAZAM (CANADA ONLY)

- 10 mg PO daily, increasing every 5–7 days until seizures are controlled, side effects become intolerable, or a maximum dose of 80 mg is reached
- daily doses up to 30 mg may be taken as a single dose at bedtime; if the daily dose is divided, the largest portion should be given at bedtime

CLONAZEPAM

- start with 0.5 mg PO HS for 7 days, as clonazepam is very sedating
- increase the dosage by 0.5 mg every 3–5 days (given BID) until seizures are controlled, side effects become intolerable, or a maximum daily dosage of 20 mg PO is reached (usual dosage is 4–6 mg/d)
- largest dose should be given at bedtime if doses are not equally divided

NITRAZEPAM

- start with 2.5 mg PO TID, increasing the dosage every 3–5 days until seizures are controlled, side effect become intolerable, or a maximum dosage of 1 mg/kg/d is reached
- if doses are not equally divided, the larger dose should be given at bedtime

▶ How Long Should I Treat with My Initial Regimen?

Generalized seizures (no primary focus), partial seizures (with or without secondarily generalized tonic-clonic seizures)

- if seizures are frequent enough, use seizure frequency as a guide to determine when to increase the dosage or change drug therapy
- if not, continue therapy until steady state serum drug concentrations within the therapeutic range are achieved (see individual drug monographs)

Status epilepticus

- continue administering a benzodiazepine until a seizure has stopped
- if the patient is still experiencing seizures 1 hour after phenytoin administration, use phenobarbital

Alcohol withdrawal (treatment and prevention of seizures)

- continue administering a benzodiazepine until the seizure has stopped
- after the seizure has stopped, continue maintenance diazepam administration for 3–4 days
- for prevention of alcohol withdrawal seizures, continue the benzodiazepine therapy for 3–4 days, and at this time, diazepam administration may be stopped, as its long half-life allows it to taper itself
- continue phenytoin administration until epilepsy is ruled out

▶ *What Efficacy Parameters Should I Follow and How Frequently Do I Have to Assess My Patient?*

Generalized seizures (no primary focus), partial seizures (with or without secondarily generalized tonic-clonic seizures)

Reduction in seizure frequency

- monitor for reduction in seizure frequency (a seizure diary can be used)

Serum concentrations

- because of large interindividual and intraindividual variability of anticonvulsant drug concentrations in relation to dose, serum drug level monitoring is essential in the treatment of epilepsy
- drug level determinations are indicated in patients with poorly controlled and recurrent seizures, suspected toxicity, suspected noncompliance, hepatic or renal disease, and the addition or removal of concurrent anticonvulsants, and for establishing a baseline for monitoring long-term therapy (see individual drug monographs for specific guidelines on sampling times and ranges)
- serum drug concentration ranges may be exceeded to achieve seizure control, provided the side effects are tolerable

Status epilepticus

- cessation of seizures

Alcohol withdrawal (treatment and prevention of seizures)

- prevention or reduction of symptoms of withdrawal such as tremor, irritability, and tachycardia

▶ *Should I Add Another Drug or Substitute Therapy If My Initial Drug Therapy Fails?*

Goal is to achieve monotherapy; however, this is not always possible

Generalized seizures (no primary focus), partial seizures (with or without secondarily generalized tonic-clonic seizures)

Patient has achieved little or no seizure control with the first drug

- stop the first drug and add another first-line agent

Patient has achieved partial seizure control with the first drug

- continue the first drug, and if complete control is attained with a second drug, slowly withdraw the first agent, although some patients may be reluctant to attempt this
- reduction in polytherapy was accomplished in 80% of 90 patients, with more than 50% of these patients achieving successful monotherapy (Epilepsia 1981;22:1–10)

reduction to monotherapy also benefited more than half of the patients by improving their alertness, concentration, drive, mood, and sociability (Epilepsia 1981;22:1–10)

Status epilepticus

- if the patient is still experiencing seizures 1 hour after phenytoin administration, use phenobarbital

Alcohol withdrawal (treatment and prevention of seizures)

- continue to administer a benzodiazepine until the patient becomes sedated, and then start a maintenance dosage

▶ *How Long Should I Continue Drug Therapy?*

Generalized seizures (no primary focus), partial seizures (with or without secondarily generalized tonic-clonic seizures)

- patient should be seizure free for at least 4 years
- decision to discontinue therapy should be done with careful consideration of the patient's desire and motivation, along with an assessment of the probability of success and the risks associated with recurrence, including the possible loss of driver's license
- patients should not drive during withdrawal and for 3–4 months after, and this may make it difficult for some patients to try withdrawal
- prior to withdrawal, patients should be advised that about $^1/_3$ will experience relapse, and if this occurs, the patient and the physician will know that the drug is still necessary
- recurrence of seizures usually happens within the first 6 months
- patients at low risk can expect a 30% chance of recurrence; low-risk factors include idiopathic epilepsy, seizure onset between 2 and 35 years of age, and normal EEG; and the longer the patient has been free from seizures, the less likely they are to recur
- patients at high risk can expect a 50% chance of recurrence
- high-risk factors include partial complex seizures and seizures associated with an identifiable lesion, a history of high frequency of seizures or status epilepticus, multiple seizure types, persistence of abnormal EEG, and the development of abnormal mental functioning
- focal seizures and the persistence of a focal abnormality on the EEG are indications for continuing anticonvulsant administration for longer periods of time than is necessary in the case of generalized tonic-clonic or absence seizures
- drug withdrawal should be attempted in patients with juvenile myoclonic epilepsy but is usually not successful, and therapy probably needs to be lifelong
- drugs should be discontinued one at a time, withdrawing the least effective or most toxic first
- dosage should be decreased slowly over 3–6 months until the drug is completely withdrawn
- allow a new steady state condition to be reached between dosage reductions
- if the patient remains seizure free for 1 month, the second drug is discontinued in the same manner, and so on
- if seizures recur, drug therapy should be restarted with the last agent withdrawn

Status epilepticus

- continue to administer drug therapy until the seizure has stopped and then decide (as above) about the need for long-term therapy

Alcohol withdrawal (treatment and prevention of seizures)

- continue a maintenance dosage for 2–3 days, then discontinue benzodiazepine administration

- diazepam continues to be effective for 1–2 days after stopping the drug therapy owing to its long duration of action
- reinstitute a maintenance dosage if the person starts to exhibit signs and symptoms of withdrawal

Useful References

Parker WA. Epilepsy. In: Herfindal ET, Gourley DR, Hart LL, eds. Clinical Pharmacy and Therapeutics, 4th ed. Baltimore: Williams & Wilkins, 1988:570–592

Pugh CB, Garnett WR. Current issues in the treatment of epilepsy. Clin Pharm 1991;10:335–358

Winter ME, Tozer TN. Phenytoin; Levy RH, Wilensky AJ, Friel PN. Other antiepileptic drugs. In: Evans WE, Schentag JJ, Jusko WJ, eds. Applied Pharmacokinetics. Principles of Therapeutic Drug Monitoring, 2nd ed. Spokane, WA: Applied Therapeutics, 1986:493–539, 540–569

DRUG THERAPY FOR PARKINSON'S DISEASE

Ruby Grymonpre

▶ What Are My Goals of Treatment?

to restore the patient to a normal level of function for as long as possible by maintaining a balance between dopaminergic and cholinergic activity in the basal ganglia

to prevent or minimize long-term complications of Parkinson's disease

to provide the patient with the lowest possible dosage that is effective in controlling symptoms and thereby to prevent or minimize long-term complications associated with the pharmacological management of Parkinson's disease

▶ What Evidence Is Available to Support Drug Therapy for Parkinson's Disease?

Improvement in function

- in general, approximately 85% of patients with early, mild Parkinson's disease can achieve at least 50% improvement in their level of function with dopaminergic therapy (Br Med Bull 1990;46(1):124–146)

Disease progression

- there is not yet firm evidence to substantiate claims that drugs halt disease progression

▶ When Should I Consider Drug Therapy?

Parkinson's disease

Treatment is not warranted if early, mild symptoms cause no disability (clumsiness of the hands, fatigue, and sensory discomfort) • Institute treatment if disability interferes with the patient's social, emotional, or work life

- initiate therapy early when the patient has bilateral or midline involvement, without impairment of balance
- persons with preexisting cardiac or psychiatric illness are especially susceptible to the adverse effects of antiparkinsonian drugs, such as postural hypotension, mental confusion, and depression, and in these patients, the risks of side effects may outweigh the benefits of therapy

▶ What Drug Should I Use for Initial Treatment?

Parkinson's disease

Initial drug choice must be individualized, depending on the severity and presenting symptoms of Parkinson's disease and the presence or absence of other concomitant disease states

BENZTROPINE, TRIHEXYPHENIDYL, PROCYCLIDINE

- anticholinergics have been used as first-line therapy for patients with mild Parkinson's disease (tremor as the predominant symptom) and good cognitive function; however, anticholinergics are now most often used as adjuncts to levodopa therapy when tremor is a problem
- there is no difference among benztropine, trihexyphenidyl, and procyclidine with respect to efficacy; however, benztropine may have greater sedative effect than do some of the other anticholinergic agents (Clin Pharmacokinet 1987;13:141–178)
- trihexyphenidyl is more stimulating than the other agents
- benztropine is the only agent that can be given once daily, whereas trihexyphenidyl, with the exception of the sustained-release product, and procyclidine may need to be given more frequently
- decision among these agents should be based on cost, compliance issues, and the patient's response

LEVODOPA-CARBIDOPA OR LEVODOPA-BENSERAZIDE (CANADA ONLY)

- levodopa therapy should be initiated early in Parkinson's disease when symptoms interfere with the patient's social, emotional, or work life
- levodopa is the initial drug of choice and is used in conjunction with anticholinergics when tremor is a problem
- addition of a peripheral decarboxylase inhibitor (carbidopa or benserazide) allows a 60–80% reduction in the oral dose of levodopa required for therapeutic effect and reduces nausea and other peripheral effects (N Y State J Med 1987;87:147–153)
- there is clinically no difference between levodopa-carbidopa and levodopa-benserazide, and the decision about which agent to use should be based on cost and dosage flexibility (Drugs 1984;28:236–262)
- levodopa-carbidopa is available in more useful dosages and dosage forms, and in practice, most patients receive this combination
- levodopa-benserazide capsules can be opened and may be useful in patients having difficulty in swallowing tablets or capsules
- the regular levodopa-carbidopa tablets (not the sustained-release products) can be crushed and administered in a fruit-based liquid or soft food
- when capsules are opened or tablets crushed, the drug should be used immediately as levodopa oxidizes in the presence of moisture

SELEGILINE

- although there is a suggestion that selegiline halts the progression of the disease, there is no firm evidence to substantiate this claim (Drugs 1990;39:646–651)
- despite the lack of definitive evidence that selegiline delays the progression of Parkinson's disease, it has now become common to use it early in the course of treatment, either before or at the same time that levodopa administration is started
- selegiline can also be added to levodopa therapy as adjunct therapy when a patient's condition deteriorates with dosages of levodopa (with a decarboxylase inhibitor) of greater than 700 mg PO daily

BROMOCRIPTINE

- added when a patient has an unstable fluctuating pattern of response to current levodopa and selegiline therapy and when additional measures to minimize these fluctuations (e.g., reduced dosing interval of levodopa, dosage adjustments, and the use of sustained-release levodopa) have failed
- patients with dose-response fluctuations experience a smoother clinical response when bromocriptine is added, possibly because its half-life is longer than levodopa's

AMANTADINE

- in patients intolerant of other drugs for parkinsonism, amantadine can be tried; however, with the exception of a few patients, the effect is minimal and wears off quickly

VITAMINS

- there is no evidence to support the use of antioxidant vitamins (vitamin E and vitamin C) in the treatment of Parkinson's disease, and their use is not recommended (Am Fam Physician 1990;41:574–584)

▶ *What Dosage Should I Use?*

Parkinson's disease

BENZTROPINE

- 0.5 mg PO daily at bedtime
- increase the dosage at weekly intervals, on the basis of response, by 0.5 mg to a maximum dosage of 6 mg PO daily
- if tolerated, the drug may be given as 1 dose at bedtime; however, at maximum daily dosages, it is advisable to administer in divided doses if the patient experiences dose-related side effects

TRIHEXYPHENIDYL

- 1 mg PO on day 1
- increase the dosage by 2 mg increments weekly to a maximum dosage of 6–10 mg PO daily in 2 divided doses
- extended-release capsules (5 mg) should not be used as initial therapy or until establishment of an effective maintenance dosage
- extended-release capsules can be administered as a single daily dose if this is desirable for the patient
- elixir form is available for patients unable to swallow capsules or tablets

PROCYCLIDINE

- 2.5 mg PO TID
- increase the dosage at weekly intervals by 2.5 mg to a usual dosage of 5 mg 3 times a day
- if necessary, a maximum daily dosage of 45–60 mg in 3 equally divided doses may be employed

LEVODOPA-CARBIDOPA

- ½ of a scored 100 mg (levodopa)/25mg (carbidopa) tablet PO QID
- increase the dosage by ½ of a 100 mg/25 mg tablet at weekly intervals until improvement or toxicities are seen
- after the total daily dose of 200 mg with carbidopa (two 100 mg/25 mg tablets PO QID) switch to a 10:1 formulation, as only 75 mg is needed to block the peripheral dopa decarboxylase enzyme fully
- increase the dosage until a maximum of 300 mg (levodopa) PO QID is reached
- patients who have not responded to 300 mg of levodopa

(with carbidopa) PO QID are not likely to respond to higher dosages
- if the patient reaches a daily dosage of 1200 mg of levodopa (combined with at least 75 mg of carbidopa) with no response, reevaluate the diagnosis of Parkinson's disease
- patients requiring more than 700 mg of levodopa (with carbidopa) should be initiated on adjunct therapy (usually selegiline)
- in patients who find the QID dosing regimen inconvenient, a sustained-release formulation (Sinemet CR) is available and allows fewer daily dosages and reduced dose-response fluctuations
- do not start the sustained-release preparation until the patient is stabilized on the regular-release formulation because dosage adjustments are more difficult with the sustained-release formulation
- owing to a reduced bioavailability of Sinemet CR relative to Sinemet (levodopa: 0.71; carbidopa: 0.58), the daily dosage may need to be increased when switching from regular Sinemet (Neurology 1989; 39(11)(suppl 2):25–38)
- Sinemet CR has a delayed onset of activity, which is problematic for the initial morning dose when the level of function is usually at its worst; it may be useful early in therapy before morning symptoms are a major problem
- regular Sinemet tablets have a more rapid absorption rate and are recommended for the morning dose

LEVODOPA-BENSERAZIDE

- one 50 mg/12.5 mg capsule PO QID
- increase the dosage by one 50 mg/12.5 mg capsule at weekly intervals until improvement or toxicities are seen
- after a total daily dosage of 200 mg with benserazide has been achieved, further increases in benserazide dosages are not needed
- unfortunately, this preparation does not come as a 10:1 formulation

SELEGILINE

- 5 mg PO BID, with breakfast and lunch (to minimize nausea and insomnia)
- it is questionable whether higher dosages are of any benefit, and controlled studies have not been conducted on dosages greater than 10 mg PO daily (Am Fam Physician 1990;41:589–591)
- at a dosage higher than 20–25 mg, selegiline begins to lose its monoamine oxidase B selectivity and, like the nonselective monoamine oxidase inhibitors, may produce a potentially fatal hypertensive crisis if taken with food high in tyramine or with sympathomimetic medications
- after several days of treatment with selegiline, attempt to reduce the levodopa-carbidopa dosage by 10–30%
- reduction in the levodopa dosage is usually not practical unless selegiline is added late in therapy

BROMOCRIPTINE

- 1.25 mg PO daily HS for 1 week, followed by 2.5 mg PO daily HS for 1 week, 2.5 mg PO BID for 1 week, and then 2.5 mg PO TID for 1 week
- then increase by 2.5 mg PO daily every 7 days, depending on response and tolerance of side effects
- bromocriptine demonstrates a triphasic response in which, at low dosages and high dosages, the symptoms of Parkinson's disease may worsen
- there is significant variation in the optimum dosage for a given individual, ranging from 5 mg PO daily to 100 mg PO daily; however, in practice, as the dosage increases

above 30 mg daily, the chance of benefit is relatively low but the risk of side effects increases
- decrease the dosage of levodopa by 20% when stabilizing the patient on bromocriptine

AMANTADINE

- 100 mg PO daily with breakfast for 1 week, increasing to 100 mg PO BID (breakfast and lunch) thereafter
- dosage of levodopa may need to be reduced when amantadine therapy is initiated
- dosages greater than 200 mg daily are rarely necessary

▶ How Long Should I Treat with My Initial Regimen?

Parkinson's disease

- treat patients with each drug (increasing dosages weekly) until the desired effect is seen, the maximum dosage is achieved, or adverse effects become intolerable
- if a partial response (with an acceptable incidence of adverse effects) has been seen with the initial drug, continue this drug and add the next drug in the sequence

▶ What Efficacy Parameters Should I Follow and How Frequently Do I Have to Assess My Patient?

Parkinson's disease

Signs and symptoms

- assess symptoms weekly during the titration period, using one of several available evaluation scores
- evaluate for improvement or worsening of the following symptoms
- after a patient has been stabilized, assess the patient every 3 months

Tremor

- usually unilateral initially
- ''pinrolling'' or tremor of the hands
- head-bobbing and tongue and leg movement present at rest

Rigidity

- cogwheel rigidity—resistance to passive movement of joints
- speech impairment—slowed, slurred speech; monotone; hoarseness
- slowed gastrointestinal tract—drooling; dysphagia; constipation
- muscle pain or cramping

Bradykinesia

- slowness of movement, diminished spontaneity, and reduced frequency of movement
- impaired fine motor movement (difficulty in writing or buttoning a shirt)
- impaired gross movement (initiating or terminating movement)
- slowed automatic movement (''masked facies,'' dulled expressive gestures, reduced blinking reflex, and loss of arm swing)

Postural changes

- stooped, simian posture and shuffling gait

Other signs and symptoms

- seborrhea

- psychiatric disturbances (psychosis, dementia, and depression)
- sensory complaints (paresthesias and numbness)

▶ Should I Add Another Drug or Substitute Therapy If My Initial Drug Therapy Fails?

Parkinson's disease

- if a partial response (with an acceptable incidence of adverse effects) has been seen with the initial drug, continue the first drug and add another drug
- as Parkinson's disease progresses, often within 6 months to 1 year of starting therapy, the pharmacological response to levodopa deteriorates
- when adding adjuvant therapy to levodopa-carbidopa, attempt to reduce the dosage of levodopa

▶ How Long Should I Continue Drug Therapy?

Parkinson's disease

- therapy for Parkinson's disease is lifelong
- there is no role for drug holidays, as any benefit derived from drug holidays (withdrawal of antiparkinsonian therapy for 3–14 days) is usually short lived and risks include immobility, subsequent thromboembolism, aspiration and pneumonia, and severe depression
- in most cases, when another class of therapy is instituted, administration of anticholinergic drugs can be discontinued
- however, in about 20–25% of advanced cases of Parkinson's disease, the patient may benefit from long-term anticholinergic therapy in combination with levodopa, owing to severe tremor unresponsive to levodopa alone (Acta Neurol Scand Suppl 1989;126:213–219, Clin Pharmacokinet 1987;13:141–178)

Useful References

Ahlskog JE, Wilkinson JM. New concepts in the treatment of Parkinson's disease. Am Fam Physician 1990;41:574–584

Lieberman AN. Update on Parkinson disease. N Y State J Med 1987; 87:147–153

DRUG THERAPY FOR PAIN

Terry Baumann

▶ What Are My Goals of Treatment?

to eliminate the pain and suffering associated with pain as much and as quickly as possible

to use the least toxic, most effective analgesic

to titrate the dose properly and to adjust the route of administration to fit the needs of the patient and to administer for an adequate duration

to prevent pain peaks and troughs by administering medication in a round-the-clock fashion

to prevent and/or minimize side effects of analgesics

▶ What Evidence Is Available to Support Drug Therapy for Pain?

Untreated pain

- can lead to extreme anxiety, stress, and reflex reactions that can cause hypoxia, increased heart rate, and hypertension
- can lead to decreased ambulation and psychological and emotional problems

- untreated postoperative pain can lead to pulmonary dysfunction, gastrointestinal complications, metabolic dysfunction, impairment of muscle metabolism and function, and thrombus formation (Anesthesiology News 1984; 9–16)
- treatment prevents the problems mentioned above (Pharmacotherapy: A Pathophysiologic Approach 1993:924–941)

▶ *When Should I Consider Drug Therapy?*

Acute pain

- after the underlying cause is identified and treatment of that cause does not or cannot take care of the pain, treat immediately and aggressively with drug therapy
- if the underlying cause is not identified, pain should still be treated immediately and aggressively, but follow further pain symptoms so as not to mask a diagnosis (e.g., acute abdominal pain of appendicitis)

Chronic cancer pain

- chronic and persistent cancer pain should be treated in all patients

Chronic noncancer pain

- these patients often have received numerous pharmacological regimens, and simply adding another drug seldom improves pain control
- an integrated, interdisciplinary, systematic program is needed that seeks a certain function level, decreases the perception of pain, improves well-being, enhances family and social relationships, and decreases drug dependency
- unfortunately, this process may take months or even years
- when pain has not been responsive to other treatment modalities, analgesics may be appropriate

Postoperative pain

- pain should be empirically treated in all these patients
- pain serves no useful purpose in this group, and its treatment may lead to earlier ambulation with decreased risk of deep vein thrombosis and pulmonary embolism

▶ *What Drug Should I Use for Initial Treatment?*

Acute pain

Mild symptoms

ACETAMINOPHEN

- if noninflammatory pain is thought to be the cause (headache, muscle aches, and so on), acetaminophen is effective, is inexpensive, and produces little, if any, gastrointestinal toxicity

IBUPROFEN

- ibuprofen should be used if inflammation is thought to play a role (pulled muscles, toothaches, and so on) because ibuprofen has an antiinflammatory effect, whereas acetaminophen does not
- ibuprofen causes less gastric distress than does non–enteric-coated aspirin but it is more expensive
- causes more gastric distress than does acetaminophen

ASPIRIN

- aspirin can be used for inflammatory pain but causes more gastrointestinal toxicity than does acetaminophen or ibuprofen

NAPROXEN

- can also be used for its antiinflammatory effect and has a convenient BID dosing regimen

Moderate symptoms

ACETAMINOPHEN, IBUPROFEN, ASPIRIN, OR NAPROXEN WITH CODEINE, OXYCODONE, OR PROPOXYPHENE

- if treatment with nonopioid agents (see above) is ineffective after titrating rapidly to maximum dosages, add codeine, oxycodone, or propoxyphene to the above regimens
- propoxyphene may be used if true allergy to codeine exists
- propoxyphene should not be used alone becuase it produces a far better effect when used with acetaminophen or nonsteroidal antiinflammatory drugs (NSAIDs)
- oxycodone can be used instead of codeine, as it may have placebo value in patients who are convinced that a codeine product will not work (oxycodone provides no clinical advantage over codeine)
- be aware that, when acetaminophen or aspirin is used in combination products with codeine in a round-the-clock fashion, acetaminophen or aspirin toxicity may occur owing to the possible ingestion of large amounts of acetaminophen or aspirin

Severe symptoms

MORPHINE

- drug of first choice for the treatment of severe acute pain because it is as effective as other opioids with a similar adverse effect profile and comes in a large number of dosage forms

MEPERIDINE

- use if true allergy to morphine exists, but it offers no advantages over morphine and has potential additional side effects in some patients (e.g., seizures in patients with renal failure)
- is relatively ineffective orally at the dosages commonly used (50 mg PO Q4H)

HYDROMORPHONE

- there are no apparent clinical differences between hydromorphone and other narcotics
- hydromorphone is more expensive than morphine
- hydromorphone has an advantage over morphine when used parenterally in that it can be administered in smaller volumes of fluid, because of its higher potency, which may be useful for subcutaneous infusions or epidural administration when extremely high doses and small volumes are needed

BUPRENORPHINE, NALBUPHINE, BUTORPHANOL

- use only when the patient has a true allergy to meperidine and the patient does not tolerate morphine
- it has been reported that buprenorphine or nalbuphine causes less severe respiratory depression than does morphine because they are partial agonists; however, if morphine (as with any opioid) is properly titrated, there is likely little (if any) clinical difference between these drugs with regard to producing respiratory depression
- buprenorphine has a slightly longer duration of action (6 hours) than does morphine (4 hours) but is more expensive
- butorphanol can be given nasally

Cancer pain, chronic noncancer pain

Acute exacerbation

- choose drugs as for acute pain (see above)
- with patients already receiving regularly scheduled opioids, realize that dosages may have to be much higher owing to the development of tolerance

Chronic pain

MORPHINE

- drug of choice in all terminally ill patients when regular dosing with less potent agents such as acetaminophen, acetaminophen-codeine, and NSAIDs is not effective (ensure that these drugs have been used at appropriate regular intervals)
- drug of choice for chronic noncancer pain that has not been responsive to other treatment modalities and agents such as acetaminophen, acetaminophen-codeine, and NSAIDs
- morphine is as effective as other opioids with a similar adverse effect profile and comes in a large number of dosage forms

OTHER OPIOIDS

- use only if morphine is not tolerated or is ineffective despite appropriate dose titration

METHADONE

- alternative to morphine if the patient is unable to tolerate morphine
- should be used only in patients allergic to all other opioids, as it offers no advantages over morphine

FENTANYL

- fentanyl patch may be as effective as sustained-release morphine but is more difficult to titrate
- advantage of Q72H dosing
- should likely be used only after the patient has been stabilized on a regularly dosed opioid

Postoperative pain

MORPHINE

- is the drug of choice for the treatment of postoperative pain because it is as effective as other opioids with a similar adverse effect profile, comes in a large number of dosage forms
- in general, if opioids are titrated properly, there is little risk of respiratory depression

MEPERIDINE

- use if there is true allergy to morphine, but it offers no advantages over morphine
- is relatively ineffective orally at the dosages commonly used (bioavailability problem)

FENTANYL

- seldom used for postoperative pain via the IM or IV route because of its short duration of action
- opioid of choice for epidural administration because it has faster onset of action and is easier to titrate than epidural morphine because of its lipid solubility
- epidural fentanyl also produces less respiratory depression, nausea and vomiting, and itch than does epidural morphine (epidural morphine, because of its longer duration of action, produces a greater incidence of late respiratory depression)
- after epidural fentanyl administration has been stopped,

patients need to be monitored (for toxicity) only for 4 hours, whereas toxicity from epidural morphine can cause adverse effects for up to 24 hours

KETOROLAC

- the only parenteral NSAID available for postoperative pain
- can be used if the patient is unable to tolerate opioids, needs to be alert, or is at risk for developing respiratory depression from opioids (e.g., from previous experience)
- can also be used in conjunction with opioids to decrease the amount of opioids required

ACETAMINOPHEN WITH CODEINE

- after a patient no longer requires regularly dosed medications (e.g., 2–3 days postoperatively), acetaminophen with codeine may be used on an as needed basis

▶ *What Dosage Should I Use?*

Acute pain

Mild symptoms

ACETAMINOPHEN

- 500 mg PO Q4H PRN up to a maximum of 1000 mg PO Q6H

IBUPROFEN

- 400 mg PO Q4H PRN up to a maximum of 800 mg PO Q6H

ASPIRIN

- 650 mg PO Q4H PRN up to a maximum of 1000 mg PO Q6H

NAPROXEN

- 250 mg PO Q12H PRN up to a maximum of 500 mg PO Q8H

Moderate symptoms

ACETAMINOPHEN, IBUPROFEN, ASPIRIN, OR NAPROXEN WITH CODEINE, OXYCODONE, OR PROPOXYPHENE

- add 30 mg PO of codeine, 5 mg of oxycodone, or 100 mg of the napsylate salt or 65 mg of the hydrochloride salt of propoxyphene to acetaminophen or NSAID
- acetaminophen or aspirin comes in codeine- and oxycodone-containing combination products
- acetaminophen combinations with propoxyphene are available in the USA but not in Canada

Severe symptoms

Be aware that the oral route has a slightly slower onset (15–30 minutes) than does intramuscular (10–15 minutes) or intravenous (1–5 minutes) administration • Question patients frequently about the degree of pain that they are having (ideally within at most 1–2 hours after the first dose if the drug was administered via the oral or intramuscular route) • If pain is unrelieved by this time, give another dose 50% higher than the first dose • Continue this approach until pain is 75% relieved, and then maintain at this dosage for 12 hours before further adjustments are made • If the drug is being given intravenously, assess the effect of the drug within 3–5 minutes and repeat doses as needed

MORPHINE

- 20 mg PO Q4H (*not* PRN) if the patient is able to tolerate

oral agents (10 mg PO Q4H for elderly patients because of concerns about sedation and respiratory depression)
- 10 mg IM Q4H (*not* PRN) if the patient is unable to take oral medications (5 mg IM Q4H for elderly patients because of concerns about sedation and respiratory depression)
- 2.5 mg IV every 5 minutes PRN if an immediate response for severe pain is needed

MEPERIDINE

- 100 mg IM Q4H (*not* PRN) (50 mg IM Q4H for elderly patients because of concerns about sedation and respiratory depression)
- some patients may require Q3H dosing
- 25 mg IV every 5 minutes PRN if an immediate response for severe pain is needed

HYDROMORPHONE

- 4 mg PO Q4H (*not* PRN) if the patient is able to tolerate oral agents (2 mg PO Q4H [*not* PRN] for elderly patients because of concerns about sedation and respiratory depression)
- 1 mg IM Q4H if the patient is unable to take oral medications
- 0.5 mg IV every 5 minutes PRN if an immediate response for severe pain is needed

BUPRENORPHINE

- 0.3 mg IM or IV Q6H (*not* PRN) (0.15 mg IM or IV Q6H for elderly patients because of concerns about sedation and respiratory depression)

NALBUPHINE

- 10 mg IM or IV Q4H (*not* PRN) (5 mg IM or IV Q4H for elderly patients because of concerns about sedation and respiratory depression)

Cancer pain, chronic noncancer pain

Acute exacerbation

- dosages as above for severe symptoms

Chronic pain
In a patient who has received only weak opioids in the past and is experiencing pain

MORPHINE

- 10 mg PO Q4H (not PRN)
- 5 mg PO Q4H in the very frail or elderly patient because of concerns about sedation
- once pain control is achieved, switch to a sustained-release product with an immediate-release product available for breakthrough pain (see morphine monograph)

OTHER OPIOIDS

- see individual monographs and opioid equivalent chart (Table 6–1)

METHADONE

- 10 mg PO Q8H (not PRN)
- 5 mg PO Q8H in the very frail or elderly patient because of concerns about sedation

In a patient being switched from another opioid
MORPHINE

- determine the average daily requirements for the previous opioids and determine the 24 hour morphine equivalent

Table 6–1 • Opioid Equivalents*

Opioid	Equipotent Parenteral Doses (mg)	Equipotent Oral Doses (mg)	Duration (h)
morphine	10	20–30	4–5
meperidine	100	150	3–5
hydromorphone	1.3	4	4–5
buprenorphine	0.3	N/A	4–8
codeine	130	100	4–6
methadone	10	10–20	4–8
nalbuphine	10	N/A	3–6
propoxyphene	N/A	130	4–6
oxycodone	N/A	15	4–5
fentanyl	0.1	N/A	1–2

N/A = not available.
* See text discussion or specific drug monographs for starting doses.

(Table 6–1 is just a guide; after switching always adjust up or down on the basis of the patient's response)
- 24 hour requirements for morphine should be divided by 6 and given every 4 hours
- if the previous opioid dose has not been effective, the total daily dose of morphine should be increased by 25–50%

Postoperative pain
MORPHINE

In the postanesthetic care unit
- 2.5 mg IV repeated every 5 minutes PRN
- adjust the dosage on the basis of the response to each dose and titrate to achieve pain control and the desired level of sedation or respiratory rate

On the ward

Intermittent therapy
- as above for acute pain (IM or PO) but give a regular dose (*not* PRN)
- use the parenteral route initially but switch to the oral route as soon as the patient is able to take agents orally (usually 24–36 hours postoperatively)
- question the patient every 1–2 hours initially and increase the dosage on the basis of the assessment of pain relief and level of sedation (see above under acute pain)

Patient-controlled analgesia
- 1 mg/bolus with lockout of 6 minutes
- some clinicians believe that 1–2 mg/h as an infusion with patient-controlled analgesia enables patients to sleep through the night; however, evidence suggests that using a bolus with a baseline infusion may increase the amount of narcotic used and the side effects, without improving efficacy (Anaesth Intensive Care 1991;19:555–560, Anesthesiology 1992;76:362–367)
- question the patient every 1–2 hours about the degree of pain
- if pain is not controlled with bolus doses, increase the bolus dose by 25–50%
- if pain relief from a bolus is adequate but the duration of pain relief is too short, decrease the lockout period

Epidural or intrathecal administration
- can be used as an alternative to parenteral routes, but these routes should be used only by anesthetists skilled in this technique
- 8 mg epidurally as a single dose (0.2 mg intrathecally as

a single dose), with breakthrough pain treated as above with oral or parenteral opioids
- epidural morphine can also be given as a continuous infusion

MEPERIDINE

In the postanesthetic care unit
- 25 mg IV repeated every 3–5 minutes PRN
- adjust the dosage on the basis of the response to each dose and titrate to achieve pain control and a desired level of sedation or respiratory rate

On the ward

Intermittent therapy
- as above for acute pain
- question the patient frequently and increase the dosage as above for acute pain on the basis of pain relief and level of sedation

Patient-controlled analgesia
- 10 mg/bolus with lockout of 6 minutes
- evidence suggests that using a bolus with a baseline infusion may increase the chance of seizures
- question the patient every 1–2 hours about the degree of pain
- if pain is not controlled with bolus doses, increase the bolus dose by 25–50%
- if pain relief from a bolus dose is adequate but the duration of pain relief is too short, decrease the lockout period

Epidural or intrathecal administration
- not used by this route

FENTANYL
- initial epidural dose of 50–100 μg may be given with a 20 μg/h infusion
- this route should be used only by anesthetists skilled in this technique

KETOROLAC
- 60 mg IM followed by 30 mg IM Q6H (for no more than 5 days)
- 30 mg IM followed by 15 mg IM Q6H in the elderly (for no more than 5 days)

ACETAMINOPHEN WITH CODEINE
- 30 mg PO Q4H of codeine in combination with at least 325 g acetaminophen
- use 15 mg of codeine in the elderly

▶ How Long Should I Treat with My Initial Regimen?

Acute pain, chronic cancer pain, chronic noncancer pain, postoperative pain
- the maximum effect from each dose of an oral pain medication will have been achieved by 1½–2 hours, and therefore, the appropriateness of the drug and the dosage can be determined at this point
- severe pain (if being treated with parenteral [IM] opioids) should be assessed every 30–60 minutes
- when giving the drug by an IV bolus, an effect should be seen within 3–5 minutes, with maximum effect occurring in 10 minutes
- if acceptable pain control has been achieved, continue with that drug and dosage on a regular schedule for the expected duration of the pain
- if pain control is not acceptable, increase dosages by 50%

and reassess in 2 hours (see individual drug monographs for dose titration schedules)

▶ What Efficacy Parameters Should I Follow and How Frequently Do I Have to Assess My Patient?

Acute pain, chronic cancer pain, chronic noncancer pain, postoperative pain
Subjective pain evaluation
- key to achieving effective pain control is to question patients frequently about the degree of pain they are having
- frequency of pain evaluation should be based on the knowledge of how quickly the drug should work
- 10 cm visual analog score can be used to observe trends in pain control over time and can be useful
- the decision to give PRN doses or to increase the dosage should be based on the patient's assessment of the severity of pain and the duration of effect of the drug
- remember that pain is whatever the patient says it is
- when patient self-assessment is not possible, monitor agitation and heart rate

▶ Should I Add Another Drug or Substitute Therapy If My Initial Drug Therapy Fails?

Acute pain
Mild to moderate symptoms
- ensure that nonopioid agents have been titrated up to maximum allowed doses and given on a regular schedule because therapy often fails because pain medication is given on a PRN basis
- if regularly scheduled nonopioid agents fail, treat with a combination of the above with codeine and titrate appropriately
- if these combinations are ineffective, switch to morphine
Severe symptoms
- for severe pain, make sure that morphine has been titrated correctly because morphine often fails because it is improperly used or no titration has been used
- allowing the patient to control the titration using a patient-controlled analgesia device optimizes pain relief and minimizes toxicity
- in patients with acute anxiety and/or muscle spasms with proper morphine titration, add lorazepam 1 mg PO or 0.5 mg IV every 8 hours

Chronic cancer pain, chronic noncancer pain
- make sure that morphine has been titrated correctly because morphine often fails when it is improperly administered or no titration has been used
- in patients with neuropathic pain, add amitriptyline 25 mg PO at bedtime and titrate dose up to a maximum of 50 mg PO daily
- when nerve injury leads to tic-like pain, add carbamazepine 100 mg PO BID
- for bone pain, an NSAID should be added
- for spinal cord compression, corticosteroids can be added to the regimen (dexamethasone 4 mg PO or IV every 6 hours is used by most clinicians, but other corticosteroids such as prednisone could also be used)

▶ How Long Should I Continue Drug Therapy?

Acute pain
- use on a regular basis for the expected duration of pain

- acute pain should subside within days after the offending event; if this has not occurred within 1 week, further investigate the cause of the pain

Cancer pain, chronic noncancer pain

- therapy may be needed for months or years

Postoperative pain

- use on a regular basis for 48–72 hours and then use on a PRN basis when patients are being ambulated or are undergoing physical therapy
- if pain persists beyond this time, investigate for the cause

Useful References

Baumann TJ. Pain management. In: DiPiro JT, Talbert RL, Hayes PE, et al, eds. Pharmacotherapy: A Pathophysiologic Approach, 2nd ed. Norwalk CT: Appleton and Lange, 1993:924–941

Clinical Practice Guideline, Acute Pain Management: Operative or Medical Procedures and Trauma. Washington, DC: US Department of Health and Human Services, Public Health Service, Agency for Health Care Policy and Research; 1992

Clinical Practice Guideline, Management of Cancer Pain. Washington, DC: US Department of Health and Human Services, Public Health Service, Agency for Health Care Policy and Research; 1994

McEvoy GK, ed. AHFS Drug Information. Bethesda, MD: American Society of Hospital Pharmacists, 1993

Melzack R. The tragedy of needless pain. Sci Am 1990;262:27–33

Recommendations of the American Pain Society on the principles of analgesic use in the treatment of acute pain and chronic cancer pain. Clin Pharm 1990;9:601–611

Stimmel B. Pain, Analgesia, and Addiction: The Pharmacology of Pain. New York: Raven Press, 1983

Tuttle CB. Drug management of pain in cancer patients. Can Med Assoc J 1985;132:121–134

Twycross R, Lack S. Oral Morphine in Advanced Cancer. Beaconsfield, Bucks, England: Beaconsfield Publishers, 1988

DRUG THERAPY FOR MIGRAINE HEADACHE

Jerry W. Taylor

▶ What Are My Goals of Treatment?

to reduce the frequency and severity of headache
to provide total relief from a headache (may be overly ambitious, but significant relief in the level of pain the patient is experiencing is a reasonable goal)

▶ What Evidence Is Available to Support Drug Therapy for Migraine Headache?

Treatment

- abortive therapy or symptomatic management may interrupt acute attacks in up to 70–80% of patients given sumatriptan (N Engl J Med 1991;325:316–321) and 60–70% given dihydroergotamine or ergots

Prophylaxis

- cure for vascular headaches is not available
- most drugs cause a reduction in the severity and number of attacks; however, up to 25% of patients do not tolerate prophylactic agents

▶ When Should I Consider Drug Therapy?

Treatment

- treat all vascular headaches at initiation to have greatest success and to lessen the intensity and shorten the duration
- treat all infrequent severe headaches

- early treatment may abort migraine with aura if recognized in its early stages
- symptomatic therapy may also be required for patients who have breakthrough headaches while receiving prophylactic agents

Prophylaxis

- consider prophylaxis in patients with 2 headaches or more per month
- patients with severe headaches intolerant of or unresponsive to abortive therapy or with contraindications to their use
- patient with significant impairment of the quality of life, resulting in frequent absences from work or interruptions of family life
- patient with regular and predictable attacks (e.g., menstrual migraine)
- patient requiring an increased use of narcotic pain killers
- patient education is important in the management of migraine attacks, and patients should attempt to identify factors contributing to the headache (e.g., behavior, food products, and drugs) to prevent or diminish precipitating factors
- instruction on identification of the prodromal signs of impending migraine and on prompt initiation of abortive therapy at the onset of attacks is needed to be most effective

▶ What Drug Should I Use for Initial Treatment?

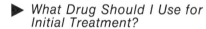

Treatment

Mild symptoms

ASPIRIN OR OTHER NONSTEROIDAL ANTIINFLAMMATORY DRUGS

- effective and safe for the treatment of mild symptoms (Am J Med 1983:75;36–42)
- caffeine in conjunction with aspirin is recommended by some clinicians, as it may increase the absorption of the aspirin and may have effects in relieving migraine of its own, but no controlled trials are available
- decision among NSAIDs for the treatment of migraine should be based on cost because no predictive measures are available to determine which agent will work

ACETAMINOPHEN

- should be used instead of aspirin if the patient has gastrointestinal intolerance to aspirin

ACETAMINOPHEN OR ASPIRIN WITH CODEINE

- in patients with infrequent, mild to moderate headaches (e.g., every 1–3 months) not effectively treated with aspirin or acetaminophen, add codeine to these agents

METOCLOPRAMIDE

- if the patient is also experiencing nausea or vomiting with the headache, add metoclopramide to the above analgesics
- metoclopramide enhances subsequent analgesic absorption as well as providing an antimigraine effect

Moderate or severe symptoms

SUMATRIPTAN

- is effective and well tolerated when given as a single subcutaneous or oral dose (JAMA 1991;265:2831–2835) but does not work in all patients and is expensive
- appears to be more effective and safer than ergotamine,

but further comparative trials are needed (Eur Neurol 1991;31:314–322)

- oral sumatriptan has been shown to be more effective than the combination of aspirin and metoclopramide (Br Med J 1991;303:1491)
- no comparative trials have been done between parenteral sumatriptan and other effective parenteral regimens (dihydroergotamine ± metoclopramide)

DIHYDROERGOTAMINE (DHE)

- is as effective as and better tolerated than (less nausea) and has only modest arterial effects when compared with ergotamine, but is only available parenterally (Headache 1990;8:857–865)
- parenteral form is especially useful in patients with concomitant nausea and vomiting
- parenteral DHE plus metoclopramide is an effective treatment for moderate to severe migraine and is less expensive than parenteral sumatriptan
- DHE can be used at home for patients who find other therapy ineffective if the patient is taught how to inject the drug subcutaneously
- nasal spray dosage form is under investigation in the USA and may be released; results of controlled trials in the treatment of migraine failed to demonstrate a benefit of the spray over placebo (Cephalalgia 1987;7:131–133); however, a recent trial has suggested some benefit (Neurology 1994;44:447–453)

ERGOTAMINE

- has the advantage over dihydroergotamine of being available as an oral, rectal, sublingual, and inhalation dosage form, but these forms are erratically absorbed (J Neurol 1991;238:S28–S35)
- ergotamine is most effective if used during the prodromal phase of the headache

PROCHLORPERAZINE

- should be used prior to the use of dihydroergotamine or ergotamine to decrease the incidence of nausea seen with these agents

METOCLOPRAMIDE

- does not have analgesic properties (J Neurol 1991; 238:S23–S27) and, therefore, should be used in conjunction with the above therapy if the patient has moderate to severe nausea and requires repeated dosing
- is likely better tolerated than prochlorperazine when given as repeated doses (Headache 1990;8:857–865)

CHLORPROMAZINE

- useful but can cause significant sedation
- experience with both chlorpromazine and metoclopramide as antimigraine agents is limited but deserves further study
- at present, neither agent is preferred over the other

MORPHINE

- may benefit the patient with migraine because relief comes with sleep and rest, which can be achieved with narcotics; however, narcotics should be avoided if at all possible
- use in the patient who fails to respond to a course of either sumatriptan or dihydroergotamine

PREDNISONE

- when a migraine continues for longer than 36–48 hours,

a short course of steroids should be used to lessen the need for narcotics

ISOMETHEPTENE MUCATE

- not as effective as ergotamine, and although safe, it likely plays little if any role in the availability of agents such as sumatriptan or dihydroergotamine

Prophylaxis
NADOLOL

- beta-blockers are as effective as other agents and less expensive than the calcium channel blockers
- propranolol, atenolol, metoprolol, and nadolol are all effective for migraine prophylaxis
- timolol and acebutolol are somewhat effective, and pindolol and oxprenolol are ineffective
- nadolol should be tried initially, as it has proven effectiveness, has the advantage over propranolol of being given once a day, and has more consistent absorption characteristics
- agents such as acebutolol and atenolol can be used if they are less expensive than nadolol

FLUNARIZINE, VERAPAMIL

- should be tried if there is contraindication to or failure of beta-blockers
- these agents are expensive but probably better tolerated than the antidepressants
- selection of preferred calcium channel blocker therapy should be based on efficacy, toxicity, and cost
- majority of the studies have been done with verapamil and flunarizine, and no comparative trials have been done
- flunarizine is more expensive than verapamil but can be given as a single daily dose; however, flunarizine does cause weight gain and somnolence in 40–50% of patients (Headache 1991;31:388–391)
- flunarizine is investigational in the USA
- toxicity profile of flunarizine likely limits its availability and wide-spread use
- during long-term therapy, extrapyramidal reactions have been reported with flunarizine (Drugs 1989;38:481–499)
- nifedipine can cause headaches, and studies have not confirmed its effectiveness (Neurology 1989;39:284–286)

AMITRIPTYLINE

- antidepressants should be used in patients not responding to or unable to tolerate beta-blockers or calcium channel blockers
- also useful if a patient experiences depression
- from clinical experience, not all tricyclic antidepressants appear to be effective
- amitriptyline has been used most extensively and appears to be effective
- nortriptyline and doxepin have also been effective and should be used if amitriptyline is effective but the patient cannot tolerate its adverse effects

NONSTEROIDAL ANTIINFLAMMATORY DRUGS

- should be tried in patients not responding to or not able to tolerate beta-blockers, antidepressants, or calcium channel blockers
- drug of choice for prophylaxis in patients with menstrual migraine
- at present, there are no predictive measures for deciding which NSAID a patient will respond to
- aspirin is considered the initial drug of choice because it is as effective as other NSAIDs and is the least expensive agent

is as effective as other NSAIDs and is the least expensive agent

- if the patient is at risk for gastrointestinal intolerance or does not tolerate enteric-coated aspirin, ibuprofen is effective, causes less gastrointestinal discomfort than does non–enteric-coated aspirin, but is more expensive than aspirin

PIZOTYLINE

- use if the above agents are not tolerated or are ineffective
- not the drug of choice because of the unwanted side effects of sedation and weight gain

METHYSERGIDE

- should be used only when above therapies have failed, because of the risk of fibrosis

PHENELZINE

- is useful in the treatment of patients subject to frequent or severe attacks of migraine who have not responded to conventional therapy

▶ What Dosage Should I Use?

Treatment

Mild symptoms

ASPIRIN

- 1000 mg PO Q4H PRN up to a maximum of 4000 mg PO daily

IBUPROFEN

- 800 mg PO Q4H PRN up to a maximum of 800 mg PO Q6H daily

NAPROXEN

- 500 mg PO Q8H PRN up to a maximum of 500 mg PO Q8H daily

ACETAMINOPHEN

- 1000 mg PO Q4H PRN up to a maximum of 4000 mg PO daily

ACETAMINOPHEN OR ASPIRIN WITH CODEINE

- add 30 mg PO of codeine to the above regimens
- doses less than 30 mg are likely ineffective
- aspirin and acetaminophen are both available in combination with codeine

METOCLOPRAMIDE

- 10 mg PO QID if the patient is able to tolerate oral medications
- administer 10 mg IV immediately prior to giving the initial dose of dihydroergotamine or ergotamine, and repeat Q8H as needed

Moderate or severe symptoms

SUMATRIPTAN

- 100 mg PO as a single dose
- 6 mg SC as a single dose in patients who either have severe symptoms or are unable to tolerate oral medications
- if the initial dose is not effective, repeated doses are not likely to be effective (N Engl J Med 1991;325: 316–321)
- if the initial dose is effective but headache returns, repeat the dose (maximum of 3 oral or 2 SC doses per 24 hours)

DIHYDROERGOTAMINE

- give 0.5 mg IV or subcutaneously (1 mg in large patients), and repeat dose of 0.5 mg at 1 hour intervals as needed
- maximum dosage should not exceed 3 mg/24 h or 6 mg/wk

ERGOTAMINE

- 1 inhalation (0.36 mg) (if an inhalation product is available), repeated in 10 minutes as needed to a maximum of 6 inhalations per 24 hours or 15 inhalations per week
- 2 mg PO or sublingually (rectally if the patient is vomiting) initially, then 1 mg repeated every 30 minutes, until the attack is aborted or a total of 6 mg has been given
- weekly dose of 10 mg should not be exceeded to avoid ergotism

PROCHLORPERAZINE

- 5 mg IV prior to the initial dose of dihydroergotamine or ergotamine

METOCLOPRAMIDE

- as above under mild symptoms

CHLORPROMAZINE

- 12.5 mg IV repeated at 20 minute intervals to a total maximum dose of 37.5 mg may be given as required

MORPHINE

- 20 mg PO Q4H if the patient is able to tolerate oral agents
- 10 mg IM Q4H if the patient is unable to take oral medications
- see drug monograph on morphine for titration schedule

PREDNISONE

- 40 mg PO daily for 4 days then taper the daily dosage by 5 mg every 2 days

Prophylaxis

NADOLOL

- 20 mg PO daily
- increase the daily dosage by 20 mg at weekly intervals until therapeutic or toxic effects appear

FLUNARIZINE

- 10 mg PO at bedtime

VERAPAMIL

- 120 mg of verapamil SR (a once-daily product sometimes given twice daily when doses exceed 240 mg/d) PO daily, increasing the dosage weekly by 120 mg daily until headaches are controlled, toxicity develops, or a maximum dosage of 480 mg PO daily is reached
- standard-release form is started at 80 mg PO Q8H, increasing the dosage weekly by 80 mg daily until headaches are controlled, toxicity develops, or a maximum dose of 360 mg/d is reached

AMITRIPTYLINE

- give 10 mg PO daily at bedtime and increase by 10 mg every 3–4 days until an effect is seen or a total dose of 50 mg is given
- dose titration increases the patient's ability to tolerate the adverse effects of amitriptyline
- leave at this dosage for 4 weeks and increase to 100 mg PO daily if there is no response to 50 mg

Nonsteroidal antiinflammatory drugs

ASPIRIN

- 650 mg PO Q12H (use enteric-coated aspirin to decrease the risk of adverse effects)

IBUPROFEN

- 400 mg PO Q8H

NAPROXEN

- 375 mg PO Q12H

PIZOTYLINE

- 0.5 mg PO TID

METHYSERGIDE

- 2 mg PO daily taken with a meal to minimize gastrointestinal discomfort
- increase the dosage gradually at weekly intervals by 2 mg daily if necessary or until it is dosed at 2 mg QID with meals

PHENELZINE

- 15 mg PO TID

▶ How Long Should I Treat with My Initial Regimen?

Treatment

- initial therapy with abortive agents should prevent headache or provide pain relief within a couple of hours
- with sumatriptan, approximately 50% of patients respond within 2 hours of an oral dose (Lancet 1991;338:782–783) and 70% of patients respond within 1 hour of SC administration
- if headaches are persistent after 1–2 hours, alternative therapy should be instituted

Prophylaxis

- prophylactic agents often require adjustment in dosage and may require several weeks to provide maximum benefit
- if tolerated, each drug should be tried for 4–6 weeks before alternative agents are tried

▶ What Efficacy Parameters Should I Follow and How Frequently Do I Have to Assess My Patient?

Treatment

Relief of pain and other symptoms such as prodrome, aura, and gastrointestinal complaints

- assess the patient hourly during the early stage of migraine attacks

Prophylaxis

Frequency and severity of headache

- patients with frequent migraine may need evaluation at 2–4 week intervals during initial dose titration, then intervals between visits may be extended in patients showing a response to treatment

▶ Should I Add Another Drug or Substitute Therapy If My Initial Drug Therapy Fails?

Treatment

- after the headache is established, the patient is unlikely to respond to other therapeutic modalities used in aborting attacks
- when headaches are established, narcotics (avoid if possible) or other sleep-producing agents may be the only effective alternative
- narcotics may be the only effective therapy in established headache but are best avoided through the appropriate use of drugs for acute onset
- it is important to initiate effective therapy early or proceed with other effective alternatives before the headache becomes entrenched

Prophylaxis

- allow an adequate trial (4–6 weeks) of prophylactic agents at appropriate dosages before abandonment
- symptomatic agents can be added in the management of breakthrough attacks
- if one prophylactic agent proves ineffective or only partially effective, discontinue therapy and try alternative choices

▶ How Long Should I Continue Drug Therapy?

Treatment

- for the acute attack, treat until relief of acute headache attacks, development of toxic effects, or maximum daily dosages have been achieved

Prophylaxis

- in the patient achieving a headache-free state, therapy should be reduced or withdrawn after 6 months to assess continued requirements
- if the patient has return of headaches, indefinite prophylactic therapy should be considered
- methysergide should not be used for longer than 6 months at a time, and after 6 months, the dosage should be tapered over 2 weeks to avoid rebound headaches, and then stopped for 1 month before continuing use if headaches recur in order to minimize the risk of fibrosis

Useful References

Taylor JW, Cleary JD, Parks BR. Primary headache disorders. In: Dipiro JT, Talbert RL, Hayes PE, et al, eds. Pharmacotherapy: A Pathophysiologic Approach, 2nd ed. Norwalk: Appleton and Lange, 1993:942–952

Watanabe MD. Headache. In: Herfindal ET, et al, eds. Clinical Pharmacy and Therapeutics, 5th ed. Baltimore: Williams & Wilkins, 1992:831–844

7 | OBSTETRICAL AND GYNECOLOGICAL CONDITIONS

DRUG THERAPY FOR BIRTH CONTROL

Deborah Stier Carson

▶ What Are My Goals of Treatment?

to provide women with effective and reversible contraception with a minimum risk of adverse effects related to estrogen or progestins

▶ What Evidence Is Available to Support Drug Therapy for Birth Control?

Efficacy of birth control

- oral contraceptives provide a reliable and reversible method of birth control; the failure rate is 0.02 pregnancies per 1200 cycles (100 woman-years) if compliance is good (Contraception 1988;37:343) and is probably 0.2 pregnancies per 1200 cycles if compliance problems are taken into account

Risk of cancer

- oral contraceptives decrease the risk of endometrial and ovarian cancer (Managing Contraceptive Pill Patients 1993:204–208)
- oral contraceptives also decrease the risk of ectopic pregnancies

▶ When Should I Consider Drug Therapy?

Hormonal contraception

- most effective form of nonpermanent birth control in women who desire birth control and will be compliant with hormonal contraception
- useful in women with dysmenorrhea or premenstrual tension and women who want to control the amount and duration of menstrual flow

Postcoital contraception

- certain oral contraceptives given within 3 days of unprotected intercourse prevent pregnancy, with a failure rate of 0.16–1.6%, depending on the time of the cycle (JAMA 1980;244:1336–1339)

▶ What Drug Should I Use for Initial Treatment?

Combination oral contraceptives contain 1 of 2 estrogens (predominantly ethinyl estradiol) plus 1 of 8 progestins (Tables 7–1 and 7–2), which differ significantly in their progestational and androgenic effects and also in the extent of their metabolism to estrogenic substances • Effects of any given oral contraceptive are a result of the specific combination of estrogen and progestin

Hormonal contraception
Most women
LOW ESTROGENIC ACTIVITY, MULTIPHASIC PRODUCTS (TRI-LEVLEN, TRIPHASIL, TRIQUILAR, JENEST, TRI-CYCLEN)

- all multiphasic preparations are reasonable first choices in most women, as they contain less progestin than do the monophasic preparations and mimic the normal cycle
- advantages of multiphasic agents, however, do not always outweigh the disadvantages (confusion regarding many colored pills, high incidence of breakthrough bleeding and spotting, less flexibility regarding missed doses, and increased incidence of benign ovarian cysts)
- women with acne, lipid abnormalities, cardiovascular risks, or metabolic abnormalities may benefit from an agent with reduced androgenic activity (Ovcon-35, Modicon, Brevicon (0.5/35), Tri-Norinyl, Synphasic, Tri-Cyclen, Desogen, Ortho-Cept), as these products contain norethindrone or desogestrel, which may have fewer cardiovascular and metabolic side effects than does levonorgestrel (Managing Contraceptive Pill Patients 1993: 128–129); however, these women can be started on a multiphasic product and evaluated after a few months to see whether these conditions have worsened or improved

LOW ESTROGENIC ACTIVITY, MONOPHASIC PRODUCTS (GENORA 1/35, NORINYL 1/35, ORTHO-NOVUM 1/35, BREVICON (1/35), ORTHO 1/35, MIN-OVRAL)

- these preparations are also reasonable first choices for an oral contraceptive because these products provide a balanced combination of estrogenic, progestational, and androgenic activity with an acceptable rate of breakthrough spotting
- monophasic combination oral contraceptives decrease the incidence of functional ovarian cysts, whereas the multiphasic oral contraceptives may not effectively suppress ovarian cysts because of the lowered progestin component

Women who have experienced a contraceptive failure or are taking interacting drugs
HIGH-ESTROGEN PRODUCTS (BREVICON, ORTHO-NOVUM 7/7/7, OR TRI-NORINYL)

- women who have experienced a contraceptive failure while properly taking a low estrogen dose oral contraceptive should be given a high-estrogen product
- women taking other drugs (rifampin, phenytoin, carbamazepine, and phenobarbital) that may reduce the efficacy of the oral contraceptive should also be started on a high-estrogen product
- although higher-dose estrogens can decrease spotting in patients taking interacting drugs, the efficacy may still be decreased but is likely better than with other single forms of birth control

Table 7–1 • Composition and Activity of Commonly Prescribed Oral Contraceptives*

Product	Composition Estrogen	μg	Progestin	mg	Relative Activities Estrogenic	Progestational	Androgenic	Spotting and BTB† (%)
50 μg Estrogen								
Ovral	e. estradiol	50	norgestrel	0.5	++++	++++	+++	4.5
Norlestrin 2.5/50	e. estradiol	50	nor. acetate	2.5	+	++++	++++	5.1
Genora, Norinyl, Ortho-Novum 1/50	mestranol	50	norethindrone	1.0	+++	+++	++	10.6
Ovcon-50	e. estradiol	50	norethindrone	1.0	++++	+++	++	11.9
Demulen 1/50	e. estradiol	50	ethy. diacetate	1.0	++	++++	++	13.9
Norlestrin 1/50	e. estradiol	50	nor. acetate	1.0	+++	+++	+++	13.6
Sub 50 μg Estrogen Monophasic								
Lo/Ovral	e. estradiol	30	norgestrel	0.3	++	++	++	9.6
Desogen, Ortho-Cept	e. estradiol	30	desogestrel	0.15	++	++++	+	9.9
Ovcon-35	e. estradiol	35	norethindrone	0.4	++++	+	+	11.0
Levlen, Nordette, Min-Ovral^C	e. estradiol	30	levonorgestrel	0.15	++	++	++	14.0
Ortho-Cyclen	e. estradiol	35	norgestimate	0.25	+++	+	+	14.3
Brevicon Modicon, Nelova 0.5/35E, Ortho 0.5/35^C	e. estradiol	35	norethindrone	0.5	++++	+	+	14.6
Genora, Nelova, Norethin, Norinyl 1 + 35, Ortho-Novum 1/35, Ortho 1/35^C	e. estradiol	35	norethindrone	1.0	+++	+++	++	14.7
Loestrin 1.5/30	e. estradiol	30	nor. acetate	1.5	+	+++++	+++	25.2
Loestrin, Minestrin 1/20^C	e. estradiol	20	nor. acetate	1.0	+	+++	+++	29.7
Demulen 1/35	e. estradiol	35	ethy. diacetate	1.0	+	++++	++	37.4
Sub 50 μg Estrogen Multiphasic								
Ortho-Novum 7/7/7	e. estradiol	35 (7)	norethindrone	0.5 (7)	++++	++	++	12.2
	e. estradiol	35 (7)	norethindrone	0.75 (7)				
	e. estradiol	35 (7)	norethindrone	1.0 (7)				
Jenest-28	e. estradiol	35 (7)	norethindrone	0.5 (7)	+++	++	++	14.1
	e. estradiol	35 (14)	norethindrone	1.0 (14)				
Tri-Levlen, Triphasil, Triquilar^C	e. estradiol	30 (6)	levonorgestrel	0.05 (6)	++	+	++	15.1
	e. estradiol	40 (5)	levonorgestrel	0.075 (5)				
	e. estradiol	30 (10)	levonorgestrel	0.125 (10)				
Tri-Norinyl, Synphasic^C	e. estradiol	35 (7)	norethindrone	0.5 (7)	++++	++	++	14.7
	e. estradiol	35 (7)	norethindrone	1.0 (9)				
	e. estradiol	35 (7)	norethindrone	0.5 (5)				
Ortho Tri-Cyclen	e. estradiol	35 (7)	norgestimate	0.180 (7)	+++	+	++	17.5
	e. estradiol	35 (7)	norgestimate	0.215 (7)				
	e. estradiol	35 (7)	norgestimate	0.250 (7)				
Ortho-Novum 10/11	e. estradiol	35 (10)	norethindrone	0.5 (10)	++++	++	++	19.6
	e. estradiol	35 (11)	norethindrone	1.0 (11)				
Progestin Only								
Ovrette	none	—	norgestrel	0.075	+	+	+	34.9
Micronor, Nor-Q.D.	none	—	norethindrone	0.35	+	+	+	42.3

*Oral contraceptives containing greater than 50 μg of estrogen are not included in this table. These products are generally not necessary to prevent conception and are associated with an increase in serious complications. Women who may need to use the higher-strength estrogen include women who have had a contraceptive failure while *properly* taking a product containing 50 μg of estrogen, women who are concomitantly taking a medication that decreases the efficacy of the estrogen, or women who have severe acne. The higher-dose estrogen products are also used to treat other conditions such as ovarian cysts, endometriosis, and dysfunctional uterine bleeding.

†Reported prevalence of breakthrough bleeding and spotting in the third cycle of use. Information should not be precisely compared.

Number in parentheses indicates the number of tablets (days) in each phase.

^C = Canadian trade name; e. estradiol = ethinyl estradiol; ethy. diacetate = ethynodiol diacetate; nor. acetate = norethindrone acetate; BTB = breakthrough bleeding; + = very low; ++ = low; +++ = moderate; ++++ = high; +++++ = very high.

Adapted from Dickey RM, ed. Managing Contraceptive Pill Patients, 7th ed. Durant, OK: Essential Medical Information Systems, Inc, 1993:130–135.

129

Table 7–2 • **Relative Biological Activity of Commonly Used Progestins***

Class Compound	Progestational Activity[1]	Estrogenic Activity[2]	Androgenic Activity[3]	Endometrial Activity[4]	Androgenic/Progestational Activity Ratio[5]
norethindrone	1.0	1.0	1.0	1.0	1.0
norethindrone acetate	1.2	1.5	1.6	0.4	1.3
ethynodiol diacetate	1.4	3.4	0.6	0.4	0.4
norethynodrel	0.3	8.3	0	na	0
levonorgestrel	5.3	0	9.4	5.1	1.6
dl-norgestrel	2.6	0	4.7	2.6	1.6
desogestrel	9.0	0	3.4	8.7	0.4
norgestimate	1.2	0	2.2	1.2	1.5
medroxyprogesterone acetate	0.3	0	0	na	0

*Calculated on the basis of norethindrone = 1.0 in activity.
[1]Based on the amount required to induce vacuoles in human endometrium or compared with stimulation by levonorgestrel.
[2]Comparative potency based on rat vaginal epithelium assay. (Norethindrone = 0.25 when ethinyl estradiol = 100. Norgestimate relative to levonorgestrel = 8.3.)
[3]Comparative potency (oral) based on rat ventral prostate assay. (Norethindrone = 1.0 when methyltestosterone = 50.)
[4]Based on estimation of the amount required to suppress bleeding for 20 days in 50% of women.
[5]Based on oral animal assays. Actual activity in women may be different and is modified by the dose of estrogen.
na = not available
Adapted from Dickey RM, ed. Managing Contraceptive Pill Patients, 7th ed. Durant, OK: Essential Medical Information Systems, Inc, 1993:128–129.

Women with absolute contraindications to estrogens

PROGESTIN ONLY PRODUCTS (NORGESTREL [OVRETTE], NORETHINDRONE [MICRONOR])

- progestin only oral contraceptives are less effective (2–3% versus 0.3–1.2% failure rate) than the combination oral contraceptives and are more likely to result in irregular spotting and bleeding and ectopic pregnancy
- their use should be considered whenever contraception is desired in women who cannot take estrogen, such as patients with systemic lupus erythematosus, varicose veins, and estrogen-induced hypertension
- can be used for women who are breast-feeding or who do not tolerate estrogen at all

PROGESTIN IMPLANTS (LEVONORGESTREL [NORPLANT])

- the levonorgestrel implant has become available in the USA, and it provides up to 5 years of effective contraception, which is not reliant on patient compliance
- efficacy of this product may be weight dependent, and side effects are similar to those of progestin only oral contraceptives
- it necessitates surgical insertion and removal and is expensive initially; however, it offers therapeutic advantages to women who desire long-term, reversible contraception, including women who cannot take estrogen and those in whom compliance is a problem

Postcoital contraception

ORAL CONTRACEPTIVE WITH HIGH ESTROGEN AND PROGESTIN COMPOSITION (OVRAL)

- these agents are effective for postcoital contraception if used within 72 hours of unprotected intercourse

▶ What Dosage Should I Use?

Hormonal contraception

- see above for product selection
- most women require no more than 35 μg of ethinyl estradiol (higher doses of estrogen increase the chance of side effects during the first 3 months) and 1 mg of norethindrone or 0.15 mg of levonorgestrel for 21 days of each 28 day cycle
- with lower doses of estrogen or progestin, spotting occurs

and missed pills are more likely to result in breakthrough ovulation

Starting time for oral contraceptives

Many products have packaging that allows the products to be taken only on a certain day • To prevent confusion, ensure that recommendations on when to start oral contraceptives take the type of packaging into account

MULTIPHASIC PRODUCTS

- in general, multiphasic oral contraceptives should be started on day 1 of menses to ensure effective first-cycle ovulation inhibition

MONOPHASIC PRODUCTS

- ovulation is inhibited as long as oral contraceptives are started by day 5 or 6 after the first day of menstrual bleeding
- although it is suggested that some oral contraceptives should be started on day 5 of the cycle, oral contraceptives can be started on the first Sunday after the menses, which ensures period-free weekends if this is desirable

Alternative dosing

- if the time of menstrual flow is inconvenient such as for athletics, honeymoon, and holidays, skipping a period is possible by starting a new 21 day package as soon as the previous one has been completed; but be aware that some breakthrough bleeding may occur
- if the woman is taking a triphasic product that has a significant increase in the progestin component during the month, she may wish to begin the new package from back to front to minimize the chance of some spotting as a result of a relative fall in progesterone levels
- if the patient experiences headaches or migraines during the week off oral contraceptives, she can consider taking oral contraceptives regularly for 3 cycles (three 21 day cycles) with 1 week off

Missed doses

- if a woman misses 1 dose, she should take it as soon as she remembers
- if a woman misses 2 doses, she should take 2 tablets for the next 2 days and use another method of birth control for the remainder of the cycle while continuing to take the oral contraceptive

- if a woman misses more than 2 doses in a row, contraception for that cycle is minimal and a new package should be begun after pregnancy is ruled out and menstruation begins

Postcoital contraception

ETHINYL ESTRADIOL–NORGESTREL (OVRAL)

- 2 tablets PO immediately and repeated in 12 hours (taken within 3 days of unprotected intercourse)

▶ *How Long Should I Treat with My Initial Regimen?*

Hormonal contraception

- unless serious problems such as heavy breakthrough bleeding, worsening headaches, and deep vein thrombosis arise, a woman should continue taking any given product for 3 months before determining what a logical product switch may be

Postcoital contraception

- 2 tablets PO taken immediately and repeated in 12 hours is all that is necessary

▶ *What Efficacy Parameters Should I Follow and How Frequently Do I Have to Assess My Patient?*

Hormonal contraception

Initial assessment

- needed for all patients prior to prescribing oral contraceptives
- obtain a complete medical, social, and family history to identify possible contraindications
- predisposing risk factors for cardiovascular, thromboembolic, and metabolic diseases (including, but not limited to, hypercholesterolemia, diabetes, hypertension, obesity, smoking, positive family history of cardiovascular disease, and diabetes) should be carefully assessed
- following are absolute contraindications: known or suspected pregnancy, as the progestins may cause fetal harm when administered to a pregnant woman; known or suspected cancer of the breast; known or suspected estrogen-dependent neoplasia or a history thereof; undiagnosed abnormal genital bleeding; active thrombophlebitis or thromboembolic disorders or a history thereof; cerebrovascular accident or a history thereof; and benign or malignant liver tumor or a history thereof
- obtain a complete history of response to previous hormonal challenges (pregnancy and previous oral contraceptive use) and characteristics of the patient's menstrual cycle
- blood pressure measurements
- Papanicolaou (Pap) smear and pelvic examination (not initially necessary in young non–sexually active patients)
- serum glucose determination, lipid profile, and liver function tests need be done only in patients with a history suggestive of a need for these tests

After the first 3 months

- schedule the first return visit after 3 cycles have been completed
- obtain a history of the menstrual cycle during oral contraceptive use (at each visit)
- patient should keep records of uterine bleeding (onset, duration, and amount as compared with bleeding before oral contraceptive use) during the first 3 months of therapy
- breast and pelvic examination need be done only yearly

Annual assessment

- if no problems exist at the end of 3 months, annual assessment is sufficient
- history of the menstrual cycle during oral contraceptive use (at each visit)
- breast and pelvic examination and Pap smear (annually)

Postcoital contraception

- next menses should begin in 2–3 weeks; if not, a pregnancy test should be ordered

▶ *Should I Add Another Drug or Substitute Therapy If My Initial Drug Therapy Fails?*

Hormonal contraception

Rational decisions for switching oral contraceptives should be based on the patient's response and adverse effects

Breakthrough bleeding or spotting

- most common reason for switching oral contraceptive is breakthrough bleeding or spotting
- for most healthy young women, spotting is not an ominous sign and may usually be managed with a watch and wait approach for several months unless spotting is a problem for the patient (Contraceptive Technology 1994: 259–260)
- in general, many cases of breakthrough bleeding can be treated by simply switching to a different oral contraceptive, regardless of estrogen or progestin activity
- however, breakthrough bleeding or spotting that continues to occur during the first 10 days of oral contraceptive use usually indicates an estrogen deficiency; therefore, switch to a product with higher estrogenic activity (see Table 7–1)
- breakthrough bleeding or spotting after the 10th day usually indicates a progestin deficiency; therefore, switch to a product with higher progestin activity (see Table 7–1)

Development of or worsening of acne, hypertension, or hair growth

- switch to a product with lower androgenic activity

Amenorrhea

- as long as pregnancy has been ruled out, switch to a lower-dose progestin product or one with higher estrogenic activity
- scanty periods or loss of withdrawal bleeding is common after long-term use of oral contraceptives, and if amenorrhea is not due to pregnancy, the addition of 20 μg of ethinyl estradiol or 0.625 mg of conjugated estrogens (Premarin) for the first 7 days of the next 2 or 3 cycles often results in a return of withdrawal bleeding for months

Contraceptive failure

- if contraceptive failure occurs while the patient is properly taking oral contraceptives, switch to a product with a higher estrogenic activity when restarting oral contraceptive use

▶ *How Long Should I Continue Drug Therapy?*

Hormonal contraception

- healthy nonsmoking women can continue to use oral contraceptives without increased risk until age 50 years
- oral contraceptives should not be used in women older than 35 years if they smoke because of markedly increased risk of cardiovascular disease

- drug-free periods ("drug holidays") from oral contraceptives are not necessary, and there is no evidence that continued use increases the risk of adverse effects

If pregnancy is desired

- if pregnancy is desired, it is currently recommended that the oral contraceptive be discontinued for 3 months before conception is attempted to allow accurate dating of pregnancy
- however, if conception occurs within the first month of discontinuing the oral contraceptive regimen, there does not appear to be an increased risk of any type of birth defects over that seen in infants born to the general population

After pregnancy

- after delivery, oral contraceptives should ideally be withheld until 4–6 weeks postpartum to allow coagulation to return to normal levels and to allow lactation to become established; however, in women who may be sexually active immediately after pregnancy (and will not use other methods of birth control), oral contraceptives should be reinstituted immediately
- if oral contraceptives are withheld for 4–6 weeks, other methods of birth control should be used during this time
- although it is controversial, it is generally considered safe to use oral contraceptives when breast-feeding if the woman is otherwise healthy and lactation is established (i.e., 4–6 weeks postpartum)

Useful References

Dickey RP, ed. Managing Contraceptive Pill Patients, 7th ed. Durant, OK: Essential Medical Information Systems, Inc, 1993.

Hatcher RA, et al, eds. Contraceptive Technology, 16th ed. New York: Irvington Publishers Inc, 1994.

DRUG THERAPY FOR LABOR INDUCTION

Glenda Meneilly

▶ What Are My Goals of Treatment?

to establish regular uterine contractions that occur every 3–5 minutes and last 60–90 seconds

to effect cervical effacement and dilation at a rate that mimics normal spontaneous labor (approximately 1 cm/h)

to deliver the fetus vaginally without increasing the risk to the mother or the fetus

▶ What Evidence Is Available to Support Drug Therapy for Labor Induction?

Improved fetal and maternal outcome

- prolonged labor is associated with an increase in maternal and fetal morbidity and mortality (Am J Obstet Gynecol 1963;85:209–222), and the use of oxytocin to prevent prolonged labor results in better fetal and maternal outcome (Am J Obstet Gynecol 1987;156:935–939)

Cervical softening

- induction of labor without cervical softening has a high failure rate
- prostaglandin administration produces effective preinduction cervical softening (Acta Obstet Gynecol Scand 1987;66:3–7)

- prostaglandins administered locally decrease the duration of labor, shorten the induction to delivery interval, decrease the oxytocin dose required subsequently, and reduce overall failure of induction (Am J Obstet Gynecol 1986;154:1275–1279)
- uterine response to oxytocin is enhanced after exposure to prostaglandin E_2 (Br Med J 1972;1:150)

▶ When Should I Consider Drug Therapy?

Induction of labor

Augmentation

- when nondrug measures such as amniotomy (artificial rupture of membranes) and nipple stimulation are unsuccessful in women with documentation of progressive dilation to at least 3 cm and effacement

Cases in which prolongation of pregnancy is dangerous to the fetus

- when fetal indications such as possible fetal demise and severe Rh isoimmunization are present

Maternal hypertension

- timing of induction depends on the severity of hypertension
- in mild chronic hypertension or pregnancy-induced hypertension, mother and fetus are monitored, with induction considered at 37–38 weeks' gestation
- induction is undertaken immediately if severe pregnancy-induced hypertension (eclampsia) or uncontrolled chronic hypertension (mean arterial pressure > 126 mmHg) is present

Maternal diabetes mellitus

- early delivery should be considered in pregnant diabetics who have poorly controlled blood glucose levels despite maximum therapy, who have progression of nephropathy or retinopathy, or who have previously delivered a macrosomic (large) fetus

Prolonged pregnancy

- induction should be undertaken at 42 weeks' gestation

Dysfunctional labor

- induction undertaken if the cervix is ripe

▶ What Drug Should I Use for Initial Treatment?

Preinduction softening and dilation of cervix
PROSTAGLANDIN E_2 GEL (CERVICAL)

- considered initial treatment if Bishop's score is 5 or less (unfavorable cervix) (Am J Obstet Gynecol 1986;154:1275–1279) in patients of gravida 1 or 2 (Table 7–3)

Induction of labor
OXYTOCIN

- use as initial treatment for Bishop's score greater than 5 (favorable cervix) or in patients of gravida 3 or greater

PROSTAGLANDIN E_2 GEL (VAGINAL)

- may be used as an alternative to oxytocin in patients with Bishop's score greater than 5
- time to induction and duration of labor are longer with prostaglandin gel (Aust N Z J Obstet Gynecol 1989;29[2]:124–128), although patient acceptance is greater (Eur J Obstet Gynecol Reprod Biol 1990;37:111–119)

▶ What Dosage Should I Use?

Preinduction softening and dilation of cervix
PROSTAGLANDIN E_2 GEL (CERVICAL)

- 0.5 mg in 2.5 mL of triacetin gel, administered into

Table 7–3 • **Bishop's Score**

Criteria	Number of Points			
	0	1	2	3
cervical dilation (cm)	0	1–2	3–4	5–6
cervical effacement (%)	0–30	40–50	60–70	>80
cervical consistency	firm	medium	soft	
cervical position	posterior	central	anterior	
ischial spines	3 cm above	2 cm above	0–1 cm above	1–2 cm below

the cervical canal just below the level of the internal cervical os

- 0.5 mg may be administered endocervically every 6 hours for a maximum of 3 doses

Induction of labor

OXYTOCIN

Preterm patient

- start with infusion rate of 1 μU/min and increase by 2 μU/min every 30 minutes; infusion rates of 20–40 μU/min may be required

Term patient, patient with favorable cervix, or patient with preexisting uterine activity

- start with infusion rate of 0.5 μU/min and increase by 1 μU/min every 30 minutes, with an infusion rate of 2–8 μU/min usually being sufficient to achieve a cervical dilation rate of 1 cm/h, and a dosage of more than 20 μU/min at term is rarely needed (Obstet Gynecol Surv 1988;43[12]:730–743)

PROSTAGLANDIN E₂ GEL (VAGINAL)

- start with 1 mg inserted into the posterior fornix of the vaginal canal
- if labor is not induced in 6 hours, a second dose of 1 or 2 mg may be inserted

▶ *How Long Should I Treat with My Initial Regimen?*

Preinduction softening and dilation of cervix

PROSTAGLANDIN E₂ GEL (CERVICAL)

- maximum of 3 doses

Induction of labor

OXYTOCIN

- infusion rate should be increased as outlined above until adequate contractions effecting a cervical dilation rate of at least 1 cm/h or the maximum infusion rate is attained

PROSTAGLANDIN E₂ GEL (VAGINAL)

- if labor is not induced in 6 hours, a second dose of 1 or 2 mg may be inserted

▶ *What Efficacy Parameters Should I Follow and How Frequently Do I Have to Assess My Patient?*

Induction of labor and cervical softening

Cervical dilation rate

- cervical status should be assessed before subsequent doses are administered

- oxytocin for induction may be started when Bishop's score is 5 or greater
- desired cervical dilation rate of 1 cm/h can be used as a guide for increasing oxytocin infusion rates

Uterine activity

- monitor every hour, and continuously for 1 hour after each insertion of gel
- monitor with every oxytocin dosage change or at least every 30 minutes
- at an effective dosage, uterine contractions occur every 3–4 minutes, with a duration of about 60 seconds
- if hyperstimulation occurs (6 contractions or more in 10 minutes for a total of 20 minutes), discontinue the oxytocin infusion, turn the patient to the left lateral position, and apply oxygen
- wait at least 15 minutes before restarting and start the infusion at ½ the previous rate, and evaluate fetal heart rate at least every 30 minutes

Fetal response

- monitor every hour, and continuously for 1 hour after each insertion of gel
- monitor with every oxytocin dosage change or at least every 30 minutes
- if fetal distress occurs (abnormal fetal heart rate pattern), manage the same as for uterine hyperstimulation
- if fetal compromise is evident (meconium staining of amniotic fluid, vaginal bleeding indicating placental abruption), prolonged induction should be avoided

▶ *Should I Add Another Drug or Substitute Therapy If My Initial Drug Therapy Fails?*

Preinduction softening and dilation of cervix

PROSTAGLANDIN E₂ GEL (CERVICAL)

- if no contractions occur after 3 doses at 6 hour intervals, oxytocin for induction should be administered
- oxytocin should not be given for at least 6 hours after the last insertion of prostaglandin cervical gel, as prostaglandins potentiate the effect of oxytocin on the uterus

Induction of labor

OXYTOCIN

- if oxytocin is not effective, reevaluate the patient, and consider cesarean section

PROSTAGLANDIN E₂ GEL (VAGINAL)

- if 2 doses of prostaglandin E₂ vaginal gel fail to induce labor, start oxytocin administration as described above
- oxytocin should not be given for at least 12 hours after the last insertion of prostaglandin vaginal gel, as prostaglandins potentiate the effect of oxytocin on the uterus

▶ *How Long Should I Continue Drug Therapy?*

Induction of labor

- if oxytocin is not successful after 10–12 hours, discontinue the infusion, allow the patient to rest, monitor the patient, and restart the infusion the next day
- this may be repeated for up to 3 days
- a 6–8 hour time limit should be used for patients with preeclampsia

Useful References

American College of Obstetricians and Gynecologists. Induction and augmentation of labor. ACOG Technical Bulletin, no. 157. Washington, DC: ACOG, 1991

Brindley BA, Sokol RJ. Induction and augmentation of labour: Basis and methods for current practice. Obstet Gynecol Surv 1988;43:730–743
Husstein P. Use of prostaglandins for induction of labor. Semin Perinatol 1991;15:173–181

DRUG THERAPY FOR LABOR INHIBITION

Glenda Meneilly

▶ What Are My Goals of Treatment?

to stop uterine contractions
to prevent progression of cervical effacement and dilation
to delay delivery of the fetus long enough (24–48 hours) to transfer the mother to a center with specialized neonatal facilities and permit acceleration of fetal lung maturity by maternal administration of glucocorticoids if gestation is less than 32 weeks

▶ What Evidence Is Available to Support Drug Therapy For Labor Inhibition?

- supporting evidence is weak owing to the lack of randomized, placebo-controlled trials of tocolytic agents
- evidence from controlled trials is poor because of the inability to diagnose preterm labor accurately and the high incidence of placebo effect in trials (Am J Obstet Gynecol 1988;95:211–222)
- in general, tocolytics stop contractions for 24–48 hours, do not improve perinatal outcome or reduce the overall rate of preterm birth, and increase maternal morbidity (Am J Obstet Gynecol 1993; 168:1247–1259)
- ritodrine has shown a trend to decreasing infant mortality in gestations of 24–27 weeks only (N Engl J Med 1992; 327:308–312)
- because perinatal morbidity and mortality are not altered, the indication for tocolysis is to delay delivery long enough to administer glucocorticoids to the mother
- glucocorticoids hasten fetal lung maturity and reduce the incidence of respiratory distress syndrome in the premature newborn (Br J Obstet Gynecol 1990;97:11–26)

▶ When Should I Consider Drug Therapy?

Premature labor

- if the onset of labor is between 24 and 32 weeks' gestation, with documented uterine contractions occurring every 7–10 minutes for 30–60 minutes, each lasting 30 seconds, and with ruptured membranes
- if membranes are ruptured, or, in the presence of intact membranes if there are documented cervical changes (cervical effacement of less than 80% or dilation of more than 2 cm)
- patient has not responded to bedrest, oral hydration, or mild sedation
- no clear cause of preterm labor, such as infection, can be determined
- use drug therapy only if there are no contraindications to the inhibition of preterm labor: major maternal illness that cannot be controlled, eclampsia or severe preeclampsia, abruptio placentae, severe fetal anomaly (incompatible with life), fetal demise, and chorioamnionitis
- tocolytics are unlikely to be successful if cervical dilation is greater than 4 cm or effacement is greater than 80%

▶ What Drug Should I Use for Initial Treatment?

Premature labor

All available agents are equal in effect, so the choice of agent is based on the route of administration, potential maternal and fetal toxicity, the cost of therapy, and overall experience with the drug

RITODRINE

- drug of choice if the patient does not have cardiac disease (arrhythmias or congestive heart failure), suspected infection, or hyperthyroidism
- greatest worldwide experience in tocolysis is with ritodrine, and ritodrine is the only drug approved by the US Food and Drug Administration for the treatment of preterm labor
- ritodrine may be given by infusion, allowing rapid onset and control of plasma concentrations; ritodrine may also be given via intramuscular injection
- highest incidence of maternal side effects occurs with ritodrine (24%), followed by magnesium (15%), then indomethacin (Am J Obstet Gynecol 1993;168:1247–1259)
- the most serious maternal side effects (arrhythmias, pulmonary edema, and hyperglycemia) are associated with ritodrine
- ritodrine causes fetal tachycardia, hyperinsulinemia, and hypoglycemia

MAGNESIUM

- drug of choice if the patient has contraindication to ritodrine
- magnesium infusions have been used for many years for the treatment of eclampsia and eclamptic seizures, but use in premature labor is limited
- magnesium sulfate may be given by intravenous infusion
- magnesium sulfate may cause neonatal respiratory depression and muscle weakness

INDOMETHACIN

- drug of choice if intravenous access is not possible (during transfer to a tertiary care center) or if polyhydramnios (excess amniotic fluid) is present
- indomethacin may be given by the oral or rectal route
- overall experience with indomethacin is limited
- indomethacin can cause premature closure of the ductus arteriosus, especially in fetuses older than 34 weeks (Am J Obstet Gynecol 1986;155:747–749)
- indomethacin causes a dose-dependent oligohydramnios owing to decreased fetal urine output, which is reversed on discontinuation of drug administration (Obstet Gynecol 1988;72:51–53)

▶ What Dosage Should I Use?

Premature labor

RITODRINE

- dilute 150 mg in 500 mL of 5% dextrose in water
- administer using a controlled infusion device at 50 μg/min
- increase by 50 μg/min every 15 minutes until uterine contractions stop, to a maximum of 350 μg/min
- once contractions stop, maintain infusion rate for 1 hour, then wean by 50 μg/min every 30 minutes to the lowest infusion rate that sustains inhibition (Am J Obstet Gynecol 1990;162:429–437)

MAGNESIUM

- add 40 g of magnesium sulfate to 1000 mL of 5% dextrose in water or $^1/_2$ normal saline
- give a 100 mL (4 g) loading dose IV over 20 minutes
- then infuse at a rate of 2 g/h, and increase the dosage every 30 minutes by 0.5 g/h until contractions are inhibited or 4 g/h is reached

INDOMETHACIN

- 50 mg PO or rectally, then 25 mg PO Q4H until contractions stop, followed by 25 mg PO Q6H (Am J Obstet Gynecol 1991;164:981–988) or 100 mg per rectum Q12H

▶ *How Long Should I Treat with My Initial Regimen?*

Premature labor

RITODRINE, MAGNESIUM, INDOMETHACIN

- continue until 12 hours after uterine activity has ceased or until 24 hours after the last dose of corticosteroid has been given
- if progressive cervical dilation or effacement occurs within 6 hours despite escalation of the dosage, consider changing to an alternative agent

▶ *What Efficacy Parameters Should I Follow and How Frequently Do I Have to Assess My Patient?*

Premature labor

Uterine activity
- monitor uterine contractions continually while intravenous dosage increases are being made, and at least every hour when a stable infusion dosage has been attained
- attempt to reduce contractions to 4 contractions per hour or fewer

Cervical dilation and effacement
- monitor cervical dilation and effacement 1–2 hours after the initiation of therapy, then no more frequently than every 12 hours
- attempt to maintain less than 4 cm dilation and less than 80% effacement

Fetal lung maturity
- for a fetus of less than 32 weeks' gestation, collect amniotic fluid to determine the lecithin/sphingomyelin ratio
- lecithin/sphingomyelin ratio of greater than 2 indicates fetal pulmonary maturity
- if amniocentesis reveals immature fetal lungs, a course of maternal glucocorticoids (dexamethasone or betamethasone) to accelerate fetal lung maturity should be considered
- 48 hours of inhibition is critical to achieve fetal lung maturity

Magnesium levels
- serum magnesium levels should be monitored every 4–6 hours, and maintained in the range of 6–8 mEq/L (3–4 mmol/L)

▶ *Should I Add Another Drug or Substitute Therapy If My Initial Drug Therapy Fails?*

Premature labor

RITODRINE

- regardless of which drug is chosen first (ritodrine or magnesium sulfate), the alternative drug successfully inhibits labor in 50–60% of cases failing to respond to the first drug (Clin Obstet Gynecol 1988;31;635–651)
- changing to another beta-mimetic, such as isoxsuprine or terbutaline, is of no benefit
- change to magnesium sulfate if progressive cervical dilation occurs within 6 hours, or intolerable side effects occur despite a reduction in infusion rate

MAGNESIUM

- change to ritodrine if progressive cervical dilation occurs within 6 hours, or intolerable side effects occur despite a reduction in the infusion rate
- if the second agent fails, combination therapy has been tried (with a high incidence of chest pain, pulmonary edema, and electrocardiographic changes)

INDOMETHACIN

- if there is no IV access, give ritodrine intramuscularly (10 mg IM, followed by 5 mg Q4H)
- titrate the dose to response and toxicity (may be increased to 10 mg Q2H) (Am J Obstet Gynecol 1988;159:323–328)
- change to ritodrine infusion when intravenous access is available

▶ *How Long Should I Continue Drug Therapy?*

Premature labor

- if membranes are ruptured, do not use drug therapy for longer than 48 hours to avoid chorioamnionitis
- if membranes are intact and gestation is less than 32 weeks, continue intensive therapy for 12 hours after contractions stop, or 24 hours after the last dose of corticosteroid has been given
- if labor begins again, restart treatment or increase the infusion rate

Useful References

Canadian Preterm Labor Investigators Groups. Treatment of preterm labor with the beta-adrenergic agonist ritodrine. N Engl J Med 1992; 327:308–312

Caritis SN, Darby MJ, Chan L. Pharmacologic treatment of preterm labor. Clin Obstet Gynecol 1988;31:635–651

Creasy RK. Preterm birth prevention: Where are we? Am J Obstet Gynecol 1993;168:1223–1230

Higby K, Xenakis EM-J, Paverstein CJ. Do tocolytic agents stop preterm labor? A critical and comprehensive review of efficacy and safety. Am J Obstet Gynecol 1993;168:1247–1259

Johnson P. Suppression of preterm labor. Current concepts. Drugs 1993;45:684–692

King JF, Grant A, Keirse MJN, Chalmers I. Beta-mimetics in preterm labour: An overview of randomized controlled trials. Br J Obstet Gynaecol 1988;95:211–222

8 | PSYCHIATRIC DISORDERS

DRUG THERAPY FOR DEPRESSION

Lyle K. Laird and Julia Vertrees

▶ What Are My Goals of Treatment?

to eliminate the target symptoms of depression, including depressed mood, irritability, sleep difficulties (usually insomnia), suicidal thoughts, guilty feelings, decreased concentration, anxiety, weight loss or gain, and somatic complaints (e.g., back pain and headaches)

to prevent the recurrence of depression after it is controlled

▶ What Evidence is Available to Support Drug Therapy for Depression?

Untreated depression

- depressive disorders tend to be recurrent, especially if left untreated; 20–50% of cases tend to be chronic, resulting in significant social impairment
- these disorders result in a markedly decreased quality of life, decreased productivity, and suicide in up to 15% of depressives

Treated depression

- reported efficacy of antidepressant drugs is well established and stable with overall response rates reported in the 65–85% range compared with responses to placebo of approximately 30% (Pharmacol Rev 1965;17:101–141, Arch Gen Psychiatry 1977;34:197–204)

Prevention of recurrences

- depressive illnesses are cyclic and therefore tend to recur; between 50% and 85% of patients with major depression have at least 1 recurrence in a lifetime (Am J Psychiatry 1986;143:18–23)
- antidepressant drugs reduce the risk of recurrence of depression (Am J Psychiatry 1985;142:469–476)

▶ When Should I Consider Drug Therapy?

Major Depressive Disorder

- if a diagnosis of a depressive disorder (bipolar or unipolar) can be made on the basis of Diagnostic and Statistical Manual, 4th ed. (DSM-IV) criteria
- target symptoms include depressed mood, irritability, sleep difficulties (usually insomnia), suicidal thoughts, guilty feelings, decreased concentration, anxiety, weight loss or gain, and somatic complaints (e.g., back pain and headaches)
- if it can be determined that the problem is not part of a normal grief process (i.e., normally a self-limiting event)
- to supplement or to facilitate psychotherapy

▶ What Drug Should I Use for Initial Treatment?

All antidepressants should be considered equally effective, and therefore, the initial drug choice depends on what the patient or patient's relatives have responded to in the past, whether concomitant disease states are present, and what side effects (Table 8–1) are acceptable or should be avoided

Major depressive disorder with no concomitant disease state

IMIPRAMINE

- imipramine is the initial drug of choice in patients without concomitant diseases because it is as effective as and less expensive than other tricyclic antidepressants
- although imipramine can cause more adverse effects than do many of the newer agents, tolerance of these adverse effects develops in many patients, and numerous patients may be effectively treated with this inexpensive drug
- useful if a sedative effect is desirable (fluoxetine is stimulating in many patients)

DESIPRAMINE

- if desipramine is less expensive than imipramine, desipramine should be chosen because it produces less sedation and anticholinergic effects than does imipramine
- clinicians often prefer this drug because it is a stimulating tricyclic antidepressant whose efficacy is thought not to decrease at higher dosages

AMITRIPTYLINE

- amitriptyline may still be the most effective drug for some patients with agitated depression owing to its sedating effect
- more sedating than imipramine

FLUOXETINE

- as effective as other antidepressants for the treatment of major depression
- if cost is not a factor, and the patient can tolerate an activating antidepressant, fluoxetine should be chosen over imipramine, as it is generally better tolerated than tricyclic antidepressants

SERTRALINE

- similar to fluoxetine
- no comparative trials between sertraline and fluoxetine (Med Lett 1992;34:47–48)
- probably inhibits cytochrome P-450 enzymes to a lesser degree than fluoxetine and, therefore, likely produces fewer drug interactions than those seen with fluoxetine
- may be less activating than fluoxetine

PAROXETINE

- similar to fluoxetine
- causes more inhibition of cytochrome P-450 enzymes than does sertraline, but less than fluoxetine (Med Lett 1993;35:24–25)

Table 8–1 • **Side Effects of Recommended Antidepressants**

	Anticholinergic Effects	Arrhythmias	Orthostatic Hypotension	Sedation	Seizures
imipramine	+ + +	+ + + +	+ + + +	+ + +	+ + +
amitriptyline	+ + + +	+ + + +	+ + + +	+ + + +	+ + +
clomipramine	+ + +	+ + + +	+ + + +	+ + +	+ + + +
desipramine	+ +	+ + +	+ + +	+ +	+ +
nortriptyline	+ + +	+ + +	+	+ +	+ +
fluoxetine	0	+	+	+	+
bupropion	0	0	0	0	+ + + +
sertraline	0	+	+	+	+
paroxetine	0	+	+	+	+

+ + + + = high; + + + = moderate; + + = low; + = very low; 0 = none.
Data from Clin Pharm 1986;5:304–318 and Drugs 1990;39:136–153.

Major depressive disorder with concomitant disease states
Congestive heart failure, low blood pressure, or orthostatic hypotension
NORTRIPTYLINE

- less potential to cause cardiovascular effects or orthostatic hypotension (Pharmacol Clin 1970;2:68–71) than with other antidepressants and should be chosen in those patients with concerns about falling (e.g., the elderly) and/or patients with orthostatic hypotension

FLUOXETINE, SERTRALINE, PAROXETINE

- if cost is not a factor, these agents can be used, as they apparently have minimal cardiovascular effects

Heart blocks (including bundle branch disease)
FLUOXETINE, SERTRALINE, PAROXETINE

- these agents appear to cause few cardiovascular effects and should be chosen in patients with heart blocks
- tricyclic antidepressants are contraindicated in patients with second- or third-degree atrioventricular blocks or left bundle branch disease (tricyclic agents can be used in patients with first-degree block or right bundle branch disease, but these patients must be evaluated and followed by a cardiologist)

BUPROPION

- bupropion is also safe in this patient population
- bupropion was thought to cause a higher incidence of seizures, but a study suggests that it is similar to that seen with other antidepressants (J Clin Psychiatry 1991; 52:450–456)
- has the disadvantage of requiring multiple daily dosing (BID or TID)

Seizure disorders
FLUOXETINE, SERTRALINE, PAROXETINE

- some antidepressants can lower the seizure threshold, and these agents appear to have a lower propensity to cause seizures than do other antidepressants that have been on the market for a longer time (e.g., tricyclic antidepressants)
- dose titration should be slow, and the usual maximum doses should be avoided
- seizure disorder should be well-controlled prior to initiating antidepressant therapy

Glaucoma
DESIPRAMINE

- if a tricyclic agent must be used, desipramine should be chosen because it produces fewer anticholinergic effects than do other tricyclic antidepressants and has a decreased risk of causing exacerbation of glaucoma (e.g., open angle glaucoma); an ophthalmologist should always be consulted for these patients
- is less expensive than fluoxetine

FLUOXETINE, SERTRALINE, PAROXETINE

- if cost is not a factor, these agents can be used, as they have no anticholinergic effects

Benign prostatic hypertrophy, chronic constipation, urinary retention
FLUOXETINE, SERTRALINE, PAROXETINE, BUPROPION, PHENELZINE, DESIPRAMINE

- all these agents have low or no anticholinergic effects

Obsessive-compulsive disorder
CLOMIPRAMINE

- should be used if the patient has depression with obsessional features, as clomipramine is effective for the treatment of obsessive-compulsive disorder

FLUOXETINE, SERTRALINE, PAROXETINE

- if the patient does not respond to or cannot tolerate clomipramine

Bipolar disorders
LITHIUM

- patients with bipolar depression or a history of bipolar disorder may not be good candidates for tricyclic antidepressants or fluoxetine and possibly other antidepressants, as these medications can cause the disorder to switch to a manic phase (Biol Psychiatry 1982;17:271–274)
- may also be used as augmentation therapy to conventional antidepressants in partial responders (J Clin Psychopharmacol 1983;3:303–307)

Depressive disorder not otherwise specified (with atypical features)
PHENELZINE

- useful in patients with atypical depression characterized either by anxiety, feeling of tension, tremor, cardiovascular or gastrointestinal symptoms, phobias, and panic attacks or by reverse vegetative symptoms such as increased sleep, increased appetite, weight gain, increased libido, and reversed diurnal variation (feeling best in the morning)

▶ *What Dosage Should I Use?*

Major depressive disorder

IMIPRAMINE, DESIPRAMINE, AMITRIPTYLINE

- 50 mg PO daily at bedtime
- increase after 3 days to 100 mg PO daily at bedtime
- increase to 150 mg PO daily at bedtime after 1 week and leave at this dosage for 10–14 days
- if target symptoms such as nervousness, somatic complaints, and appetite are not improving after 3 weeks of therapy, continue to increase the daily dosage by 50 mg at weekly intervals until a response is seen or a dosage of 300 mg PO daily has been reached

NORTRIPTYLINE

- 25 mg PO daily at bedtime
- increase after 3 days to 50 mg PO daily at bedtime
- increase to 75 mg PO daily at bedtime after 1 week and leave at this dosage for 10–14 days
- if target symptoms such as nervousness, somatic complaints, and appetite are not improving after 3 weeks of therapy, continue to increase the daily dosage by 25 mg at weekly intervals until a response is seen or a dosage of 150 mg PO daily has been reached

FLUOXETINE

- 10 mg PO daily for 2 weeks, and if there is some improvement, maintain this dosage; if not, increase to 20 mg PO daily and reevaluate in another 2 weeks
- if minimum to no change in symptoms occurs after this time, increase the dosage to 40 mg PO daily
- if some response occurs with 40 mg after another 2 weeks but not complete effect, increase the dosage to 60 mg PO daily
- if the desired effect is still not seen after another 2 weeks, consider increasing the dosage to 80 mg PO daily
- maximum adult dose is 80 mg/d (60 mg/d in geriatric patients), but studies have shown that few patients need greater than 20 mg/d for efficacy in major depression and that side effects increase with dosages of 60 mg/d or more (Psychopharmacol Bull 1987;23:164–168)
- manufacturer recommends that doses larger than 20 mg be taken in two divided doses (in the morning and at noon), but this is not necessary and even high doses can be given as a single morning dose
- studies have shown that some patients respond to 5–10 mg/d (Psychopharmacol Bull 1988;24:183–188) and that these lower dosages decrease the cost associated with fluoxetine

SERTRALINE

- 50 mg PO daily for 3–4 weeks
- if minimum to no change in symptoms occurs after this time, increase the dosage to 100 mg PO daily
- if some response occurs with 100 mg after 2 weeks, but not complete effect, increase the dosage to 150 mg PO daily
- if the desired effect is still not seen after another 2 weeks, consider increasing the dosage to 200 mg PO daily

PAROXETINE

- give 20 mg PO daily and reevaluate in 4 weeks (dosages less than 20 mg PO daily are not effective) (J Clin Psychiatry 1992;53(12):434–438)
- if minimum to no change in symptoms occurs after this time, increase the dosage to 30 mg PO daily
- if there is some response with 40 mg after 2 weeks but not complete effect, increase the dosage to 40 mg PO daily
- if the desired effect is still not seen after another 2 weeks, consider increasing the dosage to 50 mg PO daily

BUPROPION

- give 100 mg PO BID, and after 3 days, increase to 100 mg PO TID
- maximum daily dose is 450 mg with no single dose greater than 150 mg; dosing intervals should be TID (time between doses must be at least 4 hours); seek to adjust the maintenance dosage to the lowest effective dosage
- only 75 mg tablets are available in Canada
- 75 mg PO BID for 3–4 days
- increase to 75 mg PO TID for 1 week, then increase to 150 mg PO BID, and then wait for 4 weeks and evaluate

PHENELZINE

- 30 mg PO daily (15 mg PO BID) and increase by 15 mg/d at 5–7 day intervals until 60 mg PO daily is reached
- maintain this dosage for 2 weeks, and if no response occurs, increase the daily dosage by 15 mg at weekly intervals to a maximum of 90 mg PO daily (or 1 mg/kg/d, whichever is less)
- give the full daily dose by noon if possible, but at the latest, give the last dose before supper to avoid insomnia
- therapeutic trial is usually considered to be at least 45 mg/d for 4 weeks

LITHIUM

- 300 mg PO TID is the starting dose in otherwise normal, healthy adults with good renal function
- because there is much interpatient variability in response to dosages, serum concentration level, rather than dosage, is the most important monitoring variable to ensure therapeutic levels

CLOMIPRAMINE

- 50 mg PO daily at bedtime
- increase after 3 days to 100 mg PO daily at bedtime
- increase to 150 mg PO daily at bedtime after 1 week, and leave at this dosage for 10–14 days
- if target symptoms do not improve by this time, increase the daily dosage weekly by 50 mg to a maximum of 250 mg/d or until target symptoms improve
- in geriatric patients and patients with a seizure history, start with 25 mg PO at bedtime, and in general, dosages should be approximately 50% of those used in younger patients
- clomipramine has a long duration of action; hence, long-acting or sustained-release products are unnecessary and once-daily dosing is appropriate

▶ *How Long Should I Treat with My Initial Regimen?*

Major depressive disorder

- some improvement in anxiety and insomnia should be seen in the first 10 days to 2 weeks, with an increase in energy in the first 2–3 weeks
- if the response is not satisfactory after 6 weeks (4 weeks at therapeutic dosages), try a drug from a different class or consider electroconvulsive therapy, if indicated
- if target symptoms such as nervousness, somatic complaints, and appetite are not improving after 3 weeks of therapy, continue to increase the dosage of imipramine by 50 mg PO daily (25 mg for nortriptyline) and increase by 50 mg weekly (25 mg for nortriptyline) until a response

is seen or a dosage of 300 mg PO daily (150 mg PO daily for nortriptyline) has been reached
- for patients receiving fluoxetine, increase the dosage to 40 mg PO daily after 4 weeks

▶ What Efficacy Parameters Should I Follow and How Frequently Do I Have to Assess My Patient?

Major depressive disorder

Sleep disturbances
- first symptom to improve (after 10–14 days) and should be assessed weekly

Nervousness, somatic complaints, appetite, feelings of helplessness and hopelessness, and depressed mood
- tend to improve more slowly over 2–3 weeks
- close friends or relatives often notice signs of improvement before the patient is aware of changes
- adequate clinical response should not be expected for at least 4 weeks
- after they are stable, patients should be clinically assessed for target symptoms at least monthly (or weekly if clinical decompensation is suspected)

Plasma concentrations
- in general, routine determinations are considered unnecessary, as there is not a strong correlation between serum concentration and effect
- for tricyclic agents, plasma concentration determinations can be useful to assess compliance, to investigate the situation of inordinate side effects on a moderate dosage, or to monitor cases in which the maximum suggested dosage is going to be exceeded
- for the newer antidepressant drugs, plasma concentration–clinical response relationships are largely unknown
- see individual drug monographs for more specific information

▶ Should I Add Another Drug or Substitute Therapy If My Initial Drug Therapy Fails?

Major depressive disorder
- substitute drug should be tried only after a full therapeutic trial with the first drug (at least 4 weeks at therapeutic dosages) has been attempted
- adding another antidepressant to the first drug is considered polypharmacy and is not rational unless the patient has been found to be resistant to single-drug therapy
- in difficult cases, lithium augments tricyclic antidepressant therapy, and in some cases of resistant depression, a monoamine oxidase inhibitor added to a tricyclic antidepressant regimen can be beneficial (J Clin Psychiatry 1991;52:21–27)

▶ How Long Should I Continue Drug Therapy?

Major depressive disorder
- after target symptoms have been controlled and the depression has lifted, the medication should be continued for 6–9 months to ensure that the episode has run its course
- after this time, administration of antidepressants should be tapered to avoid possible withdrawal reactions such as cholinergic rebound with the tricyclic agents
- in patients with a history of repeated and perhaps increasingly frequent episodes, long-term treatment should be considered
- fluoxetine, because of its extremely long half-life (3–4

days) and its active metabolite's half-life of 7 days, is considered self-tapering and may be abruptly discontinued

Useful References

American Psychiatric Association Diagnostic and Statistical Manual of Mental Disorders, 4th ed. (DSM-IV); Washington, DC: American Psychiatric Association, 1994

Bryant SG, Brown CS. Major depressive disorders. In: Young LY, Koda-Kimble MA, eds. Applied Therapeutics: The Clinical Use of Drugs, 4th ed. Vancouver, WA: Applied Therapeutics, 1988:1231–1253

Consensus Development Panel. NIMH/NIH Consensus Development Conference Statement. Mood disorders: Pharmacologic prevention of recurrences. Am J Psychiatry 1985;142:469–476

DeVane CL. Cyclic antidepressants. In: Evans WE, Schentag JJ, Jusko WJ, eds. Applied Pharmacokinetics: Principles of Therapeutic Drug Monitoring. Spokane WA: Applied Therapeutics, 1987:852–907

DRUG THERAPY FOR PSYCHOSIS

Juan R. Avila and Patricia Marken

▶ What Are My Goals of Treatment?

to control behavior
to prevent harm to self or others
to improve thought disorder
to reduce the duration of inpatient hospitalization
to prevent or decrease the severity of future exacerbations
to return the patient to a premorbid level of functioning

▶ What Evidence Is Available to Support Drug Therapy for Psychosis?

Reduced severity and duration of psychotic episodes
- reduces acute psychotic signs and symptoms within 4–6 weeks, although the benefit can continue past that time (J Clin Psychiatry 1989;50:322–328)

Prevention of relapse and recurrence
- maintenance antipsychotic drug treatment has proved valuable in preventing psychotic relapse or recurrence and rehospitalization in patients with schizophrenia
- relapse or recurrence rate after 1–2 years of maintenance medication in responding compliant schizophrenic patients is 16–30% versus 30–86% in patients receiving placebo (Psychopharmacology: The Third Generation of Progress 1987:1103–1109)
- there are few data on the impact of drug therapy on the long-term outcome of psychosis, despite the dramatic benefits of antipsychotics over the course of several years

▶ When Should I Consider Drug Therapy?

Therapy for acute psychosis (if prompt control is required)
- for acutely psychotic and agitated patients, rapid tranquilization with antipsychotics is an option and involves giving various amounts of medication over brief intervals for up to 6 hours with the goal of calming patients who may harm themselves or others

Maintenance therapy
- maintenance treatment should be implemented if the diagnosis is a chronic disorder such as schizophrenia or schizo-affective disorder (rule out toxic, metabolic, or neurological causes)
- maintenance antipsychotic medication is often required to prevent relapse or exacerbations of acute schizophre-

nia or other psychotic illness such as acute mania, psychotic depression, and drug-induced psychotic state
- every patient with schizophrenia should receive medication unless there are compelling contraindications such as a clearly established history of lack of response during past episodes or severe adverse reactions
- antipsychotics should be started if any of the target symptoms of schizophrenia or psychosis are present, both positive and negative symptoms
- positive symptoms of schizophrenia include hallucinations, delusions, agitation or combativeness, paranoia, insomnia, ideas of reference, and associational disturbances
- negative symptoms include amotivation, poor social skills, anhedonia, alogia, poverty of speech, blunted affect, and poor grooming and hygiene
- positive symptoms of schizophrenia such as agitation, combativeness, hallucinations, insomnia, and paranoia are usually more responsive to drug therapy than are the negative symptoms

▶ What Drug Should I Use for Initial Treatment?

Despite a wide variety of different chemicals, there are no convincing data that any antipsychotic is more effective than any other, either in globally reducing psychotic symptoms or in being more effective for a particular symptom • An exception is clozapine, which has been effective in patients with treatment-resistant schizophrenia or patients with negative symptoms • Selection of an antipsychotic should be based on patient's previous therapeutic response to a specific antipsychotic or family history of response to a specific agent, differences in adverse effects of each agent, and cost

Therapy for acute psychosis (if prompt control of an acutely agitated patient is required)
If the patient previously responded to an agent with no adverse effects
- choose that agent
If there is no prior history, use a benzodiazepine and an antipsychotic agent together

LORAZEPAM
- short-term therapy with a benzodiazepine can be used to control initial agitation and decrease the need for initial high doses of antipsychotics, which decreases the possibility of adverse effects (Drugs 1992;44:981–992)
- can be given parenterally, which may be useful in patients unwilling to take oral medications

Young, otherwise healthy patient
LOXAPINE
- is a medium-potency antipsychotic with moderate anticholinergic activity and produces less sedation and orthostatic hypotension than does chlorpromazine or thioridazine and a lower incidence of acute extra-pyramidal or dystonic reactions than do high-potency agents such as haloperidol and fluphenazine
- can be given as an intramuscular injection
- young men are particularily susceptible to extrapyramidal or dystonic reactions, and therefore, it is best to avoid the high-potency agents (haloperidol) in these patients
- although for most antipsychotic agents, after control has been achieved, once-daily dosing is possible, loxapine,

with a shorter half-life than other antipsychotics, may need to be given more frequently than once daily (a once-daily dose may be tried; however, if the patient reports symptoms near the end of the dosing interval, give loxapine twice daily)

THIOTHIXENE
- is similar to loxapine, and if less expensive, choose it over loxapine
- thiothixene can be dosed once daily

Elderly patients or patients with cardiovascular or seizure disorders
HALOPERIDOL
- is a high-potency antipsychotic with low anticholinergic activity and produces less sedation and orthostatic hypotension than seen with loxapine or thiothixene but does produce a high incidence of acute extrapyramidal or dystonic reactions
- can be given as an intramuscular injection

FLUPHENAZINE
- similar to haloperidol, and if less expensive, choose it over haloperidol

If sedation is desired
CHLORPROMAZINE
- is a low-potency antipsychotic with high anticholinergic activity and produces more sedation and orthostatic hypotension than do the medium- or high-potency antipsychotics (loxapine or haloperidol) but has a low incidence of acute extrapyramidal or dystonic reactions
- can be given as an intramuscular or intravenous injection

THIORIDAZINE
- similar to chlorpromazine but no parenteral form available

Maintenance therapy
- decision as to which agent to choose is as above under therapy for acute psychosis
- if the patient is likely to be noncompliant, a depot preparation of haloperidol or fluphenazine can be used after the patient is stabilized on the oral form of these agents

▶ What Dosage Should I Use?
Oral therapy should replace parenteral therapy as soon as the patient is willing to comply with oral medication • First oral dose should be given within 12–24 hours after administration of the last parenteral dose • Check blood pressure before each dose and monitor for hypotension after each dose

Therapy for acute psychosis (if prompt control of an acutely agitated patient is required)
- preferred route is intramuscular (most rapid effect), or if the patient refuses an injection, use a liquid oral form if available because a faster response is seen with a liquid versus a tablet formulation (J Clin Psychopharmacol 1986;6:210–221)

LORAZEPAM
- 2 mg PO or IM (if the patient will not take oral medication) Q1H until the patient is settled (usually ≤4 mg)
- some clinicians recommend a maximum of 10 mg/d, but

there is no specific reason not to go higher in the absence of side effects (ataxia, sedation)

- at dosages greater than 8 mg/24 h, disinhibition and ataxia (especially in the elderly and particularly those with organic brain disease) can occur

LOXAPINE

- 50 mg PO or 25 mg IM (if the patient will not take oral medication) every 30–60 minutes until control is achieved or the patient does not tolerate the drug (usually 2–3 doses)
- start a maintenance dosage, after an adequate response occurs (see below)

THIOTHIXENE

- 10–20 mg PO or 4–10 mg IM (if the patient will not take oral medication) every 30–60 minutes until control is achieved or the patient does not tolerate the drug (usually 2–3 doses)
- start a maintenance dosage after an adequate response occurs (see below)

HALOPERIDOL

- 5–10 mg PO or 2.5–5 mg IM (if the patient will not take oral medication) every 30–60 minutes until control is achieved or the patient does not tolerate the drug (usually 2–3 doses)
- start a maintenance dosage after an adequate response occurs (see below)
- some clinicians suggest that after 20 mg IM has been administered, higher dosages may not work but the risk of adverse effects increases
- after 20 mg has been reached, consider increasing the benzodiazepine dosage or switching to a different antipsychotic agent

FLUPHENAZINE

- as above for haloperidol

CHLORPROMAZINE

- 100 mg PO or 25 mg IM (if the patient will not take oral medication) every 30–60 minutes until control is achieved or the patient does not tolerate the drug (usually 2–3 doses)
- start a maintenance dosage after an adequate response occurs (see below)

THIORIDAZINE

- 100 mg PO every 30–60 minutes until control is achieved or the patient does not tolerate the drug (usually 2–3 doses)
- start a maintenance dosage after an adequate response occurs (see below)
- no parenteral form available

Maintenance therapy

- during the first few weeks of therapy, there is no evidence that higher dosages improve psychosis faster
- higher dosages do increase the risk of adverse drug reactions and should be avoided
- several days to weeks should be allowed to determine a response before increasing the dosage
- in nonagitated or controlled patients, start with low dosages and increase the dosage every 2 weeks to minimize adverse drug reactions and to increase the patient's acceptance of medication
- initially, start with divided doses to reduce the chance or severity of adverse effects

- after the patient has become tolerant of the adverse effects, the full dose can be given at bedtime (except for loxapine)
- during the initial titration to a maintenance dosage, always provide the patient with an order for PRN benzodiazepine and an antipsychotic to be used if increased agitation occurs
- if frequent doses of PRN benzodiazepines or antipsychotics are needed, maintenance dosages may need to be increased more frequently than every 2 weeks

LORAZEPAM

- 1 mg PO TID with a 1 mg PO dose for PRN use during the day
- 1–2 mg IM Q4H PRN up to a maximum of 10 mg/24 h can also be used in patients unwilling to take the drug orally
- benzodiazepines are not used for long-term maintenance therapy and should be tapered within the first few weeks as the patient becomes less agitated (can usually start tapering after a week)

LOXAPINE

- 25 mg PO BID
- 10 mg PO BID in smaller or elderly patients
- increase the dosage every 2 weeks until an appropriate response occurs
- typical maintenance dosage is 100 mg PO daily divided into 2 doses
- maximum daily oral dose is 150 mg

THIOTHIXENE

- 5 mg PO BID
- 2 mg PO BID in smaller or elderly patients
- increase the dosage every 2 weeks until an appropriate response occurs
- typical maintenance dosage is 30 mg PO daily given as a single daily dose
- maximum daily oral dose is 60 mg

HALOPERIDOL

- 5 mg PO BID
- 2.5 mg PO BID in smaller or elderly patients
- increase the dosage every 2 weeks until an appropriate response has been seen
- typical maintenance dosage is 15 mg PO daily given as a single daily dose
- maximum daily oral dose is 100 mg
- to convert to a depot preparation, start with an IM dose of haloperidol decanoate 10–20 times the daily PO dose
- supplement the initial IM dose with an oral dose ($^1/_2$ of the previous oral dose for the first month, then $^1/_4$ of the previous oral dose for the second month) of haloperidol for breakthrough symptoms that may occur
- after the patient is stable, PRN doses may be stopped
- repeat the injection in 4 weeks, increasing the IM dose if the patient became symptomatic between injections
- IM doses can be increased to up to 500 mg; however, experience is limited with doses greater than 300 mg/mo

FLUPHENAZINE

- 5 mg PO BID
- 2.5 mg PO BID in smaller or elderly patients
- increase the dosage every 2 weeks until an appropriate response occurs
- typical maintenance dosage is 15 mg PO daily given as a single daily dose

- maximum daily oral dose is 60 mg
- to convert to a depot preparation, start with a dose of 12.5 mg IM of fluphenazine decanoate for every 10 mg of daily oral fluphenazine required
- supplement the initial IM dose with PRN doses of oral fluphenazine for breakthrough symptoms that may occur between injections
- repeat injection in 2–3 weeks, increasing the IM dose by 12.5 mg, if the patient became symptomatic between injections
- IM doses can be increased up to 100 mg; however, experience is limited with doses greater than 75 mg/2 wk

CHLORPROMAZINE

- 150 mg PO BID
- 75 mg PO BID in smaller or elderly patients
- increase the dosage every 2 weeks until an appropriate response occurs
- typical maintenance dosage is 300–400 mg PO daily given as a single daily dose
- maximum daily oral dose is 2000 mg

THIORIDAZINE

- as above for chlorpromazine
- maximum daily oral dose is 800 mg because of the risk of pigmentary retinopathy

▶ How Long Should I Treat with My Initial Regimen?

Therapy for acute psychosis (if prompt control is desired)

- in acute psychotic episodes such as in a substance abuse intoxication (with steroids, industrial hydrocarbons, glue and cleaning fluids, hallucinogens, LSD, PCP, cannabis, opioids, atropine and belladonna-containing drugs, anticholinergic agents, cocaine, and other stimulants) or brief reactive psychosis, therapy should last for the period that symptoms appear
- benzodiazepines are used to treat agitation but are used only as short-term therapy (1–2 weeks), although low-dose PRN benzodiazepines may be needed for periods of agitation
- biggest mistake clinicians make is to change drugs too quickly (i.e., within days)
- early therapeutic effect is sedation and decreased agitation, with the antipsychotic effects taking longer
- if necessary, switch to a more sedating agent; however, if the patient is calm but still very psychotic, wait at least 2–3 weeks before changing agents (preferably 4–6 weeks)

Maintenance therapy

- dosage can be increased after 2 weeks if no improvement in symptoms has been seen
- response may take up to 4–6 weeks in schizophrenia; therefore, an adequate trial should be at least 4 weeks at a standard dosage before a change to a different agent is considered (if there is a trend toward improvement at 4 weeks, continue for another 2 weeks)
- duration of therapy depends on the diagnosis, but in chronic psychosis such as schizophrenia, maintenance therapy is usually needed to maintain patient functioning

▶ What Efficacy Parameters Should I Follow and How Frequently Do I Have to Assess My Patient?

Therapy for acute psychosis (if prompt control is desired)

- titrate to decrease agitation, sedative effect, or cerebellar side effects (ataxia, slurred speech)

- initially, monitor very agitated patients continuously
- monitor vital signs and degree of agitation hourly
- should see some decrease in agitation within hours and significant improvement within 24–48 hours

Maintenance therapy

Specific target symptoms of psychosis and thought disorder (assess weekly)

- agitation and aggression, decreased sleep and appetite, hallucinations, delusions, disorganized thinking, pressured speech, absence of social drive, and restricted or blunted affect
- agitation and sleep disturbance improve within days
- hallucinations improve within weeks, and thought disorders within 1–2 months
- negative symptoms such as absence of social drive and restricted or blunted affect take weeks to months to improve and may not improve at all

Signs of decompensation

- after patients are stable, they should be monitored weekly initially for clinical signs of decompensation on an ongoing basis for as long as patients are receiving antipsychotic therapy

▶ Should I Add Another Drug or Substitute Therapy If My Initial Drug Therapy Fails?

Therapy for acute psychosis (if prompt control is desired)

- combination therapy with benzodiazepine and an antipsychotic agent is usually successful
- continue to increase to maximum doses until an effect is seen

Maintenance therapy

Clinical improvement in target symptoms (although not to optimum level) with the first drug

- ensure that an adequate trial has been given (typically 4–6 weeks at dosages within the therapeutic range; some patients require up to 8–12 weeks for full response) at typical doses of an antipsychotic agent
- increase the dosage of drug if no intolerable side effects develop
- if a positive response is seen yet intolerable side effects develop, preferably lower the dosage, or if this is ineffective, stop the drug and switch to an alternative antipsychotic agent

Little or no clinical improvement with the first drug

- evaluate the diagnosis and determine the goal of therapy and appropriateness of therapy (consider the possibility of the manic phase of a bipolar disorder or a schizoaffective disorder that may improve with lithium)
- ensure an adequate trial at a therapeutic dosage
- switch to an alternative agent from a different class of antipsychotics, and if the patient is resistant to 3 different agents, consider a trial with clozapine, which has been effective in treatment of some resistant patients
- clozapine is an atypical antipsychotic that has been used in treatment-resistant schizophrenia
- clozapine causes agranulocytosis in 1% of patients and therefore should be reserved for patients who do not tolerate or do not respond to other antipsychotics
- there is no advantage to combining different classes of antipsychotics, and monotherapy is recommended
- adjunctive or alternative therapy can be tried in treatment-resistant patients
- adjunct medications that have been tried for the treatment of resistant schizophrenia and schizoaffective dis-

order include carbamazepine (J Clin Psychiatry 1984;45: 169–171), lithium (J Clin Psychiatry 1981;42:124–128), valproic acid (Biol Psychiatry 1985;20:199–228), and benzodiazepines (Am J Psychiatry 1986;143:85–87)

▶ How Long Should I Continue Drug Therapy?

Therapy for acute psychosis (if prompt control is desired)

- for acute psychotic episodes that may be drug induced, related to mania, related to depression, or attributable to trauma, antipsychotics are used only as long as the psychosis or thought disorder is present

Maintenance therapy

- studies indicate that relapses or recurrence occurs at a constant rate, such that the probability of recurrence increases with time off medication
- there is a 50% relapse rate at 6 months and 70% at 1 year after antipsychotic drug discontinuation versus only 40% in patients receiving medication (Drugs 1992;44:981–992)
- as a rule, after the first episode, treat for 1 year; after the second episode, treat for at least 3 years; after the third episode, consider at least 5 years of maintenance therapy
- after good control has been achieved, attempt to taper the dosage of the antipsychotic to the lowest effective dosage (reduce the dosage gradually over months and observe for clinical signs of decompensation)
- after the lowest effective dosage has been reached, PRN doses can be made available to patients when they are showing signs of relapse or when they experience stressful events known to worsen symptoms
- clinical impressions suggest that elderly patients with chronic schizophrenia need less antipsychotic medication than was needed in the earlier stages of the illness (J Clin Psychiatry 1986;47[suppl 5]:17–22)
- risk of developing tardive dyskinesia increases with the length of therapy and advanced age

Useful References

Dubin WR, Weiss KJ, Dorn JM. Pharmacotherapy of psychiatric emergencies. J Clin Psychopharmacol 1986;6(4):210–221
Johnson DAW. Pharmacological treatment of patients with schizophrenia. Drugs 1990;39(4):481–488
Kane JM. The current status of neuroleptic therapy. J Clin Psychiatry 1989;50(9):322–328
Kane JM. Psychopharmacologic treatment issues. Psychiatr Med 1990; 8(1):111–124
Kane JM, Lieberman JA. Maintenance pharmacotherapy in schizophrenia. In: Meltzer HY, ed. Psychopharmacology: The Third Generation of Progress. New York: Raven, 1987:1103–1109

DRUG THERAPY FOR ANXIETY DISORDERS

Steven W. Stanislav and Patricia Marken

▶ What Are My Goals of Treatment?

to resolve or decrease symptoms that significantly interfere with the patient's ability to perform daily activities (social, occupational, family)
to help the patient develop coping skills to deal with some levels of anxiety
to prevent secondary disorders such as depression and substance abuse
to prevent suicide
to prevent relapse or recurrence of anxiety

▶ What Evidence Is Available to Support Drug Therapy for Anxiety Disorders?

Generalized anxiety disorder

- extensive research with benzodiazepines demonstrates efficacy for short-term treatment (efficacy lasting longer than 6 months is unknown) with marked improvement in about 35%, moderate improvement with residual symptoms in about 40%, and no improvement in about 25% of patients (J Clin Psychiatry 1988;8:161–167)
- buspirone has shown similar efficacy to benzodiazepines (Arch Gen Psychiatry 1988;45:444–450)
- antidepressants (doxepin, imipramine, desipramine, amitriptyline) show possible efficacy suggested from limited data; efficacy for longer than 8 weeks unknown (Arch Gen Psychiatry 1986;43:79–85, J Psychiatr Res 1988;22:7–31)

Panic disorder with or without agoraphobia

- extensive research demonstrates that alprazolam is effective in relieving spontaneous and situational panic attacks, phobic fear, avoidance behavior, anxiety, and secondary disability
- Cross-National Collaborative Panic Study showed efficacy in 47% of patients by end of week 4 compared with efficacy in 27% of patients receiving placebo (Arch Gen Psychiatry 1988;45:413–422)
- clonazepam, lorazepam, and diazepam have also shown efficacy in treating panic disorder
- studies with antidepressants (imipramine, desipramine, phenelzine, fluoxetine) show benefit; most research has been done with imipramine (Arch Gen Psychiatry 1983; 40:125–138, Behav Res Ther 1985;23:325–335, J Anxiety Dis 1988;2:77–94)

Obsessive-compulsive disorder

- extensive clinical research with clomipramine shows it to be superior to placebo and other antidepressants
- approximately 35–60% decrease in obsessions or compulsions after 8–10 weeks; however, efficacy lasting longer than 9 months is unknown (Psychiatr Ann 1989;19: 97–101)
- studies show promising results with fluoxetine with similar rates to clomipramine (J Clin Psychiatry 1989;9: 281–283)
- other selective serotonin reuptake inhibitors appear effective at the high end of dosage ranges
- limited data with buspirone suggest equivalent reduction in obsessive-compulsive disorders symptoms (either alone or in combination with fluoxetine) as with clomipramine (J Clin Psychopharmacol 1990;10:91S–100S, J Clin Psychiatry 1991;52:13–14)

▶ When Should I Consider Drug Therapy?

Generalized anxiety disorder

- there are no specific guidelines for when to initiate drug therapy; however, consider pharmacotherapy if nonpharmacological modalities are unsuccessful, if the patient is suicidal, and/or if anxiety symptoms such as keyed up feeling, muscle tension, palpitations, sweating, flushes, difficulty in concentrating, and restlessness are severe, persistent, and recurrent enough to disrupt the patient's daily life
- clinical experience suggests that concurrent psychotherapy may shorten the length of time needed for drug ther-

apy, and greater response rates may occur with combined behavioral and pharmacological therapy (Behav Res Ther 1985;23:325–335)

Panic disorder with or without agoraphobia

- unless symptoms are mild or transient, patients should be treated when patients meet the diagnostic criteria in DSM-IV (at least one attack resulting in chronic concern over having more attacks, worry about "going crazy," or significant behavioral changes)
- symptoms include shortness of breath, dizziness, palpitations, flushes, sweating, choking sensation, nausea, chest pain, and fear of dying
- if untreated, avoidance behavior tends to increase

Obsessive-compulsive disorder

- should be treated when the patient meets the diagnostic criteria in DSM-IV
- obsessions such as recurrent and persistent ideas, thoughts, impulses, or images that are experienced, at least initially, as intrusive and senseless
- compulsions such as repetitive, purposeful, and intentional behaviors that are performed in response to an obsession, in accord with certain rules, or in a stereotyped fashion
- patients are usually extremely rigid and overly preoccupied with orderliness, perfectionism, and being in control of most situations

▶ *What Drug Should I Use for Initial Treatment?*

Generalized anxiety disorder

LORAZEPAM, OXAZEPAM, CLONAZEPAM, OR OTHER BENZODIAZEPINES

- benzodiazepines have been considered first-line therapy due to extensive research and over 30 years' clinical experience
- predictors of response to benzodiazepines are acute symptoms, precipitating stress, high level of psychic and somatic anxiety, absence of or low level of depression, no previous drug treatment, good response in previous therapy, and expectation of recovery or desire for medication
- benzodiazepines have an effect immediately to within several days, whereas buspirone's effect is delayed for 2–4 weeks
- all benzodiazepines are equally effective (N Engl J Med 1993;328:1398–1405); therefore, the choice is based on the patient's previous response and cost
- agents with an intermediate duration of action (lorazepam or oxazepam) are preferred because they allow easier dose titration by both the patient and the physician
- clonazepam has an intermediate to long duration of activity (N Engl J Med 1993;328:1398–1405)
- onset of action for lorazepam is a little faster (15–45 minutes versus 45–90 minutes) than that for oxazepam (likely because it is absorbed faster) but this difference is probably not important when these agents are given long term

BUSPIRONE

- controlled studies show that buspirone is as effective as benzodiazepines in general anxiety disorders (Pharmacotherapy 1988;8:100–116)
- consider as first-line therapy if patients are newly diagnosed; when chronic anxiety is present (specific symptoms of general anxiety disorder) and there is an absence of acute precipitants; if sedation or psychomotor or cognitive impairment would be dangerous; and if there is a history of substance abuse, personality disorders, absence of panic attacks, or obsessive-compulsive disorders (J Clin Psychiatry 1990;51:3–10)
- buspirone has a slower onset of action (2–4 weeks) than do benzodiazepines
- clinical experience suggests that previous benzodiazepine responders may not respond as well to buspirone, as patients report an effect on somatic symptoms that is less dramatic than that with benzodiazepines
- buspirone appears to modulate or dampen anxiety rather than to extinguish it

IMIPRAMINE

- although not typically first-line agents, antidepressants are used in the presence of coexisting depression or dysthymia, history of substance abuse, or history of past response to antidepressants in treating similar symptoms
- imipramine allows once a day dosing, is as effective as other agents, is safe, and is less expensive than other tricyclic antidepressants
- although imipramine can cause adverse effects, many patients experience tolerance of these adverse effects, and patients can be effectively treated with this inexpensive drug

Panic disorder

ALPRAZOLAM

- only approved agent for treating panic disorders; however, other benzodiazepines may have efficacy for panic disorders (N Engl J Med 1993;328:1398–1405)
- comparative studies among alprazolam and imipramine, desipramine, and phenelzine are lacking; the superiority of one agent over another is unknown
- benzodiazepines have a faster onset of action than do antidepressants

CLONAZEPAM

- clonazepam has been equally efficacious to alprazolam (J Clin Psychiatry 1991;52:69–76)
- clonazepam has a longer duration of action than does alprazolam and can be dosed 2–3 times daily, whereas alprazolam is dosed 3–4 times daily
- some clinicians prefer clonazepam to avoid rebound anxiety when reducing or stopping alprazolam administration, although this has not been proved in clinical trials

OTHER BENZODIAZEPINES

- limited data suggest that diazepam and lorazepam may be efficacious (J Clin Psychiatry 1986;47:458–460)
- if cost is a major issue, high-dose diazepam or lorazepam can be used in place of alprazolam or clonazepam

IMIPRAMINE

- extensive research supports the use of imipramine, desipramine, and phenelzine for panic attacks, and imipramine has been superior to placebo and chlordiazepoxide (J Psychiatr Res 1988;22[1]:7–31)
- panic attacks may transiently worsen when antidepressants are started
- imipramine, desipramine, and phenelzine have minimal effects on anticipatory anxiety, and therefore, benzodiazepines should be used if symptoms are predominantly of an anticipatory type

- antidepressants may be useful in patients who are drug abusers (alcohol, and so on) because these patients are less likely to become dependent on antidepressants than on benzodiazepines
- if an antidepressant is used as initial therapy, concurrent benzodiazepine therapy may be necessary for the first 2–4 weeks (owing to lagtime for response to antidepressants)

FLUOXETINE, PAROXETINE, SERTRALINE

- fluoxetine has been shown to be effective
- dosing titration must be conservative and many patients with panic disorder do not tolerate high doses of fluoxetine
- limited data also suggest effect with paroxetine and sertraline

Obsessive-compulsive disorder

CLOMIPRAMINE

- first-line therapy owing to extensive clinical experience and research that shows greater efficacy than with tricyclic antidepressants (Pharmacotherapy 1990;10:175–197)

FLUOXETINE

- fluoxetine should be chosen for patients with inadequate response to clomipramine, hypersensitivity to clomipramine, significant cardiovascular disease (e.g., bundle branch block), or a history of past response to fluoxetine

▶ *What Dosage Should I Use?*

Generalized anxiety disorder

LORAZEPAM

- start with 0.5 mg PO BID
- if no excessive sedation occurs, increase the dosage by 0.5 mg increments every 3–4 days up to 1 mg PO TID or until symptoms are well under control

OXAZEPAM

- start with 15 mg PO BID
- if no excessive sedation occurs, increase the dosage by 15 mg increments every 3–4 days up to 30 mg PO TID or until symptoms are well under control

CLONAZEPAM

- start with 0.5 mg PO BID
- if no excessive sedation occurs, increase the dosage by 0.5 mg increments every 3–4 days up to 1 mg PO TID or until symptoms are well under control

BUSPIRONE

- start with 5 mg PO BID and, if tolerated, increase the dosage to 5 mg PO TID after 3–4 days, then increase to 10 mg PO BID after another 3–4 days if tolerated
- after 2 weeks of treatment if the patient has not improved, increase to 10 mg PO TID
- after 2 more weeks, can increase to 20 mg PO BID if the patient has still not improved
- most people who are going to respond do respond to dosages of 30 mg PO daily, although some may require 60 mg PO daily

IMIPRAMINE

- start with 25 mg PO BID
- increase after 3 days to 100 mg PO daily at bedtime
- increase to 150 mg PO daily at bedtime after 1 week and leave at this dosage for 10–14 days

- if target symptoms are not improving after 3 weeks of therapy, continue to increase the daily dosage by 50 mg at weekly intervals until a response is seen or a dosage of 300 mg PO daily has been reached

Panic disorders

ALPRAZOLAM

- goal is to prevent attacks and then to decrease the dosage if the drug is tolerated and symptoms are controlled
- 0.25 mg PO TID for 1 week
- if necessary, titrate the dose up by 0.25 mg increments to 4 mg PO daily on the basis of response and patient's ability to tolerate sedation
- QID dosing is not usually required; however, it can be used if the patient exhibits symptoms at the end of an 8 hour dosing interval
- 3–4 doses per day are needed to avoid breakthrough anxiety
- advise patients that this dosage may make them sedated and that they may have to take time off from work or school

CLONAZEPAM

- goal is to prevent attacks and then to decrease the dosage if the drug is tolerated and symptoms are controlled
- usually start with a high dose and then reduce
- 0.5 mg PO TID for 1 week
- if necessary, titrate the dose up by 0.5 mg increments to 6 mg PO daily on the basis of response and the patient's ability to tolerate sedation
- after symptoms are suppressed, can attempt to decrease the dosage and administer twice daily
- 2–3 doses per day are needed to avoid breakthrough anxiety
- advise patients that this dosage may make them sedated and that they may have to take time off from work or school

LORAZEPAM

- same as for clonazepam (see above)

IMIPRAMINE

- dosages are often lower than those needed for depression
- start with 10 mg PO daily, since clinicians have noticed that these patients do not tolerate the adverse effects as well
- after 2–3 days, increase dose to 25 mg PO daily
- titrate the dose up by 10–25 mg every 3–5 days and aim for 150 mg as the total daily dose

FLUOXETINE

- dosage titration should be conservative as many patients with panic disorder do not tolerate the adverse effects well and subsequently become noncompliant
- start with 10 mg/d
- increase dose to 20 mg PO daily after two weeks, if an adequate response has not been seen
- leave at this dose for 4–6 weeks, then increase dose to 40 mg PO daily, if an adequate response has not been seen

Obsessive-compulsive disorder

CLOMIPRAMINE

- start with 25 mg PO BID
- increase after 3 days to 100 mg PO daily at bedtime

- increase to 150 mg PO daily at bedtime after 1 week and leave at this dosage for 10–14 days
- if target symptoms do not improve by this time, increase the daily dosage weekly by 50 mg to a maximum of 250 mg/d or until improvement of target symptoms
- in geriatric patients and patients with seizure history, start with 25 mg PO at bedtime, and in general, dosages should be approximately 50% of dosages used in healthy individuals
- clomipramine has a long duration of action and once-daily dosing is appropriate

FLUOXETINE

- 10 mg PO daily for 2 weeks, and if some improvement occurs, maintain this dosage, if not, increase to 20 mg PO daily and reevaluate in another 2 weeks
- if there is minimal to no change in symptoms after this time, increase the dosage to 40 mg PO daily
- if there is some response with 40 mg after another 2 weeks but not complete effect, increase the dosage to 60 mg PO daily
- if the desired effect is still not seen after another 2 weeks, consider increasing the dosage to 80 mg PO daily
- maximum adult dosage is 80 mg/d (60 mg/d in geriatric patients), but studies have shown that few patients need greater than 20 mg/d and that side effects increase with 60 mg/d or more (Psychopharmacol Bull 1987;23:164–168)
- manufacturer recommends that dosages larger than 20 mg be taken in 2 divided doses, in the morning and at noon, but this is not necessary and even high doses can be given as a single morning dose
- some patients respond to 10 mg/d (Psychopharmacol Bull 1988;24:183–188), and these lower dosages decrease cost

▶ How Long Should I Treat with My Initial Regimen?

Generalized anxiety disorder

- symptoms of general anxiety disorder usually improve immediately to within several days with benzodiazepines
- increase the dosage of benzodiazepine every 3–4 days until improvement or adverse effects are seen
- buspirone has to be administered regularly for 2–4 weeks, and sometimes up to 6 weeks, before anxiolytic effects are apparent

Panic disorder

- symptoms of panic disorders typically take at least 3–5 weeks to improve, although 6–8 weeks is not uncommon for complete resolution of symptoms; antiphobic response may take up to 12 weeks for all drugs (J Clin Psychiatry 1986;47:27S–32S)

Obsessive-compulsive disorders

- for symptoms of obsessive-compulsive disorders (compulsive or ritualistic behavior, obsessional thoughts), studies suggest that at least 8–10 weeks of drug therapy is required for maximum response

▶ What Efficacy Parameters Should I Follow and How Frequently Do I Have to Assess My Patient?

Generalized anxiety disorder

Target symptoms

- monitor changes in increased motor or muscle tension, restlessness, and autonomic hyperactivity such as short-ness of breath, palpitations, dry mouth, nausea, vomiting, and hypervigilance
- monitor initially every 2–3 days for benzodiazepines and weekly for buspirone
- stable patients should be clinically assessed for target symptoms at least monthly or weekly if clinical decompensation is suspected

Panic disorder

Target symptoms

- monitor changes in shortness of breath, choking or smothering sensations, dizziness, palpitations or chest pain, trembling, nausea, depersonalization, tingling, and fear of impending doom
- should see initial response within several days (3–4 weeks with antidepressants)
- stable patients should be clinically assessed for target symptoms at least monthly or weekly if clinical decompensation is suspected

Obsessive-compulsive disorder

Target symptoms

- monitor changes in compulsive or ritualistic behavior and obsessional thoughts
- response is slow (3–4 weeks for initial response), and it may take 6–8 weeks to see a 50% decrease in symptoms
- stable patients should be clinically assessed for target symptoms at least monthly or weekly if clinical decompensation is suspected

▶ Should I Add Another Drug or Substitute Therapy If My Initial Drug Therapy Fails?

Generalized anxiety disorder

Clinical improvement in target symptoms (although not to optimum level) with the first drug

- reemphasize nonpharmacological therapies to reduce anxiety or stress
- ensure adequate trial period
- increase the dosage of the drug if no intolerable side effects are present

Little or no improvement with the first drug

- reconfirm the diagnosis of anxiety disorder
- ensure an adequate trial period and dosage
- switch to alternative therapy
- consider concurrent psychotherapy or behavioral therapies (especially for patients with phobic-avoidance anxiety disorders)

Panic disorders

- if the first drug fails, stop that agent and try an alternative agent

Obsessive-compulsive disorders

- if the first drug fails, stop that agent and try an alternative agent

▶ How Long Should I Continue Drug Therapy?

Generalized anxiety disorder

- chronic, yet fluctuating, clinical course of anxiety disorder raises difficult issues regarding long-term drug management
- use the lowest effective dosage for the shortest period of time; attempt periodic discontinuation

- several well-designed studies describe general anxiety disorder as a chronic illness with fluctuating levels of symptom severity, yet few long-term efficacy studies (longer than 6 months) exist and the efficacy of drug therapy beyond 6 months is unknown
- with prolonged therapy, tolerance occurs to the sedating but not the anxiolytic effect (Neurosci Biobehav Rev 1985;9:13–21)
- because of the waxing and waning nature of general anxiety disorder, attempt drug discontinuation every 6–12 months if the patient is symptom free (if the patient has a well-documented history of recurrent relapses after previous drug discontinuation, indefinite therapy may be needed)
- after medication is discontinued, relapse or recurrence may occur owing to the natural course of the illness
- patients who have a clear diagnosis of anxiety disorder and who have experienced relapse or recurrence after several previous withdrawal attempts may require indefinite drug therapy, and it is important that these patients understand that relapse is not a sign of weakness or treatment failure, but that drug therapy is therapeutic and necessary to control symptoms
- although benzodiazepine abuse is widespread and of concern when weighing the risks and benefits of long-term therapy, abuse is largely limited to individuals who primarily abuse other substances
- patients without previous substance abuse have limited risks of benzodiazepine abuse (Psychiatr Ann 1988; 18:139–145)

Panic disorder

- as is the case for general anxiety disorders, studies suggest that panic disorders are a chronic illness with waxing and waning symptoms
- no long-term follow-up studies longer than 6 months exist and the efficacy of drug therapy beyond 6 months is unknown, but patients with chronic disorders often relapse when drugs are discontinued
- some clinicians recommend at least a 6–12 month symptom-free period prior to attempting discontinuation (J Clin Psychiatry 1990;51:11–15) and then taper the drug over several months to prevent rebound symptoms
- concurrent behavioral or desensitization therapy after drug discontinuation may decrease the risk of relapse

Obsessive-compulsive disorder

- efficacy for longer than 9 months is not established; however, improvement in obsessive-compulsive disorders is maintained as long as drug therapy continues (The American Psychiatric Association Textbook of Psychiatry 1988:443–491)
- because obsessive-compulsive disorders can significantly impair one's ability to function, lifelong therapy may be indicated

Useful References

Davidson JRT. Continuation treatment of panic disorder with high-potency benzodiazepines. J Clin Psychiatry 1990;51:31–37.

Dubovsky SL. Generalized anxiety disorder: New concepts and psychopharmacologic therapies. J Clin Psychiatry 1990;51:3–32

Hayes PE, Dommisse CS. Current concepts in clinical therapeutics: Anxiety disorders I, II. Clin Pharm 1987;6:140–147, 196–215

Hollander E, Liebowitz MR, Gorman JM. Anxiety disorders. In: Talbott JA, Hales RE, Yudofsky S, eds. The American Psychiatric Association Textbook of Psychiatry. Washington, DC: American Psychiatric Press, 1988:443–491

DRUG THERAPY FOR BIPOLAR DISORDERS

Steven W. Stanislav and Patricia Marken

▶ *What Are My Goals of Treatment?*

Short-term goals

to control behavior, to stabilize mood, and to improve possible thought disorder
to prevent harm to self or others
to reduce the duration of inpatient hospitalization

Long-term goals

to prevent or attenuate the severity of future bipolar episodes and to prevent future hospitalization
to prevent dysthymia, cyclothymia, and rapid cycling
to return the patient to a premorbid level of functioning
to prevent or minimize adverse drug reactions

▶ *What Evidence is Available to Support Drug Therapy for Bipolar Affective Disorder?*

Reduction in severity and duration of manic episodes

- lithium reduces the severity and duration of manic episodes
- less convincing evidence for protective effect against depressive phase; however, clinical evidence suggests a possible benefit (Arch Gen Psychiatry 1984;41:1096–1104)

Prevention of recurrence

- lithium provides effective prophylaxis for both bipolar I (mania and depression) and II (depression with hypomania) disorders and a relapse rate approximately $2\frac{1}{2}$ times lower with lithium than with placebo (Chemotherapy in Psychiatry—Principles and Practice 1985:10–25)
- clinical experience and research with carbamazepine, although less extensive than with lithium, suggest that carbamazepine is effective in preventing recurrence of both manic and depressive episodes in 50–67% of patients (J Clin Psychiatry 1990;10:318–324)
- a moderate amount of data with valproic acid suggest possible efficacy as an alternative to lithium, carbamazepine, or lithium-carbamazepine combination (Am J Psychiatry 1990;147:431–434)

▶ *When Should I Consider Drug Therapy?*

Treatment of acute manic episode

- in all acutely manic patients requiring hospitalization

Prophylactic therapy

- use prophylactic or maintenance therapy after at least 2 well-documented episodes within 5 years (or after the first episode if the occurrence of a second episode is potentially life-threatening) (Handbook of Biological Psychiatry, Part IV 1981:225–242)
- factors favoring prophylactic therapy include potential for recurrent episode to interrupt the patient's life significantly (e.g., loss of work time and family responsibilities), ability to tolerate the drug, previous lengthy hospitalization, suicide attempt during previous episode, and positive response to drug in the past or in a first-degree relative

▶ *What Drug Should I Use for Initial Treatment?*

Treatment of acute manic episode

LORAZEPAM

- for short-term therapy in the initial stages of acute mania, lorazepam should be used, as it is available in both oral and parenteral forms and may decrease the amount of antipsychotic needed
- although clonazepam may be used (there is a suggestion that it has some specific antimanic properties), it is more expensive than lorazepam and there is little evidence that it is more effective than lorazepam

HALOPERIDOL

- antipsychotics are often also required for adequate sedation and behavioral control and are usually preferred to benzodiazepines for acutely manic patients with concurrent psychoses; however, there is some evidence that high-dose benzodiazepines may be equally efficacious with fewer adverse effects (J Clin Psychopharmacol 1985;5:109–114)
- if the patient is exhibiting psychotic symptoms, such as hearing voices, and/or is delusional, an antipsychotic should be added to the benzodiazepine
- selection of an antipsychotic should be based on patient's previous therapeutic response to a specific antipsychotic or a family history of a response to a specific agent, differences in adverse effects of each agent, and cost
- haloperidol is the most commonly used antipsychotic
- haloperidol is a high-potency antipsychotic with low anticholinergic activity, is associated with a low incidence of sedation and orthostatic hypotension (less than that seen with loxapine or thiothixene), but does have a high incidence of acute extrapyramidal or dystonic reactions
- for elderly patients or patients with cardiovascular or seizure disorders, haloperidol is a good choice

LOXAPINE

- while loxapine is not commonly used, it is a good choice in a young, otherwise healthy patient
- loxapine is a medium-potency antipsychotic with moderate anticholinergic activity and produces less sedation and orthostatic hypotension than those seen with chlorpromazine or thioridazine and a lower incidence of acute extrapyramidal or dystonic reactions than with high-potency agents such as haloperidol and fluphenazine

Prophylactic therapy (started in conjunction with therapy for acute manic episode)

No concomitant disease states

LITHIUM

- is the drug of choice because of extensive clinical experience and more controlled studies compared with those with alternative agents and should be started as soon as the acutely manic patient is willing or able to take oral agents (within 24 hours) and is medically stable (normal serum sodium level and renal function)
- drug of choice for prevention of or attenuation of recurrent bipolar episodes, although approximately 20–40% of lithium-treated patients experience relapse (Am J Psychiatry 1990;147:431–434)

CARBAMAZEPINE, VALPROIC ACID

- are alternative agents if the patient does not tolerate or has no response with lithium

- there are no direct studies comparing valproate with carbamazepine, but carbamazepine should likely be chosen first, as it has undergone more clinical testing

Concomitant disease states

Cardiovascular disease

LITHIUM

- cardiovascular disease is not always a contraindication for lithium, but avoid lithium in patients with congestive heart failure or sick sinus syndrome, as it impairs conduction (Hosp Formulary 1985;20:726–735)

Renal disease

CARBAMAZEPINE, VALPROIC ACID

- it is unclear whether preexisting renal disease increases the risk of lithium-induced nephrotoxicity; however, avoid lithium in significant renal disease (glomerulonephritis, pyelonephritis, and acute renal failure) and use carbamazepine or valproic acid

Severe dehydration

LITHIUM

- lithium may be used; however, delay therapy until fluid and electrolyte balance is restored and the patient is medically stable

Seizure disorder

CARBAMAZEPINE, VALPROIC ACID

- both agents are effective for patients with seizures and the choice depends on seizure type

▶ *What Dosage Should I Use?*

Treatment of acute manic episode

LORAZEPAM

- 2 mg PO or IM (if the patient will not take oral medication) Q1H until behavior is stabilized (usually ≤4 mg)
- some clinicians recommend a maximum of 10 mg/d, but there is no specific reason not to go higher in the absence of side effects
- at doses greater than 8 mg/24 h, disinhibition, ataxia, and other types of cerebellar toxicity can occur

HALOPERIDOL

- 5–10 mg PO or 2.5–5 mg IM (if the patient will not take oral medication) every 30–60 minutes until control is achieved or the patient does not tolerate the drug (usually 2–3 doses)
- start a maintenance dosage after an adequate response has been seen (5 mg PO BID)
- some clinicians suggest that after 20 mg IM has been administered, higher dosages may not work but the risk of adverse effects increases
- after 20 mg has been given, consider increasing the benzodiazepine dosage or switching to a different antipsychotic

LOXAPINE

- 50 mg PO or 25 mg IM (if the patient will not take medication) every 30–60 minutes until control is achieved or the patient does not tolerate the drug (usually 2–3 doses)
- start a maintenance dosage after an adequate response has been seen (50 mg PO BID)

Prophylactic therapy

Initial doses must be adjusted on the basis of serum drug concentrations and patient response (see individual drug monographs)

LITHIUM

- 300 mg PO TID is the starting dosage in normal, healthy adults with good renal function
- check level in 3–4 days and, if the serum concentration is not in the therapeutic range, increase the dose to 600 mg PO BID
- start with 300 mg PO BID in patients with estimated creatinine clearance of less than 80 mL/min, low serum sodium level, or on concurrent diuretic administration
- 300 mg PO BID in elderly patients
- because there is much interpatient variability in response to dosages, serum concentration monitoring, rather than dosage, is the most important monitoring variable to ensure therapeutic levels

CARBAMAZEPINE

- start with 200 mg PO BID
- increase the dose by 200 mg increments every week on the basis of clinical response, adverse effects, and serum concentrations
- avoid single doses greater than 400 mg to minimize gastrointestinal upset (increase dosing interval to TID or QID if needed)

VALPROIC ACID

- start with 250 mg PO BID
- increase the dosage by 250 mg every week on the basis of clinical response, adverse effects, and serum concentrations

▶ How Long Should I Treat with My Initial Regimen?

Treatment of acute manic episode

LORAZEPAM

- used as a short-term therapy until full antimanic effects of the primary drug are obtained (usually 1–2 weeks but may be up to 6 weeks)

HALOPERIDOL, LOXAPINE

- attempt to withdraw antipsychotics after there is no evidence of thought disorder, hallucinations, and delusions (usually 1–2 weeks), and then control the patient's condition with benzodiazepines and lithium
- antipsychotics are sometimes needed for maintenance therapy

Prophylactic therapy

LITHIUM, CARBAMAZEPINE, VALPROIC ACID

- continue for 5 days until concentrations are at steady state, measure serum concentration, and base further dosage adjustments on concentrations (see individual drug monographs)
- some effect may be seen in 1 week to 10 days, but it may take 2–6 weeks for full effect

▶ What Efficacy Parameters Should I Follow and How Frequently Do I Have to Assess My Patient?

Specific target symptoms of mania

- agitation; decreased sleep; rapid, pressured speech with flight of ideas for manic phase; or symptoms of depression

- agitation and sleep disturbances usually resolve within several days to weeks; however, complete mood stabilization (and resolution of thought disorder, if present) may require 6 weeks or longer
- monitor hourly for acute situation and then increase the evaluation interval to daily and then weekly

Concurrent symptoms of psychoses

- auditory or visual hallucinations and delusional or disorganized thinking
- symptoms may abate in several days (if related to acute mania) or require 6 weeks or longer for complete resolution

Lithium or carbamazepine blood concentrations

- see individual drug monographs

▶ Should I Add Another Drug or Substitute Therapy If My Initial Drug Therapy Fails?

Little or no clinical improvement with the first drug after a 6 week trial at therapeutic drug concentrations

- reconfirm the diagnosis of bipolar affective disorder
- stop the agent and switch to an alternative agent

Clinical improvement in target symptoms (although not to optimum level) with the first drug

- ensure that an adequate trial period (6 weeks) at adequate serum concentrations has been given
- continue the first drug and add an alternative agent
- antidepressants should not be used in patients with known bipolar disorder who present with symptoms of mild premanic depression (case reports exist that describe possible "switching to mania" with antidepressants)
- antidepressant therapy may be considered in severe, persistent postmanic depression; however, consider the effects of the antidepressant on clinical symptoms (e.g., many patients with postmanic depression report extreme lethargy or psychomotor retardation and may benefit from a less sedating antidepressant such as desipramine, fluoxetine, or sertraline)
- consider low-dose combination therapy of lithium and carbamazepine in patients intolerant of higher doses of either drug along (carbamazepine's syndrome of inappropriate secretion of antidiuretic hormone–like effects may decrease lithium-induced polyuria)
- although monotherapy is desired, at least 50% of patients with bipolar disorder require 2 drugs or more for stabilization (especially in mixed bipolar states or schizoaffective disorder) (J Clin Psychiatry 1988;49[11]:8–9)

▶ How Long Should I Continue Drug Therapy?

Treatment of acute manic episode

- continue drugs until symptoms have been controlled

Prophylactic therapy

- duration of therapy is not well defined
- at the minimum, treatment should continue until symptoms resolve, the patient is euthymic, and sleep normalizes (some clinicians recommend continuing therapy for several months after symptoms resolve)
- prophylactic or maintenance therapy should be continued in rapid cyclers (>4 episodes per year), and probably in patients with history of recurrent bipolar disorder (at least 1 episode per year) with marked severity and substantial disruption of functioning
- for lithium, stable patients receiving maintenance or pro-

phylactic therapy should be clinically assessed at least monthly (or weekly at the first signs of clinical decompensation) and serum levels measured every 3 months and then every 6 months when the patient has been stable for at least 1 year

- reassess the need for prophylactic therapy in patients with no signs of mania or depression for 5 years
- risk of relapse increases with the number and severity of past episodes and family history of bipolar disorders
- patients may be less responsive to lithium if the patient decompensates after lithium discontinuation

Useful References

Angst J. Bipolar disorder. In: van Praag H, Lader M, Rafaelsen OJ, Sachar EJ, eds. Handbook of Biological Psychiatry, Part IV. New York: Marcel Dekker, 1981:225–242.

Baldessarini RJ. Chemotherapy in Psychiatry—Principles and Practice. Cambridge: Harvard University Press, 1985

Post RM. Approaches to treatment-resistant bipolar affectively ill patients. Clin Neuropharmacol 1988;11:93–104

Rosenbaum JF. The course and treatment of manic-depressive illness: An update. J Clin Psychiatry 1988;49:3–26.

DRUG THERAPY FOR INSOMNIA

Jonathan A. E. Fleming

▶ What Are My Goals of Treatment?

Transient situational insomnia

to promote sleep in the short term (1–4 days) when a recurrent stressor is known to cause sleep disruption that results in daytime impairment such as fatigue, impaired work performance, and transient mood disturbances

Short-term insomnia (up to 3 weeks' duration)

to promote sleep in the short term while the patient is learning alternative, behavioral techniques such as relaxation exercises and improving sleep hygiene by eliminating daytime napping, decreasing caffeine use, and decreasing use of alcohol as a sedative (Clin Psychol Rev 1986;6:27–38)

Long-term insomnia (longer than 3 weeks' duration)

to promote sleep as a temporary measure when there is demonstrated daytime impairment from the insomnia

to buy time to exclude a medical or psychiatric disorder while maintaining optimum functioning ($1/3$–$1/2$ of patients with long-term insomnia have an underlying psychiatric disorder) (JAMA 1984;251:2410–2414)

▶ What Evidence Is Available to Support Drug Therapy for Insomnia?

Sleep efficiency

- self-report, objective (sleep laboratory studies), and placebo-controlled trials demonstrate that, in the short term, hypnotics improve sleep performance by shortening the time taken to fall asleep and decreasing the number and duration of awakenings, thus resulting in an increased total sleep time
- these improvements result in improved daytime performance and subjective well-being (J Clin Psychiatry 1988;49:349–355)

Sleep continuity

- sleep continuity (absence of arousal and awakenings) is the crucial measure of sleep quality

- duration of the sleep period may not be as important (J Clin Psychopharmacol 1990;10:76S–80S)

Untreated insomnia

- untreated, persistent insomnia for longer than a year is associated with an increased risk of developing clinical depression or an anxiety disorder (JAMA 1989;262:1479–1484)
- chronic disrupted sleep can lead to poor sleep hygiene, resulting in continued insomnia after the precipitating stress has been resolved (Psychiatr Clin North Am 1987;10:541–553)

▶ When Should I Consider Drug Therapy?

The only unambiguous indication for sleep-promoting medicines is transient and short-term insomnia (JAMA 1984;251:2410–2414)

Transient situational insomnia

- when a recurrent stressor (with first 2 daytime sleep periods of a "graveyard" shift, prior to surgery, prior to job interviews, before public speaking, and so on) is known to cause sleep disruption that results in daytime impairments

Short-term insomnia (up to 3 weeks' duration)

- while a patient is learning alternative, behavioral techniques such as relaxation exercises or improving sleep hygiene (Clin Psychol Rev 1986;6:27–38)

Long-term insomnia (longer than 3 weeks' duration)

- when there is demonstrated daytime impairment such as fatigue, impaired work performance, or transient mood disturbances, continued intermittent use of a hypnotic may be useful (provided there is demonstrable benefit)
- do not use drug therapy if there is a history of loud snoring with breath-holding and daytime somnolence, morning headache, or unexplained hypertension (consider the possibility of sleep apnea), as typically the symptoms of obstructive sleep apnea worsen when nocturnal sedatives, including alcohol, are used
- when excluding a medical or psychiatric disorder while maintaining optimum functioning ($1/3$–$1/2$ of patients with long-term insomnia have an underlying psychiatric disorder) (JAMA 1984;251:2410–2414)
- when associated with mood and anxiety disorders in which disturbed sleep is a prominent symptom

Periodic limb movement disorder

- when the limb movements have consistently caused awakenings and arousals
- this usually necessitates a sleep laboratory study, although prominent and persistent movements may be observed by the bed partner

▶ What Drug Should I Use for Initial Treatment?

Transient situational insomnia, short-term insomnia (up to 3 weeks' duration)

TEMAZEPAM, LORAZEPAM, OXAZEPAM

- all of the marketed benzodiazepines have sedative properties and can be used as hypnotics
- they differ in their pharmacokinetics, side effect profile, capacity to cause discontinuation syndromes (e.g., rebound insomnia), and cost
- lorazepam, oxazepam, and temazepam are equally effective, although there are fewer data on the use of lorazepam and oxazepam as hypnotics

- lorazepam, as with other high-potency, short-acting benzodiazepines, is associated with worse rebound effects than are less potent or longer-acting compounds (not important if being used for just a few nights)
- decision should also include cost (lorazepam and oxazepam are available as generics and are usually less expensive)
- oxazepam and temazepam are absorbed more slowly than lorazepam; however, this can be circumvented by giving the dose 15–20 minutes earlier than lorazepam would be given
- in the elderly, these short-acting agents or zopiclone (see below) is preferred

TRIAZOLAM

- with its short duration of action, triazolam is useful for the short-term management (2–3 days) of stress-related insomnia when it is important to avoid daytime sedation or effects on psychomotor performance such as jetlag
- triazolam has been removed from the market in the United Kingdom and other countries
- regulatory authorities in the USA and Canada have changed the packaging and package insert for this medication and the 0.5 mg dosage form has been removed from the market
- at doses of 0.25 mg or less, there is likely no difference between this agent and other benzodiazepines, as the spontaneously reported adverse drug reactions have occurred with doses of 0.5 mg or higher

ZOPICLONE

- newer hypnotic with fewer side effects than benzodiazepines that may be free from rebound phenomena (some studies show an absence of rebound, but some reports show its presence) and is not augmented by small amounts of alcohol
- should be used for short-term management of insomnia in patients who must avoid the amnestic effects of the benzodiazepines such as in students prior to an academic examination
- more expensive than the benzodiazepines
- may replace benzodiazepines but, because it has only recently been released, not as much data are available on safety and efficacy

ZOLPIDEM

- similar to zopiclone
- main difference between zolpidem and zopiclone is that zopiclone may cause a metallic taste

ANTIHISTAMINES

- antihistamines are available in many over the counter sleep preparations and, although these agents promote sleep, they are not as effective or as safe as benzodiazepines, they have more side effects, and compounds with long half-lives (e.g., doxylamine) are not recommended because they may cause hangover effects

BARBITURATES (e.g., SECOBARBITAL) AND NONBARBITURATE NONBENZODIAZEPINE AGENTS (e.g., ETHCHLORVYNOL), CHLORAL HYDRATE

- these agents are contraindicated in the management of insomnia because of safety factors (tolerance, lethality in overdosage, risk of abuse, and drug-drug interactions) (N Engl J Med 1990;322:239–248)
- although chloral hydrate has a clinical reputation for being effective in the elderly, tolerance of its hypnotic effect develops rapidly and its low margin of safety makes it less desirable than the benzodiazepines or zopiclone

Long-term insomnia (longer than 3 weeks' duration)

TEMAZEPAM, LORAZEPAM, OXAZEPAM, ZOPICLONE

- are all effective in the intermittent treatment of long-term insomnia
- in older patients with an anxiety disorder who are using a benzodiazepine, the dosing schedule can include a nocturnal dose to promote sleep (lorazepam or oxazepam)

CLONAZEPAM

- if insomnia is a symptom of an anxiety disorder in a young patient, the use of clonazepam, which is a long-acting benzodiazepine, may be sufficient, if given at night, both to treat the insomnia and to provide anxiolytic treatment during the day
- for Rapid Eye Movement Sleep Behavior Disorder, clonazepam is also the preferred benzodiazepine, as it appears to have specific therapeutic effects in this disorder (JAMA 1987;257:1786–1789)

IMIPRAMINE, AMITRIPTYLINE

- if insomnia is one symptom of depression, the use of a sedating antidepressant such as imipramine and amitriptyline given at night is usually sufficient both to treat the mood disorder and to improve sleep (J Affect Disord 1991;22:1256–1263)
- some antidepressants such as the monoamine oxidase inhibitors (phenelzine, tranylcypromine) and fluoxetine can cause insomnia in some patients and a hypnotic may be required during the course of antidepressant therapy to treat this side effect; however, an alternative is to switch to a sedating antidepressant

CHLORPROMAZINE

- antipsychotics are contraindicated for managing primary insomnia because of the risk of tardive dyskinesia
- for patients who require antipsychotics and who have insomnia as part of their symptom complex, a sedating phenothiazine such as chlorpromazine can be given at night

Periodic limb movement disorder

TRAZODONE

- clonazepam, temazepam (Sleep 1986;9:385–392), nitrazepam (Can J Neurol Sc 1986;13:52–54), levodopa (L-dopa) (Clin Neuropharmacol 1986;9:456–463), and trazodone (Sleep Res 1988;17:39) have demonstrated efficacy in managing this disorder
- although there are more scientific data for clonazepam and temazepam, trazodone may have an advantage over these agents in that, on the basis of clinical experience, patients do not appear to become tolerant of its effects

▶ What Dosage Should I Use?

Transient situational insomnia, short-term insomnia (up to 3 weeks' duration)

- always start with the lowest dosage form available because many patients respond to the lowest dose
- response rate to placebo in chronic insomnia is high (30–48%) so it is better to start low and increase the dose only if there is an inadequate response (J Clin Psychopharmacol 1990;10:76S–80S)
- use the doses below for 1–2 nights, and if this dose is not effective, it should be doubled (except if contraindicated)

LORAZEPAM

- 0.5 mg PO taken 40 minutes before retiring
- sublingual form has a slightly faster onset of action but, as a hypnotic, has no particular advantages over the standard oral form

OXAZEPAM

- 15 mg PO taken 1 hour before retiring circumvents the slow rate of absorption

TEMAZEPAM

- 15 mg PO taken 1–1½ hours before retiring circumvents the slow rate of absorption that is due to its hard gelatin capsule

TRIAZOLAM

- 0.125 mg PO 40 minutes before retiring

ZOPICLONE

- 7.5 mg (3.75 mg in the elderly) PO 40 minutes before retiring
- for zopiclone, the maximum dose is 11.25 mg, and exceeding this dose causes hangover and other side effects (Int Clin Psychopharmacol 1990;5[Suppl 2]:1–10)

ZOLPIDEM

- 5 mg PO 40 minutes prior to retiring
- for zolpidem, increase to 10 mg only if the lower dose is clearly ineffective

Long-term insomnia (longer than 3 weeks' duration)

OTHER DRUGS

- as above

CLONAZEPAM

- 0.25 mg PO 40 minutes before retiring
- for rapid eye movement sleep behavior disorder, start at 1 mg PO HS and increase up to 2 mg until the symptoms abate

IMIPRAMINE, AMITRIPTYLINE

- 50 mg PO 40 minutes before retiring

Periodic limb movement disorder

TRAZODONE

- start with 50 mg PO 40 minutes before retiring and increase up to a maximum of 150 mg PO HS

▶ *How Long Should I Treat with My Initial Regimen?*

Transient situational insomnia, short-term insomnia (up to 3 weeks' duration), long-term insomnia (longer than 3 weeks' duration)

- reassess the effectiveness and tolerability of each agent within 2–3 days of starting each agent

▶ *What Efficacy Parameters Should I Follow and How Frequently Do I Have to Assess My Patient?*

Transient situational insomnia, short-term insomnia (up to 3 weeks' duration)
Shortening of the time taken to fall asleep and improved sleep efficiency

- quantify through the use of a sleep diary and compare with pretreatment sleep performance

Improved daytime functioning

- quantify by comparing baseline values with changes in the symptoms (e.g., anxiety, tension, and fatigue) while the patient is receiving treatment

Long-term insomnia (longer than 3 weeks' duration)
Establishment of baseline information

- prior to starting the drug, the patient should be forewarned that only a short course of treatment will be provided, and the patient should be monitored each week, at least by telephone, to quantify efficacy and side effects
- have patients quantify their current sleep performance for 2 days in a diary, noting the time of retiring, time to fall asleep after lights out, the estimated number of awakenings and the duration and time of longest awakening, the time of awakening, and the total sleep time, as this assists in making the diagnosis and in having a baseline measure against which to assess any improvements

Initial monitoring for efficacy should be weekly at first

- ensure that the patient is following good sleep hygiene and getting up at the same time each day, avoiding naps and horizontal rests, and limiting or discontinuing caffeine, alcohol, nicotine, and or recreational drug use
- quantify and note subjective improvements in daytime performance; if none are apparent, stop the hypnotic regimen and try behavioral interventions
- particularly in the elderly, ensure that there is no impairment in coordination either on awakening during the night for washroom visits or on awakening in the morning

▶ *Should I Add Another Drug or Substitute Therapy If My Initial Drug Therapy Fails?*

Nonresponse to therapeutic doses of hypnotics

- lack of response after doubling the initial dose warrants an assessment of the patient's compliance and a reassessment of the diagnosis and drug therapy
- consider the possibility that a psychiatric disorder has been missed (e.g., major depressive episode, organic mental disorder, psychotic disorder, and so on) or that the patient has misrepresented the extent of alcohol and/or recreational drug use
- use of a cocktail of sedative hypnotics or use of the sedative side effects of another drug (e.g., methotrimeprazine) to promote sleep is not recommended, and if the patient continues to report insomnia despite adequate hypnotic doses, a referral to a sleep disorders clinic is preferred

Early morning or last third of the night insomnia

- if initial insomnia is successfully treated but the patient experiences early morning awakening, consider the development of a mood disorder or early morning insomnia caused by a short-acting hypnotic (Science 1983; 220:95–97)
- if using triazolam, switch to temazepam or oxazepam, which are longer acting and are preferred to maintain hypnotic effect during the final part of the sleep period
- escape from the hypnotic effect of triazolam (half-life, 2–5 hours) in the last third of the night is usually seen when the 0.25 mg dose is used
- increasing the dose to 0.5 mg may extend triazolam's duration of effect but also increases the risk of higher cortical impairment, particularly memory impairment, and is not recommended

Adverse effects

- if the side effects are tolerable and a satisfactory improvement in sleep performance and daytime functioning is seen, reduce the dose

- if sleep performance deteriorates or the lowest dose is already being given, change to another drug
- if the side effects are intolerable, stop the drug and change to a drug within another class (e.g., from benzodiazepine to cyclopyrrolone, such as zopiclone)

▶ How Long Should I Continue Drug Therapy?

Transient situational insomnia

- 1–4 days when a recurrent stressor is causing sleep disruption with impairment in awake functioning

Short-term insomnia (up to 3 weeks' duration)

- while the patient is being instructed in alternative, behavioral techniques for controlling insomnia
- to limit hypnotic use, educate patients about the nature of their sleep disturbance, the reduction in sleep time with age, and the limitations of hypnotics
- sleep on the nights after cessation of the hypnotic regimen is actually worse than prior to initiating treatment and this alarms the patient and suggests to the patient that he or she cannot sleep without medication
- inform the patient about rebound effects, and taper the dose prior to discontinuation and withdraw the medication at a low-stress time (e.g., on the last night of the work week or on a night preceding a day off work) while encouraging good sleep hygiene
- rebound insomnia is most apparent when high-potency, short-acting benzodiazepines (e.g., triazolam and lorazepam) are abruptly stopped; longer-acting benzodiazepines or zopiclone and zolpidem are less likely to cause rebound effects

Long-term insomnia (longer than 3 weeks' duration)

- for chronic insomnia unrelated to medical or psychiatric disorders, hypnotics should be used only infrequently and for less than 4 weeks' duration
- studies on the efficacy of long-term use of hypnotics are scant, and many sleep laboratory studies show a loss of hypnotic effect (tolerance) by the fourth week of continuous use of hypnotics, with the exception of flurazepam (Behav Med 1978;5:25–31) and zopiclone (Can J Psychiatry 1988;33:103–107), which have demonstrated continued, objective effectiveness beyond 3 months of continuous use
- about 10% of patients benefit from continuous or intermittent use of hypnotics, and long-term users often report high satisfaction with their sleep and few adverse effects (Age Ageing 1984;13:335–343)
- about 15% of long-term users show a slow deterioration of sleep within 3 weeks of stopping the medication (making it unlikely that it is rebound insomnia or a benzodiazepine withdrawal syndrome), have measurable impairments in

daytime functioning associated with sleep loss, are free from medical disorders, and do not fulfill diagnostic criteria for psychiatric disorders, despite significant levels of psychopathological change

- continued, intermittent medication use, provided there is demonstrable benefit, may be the most sensible approach
- when severe sleep disturbance and daytime symptoms persist after a course of hypnotics has been tried, the physician should reevaluate the patient and ensure that there is not a confounding medical, psychiatric, or sleep disorder
- if available, referral to a sleep disorders clinic is advisable
- noting the effects of previous trials (improvement of sleep performance, amelioration of specific daytime symptoms) is essential to deciding the next step
- if the sleep disturbance is part of a mixed, subsyndromal anxious-depressive state, patients with predominantly anxious symptoms should be treated with benzodiazepines, whereas if depressive features predominate, an antidepressant is preferred (J Affective Disord 1991;22:1256–1263)
- because these patients have chronic disorders, longer trials (6 months) are warranted
- slow taper (half of the current dosage per week) is required, and if symptoms reemerge after the taper, they should be noted and the medication administration restarted at the previously effective dosage
- repeated attempts to withdraw the drug should be undertaken at least every 6 months (Can J Cont Med Educ 1992;4:29–41)

Periodic limb movement disorder

- chronic disorder requiring long-term drug therapy
- there are no clinical studies on the long-term use of sleep-promoting medicines for this condition; however, clinical experience suggests that treatment be continued as long as it is effective
- if tolerance develops (this is rare), intermittent use (e.g., weekday nights and alternate days) or drug-free periods ("drug holidays") (taper over 1 week and stop for 2 weeks) should be tried if necessary to prevent or delay the development of tolerance

Useful References

Drugs and insomnia: The use of medications to promote sleep. JAMA 1984;251:2410–2414

DuPont RL. A practical approach to benzodiazepine discontinuation. J Psychiatr Res 1990;24(Suppl 2):81–90

Epsie C. The Psychological Treatment of Insomnia. Toronto: Wiley, 1991

Ford DE, Kamerow DB. Epidemiologic study of sleep disturbances and psychiatric disorders. An opportunity for prevention? JAMA 1989;262:1479–1484

Gillin JC, Byerley WF. The diagnosis and management of insomnia. N Engl J Med 1990;322:239–248

Krueger BR. Restless legs syndrome and periodic movements of sleep. Mayo Clin Proc 1990;65:999–1006

Spielman AJ, Caruso LS, Glovinsky PB. A behavioral perspective on insomnia treatment. Psych Clin North Am 1987;10:541–553

9 | RESPIRATORY DISEASES

DRUG THERAPY FOR ASTHMA AND CHRONIC OBSTRUCTIVE PULMONARY DISEASE

Karen F. Shalansky and Cindy Reesor Nimmo

▶ What Are My Goals of Treatment?

to control the edema, mucous hypersecretion, smooth muscle contraction, and plasma exudate that occur in the airways

to maintain normal or the best possible pulmonary airflow rates both at rest and after use of a bronchodilator

to decrease the frequency of exacerbations

to normalize the patient's lifestyle with regard to exercise tolerance and freedom from symptoms

to titrate individual control of symptoms with a minimum number of drugs and their lowest possible dosages

to prevent the development of status asthmaticus by early effective treatment

to avoid drugs that may induce bronchospasm, such as systemic or topical beta-blockers, acetylsalicylic acid (ASA), and other nonsteroidal antiinflammatory agents

to avoid external triggering factors

to ensure compliance and the proper use of inhaled preparations

▶ What Evidence Is Available to Support Drug Therapy for Asthma and COPD?

Morbidity and mortality

* increased, despite advancements in drug therapy (N Engl J Med 1992;326:501–506); this may be due to a false sense of security with beta-agonists that may cause the patient to delay seeking medical assistance
* it is hoped that optimization of the use of available therapy, with an emphasis on inhaled steroids, will reduce asthma morbidity and mortality
* damage associated with emphysema is permanent, whereas many of the pathological changes in bronchitis can, to some extent, be reversed (Chest 1990;[suppl 97]:1S–5S, 19S–23S)
* inhaled corticosteroids may slow the deterioration of asthma, and to a lesser extent chronic obstructive pulmonary disease (COPD) (Ann Intern Med 1993;118:770–778)

Reversal of bronchoconstriction

* beta$_2$-agonists and, to a lesser degree, ipratropium have demonstrated efficacy in both acute and chronic asthma (Goodman and Gilman's The Pharmacological Basis of Therapeutics 1990:632–633)
* effect also seen in patients with COPD (Arch Intern Med 1989;149:544–547)

Reduction of inflammation and bronchial hyperreactivity

* demonstrated for asthma and COPD with long-term treatment with cromolyn or corticosteroids (DICP 1987;21: 22–35, N Engl J Med 1989;321:1517–1527, Ann Intern Med 1991;114:216–223, N Engl J Med 1992;327:1928–1937)
* corticosteroids may also slow the deterioration of lung function in patients with moderate to severe dyspnea (Eur J Respir Dis 1988;70:22–26)

Prevention of exercised-induced asthma

* beta$_2$-agonists and cromolyn are effective (N Engl J Med 1994;19:1362–1367)

▶ When Should I Consider Drug Therapy?

Acute asthma or acute exacerbation of COPD

* immediate and aggressive treatment should be instituted within minutes in patients with an acute attack of a reversible obstructive pulmonary disease

Chronic asthma

* when avoidance of bronchospasm-triggering factors does not control symptoms
* when beta$_2$-agonists are required more than twice daily for 1 week, additional chronic drug therapy is needed

Exercise-induced asthma

* prophylactic therapy should be instituted prior to exercise in all patients demonstrating exercise-induced asthma

Seasonal asthma

* prophylactic therapy should be instituted in all patients demonstrating seasonal asthma, ideally prior to the season for the known offending allergen

COPD

* when symptomatic treatment is required or when avoidance of trigger factors does not control the nonspecific hyperreactivity

▶ What Drug Should I Use for Initial Treatment?

Acute asthma or acute exacerbation of COPD

SALBUTAMOL (ALBUTEROL)

* salbutamol is the first-line treatment when the goal is to achieve intermittent, short-term relief of reversible obstructive pulmonary diseases
* it is beta$_2$-selective, works quickly (within minutes), is safe in acute disease, and is inexpensive
* terbutaline may be used if it is less expensive than salbutamol

IPRATROPIUM BROMIDE

* use for severe asthma but do not use for the routine treatment of less severe asthma
* ipratropium bromide may provide additional bronchodilation and may be initiated with the first dose of the beta$_2$-agonist in patients with more severe disease
* ipratropium bromide, although providing an additional

small increment in expiratory flow rates when used with submaximum doses of beta-agonists, has never been shown to reduce other variables such as the need for admission to a hospital or to shorten duration of hospital stay
- ipratropium bromide should not be used prior to beta-agonists as there is concern that ipratropium may initially cause bronchoconstriction (Postgrad Med J 1991;67:1–3)
- in COPD, ipratropium and beta₂-agonists are equally effective for acute exacerbations (N Engl J Med 1993;328:1017–1022)

PREDNISONE

- add if significant improvement (return to at least 80% of normal lung function on the basis of pulmonary function tests) does not occur within the first 30 minutes of maximum beta₂-agonist therapy
- the corticosteroid antiinflammatory effect is delayed at least 4 hours; therefore, intravenous administration gives little if any time advantage, is significantly more expensive than oral administration, and appears to be no more effective than the oral route (JAMA 1988;260:527–529, Lancet 1986;1:181–184)

HYDROCORTISONE

- in patients who are nauseated or have oral absorption that is suspect, use parenteral hydrocortisone

Chronic asthma or COPD
SALBUTAMOL (ALBUTEROL)

- salbutamol is effective in low doses, has a low risk of side effects, and is relatively inexpensive but does not control the inflammatory component of asthma
- use as necessary for acute symptoms, but not regularly in the absence of symptoms, as continuous bronchodilator therapy leads to a greater decline in forced expiratory volume in 1 second (FEV_1) than does intermittent use (Br Med J 1991;303:1426–1431)
- on a milligram per milligram basis, fenoterol is equipotent to salbutamol; with a 200 μg/puff inhaler, a higher incidence of side effects, including hypokalemia and cardiac toxicity, has been reported (Lancet 1990;336:1396–1399, Chest 1978;73:348–351, Am Rev Respir Dis 1989;139:176–180)
- possible increase in asthmatic deaths with regular use of fenoterol (200 μg/puff) has been reported (Lancet 1989;1:917–922, Lancet 1990;336:1391–1396, N Engl J Med 1992;326:501–506), and for this reason fenoterol is not recommended
- terbutaline may be used if it is less expensive than salbutamol

BUDESONIDE, BECLOMETHASONE

- decreases inflammation, the number and severity of attacks, and the need for beta-agonist
- inhaled corticosteroids have a positive effect in both asthma and COPD (Ann Intern Med 1993;118:770–778)
- add to therapy if more than 2 beta₂-agonist inhalations are required on a daily basis or symptoms are not completely reversed by an inhaled beta₂-agonist
- add if peak expiratory flow rate (PEFR) or FEV_1 falls to 85% or less of the predicted value or best known result
- budesonide is less bioavailable than beclomethasone (Thorax 1991;46:160–164)
- in low dosages (<1000 μg/d), the impact of the difference in systemic bioavailability between these agents is likely not important

- beclomethasone in high dosage (2000 μg/d) increases urinary hydroxyproline output, which reflects an increase in bone resorption, whereas budesonide does not do this (Thorax 1991;46:160–164), but the clinical importance of this is not known
- decision between these agents should be based on cost and the patient's preference

IPRATROPIUM BROMIDE

- some clinicians recommend ipratropium as initial therapy for COPD (N Engl J Med 1993;328:1017–1022)

Exercise-induced asthma
SALBUTAMOL (ALBUTEROL)

- salbutamol is the drug of choice (N Engl J Med 1994;330:1362–1366)
- very effective, well tolerated, and less expensive than cromolyn
- salbutamol is also useful if the patient experiences breakthrough wheezing

CROMOLYN

- use if exercise-induced asthma is still a problem despite the prophylactic use of salbutamol

Seasonal asthma
CROMOLYN

- cromolyn should be tried first in patients with intermittent asthma due to allergen exposure because it is effective and has virtually no side effects

INHALED CORTICOSTEROIDS

- use if patient fails to respond to therapy with cromolyn

▶ *What Dosage Should I Use?*

Acute asthma or acute exacerbation of COPD
SALBUTAMOL (ALBUTEROL)

- 4 puffs of a metered-dose inhaler over 2 minutes, then 1 puff every minute until side effects such as tremor occur, or until breathlessness and flow rates improve
- repeat 4 puffs every 20–30 minutes for 3 doses, then every 1–2 hours until the patient is stable
- beta₂-agonists administered by a metered-dose inhaler or by nebulizer are equally effective (Chest 1987;91:804–807)
- metered-dose inhaler should be used with an aerochamber or face mask for acute asthma
- nebulizer should be used in patients who are distressed or who require oxygen to be given at the same time as the salbutamol
- 5 mg via a nebulizer every 20 minutes until side effects such as tremor occur, or until breathlessness and flow rates improve

IPRATROPIUM BROMIDE

- 0.5 mg via a nebulizer with the first dose of nebulized salbutamol, then Q4H
- 4 puffs of a metered-dose inhaler with the first dose of salbutamol, then Q4H

PREDNISONE

- 40 mg PO and continued daily if significant improvement (return to at least 80% of normal levels) does not occur within the first 30 minutes of maximum salbutamol therapy (Br Med J 1986;292:1045–1047)
- oral therapy is as efficacious in both onset and magnitude

as parenteral therapy and is much less expensive (DICP 1991;25:72–79)
- patients previously receiving high-dose maintenance corticosteroids may require greater doses of corticosteroids for treatment of an acute attack

HYDROCORTISONE

- 250 mg IV Q6H

Chronic asthma or COPD

SALBUTAMOL (ALBUTEROL)

- 2 puffs as necessary to control symptoms
- do not use regularly in the absence of symptoms

BUDESONIDE

- 200 μg inhaled BID for mild asthma, and increase to 200 μg inhaled QID during unstable periods
- 200 μg inhaled QID for patients with more severe asthma, and increase up to 1600–2000 μg/d if needed
- for patients with severe asthma, higher doses are recommended because a faster response may be seen; however, after 3–4 weeks, one may be able to reduce the dosing to a BID regimen

BECLOMETHASONE

- metered-dose inhaler in the USA contains 42 μg/puff
- metered-dose inhalers in Canada contain 50 μg/puff or 200 μg/puff (Becloforte)
- 200 μg (4 puffs of the 50 μg/puff or 1 puff of the 200 μg/puff) of the metered-dose inhaler BID is the usual starting dose for mild asthma
- 200 μg inhaled QID for patients with more severe asthma and increase up to 1600–2000 μg/d if needed
- for patients with severe asthma, higher doses are recommended because a faster response may be seen; however, after 3–4 weeks, one may be able to reduce the dosing to a BID regimen
- patients with stable asthma may be adequately controlled with BID dosing of inhaled corticosteroids; however, if the asthma becomes unstable, the patient should be switched to a TID or QID regimen (Hosp Pract 1991; April:15–26)

IPRATROPIUM BROMIDE

- 2 puffs inhaled QID

Exercise-induced asthma

SALBUTAMOL OR CROMOLYN

- inhale 1–2 puffs about 10–15 minutes prior to exercise

Seasonal asthma

CROMOLYN

- prophylaxis should be initiated 1 week prior to and continued throughout the anticipated allergen season
- 2 mg inhaled QID via a metered-dose inhaler
- 20 mg inhaled QID via a spinhaler

CORTICOSTEROIDS

- 200 μg inhaled BID

▶ *How Long Should I Treat with My Initial Regimen?*

Acute asthma or acute exacerbation of COPD

- continue frequent dosing of beta-agonists until pulmonary function returns to normal level or best result

- onset of effect with each dose is seen within 2–5 minutes after inhalation
- duration of effect is approximately 3–6 hours but may be shorter with an acute exacerbation
- dosage should then be reduced to maintenance levels (e.g., Q4–6H)
- ipratropium bromide has not been proved to offer any benefit in combination with a beta-agonist after 24 hours of initial therapy (Chest 1990;98:295–297)
- continue prednisone until significant improvement is seen (usually 48–72 hours), then taper dose over a 1 week period
- for patients with severe asthma, do not reduce prednisone until peak flows have reached optimal or previous best levels

Chronic asthma or COPD

- after control or the best result is achieved and the lowest level of effective treatment is established, the patient should be reassessed every 1–6 months, depending on the disease's severity
- deaths have often been due to failure of follow-up
- patient-specific problems such as noncompliance with therapy or lack of understanding of the disease necessitate more frequent follow-up
- requirements for substantial dose escalation should prompt immediate attention

Exercise-induced asthma

- use just prior to exercise

Seasonal asthma

- continue therapy for the duration of allergen exposure
- inhaled corticosteroids could probably be abruptly discontinued follow ing the end of the offending allergen season; however, tapering over 1 week is wise to decrease the risk of reexacerbation of disease

▶ *What Efficacy Parameters Should I Follow and How Frequently Do I Have to Assess My Patient?*

Acute asthma or acute exacerbation of COPD

For severe acute asthma, assess the patient after each dose of inhaled bronchodilator and until improvement is seen • Assess heart rate, degree of respiratory distress, and presence of cyanosis • Perform pulmonary function tests

Peak expiratory flow rate

- should be measured before treatment if possible
- measured after treatment to assess the effect of treatment
- patients with an acute attack should be given a peak flow gauge and should record PEFR at least twice daily

Forced expiratory volume in 1 second

- assess once to determine the reversibility of bronchoconstriction
- reversibility is indicated by an increase of 15–20% in FEV_1 after bronchodilator administration

Arterial blood gases

- measure if the patient has a PEFR less than 40% of predicted, the FEV_1 is less than 1.2 L, or the patient is not responding to treatment
- repeated measurements should be done if there is initial elevation of carbon dioxide partial pressure or the patient experiences fatigue

Chronic asthma or COPD

Frequency of beta$_2$-agonist use as needed • Pulmonary function tests

- pulmonary function tests can be used to assess the effectiveness of long-term therapy; however, some patients given bronchodilators (salbutamol, ipratropium bromide, theophylline) do not have a demonstrable effect on pulmonary function test results but become clinically improved (increase in the distance that the patient can walk and decreases in the use of PRN medications; fewer reports of shortness of breath, chest tightness, and wheezing)
- patients placed on either oral or inhaled corticosteroids should have these medications continued only if a positive measurable response is seen after institution of these agents

Peak expiratory flow rate

- a peak flowmeter should be used by patients who experience severe attacks with little warning and patients who have symptoms of breathlessness or chest tightness repeatedly or who require regular Q6H to Q8H beta$_2$-agonist administration (J Allergy Clin Immunol 1990;85:1098–1111)
- establish best PEFR early in therapy
- usually measured on waking and before bed and before and after beta$_2$-agonist administration (minimum of twice daily [i.e., AM and PM]) and is the best of 3 measurements on each occasion
- daily variation should be less than 20% and ideally less than 10%
- patients should be instructed to double the dose of inhaled corticosteroids if PEFR is less than 75% of the best value, start a short course of oral steroids if PEFR is less than 50% of the best value, and call the physician if PEFR is less than 25% of best results (Postgrad Med J 1991;67:1–3)

Exercise-induced asthma

- evaluate the incidence of bronchospasm associated with exercise

Seasonal asthma

- as above for chronic asthma

▶ *Should I Add Another Drug or Substitute Therapy If My Initial Drug Therapy Fails?*

Acute asthma or acute exacerbation of COPD

THEOPHYLLINE, AMINOPHYLLINE

- add as a third-line agent only if the patient fails to improve after the first 12 hours with initial treatment with salbutamol, ipratropium bromide, and prednisone or cannot tolerate maximal salbutamol therapy and heart rate is less than 120 bpm
- benefit is small and the risk or side effects are substantial (Chest 1990;98:1–3)

INTRAVENOUS SALBUTAMOL (CANADA) OR SUBCUTANEOUS TERBUTALINE (USA)

- add only if the patient fails to respond to initial treatment and cardiac monitoring is available

INTUBATION

- should be considered if the blood carbon dioxide level is rising, acidosis develops, or the patient becomes exhausted

Chronic asthma or COPD

IPRATROPIUM BROMIDE

- added only after progression from beta-agonists to high-dose inhaled steroids has failed to control asthmatic symptoms
- ipratropium bromide appears to be more effective in COPD than in asthma (Arch Intern Med 1989;149:544–547); however, beta-adrenergic agents and anticholinergic agents have been found to be equivalent when large doses are used (Arch Intern Med 1993;153:814–828)

THEOPHYLLINE

- should be tried only in patients not responding to inhaled corticosteroids
- for nocturnal asthma, the first-line prophylactic treatment is inhaled corticosteroids and only if symptoms are still present should theophylline be added
- for COPD, some patients derive subjective improvement from theophylline that is not achieved with inhaled bronchodilators (Chest 1990;97:19S–23S, Chest 1985;88:112S–117S)

CROMOLYN

- minimal antiinflammatory activity in comparison with that of high-dose inhaled corticosteroids
- use only in asthmatic patients receiving a beta$_2$-agonist and inhaled corticosteroids who are experiencing major side effects
- in many cases, cromolyn is ineffective for the treatment of chronic asthma in adults

PREDNISONE

- use only if symptoms remain uncontrolled with maximally tolerated doses of inhalers

Exercise-induced asthma

- if salbutamol is not effective, use cromolyn and vice versa

Seasonal asthma

- as above for chronic asthma

▶ *How Long Should I Continue Drug Therapy?*

Acute asthma or acute exacerbation of COPD

- aggressive therapy must be continued until blood gas values and pulmonary function test results return to normal levels or the best achievable result is obtained

Discharge from the hospital should be considered in the following situations:

- PEFR or FEV$_1$ has increased to greater than 50% of the predicted or best result
- improvement is considered to be maintained
- patient compliance with corticosteroid treatment for the duration of the exacerbation is assured
- follow-up assessment is scheduled within a few days (J Allergy Clin Immunol 1990;85:1098–1111)

Chronic asthma

- therapy may be required indefinitely; however, consider dosage tapering every 6–12 months and possible withdrawal depending on the disease's severity
- between 30% and 70% of children markedly improve or become symptom free by early adulthood; however, remissions are less frequent in older patients
- patients with less frequent attacks and normal pulmonary

function test results during the initial assessment also have increased remission rates
- first agents to reduce or discontinue in a patient with controlled asthma should be oral corticosteroids, then theophylline and/or ipratropium bromide

Chronic COPD
- therapy for COPD is generally required indefinitely

Exercise-induced asthma
- use just prior to exercise

Seasonal asthma
- continue therapy for the duration of allergen exposure

Useful References

Ferguson GT, Cherniak RM. Management of chronic obstructive pulmonary disease. N Engl J Med 1993;328:1017–1022
Hargreave FE, Dolovich J, Newhouse MT. The assessment and treatment of asthma: A conference report. J Allergy Clin Immunol 1990;85: 1098–1111
McFadden ER, Gilbert IA. Asthma. N Engl J Med 1992;327:1928–1937

10

RHEUMATIC DISEASES

DRUG THERAPY FOR RHEUMATOID ARTHRITIS AND OSTEOARTHRITIS

Kelly W. Jones

▶ What Are My Goals of Treatment?
to preserve quality of life
to reduce joint pain and inflammation
to preserve joint function and the ability to perform activities of daily living
to prevent deformity

▶ What Evidence Is Available to Support Drug Therapy for Rheumatoid Arthritis and Osteoarthritis?

Rheumatoid arthritis
- rheumatologists in general believe that the overall treatment of rheumatoid arthritis is better today, but there is lack of convincing evidence that the drugs alter the outcome of the disease process
- growing concern among rheumatologists is the underestimation of morbidity and mortality with rheumatoid arthritis (Ann Intern Med 1987;106:304–312)
- there is no good evidence to date that disease-modifying antirheumatic agents used to treat rheumatoid arthritis induce remission of the disease (Ann Intern Med 1991;115:825–826)
- some studies show that sequential long-term use of disease-modifying antirheumatic drugs, when added to non-steroidal antiinflammatory drugs (NSAIDs) and/or corticosteroids, prevents joint destruction and disability in only a few patients (18%) (Lancet 1987;1:1108–1111, Arthritis Rheum 1989;32[suppl 4]:S62)
- there is considerable interest in finding new therapies, particularly combinations of disease-modifying antirheumatic drug therapy, to improve the long-term outcome of the disease (Arthritis Rheum 1990;33:113–119)
- intramuscular gold, azathioprine, and cyclophosphamide prevent the progression of damage

Osteoarthritis
- no drugs have been shown to prevent the progression of osteoarthritis

- acetaminophen and NSAIDs reduce pain (N Engl J Med 1991;325:87–91)
- one trial (Lancet 1989;2:519–521) suggests that patients given NSAIDs may experience worsening of osteoarthritis as compared with patients given placebo and other analgesics, and NSAIDs are being questioned for the treatment of osteoarthritis

▶ When Should I Consider Drug Therapy?

Rheumatoid arthritis
- drug therapy should begin soon after the definitive diagnosis has been made or within 2 months of the onset of symptoms
- when mild symptoms are present, therapy must be started to try to prevent progression of the disease to more severe symptoms, radiographic changes, and eventual swelling and cartilage loss that is irreversible (N Engl J Med 1990;322:1277–1289)
- evidence is clear that joint destruction occurs early in the disease process and more aggressive therapy needs to be considered before overt destruction occurs (N Engl J Med 1990;322:1277–1289)
- if a patient has developed loss of function and deformity occurs, therapy becomes less useful because of the irreversible destruction of the joint
- in patients with advanced disease, inflammatory disease may continue to be present and, if present, should be treated
- for less-threatening symptoms, physical therapy, occupational therapy, and reconstructive joint surgery provide the best overall results functionally

Osteoarthritis
- when symptoms are not controlled with weight loss and/ or physical or occupational therapy

▶ What Drug Should I Use for Initial Treatment?

Rheumatoid arthritis (nonerosive)
NSAIDs, INCLUDING ASPIRIN

- initial drugs of choice for rheumatoid arthritis are NSAIDs, including aspirin

- at present, there are no predictive measures for deciding to which NSAID a patient will respond
- all agents (when given in sufficient doses) decrease swelling, relieve pain, and increase movement
- there is no evidence to suggest that any NSAID is protective of cartilage and joint
- the least toxic agents are usually considered to be enteric-coated aspirin, ibuprofen, and salsalate and the most toxic are indomethacin, tolmetin, and meclofenamic acid (Arthritis Rheum 1991;34:1353–1360)
- there is mounting evidence, however, that cyclooxygenase is an isoenzyme and not a true enzyme and that certain NSAIDs may work only on certain isoenzymes, explaining the variability in response (DICP 1989;23: 76–85)
- decision among agents should be on the basis of the presence of concomitant diseases and cost

No concomitant diseases

ASPIRIN

- enteric-coated aspirin is considered the first-line drug of choice because it is as effective as other NSAIDs, is the least expensive agent, and is effective when given on a Q12H schedule
- at high dosages, zero-order kinetics prevail and aspirin can be given Q12H

IBUPROFEN

- is also a reasonable first-line agent because of its low cost and low adverse effect profile in high antiinflammatory dosages

OTHER NSAIDs

- should be chosen if the patient does not tolerate aspirin or ibuprofen or when neither agent is effective
- choice among NSAIDs in patients with no concomitant diseases should be based on cost
- do not start with indomethacin owing to the high incidence of adverse effects and drug interactions with this drug
- do not start with piroxicam or tenoxicam, especially when acute pain is present, because the long half-lives of these agents do not allow for rapid dosing flexibility and they should be used only for maintenance therapy
- sustained-release NSAIDs are as effective as regular-release NSAIDs, but more long-term trials are needed before any definitive statements can be made about differences in efficacy or toxicity

Gastric ulcers or gastrointestinal intolerance to enteric-coated aspirin

IBUPROFEN

- patients with a history of gastric ulcerations are at high risk for significant morbidity and mortality from the use of NSAIDs, and in patients with a history of peptic ulcer disease, ibuprofen along with the nonacetylated salicylates is thought to be least toxic to the gastrointestinal tract
- some references suggest that there is no clear evidence that NSAIDs vary in the incidence of gastrointestinal side effects (N Engl J Med 1991;324:1716–1725), but trends suggest that plain aspirin, tolmetin, indomethacin, and possibly ketoprofen have the highest incidence of toxicity (Clin Pharm 1992;11:690–713)
- high-dose NSAIDs, debilitating disease, advanced age, and alcohol and tobacco use predispose patients to gastric adverse effects (Clin Pharm 1992;11:690–713)

- if patients are at risk, use misoprostol 100 μg PO QID
- misoprostol has been effective in preventing NSAID ulceration (Lancet 1988;2:1277–1280), and other agents have generally been no better than placebo (Mayo Clin Proc 1992;67:354–364)
- there is no evidence that misoprostol prevents ulcer complications and death (Am J Gastroenterol 1991;86: 264–266)

Hepatic disease (medical history, alcohol abuse, and so on)

- naproxen, ibuprofen, tolmetin, and piroxicam are less likely to produce elevated liver function tests; therefore, choose whichever is the least expensive

Elderly patients (older than 60 years); patients receiving diuretics; and patients with hypovolemia, gout history, or congestive heart failure

- these patients are at greatest risk for developing NSAID-induced renal dysfunction
- all NSAIDs have the potential to cause adverse renal effects (N Engl J Med 1991;324:1716–1725)
- in studies with small samples, sulindac and piroxicam generally had the least effect on the kidney (Drug Intell Clin Pharm 1989;23:76–83, Ann Intern Med 1990;112: 568–576)
- approximate order of nephrotoxicity: fenoprofen > indomethacin > ibuprofen = flurbiprofen = mefenamic acid = naproxen = diclofenac > tolmetin = piroxicam > sulindac

Allergy to aspirin or patients with the classic triad of rhinosinusitis, nasal polyps, and asthma

- these patients are also allergic to NSAIDs, as these reactions are related to prostaglandin inhibition, which in turn leads to the release of histamine in the respiratory tract
- it is best to make an assessment of the actual allergic reaction to aspirin before starting the patient on NSAID therapy
- if patients are truly allergic to aspirin, avoid NSAIDs, use acetaminophen to relieve pain, then add the disease-modifying agents

Hypertension

ASPIRIN AND SULINDAC

- among NSAIDs, aspirin and sulindac appear to have the least hypertensive effect (Ann Intern Med 1994;121: 289–300); however, all NSAIDs likely have the potential to worsen blood pressure control and blood pressure should be measured at every follow-up visit in patients who are hypertensive or borderline hypertensive
- avoid NSAIDs, if possible, in patients with hypertension
- in patients who must use NSAIDs ensure the lowest effective dose is being used

Headaches

- patients with frequent headaches should not be given indomethacin, naproxen, tolmetin, or diclofenac, as these agents may produce headaches and can cause other central nervous system symptoms

Patients taking lithium

SULINDAC AND ASPIRIN

- are the least likely to decrease lithium clearance and cause lithium toxicity (DICP 1989;23:76–85)

Patients taking anticoagulants (other than aspirin and warfarin for cardiovascular disease)

IBUPROFEN, DICLOFENAC, TOLMETIN

- should be the only NSAIDs used in patients taking oral anticoagulants because of their short effect on platelets compared with that of other agents (DICP Ann Pharmacotherapy 1989;23:76–85)

Patients in whom compliance is a problem

PIROXICAM, TENOXICAM, NABUMETONE, OXAPROZIN

- use these agents only after arthritis pain has been initially controlled with another drug
- useful in patients who have a history of noncompliance (once-daily dosing); however, once-daily dosing may not be preferred in patients with arthritis pain, as these patients may want to dose more than once per day (DICP Ann Pharmacother 1989;23:76–85)
- most regular-release NSAIDs, including aspirin, can be taken on a Q12H basis when being used to treat arthritic conditions, and therefore, the only advantage that once-daily NSAIDs provide is once- versus twice-daily dosing
- decision among these agents should be on the basis of cost

SUSTAINED-RELEASE NSAIDs

- can be used once daily, preferably in the evening to attempt reduction in morning stiffness, and should be chosen if less expensive than either piroxicam, tenoxicam, nabumetone, or oxaprozin

Rheumatoid arthritis (erosive)

NSAIDs PLUS DISEASE-MODIFYING ANTIRHEUMATIC DRUGS

- if the disease is progressive, disease-modifying antirheumatic drugs should be added to NSAID therapy to decrease the progression of the disease

Mild disease

PREDNISONE

- because disease-modifying antirheumatic drugs are classically slow in onset of action, corticosteroids should be used when a regimen of disease-modifying drugs is initiated and then tapered and discontinued when disease activity is controlled
- systemic corticosteroids are also useful short term when patients have disease flares
- should also be used when the patient's symptoms are severe and are disrupting the quality of life
- prednisone is useful in patients when systemic manifestations of rheumatoid arthritis such as vasculitis, pericarditis, and scleritis become clinically important

HYDROXYCHLOROQUINE

- is effective for mild disease and is well tolerated
- not as effective as gold but better tolerated
- should be used if the diagnosis of rheumatoid arthritis versus systemic lupus erythematosus is uncertain because this agent can be used to treat both conditions

GOLD (ORAL)

- if the patient will be compliant with office visits and laboratory work

Moderate disease

PREDNISONE

- see above under mild disease

SULFASALAZINE

- should be used instead of gold in patients who have moderate disease who are classically noncompliant with office visits and follow-up laboratory work and in patients who fail to respond to 6 months of gold therapy
- generally better tolerated than intramuscular gold

Severe disease

PREDNISONE

- see above under mild disease

METHOTREXATE

- although more experience has been obtained with intramuscular gold, methotrexate should be chosen, as it has a longer duration of effectiveness and it is likely better tolerated than gold
- has a faster onset than other disease-modifying agents, with disease suppression being seen in 2–6 weeks rather than up to 12 weeks with other agents
- it is important that, when patients begin methotrexate therapy, their NSAID therapy not be stopped and started (i.e., be consistent) owing to the potential for a drug interaction with methotrexate (NSAIDs increase the serum concentrations of methotrexate)

GOLD (INJECTABLE)

- should be chosen over methotrexate in women who are sexually active and who may not be compliant with an effective form of birth control because methotrexate is teratogenic
- injectable gold is more effective than oral gold (Arthritis Rheum 1990;33:1449–1461)

AZATHIOPRINE

- as a third-line agent after gold and methotrexate
- azathioprine should be chosen before penicillamine because it works more quickly than penicillamine (8–10 weeks versus 6 months) and penicillamine has a number of toxicities that may not be reversible on discontinuation of the drug administration

PENICILLAMINE

- after failure with azathioprine

CYCLOSPORINE

- reserved for patients who fail to respond to the above therapy
- effective for severe disease, but is expensive and can cause renal toxicities and worsening of hypertension

CYCLOPHOSPHAMIDE

- use in patients with serious systemic complications such as vasculitis

Osteoarthritis

ACETAMINOPHEN

- acetaminophen is the initial drug of choice because it has been shown to be as effective as ibuprofen (N Engl J Med 1991;325:87–91), has few toxicities, and is less expensive than NSAIDs

NSAIDs, INCLUDING ASPIRIN

- in patients who do not tolerate or receive effect from acetaminophen
- at present, there are no predictive measures for deciding which NSAID a patient will respond to
- all NSAIDs when given in sufficient dosages decrease swelling, relieve pain, and increase movement

▶ *What Dosage Should I Use?*

Rheumatoid arthritis (nonerosive)

In general, when used long term, most of the shorter-acting NSAIDs can be dosed, if tolerated, twice daily

ASPIRIN

- 1950 mg PO Q12H as enteric coated up to a maximum of 5400 mg PO daily
- at high dosages, enteric-coated aspirin exhibits zero-order elimination and it can be dosed twice daily

IBUPROFEN

- 800 mg PO Q8H up to a maximum of 3200 mg PO daily

NAPROXEN

- 500 mg PO Q12H up to a maximum of 1500 mg PO daily
- 550 mg PO Q12H up to a maximum of 1650 mg PO daily (naproxen sodium)

TOLMETIN

- 400 mg PO Q8H up to a maximum of 2000 mg PO daily

PIROXICAM

- 10 mg PO at HS to a maximum of 20 mg PO at HS

TENOXICAM

- 10 mg PO at HS

SULINDAC

- 150 mg PO Q12H up to a maximum of 400 mg PO daily

INDOMETHACIN

- 25 mg PO Q8H up to a maximum of 200 mg PO daily

FLURBIPROFEN

- 100 mg PO Q12H up to a maximum of 300 mg PO daily

DICLOFENAC

- 75 mg PO Q12H up to a maximum of 200 mg PO daily

KETOPROFEN

- 75 mg PO Q8H up to a maximum of 300 mg PO daily

ETODOLAC

- 400 mg PO Q12H up to a maximum of 1200 mg PO daily

NABUMETONE

- 1000 mg PO at HS to a maximum of 2000 mg PO daily, split doses greater than 1000 mg

OXAPROZIN

- 1200 mg PO at HS to a maximum of 1800 mg PO daily, split doses greater than 1200 mg

Rheumatoid arthritis (erosive)

PREDNISONE

- 5 mg PO daily

- increase the dosage to 7.5 mg PO daily if 5 mg is not effective
- higher dosages are usually avoided owing to concerns about toxicity (N Engl J Med 1990;322:1277–1289)

HYDROXYCHLOROQUINE

- give 6 mg/kg PO daily up to a maximum of 400 mg/d, and assess effectiveness in 12 weeks

GOLD (ORAL)

- 6 mg PO daily as a single dose or in divided doses twice daily
- splitting the dose may help the patient tolerate the gastrointestinal side effects
- if there is no response in 6 months, increase the dosage to 9 mg daily (3 mg PO TID) for 3 months
- if the patient does not respond to 3 months of 9 mg daily, discontinue the drug administration

SULFASALAZINE

- 500 mg PO BID of the enteric-coated product for 2 weeks, then increase to 1000 mg PO BID for 2 weeks, and if necessary, increase to 1500 mg PO BID at 6 weeks

METHOTREXATE

- 7.5 mg PO weekly, with the entire dose administered as a single daily dose
- increase the dosage every 6 weeks (by 2.5 mg) on the basis of the patient's response up to a maximum of 20 mg/wk

GOLD (INJECTABLE)

- give a 10 mg IM test dose followed 1 week later with 25 mg IM and increase to 50 mg IM weekly (see drug monograph on gold complexes for further dosage adjustment recommendations)

AZATHIOPRINE

- 1.5 mg/kg PO daily (100 mg/d) as a single dose in the evening and increase by 0.5 mg/kg/d every 3 months until 2.5 mg/kg/d (150 mg/d) is reached

PENICILLAMINE

- administer 250 mg PO daily for 2 months and increase to 500 mg PO daily for 2 months, then increase to 750 mg/d
- available as capsules and tablets, and the choice is based on the patient's preference
- at dosages greater than 500 mg daily, split the dose (e.g., 500 mg AM, 250 mg PM)
- dosages greater than 1 g daily do not increase efficacy to any significant degree (Med Clin North Am 1986;70: 285–304)

CYCLOSPORINE

- start with 5 mg/kg/d divided into 2 doses
- decrease the dosage by 50% if hypertension or nephrotoxicity develops
- some patients have successfully been treated with 3 mg/kg/d (Crit Care Med 1990;18:132–137)

CYCLOPHOSPHAMIDE

- give 1 mg/kg PO daily and increase to 2 mg/kg PO daily after 6 weeks

Osteoarthritis

ACETAMINOPHEN

- start with 500 mg PO Q6H and adjust dose to a maximum of 1000 mg PO Q6H

NSAIDs

- in general, use approximately 50% of the starting dosage used in rheumatoid arthritis (see above)

▶ *How Long Should I Treat with My Initial Regimen?*

Rheumatoid arthritis (nonerosive)

NSAIDs

- it is important to be aware of the onset of antiinflammatory action
- this time frame can be 7 days with some drugs (ibuprofen, tolmetin, diclofenac, and ketoprofen) and 14 days with other drugs (sulindac, flurbiprofen, naproxen, and piroxicam)
- if the initial dosage does not work within 7 days after starting the drug, increase to the maximum dosage
- if maximum dosages have not worked within another 7 days, a change in therapy to another NSAID is appropriate
- give the drug a total of 14 days to work
- it is important that the patient is educated about what to expect in terms of onset of relief
- patients should be told that their pain will not go away with 1 dose or with 2 days of therapy, but that by 2 weeks, they should be experiencing significant relief
- when changing therapy, there is little support for selecting an NSAID from another class
- simply switch to any agent with a short half-life
- for example, if antiinflammatory dosages of ibuprofen fail after 2 weeks of therapy, switch the patient to diclofenac for 2 weeks at a dosage of 75 mg BID

Rheumatoid arthritis (erosive)

PREDNISONE

- give for morning stiffness until disease-modifying agents start to work

HYDROXYCHLOROQUINE

- use for at least 6 months before therapy is discontinued
- if the patient can tolerate the trial, continue for 9 months

SULFASALAZINE

- this drug should be given at least a 3 month trial at 3 g/d before resorting to other therapies
- improvement should be noted by 8 weeks
- sulfasalazine can be used indefinitely as long as the patient tolerates the drug and is receiving relief from the drug

GOLD (INJECTABLE)

- gold therapy should be given at least a 6 month trial before switching to another therapy
- it is important to try a 1 g cumulative dose trial before stopping administration
- gold therapy can be continued indefinitely if it is tolerated, but many patients fail therapy owing to side effects or loss of effectiveness

METHOTREXATE

- increase the dosage by 2.5 mg PO weekly every 6 weeks until a response is seen or a total weekly dose is 20 mg

AZATHIOPRINE

- give a 12 week trial on the maximum dosage (Clin Pharm 1987;6:475–491), and if there is no response, stop the drug administration

- treatment with this agent can continue indefinitely, but studies show that toxicity is the limiting factor

PENICILLAMINE

- a response requires 4–6 months of treatment total
- continue therapy as long as the drug is tolerated and effective (Med Clin North Am 1986;70:285–304)
- up to 50% of patients stop therapy with penicillamine after 1 year owing to the drug's toxicity or loss of effect

CYCLOSPORINE

- onset of effect is 8 weeks, and a peak effect is seen in 6 months

CYCLOPHOSPHAMIDE

- stop the drug administration if there is no response by 4 months
- treatment with this agent can continue indefinitely, but studies show that toxicity is the limiting factor

Osteoarthritis

ACETAMINOPHEN, NSAIDs

- use acetaminophen for 1 month, in conjunction with other measures (e.g., physiotherapy) before switching to NSAIDs

▶ *What Efficacy Parameters Should I Follow and How Frequently Do I Have to Assess My Patient?*

Rheumatoid arthritis

Joint tenderness count, sedimentation rate measurements, grip strength, duration of morning stiffness, time to onset of fatigue, and patient's report of specific symptoms

- patient's symptoms and X-rays should be assessed monthly for the first 2 months, and after the disease is under control, the patient can be assessed every 3 months for 6 months then every 6 months
- these measures should be used to guide starting and stopping drug therapy
- one study found that clinical and laboratory measures of physical well-being appeared to be unrelated to psychological and social measures of well-being (J Rheumatol 1991;18:650–653)
- it is important to include the patient's self-assessment of the drug's effect on the patient's ability to function and well-being

Osteoarthritis

- patient should be assessed for duration of pain, level of physical activity, duration of morning stiffness, range of motion, and palpation of affected joints
- patient symptoms should be assessed monthly for the first 2 months, especially when new agents are tried, and after under control, patient can be assessed at every physician visit
- rarely does osteoarthritis present as the sole disease process in a patient
- no laboratory abnormalities are associated with osteoarthritis

▶ *Should I Add Another Drug or Substitute Therapy If My Initial Drug Therapy Fails?*

Rheumatoid arthritis

- NSAIDs, if tolerated, should be continued when disease-modifying agents are added

- prednisone should be added to the disease-modifying agents when they are started and continued until these agents take effect
- while combination therapy of 1, 2, or 3 of the disease-modifying agents has been used, there is little evidence to support this; however, trials are presently ongoing

Osteoarthritis

- if the patient achieves some symptom control with acetaminophen, continue the acetaminophen and add an NSAID for PRN use (i.e., when symptoms are worse) or on a regular basis

▶ How Long Should I Continue Drug Therapy?

Rheumatoid arthritis

- therapy usually lasts a lifetime, depending on the rate of remissions and flares
- clinician cannot predict which patients will do well and which will deteriorate, with rapidly progressive crippling arthritis
- after pain control is achieved with the NSAID, decrease the daily dosage by 25% every 1–2 weeks until the minimum effective dose is identified (once-daily dosing or PRN dosing may be all that is required)
- predictive factors for a poor prognosis include high serum rheumatoid factor levels, concomitant vasculitis, onset before age 30 years, male gender, and extraarticular manifestations
- 70–80% of patients may follow a cyclic course of remissions and flares
- during remission, the lowest effective doses of medications can be used to maintain control
- 10% experience 1–2 episodes, then achieve a long-lasting remission for several years
- 3–10% have progressive disease with no remission and generally respond poorly to treatment

Osteoarthritis

- therapy should be continued as long as the drug is effective
- use on a regular basis when pain affects the quality of life
- try to decrease the dosage of acetaminophen or NSAIDs to the lowest effective level
- after pain control is achieved, decrease the daily dosage by 25% every 1–2 weeks until the minimum effective dosage is identified (once-daily dosing or PRN dosing may be all that is required)

Useful References

Clair WE, Polisson RP. Therapeutic approaches to the treatment of rheumatoid disease. Med Clin North Am 1986;70:285–304

Harris ED. Rheumatoid arthritis: Pathophysiology and implications for therapy. N Engl J Med 1990;322:1277–1289

Pugh MC, Pugh CB. Disease modifying drugs for rheumatoid arthritis. Clin Pharm 1987;6:475–491

DRUG THERAPY FOR OSTEOPOROSIS

Deborah Stier Carson

▶ What Are My Goals of Treatment?

to prevent primary and secondary osteoporosis associated with menopause, aging, chronic immobility, chronic use of sytemic glucocorticoids, and hypothyroidism

to increase total bone mass or rebuild new bone, particularly the trabecular plates, in patients with established osteoporosis

to prevent osteoporotic fractures by maximizing peak bone mass during growth

to alleviate disease-related pain and to increase activity and mobility

▶ What Evidence Is Available to Support Drug Therapy for Osteoporosis?

Prevention of osteoporosis

- hormone replacement therapy in postmenopausal women prevents osteoporosis, decreases vertebral and other fractures, and prevents further loss of height (JAMA 1984;252:799–802)
- adequate calcium intake and exercise premenopausally improve bone density, thus decreasing the risk of osteoporosis later in life
- bone loss can be slowed by calcium supplementation and exercise in postmenopausal women but not as effectively as by hormonal replacement (N Engl J Med 1991;325:1189–1195)
- synthetic 1,25-dihydroxycholecalciferol (calcitriol, Rocaltrol) can improve calcium balance and reduce bone loss and vertebral fractures, particularly in postmenopausal women who have calcium malabsorption (Metabolism 1990;39[suppl 1]:30–34, 35–38, 43–49)
- long-term use of thiazide diuretics increases serum calcium levels, is associated with increased bone density, and decreases hip fractures in men and women (Br Med J 1990;301:1303–1305)

Replacement of bone loss

- addition of a progestin to estrogen replacement may actually increase bone mass by promoting new bone formation on the basis of at least 3 studies (Obstet Gynecol 1979;53:277–281, Lancet 1981;1:459–461, Postgrad Med J 1978;54[Suppl 2]:47–49) and has been shown to reduce the rate of hip fracture (N Engl J Med 1987;817:1169–1174)
- there is little evidence to suggest that estrogen therapy can replace significant bone loss after it has occurred, and estrogen appears to be less effective at preventing bone loss after the age of 65 or 70 years
- other studies reported that progesterone alone may also be useful in increasing bone formation (J Clin Endocrinol Metab 1990;71[4]:836–841)
- calcitonin (salmon) (Calcimar), the only treatment approved by the US Food and Drug Administration (FDA) for established osteoporosis with bone biopsy–proven high turnover, can increase bone mineral content, increase femoral bone density, and alleviate disease-related pain (Calcif Tissue Int 1986;381:3–8, Curr Ther Res 1985;38:455–464, Metabolism 1985;34:124–129)
- preliminary data with intermittent etidronate administration were favorable (N Engl J Med 1990;322:1265–1271, N Engl J Med 1990;323:73–79); however, follow-up data were not encouraging and etidronate did not receive FDA approval for osteoporosis (newer data have shown benefit and etidronate may receive approval)
- calcitriol has reduced the rate of new vertebral fractures in women with postmenopausal osteoporosis (N Engl J Med 1992;326:357–362)
- although sodium fluoride stimulates bone formation and increases cancellous bone mass, it may decrease cortical bone mineral density and increase skeletal fragility (N Engl J Med 1990;322:802–809)

▶ When Should I Consider Drug Therapy?

Prevention of osteoporosis or bone loss

- all perimenopausal and postmenopausal women deserve to have hormone replacement considered, particularly women who are at high risk for developing postmenopausal osteoporosis (risk factors such as small stature, sedentary lifestyle, Caucasian and Asian ancestry, low weight, and hereditary predisposition)
- hormone replacement therapy is most successful if begun as soon as possible after clinical menopause (Orthop Clin North Am 1990;21:109–124)
- after the age of 65 or 70 years, estrogen (on a per milligram basis) is less effective in preventing bone loss but should still be considered unless otherwise contraindicated
- patients with low calcium intake, especially elderly patients

Treatment of osteoporosis (low bone mass and fractures)

- all patients with a history of osteoporotic compression fractures (Am J Med 1983;75:899–901)
- all patients with low bone mass regardless of whether they have experienced osteoporotic compression fractures
- all patients with steroid- or ethanol-induced osteoporosis or chronic immobility (Orthop Clin North Am 1990; 21:109–124)

▶ What Drug Should I Use for Initial Treatment?

Prevention of osteoporosis or bone loss and treatment of osteoporosis (low bone mass and fractures)

ESTROGEN

- estrogen prevents type 1 osteoporosis in women, decreases vertebral and other fractures, and prevents further loss of height (JAMA 1984;252:799–802, N Engl J Med 1987;817:1169–1174); however, the major effect is in the first 10–15 years after menopause
- estrogens are the only treatment that prevents menopausal symptoms and decreases cardiovascular risk (N Engl J Med, 1991;325:756–762)
- oral and transdermal estrogens appear to be equally effective, and the decision should be based on the patient's preference
- transdermal estrogen is more expensive than oral therapy
- transdermal estrogen may be safer if the patient has a history of clotting disorders (in general, estrogen therapy is not recommended for patients with active disease) or hypertension, as nonoral administration avoids the first-pass hepatic effects, thereby possibly avoiding alterations in renin substrate and coagulation factors
- data to date do not support the beneficial effects of transdermal estrogen on plasma lipids or in achieving decreased cardiovascular risk (Drugs 1990;39:203–217)

MEDROXYPROGESTERONE

- cyclic medroxyprogesterone, in addition to estrogen, should be recommended, particularly in women with an intact uterus to prevent endometrial cancer from unopposed estrogen stimulation
- in women unwilling to accept the resumption of menstruation, continuous estrogen and medroxyprogesterone administration can be prescribed; however, there are few data on continuous use regarding the risk of endometrial cancer and effects on plasma lipids and lipoproteins (Am J Med 1990;162:1534–1542, Obstet Gynecol 1990;75[suppl 4]:59S–76S)

- although it is not recommended, unopposed estrogen therapy provides a positive reduction in cardiovascular disease that outweighs the increased risk of endometrial cancer from unopposed estrogen therapy (N Engl J Med 1991;325:800–802)
- in women without an intact uterus, medroxyprogesterone should be added to estrogen therapy only if bone density is low (some progestins may promote new bone formation)
- levonorgestrel and norgestrel tend to be androgenic, and their use is not recommended for postmenopausal therapy

CALCIUM

- calcium supplements should be used if the daily intake of calcium is below the recommended dietary allowance (approximately 1500 mg/d of elemental calcium in postmenopausal women)

VITAMIN D

- should be used if there is evidence of calcium malabsorption, low dietary intake of vitamin D (200 IU/d), or low or no exposure to sunlight

CALCITONIN

- is the only FDA-approved treatment for established osteoporosis, and can be added to the above regimen; however, consideration should be given to cost, convenience, and perceived benefit before therapy is initiated
- although calcitonin is relatively safe and has few side effects, it is expensive, it necessitates parenteral administration, and lasting benefits have not been established
- it should be considered only in patients who cannot take hormonal therapy or in patients who have significant pain from osteoporosis because in low doses calcitonin may provide pain relief
- calcitonin (human) (versus calcitonin [salmon]) is available in the USA and is less immunogenic, but the clinical relevance of this is unknown

ETIDRONATE

- although the data about etidronate efficacy are controversial (N Engl J Med 1990;323:124–125), it can be considered in patients with a severe decrease in bone density who cannot use hormone replacement or are elderly and do not want to use hormone replacement
- should be used only by clinicians familiar with its use

CALCITRIOL

- data to date for the use of this agent to treat osteoporosis are insufficient and conflicting, and this agent cannot be routinely recommended at this time
- although the newer data are encouraging, the most appropriate and safe combination of calcitriol and calcium intake has not been determined, and at present, the use of calcitriol should be considered experimental (N Engl J Med 1992;326:406–407)

▶ What Route and Dosage Should I Use?

Prevention of osteoporosis or bone loss and treatment of osteoporosis (low bone mass and fractures)

ESTROGEN

Oral

- 0.625 mg of conjugated equine estrogen or equivalent estrogen preparation PO daily in patients with an intact uterus
- 0.625 mg of conjugated equine estrogen or equivalent

estrogen preparation PO daily in patients with or without an intact uterus

- if breast tenderness develops, give estrogen just for the first 25 days of each month
- any estrogen dose less than or equivalent to 0.625 mg of conjugated equine estrogen may not be sufficient to prevent bone loss (data suggest that doses of <0.625 mg are effective if calcium intake is good)
- if the woman is close to the perimenopausal period and retains some ability to produce estradiol, 0.625 mg of conjugated equine estrogen may not be tolerated
- lower dose (0.325 mg) may be necessary initially, but an attempt to increase to 0.625 mg/d of conjugated equine estrogen should be tried within 3–6 months

Transdermal

- estradiol 4 mg (Estraderm 0.05 mg/24 h) transdermal patch applied twice weekly; if breast tenderness develops, give for only 3 weeks each month
- change the patch on same days of the week (e.g., every 3–4 days)

MEDROXYPROGESTERONE

- 10 mg PO daily for 12 consecutive days each calendar month (usually day 1–12) in women who have an intact uterus
- 10 mg dose likely has a greater effect on the endometrium; however, if it is not tolerated, 5 mg PO daily may be used
- 2.5 mg PO daily in combination with estrogen can be used to reduce cyclic withdrawal bleeding
- continuous progestin administration reduces cyclic withdrawal bleeding; however, many women still experience irregular spotting and bleeding for up to 12 months
- indicators such as lipid profiles, blood glucose levels and blood pressure suggest that a continuous regimen is as safe as cyclic regimens for the prevention of osteoporosis and cardiovascular disease, but no long-term data are available

CALCIUM

- enough to ensure a total intake of 1000–1500 mg PO daily of elemental calcium

VITAMIN D

- enough to ensure a total intake of 400 IU PO daily

CALCITONIN (SALMON/HUMAN)

- 100 units SC or IM once daily of calcitonin (salmon), or if the patient is allergic to calcitonin (salmon), give calcitonin (human) at 0.5 mg SC daily
- calcitonin (salmon) dosages as low as 20 units SC daily or 50 units every other day have demonstrated some ability to increase bone mineralization, but the response is diminished as the dosage is reduced
- calcitonin (salmon) is more potent, on a weight basis and has a longer duration of action than does calcitonin (human) (AHFS Drug Information 1994:2077; Calcitonin, 2076–2079), and as expected, hypersensitivity to calcitonin (salmon) is greater than to calcitonin (human)
- because there is no evidence of differences in efficacy and calcitonin (human) is more expensive, calcitonin (human) should be used only when there is a proven allergy to calcitonin (salmon)

ETIDRONATE

- 400 mg PO daily for 2 weeks then stop for 13 weeks, then continue to repeat this cycle

▶ How Long Should I Treat with My Initial Regimen?

Prevention of osteoporosis or bone loss and treatment of osteoporosis (low bone mass and fractures)

- therapy should be continued indefinitely; however, initially, the drug therapy should be assessed with regard to patient tolerability of each agent every 2–3 weeks

▶ What Efficacy Parameters Should I Follow and How Frequently Do I Have to Assess My Patient?

Prevention of osteoporosis or bone loss, and treatment of osteoporosis (low bone mass and fractures)

Uterine bleeding

- any abnormal or undiagnosed bleeding must be investigated
- if breakthrough bleeding (2 episodes or more) occurs while the patient is taking a cyclic regimen of estrogen and progestin, or the bleeding is heavier than premenopausal menstrual bleeding, an endometrial biopsy is indicated to rule out endometrial hyperplasia or cancer
- if regular withdrawal bleeding occurs around days 7–9 of medroxyprogesterone administration or if the onset of bleeding has varied by 5–6 days, increase medroxyprogesterone dose if it is presently at 5 mg or less
- if the dose is greater than 5 mg, a biopsy should be done

Breast and pelvic examination

- yearly examination with a mammogram at least every 2–3 years

Incidence of fractures or pain

- assess at each follow-up examination

Bone density

- not recommended for everyone because of expense
- recommended for cases of early menopause (medical or surgical) or with a history of osteoporosis

Serum calcium concentrations

- not recommended, as serum calcium levels are usually normal, and routine measurement is not recommended for hormone therapy/calcium replacement

▶ Should I Add Another Drug or Substitute Therapy If My Initial Drug Therapy Fails?

Prevention of osteoporosis or bone loss and treatment of osteoporosis (low bone mass and fractures)

- equivalent doses of other estrogens may be used
- calcitonin should be considered only in patients who cannot take hormonal therapy or in patients who have significant pain from osteoporosis because in low doses calcitonin may provide pain relief

▶ How Long Should I Continue Drug Therapy?

Prevention of osteoporosis or bone loss and treatment of osteoporosis (low bone mass and fractures)

- best duration of hormonal therapy or calcium replacement is unknown, but with available data, 10 years seems reasonable
- because bone loss resumes immediately after discontinuation of therapy, patients who have tolerated therapy and who are willing to remain on treatment can continue indefinitely
- calcitonin (salmon) administration should be continued for 18–24 months, and studies using calcitonin have dem-

onstrated a plateau effect on bone mass after 1–2 years of therapy

Useful References

Christiansen C. Prevention and treatment of osteoporosis with hormone replacement therapy. Int J Fertil 1993;38(suppl):45–54
Jones KP. Estrogens and progestins: What to use and how to use it. Clin Obstet Gynecol 1992;35:871–883
Riggs BL, Melton LJ. The prevention and treatment of osteoporosis. N Engl J Med 1992;327:620–627

DRUG THERAPY FOR GOUT

C. Wayne Weart

▶ What Are My Goals of Treatment?

to treat an acute gouty attack
to lower elevated serum uric acid concentrations
to prevent recurrent acute gouty attacks
to prevent or resolve the sequelae of urate deposition in tissues, such as tophi, gouty nephropathy, nephrolithiasis, and bone erosions
to avoid, when possible, drugs that may increase serum uric acid levels in patients with gout who are susceptible to alcohol, diuretics, and low-dose salicylates

▶ What Evidence Is Available to Support Drug Therapy for Gout?

Decreased pain associated with an acute attack of gout

- colchicine (Aust N Z J Med 1987;17:301–304), NSAIDs, or corticosteroids are effective for the symptomatic treatment of acute gouty attacks

Decreased recurrence of gouty attacks and prevention of complications

- low-dose colchicine maintenance therapy reduces the risk of mobilization gout (e.g., precipitated by allopurinol) and prevents recurrent acute gouty attacks (Pharmacotherapy 1991;11:196–211)
- uric acid–lowering therapy with allopurinol, probenecid, or sulfinpyrazone may prevent recurrent gouty attacks, prevent tophaceous gout, and gradually dissolve urate deposits (the greater the serum uric acid level, the greater the risk) (Primer on Rheumatic Diseases 1988:202–206)
- allopurinol may prevent gouty nephropathy or nephrolithiasis due to either uric acid or calcium stones (Arch Intern Med 1985;145:1492–1502)

▶ When Should I Consider Drug Therapy?

Treatment of acute attack

- drug therapy should be used for all episodes of acute gouty attacks in an attempt to decrease pain

Prophylactic therapy

- all patients with a history of severe, frequent recurrent episodes of acute gouty arthritis should be given the option of prophylactic therapy
- patients with serum uric acid concentrations of 12–13 mg/dL (700 μmol/L) or greater, especially if this is associated with chronic renal failure, as these patients are at an increased risk for acute gouty attacks, gouty nephropathy, nephrolithiasis, or tophaceous gout
- in all patients with chronic tophaceous gout

▶ What Drug Should I Use for Initial Treatment?

Treatment of acute attack

INDOMETHACIN

- initial drug of choice for the acute attack, as it is generally better tolerated than colchicine because most patients experience gastrointestinal toxicity when given colchicine (Aust N Z J Med 1987;17:301–304)
- some patients, including those for whom therapy is delayed several days after the onset of an acute attack, get more effect from indomethacin than from colchicine (Primer on Rheumatic Diseases 1988:202–206)
- other NSAIDs have been used (e.g., naproxen and ibuprofen) with apparently similar efficacy, but experience is much less extensive to date
- other NSAIDs should be tried if the patient cannot tolerate indomethacin (Pharmacotherapy: A Pathophysiologic Approach 1989:912–917)

PREDNISONE

- used when indomethacin or other NSAIDs are not effective or are poorly tolerated
- initial drug of choice in patients with a history of aspirin allergy and/or renal failure, as these patients are at risk for NSAID-induced nephrotoxicity (Semin Arthritis Rheum 1990;19:329–336)
- some authors suggest that colchicine 0.6 mg PO BID should be added during and following therapy to decrease the risk of rebound of the gouty attack; however, this is not always needed (Semin Arthritis Rheum 1990;19: 329–336)
- if just 1 joint is affected (especially the knee or ankle), intraarticular injections should be considered

HYDROCORTISONE

- if gout occurs while patient is taking nothing by mouth (e.g., after surgery)

COLCHICINE

- use in patients with a history of heart failure, active peptic ulcer disease, and severe hypertension, as these patients should not take prednisone or NSAIDs
- colchicine produces a high incidence (80–100%) of gastrointestinal side effects (e.g., diarrhea)

Prophylactic therapy

ALLOPURINOL

- patients who excrete greater than 600 mg/24 h of uric acid (on a low-purine diet) on the basis of a 24 hour urine collection or have reduced renal function (glomerular filtration rate < 50 mL/min) or a history of nephrolithiasis and are deemed candidates for uric acid–lowering therapy should be treated with allopurinol
- allopurinol is chosen in these patients rather than a uricosuric agent such as probenecid because allopurinol is a xanthine oxidase inhibitor and decreases serum uric acid levels by inhibiting uric acid synthesis
- no need to discontinue uric acid–lowering therapy during an acute gouty attack after it has been initiated; however, initial uric acid–lowering therapy should not be started until 2–3 weeks after an attack

PROBENECID

- patients who excrete less than 600 mg/24 h of uric acid, have good renal function (glomerular filtration rate > 50 mL/min) and no history of nephrolithiasis, and are

deemed candidates for uric acid–lowering therapy can be treated with either probenecid or allopurinol
- probenecid and allopurinol are the preferred agents and are considered equally effective in these patients, and the choice largely depends on the patient's preference (cost or frequency of administration) and adverse effects

SULFINPYRAZONE

- use only if uricosuric therapy is required and the patient cannot use probenecid
- probenecid is the preferred agent in patients who excrete less than 700 mg/24 h of uric acid, as it has fewer adverse gastrointestinal and hematological effects than does sulfinpyrazone
- no real advantages over other agents and is generally not used

COLCHICINE

- low-dose prophylactic therapy should be used in patients with preexisting tophaceous gout, those with a long history of recurrent gouty attacks, or those with significantly elevated serum uric acid levels (>12–13 mg/dL) who are begun on uric acid–lowering therapy to prevent mobilization gout

▶ *What Dose Should I Use?*
Treatment of acute attack
INDOMETHACIN

- 50 mg PO TID until a significant response occurs, then reduce the dosage to 25 mg PO TID until the attack has fully resolved

PREDNISONE

- 40 mg PO daily for 3–4 days, then taper down by 5 mg/d

HYDROCORTISONE

- 250 mg IV Q6H, and switch to oral prednisone when the patient can take oral medications

COLCHICINE

- 1.2 mg PO and repeat Q12H until patient gets pain relief, experiences nausea and/or diarrhea, or a total of three 1.2 mg doses have been given
- many clinicians suggest giving 1.2 mg PO followed by 0.6 mg every 1–2 hours until pain relief occurs, gastrointestinal symptoms occur, or a total dose of 7 mg is reached; however, colchicine does not produce immediate (within 6–12 hours) pain relief and thus all patients will reach, using every-hour dosing method, doses at which toxicity occurs (Aust N Z J Med 1987;17:301–304)
- parenteral colchicine should not be used owing to its high risk of severe local irritation, central nervous system effects, and agranulocytosis

Prophylactic therapy
Wait 2–3 weeks after an acute gouty attack to initiate therapy to lower uric acid concentrations, as urate-lowering therapy may exacerbate the acute gouty attack

ALLOPURINOL

- give 100 mg PO daily, and gradually increase the dosage weekly by 100 mg daily until the serum uric acid level is less than 6 mg/dL or the total daily dose reaches 800 mg
- often 100–200 mg PO daily is effective and produces little toxicity

- doses greater than 300 mg PO daily should be divided for twice-daily administration
- slow dosage titration is generally recommended to prevent or minimize the risk of mobilization gout

PROBENECID

- give 250 mg PO BID, and increase the dosage weekly by 250 mg daily until the serum uric acid concentration is less than 6 mg/dL or the total daily dose reaches 3 g
- slow dosage titration is recommended to prevent or minimize the risk of mobilization gout and to avoid sudden excretion of large amounts of uric acid through the kidney

SULFINPYRAZONE

- give 100 mg PO daily, and gradually increase the dosage by 100 mg weekly until the serum uric acid concentration is less than 6 mg/dL or the total daily dose reaches 800 mg
- slow dosage titration is recommended to prevent or minimize the risk of mobilization gout and to avoid sudden excretion of large amounts of uric acid through the kidney

COLCHICINE

- a dose of 0.6 mg PO daily can be used because of the long duration of activity for colchicine
- if the patient develops symptoms during the prophylactic period while on 0.6 mg PO daily, increase the dose to 0.6 mg PO BID

▶ *How Long Should I Treat with My Initial Regimen?*
Treatment of acute attack
INDOMETHACIN

- give full dosage (50 mg PO TID) until a significant response occurs (typically 2–3 days), and then reduce the dosage (25 mg PO TID) and continue drug therapy until the attack is fully resolved (typically 7–10 days)

PREDNISONE

- give full dosage for 3–4 days, and then taper by 5 mg daily over the next 8 days

COLCHICINE

- because colchicine is excreted slowly, its toxicity is dose related, and the effect is prolonged
- give colchicine on day 1 only and then start again on day 7 if prophylactic therapy is needed

Prophylactic therapy
ALLOPURINOL, PROBENECID, SULFINPYRAZONE

- uric acid–lowering therapy with either uricosurics or allopurinol should be continued indefinitely unless the patient has lost a significant amount of weight and the serum uric acid level remains less than 6 mg/dL when therapy is discontinued

COLCHICINE

- use colchicine for 12 months if the patient had a uric acid level of 12–13 mg/dL (700 μmol/L) or greater and tophi, and stop after this time if the uric acid level has been decreased and and no attacks have occurred
- use colchicine for 3–6 months if the serum uric acid level is less than 12 mg/dL and there are no tophi
- in patients receiving colchicine for the prevention of mobilization gout and in patients receiving allopurinol, probenecid, or sulfinpyrazone, stop colchicine administra-

tion after serum uric acid concentrations have been in the desired range for 3 months

▶ What Efficacy Parameters Should I Follow and How Frequently Do I Have to Assess My Patient?

Treatment of acute attack

Symptoms

- reduction in pain and swelling typically occurs within 12–48 hours with agents used for treatment of acute attacks; however, if the attack is already established (e.g., 48 hours), response to treatment is slower

Prophylactic therapy

Serum uric acid level (in patients receiving uric acid–lowering therapy)

- measure at initiation of treatment and repeat weekly until an appropriate dosage has been determined to reduce the serum uric acid level below 6 mg/dL
- measure every 6–12 months after serum uric acid levels are stable

Number of attacks

- number of acute gouty attacks should decrease

▶ Should I Add Another Drug or Substitute Therapy If My Initial Drug Therapy Fails?

Treatment of acute attack

- if any agent fails (i.e., no response after 24 hours) or is not tolerated, the alternative agent should be tried

Prophylactic therapy

- although not often necessary, a few patients with severe elevations in uric acid levels may require combination therapy with allopurinol and a uricosuric agent and colchicine (i.e., patients who have not achieved a serum uric acid level of <6 mg/dL with maximum recommended doses of either class of urate-lowering agent)

▶ How Long Should I Continue Drug Therapy?

Treatment of acute attack

- indomethacin should be given until the attack is fully resolved
- colchicine need be given only until pain is under control or a total dose of 4.8 mg has been reached

Prophylactic therapy

- uric acid–lowering therapy is usually continued indefinitely, but consideration should be given to reduced dosage of allopurinol for aging patients, those with reduced renal function, or those obese patients who have successfully attained ideal body weight
- generally not able to withdraw uric acid–lowering therapy but may be able to reduce dosage as long as the serum uric acid level is maintained below 6 mg/dL

Useful References

Becker MA. Pathogenesis of hyperuricemia. In: Primer on the Rheumatic Diseases, 9th ed. Atlanta: Arthritis Foundation, 1988:195–198

German DC, Holmes EW. Hyperuricemia gout. Med Clin North Am 1986;70:419–436

Hawkins DW. Gout and hyperuricemia. In DiPiro JT, Talbert RL, Hayes PE, eds. Pharmacotherapy: A Pathophysiologic Approach. New York: Elsevier, 1989:912–917

Levy M, Spino M, Read SE. Colchicine: A state of the art review. Pharmacotherapy 1991;11:196–211

McCarty DJ. Intractable gouty arthritis. Hosp Pract 1987;22:191–209

Paulus HE, Schlosstein LH, Godfrey RG, et al. Prophylactic colchicine therapy of intercritical gout. Arthritis Rheum 1974;17:609–614

Rundles W. The development of allopurinol. Arch Intern Med 1985;145:1492–1502

Simkin PA. Management of gout. Ann Intern Med 1979;90:812–816

Tate G, Schumacher HR. Clinical features. In: Primer on the Rheumatic Diseases, 9th ed. Atlanta: Arthritis Foundation, 1988:198–202

Wallace SL, Singer JZ. Treatment. In: Primer on the Rheumatic Diseases, 9th ed. Atlanta: Arthritis Foundation, 1988:202–206

Wallace SL, Singer JZ. Therapy in gout. Rheum Dis Clin North Am 1988;14:441–457

Wallace SL, Singer ZS. Review: Systemic toxicity associated with the intravenous administration of colchicine—Guidelines for use. J Rheumatol 1988;15:495–499

Wisner DE, Simkin PA. Management of gout and hyperuricemia. Prim Care 1984;11(2):283–294

11 | DRUG-INDUCED ADVERSE REACTIONS

DRUG-INDUCED SKIN RASH

Otto L. A. Schlappner

▶ My Patient Has a Skin Rash, How Do I Determine If This Is Drug Induced?

Do a thorough drug history

- review all drugs (prescription and nonprescription) that the patient has started within the past 4–8 weeks
- some drugs may not cause a reaction for up to 8 weeks; however, the majority of the drugs that do induce a reaction do so within 1 week
- suspect any drug, but usually consider those started recently

Do a thorough allergy history

- question the patient as to previous drug, food, and contact allergies and possible drug cross-reactions and photosensitivity

For example

- salicylate allergies can be induced by salicylates that are present in many foods
- antihistamine contact allergies can be reactivated by oral antihistamines
- phototoxic dermatitis (when systemically administered

drugs absorb energy from the sunlight through the skin and this energy is transmitted to surrounding tissue, inducing an acute, erythematous, dermatitis-like sunburn) can occur after the administration of tetracyclines, nalidixic acid, phenothiazines, and sulfonamides
- previous allergies to certain drugs or cross-reacting drugs usually recur on either systemic or topical readministration

Ask whether the patient has had a recent systemic viral illness
- certain drugs, such as ampicillin, tend to cause a high incidence of morbilliform eruptions in patients with mononucleosis
- there also appears to be an increase in the frequency of erythema multiforme and maculopapular eruptions in patients with acute bacterial or viral infectious diseases (may in part be due to the use of antipyretics, antiinflammatory drugs, and antibiotics)

Assess when the rash started
- make a ''drug calendar'' with the dates of the skin rash
- drug-induced skin rashes resolve with discontinuation of the drug administration and usually recur on reintroduction of the drug

Assess the type of skin rash
- the type of skin rash can give clues to a drug-induced rash
- for example, penicillins, sulfonamides, and phenytoin induce a maculopapular rash, whereas phenolphthalein induces fixed eruptions

Perform blood count and skin biopsy
- one can look for blood or tissue eosinophilia by doing a white blood cell count (with differential count) or a skin biopsy, but this is not usually warranted
- may be useful if there are other possible reasons for a skin rash (viral or infectious cause, and so on)

▶ *What Drugs Are Most Likely to Cause Skin Rash?*

All drugs have the potential to cause a skin rash • In order of their likelihood of causing a skin rash, the following are the drugs most commonly involved

PENICILLINS AND CEPHALOSPORINS
- mostly macular, maculopapular, and urticarial skin rashes

SULFONAMIDES AND POTENTIALLY CROSS-REACTING DRUGS (THIAZIDES AND SULFONYLUREAS)
- macular, maculopapular, and urticarial rash; erythema multiforme; erythroderma; exfoliative dermatitis; and also photodermatitis
- rarely, erythema nodosum and toxic epidermal necrolysis (<1%)

NONSTEROIDAL ANTIINFLAMMATORY DRUGS
- with aspirin, mostly urticaria and more rarely purpura, scarlatiniform erythema, erythema multiforme, and fixed eruptions
- with other nonsteroidal antiinflammatory drugs, there is pruritus, urticaria, erythematous rashes, erythema multiforme, vesiculobullous eruptions, fixed eruptions, purpura, vasculitis, photosensitivity dermatitis, exfoliative erythroderma and toxic epidermal necrolysis, pseudoporphyria and stomatitis, and exacerbation of psoriasis

OPIOIDS
- pruritus, urticaria, erythematous rashes, and complications at injection sites such as abscesses, hyperpigmentation, and scarring

ISONIAZID
- acneiform eruptions and, rarely, other eruptions such as urticaria, purpura, and exfoliative dermatitis

ETHIONAMIDE
- eczematous and acneiform eruptions and sometimes stomatitis

RIFAMPIN
- rarely causes epidermal necrolysis, pemphigus, and porphyria cutanea tarda

CARBAMAZEPINE
- causes erythematous, urticarial, and purpuric rashes in about 3% of patients
- also reported are toxic epidermal necrolysis, exfoliative dermatitis, and lupus erythematosus–like syndrome and erythema multiforme

PHENYTOIN
- commonly causes maculopapular and erythematous rashes
- cutaneous plaques and nodules, exfoliative dermatitis, and toxic epidermal necrolysis
- gingival hyperplasia is a well-known common side effect

VALPROIC ACID
- transient rashes and stomatitis

HYDRALAZINE
- lupus erythematosus–like syndrome with occasional orogenital ulcerations and leg ulcers

PROCAINAMIDE
- lupus erythematosus–like syndrome with urticarial vasculitis

ANTISERA AND VACCINES
- can cause both early and late hypersensitivity reactions with urticaria, asthma, anaphylaxis, and serum sickness
- with serum sickness, there can be erythema of the fingers, toes, palms, and soles, with a subsequent morbilliform eruption
- local reactions include erythema, swelling, tenderness, itching, eczema, inflammatory nodules, and necrosis

ALLOPURINOL
- scarlet fever and measles-like (scarlatiniform and morbilliform) rashes occur acutely, as well as urticaria, generalized exfoliative dermatitis, and rarely, toxic epidermal necrolysis
- can also potentiate the risk of ampicillin reactions
- eruptions are more common in patients with poor renal function

PENICILLAMINE
- acute urticarial and morbilliform rashes occur within the first few weeks
- on withdrawal of the drug administration, there is clearing of the eruption, and reexposure to the drug may not lead to a recurrence of the eruption

- drug-induced pemphigus foliaceus, pemphigus vulgaris, or pemphigus erythematosus occurs in less than 7% of patients receiving the drug
- oral blistering can occur, as can erosive vulvovaginitis
- bullous pemphigoid–like reactions, cicatricial pemphigoid, systemic lupus erythematosus, dermatomyositis, myasthenia gravis, morphea, and systemic sclerosis have been reported
- other manifestations include induction or exacerbation of a lichen planus–like reaction, blistering, and erosions of the mouth, tongue, and lip

GOLD SALTS

- pruritic rashes and mouth ulcers are common
- generalized exfoliative dermatitis and erythema multiforme–like eruptions, and pityriasis rosea–like, lichen planus–like, and nummular eczema–like reactions are seen
- less common reactions include toxic epidermal necrolysis, polyarteritis, and lupus erythematosus–like syndromes
- loss of taste, metallic taste, stomatitis, and glossitis have also been reported

▶ *What Are the Characteristics of Drug-Induced Skin Rashes?*

Erythematous, macular, and maculopapular eruptions (may also be annular)

- occur in 50% of patients with a drug-induced skin rash

Urticaria, angioedema

- occur in 25% of patients with a skin rash

Photosensitivity reactions

- most often noted on sun-exposed skin as pruritus, erythema, papules, nodules, plaques, or bullae
- also sunburn-like eczematous eruptions

Vascular reactions

- vascular reactions with allergic vasculitis, periarteritis nodosa, livedo reticularis, erythema nodosum, hemorrhagic infarcts, petechiae, ecchymoses, purpura (flat and palpable), toxic epidermal necrolysis, vesiculobullous eruptions, erythematous eruptions, lichenoid or lichen planus–like eruptions, and pigmentary changes can be seen

Exfoliative dermatitis

- exfoliative dermatitis can follow a maculopapular or erythematous eruption

Fixed eruption

- sharply demarcated erythema recurring in the same site

Angioneurotic edema or giant urticaria

- may also develop, as may serum sickness with fever or arthralgias

Toxic epidermal necrolysis

- is life threatening and may be preceded by erythema of the skin, erythema multiforme, or a maculopapular eruption

▶ *How Do I Treat the Skin Rash?*

Drug administration cessation

- unless the condition being treated is life-threatening, always stop administration of the suspected drug and use an alternative agent

Treatment
Mild or asymptomatic rash

- no treatment is necessary

Vesicular, bullous, exudative, or eroded rash

- lukewarm saline or oatmeal baths for 15–20 minutes BID or TID may be useful (1 cup of salt or 42 g of colloidal oatmeal [Aveeno] per lukewarm tub of water)
- icy cold wet compresses applied to very itchy areas for 2–3 minutes usually relieve the itch immediately

Pruritic rash
TOPICAL STEROIDS

- apply topical steroids (betamethasone valerate 0.1%) sparingly to all involved skin areas and rub in well 3 times daily
- if the eruption is acute and itchy, vesicular, or exudative, apply every 2 hours until there is improvement
- lotions or creams should be used for vesicular or wet lesions, whereas ointments should be applied to dry lesions
- topical preparations should be applied after compresses or baths

ORAL ANTIHISTAMINES

- patients who are uncomfortable or itchy should receive oral antihistamines, preferably regularly (not on a PRN basis)
- chlorpheniramine is likely the initial drug of choice because it is much less expensive than the newer agents and is convenient to take, as it can be given once daily (Clin Pharmacokinet 1991;21:372–393)
- chlorpheniramine is rapid acting, causes less sedation, and produces fewer anticholinergic effects than do agents such as diphenhydramine and hydroxyzine
- if sedation is a problem with chlorpheniramine (seen with 20% of patients), switch to a nonsedating agent such as astemizole, loratadine, or terfenadine, whichever is the least expensive
- if sedation is required (may be desirable in an acute allergic reaction), diphenhydramine or hydroxyzine should be used, as these are effective and sedating

TOPICAL ANTIHISTAMINES

- topical antihistamines are not effective; however, in some cases, patients may request a topical preparation and an agent such as diphenhydramine/calamine (Caladryl) may be tried (may have a large placebo effect)

PREDNISONE

- in patients who are very uncomfortable or itchy, patients who have severe reactions, or patients for whom topical treatment might be slow in leading to improvement or resolution, a short course of prednisone 40 mg PO daily should be tried
- after improvement sets in, usually within 3 days, prednisone can be tapered by 5 mg/d

TOPICAL ANTIBIOTICS

- in skin reactions that lead to denudation, application of topical antibiotics, such as mupirocin, in conjunction with keeping the skin clean with soap and water, should be done to prevent secondary infections

▶ *How Quickly Should My Patient Respond and What Should I Monitor with Regard to the Efficacy of My Treatment?*

Response is variable

- if administration of the offending drug has been stopped,

improvement may begin within hours or may take 30 days or longer

- sulfonamide or allopurinol rashes may take 2 weeks to clear versus 2–3 days for penicillin rashes
- drug rashes on Caucasian patients tend to improve faster than those on Oriental patients, likely owing to differences in drug metabolism
- in time, the acuteness of the eruption fades, no new lesions develop, and itching (if present) decreases
- scaling and desquamation may occur as the skin heals and peels
- postinflammatory hyperpigmentation or hypopigmentation can also result

▶ Do I Have to Stop Administration of the Drug That Is Causing the Skin Rash?

Administration of the drug should be stopped in most cases

- except when the drug is needed for a life-threatening situation, it is mandatory to stop the drug therapy to allow the eruption to fade and to alleviate discomfort, anxiety, and cosmetic changes
- minor skin rash, after a few hours or days, can become a severe, widespread, maculopapular reaction, which in turn can (rarely) progress to bullous erythema multiforme or even toxic epidermal necrolysis
- in addition, an allergic urticaria can be a cutaneous manifestation of anaphylaxis, which may present at the same time or after the onset of urticaria
- after the drug administration has been stopped, evaluate the patient daily to ensure that the rash is improving
- if the drug is necessary for treating a serious or life-threatening illness and no alternative drug can be used, the drug therapy can be continued and the patient can be treated symptomatically as above

Administration of the drug should be avoided in the future

- regardless of when during the course of therapy a drug rash occurred (early or late), the drug should probably be avoided in the future because there is an increased likelihood that a similar or worse reaction will occur
- if the drug is to be reused, the clinician and the patient should be aware of the potential for a more severe reaction and the patient should be told to seek immediate medical attention if symptoms recur

Useful References

Breathnach SM. Chapter 74. In: Champion RH, Burton JL, Ebling FJG, eds. Rook, Wilkinson, Ebling; Textbook of Dermatology, 5th ed. Cambridge, MA: Blackwell, 1992:2961–3035

Breathnach SM, Hinter H. Adverse Drug Reactions and the Skin. Cambridge, MA: Blackwell, 1992.

Bruinsma WA. A guide to drug eruptions: The European File of side effects. In: Dermatology, 5th ed. Oosthuizen, The Netherlands: The File of Medicine, 1990

DRUG-INDUCED ANAPHYLAXIS

Robert Schellenberg

▶ My Patient Has Shortness of Breath and Difficulty in Swallowing, How Do I Determine If This Is Drug Induced?

Discontinue administration of all drugs immediately

- while evaluating the patient, discontinue the administration of all drugs immediately and initiate treatment for anaphylaxis

Do a thorough and accurate history

- anaphylaxis to drugs usually occurs within 20 minutes of administration
- some non–immunoglobulin E (IgE)–mediated anaphylactoid responses (e.g., to acetylsalicylic acid [ASA] or metabisulfite) may be delayed 2–6 hours

▶ What Drugs Are Most Likely to Cause Anaphylaxis?

Any drug is possible

- most common are penicillins, cephalosporins, imipenem, sulfa drugs, acetylsalicylic acid and other nonsteroidal antiinflammatory drugs (cross-reactivity high), dextran, protamine, streptokinase, any injectable or oral drugs containing metabisulfites, and radiocontrast material

▶ What Are the Characteristics of Drug-Induced Anaphylaxis?

Clinical manifestations

- identical to anaphylaxis from any cause
- life-threatening symptoms include laryngeal edema, severe bronchospasm, systemic hypotension, and arrhythmias
- pruritus, flushing, urticaria, angiodema, and paresthesias are common and may precede more serious symptoms
- gastrointestinal manifestations such as nausea, vomiting, and diarrhea may also occur

▶ How Do I Treat Anaphylaxis?

Drug therapy

EPINEPHRINE

- give epinephrine while ensuring an adequate airway, as epinephrine may immediately decrease angioedema
- (1 : 1000 solution) 0.5 mL SC every 5–10 minutes as necessary to maintain blood pressure or a patent airway
- for nonresponding, severe, or prolonged hypotension, give 0.5 mg (5 mL of 1 : 10,000 solution) IV and repeat every 5–20 minutes as needed

Adequate airway

- intubation or tracheostomy may be required if ventilation is inadequate

Intravenous fluids

- if the patient is hypotensive, place the patient in a supine position with legs and hips elevated
- give 1–2 L of normal saline rapidly if the patient is hypotensive
- colloid is beneficial if hypotension is protracted

Other measures after the above have been instituted

- diphenhydramine 50 mg IV over 5 minutes or IM if there is no IV access
- if the patient is bronchospastic, give oxygen 6 L/min by mask and nebulized salbutamol 5 mg in 5 mL of normal saline every 20 minutes until bronchospasm disappears
- if there is evidence of adequate filling pressures (normal central venous pressure) but cardiac output is still decreased, give dobutamine (initially, 5 μg/kg/min IV) and titrate according to response
- IV corticosteroids (hydrocortisone 1000 mg or methylprednisolone 250 mg) should be given if shock is not readily reversible

▶ *How Quickly Should My Patient Respond and What Should I Monitor with Regard to the Efficacy of My Treatment?*

Within 10 minutes

- most patients respond within 10 minutes of the initiation of therapy, although some reactions are protracted and some patients may experience relapse

Monitor vital signs

- monitor blood pressure, heart rate and rhythm, and signs of respiratory compromise continuously
- if anaphylaxis is prolonged, consider central venous pressure monitoring

▶ *Do I Have to Stop Administration of the Drug That Is Causing the Anaphylaxis?*

All drugs should be stopped immediately if an anaphylactic reaction is suspected

▶ *How Long Should I Treat the Anaphylaxis?*

Until vital signs have stabilized and there is no evidence of cardiac or respiratory compromise

- for mild symptoms responding quickly to treatment and cases involving a known causative agent that is metabolized or excreted rapidly, continue monitoring in a supervised setting for a minimum of 2 hours after complete resolution of symptoms
- when anaphylaxis is caused by a long-acting drug, the patient should be monitored in a supervised setting for 24 hours

▶ *What Do I Do If I Must Use a Drug That Has Caused an Allergic Reaction or Anaphylaxis in the Past?*

In all cases, search for a chemically dissimilar alternative

- if at all possible, use a chemically dissimilar alternative

For cases of previous reactions to radiocontrast material

Mild reaction

- pretreat with prednisone 50 mg PO Q6H for 4 doses prior to the procedure and diphenhydramine 50 mg IM 20 minutes prior to the procedure

Severe reaction

- use a nonionic preparation plus pretreat with prednisone 50 mg PO Q6H for 4 doses prior to the procedure and diphenhydramine 50 mg IM 20 minutes prior to the procedure

For cases of previous reaction to beta-lactams

- all patients with a history of an allergic reaction that suggests an IgE-mediated reaction should receive skin tests
- reliable skin tests are available only for penicillin G (major and minor determinants)
- if the penicillin skin test is positive, there is a significant risk of reaction to cephalosporins and imipenem
- skin tests have a high predictive value (J Allergy Clin Immunol 1981;68:171–180) regarding IgE-mediated reactions but are not helpful for assessment of non–IgE-mediated reactions, including the delayed maculopapular rash (usual onset 7–10 days after starting penicillin), interstitial nephritis, and serum sickness

Skin test

- give 0.02 mL intradermally, and a positive test result is a wheal and flare developing within 10 minutes

Negative skin test result

- have epinephrine on hand, and start IV beta-lactam administration slowly; if there is no reaction after 5 minutes, speed up and infuse the rest of the drug over 40–45 minutes
- monitor blood pressure, heart rate, presence of breathing difficulty, and urticaria
- severe reactions usually occur in the first 20 minutes and often within the first couple of minutes

Positive skin test result

- desensitization is required
- temporary desensitization in patients with IgE antibodies against a drug can be accomplished by incremental dosage increases, beginning with small amounts
- for beta-lactam antibiotics, a starting dose of 0.01 mg is given PO or SC (the route likely does not matter), and double the dose every 15 minutes while constantly monitoring for a reaction
- after a therapeutic dose (1 g) is achieved (after 3–4 hours), regular dosing can be commenced
- desensitization does not confer protection for future treatment courses of these drugs
- reassessment is required prior to each future use

Useful References

Bochner BS, Lichtenstein LM. Anaphylaxis. N Engl J Med 1991;324: 1785–1790

Greenberger PA, Patterson R, Tapio CM. Prophylaxis against repeated radiocontrast media reactions in 857 cases. Arch Intern Med 1985; 145:2197–2200

Marquardt DL, Wasserman SI. Anaphylaxis. In: Middleton E Jr, Reed CE, Ellis EF, et al, eds. Allergy. Principles and Practice, 4th ed. St Louis: Mosby, 1993:1525–1536

Stark BJ, Sullivan TJ. Biphasic and protracted anaphylaxis. J Allergy Clin Immunol 1986;78:76

Sullivan TJ, Wedner HJ, Shatz GS, et al. Skin testing to detect penicillin allergy. J Allergy Clin Immunol 1981;68:171–180

Weiss ME, Adkinson NF. Immediate hypersensitivity reactions to penicillin and related antibiotics. Clin Allergy 1988;18:515–540

DRUG-INDUCED DIARRHEA

James McCormack

▶ *My Patient Has Diarrhea, How Do I Determine If This Is Drug Induced?*

Do a thorough drug history

- document all prescription and nonprescription medications
- if the patient is in a hospital, check the medication administration records for both regular and PRN orders
- for some patients, laxative abuse should also be considered

▶ *What Drugs Are Most Likely to Cause Diarrhea?*

Laxatives (stimulants, stool softeners, and so on) and antacids (especially magnesium containing)

- most common drugs to cause diarrhea
- often given regularly in the hospital and extended care setting, even in the presence of diarrhea, so check medication administration records

Sorbitol-containing drug products

- many liquid dosage forms contain sorbitol as a sweetening

agent, and when consumed in normal dosages, many of these products contain sufficient sorbitol to produce diarrhea
- check the sorbitol content of any liquid dosage products in the patient's drug regimen (Can J Hosp Pharm 1991; 44:297–300)

Antibiotics
- common cause of diarrhea
- all antibiotics have been linked to the development of pseudomembranous colitis, with the most commonly implicated antibiotics being clindamycin, ampicillin, and cephalosporins
- if the patient has received antibiotics only in the previous 1–2 days, *Clostridium difficile* infection is unlikely and diarrhea has probably resulted from a mild irritant action caused by the antibiotic

Other drugs
- Reserpine, methyldopa, quinidine, digoxin, colchicine, sorbitol, theophylline, any of the cholinergic agents (e.g., bethanechol), and misoprostol
- Consider all drugs that have been started or have had a dosage increase in the previous 2–3 days

▶ *What Are the Characteristics of Drug-Induced Diarrhea?*

Laxatives (stimulants, stool softeners, and so on), antacids (especially magnesium containing), and other drugs
- usually characterized by frequent watery diarrhea that generally (>95% of the time) is not bloody

Sorbitol-containing drug products
- usually characterized by frequent watery diarrhea

Antibiotics
- patients who are currently receiving or have received antibiotics in the previous 4–8 weeks should be considered to potentially have *C. difficile* infection
- this infection commonly presents with mild to moderate diarrhea, usually with lower abdominal cramping
- the worst presentation of *C. difficile* infection is pseudomembranous colitis and a typical patient with this condition will have profuse greenish, watery, foul-smelling diarrhea; a temperature of 39–41°C (102.2–105.8°F); abdominal tenderness; leukocytosis; and hypoalbuminemia

▶ *How Do I Treat the Diarrhea?*

Laxatives (stimulants, stool softeners, and so on), antacids (especially magnesium containing), other drugs, and antibiotics if *C. difficile* infection is not suspected
- stop the administration or decrease the dosage of suspected drugs
- reevaluate the need for the suspected drugs, and if possible, stop the administration or decrease the dosage
- if regularly dosed antacids are required, alternate an aluminum-magnesium product with an aluminum or calcium only preparation and titrate the dose on the basis of stool frequency and consistency

Sorbitol-containing dosage forms
- if possible, obtain the liquid dosage form from a manufacturer that does not utilize sorbitol as the sweetening agent
- alternatively, use the solid oral dosage form of the drug

Antibiotics (if *C. difficile* infection is suspected)
- do stool cultures for *C. difficile;* isolation of the organism takes 36–48 hours

- do stool tests for *C. difficile* toxin; results can be obtained almost immediately if necessary
- sigmoidoscopy is not necessary in most cases, as many patients do not have positive findings either because lesions are missed or they are not present

Mild symptoms (limited to increased stool frequency and no severe abdominal pain, blood in the stool, or fever)
- stop the administration of the offending antibiotic and treat with supportive fluid and electrolyte replacement
- drug therapy for mild symptoms is not usually indicated unless the patient is elderly or debilitated

Asymptomatic patients with positive test results for the toxin or a positive culture for *C. difficile*
- do not require drug therapy
- up to 20% of hospitalized patients are asymptomatic carriers (JAMA 1993;269:71–75)
- correct fluid and electrolyte abnormalities as required

If the patient has not improved within 72 hours; if antibiotic therapy for an infection must be continued; if severe symptoms such as high fever, abdominal tenderness, and signs and symptoms of peritoneal inflammation are present; or if the patient is symptomatic and has a positive test result for toxin and/or positive culture
- start drug therapy immediately, along with replacement of fluid and electrolytes

METRONIDAZOLE
- 250 mg PO Q6H for at least 7 days (therapy longer than 10 days is rarely needed)
- recommended initial treatment of choice for *C. difficile* infection, as it is much less expensive than and as effective as vancomycin (Lancet 1983;2:1043–1046, N Engl J Med 1994;330:257–262)

VANCOMYCIN
- 125 mg PO Q6H for at least 7 days (therapy longer than 10 days is rarely needed)
- use in patients with proven metronidazole-resistant *C. difficile* organisms or in patients who do not respond adequately to metronidazole
- some clinicians suggest that vancomycin is the drug of choice in patients who are seriously ill because some *C. difficile* organisms are resistant to metronidazole (JAMA 1993;269:71–75)
- vancomycin 500 mg PO Q6H is no more effective than 125 mg PO Q6H (Am J Med 1989;86:15–19)
- unless patients are anephric, determination of vancomycin serum levels is not required because there is limited oral absorption
- if the patient is pregnant, use vancomycin because there is concern about possible teratogenicity with metronidazole and vancomycin has virtually no systemic absorption

ANTIPERISTALTICS
- narcotics or other drugs with antiperistaltic activity should *not* be used because the *C. difficile* toxin is retained longer and can therefore cause more damage and prolong the illness

If a patient with severe illness has gastrointestinal obstruction or ileus
METRONIDAZOLE
- patients who cannot receive oral therapy can be treated adequately with parenteral metronidazole 500 mg IV Q8H (N Engl J Med 1994;330:257–262)

▶ How Quickly Should My Patient Respond?

Laxatives (stimulants, stool softeners, and so on), antacids (especially magnesium containing), sorbitol-containing drug products, and other drugs

- within 1–2 days after administration of the drug has been stopped or the dosage has been decreased

Antibiotics (if *C. difficile* infection is suspected)

- should see a decrease in fever, diarrhea, and cramps within 48 hours
- if the patient does not adequately respond within 96 hours, consider alternative therapy (e.g., vancomycin instead of metronidazole)
- fever and diarrhea may take up to 1 week to resolve completely
- relapses can occur in up to 20% of patients, and these patients can be retreated with either metronidazole or vancomycin
- as antibiotic resistance is not commonly the reason for relapses, the use of vancomycin for relapses after metronidazole treatment is not necessarily rational

▶ What Should I Monitor with Regard to the Efficacy of My Treatment?

Laxatives (stimulants, stool softeners, and so on), antacids (especially magnesium containing), sorbitol-containing drug products, and other drugs

Stool frequency
- monitor stool frequency daily until the frequency is back to normal (ask patients about their normal frequency)

Antibiotics (if *C. difficile* infection is suspected)

Cultures or tests for toxins
- repeated cultures are not useful in most cases because patients may become asymptomatic, yet be chronic carriers
- successful treatment is characterized by resolution of symptoms
- if the patient has not adequately responded, repeated cultures may be useful to identify resistant organisms

▶ Do I Have to Stop Administration of the Drug That Is Causing the Diarrhea?

Laxatives (stimulants, stool softeners, and so on), antacids (especially magnesium containing), and other drugs

- if possible, reduce the dosage or stop administration of the suspected drug
- if you cannot stop therapy with the suspected drug or decrease the dosage, continue therapy, and in many instances, the diarrhea is self-limiting and/or decreases over time
- if diarrhea becomes clinically important, consider alternative drug therapy

Sorbitol-containing drug products

- obtain the liquid dosage form from a manufacturer that does not use sorbitol as the sweetening agent
- use the solid oral dosage forms (tablets or capsules)

Antibiotics (if *C. difficile* infection is suspected)

- stop the antibiotic administration if possible
- if the antibiotic administration needs to be continued, drug therapy for *C. difficile* infection should be started immediately, even in patients with mild symptoms
- no evidence is available to suggest that switching to a different antibiotic has any benefit, and almost all antibiotics have been shown to cause *C. difficile* infection

Useful References

Fekety R, Shah AB. Diagnosis and treatment of *Clostridium difficile* colitis. JAMA 1993;269:71–75
Greenwood JK, Brown G. Sorbitol-induced diarrhea in the tube-fed patient. Can J Hosp Pharm 1991;44:297–300
Kelly CP, Pothoulakis C, LaMont JT. *Clostridium difficile* colitis. N Engl J Med 1994; 330:257–262

DRUG-INDUCED CONSTIPATION

Leslie Mathews

▶ My Patient Has Constipation, How Do I Determine If This Is Drug Induced?

All drugs

Do a thorough drug history
- note all prescription and nonprescription medications, both those with regularly scheduled administration and those given on a PRN basis, the date of initiation, the dosage, and the indication
- compare the symptoms of constipation before and after initiation of the offending drug therapy
- compare the onset of symptoms with changes in drug therapy

Laxative abuse

- consider laxative abuse when a patient admits to regular use of stimulant laxatives (e.g., castor oil, phenolphthalein, senna, cascara, and bisacodyl) and/or regular use of enemas and/or reports a need to increase the dosage to maintain regular bowel movements

▶ What Drugs Are Most Likely to Cause Constipation?

- narcotic analgesics, aluminum hydroxide–containing antacids, anticholinergic agents and agents with anticholinergic properties (antidepressants, antihistamines, antipsychotics, and antiparkinsonian agents), barium sulfate, cholestyramine, muscle relaxants, iron preparations, verapamil, and antidiarrheal agents

▶ What Are the Characteristics of Drug-Induced Constipation?

All drugs

- decreased frequency of stool (<3 bowel movements per week); the presence of hard, dry stools that are difficult to pass; and abdominal discomfort
- spurious diarrhea can occur with fecal impaction

Laxative abuse

- suspect laxative abuse when a patient has any combination of the following symptoms: dehydration, hypokalemia, hypocalcemia, hypermagnesemia, metabolic alkalosis, evidence of malabsorption, spurious diarrhea, vomiting, edema, abdominal pain, finger clubbing, weakness, and weight loss (Hosp Pharm 1988;23:565–573)
- to confirm suspicion, collect and analyze urine samples for 3 successive days
- surreptitious laxative use can be confirmed with urine screens to detect phenolphthalein, bisacodyl, senna, and danthron, which are identifiable in urine for 32 hours after a single dose (Hosp Pharm 1988;23:565–573)
- after use of anthraquinones for 4–12 months, melanosis coli (a dark discoloration of the bowel, mainly in the

cecum and rectum) can be detected by sigmoidoscopic examination

- after several years of stimulant laxative use, the colon on radiographic examination appears dilated and smooth, lacks haustral markings, and appears similar to that found with ulcerative colitis

▶ How Do I Treat the Constipation?

Prevention of constipation

- constipation is more easily prevented than treated
- when initiating treatment with any potentially constipating drug therapy, increase the dietary fiber and fluid intake whenever possible
- for anticipated long-term therapy with constipating drugs (especially narcotics), initiate prophylaxis with a fiber and bulk-forming laxative (1 teaspoon of psyllium hydrophilic mucilloid in 250 mL of fluid BID)
- if bulk-forming laxatives are contraindicated or ineffective after a 2–3 day trial, initiate stimulant laxative therapy (bisacodyl 5 mg PO daily) and titrate the dose according to response
- other effective stimulant laxatives include Senokot 15 mg PO daily or cascara aromatic fluid extract 5 mL PO daily
- if long-term use of both constipating drug therapy and a stimulant laxative is anticipated, the use of lactulose 30 mL daily, titrated to response, in place of the stimulant laxative has less long-term toxicity
- addition of docusate to any of the above therapies is questionable because evidence of effectiveness is lacking (J Chronic Dis 1976;29:59–63, Geriatrics 1991;46:84–86) and adverse effects are possible with regular use

Treatment of constipation

- discontinue or decrease the dosage of constipating medication whenever possible
- because the effect is often dose dependent, adjusting the dosage downward, while still maintaining therapeutic efficacy, may eliminate the problem of constipation
- change to a less constipating drug if a reasonable alternative exists (e.g., verapamil is more constipating than diltiazem or nifedipine) (Hosp Pract 1990;25:89–100)
- use bulk-forming laxatives as long as there are no contraindications or the patient has fluid restrictions, otherwise use lactulose
- glycerin suppositories and/or enema solutions (tap water, sodium phosphate [Fleet], saline) may be required as a single dose for fecal impaction when constipation is resistant to oral laxatives

Treatment of laxative abuse

- goal is eventually to stop all laxative use (with the exception of the bulk-forming laxatives)
- to attain this goal, counsel the patient on general measures to prevent and treat constipation
- correct any misconceptions about bowel function (e.g., you will not become "toxic" without a daily bowel movement)
- treat any underlying causes of constipation (e.g., hemorrhoids and depression)
- arrange psychiatric counseling, if indicated
- with less serious cases (e.g., short-term abuse and no evidence to suggest significant colon injury), discontinue the administration of all laxatives immediately, prescribe a bulk-forming laxative, and advise the patient not to expect a bowel movement for a few days
- for more serious cases (atonic colon), wean the patient from stimulants, using the minimum effective dosage;

reduce the dosage weekly; increase dietary fiber intake; and add a bulk-forming laxative

- substitute a low dosage (30 mL daily) of lactulose or 30 mL of magnesium hydroxide for the stimulant laxative if constipation relapses while weaning the patient from stimulants

▶ How Quickly Should My Patient Respond and What Should I Monitor with Regard to the Efficacy of My Treatment?

Prevention of constipation

- patients should maintain a normal frequency of bowel movements

Treatment of constipation

- response time varies depending on the agent used and the severity of constipation
- bulk-forming laxatives produce a soft, bulky stool within 2–3 days; however, with more severe and chronic constipation, full effects may be delayed for up to 4 weeks
- stimulants produce soft formed or semiliquid stool within 6–24 hours
- suppositories initiate defecation within 60 minutes
- lactulose produces a soft or semiliquid stool within 6–24 hours, with full effects occurring by 24–48 hours
- advise the patient to report the presence of abdominal discomfort, hard or dry stool, or need for straining
- in hospitalized patients, check stool charts and/or question the patient or the nurse about abdominal discomfort and the frequency and consistency of stool
- if treatment is ineffective, do an abdominal examination to detect distention or tenderness and a rectal examination to detect impaction

Treatment of laxative abuse

- full effect from bulk-forming laxatives may take several weeks
- lactulose should produce a soft or semifluid stool in 6–24 hours, with full effects occurring within 48 hours
- magnesium hydroxide produces 1 bowel movement or more within 6–12 hours
- glycerin suppository should cause an effect within 15–60 minutes
- sodium phosphate enema produces a watery evacuation within 5–30 minutes, depending on the retention time

▶ How Long Should I Treat the Constipation?

Prevention of constipation

- patients should receive therapy until administration of the constipating drug is stopped

Treatment of constipation

- treat until regular bowel habits are attained and then continue therapy until administration of the constipating drug is stopped
- an attempt to decrease the dosage of the laxative can be made after 2–3 months to determine whether tolerance to the constipating effects of a constipating drug has developed

Treatment of laxative abuse

- after satisfactory bowel function has returned, periodic bouts of acute or painful constipation can be treated with oral magnesium hydroxide or glycerin suppositories

Useful References

Oster JR, Materson BJ, Rogers AI. Laxative abuse syndrome. Am J Gastroenterol 1980;74:451–458

Portenoy RK. Constipation in the cancer patient. Med Clin North Am 1987;71:303–311

Tremaine WJ. Chronic constipation: Causes and management. Hosp Pract 1990;25:89–100

DRUG-INDUCED NAUSEA AND VOMITING

Lynne Nakashima

▶ My Patient Has Nausea and Is Vomiting, How Do I Determine If This Is Drug Induced?

Do a thorough drug history

- document all prescription and nonprescription medications
- if the patient is in a hospital, check the medication administration records for both regular and PRN orders
- if serum concentrations are routinely monitored, document serum drug concentrations for any drugs that can cause nausea and vomiting

▶ What Drugs Are Most Likely to Cause Nausea and Vomiting?

Non-antineoplastic agents

- opioids, theophylline, digoxin, antibiotics (e.g., tetracycline and erythromycin), anticholinergics, alcohol, ipecac, and so on
- virtually all drugs have the potential to cause nausea and vomiting, depending on the dose administered

Antineoplastic agents

- emetogenic potential varies among the different agents, with doses and route of administration, and with the patients' responses
- high emetogenic potential drugs: cisplatin, cyclophosphamide, dacarbazine, dactinomycin, mechlorethamine, and streptozocin (Recent Results Cancer Res 1991;121:68–85)
- moderate emetogenic potential drugs: carmustine, cytarabine, daunorubicin, doxorubicin, lomustine, procarbazine, and carboplatin
- low emetogenic potential drugs: fluorouracil (5-fluorouracil), bleomycin, chlorambucil, etoposide, hydroxyurea, methotrexate, mitomycin, vinblastine, vincristine, and vindesine

▶ What Are the Characteristics of Drug-Induced Nausea and Vomiting?

- usually characterized by acute onset of nausea, retching, and vomiting
- may have delayed onset (1–7 days) after antineoplastic drug therapy

▶ When Should I Use Prophylactic Measures?

Non-antineoplastic agents

- in general, prophylactic measures are not used
- in patients receiving opioids, prophylactic therapy should be used in patients who are at high risk for aspiration owing to an inability to rid the mouth rapidly of vomitus (e.g., highly sedated patients), patients with debilitating neurological disease, and patients who have recently undergone oral surgery (especially those who have their jaws occluded by wires)

Antineoplastic agents

- whenever the patient is receiving highly emetogenic cancer chemotherapy
- it is important to prevent anticipatory nausea and vomiting because nausea and vomiting usually worsen with each cycle and up to 30% of patients refuse further treatment because of intolerable nausea and vomiting

▶ How Do I Treat Drug-Induced Nausea and Vomiting?

Non-antineoplastic agents

Use nondrug measures

- limit oral intake to small frequent amounts of any noncarbonated liquid
- have the patient lie down and keep head movement to a minimum
- advance the diet slowly and as tolerated, ensure adequate hydration, and restrict activity to minimize vetibular disturbances
- relaxation techniques may be useful

If possible, stop the administration of or decrease the dosage of the suspected causative drugs

- reevaluate the need for the suspected causative drugs and the dosage being used, as nausea and vomiting may indicate a toxic dose

If the dosage of suspected drugs cannot be decreased or discontinued

- try an agent such as prochlorperazine, perphenazine, or thiethylperazine
- these agents are likely equally effective, and the decision among them should be based on cost and availability (these agents likely cause less sedation than does dimenhydrinate)
- if sedation is desired, choose dimenhydrinate over these agents
- give 5 mg of prochlorperazine or thiethylperazine (4 mg for perphenazine) PO ½ hour before the dose of the suspected agent
- continue oral therapy Q6H PRN
- if the oral route is not tolerated, a trial of a 25 mg prochlorperazine rectal suppository Q6H is warranted before using parenteral formulations
- if nausea and vomiting are not controlled, first try increasing the dosage of prochlorperazine to 10 mg (8 mg for perphenazine) PO Q6H around the clock or switch to parenteral therapy (10 mg IV or IM Q6H for prochlorperazine, 5 mg IV or IM Q6H for perphenazine, or 10 mg IM Q6H for thiethylperazine)
- if nausea and vomiting continue, reassess the patient and consider a full workup for the cause of nausea and vomiting and treat appropriately
- if no other underlying causes are determined, a trial of haloperidol 1 mg PO, or IM if oral therapy not tolerated, may be useful

Antineoplastic agents

- prophylactic therapy should be used for chemotherapy that includes either a high or moderate emetogenic drug
- for drugs with low emetogenic potential, prophylactic therapy should be used in patients who experienced nausea or vomiting with a previous course of these drugs
- see section on drug therapy for nausea and vomiting for specific recommendations and doses

▶ *How Quickly Should My Patient Respond and What Should I Monitor with Regard to the Efficacy of My Treatment?*

Control should be obtained within the first 12–24 hours

- if the patient does not respond, first increase the dosage while monitoring for side effects, then if a response is still not obtained, change to a different drug
- for patients receiving antineoplastic therapy, combination therapy is often most effective

Frequency of assessment depends on the severity and frequency of nausea and vomiting

Number and severity of vomiting episodes
- determine the time of occurrence during the day, its force, a description of vomitus, and associated symptoms

Fluid balance
- only needed if vomiting occurs for a prolonged period
- assess jugular venous pressure and orthostatic changes in blood pressure and heart rate; any decrease in upright diastolic pressure plus a rise in heart rate of 20 bpm or greater is abnormal
- oliguria
- weight
- rising values of hematocrit, creatinine, urea, sodium, and bicarbonate plus decreasing potassium and chloride levels are an indication of dehydration

▶ *Do I Have to Stop Administration of the Drug That Is Causing the Nausea and Vomiting?*

- in some cases, a reduction in dosage helps to alleviate the symptoms of nausea and vomiting

- for chemotherapy-induced nausea and vomiting, the symptoms of nausea and vomiting can usually be controlled with prophylactic antiemetic regimens and it is imperative to continue antineoplastic agent treatment of the disease state

▶ *How Long Should I Treat the Nausea and Vomiting?*

- in general, treatment should last only until symptoms are resolved and either the causative agent is stopped or the dosage reduced to a tolerable level
- for chemotherapy-induced nausea and vomiting, delayed symptoms may occur up to 1 week after the last dose of chemotherapy and treatment should last for up to 1 week after chemotherapy, depending on the patient
- tolerance to narcotics develops in about 1 week, and antiemetic therapy can usually be discontinued or tapered at this time
- if nausea persists with the first narcotic agent, consider changing to another narcotic rather than treating with an antiemetic agent

Useful References

Martin JK, Norwood MB. Pharmacist management of antiemetic therapy under protocol in an oncology clinic. Am J Hosp Pharm 1988; 45:1322–1328

Merrifield KR, Chaffee BJ. Recent advances in the management of nausea and vomiting caused by antineoplastic agents. Clin Pharm 1989;8: 187–199

Tortorice PV, O'Connell MB. Management of chemotherapy-induced nausea and vomiting. Pharmacotherapy 1990;10(2):129–145

Triozzi PL, Laszlo J. Optimum management of nausea and vomiting in cancer chemotherapy. Drugs 1987;34:136–149

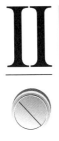

II

Drug Monographs

ACEBUTOLOL

Robert Rangno and James McCormack

USA (Sectral)
CANADA (Sectral, Monitan)

▶ When Should I Use This Drug?

Consider an alternative agent

- acebutolol is more beta$_1$-selective than nadolol but less selective than atenolol
- acebutolol has more intrinsic sympathomimetic activity (ISA) than does nadolol or atenolol but less than pindolol
- agents with ISA should theoretically produce less bradycardia; however, if bradycardia is a problem with beta-blockers, it is likely best just to reduce the dosage
- usually recommended to be dosed twice daily, which is a disadvantage compared with the once-daily dosing of atenolol or nadolol
- offers no proven clinical advantages over atenolol and nadolol and should be chosen over these agents only if acebutolol is less expensive (not available as a generic agent)
- reported to have fewer effects on lipids than do some other beta-blockers but the lipid changes with all beta-blockers are usually slight, are short lived, and have no proven adverse consequence
- propranolol has been shown to reverse atherosclerosis despite the fact that it increases serum lipid levels (J Hypertens 1991; 9(Suppl) S21)

ACETAMINOPHEN

Terry Baumann and Jerry Taylor

USA (Tylenol, various products)
CANADA (Tylenol, various products)

▶ When Should I Use This Drug?

Acute pain (mild to moderate), general aches and pain

- for mild to moderate acute pain if the pain is thought to have a noninflammatory origin (headache, muscle aches), as acetaminophen is effective, is inexpensive, and produces little, if any, gastrointestinal toxicities

Cancer pain, chronic noncancer pain

- acetaminophen is useful, in conjunction with codeine, for moderate symptoms if treatment with nonopioid agents is ineffective at maximum doses
- be aware that, when acetaminophen is used in combination products with codeine in a round-the-clock fashion, acetaminophen toxicity may occur owing to the possible ingestion of large amounts of acetaminophen

Postoperative pain

- after the patient no longer requires regularly dosed medications (e.g., 2–3 days postoperatively), acetaminophen with codeine may be used on a PRN basis

Osteoarthritis

- acetaminophen is the initial drug of choice because for many patients it is as effective as ibuprofen (N Engl J Med 1991; 325:87–91), has fewer toxicities than NSAIDs, and is less expensive

Migraine

- use instead of aspirin for mild symptoms if the patient has gastrointestinal intolerance to aspirin

Fever

- minor fever should not be treated, as it does not cause any damage and may trigger immune defenses
- if a fever makes the patient uncomfortable, acetaminophen may be used transiently to reduce the fever
- acetaminophen is tolerated better than aspirin

▶ When Should I Not Use This Drug?

Severe pain

- not effective for severe pain by itself but may be useful when combined with an opioid
- use regularly dosed morphine or another opioid for severe pain

Rheumatoid arthritis

- acetaminophen has only weak antiinflammatory activity

▶ What Contraindications Are There to the Use of This Drug?

- Intolerance of or allergic reaction to acetaminophen

▶ What Drug Interactions Are Clinically Important?

- None

▶ What Route and Dosage Should I Use?

How to administer

- orally—may be given with food or milk or on an empty stomach
- parenterally—not available

Acute pain, general aches and pain

- 500 mg PO Q4H to a maximum of 1000 mg PO Q6H

Cancer pain, chronic noncancer pain

- 325–650 mg PO Q4H in conjunction with 30 mg of codeine, if required

Postoperative pain

- 325 mg PO Q4H in conjunction with 30 mg of codeine, if required

Osteoarthritis

- start with 500 mg PO Q6H and adjust dose up to a maximum of 1000 mg PO Q6H

Migraine

- 1000 mg PO Q4H PRN up to a maximum dose of 4000 mg PO daily

Fever

- 500 mg PO Q4H up to a maximum dose of 4000 mg PO daily

▶ Dosage Adjustment for Renal or Hepatic Dysfunction

- dosage adjustment is usually not required if the dose is titrated properly
- consider a maximum daily dose of 2000 mg in a patient with liver dysfunction

▶ What Should I Monitor with Regard to Efficacy and Toxicity?

Efficacy

Acute pain, general aches and pain, chronic cancer pain, chronic noncancer pain, postoperative pain, migraine

Subjective pain evaluation

- key to achieving effective pain control is to question patients frequently about the degree of pain they are having
- frequency of pain evaluation should be based on the knowledge of how quickly the drug should work
- decision to give PRN doses or to increase the dosage should be based on the patient's assessment of the pain's severity
- remember that pain is whatever the patient says it is
- when self-assessment by the patient is not possible, monitor agitation and heart rate

Osteoarthritis

- pain and the ability to conduct normal daily activities are important variables to follow when assessing the patient

Fever

- patient's comfort and reduction in fever

Toxicity

Hepatic necrosis (after overdose)

- dose-dependent hepatic necrosis can be fatal in overdoses of 150 mg/kg or more
- can be seen at lower doses in patients also receiving enzyme-inducing drugs
- overdose treatment is mainly symptomatic (gastric lavage, respiratory support, and fluid administration); however, oral acetylcysteine, which may replenish glutathione stores (which interact with toxic metabolites that cause liver toxicity), should be administered
- amount of acetylcysteine to be administered can be determined by an acetaminophen level and a nomogram relating concentration and probable hepatic toxicity; however, acetylcysteine should not be withheld pending this determination
- 140 mg/kg PO of acetylcysteine should be administered as soon as possible, followed by 70 mg/kg every 4 hours for 17 doses or as indicated by the nomogram
- nausea, vomiting, and abdominal pain usually occur 2–3 hours after ingestion of acetaminophen
- characteristic signs of acetaminophen overdose are cyanosis of skin, mucosa, and fingernails

Hepatotoxicity

- while acetaminophen can cause hepatotoxicity, it rarely occurs except in overdose
- hepatotoxicity can be potentiated by chronic alcoholism
- no routine monitoring is recommended
- in comparison to the overall toxicities seen with NSAIDs, acetaminophen is considerably safer to use long-term
- consider a maximum daily dose of 2000 mg in a patient who is an alcoholic or who has liver dysfunction

Anemia, renal damage

- can occur, but no guidelines on monitoring are available
- patients on chronic therapy should have serum creatinine measured 1–2 times per year

▶ How Long Do I Treat Patients with This Drug?

Acute pain, general aches and pain

- use on a regular basis for the duration of pain
- acute pain should subside within days after the offending event; if this has not occurred within 1 week, further investigate the cause of the pain

Cancer pain, chronic noncancer pain

- therapy may be needed for months or years

Postoperative pain

- use on a regular basis for 48–72 hours, and then use on a PRN basis when patients are being ambulated

Osteoarthritis

- after pain control is achieved, decrease the daily dosage by 25% every 1–2 weeks until the minimum effective dose is identified (once daily dosing or PRN dosing may be all that is required)
- therapy should be continued as long as the drug is effective

Migraine

- initial therapy with acetaminophen should prevent pain or provide pain relief within a couple of hours
- if headaches are persistent after 1–2 hours, alternative therapy should be instituted

Fever

- if therapy is required for longer than 2–3 days, reevaluate the reason for fever

▶ How Do I Decrease or Stop the Administration of This Drug?

- unless it is combined with codeine, administration of acetaminophen may be stopped abruptly

▶ What Should I Tell My Patients About This Drug?

- if you are self-administering for longer than 10 days, seek medical advice

- keep away from children, as even small accidental doses (150 mg/kg) can cause severe toxicity or death
- if you notice nausea, vomiting, or abdominal pains, seek medical advice

▶ Therapeutic Tips

- most effective when used with opiates
- acetaminophen has been shown to be as effective as ibuprofen (N Engl J Med 1991;325:87–91) for osteoarthritis, has fewer and less severe toxicities than NSAIDs, and is less expensive than NSAIDs

Useful References

See Morphine

ACETOHEXAMIDE

Christy Silvius Scott

USA (Dymelor, generic)
CANADA (Dimelor)

▶ When Should I Use This Drug?

Consider an alternative agent

- offers no advantages over other oral hypoglycemics
- it must be given more frequently than once daily; the active metabolite (hydroxyhexamide) provides most of the action, and accumulates in renal dysfunction

Useful Reference

Gerich JE. Oral hypoglycemic agents. N Engl J Med 1989;321:1231–1245

ACYCLOVIR

Ann Beardsell

USA (Zovirax)
CANADA (Zovirax)

▶ When Should I Use This Drug?

Mucosal and cutaneous herpes simplex

- drug of choice for use in immunocompetent patients with moderate to severe mucocutaneous herpes simplex virus (HSV) type 1 and HSV-2 infection
- drug of choice for the treatment of initial and recurrent HSV-1 and HSV-2 infections in immunocompromised patients (Med Lett 1992;34:31–36)
- decreases the duration of viral shedding, pain, itching, and positive cultures and the time required for crusting and healing of lesions

Genital herpes

- drug of choice for severe first episode in immunocompetent and immunocompromised patients
- should be used as prophylaxis for recurrent episodes in selected patients (those with poor immune status, severe recurrent episodes, and >6 episodes per year)
- not to be used in patients with mild episodes that can be managed with symptomatic support and counseling (Antimicrob Agents Chemother 1987;31:361–367)

Herpes simplex encephalitis

- drug of choice in patients older than 6 months (Med Lett 1992; 34:31–36)

Herpes zoster (reactivation of chickenpox—shingles)

- drug of choice for acute episodes (particularly in immunocompromised patients) of cutaneous and disseminated infections (including encephalitis)

Varicella-zoster virus infection (primary infection—chickenpox)

- acyclovir decreases pain and speeds healing to a mild degree in immunocompetent patients (Ann Intern Med 1988;108:221–237)
- drug of choice in immunocompromised patients (Ann Intern Med 1988;108:221–237)

▶ *When Should I Not Use This Drug?*

Topically in immunocompetent patients

- this route of administration has not been effective in the treatment of any HSV infections in immunocompetent patients (Can Fam Physician 1991;37:92–98, N Engl J Med 1986;314:749–757)
- in immunocompromised patients, oral or parenteral therapy should be chosen, as acyclovir given by these routes has a demonstrable effect

▶ *What Contraindications Are There to the Use of This Drug?*

- Intolerance of or allergic reaction to acyclovir

▶ *What Drug Interactions Are Clinically Important?*

Drugs that may increase the effect of acyclovir

PROBENICID

- blocks the renal clearance of acyclovir and should be avoided

ZIDOVUDINE

- may result in drowsiness and lethargy, although this can also be caused by the human immunodeficiency virus (HIV) disease itself
- this interaction is more likely with IV acyclovir, but patients should be monitored for unusual drowsiness when taking either oral or parenteral acyclovir

NEPHROTOXIC DRUGS (AMINOGLYCOSIDES, AMPHOTERICIN B, FUROSEMIDE)

- patients are at greater risk for nephrotoxicity when these agents are used together with acyclovir
- monitor serum urea and creatinine levels 3 times weekly
- if the serum creatinine level rises no more than 25% over baseline values, no dosage changes are needed, but be alert for further increases
- if an increase in the serum creatinine level of 50% over baseline values occurs, the need for continued therapy with these agents should be reassessed and discontinuation of therapy and the use of alternative nonnephrotoxic agents to complete the treatment course are advised

METHOTREXATE

- parenteral acyclovir can have encephalopathic effects
- in patients with a prior history of neurological reactions to intrathecal methotrexate, the risk of this adverse effect may be increased
- no dosage adjustments are needed; just be aware of the potential for the adverse effect and use acyclovir only for a severe outbreak during chemotherapy

Drugs that may decrease the effect of acyclovir

- none

Drugs that may have their effect increased by acyclovir

- none

Drugs that may have their effect decreased by acyclovir

- none

▶ *What Route and Dosage Should I Use?*

How to administer

- orally—can be taken with food or milk or on an empty stomach
- parenterally—administer IV acyclovir over at least 1 hour at a maximum concentration of 10 mg/mL

Mucosal and cutaneous herpes simplex

- 400 mg PO TID (some clinicians recommend 200 mg PO five times daily) for the initial infection or recurrent, intermittent episodes

Genital herpes

- 400 mg PO TID (some clinicians recommend 200 mg PO five times daily) for the first or a recurrent episode

- 400 mg PO 5 times daily for the initial infection if rectal herpes is present
- 5 mg/kg IV Q8H or 400 mg PO 5 times daily (if the patient can take oral medication) for immunocompromised patients
- for prophylaxis, start with 200 mg PO BID, and if this is not effective, increase the dosage to as much as 400 mg PO 5 times daily

Herpes simplex encephalitis

- 10 mg/kg IV Q8H

Herpes zoster

- 800 mg PO 5 times daily
- 10 mg/kg IV Q8H initially if the episode is severe and the patient is immunocompromised

Varicella-zoster virus infection

- 800 mg PO QID
- 10 mg/kg IV Q8H if the patient is immunocompromised

Dosage adjustments for renal dysfunction

- renally eliminated

Normal Dosing Interval	$C_{cr} > 60$ mL/min or 1 mL/s	C_{cr} 30–60 mL/min or 0.5–1 mL/s	$C_{cr} < 30$ mL/min or 0.5 mL/s
3–5 times per day	no adjustment needed	no adjustment needed	2 times per day
Q8H	no adjustment needed	Q12H	Q24H

▶ *What Should I Monitor with Regard to Efficacy and Toxicity?*

Efficacy

Mucosal and cutaneous herpes simplex, genital herpes, herpes zoster, varicella-zoster virus infection

- for treatment of acute infections, efficacy is monitored by the progressive drying and crusting of skin lesions
- reevaluate at 7–10 days to ensure that clinical resolution has occurred
- follow-up viral cultures are unnecessary, except in patients who have persistent mucocutaneous lesions caused by HSV despite appropriate treatment with acyclovir, and in such patients, the possibility of acyclovir-resistant HIV should be excluded
- treatment failure suggests possible acyclovir-resistant strains

Prophylaxis

- evaluate the frequency of recurrent infections
- frequent recurrences suggest possible acyclovir-resistant strains

Herpes simplex encephalitis

- improvement in mental status indicates response to therapy

Toxicity

- is minimal but can occur

Neurological effects

- headache and lethargy are more common with long-term use as compared with short-term use
- manage headaches symptomatically with mild analgesics and weigh the benefits and risks if headache becomes debilitating

Gastrointestinal effects

- nausea, vomiting, and diarrhea are common, especially in patients being treated with high doses orally
- uncommon with parenteral administration
- treat symptomatically

Renal effects

- preexisting severe renal disease, dehydration, and concomitant use of nephrotoxic drugs with acyclovir increases the risk of renal impairment
- renal impairment caused by acyclovir crystallization in the renal tubules may occur in some patients who are receiving parenteral acyclovir that is administered by rapid IV injection or infusion over less than 10 minutes, who are dehydrated, and who have low urine output

- to prevent this, administer IV acyclovir over at least 1 hour with a maximum concentration of 7 mg/mL, maintaining adequate hydration (do not administer by direct IV push)
- monitor serum urea and creatinine levels 3 times weekly

▶ *How Long Do I Treat Patients with This Drug?*

Mucosal and cutaneous herpes simplex

- treat infection for 7 days (10 days if lesions heal slowly)
- treat recurrent episodes for 5 days

Genital herpes

- treat initial infection for 7 days (10 days if lesions heal slowly)
- treat recurrent episodes for 5 days
- for prophylaxis, stop treatment after 6–9 months to determine whether the frequency or severity is still sufficient to warrant prevention (Antimicrob Agents Chemother 1987;31:361–367)
- in immunocompromised patients, prophylactic treatment should likely continue indefinitely

Herpes simplex encephalitis

- 14 days (21 days if improvement is slow)

Herpes zoster

- treat infection for 7 days (10 days if lesions heal slowly)

Varicella-zoster virus infection

- 5 days; 7 days if the patient is immunocompromised

▶ *How Do I Decrease or Stop the Administration of This Drug?*

- may be stopped abruptly

▶ *What Should I Tell My Patients About This Drug?*

- begin using this medication as soon as symptoms begin to appear (this is especially important when the patient is immunocompromised)
- medication may be taken with food
- take medication exactly as prescribed, and do not stop therapy early or take beyond the recommended duration
- women with genital herpes are at higher risk for cervical cancer and, therefore, should have yearly Papanicolaou's smears done

▶ *Therapeutic Tips*

- treatment of acute episodes should begin as soon as possible, as early as the initial tingling and before the development of vesicles, for best response
- patients who have recurrent infections but are not taking acyclovir prophylactically should keep a supply on hand to initiate prompt treatment

ADENOSINE

James Tisdale

USA (Adenocard)
CANADA (not available)

▶ *When Should I Use This Drug?*

Atrioventricular nodal reentrant tachycardia

- adenosine is considered the drug of choice for the acute termination of atrioventricular nodal reentrant tachycardia because of its short half-life and significantly lower incidence of hypotension in comparison with verapamil (Ann Intern Med 1991;114:513–515, JAMA 1992;268:2199–2241)

Diagnosis or management of wide QRS complex tachycardias

- adenosine should be used in patients with wide complex QRS tachycardias of uncertain origin that do not respond to lidocaine (JAMA 1992;268:2199–2241)

▶ *When Should I Not Use This Drug?*

Atrial fibrillation or flutter

- adenosine is effective only for the termination of tachycardias that are sustained by conduction through the atrioventricular

(AV) node and therefore is not effective for the termination of atrial fibrillation or flutter

Atrial tachycardia

- adenosine is ineffective for the termination of atrial tachycardia

Ventricular arrhythmias

- adenosine is ineffective for the termination of ventricular arrhythmias

▶ *What Contraindications Are There to the Use of This Drug?*

Intolerance of or allergic reaction to adenosine

Asthma

- adenosine should not be used in patients with asthma or bronchospasm, as it may result in bronchoconstriction and asthma exacerbation (Drugs 1991;41:596–624)

▶ *What Drug Interactions Are Clinically Important?*

Drugs that may increase the effect or toxicity of adenosine

DIPYRIDAMOLE

- dipyridamole blocks the cellular uptake of adenosine and inhibits its metabolism in blood
- patients receiving dipyridamole may respond to unusually low doses of adenosine
- for patients taking dipyridamole: start with 1 mg IV adenosine administered over 1–2 seconds; if no response occurs in 2 minutes, administer 3 mg IV over 1–2 seconds; if no response occurs in 2 minutes, administer 6 mg IV over 1–2 seconds

Drugs that may decrease the effect or toxicity of adenosine

THEOPHYLLINE AND OTHER METHYLXANTHINES

- methylxanthine compounds inhibit the effects of adenosine, perhaps by competitively blocking adenosine-sensitive receptors
- patients receiving methylxanthine compounds may require unusually high doses of adenosine or may not respond at all
- use an initial dose of 12 mg of adenosine rather than 6 mg

Drugs that may have their effect or toxicity increased by adenosine

- none

Drugs that may have their effect or toxicity decreased by adenosine

- none

▶ *What Route and Dosage Should I Use?*

How to administer

- orally—unavailable
- parenterally—as an IV bolus

Atrioventricular nodal reentrant tachycardia, diagnosis or management of wide QRS complex tachycardias

- 6 mg IV administered over 1–2 seconds, followed by a normal saline flush
- if no response occurs within 2 minutes, administer 12 mg IV over 1–2 seconds, followed by a normal saline flush
- if no response occurs within 2 minutes, administer an additional 12 mg IV over 1–2 seconds, followed by a normal saline flush
- if still no response occurs, further investigate the cause of arrhythmia

Dosage adjustments for renal or hepatic dysfunction

- metabolized in the blood
- dosage adjustment for renal or hepatic dysfunction is not necessary

▶ *What Should I Monitor with Regard to Efficacy and Toxicity?*

Efficacy

Atrioventricular nodal reentrant tachycardia, diagnosis or management of wide QRS complex tachycardias

- monitor the electrocardiogram (ECG) continuously during the drug administration for termination or continuation of tachycardia
- relief of the symptoms associated with tachycardia (shortness of breath, palpitations, dizziness, chest pain) should occur with the resolution of arrhythmia

Toxicity

Facial flushing and dyspnea

- have been reported to occur in 15–100% of patients
- adenosine may actually cause prolonged worsening of breathing in asthmatic patients (its use is contraindicated in asthma)
- adverse effects of adenosine usually last less than 1 minute (half-life < 10 seconds)

Nonischemic chest pressure

- is commonly seen but is usually transient and does not necessitate treatment
- is not associated with ECG changes

Bradycardia, atrioventricular block

- watch for the following after termination of paroxysmal supraventricular tachycardia (PSVT): atrial fibrillation, atrial tachycardia, ventricular premature beats, and ventricular tachycardia
- atrial fibrillation lasting several hours after termination of PSVT has been reported
- treat the atrial fibrillation if the patient is symptomatic

▶ *How Long Do I Treat Patients with This Drug?*

Atrioventricular nodal reentrant tachycardia, diagnosis or management of wide QRS complex tachycardias

- discontinue treatment after tachycardia has been terminated or after the diagnosis of wide QRS complex tachycardia has been made
- maximum of 3 doses should be given
- if arrhythmia persists after 3 doses, reconsider the origin of arrhythmia

▶ *How Do I Decrease or Stop the Administration of This Drug?*

- may be stopped abruptly

▶ *What Should I Tell My Patients About This Drug?*

- it may cause facial flushing, shortness of breath, chest pressure, or nausea
- any side effects are likely to be short lived

▶ *Therapeutic Tips*

- adenosine therapy is not effective for the termination of atrial fibrillation, atrial flutter, atrial tachycardia, or ventricular arrhythmias and should not be administered to patients with these arrhythmias

Useful References

Parker RB, McCollam PL. Adenosine in the episodic treatment of paroxysmal supraventricular tachycardia. Clin Pharm 1990;9:261–271

Faulds D, Chrisp P, Buckley MM-T. Adenosine. An evaluation of its use in cardiac diagnostic procedures, and in the treatment of paroxysmal supraventricular tachycardia. Drugs 1991;41:596–624

DiMarco JP, Miles W, Akhtar M, et al. Adenosine for paroxysmal supraventricular tachycardia: Dose ranging and comparison with verapamil. Assessment in placebo-controlled, multicenter trials. Ann Intern Med 1990;113:104–110

Rankin AC, McGovern BA. Adenosine or verapamil for the acute treatment of supraventricular tachycardia? Ann Intern Med 1991;114:513–515

ALLOPURINOL

C. Wayne Weart

USA (Zyloprim, Lopurin, Zurinol, generic)
CANADA (Alloprin, Apo-Allopurinol, Novapurol, Purinol, Zyloprim)

▶ *When Should I Use This Drug?*

Prophylaxis of acute gouty arthritis and chronic tophaceous gout

- patients who excrete greater than 600 mg/24 h of uric acid (on a low-purine diet) based on a 24 hour urine collection, have reduced renal function (glomerular filtration rate < 50 mL/min), or have a history of nephrolithiasis and are deemed candidates for uric acid–lowering therapy
- allopurinol is chosen in these patients rather than a uricosuric agent such as probenecid because allopurinol is a xanthine oxidase inhibitor and decreases the serum uric acid level by inhibiting uric acid synthesis

Patients undergoing short courses of intense chemotherapy for malignancies (including leukemia and lymphoma)

- allopurinol prevents uric acid nephropathy during short courses of intense chemotherapy

Prevention of recurrent calcium oxalate stones in patients with hyperuricemia

- patients with a history of calcium oxalate stones should receive prophylactic allopurinol

▶ *When Should I Not Use This Drug?*

Acute attack of gout

- do not initiate therapy with allopurinol in a patient with an acute gouty attack until the acute attack has resolved
- there is no need to discontinue uric acid–lowering therapy during an acute gouty attack after it has been initiated; however, initial uric acid–lowering therapy should not be started during an attack

▶ *What Contraindications Are There to the Use of This Drug?*

- intolerance of or allergic reaction to allopurinol

▶ *What Drug Interactions Are Clinically Important?*

Drugs that may increase the effect or toxicity of allopurinol

AMPICILLIN, AMOXICILLIN

- concurrent administration of allopurinol and ampicillin or amoxicillin appears to increase the risk of skin reactions 2-3–fold (J Clin Pharmacol 1981;21:456–458)
- do not use allopurinol with these agents; use erythromycin or a cephalosporin with allopurinol

Drugs that may decrease the effect of allopurinol

- none

Drugs that may have their effect or toxicity increased by allopurinol

WARFARIN

- data are conflicting, but the possibility of an enhanced anticoagulant effect should not be overlooked
- use alternative agents if possible
- if not, monitor INR every 2 days until the full extent of interaction is seen and adjust the dosage as for a warfarin dosage change
- monitor INR every 2 days when the administration of an interacting drug is discontinued and adjust as for a warfarin dosage change

CYCLOPHOSPHAMIDE

- allopurinol may increase the risk of myelosuppression from cyclophosphamide and possibly the risk of infection or bleeding
- do not use together

THEOPHYLLINE

- large doses (>600 mg/d) of allopurinol may reduce the clearance of theophylline and lead to toxicity
- monitor serum theophylline levels; measure every 2 days until the extent of any interaction is known and adjust the dosage of theophylline accordingly

THIOPURINES

- allopurinol inhibits the metabolism of azathioprine and mercaptopurine, which enhances the effect of these chemotherapeutic agents
- reduce the dosage of either of these thiopurines by 25%

ANGIOTENSIN CONVERTING ENZYME INHIBITORS

- allopurinol may increase the risk of allergic reactions in patients receiving angiotensin converting enzyme inhibitors

Drugs that may have their effect decreased by allopurinol

- none

▶ *What Route and Dosage Should I Use?*

How to administer

- orally—take with food or milk
- parenterally—not available

Prophylaxis of acute gouty arthritis

- give 100 mg PO daily and increase the dosage weekly in 100 mg/d increments until the serum uric acid level is less than 6 mg/dL or a total dose of 800 mg/d is reached
- dosages greater than 300 mg daily should be divided and given twice daily

Patients undergoing short courses of intense chemotherapy for malignancies (including leukemia and lymphoma)

- 300 mg PO BID for 2–3 days along with adequate or increased fluid intake

Prevention of recurrent calcium oxalate renal stones in patients with hyperuricemia

- give 300 mg PO daily; the dosage is adjusted to normalize or reduce urine concentrations of uric acid
- increased fluid intake is also required (i.e., 2–3 L/d)

Dosage adjustments for renal or hepatic dysfunction

- renally eliminated

Normal Dosing Interval	$C_{cr} > 60$ mL/min or 1 mL/s	C_{cr} 30–60 mL/min or 0.5–1 mL/s	$C_{cr} < 30$ ml/min or 0.5 mL/s
Q24H	no adjustment needed	reduce dosage by 50%	decrease dosage by 75%

▶ *What Should I Monitor with Regard to Efficacy and Toxicity?*

Efficacy

Prophylaxis of acute gouty arthritis

Serum uric acid level

- measure baseline level and repeat weekly until the appropriate dosage has been determined to reduce the serum uric acid below 6 mg/dL
- after stable, measure the serum uric acid level every 6–12 months

Number of attacks

- number of acute gouty attacks should decrease

Patients undergoing short courses of intense chemotherapy for malignancies (including leukemia and lymphoma)

- serum uric acid level monitoring is not required

Prevention of recurrent calcium oxalate stones in patients with hyperuricemia

- monitor serum and 24 hour urine uric acid levels

Toxicity

Serum creatinine level

- measure yearly (twice a year in the elderly)
- as renal function declines, evaluate the dosage required to maintain serum uric acid levels at less than 6 mg/dL

Allergic reactions

- caution the patient about rash and the need to discontinue therapy at the first sign of rash
- risk of potentially fatal drug reactions (toxic epidermal necrolysis), especially with higher dosages in patients with reduced renal or hepatic function

Hepatic toxicity

- can cause fatal hepatic necrosis
- uncommon and unpredictable
- tell patients that it has the potential to cause this effect and tell them to contact the physician if they experience jaundice or unexplained fatigue

▶ *How Long Do I Treat Patients with This Drug?*

Prophylaxis of acute gouty arthritis

- uric acid–lowering therapy is usually continued indefinitely but consideration should be given to a reduced dosage of allopurinol as patients age or have a reduction in renal function or in obese patients who have successfully attained ideal body weight
- generally not able to withdraw uric acid–lowering therapy but may be able to reduce the dosage as long as the serum uric acid level is maintained below 6 mg/dL

Patients undergoing short courses of intense chemotherapy for malignancies (including leukemia and lymphoma)

- 3 days

Prevention of recurrent calcium oxalate stones in patients with hyperuricemia

- indefinitely, unless the cause of the hyperuricemia is corrected

▶ *How Do I Decrease or Stop the Administration of This Drug?*

- may be stopped abruptly

▶ *What Should I Tell My Patients About This Drug?*

- maintain an adequate fluid intake, enough to produce at least 2 L of urine output per day to minimize the risk of renal stone formation
- allopurinol may be taken with food to reduce gastrointestinal effects
- tell your physician if you experience a rash, jaundice, fatigue, painful urination, blood in the urine, irritation of the eyes, or swelling of the lips or mouth, as this may indicate a potential adverse effect of allopurinol

▶ *Therapeutic Tips*

- start allopurinol therapy with low doses (100 mg/d) and gradually increase the dosage
- ensure that the dosage is adjusted for renal function
- low-dose colchicine should be given concurrently for the first 3 months to reduce the risk of mobilization gout
- consider the possibility of drug-induced hyperuricemia or rarely drug-induced gout (e.g., alcohol, thiazide and loop diuretics, penicillins, low-dose aspirin, niacin, and other drugs may increase the serum uric acid concentrations)

Useful References

Hawkins DW. Gout and hyperuricemia. In: DiPiro JT, Talbert RL, Hayes PE, et al, eds. Pharmacotherapy: A Pathophysiologic Approach. New York: Elsevier, 1989:912–917

Rundles W. The development of allopurinol. Arch Intern Med 1985; 145:1492–1502

Simkin PA. Management of gout. Ann Intern Med 1979;90:812–816

Wallace SL, Singer JZ. Treatment. In: Schumacher HR, Jr, ed. Primer on Rheumatic Diseases, 9th ed. Atlanta: Arthritis Foundation. 1988: 202–206

Wallace SL, Singer JZ. Therapy in gout. Rheum Dis Clin North Am 1988;14:441–457

Wisner DE, Simkin PA. Management of gout and hyperuricemia. Prim Care 1984;11:283–294

ALPRAZOLAM

Steven Stanislav and Patricia Marken

USA (Xanax)
CANADA (Xanax)

▶ *When Should I Use This Drug?*

Panic disorder

- only approved agent for treating panic disorder; however, other benzodiazepines may have efficacy for panic disorder
- comparative studies of alprazolam and imipramine, desipramine, or phenelzine are lacking; superiority of one agent over another is unknown
- clonazepam has been shown to be as efficacious as alprazolam (J Clin Psychiatry 1991;52[2]:69–76)

- clonazepam has a longer duration of action than does alprazolam and can be dosed 2–3 times daily, whereas alprazolam is dosed 3–4 times daily

▶ When Should I Not Use This Drug?

Sleep disorder

- alprazolam is effective but there are insufficient data and no special properties to warrant its preferred use as a primary hypnotic (Psychopharmacology 1981;75:258–261)
- sedative effect can be used by nocturnal dosing for patients who have insomnia as part of their symptom complex (J Affective Disord 1990;18:67–73, J Clin Psychopharmacol 1990;10:112–118)

Depressive disorder

- no longer recommended for depressive disorders
- it was originally thought that high doses may have an antidepressant effect, but alprazolam has fallen out of favor for treating depression

General anxiety disorder

- although alprazolam is effective, it provides no advantages over less expensive agents such as lorazepam and oxazepam

▶ What Contraindications Are There to the Use of This Drug?

see Lorazepam

▶ What Drug Interactions Are Clinically Important?

see Lorazepam

▶ What Route and Dosage Should I Use?

How to administer

- orally—may be taken with food or milk or on an empty stomach
- parenterally—not available

Panic disorder

- goal is to prevent attacks, then decrease the dosage if it is tolerated and symptoms are controlled
- 0.25 mg PO TID for 1 week
- advise the patient that this dosage may make him or her sedated and that he or she may have to take time off from work or school
- if necessary, titrate the dose up by 0.25 mg increments to 4–7 mg PO daily on the basis of the patient's response and ability to tolerate sedation
- QID dosing is not usually required; however, it can be used if the patient exhibits symptoms at the end of an 8 hour dosing interval
- after symptoms are suppressed, one can attempt to decrease the dosage and administer 3 times daily
- 3–4 doses per day are needed to avoid breakthrough anxiety

Dosage adjustments for renal or hepatic dysfunction

- hepatically metabolized
- no dosage guidelines for adjustments for organ dysfunction are available; however, always start with the lowest dose and titrate to response

▶ What Should I Monitor with Regard to Efficacy and Toxicity?

Efficacy

Panic disorder

Target symptoms

- monitor changes in shortness of breath, choking or smothering sensations, dizziness, palpitations or chest pain, trembling, nausea, depersonalization, tingling, and fear of impending doom
- should see an initial response within several days
- stable patients should be clinically assessed for target symptoms at least monthly or weekly if clinical decompensation is suspected

Toxicity

see Lorazepam

Sedation

- significant daytime sedation with psychomotor impairment can occur at the initiation of treatment
- patients should be cautioned about engaging in complex tasks such as driving

Withdrawal reactions

- after high-dose therapy, marked withdrawal reactions can occur, even when the dosage is tapered slowly (J Clin Psychiatry 1990;51:206–209)

▶ How Long Do I Treat Patients with This Drug?

Panic disorder

- studies suggest that, as is the case for general anxiety disorder, panic disorder is a chronic illness with waxing and waning symptoms
- no long-term follow-up studies longer than 6 months exist, and the efficacy of drug therapy beyond 6 months is unknown, but long-term patients do experience relapse when drug administration is discontinued
- some clinicians recommend at least a 6–12 month symptom-free period before attempting discontinuation of therapy (J Clin Psychiatry 1990;51:11–15)
- concurrent behavioral or desensitization therapy after drug discontinuation may decrease the risk of relapse

▶ How Do I Decrease or Stop the Administration of This Drug?

- decrease the dosage by approximately 10% per week (e.g., decrease the daily dosage by 0.25 mg weekly)
- after the dosage is down to 2 mg PO daily, decrease the daily dosage by 0.25 mg every 2–3 weeks
- weekly telephone evaluations are advised

▶ What Should I Tell My Patients About This Drug?

see Lorazepam

▶ Therapeutic Tips

- do not use as a "stand alone" hypnotic
- can be useful as a short-acting agent in the premenstrual syndrome to decrease irritability
- rearrange dosing times to match the times of day when panic attacks tend to occur

Useful References

Bonnet MH, Kramer M, Roth T. A dose response study of the hypnotic effectiveness of alprazolam and diazepam in normal subjects. Psychopharmacology 1981;75:258–261

Risse SC, Whitters A, Burke J, et al. Severe withdrawal symptoms after discontinuation of alprazolam in eight patients with combat-induced posttraumatic stress disorder. J Clin Psychiatry 1990;51:206–209

AMANTADINE

Ruby Grymonpre

USA (Symadine, Symmetrel)
CANADA (Symmetrel)

▶ When Should I Use This Drug?

Parkinson's disease

- in patients intolerant of other drugs for parkinsonism, amantadine can be tried; however, except for a few patients, the effect is minimal and wears off quickly

Influenza prophylaxis or treatment

- amantadine can be used to treat only influenza A (not influenza B)
- amantadine should be considered in high-risk patients if the influenza vaccine is not available or in patients who cannot take the vaccine
- give as soon as the outbreak starts
- if patients are vaccinated after local outbreaks (of influenza A only), chemoprophylaxis with amantadine should be given for 2 weeks, as this is the time required to develop immunity

- must be given within 48 hours of the onset of symptoms to be effective (Antimicrob Agents Chemother 1983;23:577–582)

▶ When Should I Not Use This Drug?

When other agents have not been tried

- as initial single therapy in early, minimally symptomatic Parkinson's disease (modest efficacy with about 65% response rate and a greater incidence of side effects as compared to levodopa/carbidopa (Br Med Bull 1990;46:124–146)

▶ What Contraindications Are There to the Use of This Drug?

- Intolerance of or allergic reaction to amantadine

▶ What Drug Interactions Are Clinically Important?

Drugs that may increase the effect or toxicity of amantadine

PHENOTHIAZINES, ANTICHOLINERGICS, MEPERIDINE, TRICYCLIC ANTIDEPRESSANTS, QUINIDINE, DISOPYRAMIDE, OR SOME ANTIHISTAMINES

- may result in additive anticholinergic adverse effects (e.g., xerostomia, blurred vision, constipation, and confusion); therefore, use the lowest effective dosages of both agents

Drugs that may decrease the effect of amantadine

- none

Drugs that may have their effect or toxicity increased by amantadine

- none

Drugs that may have their effect decreased by amantadine

- none

▶ What Route and Dosage Should I Use?

How to administer

- orally—with meals (breakfast and lunch)
- parenterally—not available

Parkinson's disease

- 100 mg PO daily with breakfast for 1 week, increasing to 100 mg PO BID (breakfast and lunch) thereafter
- dosage of levodopa may need to be reduced when amantadine therapy is initiated
- dosages greater than 200 mg daily are rarely necessary

Influenza prophylaxis or treatment

- 200 mg PO daily is usually recommended, starting at the time of exposure or outbreak
- 100 mg daily may also be effective and can be used if patients do not tolerate the higher dose
- 200 mg PO daily is used for treatment

Dosage adjustments for renal or hepatic dysfunction

- renally eliminated

Normal Dosing Interval	$C_{cr} > 60$ mL/min or 1 mL/s	C_{cr} 30–60 mL/min or 0.5–1 mL/s	$C_{cr} < 30$ mL/min or 0.5 mL/s
BID	no adjustment needed	z100 mg daily	100 mg Q 2 days (200 mg Q 7 days if $C_{cr} < 15$ ml/min)

▶ What Should I Monitor with Regard to Efficacy and Toxicity?

Efficacy

Parkinson's disease

Signs and symptoms

- assess symptoms weekly during the titration period

- after the patient has been stabilized, assess the patient every 3 months

Influenza prophylaxis or treatment

- assess for the signs and symptoms of influenza infection
- for treatment, assess temperature, muscle aches and pains, and weakness

Toxicity

Anticholinergic effects

Dry mouth

- increase fluid intake and/or use sugarless chewing gum or hard candies
- perform scrupulous oral hygeine, and use saliva substitutes

Constipation

- increase exercise, increase fluid and fiber intake in the diet, and if needed, use a laxative

Blurred vision, urinary hesitancy

- dose related and may resolve with a dosage reduction
- if persistent or severe, may need to stop the drug

Ankle edema (not common)

- occurs in 5–10% of patients (Adverse Drug React Bull 1990;145:544–547)
- often occurs with livedo reticularis
- more common in women
- not associated with congestive heart failure
- not a serious effect, and if amantadine is providing benefit, leg elevation, diuretic therapy, and dosage reduction may be attempted
- otherwise, it is advisable to discontinue drug administration if this occurs

Orthostatic hypotension

- treatment of orthostatic hypotension includes the patient rising slowly from supine or sitting positions and wearing support stockings
- dose related and may resolve with a dosage reduction
- if persistent or severe, may need to stop the drug

Gastrointestinal side effects

- nausea, vomiting, cramps, and diarrhea
- can be minimized by taking the drug with food

Livedo reticularis

- small vessel disease, discoloring the skin in a reddish-blue to purple blotchy pattern, affecting especially the legs (although it may also affect the upper extremities)
- occurs in 50–55% of patients receiving amantadine (Adverse Drug React Bull 1990;145:544–547) and in women about twice as often as in men (Drug Intell Clin Pharm 1987;21:10–21)
- may occur at a higher frequency when dosages exceed 200 mg/d
- may appear any time from 2 weeks to 20 months of treatment, although it appears most frequently between 3 and 6 months
- benign and asymptomatic side effect; however, it is advisable to discontinue drug administration if it occurs unless there is clear evidence of benefit
- disappears within 2–4 weeks after therapy is withdrawn

Central nervous system effects

- confusion, insomnia, nervousness, dizziness, and depression
- these reactions may be dose related, so if they occur, decrease the dosage of amantadine
- in patients with psychiatric illness, monitor for a recurrence of psychiatric episodes (including dementia, depression, and psychosis)
- seizures have also been reported at high dosages and in patients with renal impairment

Laboratory values

- may cause mild elevations in blood urea nitrogen and alkaline phosphatase levels (not clinically important)

Glaucoma

- monitor intraocular pressure annually, and ask the patient to report any visual disturbances and/or eye pain

Cardiovascular effects

- monitor heart rate, blood pressure (with the patient lying and standing), and the presence of any chest pain, especially in older patients or patients with cardiac disease or those taking antihypertensive medication
- monitor weekly while titrating the dose and then every 3 months afterward

▶ *How Long Do I Treat Patients with This Drug?*

Parkinson's disease

- use the drug until efficacy declines (usually after 30–60 days of treatment)
- drug efficacy may return if amantadine therapy is resumed after 2–3 weeks

Influenza prophylaxis or treatment

- for prophylaxis, use for 6–12 weeks (the duration of prevention depends on the duration of the outbreak)
- for treatment, continue for 48 hours after the disappearance of symptoms

▶ *How Do I Decrease or Stop the Administration of This Drug?*

- amantadine should not be discontinued abruptly if being used for parkinsonism
- reduce the dosage by 100 mg on alternate days at weekly intervals
- some patients require dosage reductions of less than 100 mg (for these patients the syrup form [50 mg/mL] is helpful)

▶ *What Should I Tell My Patients About This Drug?*

- it is best to take the last dose of this drug before 4 PM to avoid sleep disturbances
- contact your physician if symptoms do not improve within the next day or two
- central nervous system effects and additive effects of over the counter preparations are possible
- amantadine confers increased protection against influenza A infection

▶ *Therapeutic Tips*

- ensure that the drug dosage is adjusted for renal function, especially in the elderly
- swallowing the large amantadine caplets may be difficult, especially if dysphagia is present (amantadine syrup is a useful alternative)

Useful References

Berg MJ, Ebert B, Willis DK, et al. Parkinsonism—Drug treatment: Part 1. Drug Intell Clin Pharm 1987;21:10–21
Robertson DRC, George CF. Adverse effects and long-term problems of antiparkinsonian therapy. Adverse Drug React Bull 1990;145:544–547

AMIKACIN

David Guay and Ann Beardsell

USA (Amikin)
CANADA (Amikin)

▶ *When Should I Use This Drug?*

see antibiotic susceptibility chart (Table 4–1 in Chapter 4)

Upper urinary tract infection (pyelonephritis), acute or chronic bacterial prostatitis, pneumonia, intraabdominal infection, endocarditis, cellulitis, acute or chronic osteomyelitis, meningitis, gram-negative shock, febrile neutropenia

- amikacin should be used in these infections only if they are documented to be caused by organisms resistant to gentamicin and tobramycin and sensitive to amikacin
- amikacin is usually much more expensive than gentamicin or tobramycin

▶ *When Should I Not Use This Drug?*

see Gentamicin

Mycobacterium avium **infection**

- although amikacin is the only aminoglycoside with useful activity against this organism (Antimicrob Agents Chemother 1984;26: 841–844), amikacin has not provided additional benefit in multidrug regimens (Clin Infect Dis 1993;17:7–20) and is associated with significant inconvenience (IV therapy) and potential toxicity

▶ *What Contraindications Are There to the Use Of This Drug?*

see Gentamicin

▶ *What Drug Interactions Are Clinically Important?*

see Gentamicin

▶ *What Route and Dosage Should I Use?*

How to administer

- parenterally—dilute in 100 mL of saline or 5% dextrose in water and infuse over 30 minutes
- can be given intramuscularly, if the intravenous route is not available

Dosages depend on the patient's size, the severity of illness, and renal function • Round the dosage up to the nearest 50 mg dose (e.g., 200, 250, 300 mg) for ease of administration

Upper urinary tract infection (pyelonephritis), acute or chronic bacterial prostatitis, pneumonia, intraabdominal infections, endocarditis

- 5 mg/kg IV Q8H

Meningitis

- 5 mg/kg IV Q8H plus 10 mg intrathecally or intraventricularly Q24H if the patient fails to respond to IV therapy

Gram-negative shock

- 5 mg/kg IV Q8H

Febrile neutropenia

- 5 mg/kg IV Q8H

Dosage adjustments for renal or hepatic dysfunction

- renally eliminated

Normal Dosing Interval	C_{cr} >60 mL/min or 1 mL/s	C_{cr} 30–60 mL/min or 0.5-1 mL/s	C_{cr} <30 mL/min or 0.5 mL/s
Q8H	no adjustment needed	Q12H	Q24H

▶ *What Should I Monitor with Regard to Efficacy and Toxicity?*

Efficacy

- for antibiotic administration monitoring guidelines, see specific section on drug therapy

Toxicity

see Gentamicin

Desired serum concentrations

- 5–10 mg/L (predose) and 20–30 mg/L (postdose)
- remember that these ranges are guidelines and patients may require higher or lower concentrations, depending on the clinical course and toxicity
- prior to ordering any serum concentration determinations, ensure that patients are receiving an appropriate dosage for their age, weight, renal function, and disease state
- for further information on serum concentration measurement, see drug monograph on gentamicin

▶ *How Long Do I Treat Patients with This Drug?*

see Gentamicin

▶ *How Do I Decrease or Stop the Administration of This Drug?*

- may be stopped abruptly

▶ *What Should I Tell My Patients About This Drug?*

see Gentamicin

▶ *Therapeutic Tips*

- ensure that the organism's sensitivity mandates the use of amikacin rather than gentamicin or tobramycin
- serum concentrations are not required in patients receiving amikacin for *Mycobacterium avium*

AMILORIDE

Ian Petterson

USA (Midamor);
amiloride/hydrochlorothiazide combination: Moduretic
CANADA (Midamor);
amiloride/hydrochlorothiazide combination: Moduret, Apo-Amilzide, Novamilor, Nu-Amilzide)

▶ *When Should I Use This Drug?*

Chronic (noncrisis) hypertension

- when given alone, amiloride produces only a modest lowering of blood pressure, although it has more of an effect than does triamterene
- blood pressure reduction is additive with thiazide diuretics
- use in combination with thiazide diuretics only to prevent or treat hypokalemia
- use only for documented hypokalemia or high risk of adverse effects from hypokalemia (e.g., patients with cardiac arrhythmias, muscle weakness, and concomitant digoxin therapy)

Hypokalemia (prevention or treatment of hypokalemia associated with the use of kaliuretic diuretics)

- likely more effective than oral potassium supplementation or triamterene for the treatment of hypokalemia due to the use of thiazide or loop diuretics
- causes less severe adverse effects than does spironolactone, especially when spironolactone is used in high doses
- useful for patients who have diuretic-induced hypokalemia and cannot tolerate potassium supplementation or for whom supplements are not successful in correcting the hypokalemia
- useful in the prevention of hypokalemia when the consequence of low potassium represents a significant risk of toxicity to the patient (e.g., digoxin therapy, arrhythmias, and myasthenia gravis)

Hypomagnesemia (associated with the use of kaliuretic diuretics)

- maintains magnesium as well as potassium levels (Drugs 1984; 28[suppl 1]:161–166)

Primary hyperaldosteronism

- corrects hypertension and electrolyte abnormalities associated with primary hyperaldosteronism but is not as effective as spironolactone (Clin Pharm Ther 1980;27:317–323)
- should be used only if spironolactone is unsuccessful or not tolerated

Edema of heart failure and cirrhosis

- amiloride should be used only in combination with a more effective diuretic (thiazide or loop), as it has limited natriuretic activity

▶ *When Should I Not Use This Drug?*

Patients taking other potassium-sparing agents (potassium-sparing diuretic or angiotensin converting enzyme inhibitor)

- risk of hyperkalemia and inappropriate duplication of therapy
- use only if the patient is still hypokalemic despite maximum doses of other potassium-sparing agents

Single-agent diuretic

- is not effective as a single agent and should always be combined with either furosemide or hydrochlorothiazide

▶ *What Contraindications Are There to the Use of This Drug?*

Intolerance of or allergic reaction to amiloride

Moderate to severe renal insufficiency (C_{cr} <30 mL/min)

- drug is ineffective and risk of hyperkalemia increases as renal function decreases

Hyperkalemia (potassium level >5 mmol/L)

- risk of life-threatening hyperkalemia

Diabetic nephropathy

- increased risk of hyperkalemia

▶ *What Drug Interactions Are Clinically Important?*

Drugs that may increase the effect of amiloride

POTASSIUM-SPARING DIURETICS OR POTASSIUM SUPPLEMENTS

- risk of hyperkalemia is increased when other potassium-sparing diuretics or potassium supplements are used concurrently with amiloride

ANGIOTENSIN CONVERTING ENZYME INHIBITORS (CAPTOPRIL, ENALAPRIL, LISINOPRIL)

- little reason to use amiloride with angiotensin converting enzyme inhibitors because both drugs are effective potassium-sparing agents
- risk of hyperkalemia is increased when both agents are used together

NONSTEROIDAL ANTIINFLAMMATORY DRUGS

- possible increased serum potassium level due to decreased glomerular filtration rate
- not usually clinically important unless the patient has poor renal function

Drugs that may decrease the effect of amiloride

NONSTEROIDAL ANTIINFLAMMATORY DRUGS

- avoid combination if possible, and if not, monitor serum creatinine, potassium, and weight at baseline and every 4 days for 2–3 weeks, then every 2 weeks for 8 weeks, then every month for 3 months, and then as needed (J Musculoskel Med 1991; 8[8]:31–46)

Drugs that may have their effect increased by amiloride

LITHIUM

- amiloride may reduce lithium's renal clearance, leading to possible toxicity, although amiloride is less likely to do this than other diuretics
- toxicity due to increased lithium levels can be life threatening
- monitor the lithium level as for a dosage change of lithium (after 5 days) after initiating amiloride therapy or earlier if symptoms of toxicity are seen
- adjust the lithium dosage on the basis of lithium levels
- new steady state should be achieved in 5–7 days
- if already at the upper end of lithium's therapeutic range, empirically decrease the lithium dosage by 30%

Drugs that may have their effect decreased by amiloride

DIGOXIN

- may alter its clearance or diminish its inotropic effect
- control of atrial fibrillation by digoxin may be lost when amiloride therapy is added

▶ *What Route and Dosage Should I Use?*

How to administer

- orally—take with food to minimize gastrointestinal upset
- parenterally—not available

Chronic (noncrisis) hypertension, hypokalemia, hypomagnesemia, primary hyperaldosteronism, edema of heart failure and cirrhosis

- 2.5 mg PO daily as a starting dose and titrate to effect

- if a greater effect is required, the dosage may be increased by 2.5 mg/d at weekly intervals to a maximum of 20 mg/d (dosages greater than 10 mg/d are rarely required)
- when amiloride is used in combination with a thiazide, dosages of each drug should be optimized separately; then if the fixed combination is appropriate, therapy can be switched to a combination product

▶ *What Should I Monitor with Regard to Efficacy and Toxicity?*

Efficacy

see Spironolactone

Toxicity

Hyperkalemia

- in the case of a large dose or suspected decreased renal function, monitor serum potassium levels every 3–4 days until maximum effect is seen in 7–14 days; otherwise, monitor serum potassium levels 2 weeks after starting or increasing the dosage
- hyperkalemia is of great concern if the potassium level is greater than 6 mmol/L or has risen dramatically since the initiation of therapy
- 10% incidence in the elderly or in patients with diabetes or renal dysfunction
- approximately 1–2% occurrence with concurrent thiazide use
- stop drug administration if the patient becomes hyperkalemic, but realize that potassium levels may still rise for up to 3 days
- if electrocardiographic changes occur, regardless of the potassium level, the drug administration should be stopped
- if mild hyperkalemia develops (potassium level of 5–5.9 mmol/L), decrease the dosage by 50%
- if the potassium level is unchanged in 3 days, decrease the dosage further and reevaluate need for amiloride

Gastrointestinal effects

- 3–8% of patients have gastrointestinal complaints; therefore, the patient should take drug with food

Renal function

- increased serum urea and creatinine levels may occasionally be seen but are likely not indicative of nephrotoxity but are due to hypovolemia and decreased glomerular filtration rate, indicating excess diuretic use
- monitor baseline urea and creatinine levels every 3–4 months thereafter for patients with initial diminished function

▶ *How Long Do I Treat Patients with This Drug?*

see Spironolactone

▶ *How Do I Decrease or Stop the Administration of This Drug?*

- may be stopped abruptly

▶ *What Should I Tell My Patients About This Drug?*

- because this drug helps maintain your potassium balance you should avoid any potassium supplements
- you may experience some nausea or stomach upset but taking it with food should alleviate this (if it persists contact your physician as it may indicate an electrolyte abnormality)
- avoid the use of aspirin or nonsteroidal antiinflammatory drugs without first consulting your physician, as these drugs may decrease the effect of the amiloride (use acetaminophen)

▶ *Therapeutic Tips*

- avoid in renal dysfunction (C_{cr} <30 mL/min) because of risk of serious hyperkalemia
- do not start with a fixed combination product (e.g., amiloride-hydrochlorothiazide [Moduret])
- titrate the dose of each drug separately and then use a combination if appropriate
- may be able to decrease the dosage of a concurrently administered diuretic
- do not use in combination with other potassium-sparing agents, potassium supplements, or angiotensin converting enzyme inhibitors

- if hyperkalemia develops, this likely indicates that there is overt renal failure or that the drug was not needed

Useful References

Nader C, Thompson JR, Alpern RJ. Complications of diuretic use. Semin Nephrol 1988;8:365–387

Krishna GG, Shulman MD, Narins RG. Clinical use of potassium sparing diuretics. Semin Nephrol 1988;8:354–364

Ryan MP. Magnesium and potassium-sparing diuretics. Magnesium 1986; 5:282–292

Dyckner T, Wester P. Potassium-sparing diuretics. Acta Med Scand 1985; 707(suppl):79–83

AMINOPHYLLINE

Karen Shalansky and Cindy Reeser Nimmo

USA (Aminophylline, Phyllocontin, Truphylline)
CANADA (Phyllocontin)

▶ *When Should I Use This Drug?*

Acute asthma or acute exacerbation of chronic obstructive pulmonary disease

- add as a third-line agent only if the patient fails to improve after the first 12 hours of initial treatment with salbutamol, ipratropium bromide, or prednisone or cannot tolerate maximum salbutamol therapy and the heart rate is less than 120 bpm
- benefit is small and the risks and side effects are substantial (Chest 1990;98:1–3)
- some clinicians suggest that aminophylline is of no benefit in acute asthma when appropriate doses of beta$_2$-agonist, ipratropium bromide, and corticosteroids have been tried and that theophylline only increases the risk of toxicity (Chest 1990;98:1–3)
- parenteral aminophylline should be used only when patients cannot take or tolerate oral medications

▶ *When Should I Not Use This Drug?*

Chronic asthma or chronic obstructive pulmonary disease

- aminophylline sustained-release products offer no advantage over oral theophylline products unless they are less expensive

▶ *What Contraindications Are There to the Use of This Drug?*

see Theophylline

▶ *What Drug Interactions Are Clinically Important?*

see Theophylline

▶ *What Route and Dosage Should I Use?*

see Theophylline

- aminophylline contains 80% by weight anhydrous theophylline
- multiply the theophylline dose by 1.25 for the equivalent aminophylline dose

Conversion from intravenous aminophylline to oral theophylline

- take the hourly infusion rate of aminophylline, multiply by 10, and give this dose as a sustained-release preparation every 12 hours (e.g., if the aminophylline infusion is 30 mg/h, give sustained-release theophylline 300 mg Q12H)
- stop the infusion and start the sustained-release preparation at the same time

▶ *What Should I Monitor with Regard to Efficacy and Toxicity?*

see Theophylline

▶ *How Long Do I Treat Patients with This Drug?*

see Theophylline

▶ *How Do I Decrease or Stop the Administration of This Drug?*

- may be stopped abruptly

▶ *What Should I Tell My Patient About This Drug?*

see Theophylline

▶ *Therapeutic Tips*

see Theophylline

Useful References

Hendeles L, Weinberger M. Theophylline. "A state of the art" review. Pharmacotherapy 1983;3:2–44

Ellis E, Hendeles L. Theophylline. In: Taylor WJ, Caviness MHD, eds. A textbook for the Clinical Application of Therapeutic Drug Monitoring. Irving, TX: Abbott Laboratories, 1986:185–201

AMIODARONE

James Tisdale

USA (Cordarone)

CANADA (Cordarone)

▶ *When Should I Use This Drug?*

Amiodarone should not be used without consulting a cardiologist or a cardiac electrophysiologist

Ventricular tachycardia

- recurrent, symptomatic ventricular tachycardia in patients who have failed to respond to or to tolerate other antiarrhythmic agents
- survivors of an episode of sudden cardiac death in whom other antiarrhythmic agents have failed to suppress ventricular tachycardia or fibrillation during electrophysiological (EP) testing and who do not desire nonpharmacological therapy, such as an automatic implantable cardioverter-defibrillator
- survivors of an episode of sudden cardiac death in whom ventricular tachycardia is not inducible during EP testing and who do not desire nonpharmacological therapy such as an automatic implantable cardioverter-defibrillator

Supraventricular arrhythmias

- recurrent, symptomatic supraventricular arrhythmias (atrial fibrillation or flutter, atrioventricular [AV] nodal reentrant tachycardia, Wolff-Parkinson-White syndrome) in patients who have failed to respond to or to tolerate other available antiarrhythmic agents (some clinicians recommend amiodarone as first-line therapy)

▶ *When Should I Not Use This Drug?*

Patients with asymptomatic cardiac arrhythmias

- treatment of asymptomatic arrhythmias with any drugs has not proved beneficial

▶ *What Contraindications Are There to the Use of This Drug?*

Intolerance of or allergic reaction to amiodarone

Patients with marked sinus bradycardia

- amiodarone may depress sinus node function and worsen bradycardia and should not be used in patients with sinus bradycardia unless a functioning pacemaker is present

Patients with second- or third-degree atrioventricular block

- amiodarone depresses conduction through the AV node and should not be used in patients with second- or third-degree AV block unless a functioning pacemaker is present

▶ *What Drug Interactions Are Clinically Important?*

Drugs that may increase the effect or toxicity of amiodarone

- none

Drugs that may decrease the effect or toxicity of amiodarone

- none

Drugs that may have their effect or toxicity increased by amiodarone

DIGOXIN

- amiodarone increases the bioavailability and decreases the renal and nonrenal clearance of digoxin, and serum digoxin concentrations increase by approximately 60% when digoxin is taken in combination with amiodarone
- when amiodarone therapy is initiated in patients receiving digoxin, the dosage of digoxin should be empirically decreased by 50%
- if digoxin toxicity is suspected, measure a digoxin serum concentration

WARFARIN

- amiodarone inhibits the hepatic metabolism of warfarin, and this effect may be dependent on the amiodarone dosage
- when amiodarone therapy is initiated in patients receiving warfarin, the warfarin dosage should be decreased by $1/3$ in patients receiving amiodarone 200 mg daily, by $1/2$ in patients receiving amiodarone 400 mg daily, and by $2/3$ in patients receiving amiodarone greater than 400 mg daily (Clin Pharmacokinet 1989;17:130–140)
- monitor the INR every 2 days until the full extent of interaction is seen, and adjust the dosage as for a warfarin dosage change

QUINIDINE

- amiodarone therapy in patients receiving quinidine results in increased serum quinidine concentrations
- when amiodarone therapy is initiated in patients receiving quinidine, the dosage of quinidine should be reduced by 50% and a serum quinidine concentration should be determined 3 days after the initiation of amiodarone therapy
- electrocardiogram (ECG) should be monitored daily for 5 days after the initiation of amiodarone therapy for an increase in QT interval of greater than 25% and if this occurs, stop the interacting drug

PROCAINAMIDE

- amiodarone therapy in patients receiving procainamide results in decreased renal clearance of procainamide
- when amiodarone therapy is initiated in patients receiving procainamide, the procainamide dosage should be decreased by 20–25% and a serum procainamide and *N*-acetylprocainamide concentration should be obtained 3 days after the initiation of amiodarone therapy
- ECG should be monitored daily for 3 days for an increase in QT interval of greater than 25% and if this occurs, stop the interacting drug

FLECAINIDE

- amiodarone therapy in patients receiving flecainide results in increased serum flecainide concentrations
- when amiodarone therapy is initiated in patients receiving flecainide, the flecainide dosage should be decreased by 50% and a serum flecainide concentration should be determined 2 weeks after the initiation of amiodarone therapy

PHENYTOIN

- amiodarone inhibits the hepatic metabolism of phenytoin
- magnitude of this interaction is variable and difficult to predict
- monitor serum phenytoin concentrations weekly until a new steady state is established or until symptoms of toxicity occur, and adjust the dosage accordingly

Drugs that may have their effect or toxicity decreased by amiodarone

- none

▶ *What Route and Dosage Should I Use?*

How to administer

- orally—with or without food
- parenterally—not available

Ventricular tachycardia, supraventricular arrhythmias

Loading regimens

- reasonable approach to amiodarone loading is 1000 mg PO daily (400, 400, and 200 mg divided Q8H) for 1 week, 800 mg PO daily (400 and 400 mg divided Q12H) for 1 week, and then 600 mg PO daily (400 and 200 mg divided Q12H) for 2 weeks
- several amiodarone loading regimens have been described in the literature (Am Heart J 1983;106:951–956, Circulation 1986;

73:1231–1238, Am Heart J 1990;120:1356–1363), with high dosages for 5–14 days followed by tapering dosages until a maintenance dosage of 100–400 mg daily is achieved; however, the merits of the various regimens are unknown

Maintenance dosage

- 400 mg PO daily for the treatment of ventricular arrhythmias
- 200 mg PO daily for the treatment of supraventricular arrhythmias

Dosage adjustments for renal or hepatic dysfunction

- hepatically metabolized
- no dosage adjustments required for renal or hepatic impairment

▶ What Should I Monitor with Regard to Efficacy and Toxicity?

Efficacy

Ventricular tachycardia, supraventricular arrhythmias

Serum concentrations

- therapeutic range of amiodarone and desethylamiodarone together is usually quoted as 1–2.5 mg/L
- range of serum amiodarone concentrations required for efficacy varies widely among patients
- if therapeutic monitoring is performed, use the method of monitoring target serum amiodarone concentrations (Clin Pharmacokinet 1991;20:151–166) (see drug monograph on quinidine)

Electrocardiography or Holter monitoring

- presence or absence of arrhythmia and reduced frequency of arrhythmia episodes

Vital signs

- symptoms associated with arrhythmia (palpitations, shortness of breath, chest pain, or syncope)

Toxicity

Thyroid function

- amiodarone may cause clinical hyperthyroidism or hypothyroidism
- patients should have thyroid function tests performed prior to the initiation of therapy
- frequent serial thyroid function tests are not necessary, but thyroid function tests should be performed if signs or symptoms of hyperthyroidism or hypothyroidism develop
- amiodarone therapy should be discontinued if patients experience clinical hyperthyroidism or hypothyroidism that is unresponsive to medical therapy

Congestive heart failure

- patients with left ventricular dysfunction who are receiving amiodarone should be monitored for symptoms of worsening heart failure
- amiodarone therapy should be discontinued if symptoms of worsening congestive heart failure develop

Cardiac arrhythmias

- ECG should be monitored at baseline, at 2 months after the initiation of therapy, and every 6 months thereafter for the development of new arrhythmias, increase in QT interval of greater than 50%, and sinus bradycardia or AV block
- if QT interval increases to between 25 and 50%, decrease the dose by 50%
- if the QT interval increases by greater than 50%, stop drug
- amiodarone therapy should be discontinued if new cardiac arrhythmias develop

Pulmonary effects

- amiodarone may cause pneumonitis or pulmonary fibrosis
- patients should undergo a baseline chest X-ray and pulmonary function tests prior to initiating amiodarone therapy
- regular serial chest X-rays and pulmonary function tests are not necessary but should be performed if cough or dyspnea develops
- amiodarone therapy should be discontinued if pulmonary toxicity develops
- in addition to stopping amiodarone, prednisone 60 mg daily may be used if symptoms warrant immediate resolution and tapered down and discontinued over 2–6 months

Gastrointestinal effects

- patients should be monitored for nausea, constipation, and anorexia, which have been reported in 5–80% of patients receiving amiodarone
- dosage reduction of 50% may alleviate gastrointestinal adverse effects
- discontinuation of therapy is usually not required

Liver

- amiodarone may cause transient, asymptomatic elevations in liver enzymes and cause hepatitis in approximately 0.3% of patients
- baseline liver function test results should be obtained prior to the initiation of amiodarone therapy and every 6 months during therapy
- discontinuation of amiodarone therapy is not required unless evidence of cholestatic injury or hepatomegaly develops
- asymptomatic elevations in liver function test results often normalize over several weeks without discontinuation of therapy

Neurological findings

- patients should be monitored for tremor, which may occur in up to 39% of patients
- in addition, patients should be monitored for ataxia (incidence of approximately 37%) and peripheral neuropathy (incidence of approximately 6–10%)
- in patients who experience neurological toxicity, the dosage of amiodarone should be decreased, and if symptoms do not resolve, discontinuation of therapy is warranted
- to minimize the risk of central nervous system toxicity, the sum of plasma amiodarone and desethylamiodarone concentrations should be maintained below 2.5 mg/L (Clin Pharmacokinet 1991;20:151–166)

Ocular findings

- amiodarone therapy results in bilateral symmetrical corneal microdeposits in nearly 100% of patients
- although these microdeposits are usually asymptomatic, some patients have blurred vision, photophobia, and blue-green halos around objects
- patients should have baseline ophthalmological examinations prior to the initiation of therapy and on the development of symptoms
- discontinuation of therapy is not required unless visual disturbances occur

Dermatological effects

- patients receiving amiodarone should be warned that photosensitivity (incidence of approximately 5–20%) and blue-gray discoloration of the skin (incidence of approximately 1–7%) may occur
- discontinuation of therapy is usually not required

▶ How Long Do I Treat Patients with This Drug?

Ventricular tachycardia, supraventricular arrhythmias

- because amiodarone therapy is required in patients with serious symptomatic cardiac arrhythmias refractory to other forms of therapy and because many patients receiving the drug are at risk for sudden cardiac death due to arrhythmias, amiodarone therapy is required indefinitely

▶ How Do I Decrease or Stop the Administration of This Drug?

- may be stopped abruptly because of amiodarone's extremely long half-life

▶ What Should I Tell My Patient About This Drug?

- contact your physician if you have shortness of breath, coughing, fever, chest pain, palpitations, dizziness, tremors, difficulty in walking, numbness of the hands or feet, nausea, anorexia, or disturbances in vision
- avoid the sun if possible, and if not possible, use a sunscreen (at least sun protection factor [SPF] 15) when spending time in the sun

▶ Therapeutic Tips

- range of serum amiodarone concentrations required for efficacy varies widely among patients, and therefore, the therapeutic range is of relatively little use in monitoring the efficacy of amiodarone

Useful References

Greene HL. The efficacy of amiodarone in the treatment of ventricular tachycardia or ventricular fibrillation. Prog Cardiovasc Dis 1989; 31:319–354

Kopelman HA, Horowitz LN. Efficacy and toxicity of amiodarone for the treatment of supraventricular tachycardia. Prog Cardiovasc Dis 1989;31:355–366

Lesko LJ. Pharmacokinetic drug interactions with amiodarone. Clin Pharmacokinet 1989;17:130–140

Wilson JS, Podrid PJ. Side effects from amiodarone. Am Heart J 1991; 121;158–171

AMITRIPTYLINE

Lyle K. Laird and Julia Vertrees

USA (Elavil, Endep, Enovil, others)
CANADA (Apo-Amitriptyline, Elavil, Levate, Novotriptyn)

▶ *When Should I Use This Drug?*

Major depression, dysthymia, panic disorder, generalized anxiety disorder, chronic pain syndromes

- although amitriptyline is often one of the first choices in the pharmacotherapy of depressive illnesses and is as effective as other antidepressants in treating depression, it causes the highest incidence of anticholinergic adverse effects and sedation
- as initial therapy, imipramine should be chosen over amitriptyline; however, if a patient has had a good response with amitriptyline and no adverse effects, continue the therapy
- may still be the most effective drug for some patients with agitated depression owing to its sedative properties

Migraine prophylaxis

- useful for prophylaxis in patients with tension-type headaches, mixed headache syndrome, or migraine both with and without depressive features
- is effective in preventing migraine headaches and is often used as an alternative drug of choice when beta-blockers cannot be used
- imipramine does not appear to be as effective as amitriptyline for migraine prophylaxis

▶ *When Should I Not Use This Drug?*

see Imipramine

▶ *What Contraindications Are There to the Use of This Drug?*

see Imipramine

Pregnancy

- adequate human studies have not been done

▶ *What Drug Interactions Are Clinically Important?*

see Imipramine

▶ *What Route and Dosage Should I Use?*

How to administer

- orally—can be given with food or on an empty stomach
- parenterally—intramuscular form available but is painful and has not been shown to work faster

Major depression, dysthymia, general anxiety disorders

- 50 mg PO daily at bedtime
- increase after 3 days to 100 mg PO daily at bedtime
- increase to 150 mg PO daily at bedtime after 1 week and leave at this dosage for 10–14 days
- if target symptoms are not improving after 3 weeks of therapy, continue to increase the daily dose by 50 mg at weekly intervals until a response is seen or a dosage of 300 mg PO daily has been reached
- in geriatric patients and patients with a seizure history, start with 25 mg PO at bedtime, and in general, dosages should be approximately 50% of those used in younger patients

- amitriptyline has a long duration of action; hence, long-acting or sustained-release products are unnecessary and once-daily dosing is appropriate in adults
- after the patient has experienced a therapeutic response, the dosage should be maintained at this level for 6–9 months because relapses may occur if a dosage reduction is attempted

Panic disorder, chronic pain syndromes

- dosages are often lower than those cited above
- start with 10 mg PO daily, as clinicians have noticed that these patients do not tolerate the adverse effects as well
- for panic disorders, titrate the dose up by 10–25 mg/wk and aim for a maximum of 150 mg as the total daily dose
- in chronic pain syndromes, the usual effective dosage range is 25–50 mg PO daily and amitriptyline is generally used as adjuvant therapy

Migraine prophylaxis

- give 10 mg PO daily at bedtime and increase by 10 mg every 3–4 days until an effect is seen or a total dose of 50 mg is given
- leave at this dosage for 4 weeks before considering the drug ineffective

Dosage adjustments for renal or hepatic dysfunction

- hepatically metabolized
- in patients with decreased renal or hepatic function, start with low doses as for geriatric patients

▶ *What Should I Monitor with Regard to Efficacy and Toxicity?*

Efficacy

see Imipramine

Plasma concentration

- there is no benefit to be derived from routine monitoring of amitriptyline serum concentrations (Applied Pharmacokinetics: Principles of Therapeutic Drug Monitoring 1987:852–907)

Migraine prophylaxis • Frequency and severity of headache

- the patient with frequent migraine may need evaluation at 2–4 week intervals during the initial dose titration, then the time between follow-up visits may be extended in patients showing response to treatment

Toxicity

see Imipramine

- amitriptyline and doxepin cause the highest incidence of sedation and anticholinergic effects among the tricyclic antidepressants

▶ *How Long Do I Treat Patients with This Drug?*

see Imipramine

Migraine prophylaxis

- 4 week trial period should be used before the drug is considered ineffective
- in the patient achieving a headache-free state, therapy should be reduced or withdrawn after 6 months to assess continued requirements
- if patient has return of headaches, continual prophylactic therapy should be considered

▶ *How Do I Stop or Decrease the Administration of This Drug?*

see Imipramine

▶ *What Should I Tell My Patients About This Drug?*

see Imipramine

▶ *Therapeutic Tips*

see Imipramine

Useful References

Bryant SG, Brown CS. Major depressive disorders. In: Young LY, Koda-Kimble MA, eds. Applied Therapeutics: The Clinical Use of Drugs, 4th ed. Vancouver, WA: Applied Therapeutics, 1988:1231–1253

Wells BG, Hayes PE. Depressive illness. In: DiPiro JT, Talbert RL, Hayes PE, et al, eds. Pharmacotherapy: A Pathophysiologic Approach. New York: Elsevier, 1989:748–764

Applied Pharmacokinetics: Principles of Therapeutic Drug Monitoring. Spokane, WA: Applied Therapeutics, 1987:852–907

AMOXAPINE

Lyle K. Laird and Julia Vertrees

USA (Asendin, others)
CANADA (Asendin)

▶ When Should I Use This Drug?

Consider an alternative agent

- amoxapine is no more effective than other antidepressants and does not work any faster than other antidepressants
- amoxapine has some antipsychotic properties; however, if a patient is psychotic and depressed, use a combination of an antipsychotic and an antidepressant, which allows better dosage adjustment
- offers no advantages over the other antidepressants and may cause tardive dyskinesia

AMOXICILLIN

John Rotschafer and Kyle Vance-Bryan

USA (Amoxil, Larotid, Polymox, Robamox, Trimox, Wymox, Sumox, Utimox)
CANADA (Amoxican, Apo-Amoxi, Moxilean, Novamoxin, Penamox, Polymox)

▶ When Should I Use This Drug?

see antibiotic susceptibility chart (Table 4–1 in Chapter 4)

Otitis media

- amoxicillin is the drug of choice for the initial treatment of acute otitis media because it is inexpensive and causes fewer adverse effects than does trimethoprim-sulfamethoxazole
- trimethoprim-sulfamethoxazole can be chosen over amoxicillin in patients who require BID dosing (versus TID dosing for amoxicillin) or are penicillin allergic
- although some clinicians suggest that guidelines for antibiotic use be set by the frequency of beta-lactamase–producing organisms, this information is not readily available because cultures of the middle ear are rarely done

Sinusitis, acute mastoiditis, acute exacerbations of chronic bronchitis

- as above for otitis media

Pneumonia

- for the treatment of mild to moderate community-acquired pneumonia, amoxicillin can be used in patients with a history of intolerance of erythromycin
- amoxicillin covers most common pathogens, with the exception of *Mycoplasma, Legionella,* and *Chlamydia*

Lower urinary tract infection (cystitis), asymptomatic bacteriuria, catheter-related infection

- amoxicillin is useful for these infections in patients allergic to trimethoprim-sulfamethoxazole (trimethoprim-sulfamethoxazole has convenient twice-daily dosing versus TID dosing for amoxicillin)

Animal bites (including cat, dog, rat, raccoon, skunk, and bat)

- empirical drug of choice for these infections is usually amoxicillin-clavulanate (covers staphylococci better than amoxicillin alone does)
- therapy should be based on a culture and Gram stain of the infected site (if staphylococci are present or suspected, choose amoxicillin-clavulanate; otherwise, use amoxicillin)

Bacterial endocarditis prophylaxis

- amoxicillin is the drug of choice for patients who are undergoing dental, oral, or respiratory tract procedures and who are able to tolerate oral agents

- use amoxicillin instead of penicillin V because it is better absorbed from the gastrointestinal tract and provides higher, more sustained serum concentrations

▶ When Should I Not Use This Drug?

Cellulitis

- use cloxacillin or nafcillin because most staphylococcal organisms produce beta-lactamases and are not sensitive to amoxicillin

Lyme disease

- tetracycline is the drug of choice for the treatment of the early stages of the disease, and ceftriaxone is recommended in late disease, especially if patients have neurological complications

Chronic mastoiditis

- usually a polymicrobial infection that necessitates surgery; base therapy on the results of cultures and sensitivity studies

Shigellosis

- use ciprofloxacin or norfloxacin

Infections caused by *Klebsiella pneumoniae, Staphylococcus aureus, Pseudomonas* spp., *Acinetobacter* spp., *Enterobacter* spp., *Serratia marcescens, Citrobacter* spp., *Bacteroides fragilis,* beta-lactamase–producing strains of *Haemophilus influenzae,* and *Moraxella (Branhamella) catarrhalis*

- amoxicillin is not active against these organisms

▶ What Contraindications Are There to the Use of This Drug?

see Penicillin

▶ What Drug Interactions Are Clinically Important?

see Penicillin

▶ What Route and Dosage Should I Use?

How to administer

- orally—may take with food or milk or on an empty stomach
- parenterally—not available

Sinusitis, otitis media, acute mastoiditis, acute exacerbations of chronic bronchitis, pneumonia, lower urinary tract infection (cystitis), asymptomatic bacteriuria, catheter-related infection, animal bites (including cat, dog, rat, raccoon, skunk, and bat)

- 500 mg PO TID

Bacterial endocarditis prophylaxis

- 3 g PO 1 hour before the procedure and 1.5 g PO 6 hours after the first dose

Dosage adjustments for renal or hepatic dysfunction

- renally eliminated

Normal Dosing Interval	C_{cr} >60 mL/min or 1 mL/s	C_{cr} 30–60 mL/min or 0.5-1 mL/s	C_{cr} <30 mL/min or 0.5 mL/s
Q8H	no adjustment needed	Q12H	Q24H

▶ What Should I Monitor with Regard to Efficacy and Toxicity?

Efficacy

- for antibiotic monitoring guidelines, see specific section on drug therapy

Toxicity

see Ampicillin

▶ How Long Do I Treat Patients with This Drug?

Sinusitis, otitis media, acute mastoiditis, acute exacerbations of chronic bronchitis

- usual duration of therapy is 7 days or 4–5 days after the patient has become afebrile and clinically improved

Pneumonia

- if the patient responds rapidly, a 10 day course of therapy is sufficient

Lower urinary tract infection (cystitis)

- single high-dose therapy is likely effective; however, with 3 day therapy, patients take antibiotics for the duration of their symptoms and there may be a slightly lower relapse rate
- patients should be instructed to telephone or return to the physician if no response is seen after a 3 day treatment

Asymptomatic bacteriuria

- treat for 3 days, 7 days if pregnant (Ann Intern Med 1991;114: 713–719)

Catheter-related infection

- treat for 5 days (Geriatrics 1988;43[8]:43–48)

Animal bites (including cat, dog, rat, raccoon, skunk, and bat)

- usual duration of therapy is 7–14 days or 4–5 days after the patient has become afebrile and clinically improved

Bacterial endocarditis prophylaxis

- 2 doses

▶ How Do I Stop or Decrease the Administration of This Drug?

- may be stopped abruptly

▶ What Should I Tell My Patients About This Drug?

see Penicillin

▶ Therapeutic Tips

see Penicillin

Useful References

Wright AJ, Wilkowske CJ. The penicillins. Mayo Clin Proc 1987;62:806–820

AMOXICILLIN-CLAVULANATE

John Rotschafer, Kyle Vance-Bryan, and Rick Zabinski

USA (Augmentin)
CANADA (Clavulin)

▶ When Should I Use This Drug?

see antibiotic susceptibility chart (Table 4–1 in Chapter 4)

The addition of clavulanic acid extends the activity of amoxicillin to include beta-lactamase–producing strains of *Haemophilus influenzae, Escherichia coli, Proteus* spp., *Klebsiella pneumoniae, Staphylococcus aureus* or *S. epidermidis* (but not methicillin-resistant strains), *Moraxella (Branhamella) catarrhalis, Neisseria gonorrhoeae,* and *Legionella pneumophila*

Otitis media

- amoxicillin is the drug of choice for the initial treatment of acute otitis media because it is less expensive than amoxicillin-clavulanate
- use of amoxicillin-clavulanate is limited by its high cost and its tendency to produce diarrhea
- amoxicillin-clavulanate or cefixime (the decision between these agents should be based on cost and tolerability) should be chosen after 2–3 failures with amoxicillin or trimethoprim-sulfamethoxazole
- amoxicillin-clavulanate is chosen over cefaclor, as it does not appear to be associated with serum sickness, which can occur with cefaclor
- erythromycin ethylsuccinate-sulfisoxazole is usually slightly less expensive than amoxicillin-clavulinate; however, it is likely less well tolerated (abdominal pain)
- although some clinicians suggest that guidelines for antibiotic use be guided by the frequency of beta-lactamase–producing organisms, this information is not readily available because cultures of the middle ear are rarely done

Pneumonia

- useful agent for mild to moderately ill patients with pneumonia in which a sputum Gram stain shows gram-negative coccobacilli (*H. influenzae*)
- in many areas, the rate of ampicillin-resistant *H. influenzae* is too high to warrant the empirical use of amoxicillin in patients with a potentially life-threatening infection (pneumonia)
- even in areas with a low incidence, agents with activity against ampicillin-resistant *H. influenzae* (amoxicillin-clavulanate, cefuroxime axetil) should be used until culture and sensitivity testing results are known
- this agent also has good activity against other gram-negative organisms that may be present (e.g., *Klebsiella*)
- decision between cefuroxime axetil and amoxicillin-clavulanate should be based on cost

Sinusitis, acute mastoiditis, acute exacerbations of chronic bronchitis

- as above for otitis media

Animal bites (including cat, dog, rat, raccoon, skunk, and bat), human bite wounds

- can be used as it covers most of the potential organisms; however, it is usually more expensive than cloxacillin-penicillin and has not been demonstrated to be superior to this combination
- use if less expensive than the cloxacillin-penicillin combination

▶ When Should I Not Use This Drug?

First episodes of otitis media

- amoxicillin or trimethoprim-sulfamethoxazole should be tried initially before using a more expensive agent such as amoxicillin-clavulanate

Cellulitis

- use cloxacillin or nafcillin because these agents are less expensive than amoxicillin-clavulanate and are just as effective if staphylococcal or streptocococcal organisms are present

▶ What Contraindications Are There to the Use of This Drug?

- intolerance of or allergic reaction to penicillins or clavulanate

see Penicillin

▶ What Drug Interactions Are Clinically Important?

see Penicillin

▶ What Route and Dosage Should I Use?

How to administer

- orally—may take with food or milk or on an empty stomach

Sinusitis, otitis media, acute mastoiditis, acute exacerbations of chronic bronchitis, pneumonia, animal bites (including cat, dog, rat, raccoon, skunk, and bat), human bite wounds

- 500 mg PO TID

Dosage adjustments for renal or hepatic dysfunction

- renally eliminated

Normal Dosing Interval	C_{cr} >60 mL/min or 1 mL/s	C_{cr} 30–60 mL/min or 0.5–1 mL/s	C_{cr} <30 mL/min or 0.5 mL/s
Q8H	no adjustment needed	Q12H	Q24H

▶ What Should I Monitor with Regard to Efficacy and Toxicity?

Efficacy

- for antibiotic administration monitoring guidelines, see specific section on drug therapy

Toxicity

see Ampicillin

▶ How Long Do I Treat Patients with This Drug?

Sinusitis, otitis media, acute mastoiditis, acute exacerbations of chronic bronchitis

- usual duration of therapy is 7–14 days or 4–5 days after the patient has become afebrile and clinically improved

Pneumonia

- if the patient responds rapidly, a 10 day course of therapy is sufficient

Animal bites (including cat, dog, rat, raccoon, skunk, and bat), human bite wounds

- usual duration of therapy is 7–14 days or 4–5 days after the patient has become afebrile and clinically improved

▶ How Do I Decrease or Stop the Administration of This Drug?

- may be stopped abruptly

▶ What Should I Tell My Patients About This Drug?

see Penicillin

▶ Therapeutic Tips

see Penicillin

Useful References

Wright AJ, Wilkowske CJ. The penicillins. Mayo Clin Proc 1987;62:806–820

AMPHOTERICIN B

Peter Jewesson

USA (Fungizone)
CANADA (Fungizone)

▶ When Should I Use This Drug?

Systemic blastomycosis, histoplasmosis, mucormycosis, sporotrichosis, aspergillosis, and paracoccidioidomycosis

- drug of choice for these infections if rapidly progressing and life-threatening
- with availability of alternative, less toxic agents (e.g., fluconazole) and experimental delivery forms (e.g., liposomal amphotericin B), the role of amphotericin B will change as clinical experience with newer modalities increases

Disseminated candidiasis, cryptococcosis

- drug of choice; however, when fungal resistance is suspected or the infection is considered severe, flucytosine should be added to amphotericin

Cryptococcal meningitis

- amphotericin in combination with flucytosine has been shown to be the treatment of choice in non-AIDS patients (N Engl J Med 1979;301:126) but it is unclear whether it is more effective than amphotericin B alone in AIDS patients (Ann Intern Med 1990;113:183; N Engl J Med 1992;326:83–89)
- add flucytosine to amphotericin B unless there are significant cytopenias, renal impairment or a history of hypersensitivity reactions to flucytosine

Coccidioidomycosis

- drug of choice for severe infections
- use ketoconazole in less severe infections because it is less toxic and less expensive

Empiric therapy in persistently febrile neutropenic patients

- in patient still febrile after 48 hours of appropriate broad spectrum antibacterial therapy or even earlier if systemic fungal infection is suspected (Arch Intern Med 1990;150:2258–2264)

Candida cystitis

- use amphotericin B irrigation if patient is anuric

- also use in patient with a potential fungemia who meets the criteria for systemic amphotericin B therapy

▶ When Should I Not Use This Drug?

Mild fungal infections (e.g., thrush in a non-neutropenic host)

- known to be responsive to less toxic agents such as ketoconazole or fluconazole as risks of toxicity outweigh the benefits

Secondary prevention of cryptococcal meningitis

- fluconazole is now the drug of choice in the secondary prevention (i.e., prophylaxis) of cryptococcal meningitis
- fluconazole, 200 mg PO, daily is clearly the preferred approach (N Engl J Med 1992;326:793–798; N Engl J Med 1991;324:580–584), despite its cost and potential drug interactions, because it has greater efficacy, convenience (once daily oral vs. IV dosing), and tolerance compared with amphotericin B

▶ What Contraindications Are There to the Use of This Drug?

intolerance or allergic reactions to amphotericin B

severe amphotericin-induced hypotension—hypotension is usually infusion rate–related; however, if it is severe despite infusion rate adjustment, amphotericin should be avoided

severe renal dysfunction—amphotericin should be avoided in patients with CrCl < 30 mL/min

▶ What Drug Interactions Are Clinically Important?

Drugs that may increase the effect or toxicity of amphotericin B

CORTICOSTEROIDS

- corticosteroids may enhance potassium depletion caused by amphotericin
- monitor serum potassium concentrations twice weekly and keep potassium in the normal physiological range
- may be useful to place all patients on 40–80 mEq of potassium replacement daily while patient is receiving this combination

DIURETICS, AMINOGLYCOSIDES, VANCOMYCIN, CISPLATIN

- increased probability of nephrotoxicity
- no change in monitoring frequency; just be aware of the potential for toxicity

Drugs that may decrease the effect of amphotericin B

- none

Drugs that may have their effect or toxicity increased by amphotericin B

DIGOXIN

- amphotericin B–induced hypokalemia can increase the risk of digoxin toxicity

Drugs that may have their effect decreased by amphotericin B

- none

▶ What Route and Dosage Should I Use?

How to administer

Parenterally

- for peripheral lines the manufacturer recommends diluting amphotericin B in D_5W to 0.1 mg/mL (precipitates in saline)
- concentrations up to 1.4 mg/mL in D_5W are stable in vitro and may be useful for volume-overloaded patients (this concentration must be given via a central line)
- infuse over 2–6 hours daily (2 hours if central line and if patient has no preexisting cardiac dysfunction or electrolyte imbalances)
- individualize infusion duration to reduce delivery time, potential for infusion-related incompatibilities, and need for additional IV lines
- to determine minimum tolerated infusion duration, reduce duration of infusion by 30 minutes daily (to a minimum of 2 hours) until intolerance demonstrated (e.g., fever and chills, hypotension, nausea and vomiting, etc.), then increase by 30 minutes and administer further doses over this period

Topical regimens

- 5–50 mg of amphotericin B in 1000 mL of sterile water for continuous irrigation or 25–50 mg/L in 100–200 mL for intermittent instillation into bladder (dose and choice of regimen are controversial)

Intrathecal injection

- 0.25–0.5 mg in 5 mL $D_{10}W$ into lumbar puncture site following a 25-mg hydrocortisone LP injection while patient is in Trendelenburg position
- intrathecal amphotericin B is usually not indicated because of significant risks of complications and should be used only if agents such as fluconazole cannot be used

Systemic fungal infections

- optimal parenteral dosage regimen (dilution characteristics, rate of infusion, daily and total dose) remain controversial
- while a test dose is often recommended, it is not a good predictor of a severe reaction and the indication for amphotericin B is usually severe enough to warrant
- a common maintenance dose is 0.6 mg/kg/day
- a daily dose of 1.0 mg/kg/day can be given for severe infections (as tolerated by patient)
- doses up to 1.5 mg/kg have been used for uncommon resistant infections (*Fusarium* spp.)
- since amphotericin has a serum elimination $t_{1/2}$ of about 24 hours, a dosing interval of every two days is probably adequate for the treatment of less severe infections, facilitates outpatient therapy, and could be used if the patient is past the acute phase of the infection
- the total recommended dose/duration of therapy is indicated below

Blastomycosis

- 2 g total dose

Histoplasmosis

- 2–3 weeks for prolonged or severe pulmonary histoplasmosis
- 2–3 g total dose for disseminated or chronic pulmonary histoplasmosis

Mucormycosis

- 30–40 mg/kg over 2–3 months

Sporotrichosis

- 2–3 months

Aspergillosis

- 4–12 weeks

Paracoccidioidomycosis

- 4–12 weeks

Disseminated candidiasis

- 6–12 weeks or longer

Cryptococcal meningitis

- continue 0.7 mg/kg IV daily until there is marked improvement (usually 2–3 weeks), then complete 10-week course with fluconazole, 400 mg PO daily (N Engl J Med 1992;327:565)

Coccidioidomycosis

- 1 g total dose

Empiric therapy in persistently febrile neutropenic patients

- if no documented fungal infection, continue until patient afebrile for 2 days and resolution of severe neutropenia (granulocytes > 0.5 G/L) (Arch Intern Med 1990;150:2258–2264)

Candida cystitis

- start with an intermittent dose of 25 mg in 100–200 mL every 6 hours with tube clamping for at least 60 minutes
- if this is ineffective increase dose to 50 mg

Dosage adjustments for renal/liver dysfunction

- eliminated by biliary tract and other unknown routes

Normal Dosing Interval	C_{cr} >60 mL/min or 1.0 mL/s	C_{cr} 30–60 mL/min or 0.5–1.0 mL/s	C_{cr} <30 mL/min or 0.5 mL/s
Q24H	no adjustment needed	extend interval to Q2days	avoid drug if possible

▶ *What Should I Monitor with Regard to Efficacy and Toxicity?*

Efficacy

Blastomycosis, histoplasmosis, mucormycosis, sporotrichosis, aspergillosis, and paracoccidioidomycosis, disseminated candidiasis, coccidioidomycosis, empiric therapy in persistently febrile neutropenic patients

Signs and symptoms

- serial monitoring to identify resolution of clinical signs and symptoms
- reduced fever, healed ulcerations and erosions, stabilized blood pressure
- resolution of any positive funduscopic examination features (exudates, hemorrhages, inflammation)

Microbiology

- if originally positive, repeat cultures if sterile body sites should become negative

Candida cystitis

- repeat urine culture within 48 hours of discontinuing treatment course to confirm absence of fungal growth

Toxicity

Hypotension

- occasionally observed with first few doses, and, if severe, discontinue drug
- monitor blood pressure prior to and at 5 minutes, 15 minutes, and 30 minutes during infusion on days 1, 2, 3 and continue during subsequent infusions until no changes in blood pressures are observed with the infusion

Fever and rigors

- common during first week but diminish thereafter
- if severe, discontinue infusion and should subside within 4 hours, or give meperidine 25–50 mg IV over 5–10 minutes if chills do not resolve within 15 minutes of stopping infusion
- control with premedications if needed
- 30 minutes prior to infusion, premedicate with aspirin or acetaminophen, 650 mg PO/PR, and repeat Q3H × 2 doses if required (while there is no gold standard regimen, this one has been used with success)
- add diphenhydramine, 50 mg PO/PR, to above regimen if unsuccessful

Anorexia, nausea, and vomiting

- common during first week but diminish thereafter
- control with premedications

Anemia

- >75% of patients demonstrate reduced hematocrit
- iron supplementation will not reverse anemia; transfusion provides only temporary benefit; erythropoietin may be helpful
- monitor hemoglobin twice weekly
- discontinue therapy if severe

Hypokalemia

- results from renal tubular defect
- supplement therapy for all patients with minimum of 40 mmol potassium chloride (not in same IV bag) daily and adjust according to serum potassium concentration
- monitor serum potassium concentrations at least twice weekly

Nephrotoxicity

- observed in most patients but varies in severity

- 15% of patients receiving 2 g total dose and 80% of patients receiving >5 g total dose will have permanent renal damage (severe in latter group)
- results from vasoconstriction and direct toxic effect on renal tubular cell membranes
- if serum creatinine exceeds 2.5 mg/dL (220 umol/L), reduce dose by 50% or to alternate-day therapy (same dose every 48 h) or discontinue drug if alternative drugs are available and acceptable
- monitor serum creatinine concentrations three times weekly
- keep patient well hydrated

Phlebitis

- common
- avoid by administering by central line
- if peripheral line used, adjust concentration to less than 0.1 mg/mL and/or pH to 6.0–6.5 and/or add heparin 0.5 U/mL to IV bag

Pulmonary reactions (acute dyspnea, hypoxemia, interstitial infiltrates)

- occur when coadministered with leukocyte transfusions

▶ *How Long Do I Treat Patients with This Drug?*

Systemic fungal infections

- continue therapy until appropriate dose/duration is reached and therapeutic response has been achieved

▶ *How Do I Decrease or Stop the Administration of This Drug?*

- may be stopped abruptly

▶ *What Should I Tell My Patient About This Drug?*

- drug is toxic but considered to be the standard for the treatment of serious fungal infections
- intensive monitoring will be undertaken to attempt to minimize adverse reactions and ensure adequate therapeutic response
- alert hospital staff regarding any adverse reactions during or following the infusion

▶ *Therapeutic Tips*

- ensure benefits of therapy outweigh risk of toxicity before embarking on a treatment course
- expect that all patients will develop some form of drug-related toxicity and be prepared to interrupt therapy if needed
- an I.D. consult (or alternative available specialist) recommended in patients requiring (or suspected to require) amphotericin B
- use with caution in pregnant women; no known teratogenicity; however, typical toxicities can be expected in both mother and fetus
- intranasal or aerosolized amphotericin has been used experimentally as a prophylactic agent to prevent invasive aspergillosis; however, no controlled trials have been performed

Useful References

Bennett JE. Antifungal Agents. In: Mandell GL, Douglas RG Jr, Bennett JE, eds. Principles and Practice of Infectious Diseases, 3rd ed. New York: Churchill Livingstone, 1990:361–370.
Hoeprich PD, Rinaldi MG. Candidosis. In: Hoeprich PD, Jordan MC. Infectious Diseases, 4th ed. Philadelphia: JB Lippincott, 1989;465–481.

AMPICILLIN

John Rotschafer, Kyle Vance-Bryan, and Rick Zabinski

USA (A-Cillin, Alpen-N, Amcill, Amperil, Omnipen, Pensyn, Penbritine, Polycillin)
CANADA (Amcill, Ampicin, Apo-Ampi, Biosan, Novo Ampicillin, Penbritin)

▶ *When Should I Use This Drug?*

see antibiotic susceptibility chart (Table 4–1 in Chapter 4)

Upper urinary tract infections

- drug of choice (in combination with gentamicin) if patients have severe systemic pyelonephritis or if the sensitivities of organisms are not known

- ampicillin and gentamicin have activity against organisms that commonly cause urinary tract infection: *Escherichia coli, Proteus* sp., *Klebsiella-Enterobacter* sp., *Pseudomonas aeruginosa,* and *Enterococcus*

Pneumonias

- useful in patients with pneumonia after it is proved to be caused by sensitive strains of *Haemophilus influenzae* and/or *Streptococcus pneumoniae*
- in many areas, the rate of ampicillin-resistant *H. influenzae* is too high to warrant the empirical use of ampicillin in patients with a potentially life-threatening infection
- even in areas with a low incidence of *H. influenzae*, agents with activity against ampicillin-resistant *H. influenzae* (cefuroxime) should be used until culture and sensitivity testing results are known
- if pneumonia is caused by *S. pneumoniae* alone, use penicillin G

Meningitis

- ampicillin covers *S. pneumoniae* and *Neisseria meningitidis, Listeria monocytogenes,* and ampicillin-sensitive *H. influenzae,* which are the most common organisms in the adult patient population
- useful as empirical therapy in combination with chloramphenicol if the cerebrospinal fluid Gram stain is not yet available or the Gram stain shows no organisms
- use in conjunction with cefotaxime or ceftriaxone, especially in adults 50 years or older or patients with a history of head injury, concurrent sinusitis, otitis media, pneumonia or epiglottitis, diabetes, alcoholism, or hypogammaglobulinemia, as these agents are necessary to cover ampicillin-resistant *H. influenzae* and other gram-negative organisms that may be present in this population (Infect Dis Clin North Am 1990;4:645–659)

Endocarditis

- useful (in combination with gentamicin), if endocarditis is caused by susceptible strains of *Streptococcus faecalis* (penicillin G is also effective)

Bacterial endocarditis prophylaxis

- drug of choice for bacterial endocarditis prophylaxis in patients unable to take oral medications
- used in conjunction with gentamicin for genitourinary or gastrointestinal procedures

Intraabdominal infections

- drug of choice in conjunction with cefotaxime or ceftriaxone for spontaneous bacterial peritonitis in cirrhotics, as this regimen covers enterococci, Enterobacteriaceae, and aerobic streptococci
- ampicillin plus an aminoglycoside may be used; however, some studies suggest that there is an increased incidence of nephrotoxicity in cirrhotic patients receiving aminoglycosides, but this is not yet clearly delineated (Gastroenterology 1982;82:97–105, Hepatology 1985;5:457–462)
- add ampicillin to regimens (e.g., metronidazole and gentamicin) for other intraabdominal infections if enterococcus is the predominant organism seen on culture

▶ *When Should I Not Use This Drug?*

Oral administration

- oral ampicillin is not recommended (use amoxicillin) because amoxicillin is better absorbed, can be taken with food, is given TID versus QID, and has fewer side effects

Shigellosis

- fluoroquinolones are now the drugs of choice

Streptococcus pneumoniae

- use penicillin because it is less expensive

Soft tissue infections

- use cloxacillin/nafcillin or cefazolin because most staphylococcal organisms produce beta-lactamases and are not sensitive to ampicillin

Intraabdominal infections

- unless enterococci are proven or suspected

***Klebsiella pneumoniae, Staphylococcus aureus, Pseudomonas* spp., *Acinetobacter* spp., *Enterobacter* spp., *Serratia marcescens, Citrobacter* spp., and *Bacteroides fragilis* infections**

- ampicillin is inactive against many strains of these organisms

▶ *What Contraindications Are There to the Use of This Drug?*

see Penicillin

▶ *What Drug Interactions Are Clinically Important?*

see Penicillin

▶ *What Route and Dosage Should I Use?*

How to administer

- orally—use amoxicillin instead of ampicillin
- parenterally—administer intravenously in 100 mL of IV fluid (normal saline or 5% dextrose in water) and infuse over 30 minutes

Upper urinary tract infections, pneumonias, intraabdominal infections

- 1 g IV Q6H for mild to moderate infections
- 2 g IV Q6H for severe infections

Meningitis, endocarditis

- 2 g IV Q4H

Bacterial endocarditis prophylaxis

- 2 g IV or IM 30 minutes before the procedure or at induction of anesthesia and 1 g IV or IM 6 hours after the first dose

Dosage adjustments for renal or hepatic dysfunction

- renally eliminated

Normal Dosing Interval	$C_{cr} > 60$ mL/min or 1 mL/s	C_{cr} 30–60 mL/min or 0.5–1 mL/s	$C_{cr} < 30$ mL/min or 0.5 mL/s
Q4H	no adjustment needed	Q6H	Q8H
Q6H	no adjustment needed	Q8H	Q12H

▶ *What Should I Monitor with Regard to Efficacy and Toxicity?*

Efficacy

- for antibiotic monitoring guidelines, see specific section on drug therapy

Toxicity

see Penicillin

▶ *How Long Do I Treat Patients with This Drug?*

Upper urinary tract infections

- 14 days of IV and PO therapy
- consider switching to oral amoxicillin (500 mg PO Q8H) after the patient has become afebrile and has clinically improved for 1–2 days

Pneumonias

- usual duration of therapy is 10 days or 4–5 days after the patient has become afebrile and has clinically improved
- consider switching to oral amoxicillin (500 mg PO Q8H) after the patient has become afebrile and has clinically improved for 1–2 days

Meningitis

- 10 days for patients who respond quickly if meningitis is caused by *N. meningitidis* or *H. influenzae;* however, treat for 14 days if the patient responds slowly

Endocarditis

- 4 weeks

Bacterial endocarditis prophylaxis

- 2 doses

Intraabdominal infections

- treatment should continue for 10 days; however, extend therapy if the patient has not been asymptomatic for 72 hours

▶ *How Do I Decrease or Stop the Administration of This Drug?*

- may be stopped abruptly

▶ *What Should I Tell My Patients About This Drug?*

see Penicillin

▶ *Therapeutic Tips*

- instead of oral ampicillin use oral amoxicillin because it has better absorption, causes less diarrhea and skin rash, can be given via TID versus QID dosing, may be given with food, and when given TID, is usually less expensive than ampicillin

see Penicillin

Useful References

Wright AJ, Wilkowske CJ. The penicillins. Mayo Clin Proc 1987;62:806–820

AMPICILLIN-SULBACTAM

John Rotschafer, Kyle Vance-Bryan, and Rick Zabinski

USA (Unasyn)
CANADA (not available)

▶ *When Should I Use This Drug?*

Consider an alternative agent

- limited clinical usefulness as empirical therapy for acute infections because there are equally efficacious, less expensive agents available
- may be of value for infection due to beta-lactamase–producing enterococci

Useful References

Wright AJ, Wilkowske CJ. The penicillins. Mayo Clin Proc 1987;62:806–820
Campoli-Richards DM, Brogden RN. Sulbactam/ampicillin: A review of its antibacterial activity, pharmacokinetic properties, and therapeutic use. Drugs 1987;33:577–609

ANTACIDS (aluminum-magnesium combinations)

James McCormack

USA (multiple products)
CANADA (multiple products)

Products that contain aluminum-magnesium combination

Some of these products contain simethicone, which plays little if any role in the treatment of peptic ulcer disease or gastroesophageal reflux. Product formulations occasionally vary between countries

Suspensions—brand name (the number in parentheses indicates the approximate acid-neutralizing capacity in milliequivalents per 5 mL of suspension)

Alamag (13)
Amphojel 500 (32)
Diovol (13)
Diovol Ex (27)
Gaviscon (4)
Gelusil extra strength (32)
Kudrox (25)
Maalox (14)
Maalox TC (27)
Mylanta (12)
Mylanta-II (19)
Mylanta double strength (32)
Riopan (10)

Riopan plus (28)
Univol (13)

Tablets—brand name (the number in parentheses indicates the approximate acid-neutralizing capacity in milliequivalents per tablet)
Camalox (17)
Diovol (11)
Diovol Ex (28)
Gaviscon extra strength relief formula (8)
Gelusil (11)
Gelusil-400 (20)
Gelusil extra strength (20)
Maalox (23)
Mylanta (8)
Mylanta-II (19)
Rulox No. 1 (10)
Rulox No. 2 (23)

Products containing only aluminum hydroxide

Suspensions—brand name (the number in parentheses indicates the approximate acid-neutralizing capacity in milliequivalents per 5 mL of suspension)
AlternaGEL (16)
Amphojel (10)
Basaljel (14)

▶ When Should I Use This Drug?

Dyspepsia associated with or without duodenal or gastric ulcers, gastro-esophageal reflux

- useful for acute upper gastrointestinal symptoms associated with these conditions
- choice among antacids should be based on cost for equivalent acid-neutralizing ability
- initially, use a combination containing aluminum and magnesium (with low sodium levels) to minimize gastrointestinal adverse effects
- most aluminum-magnesium antacids are low in sodium (check the content of individual products)
- aluminum causes constipation, and magnesium causes diarrhea
- products containing sodium bicarbonate, calcium carbonate, or simethicone offer no advantages over aluminum-magnesium combination products

▶ When Should I Not Use This Drug?

Duodenal or gastric ulcers

- although daily antacid doses equivalent to 180–200 mEq of neutralizing activity divided into 4 doses are as effective as other agents for the treatment of peptic ulcer disease (Scand J Gastroenterol 1986;21:385–391), antacids are generally more expensive, need to be given 4 times daily, and are usually associated with a higher incidence of gastrointestinal adverse effects than are H$_2$ antagonists

Stress ulcer prophylaxis

- although antacids are effective, use H$_2$ antagonists or sucralfate because they produce less toxicity and usually require less frequent administration

Combination with other antiulcer medications, except for use on an as needed basis

- no studies support combination therapy of regularly dosed upper gastrointestinal drugs for the treatment of peptic ulcer disease, and combination therapy increases the cost and the chance of adverse effects (Lancet 1988;1:1383–1385, N Engl J Med 1991; 325:1017–1025, Am J Gastroenterol 1993;88:675–679)

Hyperphosphatemia

- calcium carbonate–containing antacids have been shown to be as effective as, if not more effective than, aluminum hydroxide products in the treatment of hyperphosphatemia due to chronic renal failure (N Engl J Med 1991;324:527–531)
- aluminum hydroxide–containing antacids, although effective, are not recommended because of the concerns about aluminum

toxicity in this patient population (Ann Clin Biochem 1987; 24:337–344, N Engl J Med 1991;324:527–531)

▶ What Contraindications Are There to the Use of This Drug?

- none

▶ What Drug Interactions Are Clinically Important?

Drugs that may increase the effect or toxicity of antacids

- none

Drugs that may decrease the effect of antacids

- none

Drugs that may have their effect or toxicity increased by antacids

- none

Drugs that may have their effect decreased by antacids

H$_2$ ANTAGONIST, SUCRALFATE, TETRACYCLINE

- antacids decrease the absorption of many drugs
- do not take antacids within 1 hour of the administration of other drugs

▶ What Route and Dosage Should I Use?

How to administer

- orally—can be given with food or on an empty stomach

Dyspepsia associated with or without duodenal or gastric ulcers, gastro-esophageal reflux

- usual dose is 30 mL of the regular-strength antacids or 15 mL of the double- or extra-strength antacids as needed for symptoms up to 6 times per day
- usual tablet dose is 2 tablets of regular-strength antacids or 1 tablet of the double- or extra-strength antacids as needed for symptoms up to 6 times per day

Dosage adjustments for renal or hepatic dysfunction

- magnesium and aluminum are renally eliminated
- dosage adjustments for PRN use are not required if the drug is being used only occasionally
- if the drug is used regularly, avoid in patients with an estimated creatinine clearance of less than 30 mL/min (0.5 mL/s) because of concern about increased serum magnesium and aluminum levels

▶ What Should I Monitor with Regard to Efficacy and Toxicity?

Efficacy

Dyspepsia associated with or without duodenal or gastric ulcers, gastroesophageal reflux

- relief of symptoms such as epigastric pain or discomfort; belching; sensations of burning, bloating, and fullness; and nausea and vomiting

Toxicity

Gastrointestinal effects

Diarrhea

- most common adverse effect with aluminum-magnesium antacids
- if diarrhea occurs, use an agent with a higher aluminum hydroxide content
- if a higher aluminum content antacid is not available, alternate doses of an aluminum-magnesium antacid with an aluminum only product

Constipation

- if constipation occurs, use an agent with a higher magnesium content

▶ How Long Do I Treat Patients with This Drug?

Dyspepsia associated with or without duodenal or gastric ulcers, gastroesophageal reflux

- treat for 2 weeks, and if symptoms resolve, stop therapy

- if symptoms are still present, evaluate the cause (Am Fam Physician 1987;35:222–230)

▶ How Do I Decrease or Stop the Administration of This Drug?

- may be stopped abruptly

▶ What Should I Tell My Patients About This Drug?

- it may take several days for this drug to relieve stomach pain
- if no relief of symptoms is seen in 7 days, contact your physician
- this drug interacts with many medications; therefore, take all other medications 1 hour before or 1 hour after taking antacids
- contact your physician if you develop any excessive constipation or diarrhea

▶ Therapeutic Tips

- if diarrhea occurs with proper doses of aluminum-magnesium combination ant-acids, try using alternating doses of an aluminum-containing antacid and the aluminum-magnesium combination

ASPIRIN

Kelly Jones, Terry Baumann, and Jerry Taylor

USA (various generic aspirin, various generic buffered and enteric-coated aspirin)
CANADA (Entrophen, various generic aspirin, various generic buffered and enteric-coated aspirin)

▶ When Should I Use This Drug?

Rheumatoid arthritis

- enteric-coated aspirin is the nonsteroidal antiinflammatory drug (NSAID) to which all other drugs are compared
- many rheumatologists try enteric-coated aspirin as first-line treatment of rheumatoid arthritis because of cost benefits
- enteric-coated aspirin is likely as well tolerated as other NSAIDs
- if gastrointestinal intolerance occurs with enteric-coated aspirin, ibuprofen should be chosen, as it is the next least expensive agent
- aspirin is the preferred agent in patients taking lithium, as aspirin and sulindac are the NSAIDs least likely to decrease lithium clearance and increase lithium toxicity (DICP 1989;23:76–85)
- patients receiving concomitant anticoagulant therapy should be treated with ibuprofen (except if aspirin is being used for cardiovascular prophylaxis), which appears to be safer in patients taking anticoagulants than other NSAIDs (J Am Board Fam Pract 1989;2:257–271, Drug Intell Clin Pharm 1989;23:76–85)

Osteoarthritis

- all NSAIDs, including aspirin, are effective for osteoarthritis and should be considered if maximal doses (4 g/d) of acetaminophen are ineffective
- decision among NSAIDs should be based on cost because no predictive measures are available to determine which agent will work

Acute pain, general aches and pains, bone pain, dysmenorrhea

- aspirin can be used for inflammatory pain but non–enteric-coated aspirin causes more gastrointestinal toxicity than does acetaminophen or ibuprofen
- aspirin is usually slightly less expensive than ibuprofen
- non–enteric-coated aspirin causes more gastric distress than does acetaminophen

Cancer pain, chronic noncancer pain

- aspirin is useful, in conjunction with codeine, for moderate symptoms if treatment with nonopioid agents is ineffective after titrating rapidly to maximum doses
- be aware that, when aspirin is used in combination products with codeine in a round-the-clock fashion, aspirin toxicity may occur from the possible ingestion of large amounts of aspirin

Migraine treatment

- aspirin is effective and safe for the treatment of mild symptoms

- caffeine in conjunction with aspirin is recommended by some clinicians, as it may increase the absorption of the aspirin and may have effects of its own in relieving migraine, but no controlled trials are available
- decision among NSAIDs for the treatment of migraine should be based on cost because no predictive measures are available to determine which agent will work

Migraine prophylaxis

- NSAIDs should be tried in patients not responding to or not able to tolerate beta-blockers, antidepressants, and calcium channel blockers
- drug of choice for prophylaxis in patients with menstrual migraine
- at present, there are no predictive measures for deciding which NSAID a patient will respond to
- aspirin is considered the first-line drug of choice because it is as effective as other NSAIDs and is the least expensive agent
- if the patient is at risk for gastrointestinal intolerance or does not tolerate enteric-coated aspirin, ibuprofen is effective, causes less gastrointestinal tolerance than does non–enteric-coated aspirin, but is more expensive than aspirin

Chronic stable angina

- all patients with proven chronic stable angina (men and women) should be treated with daily aspirin, as aspirin decreases mortality from myocardial infarction and other thromboembolic events (Cardiology 1990;77[suppl 2]:99–109, Lancet 1988;2:349–360, N Engl J Med 1992;327:175–181)

Unstable angina

- all patients with strongly suspected or proven unstable angina should receive an oral aspirin tablet (N Engl J Med 1988; 319:1105–1111), as it has been shown to decrease mortality in unstable angina (N Engl J Med 1983;309:396–403) and its beneficial effects have been confirmed in subsequent studies (N Engl J Med 1985;313:1369–1375, N Engl J Med 1988;319:1105–1111)
- aspirin decreases the progression of unstable angina to myocardial infarction (N Engl J Med 1985;313:1369–1375, N Engl J Med 1983;309:396–403, N Engl J Med 1988;319:1105–1111)

Acute myocardial infarction

- aspirin therapy should be given early to all patients
- routine use of heparin rather than aspirin to reduce mortality or reinfarction after streptokinase cannot be recommended at this time (Chest 1992;102:456S–481S, Lancet 1988;2:349–360)
- aspirin can be used in patients who will require warfarin long term as evidenced by a pilot study of ischemic heart disease (Eur Heart J 1988;836–843) and mechanical heart valves (Can J Cardiol 1991;7[suppl A]:95A)
- aspirin should be continued in all patients indefinitely unless a contraindication exists

Coronary artery bypass

- increases graft patency when compared with placebo (N Engl J Med 1992;327:175–181)

Transient ischemic attacks

- agent of choice because of its antiplatelet activity, low cost, and efficacy (Pharmacotherapy: A Pathophysiologic Approach, 2nd ed. 1988)
- although ticlopidine was shown to be slightly more effective than aspirin (13% incidence of stroke with aspirin versus 10% with ticlopidine), ticlopidine had a higher incidence of adverse effects (diarrhea, rash, and severe neutropenia) (N Engl J Med 1989; 321:501–507)
- ticlopidine is far more expensive and less convenient to take than aspirin

Completed stroke

- drug of choice for male patients after a completed stroke
- aspirin is effective, is well tolerated, and is inexpensive
- in women, there is a suggestion that ticlopidine is slightly more effective (Neurology 1992;42:111–115)

- some clinicians suggest that ticlopidine should be used in patients with significant neurological deficit

Mechanical prosthetic valves

- use aspirin if warfarin is contraindicated, and use in addition to warfarin if the patient experiences systemic embolism while receiving adequate warfarin therapy (Chest 1992;102[suppl]: 445S–455S)

▶ *When Should I Not Use This Drug?*

Combination with other NSAIDs

- combinations of NSAIDs provide no increase in effectiveness compared with that with maximum doses of single agents and significantly increase the risk of adverse effects (this does not apply to patients taking aspirin for stroke or MI prophylaxis)

Severe pain

- not effective for severe pain

Asymptomatic patients for prevention of myocardial infarction or stroke (primary prevention)

- no current evidence supports the routine use of aspirin or other drugs to reduce the incidence of myocardial infarction or stroke (Can Med Assoc J 1991;145:1091–1095, N Engl J Med 1992;327: 175–181)

▶ *What Contraindications Are There to the Use of This Drug?*

Intolerance of or allergic reaction to aspirin

- allergic reactions do occur with NSAIDs as a class and are cross-reactive with aspirin
- patients who are allergic to aspirin or who have the classic rhino-sinusitis, nasal polyps, and asthma triad should avoid aspirin and other NSAIDs
- hypersensitivity reactions can range from fever, rash, headache, abdominal pain, and nausea and vomiting to liver damage and aseptic meningitis (may occur within 48 hours)

Systemic lupus erythematosus

- should not take aspirin owing to the association of hypersensitivity reactions with ibuprofen (J Am Board Fam Pract 1989; 2:257–271, Clin Pharm 1982;1:561–565)

Reye's syndrome

- do not use in children, especially in those who have recently had influenza or chickenpox because of the association with Reye's syndrome

▶ *What Drug Interactions Are Clinically Important?*

Drugs that may increase the effect or toxicity of aspirin

HEPARIN, WARFARIN

- aspirin affects platelet function and can increase the risk of hemorrhage
- use acetaminophen or narcotic analgesics if possible
- after myocardial infarction, low-dose aspirin therapy can be used in combination with warfarin, as the benefit outweighs the risk
- in patients who require high-dose aspirin or NSAIDs to adequately control a life-altering disease (e.g., rheumatoid arthritis), the combination of an NSAID and warfarin can be used; however, keep partial thromboplastin time and/or INR at the lower limit of normal levels and make the patient aware of the potential for bleeding

DIURETICS

- diuretics plus NSAIDs increases the risk of renal failure
- avoid this combination if possible, and if not, monitor serum creatinine, potassium, and weight levels at baseline and every 4 days for 2–3 weeks, then every 2 weeks for 8 weeks, then every month for 3 months, and then as needed (J Musculoskel Med 1991;8[8]:31–46)

PROBENECID

- decreases renal clearance of NSAIDs; therefore, reduce the dosages of NSAID and monitor as for a dosage change

Drugs that may decrease the effect of aspirin

CHOLESTYRAMINE

- binds NSAIDs and decreases absorption; therefore, separate the time of administration by 4 hours

Drugs that may have their effect or toxicity increased by aspirin

POTASSIUM-SPARING DIURETICS

- avoid combination with aspirin if possible, and if not, monitor serum creatinine, potassium, and weight levels at baseline and every 4 days for 2–3 weeks, then every 2 weeks for 8 weeks, then every month for 3 months, and then as needed (J Musculoskel Med 1991;8[8]:31–46)

METHOTREXATE

- NSAIDs decrease the clearance of methotrexate and increase the risk of toxicity
- no problem if using doses for rheumatoid arthritis, but the combination must not be used when high doses (for chemotherapy) of methotrexate are being used
- it is important that, when a patient begins methotrexate therapy, their NSAID therapy not be stopped and started (i.e., be consistent) owing to the potential for drug interaction

Drugs that may have their effect decreased by aspirin

ANTIHYPERTENSIVES

- NSAIDs can reduce the hypotensive effect by causing salt and water retention
- among NSAIDs, aspirin and sulindac appear to have the least hypertensive effect (Ann Intern Med 1994;121:289–300); however, all NSAIDs likely have the potential to worsen blood pressure control and blood pressure should be measured at every follow-up visit in patients who are hypertensive or borderline hypertensive
- avoid NSAIDs, if possible, in patients with hypertension
- in patients who must use NSAIDs ensure the lowest effective dose is being used

DIURETICS

- NSAIDs may oppose the diuretic and natriuretic effects of diuretics and increased doses of diuretics may be required
- avoid combination if at all possible
- in patients who must use NSAIDs, ensure the lowest effective dose is being used

▶ *What Route and Dosage Should I Use?*

How to administer

- orally—take with food or milk
- parenterally—not available
- rectally—can be administered rectally

Rheumatoid arthritis

- 1950 mg PO Q12H as enteric-coated tablets up to a maximum of 5400 mg PO daily
- at high doses, enteric-coated aspirin exhibits zero-order elimination and it can be dosed twice daily

Osteoarthritis

- 975 mg PO Q12H as enteric-coated tablets

Acute pain, general aches and pain, bone pain, dysmenorrhea

- 325–650 mg PO or rectally Q4H as needed up to a maximum of 4000 mg PO daily

Cancer pain, chronic noncancer pain

- 325–650 mg PO Q4H in conjunction with 30 mg of codeine, if required

Migraine treatment

- 1000 mg PO Q4H PRN up to a maximum of 4000 mg PO daily

Migraine prophylaxis

- 650 mg PO Q12H (use enteric-coated aspirin to decrease the risk of adverse effects)

Chronic stable angina, unstable angina, acute myocardial infarction, coronary artery bypass, transient ischemic attacks, mechanical prosthetic valves

- 325 mg (enteric coated) PO daily (Br Med J 1988;296:316)
- although low-dose aspirin (30–75 mg PO daily) has been shown to be effective (N Engl J Med 1991;325:1261–1266, Lancet 1991;338:1345–1349) these dosage forms are sometimes difficult to find and may be more expensive than the 325 mg dose
- if 325 mg is not well tolerated use lower dose version or give 325 mg PO every other day
- start therapy at time of suspected diagnosis with angina or transient ischemic attacks
- start therapy as soon as possible after suspected myocardial infarction
- start therapy within 6–12 hours after surgery (if begun before surgery, the incidence of perioperative bleeding is higher) (N Engl J Med 1992;327:175–181)

Dosage adjustments for renal or hepatic dysfunction

- renal and hepatic elimination

Normal Dosing Interval	C$_{cr}$ > 60 mL/min or 1 mL/s	C$_{cr}$ 30–60 mL/min or 0.5–1 mL/s	C$_{cr}$ < 30 mL/min or 0.5 mL/s
Q4H	no dosage adjustment needed	Q6H	avoid
Q12H	no dosage adjustment needed	Q24H	avoid

▶ *What Should I Monitor with Regard to Efficacy and Toxicity?*

Efficacy

Rheumatoid arthritis

- patient's self-assessment is important in making a clinical decision about whether to try another NSAID
- pain and the ability to conduct normal daily activities are important variables to follow when assessing NSAID efficacy

Osteoarthritis

- pain and the ability to conduct normal activities are important variables to follow when assessing NSAID therapy

Acute pain, general aches and pain, bone pain, dysmenorrhea, cancer pain, chronic noncancer pain

- key to achieving effective pain control is to question patients frequently about the degree of pain they are having
- frequency of pain evaluation should be based on the knowledge of how quickly the drug should work
- decision to give PRN doses or to increase the dosage should be based on the patients' assessment of the pain severity
- remember, pain is whatever the patient says it is
- when a patient's self-assessment is not possible, monitor agitation and heart rate

Migraine treatment

- relief or decrease in the amount of pain within 1–2 hours

Migraine prophylaxis

- evaluate frequency and severity of headache
- patient with frequent migraine may need evaluation at 2–4 week intervals during the initial dose titration, then visits may be extended in patients showing response to treatment

Chronic stable angina

- aspirin does not affect symptoms; therefore, evaluation is limited to the incidence of myocardial infarction

Unstable angina

- relief of chest pain and decreased frequency of chest pain
- incidence of myocardial infarction

Acute myocardial infarction

- relief of chest pain and decreased frequency of chest pain
- reduced incidence of reinfarction

Coronary artery bypass

- occlusion of graft

Occurrence of transient ischemic attacks

- assess the patient monthly initially and tell the patient to contact the physician if any future transient ischemic attacks occur (loss of vision in one eye, dizziness, weakness on one side, numbness in face, arm, or leg)
- if no transient ischemic attacks occur during the first 3 months, assess every 6 months thereafter

Mechanical prosthetic valves

- evidence of transient ischemic attacks or stroke

Toxicity

Salicylism

- excessive salicylate ingestion causes tinnitus, tachypnea, and vomiting
- if this occurs, aspirin should be stopped and restarted at 50% of the previous dose once symptoms have resolved
- if symptoms are intolerable or do not go away with dosage reduction, stop aspirin and use ibuprofen

see Ibuprofen

▶ *How Long Do I Treat Patients with This Drug?*

Rheumatoid arthritis

- if the initial dosage does not work within 7 days after starting the drug therapy, increase to the maximum dosage
- if maximum dosages have not worked within another 7 days, a change in therapy to another NSAID is appropriate
- give the drug a total of 14 days to work
- treatment of rheumatoid arthritis with aspirin or any other NSAID is indefinite
- try to decrease the dosage to the lowest effective level, and the dosage can be decreased during times of disease inactivity to the lowest possible amount to maintain control
- NSAIDs should not be stopped when other second- or third-line agents are added to the treatment of rheumatoid arthritis

Osteoarthritis

- therapy should be continued as long as the drug is effective
- use on a regular basis when pain affects the quality of life
- after pain control is achieved, decrease the daily dosage by 25% every 1–2 weeks until the minimum effective dosage is identified

Acute pain, general aches and pain, bone pain, dysmenorrhea

- use on a regular basis for the duration of the pain
- acute pain should subside within days after the offending event; if this has not occurred within 1 week, further investigate the cause of the pain

Cancer pain, chronic noncancer pain

- therapy may be needed for months or years

Migraine treatment

- initial therapy with aspirin should prevent pain or provide pain relief within a couple of hours
- if headaches are persistent after 1–2 hours, alternative therapy should be instituted

Migraine prophylaxis

- use of prophylactic agents often necessitates adjustment in dosage and may need to be given for several weeks to provide maximum benefit
- if the patient achieves a headache-free state, therapy should be reduced or withdrawn after 6 months to assess continued requirements

Chronic stable angina, unstable angina, acute myocardial infarction, coronary artery bypass, transient ischemic attacks, mechanical prosthetic valves

- treatment should be considered indefinitely

▶ *How Do I Decrease or Stop the Administration of This Drug?*

- may be stopped abruptly if needed

▶ What Should I Tell My Patients About This Drug?

- it is important to be educated about what to expect in terms of onset of relief
- rheumatoid arthritis pain will not go away with 1 dose or with 2 days of therapy, but by 2 weeks, you should experience significant relief
- avoid concomitant use of other NSAIDs, especially over the counter products containing ibuprofen or aspirin
- do not use enteric-coated tablets for acute pain (have a delayed onset of action)
- take aspirin with food, milk, or antacids if gastrointestinal upset occurs and tell your physician of any gastrointestinal intolerance
- notify your physician of any rash, unusual fever, edema, black stools, or weight gain
- take with a full glass of water to prevent esophageal lodging and to facilitate dissolution of the drug
- do not take aspirin if there is a strong vinegar odor from the tablets
- decide whether to use long-acting aspirin preparations because they are expensive
- if self-administering for acute pain for longer than 10 days, seek medical advice

▶ Therapeutic Tips

- use of enteric-coated aspirin may reduce direct local irritation of the gastrointestinal mucosa
- if there is no response, consider a non–enteric-coated product, as some patients may not get an effect from enteric-coated aspirin (especially some generic brands)
- for rheumatoid arthritis, use higher dosages initially and decrease to the lowest effective dosage
- give a 14 day trial at maximum dosages (3.2 g/d) before changing agents
- concurrent administration of acetaminophen (4 g/d) augments the analgesic effects of aspirin without increasing toxicity
- do not use two NSAIDs concomitantly because this may increase toxicity and may reduce the serum concentrations of both agents
- be aware that when aspirin is used in combination products with codeine in a round-the-clock fashion, aspirin toxicity may occur owing to the possible ingestion of large amounts of aspirin

Useful References

Levy RA, Smith DL. Clinical differences among nonsteroidal antiinflammatory drugs: Implications for therapeutic substitution in ambulatory patients. DICP, Ann Pharmacother 1989;23:76–85

Miller LG, Prichard JG. Selecting nonsteroidal anti-inflammatory drugs: Pharmacologic and clinical considerations. J Am Board Fam Pract 1989;2:257–271

Roth SH, Bennett RE. Nonsteroidal anti-inflammatory drug gastropathy. Arch Intern Med 1987;147:2093–2099

ASTEMIZOLE

Penny Miller

USA (Hismanal)
CANADA (Hismanal)

▶ When Should I Use This Drug?

Seasonal allergic rhinitis, chronic (perennial) rhinitis, chronic dermatological allergies (atopic dermatitis, chronic urticaria, pruritus of unknown cause)

- all antihistamines are considered to have relatively the same efficacy in preventing or treating allergic reactions; however, there is great interpatient variation in the response to a given antihistamine
- selection of any particular antihistamine is based on the degree of sedation and anticholinergic effects, plus the convenience of dosing and cost
- astemizole is useful if the patient has sedative effects or would be sensitive to the sedative effects from less expensive antihistamines such as chlorpheniramine
- choice among astemizole, terfenadine, and loratadine should be based on cost
- astemizole has a slow onset of action (3–4 days)

- does not impair psychomotor activity or potentiate ethanol's central nervous system (CNS) effects such as sedation, decreased visual discrimination, and slowed reaction times
- does not lower the seizure threshold (unlike the case with diphenhydramine or chlorpheniramine)
- demonstrates little or no anticholinergic side effects (antihistaminic effects are responsible for the relief of allergic symptoms)

▶ When Should I Not Use This Drug?

Acute allergic reactions

- do not use for acute allergic reactions if a rapid onset of action is desired because it has a slow onset of action and relief of symptoms can take up to 5 days

Common cold

- for the symptoms of sneezing and runny nose, astemizole is not effective because it has little or no anticholinergic effects

Anaphylaxis and angioedema

- not useful because of the slow onset of action

▶ What Contraindications Are There to the Use of This Drug?

- intolerance of or allergic reaction to astemizole
- severe hepatic dysfunction
- heart disease (patients susceptible to prolonged QT intervals) or metabolic disease (disturbances in electrolyte levels)

▶ What Drug Interactions Are Clinically Important?

see Terfenadine

▶ What Route and Dosage Should I Use?

How to administer

- orally—take on an empty stomach or with food or milk (Clin Pharmacokinet 1991;21:372—393)
- parenterally—not available

Seasonal allergic rhinitis, chronic (perennial) rhinitis, chronic dermatological allergies (atopic dermatitis, chronic urticaria, pruritus of unknown cause)

- 10 mg PO daily
- 10 mg PO daily is the maximum recommended dosage

Dosage adjustments for renal or hepatic dysfunction

- hepatically metabolized
- no dosage adjustments are required; titrate the dose up to an effect
- avoid using in patients with hepatic dysfunction

▶ What Should I Monitor with Regard to Efficacy and Toxicity?

Efficacy

see Chlorpheniramine

Toxicity

Mild fatigue, headache, dry mouth, and sedation

- can occur but less often than with chlorpheniramine and is likely not clinically significant

Weight gain

- because it is a serotonin antagonist, weight gain of 1.3–3.1 kg after 8 weeks of use has occurred (Br J Clin Pharmacol 1984; 18:1–8)

Cardiac arrhythmias

- serious cardiac arrhythmias (ventricular tachycardia, torsades de pointes, ventricular fibrillation) and QT prolongation, hypotension, palpitations, and syncope have occurred with dosages 2 or 3 times above the recommended levels and at normal dosages in patients with significant hepatic dysfunction and/or with concomitant administration of drugs that inhibit hepatic metabolism
- avoid the use of this drug in patients who have hepatic dysfunction or are taking interacting drugs, and do not exceed recommended dosages

▶ How Long Do I Treat Patients with This Drug?

see Chlorpheniramine

▶ How Do I Decrease or Stop the Administration of This Drug?

- may be stopped abruptly, as its long half-life allows for its own titration and an effect can be seen for a few days after stopping administration of the drug

▶ What Should I Tell My Patients About This Drug?

- there is a lag period of 3–5 days for symptoms to be maximally alleviated
- allergy skin tests can be inhibited for longer than 1 month after taking a dose
- weight gain of 1.3–3.1 kg after 8 weeks' use has occurred, as this drug can stimulate one's appetite
- episodes of syncope, dizziness, chest pain, shortness of breath, and/or palpitations should be reported to your physician
- do not exceed the recommended dosage of 10 mg PO daily

▶ Therapeutic Tips

- therapeutic effect is seen for up to 3 days after stopping administration of the medication owing to its long half-life
- it was initially thought that food decreased the absorption of astemizole; however, studies have shown this not to be true (Clin Pharmacokinet 1991;21:372–393)
- allergy skin tests can be inhibited for longer than 1 month after taking a dose
- unlike the case with diphenhydramine and chlorpheniramine, there is no additive CNS depression when this drug is combined with alcohol or other CNS depressants

Useful References

Mann KV, Crowe JP, Tietze KJ. Drug reviews. Non-sedating histamine H1 receptor antagonists. Clin Pharm 1989;8:331–344

Sutherland D. Antihistamine agents—New options or just more drugs? On Continuing Practice 1991;18:31–36

Estelle F, Simmons R, Simons KJ. Pharmacokinetic optimization of histamine H1-receptor antagonist therapy. Clin Pharmacokinet 1991;21:372–393

ATENOLOL

Robert Rangno and James McCormack

USA (Tenormin, generic)
CANADA (Tenormin, Apo-Atenol, Novo-Atenol, Nu-Atenol)

▶ When Should I Use This Drug?

Atenolol should be chosen over nadolol if it is less expensive than nadolol, if a beta$_1$-selective agent is required (e.g., in patients with cold extremities), or if a parenteral agent is required (e.g., immediately after a myocardial infarction)

see Nadolol

▶ When Should I Not Use This Drug?

see Nadolol

▶ What Contraindications Are There to the Use of This Drug?

see Nadolol

▶ What Drug Interactions Are Clinically Important?

see Nadolol

▶ What Route and Dosage Should I Use?

How to administer

- orally—should be given with food
- parenterally—administer over 5 minutes (not available in Canada)

Acute (crisis) hypertension

- 100 mg PO daily given immediately

Chronic (noncrisis) hypertension

- 25 mg PO daily
- increase the dosage every 4 weeks by 25 mg PO daily until an effect is seen
- dosage increases up to 100 mg PO daily may be necessary in some patients, but no benefit is likely to result from further increases

Chronic stable angina

- 50 mg PO daily is given for the initial treatment of angina
- increases of 50 mg daily can be made every 3 days until symptoms are controlled or a maximum dosage of 200 mg PO daily is reached
- can also be titrated until exercise-induced heart rate is decreased by 15%

Unstable angina, myocardial infarction

- give 5 mg IV over 5 minutes, and follow with another 5 mg IV 10 minutes later unless heart rate is <60 bpm or systolic blood pressure is <100 mmHg
- patients who tolerate the IV doses should receive 50 mg PO 2 hours after the last IV dose and again in 12 hours
- a dosage of 100 mg PO daily is continued until the patient is discharged from the hospital unless side effects or contraindications occur

Atrial flutter or fibrillation, atrioventricular nodal reentrant tachycardia

- 5 mg IV over 5 minutes and if tolerated (systolic blood pressure >100 mm Hg, heart rate >60 bpm) give a second dose of 5 mg IV 10 minutes later (IV atenolol is not available in Canada)
- do not push IV dose until a response is seen, as beta-blockers do not always work and can precipitate asystole
- parenteral route is used if the patient is symptomatic and the goal is to control the ventricular rate rapidly
- if the patient is not symptomatic and rapid rate control is desired, start with 25 mg PO daily and increase every 2–3 days by 25 mg PO daily until the heart rate is controlled or a maximum dose of 200 mg/d is reached

Ventricular arrhythmias

- give 50 mg PO daily (25 mg PO daily in patients with low blood pressure, patients with a heart rate of <60 bpm, or those receiving concomitant therapy with agents that depress the function of the sinoatrial or atrioventricular nodes), and increase every 2–3 days until beta-blockade is achieved (resting heart rate and heart rate during exercise is suppressed) or a dosage of 100 mg PO daily is reached

Migraine prophylaxis

- 25 mg PO daily
- increase the daily dosage by 25 mg at weekly intervals until therapeutic or toxic effects appears

Esophageal varices rebleeding and portal hypertension

- start with 25 mg PO daily and increase every 2–3 days by 25 mg PO daily until the resting heart rate is reduced by 20–25% or a maximum dosage of 200 mg/d is reached

Thyrotoxicosis, alcohol withdrawal syndrome

- give 25 mg PO and repeat at 2 hour intervals until blood pressure and heart rate are controlled

Situational anxiety, such as performance anxiety in musicians

- 25 mg PO at least 1 hour before the precipitating event

Benign familial tremor

- 25 mg PO daily
- increase the daily dosage by 25 mg PO daily at weekly intervals until therapeutic or toxic effects appear

Dosage adjustment for renal or hepatic dysfunction

- renally eliminated
- in general, even in patients with normal renal function, start with a low dosage and titrate up to an effect

Normal Dosing Interval	$C_{cr} > 60$ mL/min or 1 mL/s	C_{cr} 30–60 mL/min or 0.5–1 mL/s	$C_{cr} < 30$ mL/min or 0.5 mL/s
Q24H	no adjustment needed	decrease dosage by 50%	decrease dosage by 75%

▶ **What Should I Monitor with Regard to Efficacy and Toxicity?**

see Nadolol

▶ **How Do I Decrease or Stop the Administration of This Drug?**

see Nadolol

▶ **What Do I Tell My Patients About This Drug?**

see Nadolol

▶ **Therapeutic Tips**

- patients rarely require more than 100 mg/d; these patients can be identified by having inadequately blocked exercise-induced tachycardia; however, confirm the patient's compliance before increasing the dosage
- dosages greater than 100 mg/d are unlikely to retain true beta$_1$-selectivity

Useful Reference

Heel RC, Brogden RN, Speight TM, Avery GS: Atenolol: A review of its pharmacological properties and therapeutic efficacy in angina pectoris and hypertension. Drugs 1979;17:425–460

AZATHIOPRINE

Kelly Jones and Scott Whittaker

USA (Imuran)
CANADA (Imuran)

▶ **When Should I Use This Drug?**

Severe rheumatoid arthritis

- as a third-line agent after gold and methotrexate because of concern about the development of neoplasms (non-Hodgkin's lymphoma, squamous cell skin cancer, adenocarcinoma of the lung) (Arthritis Rheum 1972;15:183–186)
- azathioprine should be chosen before penicillamine because it works more quickly than penicillamine (8–10 weeks versus 6 months), and penicillamine has a number of toxicities that may not be reversible on discontinuation of the drug administration

Crohn's disease

- chronic, unresponsive Crohn's disease has been successfully treated with azathioprine and its active metabolite, 6-mercapto-purine
- it is essential to recognize that these medications take months for onset of effect, and hence these medications have no role in acute, severe disease
- initial reports showed no efficacy of azathioprine, but these studies were criticized because only a 17 week treatment period was used (Gastroenterology 1981;80:193–196)
- in other studies using a 1–2 year treatment period, the drugs were effective (N Engl J Med 1980;302:981–987)
- these antimetabolites are most often used in concert with other medications, particularly steroids, and may have some steroid-sparing effect
- in general, these drugs are used as a last resort, owing to the known side effects, especially pancreatitis, leukopenia, and the potential long-term oncogenic effects

▶ **When Should I Not Use This Drug?**

Mild to moderate nonprogressive disease

- other agents are available that are effective and less toxic

▶ **What Contraindications Are There to the Use of This Drug?**

Intolerance of or allergic reaction to azathioprine

Strong family history of non-Hodgkin's lymphomas

- there has been an associated risk with inducing non-Hodgkin's lymphoma with azathioprine
- risk of cancer is increased with rheumatoid arthritis, and the use of azathioprine additionally increases this risk (Am J Med 1985;78[1A]:44–49)

Previous treatment with alkylating agents such as chlorambucil and cyclophosphamide

- there is an increased risk of neoplasia

Hepatic disease

- increased risk of hepatotoxicity

▶ **What Drug Interactions Are Clinically Important?**

Drugs that may increase the effect or toxicity of azathioprine

ALLOPURINOL

- xanthine oxidase is involved in the metabolism of azathioprine, and allopurinol can increase serum levels of azathioprine
- dosage of azathioprine should be empirically reduced by 25% if allopurinol administration is started (JAMA 1988;259:2446–2449)

Drugs that may decrease the effect of azathioprine

- none

Drugs that may have their effect or toxicity increased by azathioprine

- none

Drugs that may have their effect or toxicity decreased by azathioprine

- none

▶ **What Route and Dosage Should I Use?**

How to administer

- orally—take with food

Severe rheumatoid arthritis

- 1.5 mg/kg PO daily (100 mg/d) as a single dose in the evening and increase by 0.5 mg/kg/d every 3 months until 2.5 mg/kg/d (150 mg/d) is reached
- can be divided into twice-daily dosing if gastrointestinal upset occurs

Crohn's disease

- start at 50 mg PO daily
- increase to 75 mg/d or even 100 mg/d (or 2 mg/kg) if the initial dosage is not effective after 3 months

Dosage adjustments for renal or hepatic dysfunction

- hepatically metabolized to 6-mercaptopurine
- avoid in liver failure

Normal Dosing Interval	$C_{cr} > 60$ mL/min or 1 mL/s	C_{cr} 30–60 mL/min or 0.5–1 mL/s	$C_{cr} < 30$ mL/min or 0.5 mL/s
Q24H	no adjustment needed	no adjustment needed	decrease dosage by 50%

▶ **What Should I Monitor with Regard to Efficacy and Toxicity?**

Efficacy

Rheumatoid arthritis

Joint tenderness count, sedimentation rate measurements, grip strength, duration of morning stiffness, time to onset of fatigue, and patient's report on specific functions

- patient should be assessed monthly for the first 2 months, and after symptoms are under control, the patient can be assessed every 3 months for 6 months, then every 6 months

- these measures should be used to guide the initiation and discontinuation of drug therapy
- in one study, clinical and laboratory measures of physical well-being appeared to be unrelated to psychological and social measures of well-being (J Rheumatol 1991;18:650–653)
- it is important to include the patients' self-assessment of the drug on their function and well-being

Crohn's disease

- these medications take months for onset of effect

Signs and symptoms

- diarrhea, abdominal pain, fever, abdominal distention and tenderness, size of mass (if present), and appetite

Toxicity

Hematological effects

- most common toxicity that is dose related—thrombocytopenia, leukopenia (most common), and macrocytic anemia
- do baseline complete blood count and platelet counts, then weekly for 2 months, then every 2 weeks for 2 months, and then every month for the duration of treatment
- discontinue the drug administration if the leukocyte count is less than 3500/mm^3, the granulocyte count is less than 1000/mm^3, or the platelet counts decrease to less than 100,000/mm^3
- administration of the drug can be restarted at 50–75% of the previous dosage after blood counts have recovered (usually 3 weeks) (Clin Pharm 1987;6:475–491)

Hepatotoxicity

- occurs in fewer than 1% of patients
- biliary stasis, jaundice, and portal hypertension
- perform baseline liver enzyme test, and repeat monthly
- discontinue if liver enzyme levels are greater than 3 times baseline values

Gastrointestinal effects

- nausea, vomiting, diarrhea, and anorexia
- dose related; therefore, divide dose and give with meals if gastrointestinal side effects occur

Hypersensitivity syndrome

- can manifest in many different forms: fever, arthralgias, myalgias, various skin eruptions (urticaria, exanthematous eruptions), headache, interstitial nephritis, pneumonitis, dyspnea, cough, nausea, vomiting, cholestatic jaundice, pancreatitis, hepatocellular damage, and hypotension
- mild hypotension on the first dose may predict worse hypotension on the second dose; the syndrome mimics septic shock
- these symptoms usually occur after several days of treatment and resolve a few days after discontinuation of the drug administration (Am J Med 1988;84:960–963)

▶ *How Long Do I Treat Patients with This Drug?*

Rheumatoid arthritis

- give a 12 week trial on the maximum dose (Clin Pharm 1987; 6:475–491), and if there is no response, stop the drug administration
- treatment with this agent is indefinite, but studies show that toxicity is the limiting factor

Crohn's disease

- treatment with this agent is indefinite

▶ *How Do I Decrease or Stop the Administration of This Drug?*

- may be stopped abruptly

▶ *What Should I Tell My Patients About This Drug?*

- counsel the patient about the use of proper contraception (for both partners)
- patients should report any unusual bleeding, headaches, sore throats, unusual lumps or masses, stomach pain, yellow skin, sores in mouth, and darkened urine
- always make sure to keep follow-up appointments for close monitoring

▶ *Therapeutic Tips*

- for rheumatoid arthritis azathioprine is considered a third-line agent
- a reliable patient is essential for compliance and close follow-up

Useful References

Pugh MC, Pugh CB. Current concepts in clinical therapeutics: Disease-modifying drugs for rheumatoid arthritis. Clin Pharm 1987;6:475–491
Weinblatt ME, Maier AL. Newer immunosuppressive therapies for rheumatoid arthritis. Crit Care Med 1990;18(2):S126–131
Wilder RL. Treatment of the patient with rheumatoid arthritis refractory to standard therapy. JAMA 1988;259:2446–2449

AZTREONAM

James McCormack

USA (Azactam)
CANADA (not available)

▶ *When Should I Use This Drug?*

see antibiotic susceptibility chart (Table 4–1 in Chapter 4)

Pneumonia, sepsis, osteomyelitis, cellulitis, intraabdominal infections, urinary tract infections, endocarditis

- may be used if these infections are caused by gram-negative organisms sensitive to aztreonam
- should be used only if it is less expensive than other potentially useful agents (quinolones, penicillins, cephalosporins)

Alternative to aminoglycoside therapy

- can be used for the treatment of gram-negative infections as an alternative to aminoglycosides if they are contraindicated
- should be used as an alternative only if it is less expensive than other agents that could also potentially be used (quinolones, penicillins, cephalosporins)

▶ *When Should I Not Use This Drug?*

Infections caused by gram-positive and/or anaerobic organisms

- aztreonam is not active against these organisms

▶ *What Contraindications Are There to the Use of This Drug?*

Intolerance of or allergic reaction to aztreonam or penicillins

- cross-reactivity with penicillins is rare
- if the patient states an allergy to penicillins or cephalosporins, check whether the patient has actual allergic symptoms
- in patients reporting a rash-type allergy, aztreonam can usually be given
- in patients reporting an immediate hypersensitivity reaction to penicillins, aztreonam can be used, but a physician must evaluate the patient closely (i.e., be at the bedside and have epinephrine available) during the administration of the first dose

▶ *What Drug Interactions Are Clinically Important?*

- none

▶ *What Route and Dosage Should I Use?*

How to administer

Orally

- not available

Parenterally

- may be given intravenously or intramuscularly
- to give intravenously, dilute in 50–100 mL of sterile water, normal saline, or 5% dextrose in water and infuse in over 20–60 minutes
- may also be given undiluted by IV push over 3–5 minutes

Pneumonia, sepsis, osteomyelitis, cellulitis, intraabdominal infections, urinary tract infections, endocarditis, alternative to aminoglycoside therapy

- 1000 mg IV or IM Q12H for lower urinary tract infections
- 1000 mg IV Q8H for mildly or moderately ill patients
- 2000 mg IV Q8H for severely ill patients

Dosage adjustments for renal or hepatic dysfunction

- 75% renally eliminated

Normal Dosing Interval	$C_{cr} > 60$ mL/min or 1 mL/s	C_{cr} 30–60 mL/min or 0.5–1 mL/s	$C_{cr} < 30$ mL/min or 0.5 mL/s
Q8H	no adjustment needed	no adjustment needed	Q12H

▶ What Should I Monitor with Regard to Efficacy and Toxicity?

Efficacy

- for antibiotic administration monitoring guidelines, see specific section on drug therapy

Toxicity

Allergic reactions (rash, anaphylaxis, and so on)

- occur in fewer than 1% of patients
- question the patient daily about these symptoms
- if these reactions occur, stop the drug

Gastrointestinal symptoms

- diarrhea, nausea, vomiting, and colitis have been reported in about 1–2% of patients
- if these effects are severe, aztreonam therapy should be discontinued
- for specific treatment of drug-induced diarrhea or nausea and vomiting, see Chapter 3

▶ How Long Do I Treat Patients with This Drug?

- for antibiotic administration duration, see specific section on drug therapy

▶ How Do I Decrease or Stop the Administration of This Drug?

- may be stopped abruptly

▶ What Should I Tell My Patients About This Drug?

- this agent is somewhat related to penicillins and cephalosporins
- have you ever had a severe allergic reaction to a penicillin or cephalosporin? and if so, describe the reaction and how long ago it happened
- if you have a rash, itching, wheezing, or difficulty in breathing, please notify a nurse or physician
- aztreonam can cause diarrhea, and if the diarrhea is severe, contact your physician

▶ Therapeutic Tips

- ensure that the dosage is adjusted for renal dysfunction
- use this drug only if it is less expensive than other potential alternative agents (penicillins, cephalosporins, or quinolones)

BACAMPICILLIN

John Rotschafer, Kyle Vance-Bryan, and Rick Zabinski

USA (Spectrobid)
CANADA (Penglobe)

▶ When Should I Use This Drug?

Consider an alternative agent

- identical indications to those for amoxicillin
- use amoxicillin instead of bacampicillin because amoxicillin is less expensive

Useful Reference

Wright AJ, Wilkowske CJ. The penicillins. Mayo Clin Proc 1987;62:806–820.

BECLOMETHASONE DIPROPIONATE

Karen Shalansky and Cindy Reeser Nimmo

USA (Beclovent, Vanceril)
CANADA (Beclodisk, Becloforte, Beclovent, Beclovent Rotahaler, Vanceril)

▶ When Should I Use This Drug?

Chronic asthma or chronic obstructive pulmonary disease

- inhaled corticosteroids are the drugs of choice in patients requiring stepwise progression of therapy from PRN use of beta$_2$-agonists
- inhaled corticosteroids decrease inflammation and decrease the number and severity of attacks and the need for beta-agonists
- inhaled corticosteroids have a positive effect in both asthma and chronic obstructive pulmonary disease (Ann Intern Med 1993;118:770–778)
- add to therapy if more than 2 beta$_2$-agonist inhalations are required daily or if symptoms are not completely reversed by an inhaled beta$_2$-agonist
- add if the peak expiratory flow rate or forced expiratory volume in 1 second falls to 85% or less of the predicted value or best known result
- use in all patients receiving regular doses of an oral corticosteroid (except for acute attack); high-dose inhaled corticosteroids should be given, as they may allow a reduction or discontinuation of oral corticosteroid therapy
- powder inhalation products contain lactose, which may occasionally cause a cough when it is on the back of the throat
- surfactants in the aerosolized inhalers can cause bronchospasm in some patients
- budesonide has less systemic bioavailability than does beclomethasone (Thorax 1991;46:160–164)
- in low dosages (<1000 μg/d), the impact of this difference in systemic bioavailability between these agents is likely not important
- beclomethasone in high dosage (2000 μg/d) increases urinary hydroxyproline output, which reflects an increase in bone resorption, whereas budesonide does not produce this effect (Thorax 1991;46:160–164)
- decision about using this agent or budesonide should be based on cost and the patient's inhaler preference

Seasonal asthma

- second-line drug after cromolyn sodium therapy has failed in patients with asthma due to allergen exposure, because cromolyn sodium is associated with a lower incidence of adverse effects

▶ When Should I Not Use This Drug?

Acute asthma

- studies are presently ongoing to evaluate the role of inhaled corticosteroids in acute asthma; however, at present, they are not recommended in patients requiring medical attention for acute asthma

▶ What Contraindications Are There to the Use of This Drug?

Intolerance of or allergic reaction to inhaled beclomethasone

- aerosolized inhalers contain fluorocarbons and oleic acid
- powder inhalation products contain lactose

Untreated fungal, bacterial, or viral infections or active or quiescent pulmonary tuberculosis

- high dosages (>1000 μg/d) of inhaled corticosteroids may depress the body's immune system and its ability to fight infections
- if the infection is treated, this is likely not a problem

▶ What Drug Interactions Are Clinically Important?

- none

▶ What Route and Dosage Should I Use?

Available as a metered-dose inhaler and diskhaler (not available in the USA)

- dry powder inhalers require the following minimum inspiratory flow rates to be effective: spinhaler, 200 L/min; rotahaler, 120 L/min; diskhaler, <60 L/min; turbuhaler, 30 L/min

- diskhaler and turbuhaler have the advantage of not being affected by the humidity
- turbuhaler has the advantage of containing the drug without excipients
- all patients require teaching of proper inhaler technique and periodic reinforcement of correct technique

Chronic asthma or chronic obstructive pulmonary disease

Metered-dose inhaler

- metered-dose inhaler in the USA contains 42 μg/puff
- metered-dose inhalers in Canada contain 50 μg/puff or 200 μg/puff (Becloforte)
- 200 μg (4 puffs of the 50 μg/puff or 1 puff of the 200 μg/puff) of the metered-dose inhaler BID is the usual starting dose for mild asthma
- administer 200 μg inhaled QID for patients with more severe asthma and increase up to 1600–2000 μg/d if needed
- for patients with severe asthma, higher doses are recommended because a faster response may be seen; however, after 3–4 weeks one may be able to reduce the dosing to a BID regimen
- patients with stable asthma may be adequately controlled with BID dosing of inhaled corticosteroids; however, if the asthma becomes unstable, the patient should be switched to a TID or QID regimen (Hosp Pract 1991;April:15–26)

Diskhaler or Rotahaler

- may be preferred to a metered-dose inhaler in patients who have difficulty using a metered-dose inhaler

Converting from systemic oral corticosteroids

- initiate inhaled corticosteroid administration at 200 μg QID for 10 days, then taper oral corticosteroid as tolerated

Seasonal asthma

- 200 μg inhaled BID
- prophylaxis should be initiated 1 week prior to and continued throughout the anticipated allergen season

▶ *What Should I Monitor with Regard to Efficacy and Toxicity?*

Efficacy

see Budesonide for efficacy parameters

Toxicity

Oropharyngeal candidiasis

- dose-dependent adverse effect, which usually responds to topical antifungal therapy or a temporary reduction in dosage
- may be minimized through the use of an extender device and gargling with water after each inhalation
- frequency of oral candidiasis with high-dose inhalers is similar to that with low-dose inhalers

Dysphonia

- dose-dependent adverse effect
- usually responds to a reduction in dosage but may recur after the dosage is increased
- may be minimized through the use of an extender device and gargling with water after each inhalation

Mild hypothalamic-pituitary-adrenal axis suppression

- patients receiving equal to or greater than 1600 μg/d are at greatest risk and should be treated similarly to patients receiving long-term oral corticosteroids (J Allergy Clin Immunol 1988;82:297–306)
- potential for side effects may increase with concomitant oral and inhaled corticosteroid therapy

▶ *How Long Do I Treat Patients with This Drug?*

see Budesonide

▶ *How Do I Decrease or Stop the Administration of This Drug?*

see Budesonide

▶ *What Should I Tell My Patients About This Drug?*

- inhaled corticosteroid is used to prevent bronchospasm and does not relieve an attack that has already started

- although it is generally recommended to precede corticosteroid inhalation with inhalation of a bronchodilator, this practice has not been shown to increase the delivery of the drug to the lungs or to increase the efficacy of the corticosteroid
- compliance with regular therapy is essential to maintain control of asthma
- use the inhaler exactly as directed

Metered-dose inhaler

1. place the canister firmly into the outer shell
2. shake well and remove the cap
3. exhale to a normal relaxed expiration
4. place the tip of the mouthpiece—either 2 fingerbreadths in front of widely opened mouth or between the teeth and lips
5. breathe in slowly, and at the same time, press the canister to release 1 puff of the drug
6. continue to inhale as deeply as possible—hold the breath for as long as confortable (5–10 seconds)
7. breathe out to a normal relaxed resting position
8. if a second inhalation is prescribed, the same procedure is repeated with the second puff, 30 seconds after the first

Extension device (e.g., Aerochamber) (for use with metered-dose inhaler)

1. remove the mouthpiece covers from the inhaler and extension device
2. shake the inhaler well and insert into the appropriate opening on the extension device
3. exhale to a normal relaxed expiration, and then place the mouthpiece of the extension device between the teeth and lips—do not cover the small holes on either side of the mouthpiece
4. activate the metered-dose inhaler into the extension device
5. breathe in slowly and deeply—hold your breath for 5–10 seconds—breathe out slowly to a normal relaxed resting position
6. if you are unable to take a deep breath, breathe in and out normally for 3 or 4 breaths
7. if a second inhalation is prescribed, the same procedure is repeated with the second puff, at least 30 seconds after the first

Rotahaler

1. hold the rotahaler by the mouthpiece and twist the barrel until it stops
2. press a rotacap into the raised square hole with the clear end pointed down
3. keep the barrel level with the white dot marked on the side and twist the barrel in the opposite direction to pierce the capsule
4. exhale to a normal expiration
5. place the mouthpiece between the teeth and lips and tilt the head back
6. breathe in quickly—hold the breath for as long as possible (5–10 seconds)
7. if a second inhalation is prescribed, repeat the procedure after 30 seconds

Diskhaler

1. remove the outer blue cover
2. grasp the white cartridge and gently pull—squeeze the ribbed sides to remove cartridge unit
3. place the disk on the cartridge wheel with the numbers face up; slide the cartridge back into the body
4. gently push in and pull out the loaded cartridge—the disk will rotate—continue this step until the number 8 appears in the indicator window
5. lift the rear edge of the diskhaler lid to a 90 degree angle—this pierces both the top and bottom of the blister
6. exhale to a normal relaxed expiration
7. keeping the disk level, place the mouthpiece between the teeth and lips
8. breathe in quickly—hold your breath for as long as possible (5–10 seconds)

9. if a second inhalation is prescribed, repeat steps 4–8 (the next blister to appear should be number 7) 30 seconds after the previous inhalation
10. each disk has 8 blisters of drug—to replace a disk, follow steps 1–3, removing the old disk

▶ *Therapeutic Tips*

- patients taking high-dose (≥1600 μg/d) inhaled corticosteroids may require supplemental systemic corticosteroids during periods of stress (e.g., infection and surgery)
- high-dose corticosteroids are best administered through an extender device to maximize drug delivery and to minimize the development of oropharyngeal candidiasis
- inhaled corticosteroids do not have to be given after an inhaled dose of salbutamol and should be used only in conjunction with salbutamol when salbutamol is needed for symptom relief
- high-dose inhaled corticosteroids produce a faster response than does low-dose therapy
- higher dosages of inhaled corticosteroids are required to normalize pulmonary function than to relieve symptoms

Useful References

Johnson CE. Aerosol corticosteroids for the treatment of asthma. DICP 1987;21:784–790.

Smith MJ. The place of high-dose inhaled corticosteroids in asthma therapy. Drugs 1987;33:423–429

Kongig P. Inhaled corticosteroids—Their present and future role in the management of asthma. J Allergy Clin Immunol 1988;82:297–306

BENAZEPRIL

Jack Onrot and James McCormack

USA (Lotensin)
CANADA (Lotensin)

▶ *When Should I Use This Drug?*

see Enalapril

▶ *When Should I Not Use This Drug?*

see Enalapril

▶ *What Contraindications Are There to the Use of This Drug?*

see Captopril

▶ *What Drug Interactions Are Clinically Important?*

see Captopril

▶ *What Route and Dosage Should I Use?*

How to administer

- orally—can be administered with or without food
- parenterally—not available

Congestive heart failure

- 5 mg PO daily
- rapidity of dosage escalation depends on the severity of symptoms
- dosage may be increased daily if necessary
- no value of exceeding a total daily dose of 40 mg

Chronic (noncrisis) hypertension

- 5 mg PO daily
- increase the dosage by 5 mg PO daily every 4 weeks until adequate blood pressure is achieved or a daily dose of 20 mg is reached
- limited value in exceeding a total daily dose of 20 mg (dosages as high as 40 mg PO daily have been used)
- for some patients, the antihypertensive effect may be diminished before 24 hours and twice-daily dosing may be required (Inpharma 1993;881:5)

Dosage adjustments for renal or hepatic dysfunction

- predominantly renally eliminated (some biliary elimination)

- titrate the dose in response to the clinical effect and not on the basis of concurrent renal or hepatic function

▶ *What Should I Monitor with Regard to Efficacy and Toxicity?*

see Captopril

▶ *How Long Do I Treat Patients with This Drug?*

see Captopril

▶ *How Do I Decrease or Stop the Administration of This Drug?*

see Captopril

▶ *What Should I Tell My Patients About This Drug?*

see Captopril

▶ *Therapeutic Tips*

see Captopril

BENDROFLUMETHIAZIDE (BENDROFLUAZIDE)

Ian Petterson

USA (Naturetin)
CANADA (Naturetin)

▶ *When Should I Use This Drug?*

Decision among the different thiazide diuretics should be based on cost, as there is little, if any, difference in clinical effect among these agents • Although bendroflumethiazide is more potent, this confers no benefit, as thiazide diuretics are all given once daily and are well tolerated

see Hydrochlorothiazide

▶ *When Should I Not Use This Drug?*

see Hydrochlorothiazide

▶ *What Contraindications Are There to the Use of This Drug?*

see Hydrochlorothiazide

▶ *What Drug Interactions Are Clinically Important?*

see Hydrochlorothiazide

▶ *What Route and Dosage Should I Use?*

How to administer

- orally—may be given with food or on an empty stomach
- parenterally—not available

Chronic (noncrisis) hypertension

- 1.25 mg PO daily
- dosage may be increased every 2–4 weeks if the current dosage is not adequately controlling blood pressure
- dosage should rarely exceed 2.5 mg and never exceed 5 mg daily, as there is no greater hypotensive effect and there is an increased incidence of adverse reactions

Congestive heart failure

- 1.25 mg PO daily
- dosage may be increased every 2 weeks if the current dosage is not adequately controlling the edema
- in cardiac failure, thiazide diuretics are effective in potentiating the diuretic effect of loop diuretics (furosemide) but start with low dosages (1.25 mg daily) and be aware of possible profound dehydration and electrolyte disturbances with standard dosages (Ann Intern Med 1991;114:886–894)

Cirrhosis

- 1.25 mg PO daily
- in cirrhosis, if an effect is not seen with 5 mg daily, the addition of low-dose spironolactone has an additive effect and reverses hypokalemia

Dosage adjustments for renal or hepatic dysfunction

- renally eliminated
- no adjustment is needed for renal impairment, except avoid administration of the drug in patients with moderate to severe renal function (creatinine clearance < 30 mL/min) as effectiveness is lost

▶ What Should I Monitor with Regard to Efficacy and Toxicity?

see Hydrochlorothiazide

▶ How Long Do I Treat Patients with This Drug?

see Hydrochlorothiazide

▶ How Do I Decrease or Stop the Administration of This Drug?

see Hydrochlorothiazide

▶ What Should I Tell My Patients About This Drug?

see Hydrochlorothiazide

▶ Therapeutic Tips

see Hydrochlorothiazide

Useful References

Nader C, Thompson JR, Alpern RJ. Complications of diuretic use. Semin Nephrol 1988;8:365–387
Black HR. Metabolic considerations in the choice of therapy for the patient with hypertension. Am Heart J 1991;121:707–715
Freis ED. Critique of the clinical importance of diuretic induced hypokalemia and elevated cholesterol levels. Arch Intern Med 1989;149:2640–2648

BENZTROPINE

Ruby Grymonpre

USA (Cogentin)
CANADA (Cogentin)

▶ When Should I Use This Drug?

Parkinson's disease

- anticholinergics have been used as first-line therapy for patients with mild Parkinson's disease (tremor as the predominant symptom) and good cognitive function; however, anticholinergics are now most often used as adjuncts to levodopa therapy when tremor is a problem
- there is no difference among benztropine, trihexyphenidyl, procyclidine, and biperiden with respect to efficacy; however, benztropine may have a greater sedative effect than some of the other anticholinergic agents (Clin Pharmacokinet 1987;13:141–178)
- trihexyphenidyl is more stimulating than the other agents
- benztropine is the only agent that can be given once daily, whereas trihexyphenidyl, with the exception of the sustained-release product, and procyclidine may need to be given more frequently
- decision among these agents should be based on cost, compliance issues, and the patient's response

▶ When Should I Not Use This Drug?

Initial single therapy

- as an initial single drug for the treatment of Parkinson's disease (with the exceptions noted above) as benztropine only produces modest improvement of symptoms in 10–25% of patients and causes a greater frequency of side effects than other effective therapy (Br Med Bull 1990;46:124–146

Treatment of sialorrhea

- commonly associated with Parkinson's disease (this symptom is due to a reduced swallowing ability and head drooping and not a cholinergic excess)
- levodopa is a more rational therapy for this problem

▶ What Contraindications Are There to the Use of This Drug?

Intolerance of or allergic reaction to benztropine

Narrow angle glaucoma, urinary obstruction (e.g., prostatic enlargement and bladder neck obstruction), obstruction of the gastrointestinal tract (e.g., pyloric or duodenal obstruction)

- owing to exacerbations of these disease states caused by anticholinergic effect

▶ What Drug Interactions Are Clinically Important?

Drugs that may increase the effect or toxicity of benztropine

PHENOTHIAZINES, AMANTADINE, MEPERIDINE, TRICYCLIC ANTIDEPRESSANTS, QUINIDINE, DISOPYRAMIDE, OR SOME ANTIHISTAMINES

- may result in additive anticholinergic adverse effects (e.g., xerostomia, blurred vision, constipation, and confusion); therefore, use the lowest effective dosages of both agents

Drugs that may decrease the effect of benztropine

ANTACIDS

- decrease the extent of absorption of oral anticholinergics
- oral anticholinergics should be administered at least 1 hour before antacid administration

Drugs that may have their effect or toxicity increased by benztropine

POTASSIUM SUPPLEMENTS

- anticholinergics may slow gastrointestinal motility and allow wax matrix potassium supplements (Slow-K) to cause gastric irritation or erosion
- use microencapsulated potassium supplement (Micro-K)

Drugs that may have their effect decreased by benztropine

LEVODOPA

- by inhibiting gastrointestinal motility, antimuscarinics can decrease the extent of levodopa absorption, but this is usually not a clinical problem
- when anticholinergic therapy is being discontinued, levodopa toxicity may occur

KETOCONAZOLE

- by increasing gastric pH, anticholinergics may decrease ketoconazole absorption
- anticholinergics should be given at least 2 hours after ketoconazole administration

▶ What Route and Dosage Should I Use?

How to administer

- orally—food probably decreases absorption (ensure that the drug is taken consistently either with food or milk or on an empty stomach)
- parenterally—can be administered intravenously or intramuscularly and the onset of action is the same (IV administration is rarely necessary)

Parkinson's disease

- 0.5 mg PO daily at bedtime
- increase the dosage at weekly intervals, based on response, by 0.5 mg to a maximum dosage of 6 mg PO daily
- if tolerated, the drug may be given as 1 dose at bedtime; however, at maximum daily dosages, it is advisable to administer in divided doses if the patient experiences dose-related side effects

Dosage adjustments for renal or hepatic dysfunction

- unknown
- no dosage adjustment is required; just start with a low dosage and titrate up to effect or toxicity

▶ What Should I Monitor with Regard to Efficacy and Toxicity?

Efficacy

Parkinson's disease

Signs and symptoms

- assess symptoms weekly during the titration period
- after the patient has been stabilized, assess the patient every 3 months

Toxicity

Anticholinergic effects

Dry mouth

- increase fluid intake and/or use sugarless chewing gum or hard candies
- perform scrupulous oral hygeine; use saliva substitutes

Constipation

- increase exercise, fluid intake, and the amount of fiber in the diet, and if needed, use a laxative

Orthostatic hypotension

- treatment of orthostasis includes rising slowly from supine or sitting positions and wearing support stockings
- is dose related and may resolve with a dosage reduction
- if persistent or severe, may need to stop administration of the drug

Blurred vision, urinary hesitancy

- is dose related and may resolve with dosage reduction
- if persistent or severe, may need to stop administration of the drug

Central nervous system effects

- confusion, sedation, delusions, and hallucinations
- these reactions may be dose related, so if they occur, decrease the dosage of benztropine
- in patients with psychiatric illness, monitor for a recurrence of psychiatric episodes (including dementia, depression, and psychosis)

Cardiovascular effects

- monitor heart rate, blood pressure (with the patient lying and standing), and the presence of any chest pain, especially in older patients or patients who have cardiac disease or are receiving antihypertensive medication
- monitor weekly while titrating the dose and then every 3 months afterward

▶ How Long Do I Treat Patients with This Drug?

Parkinson's disease

- in most cases, when another class of therapy is instituted, anticholinergic drug therapy can be discontinued
- however, in about 20–25% of advanced cases of Parkinson's disease, the patient may benefit from long-term anticholinergic therapy in combination with levodopa, because severe tremors are unresponsive to levodopa alone (Acta Neurol Scand Suppl 1989;126:213–219, Clin Pharmacokinet 1987;13:141–178)

▶ How Do I Decrease or Stop the Administration of This Drug?

- benztropine administration should not be discontinued abruptly because marked worsening of parkinsonian symptoms may occur
- taper the dosage by 30% every 7 days

▶ What Should I Tell My Patients About This Drug?

- contact your physician if symptoms do not improve over the next 1–2 days
- this drug can cause dry mouth, constipation, problems with urination, palpitations, and confusion, and if any of these symptoms occur and are bothersome, contact your physician
- some of these problems may be worsened by ingredients in cough and cold medications; therefore, check with your physician or pharmacist before using these agents

▶ Therapeutic Tips

- use of anticholinergic agents is declining owing to the effects of this class of drugs on cognitive function
- monitor cognitive status in elderly patients and patients with impaired cognitive function
- although all anticholinergic agents are considered equivalent at equipotent dosages, patients who do not respond to one anticholinergic may benefit from a different anticholinergic agent
- patients who are maintained on nothing by mouth (NPO) status near the time of surgery and cannot take levodopa may be treated with injectable (IM) benztropine if symptoms are a problem

BETAXOLOL

Robert Rangno and James McCormack

USA (Kerlone)
CANADA (not available)

▶ When Should I Use This Drug?

Consider an alternative agent

- provides no clinical advantages over other beta-blockers (Med Lett 1990;32:61–62)

BIPERIDEN

Ruby Grymonpre

USA (Akineton)
CANADA (Akineton)

▶ When Should I Use This Drug?

Consider an alternative agent

- biperiden is chemically related to trihexyphenidyl
- biperiden is not a recommended antiparkinsonian agent, as there has been greater clinical experience with trihexyphenidyl and there appears to be no real advantage in using biperiden over trihexyphenidyl

BISACODYL

Leslie Mathews

USA (Dulcolax, Bisco-Lax, Delco-lax, Carter's Little Pills, Bisac-Evac)
CANADA (Dulcolax, Bisacolax, Evac-Q-Kwik suppository; combination: Dulcodos, Royvac)

▶ When Should I Use This Drug?

Acute constipation

- when bulk-forming laxatives or osmotic laxatives are ineffective or contraindicated
- to provide a more rapid effect than that with a bulk-forming laxative
- all stimulant laxatives are equally effective and are less expensive than agents such as lactulose
- although some authors advocate the use of senna over any of the other stimulants, claiming that it is the mildest and that standardized senna is the most physiological of all the nonfiber laxatives (Pharmacology 1988;36[suppl 1]:230–236), there are no good studies to confirm or deny these claims
- should be used only short term, as other agents are safer and more effective for long-term treatment
- decision about which stimulant laxative (bisacodyl, senna, cascara sagrada) to use should be based on availability and cost

Chronic constipation

- occasional use in patients with an absent or poor defecation reflex or severely delayed gut transit or in patients with severe debilitation or terminal illness (if long-term use is required, use lactulose)
- useful for bedridden, anorexic patients who are unable to tolerate fluids (and therefore bulk-forming laxatives cannot be used)
- patients with neurogenic constipation (e.g., patients with spinal cord injury or multiple sclerosis) often require stimulation of the

gut, frequently in conjunction with the use of stool softeners and regular stimulation of the rectal mucosa with suppositories and/or enemas to prevent fecal impaction

Bowel preparation

- bisacodyl suppositories or enemas used before diagnostic procedures or colorectal surgery in conjunction with osmotic laxatives
- use when polyethylene glycol–electrolyte solution (GoLYTELY) is contraindicated, as bisacodyl can cause mucosal injury and interfere with the interpretation of sigmoidoscopy or barium enema results (Young LY, Kod a-Kimble MA, eds. Applied Therapeutics: The Clinical Use of Drugs, 4th ed. Vancouver, WA:1988:101–122)

▶ *When Should I Not Use This Drug?*

Long-term use for chronic constipation

- bulk-forming laxatives or lactulose is safer for regular use
- only occasional, limited use (up to 7 days) is acceptable
- can cause significant fluid and electrolyte imbalance and can lead to dependence, abuse, nutritional problems, and possible bowel injury

Pregnancy

- avoid use owing to the potential for fluid and electrolyte disturbances with diarrhea
- safety in pregnancy is not established

Hard and dry stool

- suppositories may be ineffective (Pharm Bull 1987;21:1–7)

▶ *What Contraindications Are There to the Use of This Drug?*

Intolerance of or allergic reaction to bisacodyl

Symptoms of acute abdomen or intestinal obstruction

- stimulation of the gut in this situation could potentially produce increased inflammation, pain, obstruction, or rupture

Anorectal fissures, ulcerated hemorrhoids

- enemas and suppositories are contraindicated because of the potential for worsening these conditions

▶ *What Drug Interactions Are Clinically Important?*

- none

▶ *What Route and Dosage Should I Use?*

How to administer

Orally

- take with a full glass of water

Rectally

- remove the wrapper, moisten the suppository with lukewarm water, and insert the tapered end high and against the wall of the rectum
- to administer an enema, the patient lies on the left side or in knee-chest position and gently inserts the prelubricated nozzle into rectum toward navel and squeezes the bottle slowly
- patient should remain reclining until abdominal cramping is felt, at which time rectal contents can be expelled

Acute constipation, chronic constipation

- 5 mg PO daily
- increase the dosage as needed after 24 hours by 5 mg to a maximum of 15 mg PO daily

Bowel preparation

- 10 mg PO the night before examination
- one suppository or 1 enema (10 mg) once on the morning of the examination

▶ *What Should I Monitor with Regard to Efficacy and Toxicity?*

Efficacy

Acute constipation, chronic constipation, bowel preparation

- oral treatment produces soft or semiliquid stool in 6–24 hours

- rectal administration of a suppository or microenema stimulates the rectal mucosa, initiating defecation within 15–60 minutes
- question the patient about the frequency and consistency of stools and/or check stool charts if the patient is hospitalized
- if acute constipation persists after 1 week without explanation, investigate for gastrointestinal pathological changes

Toxicity

Gastrointestinal symptoms (diarrhea, abdominal cramping)

- discontinue administration for diarrhea or severe cramping
- decrease the dose for milder cramping

Anorectal symptoms with suppositories or enemas

- irritation and burning are common
- proctitis, sloughing of epithelium, fissures, and tenesmus can occur, particularly with prolonged use
- question the patient about these effects; discontinue administration for significant irritation

Fluid and electrolyte loss (dehydration, hypokalemia)

- can occur with prolonged or acute diarrhea
- discontinue drug administration if fluid and electrolyte losses occur
- monitor for signs of dehydration
- monitor fluid and electrolyte levels, and replace serum electrolytes and fluid daily until losses are resolved

Endocrine or metabolic symptoms (metabolic acidosis or alkalosis, weight loss, weakness, malabsorption of nutrients, protein-losing enteropathy)

- are rare, but can occur with abuse of large doses long term (Hosp Pharm 1988;23:565–573)
- if surreptitious abuse is suspected, do a urine screen for bisacodyl
- discontinue administration or wean as for laxative abuse

Cathartic colon

- prolonged use over several years may inflict neuromuscular injury, especially of the ascending colon, resulting in a sluggish or nonfunctioning bowel (Postgrad Med 1988;83:339–349, Dis Col Rectum 1973;16:455–458, Gut 1968;9:139–143)

▶ *How Long Do I Treat Patients with This Drug?*

Acute constipation, chronic constipation

- discontinue as soon as possible
- limit use to a maximum of 7 days, with a few exceptions (e.g., long-term opiate use in terminal illness or neurogenic constipation)
- laxative abusers may have to be weaned gradually over several weeks or months

▶ *How Do I Decrease or Stop the Administration of This Drug?*

- administration may be stopped abruptly but long-term users may need to be weaned gradually

▶ *What Should I Tell My Patients About This Drug?*

- discontinue for diarrhea or relief of constipation
- decrease the dosage by 50% for persistent abdominal cramps
- notify your physician if constipation persists after 1 week of use
- prolonged use can cause serious side effects and lead to laxative dependency and loss of normal bowel function
- complete bowel emptying can occur
- you may not have another bowel movement for 2–3 days after use
- take at bedtime to produce effects by morning
- do not chew or crush tablets (swallow whole)
- do not take tablets within 1 hour of drinking milk or taking an antacid
- suppositories or enemas may cause a burning sensation; therefore, stop use for anal swelling or pain
- insert suppository against wall of rectum rather than into stool and defecation will occur within an hour

▶ *Therapeutic Tips*

- tablets are enteric coated to prevent gastric irritation and cramping; therefore, chewing, crushing, or using an antacid H_2 blocker or milk concurrently may cause severe cramping or nausea

Useful References

Tedesco FJ. Laxative use in constipation. Am J Gastroenterol 1985;80: 303–309

Rousseau P. Treatment of constipation in the elderly. Postgrad Med 1988;83:339–349

Young, LY, Kod a-Kimble MA, eds. Applied Therapeutics: The Clinical Use of Drugs, 4th ed. Vancouver, WA: Applied Therapeutics, 1988: 101–122

BITOLTEROL

Karen Shalansky and Cindy Reesor Nimmo

USA (Tornalate)
CANADA (not available)

▶ *When Should I Use This Drug?*

Consider an alternative agent

- is a long-acting beta$_2$-agonist that provides no apparent clinical advantage over other available agents, unless it is being used on a regular basis (beta-agonists should primarily be used for symptomatic relief)
- a long-acting beta$_2$-agonist could be considered in a patient who continues to have nighttime symptoms/awakenings despite optimal use of inhaled corticosteroids and a dose of salbutamol at bedtime (N Engl J Med 1992;327:1420–1425)

BRETYLIUM TOSYLATE

James Tisdale

USA (Bretylol, bretylium tosylate)
CANADA (Bretylate, bretylium tosylate)

▶ *When Should I Use This Drug?*

Ventricular tachycardia

- bretylium tosylate should be used for the treatment of acute sustained or symptomatic ventricular tachycardia that has not responded to therapeutic dosages of lidocaine or procainamide (JAMA 1992;268:2199–2241)

Ventricular fibrillation

- bretylium tosylate should be used for the treatment of acute ventricular fibrillation that has not responded to therapeutic dosages of lidocaine (JAMA 1992;268:2199–2241)

▶ *When Should I Not Use This Drug?*

Asymptomatic ventricular arrhythmias

- no evidence that treatment is beneficial

Supraventricular arrhythmias

- bretylium tosylate is not effective for the treatment of supraventricular arrhythmias

Prophylaxis of ventricular fibrillation after myocardial infarction

- bretylium should not be used for routine prophylaxis of ventricular fibrillation after myocardial infarction

▶ *What Contraindications Are There to the Use of This Drug?*

Intolerance of or allergic reaction to bretylium

Severe hypotension

- bretylium tosylate should be used only in patients with severe hypotension when other agents have failed and vasopressor agents are available, as the sympatholytic effects of the drug may further decrease blood pressure

Severe aortic stenosis, pulmonary hypertension

- bretylium tosylate should not be used in patients with severe aortic stenosis or pulmonary hypertension with a fixed cardiac output, as they may not be able to compensate for the peripheral vasodilation caused by the drug

▶ *What Drug Interactions Are Clinically Important?*

- none

▶ *What Route and Dosage Should I Use?*

How to administer

- orally—unavailable
- parenterally—by intermittent bolus or continuous infusion

Ventricular tachycardia, ventricular fibrillation

Loading dose

- for hemodynamically unstable ventricular tachycardia or ventricular fibrillation, the initial loading dose should be 5 mg/kg administered undiluted, by rapid injection
- if there is no response in 3–5 minutes for ventricular fibrillation or 5–15 minutes for ventricular tachycardia, administer 10 mg/kg undiluted, by rapid injection
- if there is no response in several minutes, administer an additional dose of 10 mg/kg undiluted, by rapid IV injection
- for hemodynamically stable ventricular tachycardia, administer 5 mg/kg diluted approximately 4-fold in 5% dextrose in water or normal saline and administer over 15–30 minutes
- if there is no response in 1 hour, administer an additional dose of 10 mg/kg diluted 4-fold in 5% dextrose in water or normal saline and administer over 15–30 minutes

Maintenance dose

- initial maintenance dose should be 2 mg/min by continuous IV infusion

Dosage adjustments for renal or hepatic dysfunction

- renally eliminated
- in patients with estimated creatinine clearance less than 25 mL/min, initiate maintenance infusions at 1 mg/min

▶ *What Should I Monitor with Regard to Efficacy and Toxicity?*

Efficacy

Ventricular tachycardia, ventricular fibrillation

Intermittent electrocardiograms

- continuous electrocardiographic evaluation for persistence or recurrence of ventricular tachycardia or fibrillation

Symptoms

- monitor continuously for shortness of breath, hypotension, palpitations, chest pain, and dizziness

Toxicity

Hypotension and postural hypotension

- monitor blood pressure continuously during the loading bolus and for the entire duration of the maintenance infusion
- bretylium tosylate–induced hypotension should be treated with intravenous fluids if the patient is hypovolemic
- infusions of dopamine or norepinephrine may be used if bretylium tosylate therapy cannot be discontinued
- hypotension requiring discontinuation of therapy occurs in approximately 10% of patients receiving bretylium tosylate

Nausea and vomiting

- is often a result of rapid administration and often resolves without drug discontinuation
- if continued bretylium therapy is required, antiemetics may be tried but their benefit is unproved

Diarrhea, flushing, dyspnea, diaphoresis

▶ *How Long Do I Treat Patients with This Drug?*

Ventricular tachycardia, ventricular fibrillation

- intravenous bretylium tosylate therapy should be continued until the underlying cause of the arrhythmia is identified and corrected
- if no underlying cause of arrhythmia is identified, or if an identified underlying cause is not corrected, bretylium tosylate therapy

should be continued until the patient is stabilized on oral antiarrhythmic drug therapy (as recommended by a cardiologist or an electrophysiologist)

▶ How Do I Decrease or Stop the Administration of This Drug?

- may be stopped abruptly

▶ What Should I Tell My Patients About This Drug?

- this drug may cause nausea and vomiting or dizziness if the patient sits up rapidly

▶ Therapeutic Tips

- bretylium tosylate causes an initial release of norepinephrine from adrenergic nerve endings, followed by blockade of reuptake of norepinephrine into adrenergic nerve endings, and therefore, during the first 20–30 minutes of a bretylium tosylate infusion, heart rate and blood pressure may increase
- after this period, heart rate and blood pressure usually decrease
- although bretylium tosylate is administered by continuous intravenous infusion, the half-life of the drug is 5–10 hours in patients with normal renal function and is considerably longer in patients with renal dysfunction; therefore, hypotension and other adverse effects may persist for several hours after discontinuation of therapy

Useful References

Anderson JL. Bretylium tosylate: Profile of the only available class III antiarrhythmic agent. Clin Ther 1985;7:205–224

Narang PK, Adir J, Josselson J, et al. Pharmacokinetics of bretylium in man after intravenous administration. J Pharmacokinet Biopharm 1980; 8:363–372

Holder DA, Sniderman AD, Fraser G, et al. Experience with bretylium tosylate by a hospital cardiac arrest team. Circulation 1977;55:541–544

BROMOCRIPTINE

Ruby Grymonpre

USA (Parlodel)
CANADA (Parlodel)

▶ When Should I Use This Drug?

Parkinson's disease

- added when the patient has an unstable fluctuating pattern of response to current levodopa and selegiline therapy and when additional measures to minimize these fluctuations (e.g., reduced dosing interval of levodopa, dosage adjustments, and use of sustained-release levodopa) have failed
- patients with dose-response fluctuations experience a smoother clinical response when bromocriptine is added, possibly because its half-life is longer than levodopa's half-life

Other uses

- drug withdrawal, smoking cessation, prolactin inhibition, acromegaly

▶ When Should I Not Use This Drug?

Initial single therapy

- owing to the costs and relatively high incidence of side effects associated with bromocriptine, this agent is not recommended as an initial single drug for the treatment of Parkinson's disease
- patients unresponsive to levodopa therapy should be reevaluated for Parkinson's disease before trying alternative dopaminergic agents

▶ What Contraindications Are There to the Use of This Drug?

- Intolerance of or allergic reaction to bromocriptine

▶ What Drug Interactions Are Clinically Important?

Drugs that may increase the effect or toxicity of bromocriptine

- none

Drugs that may decrease the effect of bromocriptine

- none

Drugs that may have their effect or toxicity increased by bromocriptine
ANTIHYPERTENSIVE AGENTS

- may have an additive hypotensive effect
- dosage of antihypertensive agents may need to be adjusted when these agents are used concomitantly
- treat as for a dosage change in antihypertensive therapy (e.g., assess the effect after 1–2 weeks of the combination therapy)

Drugs that may have their effect decreased by bromocriptine

- none

▶ What Route and Dosage Should I Use?

How to administer

- orally—take with food or milk
- parenterally—not available

Parkinson's disease

- 1.25 mg PO HS daily for 1 week, followed by 2.5 mg PO HS daily for 1 week, 2.5 mg PO BID for 1 week, and then 2.5 mg PO TID for 1 week
- then increase by 2.5 mg PO daily every 7 days, depending on the response and tolerance of side effects
- bromocriptine demonstrates a triphasic response in which at low dosages and high dosages the symptoms of Parkinson's disease worsen
- there is significant variation in the optimum dosage for a given individual ranging from 2.5 mg PO daily to 300 mg PO daily; however, in practice, as the dosage increases above 20 mg daily, the chance of benefit is relatively low but the risk of side effects increases

Dosage adjustments for renal or hepatic dysfunction

- hepatically metabolized
- no dosage adjustment is required; just start with low dosage and titrate up to effect or toxicity

▶ What Should I Monitor with Regard to Efficacy and Toxicity?

Efficacy

Signs and symptoms

- assess symptoms weekly during the titration period
- after the patient has been stabilized, assess the patient every 3 months

Toxicity

- 35–50% of patients do not tolerate bromocriptine, especially at dosages greater than 20 mg PO daily

Central nervous system effects

- confusion, agitation, hallucinations, delusions, sleep disturbances, and abnormal involuntary movements, including orofacial dyskinesias, facial grimacing, and choreic movements of trunk and limbs
- some degree of symptoms affects 80% of patients after 3 years of therapy
- symptoms are dose related and can be minimized with a dosage reduction
- must titrate the dose to minimize abnormal involuntary movements while maintaining optimum control of Parkinson's symptoms
- if the patient has a psychiatric illness, monitor for a recurrence of psychiatric episodes (including dementia, depression, and psychosis)

Cardiovascular effects

- orthostatic hypotension is seen especially when initiating therapy but usually decreases with continued therapy
- advise the patient to rise slowly from a supine position
- if symptoms are severe and the patient needs to wear elastic stockings and increase sodium in the diet, suspect Shy-Drager syndrome

Gastrointestinal side effects

- nausea and vomiting are seen especially when initiating therapy but usually decrease with continued therapy
- take with food or milk
- increase the dosage of bromocriptine gradually to allow tolerance of the gastrointestinal side effects and if dose titration is ineffective add domperidone 20 mg PO TID
- if the patient has had a recent gastrointestinal bleed or peptic ulcer disease, monitor for symptoms of gastrointestinal bleeding (coffee ground emesis, black tarry stools, decreased hemoglobin concentration and hematocrit, occult blood in stool, and gastric pain) annually

Pleuropulmonary fibrosis

- if patient develops chest pain or dyspnea or has decreased breath sounds or a pleural friction rub, do a chest X-ray

Rash

- erythematous rash may occur above the feet
- if bromocriptine is helping, continue therapy and treat the rash symptomatically

▶ *How Long Do I Treat Patients with This Drug?*

Parkinson's disease

- because bromocriptine is a direct dopamine agonist, efficacy is usually maintained over the long term (2 years or longer) in combination with levodopa
- as with other treatments, however, efficacy eventually decreases

▶ *How Do I Decrease or Stop the Administration of This Drug?*

- bromocriptine should not be discontinued abruptly
- when tapering therapy, reduce the dosage by 5 mg every 4 days

▶ *What Should I Tell My Patients About This Drug?*

- contact your physician if symptoms do not improve (or if symptoms worsen) over the next few days after initiation of therapy or dosing changes
- taking bromocriptine with food reduces any nausea or vomiting that you may be experiencing
- tolerance of alcohol may be decreased with concomitant use of bromocriptine, and alcohol intake should be limited

▶ *Therapeutic Tips*

- it is advisable to administer the first 1.25 mg dose of bromocriptine at bedtime with food to establish tolerance
- early combination treatment with bromocriptine to supplement the benefits of levodopa is recommended to minimize the dosage (and side effects) of each individual drug while maximizing the response to each drug
- most clinicians use this drug to treat the end-of-dose effect after the patient has tried 6 doses of levodopa a day without improvement

BUDESONIDE

Karen Shalansky and Cindy Reesor Nimmo

USA (not available)
CANADA (Pulmicort)

▶ *When Should I Use This Drug?*

Chronic asthma or chronic obstructive pulmonary disease

- drug of choice in patients requiring stepwise progression of therapy from PRN use of beta$_2$-agonists
- decreases inflammation and decreases the number and severity of attacks and the need for beta-agonists
- inhaled corticosteroids have a positive effect in both asthma and chronic obstructive pulmonary disease (Ann Intern Med 1993;188:770–778)
- add to therapy if more than 2 beta$_2$-agonist inhalations are required on a daily basis or symptoms are not completely reversed by an inhaled beta$_2$-agonist
- add if the peak expiratory flow rate or forced expiratory volume in 1 second falls to 85% or less of the predicted value or best known result

- use in all patients receiving regular doses of an oral corticosteroid (except for acute attack); high-dose inhaled corticosteroids should be given, as they may allow a reduction or discontinuation of oral corticosteroid therapy
- budesonide has less systemic bioavailability than does beclomethasone (Thorax 1991;46:160–164)
- in low dosages (<1000 μg/d), the impact of this difference in systemic bioavailability between budesonide and beclomethasone is likely not important
- beclomethasone in high dosage (2000 μg/d) increases urinary hydroxyproline output, which reflects an increase in bone resorption, whereas budesonide does not produce this effect (Thorax 1991;46:160–164)
- decision about using this agent or beclomethasone should be based on cost and the patient's inhaler preference

Seasonal asthma

- second-line drug after cromolyn sodium therapy has failed in patients with asthma owing to allergen exposure, because cromolyn sodium is associated with a lower incidence of adverse effects

▶ *When Should I Not Use This Drug?*

Acute asthma

- studies are presently ongoing to evaluate the role of inhaled corticosteroids in acute asthma; however, at present, they are not recommended in patients requiring medical attention for acute asthma

▶ *What Contraindications Are There to the Use of This Drug?*

Intolerance of or allergic reaction to inhaled budesonide

Untreated fungal, bacterial, or viral infections or active or quiescent pulmonary tuberculosis

- high dosages (>1000 μg/d) of inhaled corticosteroids may depress the body's immune system and its ability to fight infections
- if infection is treated, this is likely not a problem

▶ *What Drug Interactions Are Clinically Important?*

- none

▶ *What Route and Dosage Should I Use?*

Available as a turbuhaler

- dry powder inhalers require the following minimum inspiratory flow rates to be effective: spinhaler, 200 L/min; rotahaler, 120 L/min; diskhaler, <60 L/min; turbuhaler, 30 L/min
- diskhaler and turbuhaler have the advantage of not being affected by the humidity
- turbuhaler has the advantage of containing the drug without excipients
- all patients will require teaching of proper inhaler technique and periodic reinforcement of correct technique

Chronic asthma or chronic obstructive pulmonary disease

Turbuhaler

- 200 μg (2 inhalations of the 100 μg/inhalation or 1 inhalation of the 200 μg/inhalation) of the turbuhaler BID is the usual starting dose for mild asthma
- use 200 μg inhaled QID for patients with more severe asthma and increase up to 1600–2000 μg/d if needed
- for patients with severe asthma, higher dosages are recommended because a faster response may be seen; however, after 3–4 weeks one may be able to reduce the dose to a BID regimen
- patients with stable asthma may be adequately controlled with BID dosing of inhaled corticosteroids; however, if the asthma becomes unstable, the patient should be switched to a TID or QID regimen (Hosp Pract 1991;April:15–26)

Converting from systemic oral corticosteroids

- initiate inhaled corticosteroid administration at 200 μg QID for 10 days, then taper oral corticosteroid as tolerated

Seasonal asthma

- 200 μg inhaled BID

- prophylaxis should be initiated 1 week prior to and continued throughout the anticipated allergen season

▶ What Should I Monitor with Regard to Efficacy and Toxicity?

Efficacy

Chronic asthma, chronic obstructive pulmonary disease, seasonal asthma

- improvement occurs within 1–4 weeks of therapy, but 9–12 months may be required for normalization of airway responsiveness

Frequency of as needed beta₂-agonist use

Pulmonary function tests

- can be used to assess the effectiveness of long-term therapy
- patients receiving either oral or inhaled corticosteroids should have these medications continued only if a positive measurable response is seen after institution of these agents

Peak expiratory flow rate

- peak flowmeter should be used by patients who experience severe attacks with little warning and patients who have symptoms of breathlessness or chest tightness repeatedly or require regular Q6H to Q8H beta₂-agonist administration (J Allergy Clin Immunol 1990;85:1098–1111)
- establish best peak expiratory flow rate (PEFR) early in therapy
- usually measured on waking and before bed and before and after beta₂-agonist administration (minimum of twice daily [e.g., morning and evening]) and is the best of 3 measurements on each occasion
- daily variation should be less than 20% and ideally less than 10%
- patients should be instructed to double the dosage of inhaled corticosteroids if PEFR is less than 75% of the best value, start a short course of oral steroids if PEFR is less than 50% of the best result, and call the physician if PEFR is less than 25% of the best value (Postgrad Med J 1991;67:1–3)

Toxicity

Oropharyngeal candidiasis

- dose-dependent adverse effect, which usually responds to topical antifungal therapy or a temporary reduction in dosage
- may be minimized by gargling with water after each inhalation
- frequency of oral candidiasis with high-dose inhalers is similar to that with low-dose inhalers

Dysphonia

- dose-dependent adverse effect
- usually responds to a reduction in dosage but may reoccur after the dosage is increased
- may be minimized by gargling with water after each inhalation

Mild hypothalamic-pituitary-adrenal axis suppression

- patients receiving equal to or greater than 1600 μg/d are at greatest risk and should be treated similarly to patients receiving long-term oral corticosteroids (J Allergy Clin Immunol 1988;82:297–306)
- potential for side effects may increase with concomitant oral and inhaled corticosteroid therapy

▶ How Long Do I Treat Patients with This Drug?

Chronic asthma or chronic obstructive pulmonary disease

- continual therapy is indicated if therapy results in a significant decrease in the severity of the asthma, a reduction or discontinuation of oral corticosteroid use, or a substitution for a drug that may cause intolerable side effects
- unless a significant causative factor is identified and removed, patients treated with inhaled corticosteroids likely require the therapy indefinitely
- high dosages of inhaled corticosteroids may not need to be continued after asthma is under control
- dosages should be tapered on the basis of PEFR and symptoms (Br Med J 1991;302:738)
- after control or the best result is achieved, the dosage should be reduced to the minimum effective level

- in patients with stable asthma, an attempt should be made to reduce the dosing frequency to BID

Seasonal asthma

- inhaled corticosteroid administration could probably be abruptly discontinued after the end of the offending allergen season; however, tapering over 1 week is wise

▶ How Do I Decrease or Stop the Administration of This Drug?

- in patients receiving high-dose or long-term therapy, treatment should not be discontinued abruptly unless systemic corticosteroids are administered, as exacerbation of the asthma or withdrawal symptoms may occur
- daily dosage should be reduced weekly by 25%
- PEFRs should be consistently stable prior to decreasing the dosage and before each dosage reduction

▶ What Should I Tell My Patients About This Drug?

- inhaled corticosteroid is used to prevent bronchospasm and does not relieve an attack that has already started
- although it is generally recommended to precede corticosteroid inhalation with inhalation of a bronchodilator, this practice has not been shown to increase the delivery of the drug to the lungs or to increase the efficacy of the corticosteroid
- compliance with regular therapy is essential to maintain control of asthma
- use the inhaler exactly as directed
- patients may not be able to feel a dose administered via a turbuhaler

Turbuhaler

1. unscrew and remove the cover
2. holding the turbuhaler upright, turn the colored grip fully in 1 direction and then back again until it clicks
3. exhale to a normal relaxed expiration, and then place the mouthpiece between the teeth and lips
4. breathe in quickly and deeply through your mouth—hold your breath for 5–10 seconds—breathe out slowly to normal relaxed resting position
5. replace the cover and screw it shut
6. if the turbuhaler is dropped, the dose is lost and it must be reloaded by turning the colored grip (see step 2)

▶ *Therapeutic Tips*

- patients taking high-dose (≥1600 μg/d) inhaled corticosteroids may require supplemental systemic corticosteroids during periods of stress (e.g., infection and surgery)
- inhaled corticosteroids do not have to be given after an inhaled dose of salbutamol and should be used only in conjunction with salbutamol when salbutamol is needed for symptom relief
- high-dose inhaled corticosteroids produce a faster response than does low-dose therapy
- higher dosages of inhaled corticosteroids are required to normalize pulmonary function than to relieve symptoms

Useful References

Brogden RN, McTavish D. Budesonide. Drugs 1992;44:375–407

Johnson CE. Aerosol corticosteroids for the treatment of asthma. DICP 1987;21:784–790

Smith MJ. The place of high-dose inhaled corticosteroids in asthma therapy. Drugs 1987;33:423–429

Konig P. Inhaled corticosteroids—Their present and future role in the management of asthma. J Allergy Clin Immunol 1988;82:297–306

BULK-FORMING LAXATIVES

Leslie Mathews

Dietary Fiber

Bran and Fruit Fiber

USA (Combination: Correctol)
CANADA (Fibyrax)

Psyllium Hydrophilic Mucilloid/Ispaghula Husk

USA (Effer-Syllium, Fiberall, Hydrocil instant, Konsyl, Metamucil, Modane bulk, Naturacil; combination: Prompt, Prodiem) CANADA (Metamucil, Prodiem plain, Karacil, Fibremucilax, Fiberall, Effer-Syllium; combination: Prodiem)

Methylcellulose, Carboxymethylcellulose

USA (Cologel, combination: Disoplex)
CANADA (Citrucel)

Sterculia Gum–Karaya

Malt Soup Extract

USA (Maltsupex; combination: Syllamalt)

Calcium Polycarbophil

USA (Mitrolan, FiberCon)
CANADA (Mitrolan)

▶ When Should I Use This Drug?

Acute constipation

- bulk-forming laxatives are useful for acute constipation in patients in whom a rapid response (within hours) is not desired
- effective within 2–3 days, well tolerated, and safe for long-term use in conjunction with increased dietary fiber
- these agents do not work as rapidly as the stimulant laxatives or lactulose

Chronic constipation

- bulk-forming laxatives are the agents of choice to prevent and treat most types of constipation, especially in the elderly, and constipation related to a low-residue diet, pregnancy, acute or chronic illness, or constipating medications
- many patients respond well, requiring no alternative drug therapy (Br Med J 1990;300:1063–1065)
- safe for long-term use
- especially useful in preventing constipation in high-risk populations (hospitalized or pregnant patients, those with poor dietary habits, and patients using constipating medications)
- may need to combine with occasional osmotic or stimulant laxative and/or suppository or enema, particularly for atonic constipation
- also useful when trying to avoid strain of evacuation, as increased bulk does not necessarily mean increased straining (e.g., anorectal disorders, hernias, recovery from myocardial infarction, cerebrovascular accident, and so on)
- to maintain soft, bulky stools that are easily passed is particularly important with anorectal disease (hemorrhoids, fissures), after anorectal surgery (Dis Colon Rectum 1987;30:780–781), and in cases of myocardial infarction
- also useful to treat constipation related to irritable bowel syndrome (Gut 1987;28:1510–1513) and uncomplicated diverticular disease (Lancet 1977;1:664–666); however, efficacy in relief of other symptoms of these conditions (e.g., abdominal pain, bloating, and distention) is controversial (Am J Gastroenterol 1984; 79:1–7), but many clinicians believe that a trial is warranted (Am J Gastroenterol 1986;81:95–100)

Acute diarrhea and regulation of colostomy effluent

- absorbs water and produces a softer, bulkier mass
- use when a rapid onset is not required (onset of action is 48 hours)
- attapulgite and loperamide work faster as antidiarrheals

▶ When Should I Not Use This Drug?

Need for immediate and/or complete bowel evacuation

- for example, acute constipation with impending fecal impaction, removal of toxins, and bowel cleansing for surgery or diagnostic procedure
- bulk-forming laxatives have a relatively slow onset of action and do not facilitate thorough emptying of the colon

Neurogenic constipation

- these patients require stimulant laxatives, suppositories, or enemas to initiate bowel movements

Severe idiopathic chronic constipation

- if rectal expulsion is impossible or difficult owing to a slow colonic transit time because of generalized colonic inertia and/ or anorectal dysfunction (Lancet 1986;1:767–769)
- bulk-forming laxatives are not helpful, may aggravate symptoms, and may contribute to impaction (Hosp Pract 1990;25:89–100)
- instead institute bowel retraining using suppositories, enemas, biofeedback techniques, or surgery for severe cases

Debilitated patients with advanced disease

- fecal impaction and gastrointestinal obstruction are possible if dehydration and motility problems are present (Med Clin North Am 1987;71:305–311)
- instead use osmotics (magnesium hydroxide, lactulose), stimulants (senna, bisacodyl), suppositories (glycerin, bisacodyl), and enemas (tap water sodium phosphate [Fleet])

Constipation in chronically bedbound patients

- may exacerbate the problem by increasing bulk in an already distended colon, causing impaction or obstruction (J Gerontol Nurs 1990;16:4–11)
- importance is controversial; some studies have demonstrated successful use of bulk-forming laxatives in immobile patients (J Am Geriatr Soc 1983;31:289–293)
- lactulose should be used

Appetite suppressant in the management of obesity

- not shown to be effective

▶ What Contraindications Are There to the Use of This Drug?

Intolerance of or allergic reaction to bulk-forming laxatives

- although uncommon, anaphylaxis can occur with ingestion of psyllium hydrophilic mucilloid (Allergy Proc 1990;11:241–242)
- acute bronchospasm, rhinitis, and asthmatic attacks can occur with the inhalation of dry psyllium powder (DICP 1986;20:548)
- substitute an alternative bulk-forming laxative for psyllium

Undiagnosed abdominal pain, nausea, vomiting

- symptoms of acute abdomen or fecal impaction

Partial bowel obstruction

- for example, that related to intestinal stenosis, adhesions, or stricture
- bulk-forming laxatives may contribute to bowel obstruction
- use occasional osmotics, stimulants, or enemas instead
- depending on the severity of the obstruction, all laxatives may be contraindicated

Dysphagia, obstructive disorders of the esophagus

- bolus formation and obstruction are possible
- avoid the use of dry powder preparations in those at risk
- ensure that all bulk-forming laxatives are mixed with at least 250 mL of fluid and are ingested promptly after mixing

Significant fluid restrictions

- for example, in severe renal disease or severe debility
- obstruction of the gastrointestinal tract (esophagus, stomach, small intestine, colon) can occur if bulk-forming laxatives are taken with an inadequate amount of fluid
- use stimulant laxatives or glycerin suppositories instead

Celiac disease

- wheat bran is contraindicated
- use an alternative bulk-forming laxative (such as methylcellulose, carboxymethylcellulose sodium, Sterculia gum, malt soup extract, or calcium polycarbophil)

▶ What Drug Interactions Are Clinically Important?

- none

▶ *What Route and Dosage Should I Use?*

How to administer

Orally

- all powder and granule forms of bulk-forming laxatives should be mixed in at least 250 mL of fluid and should be ingested promptly after mixing
- other forms, if not directly mixed with water, should be taken with at least 250 mL of fluid and an additional 250 mL is recommended to increase efficacy and prevent gastrointestinal obstruction

Acute constipation, chronic constipation

- all laxatives in this class appear to be equally efficacious
- choice of product (dietary fiber, commercial powders, crystals, tablets) depends on the patient's acceptance of texture and taste (tasteless, minty, orange flavored, and so on) and excipients (low sodium, sugar free) and cost
- start with a low dosage, and increase gradually weekly over 2–4 weeks until the desired effect is obtained or the recommended maximum dosage is reached
- increase more slowly if significant cramping or bloating develops without beneficial effect

DIETARY FIBER

- start with 6 g/d PO, roughly equal to 2 tablespoons of raw bran
- increase to 10 g/d after 1 week, equivalent to 1.1 ounces of bran, 2.9 ounces of shredded wheat, or 4 slices of whole-wheat bread (Med Clin North Am 1989;73:1502–1509)
- aim for 20–30 g/d (Hosp Pract 1990;25:89–100)

Food Group	Serving Size	Amount of fiber (g)
Grains/cereals		
All-Bran 100%	1/3 cup	8.4–10.6
raw bran	3 tablespoons	5.4
whole-wheat bread	2 slices	2.6–4.6
shredded wheat	2 biscuits	4.2
corn flakes	3/4 cup	2.6
Wheaties	3/4 cup	2.6
Special K	3/4 cup	1.2
brown rice	1/3 cup	1.6
Vegetables		
baked beans	1/2 cup	9.2
peas (canned)	1/2 cup	6.7
corn	1 cob	5.2
broccoli	1/2 cup	3.2–3.5
cabbage (cooked)	1/2 cup	2.5
carrots	1/2 cup	1.0–2.8
string beans	1/2 cup	1.0–2.1
tomato	1 medium	1.0–1.9

Food Group	Serving Size	Amount of fiber (g)
Fruits		
pear (unpeeled)	1 medium	12.6
raspberries	1 cup	9.2
apple (unpeeled)	1 medium	5.6
strawberries	1 cup	2.6–3.1
banana	1 medium	2.0–3.0
peach (unpeeled)	1 medium	2.2
raisins	1/2 cup	1.1–2.0
Nuts		
peanut butter	100 g	7.6
peanuts	50 g	4.0
sunflower seeds	1/2 cup	2.1–4.2
Brazil nuts	1/2 cup	2.1–4.2

Compiled from Am J Gastroenterol 1985;80:303–309, Med Clin North Am 1989;73:1502–1509, Pocket Encyclopedia of Nutrition 1986:98.

GRAIN AND FRUIT FIBERS

- varies with product
- for Fibyrax, give 4 tablets PO daily increasing to 12 tablets PO daily

PSYLLIUM HYDROPHILIC POWDER

- varies with product
- usual dose is 1 teaspoon or package 1–3 times per day PO mixed in 240 mL of fluid for constipation
- optimum dose for irritable bowel syndrome is 20 g/d (Gut 1987;28:150–155)
- also available as crystals and wafers

METHYLCELLULOSE

- varies with product
- start with 450 mg 3 times daily mixed in 250 mL of cold fluid, gradually increase as needed to 1.8 g TID

STERCULIA GUM

- start with 5 g PO daily taken with fluid as directed, increasing to 10 g daily as needed

MALT SOUP EXTRACT

- start with 32 g PO daily in divided doses, increasing to 64 g daily as needed

CALCIUM POLYCARBOPHIL

- 2 tablets chewed and swallowed with 250 mL of fluid QID (or 4 g/d) for constipation
- 2 tablets with 250 mL of fluid every 30 minutes (maximum daily dose, 12 tablets) for severe diarrhea

▶ *What Should I Monitor with Regard to Efficacy and Toxicity?*

Efficacy

Acute constipation, chronic constipation

- produces soft formed stool in 1–5 days
- to be fully effective must be taken for 2–3 days without interruption and with an adequate amount of fluid (250–500 mL/dose)
- onset of action may be delayed in patients who have used other laxatives long term
- several weeks of use may be necessary to relieve chronic constipation

Acute diarrhea and regulation of colostomy effluent

- onset of action is up to 48 hours (Am J Med 1990;88:245–265)

Toxicity

Gastrointestinal symptoms

- abdominal bloating, cramping, and flatulence are common; nausea or vomiting is less common
- these symptoms occur particularly in the first few weeks of use but often resolve with continued use
- decrease the daily dose by a third for intolerable gastrointestinal symptoms
- to avoid or minimize these effects, increase the dosage gradually, switch to a different preparation or source of fiber, or increase the fluid intake

Esophageal obstruction (rare)

- suspect with dysphagia, coughing, choking, and drooling
- to prevent this side effect, take the bulk-forming laxative with at least 250 mL of fluid and drink powder-fluid suspensions promptly after mixing

Intestinal obstruction (uncommon)

- monitor for in high-risk patients (e.g., bedbound patients, cathartic abusers)
- X-rays may be indicated for nausea, vomiting, abdominal pain, distention, and absent bowel sounds

Allergic reactions (bronchospasm, urticaria, rhinitis, dermatitis, eye irritation, anaphylaxis)

- have occurred with psyllium after oral and inhalation exposure
- sensitization can occur with workplace exposure (e.g., nurses)

- if an allergic reaction is suspected, avoid the use of psyllium husk and use synthetic agents instead (e.g., carboxymethylcellulose sodium and calcium polycarbophil)
- hypersensitivity can be confirmed with skin testing (DICP 1986; 20:548, Allergy Proc 1990;11:241–242)

Fluid retention

- can occur with high sodium content in some preparations (e.g., carboxymethylcellulose)
- use preparation with little or no sodium content (e.g., Citrucel and Mitrolan)

▶ *How Long Do I Treat Patients with This Drug?*

Acute constipation, chronic constipation

- for at least 4–6 weeks before evaluating effectiveness
- safe to use on a regular basis indefinitely

▶ *How Do I Decrease or Stop the Administration of This Drug?*

- may be stopped abruptly

▶ *What Should I Tell My Patients About This Drug?*

- bulk-forming laxatives must be used daily for at least 2–3 days to be fully effective
- in cases of chronic, severe constipation, it may take a few weeks for complete relief
- bran is the best source of dietary fiber, either raw or processed in whole-grain cereals or breads
- sprinkle raw bran on foods or mix in fluids (e.g., milkshakes)
- other sources of dietary fiber (e.g., raisins, prunes, dried apricots, dates, beans, peas, nuts, and sweet potatoes) are beneficial as well
- mix commercial powders or crystals in 8 ounces of juice, pop, or water and drink promptly
- follow with another 8 ounces of plain fluid
- drink at least 8 ounces of fluid with each dose of tablets
- transient abdominal bloating, cramping, and flatus can occur, especially in the first week or two
- if symptoms are uncomfortable, cut back 1 dose or 1 tablespoon of bran (or its equivalent) per day
- gradually increase the dosage until the stools are soft and evacuation is comfortable
- if a skin rash, itching, hives, wheezing, or difficulty in breathing develops while taking psyllium, contact your physician immediately
- in the event of nausea, vomiting, abdominal pain, or difficulty in swallowing, contact your physician

▶ *Therapeutic Tips*

- all laxatives in this class appear to be equally efficacious
- choices are available in regard to presentation (dietary fiber, commercial powders, crystals, tablets), taste (tasteless, minty, orange flavored, and so on) and excipients (low sodium, sugar free)
- consider sodium and dextrose content when ordering products for patients with sodium or carbohydrate restrictions
- avoid use of products with aspartame (e.g., Metamucil sugar free) for patients with phenylketonuria or phenylalanine restrictions
- avoid the use of calcium polycarbophil for patients with calcium restrictions
- calcium polycarbophil tablets are preferred to psyllium suspensions by some patients because of the ease of administration and the lower incidence of flatulence (Curr Ther Res 1988;44: 770–774)
- some patients cannot tolerate enough fiber to alleviate constipation (Br Med J 1990;300:1064–1065)
- other bulk-forming laxatives in various forms can be substituted with good effect

Useful References

Taylor R. Management of constipation—high fibre diets work. Br Med J 1990;300:1063–1064

Spiller R. When fibre fails. Br Med J 1990;300:1064–1065

Tedesco FJ. Laxative use in constipation. Am J Gastroenterol 1985; 80:303–309

Natow AB, Heslin J. Pocket Encyclopedia of Nutrition. New York: Pocket Books, 1981

BUMETANIDE

Ian Petterson

USA (Bumex)
CANADA (Bumex)

▶ *When Should I Use This Drug?*

Consider an alternative agent

- there is no reason to use this drug instead of furosemide because the effects are identical and bumetanide is considerably more expensive
- although there is the suggestion that bumetanide is less ototoxic than furosemide, there are no direct comparisons between them (J Clin Pharmacol 1981;21:615–619)
- bumetanide is more potent than furosemide, and although smaller doses can be used, this offers no clinical advantages
- use furosemide if a loop diuretic is required or hydrochlorothiazide if a thiazide diuretic is needed

BUPRENORPHINE

Terry Baumann

USA (Buprenex)
CANADA (Buprenex)

▶ *When Should I Use This Drug?*

Acute pain

- use only when the patient has a true allergy to meperidine and the patient does not tolerate morphine
- although it has been reported that buprenorphine causes less severe respiratory depression than does morphine because it is a partial agonist, if morphine (as with any opioid) is properly titrated there is likely little, if any, clinical difference between these drugs with regard to respiratory depression
- has a longer duration of action (6 hours) than do morphine and nalbuphine (4 hours) but is more expensive

Postoperative pain

- drug of choice only if there is true allergy to meperidine and the patient does not tolerate morphine
- offers no advantages over morphine and is more expensive

▶ *When Should I Not Use This Drug?*

Mild to moderate pain

- unless drugs such as acetaminophen, acetaminophen-codeine, and nonsteroidal antiinflammatory drugs have been used on a regularly scheduled (not PRN) basis and are shown to be ineffective

Chronic cancer pain and chronic noncancer pain

- for moderate to severe cancer pain, use morphine, hydromorphone, methadone, or levorphanol
- only the parenteral form of buprenorphine is available
- buprenorphine may induce withdrawal symptoms in opioid-dependent patients
- dose titration may be difficult at higher dosages because upper dose limits have not been well established
- tolerance and dependence may occur if used for long periods

▶ *What Contraindications Are There to the Use of This Drug?*

Intolerance of or allergic reaction to buprenorphine

- true allergies to buprenorphine or related compounds (i. e., morphine, codeine, hydromorphone, oxymorphone, levorphanol, hydrocodone, oxycodone, butorphanol, nalbuphine) are rare
- if true allergy exists, may use meperidine or fentanyl

Severe respiratory depression

- not an absolute contraindication—just start with dosages 25% of the normal initial dose and titrate up to effect while assessing the respiratory rate and performing oximetry before each dose

▶ What Drug Interactions Are Clinically Important?

see Morphine

▶ What Route and Dosage Should I Use?

How to administer

- orally—not available
- parenterally—may be administered intramuscularly, intravenously (dilute IV buprenorphine in 10 mL of normal saline and give over at least 2 minutes); is not recommended for subcutaneous administration

Acute pain

- 0.3 mg IM Q6H (not PRN) or 0.15 mg IM Q6H (not PRN) for elderly patients because of concerns about sedation and respiratory depression
- some patients may require Q4H dosing
- question patients frequently about the degree of pain they are having (ideally, within at most 1–2 hours after the first dose if the drug was administered via the IM route)
- if pain is unrelieved by this time and there are no signs of sedation or respiratory depression, give another dose 50% higher than the first dose
- continue this approach until pain is 75% relieved, and then maintain at this dosage for 12 hours before further adjustments are made
- normal dose increments are 0.3 and 0.4 mg
- if an immediate response (within 1–5 minutes) for severe pain is needed, use intravenously as recommended for postoperative pain (see below)

Postoperative pain

In the postanesthetic care unit

- 0.3 mg IV repeated once in 30–60 minutes
- adjust the dose on the basis of the response to each dose and titrate to achieve pain control and an acceptable level of sedation or respiratory rate

On the ward

Intermittent therapy

- as above for acute pain
- question the patient frequently and increase the dose as above for acute pain on the basis of pain relief and level of sedation

Patient-controlled analgesia

- 0.05–0.1 mg/bolus with lockout of 6 minutes
- some clinicians believe that 0.1 mg/h as an infusion for patient-controlled analgesia enables patients to sleep through the night; however, evidence suggests that using a bolus with a baseline infusion may increase the amount of narcotic used and the side effects, without improving efficacy (Anaesth Intensive Care 1991;19:555–560, Anesthesiology 1992;76:362–367)
- question patients frequently about the degree of pain they are having
- if pain is not controlled with bolus doses, increase the bolus dose by 25–50%
- if pain relief from a bolus dose is adequate but the duration of pain relief is too short, decrease the lockout period

Dosage adjustments for renal or hepatic dysfunction

- renally and hepatically eliminated
- dosage adjustment is usually not required if the dose is titrated properly

▶ What Should I Monitor with Regard to Efficacy and Toxicity?

see Morphine

▶ How Long Do I Treat Patients with This Drug?

see Morphine

▶ How Do I Decrease or Stop the Administration of This Drug?

see Morphine

▶ What Should I Tell My Patients About This Drug?

see Morphine

▶ Therapeutic Tips

- because this drug has agonist and antagonist activities, it is not recommended for use with other opioids
- always prescribe buprenorphine doses at regularly scheduled intervals
- for patients who will be receiving regularly dosed narcotics for longer than 3–4 days, always consider prescribing narcotics in conjunction with a laxative and counsel the patient on the appropriate use of fluids and fiber

Useful References

see Morphine

BUPROPION

Lyle K. Laird and Julia Vertrees

USA (Wellbutrin)
CANADA (available only as compassionate release)

▶ When Should I Use This Drug?

Major depression

- bupropion is a novel-structured (aminoketone), antidepressant medication that differs both structurally and pharmacologically from the tricyclic antidepressants, monoamine oxidase inhibitors, and the other so-called second-generation antidepressant drugs
- bupropion is no more effective in the treatment of depression than any other antidepressant
- although it was initially thought that bupropion caused a high incidence of seizures, evidence suggests that it is similar to other antidepressants (0.4% incidence) with regard to seizure risk (J Clin Psychiatry 1991;52:450–456, J Clin Psychiatry 1989;50:256–261)
- bupropion is not known to cause significant autonomic, antihistaminic, or cardiovascular side effects (Pharmacotherapy 1984;4:20–34)
- it does not cause significant cardiovascular effects (including orthostatic hypotension, intracardiac conduction problems, and cardiac pump dysfunction) in medically healthy, depressed patients (J Clin Psychiatry 1983;44:176–182)
- it is apparently safe as an antidepressant in some depressed patients with preexisting cardiac disease (including left ventricular impairment, ventricular arrhythmias, and/or conduction disease) (Am J Psychiatry 1991;148:512–516)
- it is indicated for the treatment of depressive disorders that have not responded to other pharmacotherapeutic interventions
- has the disadvantage of requiring multiple daily dosing (BID or TID)
- should be used only in patients who do not respond to other antidepressants

▶ When Should I Not Use This Drug?

see Imipramine

▶ What Contraindications Are There to the Use of This Drug?

Intolerance of or allergic reaction to bupropion

Eating disorder history or current diagnosis of an eating disorder, including anorexia nervosa and bulimia nervosa

- patients with eating disorders appear to be at greater risk for seizures (J Clin Psychiatry 1989;50:256–261)

Pregnancy

- animal studies have failed to document a risk; inadequate human studies have been performed

Seizure disorders, previous head trauma, or central nervous system tumors

- can worsen seizure disorders

▶ *What Drug Interactions Are Clinically Important?*

Drugs that may increase the effect or toxicity of bupropion

ALCOHOL

- altering the alcohol use pattern or using alcohol along with bupropion may increase the risk of seizures

MONAMINE OXIDASE INHIBITORS

- concurrent use with bupropion can result in an increased incidence of adverse effects
- avoid the combination and allow at least a 2 week drug-free interval between stopping the monoamine oxidase inhibitor and starting bupropion administration

TRICYCLIC ANTIDEPRESSANTS, LITHIUM, AND ANTIPSYCHOTIC DRUGS, INCLUDING PHENOTHIAZINES, THIOXANTHENES, LOXAPINE, AND MOLINDONE

- concurrent use may lower seizure threshold
- avoid the use of more than one antidepressant
- for the other drugs, if concurrent use is necessary, start with a low dose of both agents, and titrate up to effect

Drugs that may decrease the effect of bupropion

- none

Drugs that may have their effect or toxicity increased by bupropion

- none

Drugs that may have their effect decreased by bupropion

- none

▶ *What Route and Dosage Should I Use?*

How to administer

- orally—can be given with food or on an empty stomach
- parenterally—not available

Major depression

- give 100 mg PO BID, and after 3 days, increase to 100 mg PO TID
- maximum daily dose is 450 mg with no single dose greater than 150 mg; dosing intervals should be TID (the time between doses must be at least 4 hours); seek to adjust maintenance dosage to the lowest effective level
- only 75 mg tablets are available in Canada
- 75 mg PO BID for 3–4 days
- increase to 75 mg PO TID for 1 week, then increase to 150 mg PO BID, and then wait for 4 weeks and evaluate

Dosage adjustments for renal or hepatic dysfunction

- hepatically metabolized to active metabolites
- no dosage adjustment guidelines are available
- in patients with renal or hepatic dysfunction, start with lowest available dose and titrate the dose on the basis of efficacy and toxicity

▶ *What Should I Monitor with Regard to Efficacy and Toxicity?*

Efficacy

see Imipramine

Plasma concentrations

- relationship between steady state bupropion plasma concentrations and clinical effect is not known

Toxicity

Central nervous system stimulation

- during the initiation of bupropion dosing, some agitation, motor restlessness, and insomnia may be reported
- these effects generally subside with time

Seizure

- seizure is the most clinically significant adverse effect
- incidence of seizures with bupropion may be as high as 0.4%

- seizure incidence may be decreased by limiting the total dose to 450 mg/d or less; divide the dosing so that each single dose does not exceed 150 mg
- titrate dose up slowly (see above)

Switch from depression to a manic phase

- is rare, but can occur (J Clin Psychiatry 1991;52:4–13)

▶ *How Long Do I Treat Patients with This Drug?*

see Imipramine

▶ *How Do I Decrease or Stop the Administration of This Drug?*

- after 4–6 weeks at maximally tolerated dosage (not exceeding 450 mg/d) without clinical effect, bupropion dosage should be tapered over 1–2 weeks, as tolerated, and an alternative treatment should be considered
- do not abruptly stop this medication unless toxicity (including seizure) or a hypersensitivity is suspected

▶ *What Should I Tell My Patients About This Drug?*

- take this drug as prescribed; do not increase the dosage on your own
- bupropion may be taken with food
- avoid the use of alcohol with bupropion
- tell your physician and pharmacist all medications that you are taking
- tell your physician and pharmacist if you become pregnant
- if a dose is missed, take as soon as possible and resume schedule (do not double-up on doses)
- it may take up to 4 weeks for bupropion to exert maximum antidepressant effects

▶ *Therapeutic Tips*

- if the patient has been taking a monoamine oxidase inhibitor, give at least a 2-week washout prior to starting bupropion administration
- dose titration must be gradual; the daily dosage should be divided and given on a TID schedule (with at least 4 hours between doses) with no single dose greater than 150 mg; the total daily dosage should not exceed 450 mg (to minimize the risk of seizures)
- as compared with the tricyclic antidepressants and monoamine oxidase inhibitors, bupropion has almost no cardiovascular adverse effects and may be a good choice for depressed patients with preexisting cardiac disease
- relationship between steady state bupropion plasma concentrations and clinical effect is not known
- avoid in patients with a seizure disorder
- bupropion may cause a lower incidence of sexual dysfunction compared with that with tricyclic antidepressants and monoamine oxidase inhibitors

Useful References

USP Dispensing Information. Rockville, MD: The United States Pharmacopeial Convention, 1991

Preskorn SH, Othmer SC. Evaluation of bupropion hydrochloride: The first of a new class of atypical antidepressants. Pharmacotherapy 1984;4: 20–34

Golden RN, Rudorder MV, Sherer MA, et al. Bupropion in depression I. Biochemical effects and clinical responses. Arch Gen Psychiatry 1988; 45:139–143

BUSPIRONE

Steven Stanislav and Patricia Marken

USA (BuSpar)
CANADA (BuSpar)

▶ *When Should I Use This Drug?*

Generalized anxiety disorder

- equal efficacy to benzodiazepines in controlled studies (Pharmacotherapy 1988;8:100–116)
- consider as first-line therapy if patients are newly diagnosed; when chronic anxiety is present (specific symptoms of general-

ized anxiety disorder) and there is an absence of acute precipitants; if sedation or psychomotor or cognitive impairment would be dangerous; and if there is a history of substance abuse, personality disorders, or absence of panic attacks or obsessive-compulsive disorder (J Clin Psychiatry 1990;51:3–10)

- buspirone has a slower onset of action (2–4 weeks) than do benzodiazepines
- clinical experience suggests that previous responders to benzodiazepine may not respond as well to buspirone, as patients report an effect on somatic symptoms that is less dramatic than with benzodiazepines
- buspirone appears to modulate or dampen anxiety rather than extinguish it

▶ When Should I Not Use This Drug?

Short-term or palliative anxiolytic therapy

- owing to delayed onset of effect compared with the benzodiazepines

Panic disorders, obsessive-compulsive disorders, depression

- studies have not validated buspirone effectiveness

▶ What Contraindications Are There to the Use of This Drug?

- Intolerance of or allergic reaction to buspirone

▶ What Drug Interactions Are Clinically Important?

Drugs that may increase the effect or toxicity of buspirone

MONOAMINE OXIDASE INHIBITORS

- reports of increased blood pressure with combination therapy; best to avoid concomitant use until there is further clarification

Drugs that may decrease the effect of buspirone

FLUOXETINE

- several case reports suggest that fluoxetine can increase anxiety in patients taking buspirone
- buspirone may increase the agitation that some patients experience with fluoxetine administration
- if this combination is used, look for signs of agitation within the first couple of weeks, and if agitation is seen, stop administration of one of the agents

Drugs that may have their effect or toxicity increased by buspirone

- none

Drugs that may have their effect decreased by buspirone

- none

▶ What Route and Dosage Should I Use?

How to administer

- orally—can be taken with food or milk or on an empty stomach
- parenterally—not available

Generalized anxiety disorder

- start with 5 mg PO BID, and if tolerated, increase the dosage to 5 mg PO TID after 3–4 days; then increase to 10 mg PO BID after another 3–4 days if tolerated
- after 2 weeks of treatment, if the patient has not improved, increase to 10 mg PO TID
- after 2 more weeks, can increase to 20 mg PO BID if the patient has still not improved
- most people who are going to respond will respond to dosages of 30 mg PO daily, although some may require 60 mg PO daily

Dosage adjustments for renal or hepatic dysfunction

- eliminated by hepatic metabolism and renal excretion; however, little is known about the correlations between the severity of renal or hepatic impairment and buspirone clearance
- until more conclusive data are available, it is best to avoid buspirone administration in patients with significant hepatic dysfunction (e.g., alcoholic cirrhosis) or renal dysfunction (creatinine clearance <10 mL/min)

- no dosage adjustments for minor organ dysfunction are recommended; however, always start with the lowest dose and titrate to response

▶ What Should I Monitor with Regard to Efficacy and Toxicity?

Efficacy

Generalized anxiety disorder

Target symptoms

- monitor changes in increased motor or muscle tension, restlessness, autonomic hyperactivity (shortness of breath, palpitations, dry mouth, nausea, vomiting, and so on), and hypervigilance
- monitor initially every 2–3 days for benzodiazeopines and weekly for buspirone
- after their condition is stable, patients should be clinically assessed for target symptoms at least monthly (or weekly if clinical decompensation suspected)

Toxicity

Dizziness, headache, drowsiness, nausea, and nervousness

- decrease or stop the drug administration if these symptoms increase in severity and become intolerable to the patient

▶ How Long Do I Treat Patients with This Drug?

Generalized anxiety disorder

- in contrast to benzodiazepines, buspirone has a delayed onset of action; typical response time for relief of anxiety is 2–4 weeks and as long as 6 weeks in some patients (Psychiatr Ann 1987; 17:114–120)
- discontinue drug administration if no clinical improvement occurs after at least 4 weeks of at least 20–30 mg buspirone daily (if improvement in at least 1 target symptom is seen, observe for further improvement until the end of week 6)
- use the lowest effective dose for the shortest period of time; attempt periodic discontinuation
- several well-designed studies describe generalized anxiety disorder as a chronic illness with fluctuating levels of symptom severity, yet few long-term efficacy studies (longer than 6 months) exist and the efficacy of drug therapy beyond 6 months is unknown

▶ How Do I Decrease or Stop the Administration of This Drug?

- may be stopped abruptly
- some clinicians reduce the dosage by 50% for a couple of days then stop drug

▶ What Should I Tell My Patients About This Drug?

- this drug usually takes at least 2–4 weeks, and sometimes longer, to work, and you may not notice the same euphoric or sedative effects that are typical of other agents that may have been used to treat your symptoms
- although combined use appears to be relatively safe, try to avoid or minimize your consumption of alcohol while taking this medication; alcohol may also make your symptoms worse

▶ Therapeutic Tips

- owing to its delayed onset of action, buspirone is typically not useful in acutely anxious patients (consider a short-term overlap with treatment with benzodiazepines)
- clinical experience suggests that previous benzodiazepine responders may not respond as well to buspirone
- patients report an effect that is less dramatic than that with benzodiazepines
- buspirone does not suppress the symptoms of benzodiazepine withdrawal; therefore, 2–4 weeks overlap with 20–30 mg of buspirone is recommended prior to discontinuing benzodiazepine administration (Psychiatr Ann 1988;18:139–145)
- buspirone is ineffective in managing or ameliorating insomnia associated with anxiety, and it may increase or cause insomnia
- clinicians have noticed that high doses (i.e., 60 mg) may have antiaggressive effects

Useful References

Dubovsky SL. Generalized anxiety disorder: New concepts and psychopharmacologic therapies. J Clin Psychiatry 1990;51:3–32

Hayes PE, Dommise CS. Current concepts in clinical therapeutics: Anxiety disorders I, II. Clin Pharm 1987;6:140–147, 196–215

Jann MW. Buspirone: An update on a unique anxiolytic agent. Pharmacotherapy 1988;8:100–116

BUTORPHANOL

Terry Baumann

USA (Stadol)
CANADA (Stadol)

▶ When Should I Use This Drug?

Consider an alternative agent

- offers no advantages over buprenorphine, nalbuphine, or other opioids with respect to efficacy and toxicity (Anaesthesia 1979;34:633–637)
- buprenorphine has a longer analgesic effect than does butorphanol, which allows buprenorphine to be given less frequently
- butorphanol is the only analgesic available in a nasal dosage form

CALCITONIN

Deborah Stier Carson

Calcitonin (Salmon)

USA (Calcimar)
CANADA (Calcimar)

Calcitonin (Human)

USA (Cibacalcin)
CANADA (not available)

▶ When Should I Use This Drug?

Treatment of osteoporosis

- in patients who have a history of osteoporotic compression fractures (Am J Med 1983;75:899–901)
- in postmenopausal women who cannot take estrogen because of intolerance or contraindication but who have documented high rates of bone turnover
- although calcitonin is relatively safe and has few side effects, it is expensive, it requires parenteral administration, and lasting benefits have not been established
- it should be considered only in patients who cannot take hormonal therapy or in patients who have significant pain due to osteoporosis, because in low doses calcitonin may provide pain relief
- in patients with low bone mass, regardless of whether they have experienced osteoporotic compression fractures
- in patients with steroid-induced osteoporosis (Eur J Clin Pharmacol 1987;33:35–39)

Other uses

- Paget's disease, hypercalcemia

▶ When Should I Not Use This Drug?

Treatment of osteoporosis if bone turnover is initially low

- calcitonin is of little benefit
- unfortunately, patients with low bone turnover can be identified only with a bone biopsy

Sole therapy for treatment of osteoporosis

- calcitonin should not be used alone for the treatment of established osteoporosis, but rather in conjunction with calcium and vitamin D therapy

Prevention of osteoporosis

- data to date do not support the use of calcitonin for the prevention of osteoporosis
- first-line therapy for the prevention of osteoporosis in postmenopausal women is hormonal replacement, adequate calcium intake, and exercise

▶ What Contraindications Are There to the Use of This Drug?

- intolerance of or allergic reaction to calcitonin (salmon) or calcitonin (human)

▶ What Drug Interactions Are Clinically Important?

Drugs that may increase the effect or toxicity of calcitonin

CALCIUM-CONTAINING PREPARATIONS OR VITAMIN D

- these may antagonize the treatment of hypercalcemia; therefore, do not use in combination with calcitonin when treating hypercalcemia

Drugs that may decrease the effect of calcitonin

- none

Drugs that may have their effect or toxicity increased by calcitonin

- none

Drugs that may have their effect decreased by calcitonin

- none

▶ What Route and Dosage Should I Use?

How to administer

Orally

- not available

Parenterally

- calcitonin (human) is given subcutaneously and must be reconstituted with the diluent provided and used within 6 hours
- calcitonin (salmon) can be given by an intramuscular or subcutaneous injection (if volume exceeds 2 mL, intramuscular injection in multiple sites is preferred) and is available in ready to use form but must be stored in a refrigerator

Treatment of osteoporosis

- prior to using calcitonin (salmon), a skin test should be done
- dilute 0.5 mL of 200 IU/mL to 1 mL with normal saline (0.9% sodium chloride)
- mix thoroughly and inject 1 IU (0.1 mL) intracutaneously on the flexor surface of the forearm
- if more than mild erythema or wheal occurs within 15 minutes, calcitonin (salmon) should not be used
- give calcitonin (salmon) 100 units SC or IM once daily, or if the patient is allergic to calcitonin (salmon), give calcitonin (human) at 0.5 mg SC daily
- calcitonin (salmon) dosages as low as 20 units SC daily or 50 units every other day have demonstrated some ability to increase bone mineralization, but the response is diminished as the dosage is reduced
- calcitonin (salmon) is more potent, on a weight basis, and has a longer duration of action than does calcitonin (human) (Calcitonin. AHFS Drug Information 1994;2076–2079), and as expected, hypersensitivity to calcitonin (salmon) is greater than that to calcitonin (human)
- because there is no evidence of differences in efficacy and calcitonin (human) is more expensive, calcitonin (human) should be used only when there is a proven allergy to calcitonin (salmon)

Dosage adjustments for renal or hepatic dysfunction

- no adjustments needed

▶ What Should I Monitor with Regard to Efficacy and Toxicity?

Efficacy

Treatment of osteoporosis

- positive response includes a decrease in painful symptoms, an increase in mobility, and stabilization or improvement of yearly measurements of spine or hip trabecular bone density

Toxicity

Allergic reaction

- see above discussion of a skin test

Urinary sediment

- coarse granular casts and casts containing renal tubular epithelial cells have been reported in healthy volunteers taking calcitonin (salmon); however, sediment returned to normal upon discontinuation of drug (Calcitonin. AHFS Drug Information 1994; 2076–2079)

Calcium levels

- baseline serum calcium concentration measurement and then every 6 months
- if the patient becomes hypocalcemic, decrease the dosage

▶ How Long Do I Treat Patients with This Drug?

Treatment of osteoporosis

- calcitonin administration should be continued for 18–24 months
- studies using calcitonin have demonstrated a plateau effect on bone mass after 1–2 years of therapy
- there are few rigorous studies with calcitonin and none exceeding about 2 years of follow-up, and bone density gain appears small and may start to reverse within 12–20 months, despite continued therapy (Ann Intern Med 1987;107:923–925)

▶ How Do I Decrease or Stop the Administration of This Drug?

- may be stopped abruptly

▶ What Should I Tell My Patients About This Drug?

- common side effects include diarrhea, flushing, loss of appetite, and stomach pain, but these usually disappear with continued use
- if a rash or hives appear, call your physician immediately
- thoroughly understand the proper way to administer and store the medication
- solution should be inspected for particles or discoloration

CALCIUM

Eric M. Yoshida and Angela Kim-Sing

USA (Os-Cal, Tums, Caltrate, Citracal, Posture)
CANADA (Calsan, Os-Cal, Calcium-Sandoz, Tums, Caltrate)

▶ When Should I Use This Drug?

Prevention of calcium depletion

- may be used as supplement for patients who consume a diet poor in calcium-rich foods (e.g., dairy products, leafy green vegetables, sardines, calcium-fortified foods)

Treatment of calcium deficiency

- hypocalcemia is defined as a serum ionized calcium concentration of <1.15 mmol/L or total serum calcium <2.23 mmol/L corrected according to serum albumin (add 0.2 mmol/L to the serum total calcium for every 10 g/L drop in albumin from 40 g/L)
- the need and modality of treatment depend upon whether signs and symptoms are acute/chronic or potentially life-threatening (e.g., laryngeal spasm, respiratory muscle weakness, heart failure)
- signs and symptoms of calcium deficiency in general are neuropsychiatric (e.g., confusion, depression, seizures), neuromuscular (i.e., tetany reflected by paresthesia), muscular cramps (carpopedal spasm), the Trousseau's/Chvostek's signs that detect latent tetany, dermatologic (e.g., hair loss, brittle nails, eczema, dermatitis), and cardiovascular (e.g., prolonged QT interval, hypotension)

Prevention/treatment of osteoporosis

- calcium supplements should be used if daily intake of calcium is below the recommended dietary allowance (approximately 1500 mg/d of elemental calcium)

Hyperphosphatemia secondary to chronic renal failure

- calcium carbonate–containing antacids have been shown to be as effective, if not more effective, as aluminum hydroxide in the treatment of hyperphosphatemia secondary to chronic renal failure (N Engl J Med 1991;324:527–531)
- aluminum hydroxide–containing antacids, while effective, are not recommended because of the concerns with aluminum toxicity in this patient population (Ann Clin Biochem 1987;24: 337–344, N Engl J Med 1991;324:527–531)
- in clinical practice, many nephrologists prescribe calcium and vitamin D (e.g., calcitriol) to their patients with severe renal failure

Cardioprotection during severe hyperkalemia

- parenteral calcium is recommended for cardioprotection in the acute management of severe hyperkalemia (>6.5 mEq/L or with hyperkalemic ECG changes)

Postparathyroidectomy

- hypocalcemia postparathyroidectomy may require oral supplementation following acute management; decision should be based on routine serum calcium measurements

▶ When Should I Not Use This Drug?

Cardiac arrest

- although older cardiac arrest protocols recommended parenteral calcium boluses in episodes of electromagnetic dissociation (EMD), calcium is no longer recommended except in specific situations such as hypocalcemia and hyperkalemia

▶ What Contraindications Are There to the Use of This Drug?

Intolerance or allergic reaction to calcium preparations
Parenteral administration in patients with hyperphosphatemia

- patients with hyperphosphatemia (e.g., tumor lysis syndrome, phosphate enemas) may have hypocalcemia secondary to imbalance of the serum calcium–phosphate equilibrium
- parenteral calcium administration in these circumstance may result in metastatic calcium tissue deposition. The treatment of hypocalcemia in these situations is specific to the underlying condition

Patients with hyperparathyroidism, sarcoidosis, or myeloma

- calcium should not be prescribed for patients with medical conditions that predispose to hypercalcemia

Patients with calcium kidney stones and/or hypercalciuria

- calcium supplementation should be avoided in these patients as supplementation may worsen these conditions

▶ What Drug Interactions Are Clinically Important?

Drugs that may increase effect/toxicity of calcium

VITAMIN D, THIAZIDE DIURETICS, SODIUM BICARBONATE (MILK-ALKALI SYNDROME)

- concurrent use of these drugs may increase the absorption or decrease the elimination of calcium
- after initiation of the combination of calcium and vitamin D, serum calcium should be monitored weekly initially, then every 3–6 months after the maintenance dose is established
- with thiazide diuretics and calcium, monitoring need be done only in patients who are already hypercalcemic or have a parathyroid disorder

Drugs that may decrease the effect of calcium

- none that have clinical significance in the administration of calcium supplementation, although loop diuretics (e.g., furosemide) can enhance the excretion of calcium

Drugs that may have effect/toxicity increased by calcium

DIGOXIN

- hypercalcemia can potentiate digoxin toxicity
- in the chronic administration of calcium supplementation, this should not be a problem as long as hypercalcemia is avoided
- in circumstances of acute parenteral calcium administration, patients receiving digoxin should be monitored electrocardiographically for evidence of digoxin toxicity

Drugs that may have effect decreased by calcium

FLUROQUINOLONE ANTIBIOTICS (E.G., CIPROFLOXACIN, OFLOXACIN), TETRACYCLINES, ETIDRONATE, IRON, PHENYTOIN

- oral calcium salts will decrease the absorption of these drugs if given concurrently; they should not be taken within 2 hours of a calcium dose

▶ *What Route and Dosage Should I Use?*

How to administer

- although serum calcium is measured in mmol/L (mg/dl in the USA), in practice, calcium is almost always ordered in mg (of elemental calcium)
- 1 mg of elemental calcium = 0.025 mmol = 0.05 mEq of elemental calcium
- calcium salts should be taken on an empty stomach; however, if gastrointestinal intolerance occurs, calcium may be taken with food
- oral calcium is available complexed with carbonate, citrate, glubionate, gluconate, lactate, and phosphate as single salts and combinations; also available in combination with electrolytes, vitamins, minerals, and antacids in tablets, powder, solutions, and suspensions
- if calcium is administered to bind dietary phosphate (e.g., in renal failure) then it should be taken with meals
- elemental calcium content varies with the calcium salt preparation
- dosage should be adjusted according to the amount of elemental calcium provided in each product
- calcium carbonate (40% elemental calcium) requires fewer tablets than other salts and may be the best choice
- liquid preparations (antacids) may be used but are less palatable and convenient
- bonemeal or dolomite may contain lead and should not be used as a source of calcium

Oral calcium preparations

Calcium Salt	mg of salt/tablet	Ca^{++} mg/tab	% Ca^{++}	Number of tablets to provide 1000 mg Ca^{++}
Carbonate	650	250	40%	4
	1250	500		2
Citrate	950	200	21.1%	5
Gluconate	500	45	9%	22
	650	58		17
Lactate	650	84	13%	12
Phosphate				
dibasic	500	115	23%	9
tribasic	800	304	38%	4
	1600	608	38%	2

Parenteral

- available in several formulations combined with chloride, gluceptate, gluconate, and glycerophosphate plus lactate, as single entities and in combination preparations with other minerals and electrolytes
- the most commonly used preparations are 10% calcium gluconate or chloride (note that the amount of elemental calcium per ampule in each preparation is different)
- parenteral calcium is incompatible with sodium bicarbonate and will precipitate

Parenteral calcium preparations

Calcium Salt	Ampule Volume (mL)	Elemental Calcium (mg in 10 mL)
Calcium gluconate 10%	10	90
Calcium chloride 10%	10	270
Calcium gluceptate 22%	5	180

Prevention of calcium depletion

- 1000 mg PO per day of elemental calcium for premenopausal women
- 1500 mg PO per day of elemental calcium for postmenopausal women
- 1200 mg PO per day of elemental calcium for adolescents and adults aged 11–24 years (male and female), and pregnant and lactating women over 18 years old
- 800 mg PO per day of elemental calcium for males older than 24 years
- 1600 mg PO per day of elemental calcium for pregnant adolescents

Treatment of hypocalcemia

- acutely symptomatic hypocalcemia (i.e., neurologic or cardiovascular symptoms) should be treated with an intravenous bolus of 90 mg of elemental calcium (e.g., 10 ml, or 1 ampule of 10% calcium gluconate) in 100 ml of 5% dextrose over 10 minutes
- this dose may be repeated if an unsatisfactory clinical response occurs
- these initial doses should be followed by a continuous infusion of 450–900 mg of elemental calcium (i.e., 5–10 ampules of calcium gluconate) in a liter of 5% dextrose over 6 hours
- chronic hypocalcemia may be treated with oral calcium replacement with or without vitamin D (e.g., malabsorption syndromes—both vitamin D and calcium may be deficient)
- oral doses would be similar to those under prevention and titrated based on serum calcium concentrations

Prevention/treatment of osteoporosis

- a total of 1,500 mg orally of elemental calcium (via diet and/or supplementation)

Hyperphosphatemia in end-stage renal failure

- 1250 mg of calcium carbonate (500 mg of elemental calcium) PO TID with meals is recommended
- adjust dose every two weeks based on serum phosphate concentrations

Cardioprotection during severe hyperkalemia

- 90 mg of elemental calcium (10 ml of 10% calcium gluconate) intravenously over 2 to 5 minutes should be administered
- this dose can be repeated after 5 minutes if there is no response

Postparathyroidectomy

- use doses as above under treatment of hypocalcemia

▶ *What Should I Monitor for with Regard to Efficacy and Toxicity?*

Efficacy

PREVENTION OF CALCIUM DEPLETION

- periodic review of compliance with dietary calcium replacement

Treatment of hypocalcemia

SIGNS AND SYMPTOMS

- evaluate the following every 6 hours in patients with severe hypocalcemia: neuropsychiatric (e.g., confusion, depression, seizures), neuromuscular (i.e., tetany reflected by paresthesia, muscular cramps [carpopedal spasm]), Trousseau/Chvostek signs that detect latent tetany, cardiovascular (e.g., prolonged QT intervals, hypotension)
- dermatologic (e.g., hair loss, brittle nails, eczema, dermatitis) need be evaluated only every few weeks

Serum calcium concentration (corrected for hypoalbuminemia)

- in the acute management of hypocalcemia requiring parenteral calcium, signs and symptoms of hypocalcemia should be assessed at regular intervals depending on severity
- serum calcium should be monitored every 4 hours for severe deficiency
- an increase in serum calcium of 0.25 mmol/L can be expected with every 90 mg of elemental calcium (i.e., 10 ml of 10% calcium gluconate) given

- after starting oral therapy, the serum calcium should be measured after 48 hours
- the long-term aim should be to keep the serum calcium in the lower limits of the normal range or just below normal
- serum calcium should be assessed weekly until stable, then every 2–3 months

Prevention/treatment of osteoporosis

- there are no effective monitoring parameters for monitoring the efficacy of calcium in preventing osteoporosis, although bone mass measurement (e.g., photon absorptiometry, etc.) may be of value in the initial assessment

Hyperphosphatemia in chronic renal failure

- evaluate the serum phosphate 7 days after starting oral calcium
- if the serum phosphate has not decreased, double the calcium dosage

Toxicity

Hypercalcemia

- hypercalcemia may occur with large doses of oral calcium, especially in renal failure or with the coadministration of vitamin D
- if hypercalcemia occurs, calcium (and vitamin D) should be discontinued until normocalcemia is achieved and may then be restarted at lower doses

Hypercalciuria

- hypercalciuria and renal stones are potential side effects of calcium replacement in the treatment of chronic hypoparathyroidism
- in these patients, 24-hour urine collections for calcium should be ordered every 3–6 months and vitamin D discontinued or calcium supplement decreased if the urinary calcium is >6.25 mmol (250 mg)/24 hours

Complications of parenteral calcium

- parenteral calcium may result in venous thrombosis, and if extravasation occurs, tissue calcification may occur
- the incidence of these adverse reactions is less with calcium gluconate than with calcium chloride

▶ How Long Do I Treat Patients with This Drug?

Prevention of calcium depletion

- calcium supplementation should continue until an adequate dietary intake of calcium is achieved or until risk factors for hypocalcemia are resolved

Treatment of hypocalcemia

- chronic hypocalcemia (e.g., chronic hypothyroidism, malabsorption) may require long-term oral calcium replacement
- the end-point of therapy is to maintain the serum calcium just below or at the lower limit of the normal range

Prevention/treatment of osteoporosis

- patients who have tolerated therapy and who are willing to remain on treatment can be continued on calcium supplementation indefinitely

Hyperphosphatemia in end-stage renal failure

- should be continued as long as hypophosphatemia or hypercalcemia does not occur or renal function improves

Cardioprotection during severe hyperkalemia

- usually one-time dose but may be repeated in 5–10 minutes if evidence of life-threatening electrocardiographic abnormalities persist

Postparathyroidectomy

- hypocalcemia may be only transient postparathyroidectomy, and continued use of calcium supplementation should be on the basis of serum calcium measurements (see above under treatment)

▶ How Do I Decrease or Stop This Drug?

- may be stopped abruptly

▶ What Should I Tell My Patient About This Drug?

- oral calcium supplements may cause gastrointestinal upset
- oral calcium should be taken with 8 ounces of water or juice (unless being used as a phosphate binder in renal failure)
- chewable calcium tablets should be thoroughly chewed before swallowing

▶ Therapeutic Tips

- parenteral calcium gluconate causes fewer local venous adverse effects than calcium chloride
- oral generic calcium carbonate supplements are generally inexpensive
- concomitant hypomagnesemia should always be treated (e.g., 16–40 mEq/2–5 g of magnesium sulfate intravenously over 4–6 hours) as hypocalcemia may not correct unless the serum magnesium is near normal

Useful References

Agus ZA, Wasserstein A, Goldfarb S. Disorders of calcium and magnesium homeostasis. Am J Med 1982;72:473–488

Dolan DL. Intravenous calcium before verapamil to prevent hypotension. Ann Emerg Med 1991;20:588–589

Meunier PJ. Prevention of hip fractures. Am J Med 1993;95(suppl 5A): 75S–78S

National Research Council. Recommended Dietary Allowances, 10th ed. Washington, DC: National Academy Press, 1989

Sambrook P, Birmingham J, Kelly P, Kempler S, et al. Prevention of corticosteroid osteoporosis. N Engl J Med 1993;328:1747–1752

CAPTOPRIL

Jack Onrot and James McCormack

USA (Capoten)
CANADA (Capoten, Apo-Capto, Novo-Captoril, Syn-Captopril, Nu-Capto)

▶ When Should I Use This Drug?

All angiotensin converting enzyme (ACE) inhibitors are likely equally effective, and the decision about which agent to use should be based on the convenience of administration and cost • Captopril has a relatively short half-life and should be dosed twice daily for hypertension • Enalapril and lisinopril can both be dosed once daily • Only captopril and enalapril have been shown to provide survival benefit • Although ramipril, quinapril, benazepril, and fosinopril can also be dosed once daily (for most patients), they offer no advantages over other more extensively used ACE inhibitors (Med Lett 1991; 33:83–84, Med Lett 1992;34:27–28) and should likely be chosen only if they are significantly less expensive (Drug Ther Perspect 1993;1[9]:4–7) • Captopril has a faster onset of action (30 minutes; peak effect, 60–90 minutes) than do the other available ACE inhibitors (onset, 1-2 hours; peak effect, 2–6 hours) and should be chosen over these other agents if a fast onset is desired (acute hypertension or titration in the initial treatment of congestive heart failure) • The duration of action for captopril is shorter (6–12 hours) than that for other agents (12–24 hours), and this allows easier titration, and if side effects occur, they are less prolonged than those seen with the other agents • Captopril and enalapril have caused taste disturbances, although this adverse effect has not been reported with other ACE inhibitors

Congestive heart failure

Acute pulmonary edema

- captopril is not commonly used initially to treat acute pulmonary edema
- captopril is used after diuresis has been initiated with furosemide (should not be used initially during times of rapid diuresis)
- used initially in small doses, and titrated to response
- concern exists with the use of ACE inhibitors in the context of rapid diuresis as they may cause a clinically important drop in blood pressure and an increase in serum creatinine levels
- captopril is preferred in the acute setting, over other ACE inhibitors, because its onset of action is faster (30 minutes versus 2–4 hours) and its duration of action is shorter

- the fast onset and short duration allow for easier titration, and if side effects occur, they are less prolonged
- after the patient has been stabilized, the ACE inhibitor for long-term therapy should be chosen on the basis of cost and frequency of administration

Mild to moderate heart failure

- ACE inhibitors (captopril or enalapril) prolong survival (N Engl J Med 1987;316:1429–1435, N Engl J Med 1991;325:293–302, 303–310)
- best used in conjunction with furosemide (Ann Intern Med 1984;100:777–782)
- no evidence yet exists to support the use of ACE inhibitors alone in heart failure
- also useful in patients who have had a myocardial infarction and have left ventricular dysfunction, as survival benefits have been shown (N Engl J Med 1992;327:669–677)
- in general, unless there is a contraindication, most patients with congestive heart failure should receive an ACE inhibitor

Acute (crisis) hypertension

- oral beta-blockers, nifedipine, and captopril have all been effective (Lancet 1985;2:34–35, Br J Clin Pharmacol 1986;21:377–383) in the treatment of acute (crisis) hypertension and should not be considered suboptimum to intravenous therapy
- choice among these agents should be based on which drug would ultimately be useful for long-term control and the recognition that many of these patients require more than 1 drug for adequate long-term control
- onset of action of ACE inhibitors other than captopril is likely too slow for them to be used in this condition

Chronic (noncrisis) hypertension

- ACE inhibitors are drugs of choice in patients with preexisting congestive heart failure because both conditions are treated by a single agent
- likely also useful in patients with hypertension and diabetes
- selection of a specific ACE inhibitor should be based on cost and convenience
- in patients without concomitant diseases, use ACE inhibitors only in patients who do not tolerate, do not respond to, or have contraindications to thiazide diuretics and beta-blockers because thiazide diuretics and beta-blockers have proven long-term benefit and are generally less expensive than an ACE inhibitor
- if compliance is a potential problem, once-daily therapy with an ACE inhibitor (whichever is the least expensive) should be chosen

Other uses

- diabetic nephropathy, rheumatoid arthritis

▶ When Should I Not Use This Drug?

Congestive heart failure due to aortic stenosis

- main reason for congestive heart failure in patients with aortic stenosis is obstruction and diastolic dysfunction
- ACE inhibitors cause a further drop in blood pressure in these patients

▶ What Contraindications Are There to the Use of This Drug?

Intolerance of or allergic reaction to captopril
Rapidly worsening renal failure

- use of ACE inhibitors in patients with worsening renal function should be based on an assessment of the cause of the renal impairment
- ACE inhibitors may further impair renal function in patients who require efferent renal vasoconstriction for glomerular filtration
- ACE inhibitors may increase, decrease, or have no effect on renal function, and therefore, stable renal failure is not a contraindication

Severe hypotension

- systolic blood pressure less than or equal to 85 mmHg because ACE inhibitor–induced vasodilatation may produce dangerously low perfusion pressures

Severe hyponatremia

- patients with severe hyponatremia (serum sodium level < 135 mmol/L) with associated congestive heart failure have a hyper-reninemic state and are at greatest risk for the hypotensive and renal toxic effects of ACE inhibitors (J Am Coll Cardiol 1987;10:837–855, J Am Coll Cardiol 1984;3:1035–1043)
- while it is best to correct the hyponatremia before instituting ACE inhibitor therapy the hyponatremia may be due to congestive heart failure
- if captopril needs to be started, start with a low dose (6.25 mg), water restrict the patient, and measure serum sodium daily

Bilateral renal artery stenosis, unilateral renal artery stenosis in a patient with 1 kidney

- hypotension caused by ACE inhibitors decreases renal perfusion
- ACE inhibitors interfere with reflex angiotensin II mechanisms necessary to maintain glomerular filtration in a kidney with decreased blood flow

▶ What Drug Interactions Are Clinically Important?

Drugs that may increase the effect or toxicity of captopril
DIURETICS

- after overzealous diuretic therapy with a reduction in renal blood flow, ACE inhibitors (by blocking compensating renal mechanisms) can exaggerate the rise in urea and creatinine levels and cause a reversible renal insufficiency (Ann Intern Med 1987; 106:346–354)
- patient's intravascular volume status should be normalized prior to initiating therapy with ACE inhibitors

HYDRALAZINE, NITRATES

- these can produce unacceptable hypotension when used in combination with ACE inhibitors
- in general, this combination should not be used; however, it is undergoing testing

POTASSIUM-SPARING DIURETICS, POTASSIUM SUPPLEMENTS

- ACE inhibitors interfere with aldosterone-induced potassium excretion and can lead to hyperkalemia
- the risk of hyperkalemia is enhanced by potassium-sparing diuretics or potassium supplements, especially in the context of renal insufficiency
- unless the patient remains hypokalemic when ACE inhibitors are used, this combination should be avoided

Drugs that may decrease the effect of captopril
ANTACIDS

- antacids decrease the bioavailability of captopril
- administer the antacid and captopril doses more than 2 hours apart to minimize the effect of the interaction

NONSTEROIDAL ANTIINFLAMMATORY DRUGS

- nonsteroidal antiinflammatory agents may reduce the hypotensive effect of ACE inhibitors by altering prostaglandin-mediated vasodilatation
- avoid this combination if possible, and if not, monitor serum creatinine and potassium levels and weight at baseline and every 4 days for 2–3 weeks, then every 2 weeks for 8 weeks, then every month for 3 months, and then as needed

Drugs that may have their effect or toxicity increased by captopril

- none

Drugs that may have their effect decreased by captopril

- none

▶ What Route and Dosage Should I Use?

How to administer

Orally

- should be administered on an empty stomach to prevent food from interfering with the absorption

- if this is not possible, doses should be administered consistently in relation to meals

Parenterally

- not available

Congestive heart failure

Severe heart failure with acute pulmonary edema

- give 6.25 mg PO as a single dose and assess blood pressure every 15–30 minutes for $1\frac{1}{2}$ hours
- if patients do not become hypotensive with this dose, it is unlikely that they will become hypotensive with additional doses (Eur Heart J 1992;13:1521–1527)
- if patients tolerate the 6.25 mg dose, give 6.25 mg PO BID
- double the dosage every 2–3 days until congestive heart failure is controlled or orthostatic hypotension develops (the usual maintenance dosage is 75–150 mg daily)
- maintain systolic blood pressure of greater than 90 mmHg
- optimum dosage is difficult to determine, but attempt to avoid hypotensive symptoms, avoid drops in blood pressure on standing, maintain normokalemia, and minimize adverse effects

Mild to moderate heart failure

- 6.25 mg PO BID (use a test dose as above)
- rapidity of dosage escalation depends on the severity of symptoms
- dosage may be increased daily if necessary
- no value in exceeding a total daily dosage of 150 mg
- frequent small (Q6H) doses may be required if the hypotensive effects of large doses prevent twice-daily administration (BID dosing, however, is usually appropriate)

Acute (crisis) hypertension

- give 25 mg PO and repeat every 6 hours as needed

Chronic (noncrisis) hypertension

- 6.25 mg PO BID
- increase the dosage by 12.5 mg PO daily every 4 weeks until adequate blood pressure or a maximum daily dose of 150 mg is achieved
- BID dosing is usually required for captopril

Dosage adjustments for renal or hepatic dysfunction

- renally eliminated
- titrate the dose in accord with clinical response and not on the basis of concurrent renal or hepatic function

▶ *What Should I Monitor with Regard to Efficacy and Toxicity?*

Efficacy

Congestive heart failure

Acute pulmonary edema (if captopril is used, see above under When to Use This Drug)

- look for relief of dyspnea, orthopnea, paroxysmal nocturnal dyspnea, and ankle edema
- assess jugular venous pressure, presence of peripheral edema, and liver size after each dose of furosemide
- jugular venous pressure should be normal to slightly increased (be aware that right-sided filling pressures do not always accurately reflect left-sided pressure)
- after some of the acute symptoms have decreased, assess the patient at least twice daily
- initially, assess weight daily

Mild to moderate heart failure

Signs and symptoms

- decreased dyspnea, orthopnea, paroxysmal nocturnal dyspnea, fatigue, ankle swelling, fine crackles on chest auscultation, body weight, liver size, and presence or absence of S_3 heart sounds
- jugular venous pressure should be normal to slightly increased
- after the patient is discharged from the hospital, assess within a week of discharge
- after the patient is stabilized, decrease the frequency of monitoring

- for patients with mild symptoms, assess weekly until symptoms are controlled

Urea, creatinine, and sodium levels

- these concentrations may improve if cardiac output is improved, and in patients who are hyponatremic, the serum sodium level may normalize
- in overdiuresis, urea level increases disproportionately to creatinine level increase
- monitor daily in patients with acute disease undergoing rapid diuresis
- in patients with severe chronic congestive heart failure, accept modest urea and creatinine level increases above baseline values if this is needed to maintain optimum symptom control

Acute (crisis) hypertension

Blood pressure

- preferably intraarterial blood pressure; however, if this is not available, indirect (cuff) measurements every 5 minutes until desired blood pressure is reached and then every hour, ensuring that the diastolic pressure does not go below 100 mmHg over the first 1–2 days, owing to concerns about hypoperfusion
- ideal rate of blood pressure reduction in this condition is unknown; however, the goal should be to lower pressures to the desired range (i.e., to approximately 180/110 mmHg initially) within 30 minutes to 2 hours

Electrocardiographic measurements

- continuous electrocardiographic monitoring is recommended, especially if chest pain is present, until a stable blood pressure reduction has been achieved and sustained
- this is done to look for evidence of coronary ischemia, and if this occurs, treat as for angina (also consider that blood pressure may have been lowered too far)

Chronic (noncrisis) hypertension

Blood pressure

- patients with diastolic blood pressures greater than 115 mmHg or with symptoms should be evaluated again within 48 hours to ensure that at least a 5–10 mmHg drop in blood pressure has occurred
- for patients with diastolic blood pressures less than 115 mmHg, follow-up blood pressure determinations should be done within a couple of weeks
- at each visit, do 2 blood pressure measurements, with the patient supine or sitting, after patient has been resting without conversation for 5–10 minutes
- continue to do this every 4 weeks to assess the effect of each new drug or dosage until control is achieved
- for most patients with mild hypertension, after blood pressure is controlled, blood pressure measurement 2–4 times per year is sufficient

Evidence of end-organ damage

- if blood pressure is well controlled and no other disease states exist (e.g., diabetes), measure baseline serum creatinine, blood glucose, and serum cholesterol levels and perform urinalysis
- repeat every year if other disease states are present

Toxicity

Renal function

- in patients with renal hypoperfusion (renal artery stenosis, severe volume depletion, marked hypotension, or poor cardiac output), ACE inhibitors may exaggerate renal insufficiency (Ann Intern Med 1987;106:346–354)
- in patients with chronic congestive heart failure, it is acceptable to have the urea and creatinine levels above normal (up to 2 times normal values) if this is needed to maintain optimum symptom control
- patients who are prerenal (i.e., decreased renal blood flow) require angiotensin II to maintain glomerular filtration rate
- ACE inhibitors in this setting interfere with this homeostatic mechanism and may lead to a decrease in renal function (N Engl J Med 1983;308:373–376)

- when renal insufficiency occurs, administration of ACE inhibitors should be discontinued until cardiac output can be restored to the kidneys; as urea and creatinine levels begin to fall, administration of ACE inhibitors may be restarted at lower dosages
- in patients who have severe congestive heart failure and are receiving a diuretic, check serum creatinine and urea levels every 2 days while patients are in the hospital and aggressive diuresis is being instituted
- check 1 week after discharge from the hospital
- for patients with mild congestive heart failure, check serum creatinine levels before and 4–5 days after the initiation of ACE inhibitor therapy
- repeat approximately 10 days after the initiation of therapy
- because ACE inhibitors can adversely affect renal function at any time during therapy, regular evaluation of renal function is required
- check every 2 months in patients with congestive heart failure
- check every 6 months in patients being treated for hypertension

Potassium levels

- ACE inhibitors may increase serum potassium levels
- check potassium levels every 2 days while patients are in the hospital and aggressive diuresis is being instituted
- check 1 week after discharge from the hospital
- check every 2 months in patients with congestive heart failure
- check every 6 months in patients being treated for hypertension

Blood pressure

- patient should be instructed to report any signs of hypotension (lightheadedness, weakness) during ACE inhibitor therapy
- hypotension may be encountered, so it is a good idea to warn patients that lightheadedness can occur, especially in the first 6 hours after initiating therapy or increasing the dosage
- marked hypotension is an indication for discontinuation of therapy, especially in the context of rising urea and creatinine levels and/or volume depletion
- when further ACE inhibitor effect is desired, increased dose should be titrated against falling pressure

Cough

- cough is commonly encountered (10–20%), is dose dependent in individual patients, and may necessitate discontinuation of the agent (Eur Respir J 1989;2:198–201)
- it is dry, usually worse at night, and can interfere with the patient's lifestyle
- ask the patient at each visit about the development of a dry cough
- cough may respond to decreasing the dosage
- cough is usually encountered in the same patient with different ACE inhibitors

Rash, mucosal ulcerations

- drug administration should be discontinued immediately if a rash occurs because there are reports of angioneurotic edema occurring in patients who continue to take ACE inhibitors
- captopril does not appear to produce a higher incidence of rash than does enalapril; rashes in patients receiving captopril have, on occasion, not been seen when a patient has been switched to enalapril therapy (Drug Ther Perspect 1993;[9]:4–7)

Dysgeusia

- if taste disturbances occur, stop administration of the drug and try a different agent
- has been seen only with captopril and enalapril

Proteinuria

- rare, and no monitoring is required

▶ How Long Do I Treat Patients with This Drug?

Congestive heart failure

- administration of ACE inhibitors should be continued indefinitely unless acute precipitating factors can be reversed, rendering the drug unnecessary
- because of survival benefits, patients with severe disease should not have the drug regimen discontinued unless there are adverse effects

Acute (crisis) hypertension

- drug therapy discontinuation is not advised in patients with severe to malignant hypertension or target organ damage (e.g., myocardial infarction, congestive heart failure, stroke, or renal failure); however, continual reassessment allows the hypertension to be treated with the least number of drugs at the lowest dosage that reduces the incidence of adverse effects, reduces the frequency of drug administration, and is cost effective

Chronic (noncrisis) hypertension

Stepped-down therapy, in general, should be considered in patients whose blood pressures at the previous few visits had been well controlled

- approximately 50% of patients with well-controlled blood pressures successfully undergo either a reduction in dosage or number of drugs and blood pressures remain under control for a time, but unfortunately, this period varies from patient to patient and consistent reevaluation is necessary
- this may be explained by reversal of cardiac and vascular changes that may occur after prolonged treatment with drug therapy and may be a means of "setting back the clock" of primary hypertension evolution
- as with every treatment, not everyone has blood pressure successfully respond to drug discontinuation or drug dosage reduction
- patients most likely to have a successful reduction or discontinuation of therapy may be predicted by a low pretreatment blood pressure (mild hypertension with diastolic pressure of <100 mmHg), no evidence of target organ damage, need for only monotherapy for blood pressure control, and accomplishment of weight loss, salt restriction, increased exercise, and decreased alcohol intake
- reassessment allows a reevaluation of the efficacy of nondrug measures in the treatment of hypertension such as reducing weight and reducing salt and alcohol intake

▶ How Do I Decrease or Stop the Administration of This Drug?

- for patients with congestive heart failure or any patient with toxicities, the drug regimen may be stopped abruptly
- for step-down therapy of hypertension, the dosage should be reduced by 50% with reassessment of blood pressure at 2 weeks
- if the patient is still normotensive, reduce the dosage by another 50% (i.e., to 25% of the initial dose) and recheck blood pressure in another 2 weeks
- if the blood pressure is still well controlled, stop the medication administration and recheck the blood pressure in 2 weeks
- so-called rebound hypertension does not occur if the dosage is gradually tapered, with dosage reductions of no more than 50% at 2–4 week intervals
- final dose before full drug discontinuation should be less than 1/4 the dose of the initial therapy

▶ What Should I Tell My Patients About This Drug?

- were there any allergies to ACE inhibitors in the past?
- hypotension may be encountered, so lightheadedness may occur, especially in the first 2–6 hours after initiating therapy or increasing the dosage
- skin rashes and mucosal ulcers may occur
- there may be taste alterations, and this may be temporary
- cough is the most common side effect; it is dry, is usually worse at night, and can interfere with your lifestyle
- warn patients about the cough and inquire about the cough at follow-up visits, as patients may not volunteer this common distressing symptom

▶ Therapeutic Tips

- in patients who have toxicity with ACE inhibitors, hydralazine plus isosorbide dinitrate is an alternative regimen for treating congestive heart failure
- for congestive heart failure, try to keep your patients on a regimen of ACE inhibitors because of their proven efficacy in reducing mortality

- if hyperkalemia limits therapy, reduce dosage and look for other factors that are contributing to the raised potassium levels
- ACE inhibitors and diuretics are used together for heart failure because the ACE inhibitors counteract the potassium loss from the diuretic and may also potentiate diuretic effect
- after the addition of an ACE inhibitor to a diuretic, the prior diuretic dosage may be excessive and often needs reduction
- in patients with chronic congestive heart failure, it is acceptable to have the urea and creatinine levels above normal (up to 2 times normal values) if this is needed to maintain optimum symptom control

CARBAMAZEPINE

William Parker, Steven Stanislav, and Patricia Marken

USA (Epitol, Tegretol)
CANADA (Apo-Carbamazepine, Mazepine, Novocarbamaz, Taro-Carbamazepine, Tegretol)

▶ *When Should I Use This Drug?*

Generalized seizures (no primary focus)

Tonic-clonic seizures

- if the electroencephalogram (EEG) shows partial seizures that secondarily generalize, either phenytoin or carbamazepine is the drug of choice
- if partial seizures are not present, use carbamazepine only if valproic acid is not effective or tolerated, as valproic acid is better tolerated and has fewer central nervous system (CNS) effects than do phenytoin or carbamazepine
- many clinicians prefer carbamazepine over phenytoin as initial therapy owing to fewer adverse effects, easier dose titration, and fewer cosmetic side effects than with phenytoin
- phenytoin is the drug of choice if an agent must be given parenterally (other agents are not available as parenteral agents)

Partial seizures (with or without secondarily generalized tonic-clonic seizures)

- phenytoin and carbamazepine are equally effective, and the decision between these agents is as above under generalized seizures

Trigeminal neuralgia

- useful in the symptomatic treatment of pain associated with trigeminal neuralgia and glossopharyngeal neuralgia

Prophylactic therapy for bipolar disorder (started in conjunction with acute therapy), schizoaffective disorder

- alternative agent if the patient does not tolerate or has no response with lithium
- first-line agent when a contraindication to lithium use exists or the patient cannot tolerate or is unresponsive to lithium
- consider as first choice in patient with concurrent seizure disorder that would be responsive to carbamazepine
- possible synergy with concurrent lithium therapy (J Clin Psychiatry 1988;49:13–18)
- evidence suggests prophylactic effects and a risk of relapse similar to that for lithium
- current studies are attempting to delineate subgroups with preferential response to carbamazepine (rapid cyclers)
- no direct comparative studies comparing valproate sodium with carbamazepine, but carbamazepine should likely be chosen, as it has undergone more clinical testing

Aggression

- treatment option in episodic aggressive behavior with or without coexisting seizure disorder (Psychopharmacol Bull 1980;1098–1100)

▶ *When Should I Not Use This Drug?*

Absence seizures or myoclonic seizures

- ineffective in the management of these types of seizures
- may exacerbate absence seizures
- avoid use when there is generalized synchronous, spike and wave discharges of 2.5–3 cps in association with clinical seizures, as this may aggravate these types of seizures

Status epilepticus

- drug does not prevent the generalization of epileptic discharge and is not available as a parenteral agent

Known organic cause of mania

- drug-induced mania, hyperthyroidism, severe metabolic abnormalities, tumor and so on, when these are treatable by other means

Mild, behavioral dyscontrol or psychotic agitation

- may respond equally well to temporary therapy with other agents (e.g., antipsychotics and sedative-hypnotics)

Use as a simple analgesic

- carbamazepine is not an analgesic and should not be given casually for relief of trivial facial pain or headache

▶ *What Contraindications Are There to the Use of This Drug?*

Intolerance of or allergic reaction to carbamazepine or any of the tricyclic antidepressants (these drugs are structurally related)

Patients with significant leukopenia (white blood cell count < 3000 mm³ or neutrophil count < 1500 mm³), thrombocytopenia (platelet count < 100,000/mm³), or anemia (hematocrit < 32%, hemoglobin concentration < 11 g/dL, reticulocyte count < 20,000/mm³)

- carbamazepine can cause reversible or fluctuating leukopenia and, rarely, agranulocytosis and aplastic anemia
- low-normal baseline hematological values are not an absolute contraindication; however, slower dose titration and increased laboratory monitoring are suggested if carbamazepine is used
- patients with low-normal pretreatment white blood cell and neutrophil counts should have repeated complete blood count or differential count every 2 weeks during the first 3 months of therapy (greatest risk of leukopenia exists during the initial 3 months of therapy)

Atrioventricular heart block

- carbamazepine can reduce ventricular automaticity

Within 14 days of monoamine oxidase inhibitor therapy

- increased risk of hypertensive crisis because of structural relationship to tricyclic antidepressants

Liver impairment

- can increase the risk of hepatotoxicity

Porphyria

- avoid use because carbamazepine induces hepatic cytochrome P-450 and increases hepatic heme turnover, which can exacerbate the symptoms of acute intermittent porphyria and porphyria variegata

▶ *What Drug Interactions Are Clinically Important?*

Drugs that may increase the effect or toxicity of carbamazepine

CIMETIDINE

- claimed to inhibit carbamazepine metabolism; however, 3 clinical studies have shown no effect on steady state carbamazepine concentrations

DANAZOL, DILTIAZEM, ERYTHROMYCIN, FLUOXETINE, ISONIAZID, PROPOXYPHENE, TROLEANDOMYCIN, VERAPAMIL

- usually act by inhibiting hepatic metabolism
- neurotoxicity may result from increased carbamazepine concentrations but is not life threatening
- use nifedipine in place of diltiazem or verapamil if possible
- use alternative antibiotics to erythromycin if possible
- if the inhibitor must be added for longer than 3 days, obtain a baseline serum carbamazepine concentration prior to adding inhibitor, recheck the concentration in 1 week, and reduce the dosage proportionately if concentrations are greater than 12 mg/L (50 μmol/L)

- monitor for symptoms of toxicity, and if they occur, stop the drug administration, get a repeated concentration, and adjust the dosage accordingly
- if the concentration is not available within 24 hours, restart the carbamazepine regimen at 50% of the previous dosage as long as toxicity is not present
- if no toxicity occurs, measure concentrations weekly until a new steady state has been reached
- if inhibitor administration is stopped, increase the dosage back to the preinhibitor level

MONOAMINE OXIDASE INHIBITORS

- results in gastrointestinal complaints; symptoms of CNS excitability; hyperthermia; cardiovascular events, including dysrhythmia; seizures; and coma
- most likely to occur if the carbamazepine is added to a monoamine oxidase (MAO) inhibitor regimen
- combination may be used if both carbamazepine and the MAO inhibitor are started together or if the MAO inhibitor is added to the carbamazepine regimen
- if a patient is receiving MAO inhibitor and carbamazepine is to be added, the patient should be MAO inhibitor free for at least 2 weeks prior to starting the new combination regimen (J Clin Psychopharmacol 1981;1:264–282) to allow time for new enzyme synthesis

Drugs that may decrease the effect of carbamazepine

PHENYTOIN, PHENOBARBITAL, PRIMIDONE

- these drugs usually act by inducing hepatic metabolism, and this effect is usually complete by 2–4 weeks
- dosage adjustment and increased monitoring are not required as a second antiepileptic agent is being added
- carbamazepine dose/serum concentration ratio decreases by 30–50% whenever 1 or 2 other inducing anticonvulsants (phenobarbital, phenytoin, primidone) are administered concurrently
- when carbamazepine is added to an existing anticonvulsant regimen, it may be difficult to achieve carbamazepine serum concentrations in the therapeutic range, even with carbamazepine dosages in the range of 30 mg/kg/d
- do not automatically attribute low levels to patient noncompliance; consider increased drug clearance

RIFAMPIN

- major hepatic enzyme inducer but effect on carbamazepine not established
- obtain a baseline concentration and monitor concentrations weekly until a steady state has been reached and adjust the dosage accordingly
- monitor concentration whenever a seizure occurs

Drugs that may have their effect increased by carbamazepine

- none

Drugs that have their effect decreased by carbamazepine

WARFARIN

- increases warfarin metabolism and can decrease INR
- use alternative agents if possible
- if not, monitor INR every 2 days until the full extent of the interaction is seen and adjust the dosage as for a warfarin dosage change
- monitor INR every 2 days when administration of an interacting drug is discontinued and adjust as for a warfarin dosage change

PHENYTOIN

- may decrease the steady state serum phenytoin concentration
- dosage adjustment and increased monitoring are not required if an antiepileptic drug is being added
- if interacting drugs are added, monitor serum phenytoin concentrations weekly until a steady state is established and adjust phenytoin dosage accordingly

LITHIUM

- increases the clearance of lithium

- upward adjustment in lithium dosages should be guided by the lithium level obtained after reaching a new steady state in approximately 5 days

ORAL CONTRACEPTIVES

- with concomitant use, carbamazepine may produce lower estrogen levels than expected by increasing the metabolism of estrogen to a less active form
- patients taking oral contraceptives should be started on a high-estrogen product
- although higher-dose estrogens can decrease spotting in patients taking interacting drugs, their efficacy may be decreased but they are still likely more effective than other single forms of birth control

CORTICOSTEROIDS, ISONIAZID, MEBENDAZOLE, METHADONE, THYROID HORMONES, TRICYCLIC ANTIDEPRESSANTS, MONOAMINE OXIDASE INHIBITORS, THEOPHYLLINE, DOXYCYCLINE

- carbamazepine increases the clearance of these drugs
- monitor for clinical changes and adjust the dosage if needed

▶ *What Route and Dosage Should I Use?*

How to administer

- orally—take with food or milk
- parenterally—not available

Generalized seizures (no primary focus), partial seizures (with or without secondarily generalized tonic-clonic seizures)

- 200 mg PO BID if an immediate response is needed
- if an immediate response is not needed, give 100 mg PO daily for 3 days, increase to 100 mg PO BID for 3 days, then give 100 mg PO every morning and 200 mg PO every evening for 3 days, then increase to 200 mg PO BID, as this regimen should decrease the initial gastrointestinal upset and dizziness seen with this agent
- avoid single doses greater than 400 mg to minimize gastrointestinal upset
- use serum concentrations to make further adjustments (see below)

Prophylactic therapy for bipolar disorder, schizoaffective disorder, aggression

- start with 200 mg PO BID
- increase the dose by 200 mg increments every week on the basis of clinical response, adverse effects, and serum concentrations
- avoid single doses greater than 400 mg to minimize gastrointestinal upset (increase dosing interval to TID or QID if needed)

Trigeminal neuralgia

- give 100 mg PO BID and increase the dosage in 100 mg increments until pain relief is obtained, toxicity occurs, or a maximum of 1200 mg/d is reached

Dosage adjustments for renal or hepatic dysfunction

- hepatically metabolized
- in patients with renal or hepatic disease, start with 200 mg/d and titrate to response and toxicity as above

▶ *What Should I Monitor with Regard to Efficacy and Toxicity?*

Efficacy

Generalized seizures (no primary focus), partial seizures (with or without secondarily generalized tonic-clonic seizures)

Seizure frequency

- reduction in frequency and severity of seizures

Prophylactic therapy for bipolar disorder, schizoaffective disorders, aggression

Target symptoms

- improvement in agitation; decreased sleep; rapid, pressured speech with flight of ideas for manic phase; or symptoms of depression

Symptoms of psychoses

- auditory or visual hallucinations and delusional or disorganized thinking

Trigeminal neuralgia

Pain relief

- usually see a response within 48 hours; drug should not be used preventively during periods of remission

Carbamazepine serum concentration

- 4–12 mg/L (17–50 μmol/L) for anticonvulsant effect
- serum concentration response relationships are not well defined for bipolar disorder; however, clinical reports suggest a range of 8–12 mg/L (34–50 μmol/L)
- no range defined for trigeminal neuralgia
- in general, maintain the lowest effective dosage to minimize side effects
- there is much interpatient variability in dosage requirements; therefore, serum concentration monitoring is important to monitor to ensure therapeutic levels or to minimize toxicity

Toxicity

Hematological monitoring

- no longer specified by the manufacturer, thus allowing more variability for monitoring on the basis of clinical judgment
- white blood cell count is frequently reduced by carbamazepine but usually remains in the normal range
- some patients become leukopenic but have polymorphonuclear neutrophil counts greater than 1000/mm^3 and tolerate this well
- following guidelines are suggested (DICP 1990;24:1214–1219):
- obtain complete blood count with differential leukocyte count with platelets at baseline
- patients with low-normal pretreatment white blood cell and neutrophil counts should have repeated complete blood count with differential leukocyte count every 2 weeks during the first 3 months of therapy (the greatest risk of leukopenia exists during the initial 3 months of therapy)
- check hematological values within 3 weeks of starting carbamazepine administration, as this is when most hematological abnormalities occur
- continual patient education for detection of signs or symptoms of myelosuppression (sore throat, fever, petechiae, pallor, increased bruising, fatigue)
- at first signs and symptoms of myelosuppression, discontinue the drug administration, obtain carbamazepine concentration, and determine complete blood count with differential leukocyte count and platelet count
- avoid concomitant use of other myelotoxic drugs

Gastrointestinal effects

- nausea, vomiting
- avoid by using slow titration of initial therapy, administering with food, and giving larger doses at bedtime

Neurotoxicity

- drowsiness, diplopia, blurred vision, ataxia, dizziness, nystagmus, and headache
- is usually transient; minimize by using slow titration of initial therapy, and giving larger doses at bedtime
- threshold for common side effects is 8 mg/L (34 μmol/L)
- avoid high serum levels of both lithium and carbamazepine when used together (J Clin Psychiatry 1983;44:30–31)

Hepatic effects

- elevation of liver function test results, cholestatic and hepatocellular jaundice, and hepatitis are rare
- transient elevation in liver function test results is common (usually benign and reversible on discontinuation of therapy)
- obtain baseline and follow-up liver function tests and discontinue therapy if clinical evidence of hepatotoxicity occurs and liver enzyme levels are greater than 3 times baseline values
- patients are best monitored by evaluating for the presence of extreme malaise or vomiting, yellowish pigmentation of skin or eyes, change in color of urine or stool, or severe gastrointestinal pain

▶ *How Long Do I Treat Patients with This Drug?*

Generalized seizures (no primary focus), partial seizures (with or without secondarily generalized tonic-clonic seizures)

- a 4 year seizure-free period is recommended before attempting to withdraw carbamazepine administration
- factors promoting complete withdrawal include a seizure-free period of 2–4 years, complete seizure control within 1 year of onset, an onset of seizures between 2 and 35 years of age, and a normal electroencephalogram
- patients should not drive during withdrawal and for 3–4 months after, and this may make it difficult for some patients to try withdrawal
- prior to withdrawal, patients should be advised that about 1/3 will relapse, and if this occurs, the patient and the physician will know that the drug is still necessary
- factors associated with a poor prognosis in stopping drug administration, despite a seizure-free period, include a history of a high frequency of seizures, repeated episodes of status epilepticus, multiple seizure types, and development of abnormal mental functioning

Prophylactic therapy for bipolar disorder, schizoaffective disorder, aggression

- adequate trial period is necessary to evaluate (typically, 3–4 weeks at therapeutic serum concentrations; some patients require up to 6 weeks for full response)
- duration of therapy is not well defined
- at the minimum, treatment should continue until symptoms resolve, the patient is euthymic, and sleep normalized (some clinicians recommend continuing therapy for several months after symptoms resolve)
- prophylactic or maintenance therapy should be continued in rapid cyclers (>4 episodes per year) and probably in patients with a history of recurrent bipolar disorder (at least 1 episode per year) with marked severity and substantial disruption of functioning

Trigeminal neuralgia

- some clinicians attempt to decrease the dosage or stop the drug administration at least every 3 months and do not use prophylactically during periods of remission
- other clinicians claim that withdrawal during remission may make the patient refractory to carbamazepine when symptoms recur
- maintain the lowest dosage known to be effective for the patient

▶ *How Do I Stop or Decrease the Administration of This Drug?*

- sudden withdrawal is to be avoided, especially after long-term, high-dose therapy
- withdrawal is best done over several months
- decrease the dosage by 200 mg daily each month until withdrawal is complete
- seizure relapse is most common during withdrawal or the first 3 months after withdrawal
- if seizures recur, reinstitute treatment with the same drugs used previously
- if multiple anticonvulsant therapy is present, drugs should be withdrawn 1 at a time
- for psychiatric disorders, most patients do not experience a withdrawal syndrome or rebound phenomenon on abrupt discontinuation; however, certain individuals may have increased risks of recurrence of symptoms after discontinuation (Br J Psychiatry 1986;149:498–501)
- best to taper drug; decrease the daily dosage by 100 mg every week and monitor the patient weekly for the first few weeks (monitoring for early relapse) and then monthly after that (monitoring for late relapse)

▶ *What Should I Tell My Patients About This Drug?*

- contact your physician immediately if you notice a sore throat, fever or other signs of infection, increased bruising, weakness, fatigue, or abnormal skin color

- you may experience mild drowsiness, dizziness, and nausea and vomiting the first few days after starting administration of this drug or after a dosage increase but these symptoms usually go away after a couple of weeks; however, call your physician if they persist or increase in intensity
- you may be overly sensitive to the combination of this drug with alcohol or other CNS depressants, and you should not drive or operate heavy machinery until you know how you react to these agents
- take the drug with food to minimize stomach irritation and to aid in its absorption
- do not chew controlled-release tablets

▶ Therapeutic Tips

- use of controlled-release tablets after the dose has been titrated allows most patients to be treated BID with fewer side effects
- switching brands should be done cautiously, if at all, with careful monitoring of efficacy and serum drug concentration until a steady state is apparent
- must give suspension dosage form more frequently than tablets to prevent excessive peak-trough fluctuations and resultant side effects
- changing from a BID regimen to a TID or QID schedule may increase absorption and serum concentration and improve clinical response while decreasing gastrointestinal side effects
- carbamazepine absorption tends to be capacity limited; as larger single doses are given, smaller fractions of the dose may be absorbed
- consider carbamazepine's autoinduction effects when interpreting serum levels (e.g., the serum level is likely to be lower 3–4 weeks after therapy than after the first week on the same dosage)
- serum levels should be monitored at least twice during the first month of therapy because metabolism is autoinduced
- if carbamazepine is being substituted for another anticonvulsant with known hepatic enzyme–inducing properties (phenobarbital, phenytoin), carbamazepine's half-life will be shorter than if it was being started as monotherapy, and the dosage can be increased much more rapidly
- carbamazepine can be safely used by breastfeeding mothers

Useful References

Pugh CB, Garnett WR. Current issues in the treatment of epilepsy. Clin Pharm 1991;10:335–358

Parker WA. Epilepsy. In: Herfindal ET, Gourley DR, Hart LL, eds. Clinical Pharmacy and Therapeutics, 4th ed. Baltimore: Williams & Wilkins, 1988:570–592

Levy RH, Wilensky AJ, Friel PN. Other antiepileptic drugs. In: Evans WE, Schentag JJ, Jusko WJ, eds. Applied Pharmacokinetics. Principles of Therapeutic Drug Monitoring, 2nd ed. Spokane, WA: Applied Therapeutics, 1986:540–569

Post RM, Leverich GS, Rosoff AS, Altschuler LL. Carbamazepine prophylaxis in refractory affective disorders: A focus on long-term follow-up. J Clin Psychopharmacol 1990;10(5):318–327

Ballenger JC. The clinical use of carbamazepine in affective disorders. J Clin Psychiatry 1988;49(4):13–18

CARTEOLOL

Robert Rangno and James McCormack

USA (Cartrol)
CANADA (not available)

▶ When Should I Use This Drug?

Consider an alternative agent

- nonselective beta-blocker with mild partial agonist activity
- as effective as other beta-blockers
- as with other beta-blockers with partial agonist activity, this agent may cause less bradycardia; however, the clinical benefit (if any) over that of other available agents is unknown (Med Lett 1989;31:70–71)

CASCARA

Leslie Mathews

USA (combination: Kondremul with Cascara, Nature's Remedy, Caroid tablets)
CANADA (Cascara aromatic)

▶ When Should I Use This Drug?

Acute constipation

- when bulk-forming laxatives or osmotic laxatives are ineffective or contraindicated
- to provide a more rapid effect than a bulk-forming laxative
- all stimulant laxatives are equally effective and less expensive than agents such as lactulose
- although some authors advocate the use of senna over any of the other stimulants, claiming that it is the mildest and that standardized senna is the most physiological of all the nonfiber laxatives (Pharmacology 1988;36[suppl 1]:230–236), there are no good studies to confirm or refute these claims
- should be used only acutely, as other agents are safer and more effective for long-term treatment
- decision about which stimulant laxative (bisacodyl, senna, cascara) to use should be based upon availability and cost

Chronic constipation

- occasional use in patients with an absent or poor defecation reflex or severely delayed gut transit or in patients with severe debilitation or terminal illness (if long-term therapy is required, use lactulose)
- useful for bedridden, anorexic patients who are unable to tolerate fluids (and therefore bulk-forming laxatives cannot be used)
- patients with neurogenic constipation (e.g., due to spinal cord injury and multiple sclerosis) frequently require stimulation of the gut often in conjunction with stool softeners and regular stimulation of the rectal mucosa with suppositories and/or enemas to prevent fecal impaction

▶ When Should I Not Use This Drug?

see Bisacodyl

▶ What Contraindications Are There to the Use of This Drug?

- Intolerance of or allergic reaction to cascara
see Bisacodyl

▶ What Drug Interactions Are Clinically Important?

- none

▶ What Route and Dosage Should I Use?

How to administer

- orally—take with a full glass of water
- rectally—not available

Acute constipation, chronic constipation

- most commonly used preparation is aromatic fluid extract 5 mL PO daily
- others: fluid extract 0.5–1.5 mL, bark 0.3–1 g; extract 0.2–0.4 mL

▶ What Should I Monitor with Regard to Efficacy and Toxicity?

Efficacy

see Bisacodyl

Toxicity

see Senna

▶ How Long Do I Treat Patients with This Drug?

see Bisacodyl

▶ How Do I Decrease or Stop the Administration of This Drug?

see Bisacodyl

▶ What Should I Tell My Patients About This Drug?

- discontinue with diarrhea or relief of constipation
- decrease the dose by 50% with persistent abdominal cramps
- notify your physician if constipation persists after 1 week of use

- prolonged use can cause serious side effects and lead to laxative dependency and loss of normal bowel function
- complete bowel emptying can occur
- you may not have another bowel movement for 2–3 days after use
- take at bedtime to produce effects by morning
- take each dose with a full glass of water

▶ *Therapeutic Tips*

- give dose at bedtime, especially for the elderly, to avoid nocturnal fecal incontinence
- low doses are usually effective

Useful References

Tedesco FJ. Laxative use in constipation. Am J Gastroenterol 1985; 80:303–309
Rousseau P. Treatment of constipation in the elderly. Postgrad Med 1988; 83:339–349
Godding EW. Laxatives and the special role of senna. Pharmacology 1988; 36(suppl 1):230–236

CASTOR OIL
Leslie Mathews

USA (Purge, Neoloid, Emulsoil)
CANADA (Neoloid, Ricifruit, Unisoil)

▶ *When Should I Use This Drug?*

Consider an alternative agent

- has a strong purgative action
- can cause marked cramping with therapeutic doses
- regular use can cause dehydration or electrolyte imbalance
- long-term use can cause morphological damage to the mucosa of the small intestine (Postgrad Med 1988;83:339–349) and malabsorption of nutrients (J Gerontol Nurs 1990;16:4–11)
- after use, it may take several days to produce another stool owing to complete emptying of colon
- great potential for abuse as patients attempt to maintain daily bowel movements

Useful Reference

Tedesco FJ. Laxative use in constipation. Am J Gastroenterol 1985; 80:303–309

CEFACLOR
Bruce Carleton

USA (Ceclor)
CANADA (Ceclor)

▶ *When Should I Use This Drug?*

Consider an alternative agent

- provides no clinical advantages over amoxicillin-clavulanate
- cefaclor may cause an adverse reaction resembling serum sickness in 1–2% of children, although it is more likely to cause this reaction during or after the second course of administration (Pediatr Infect Dis J 1985;4:358–361)

CEFAMANDOLE
Bruce Carleton

USA (Mandol)
CANADA (Mandol)

▶ *When Should I Use This Drug?*

Consider an alternative agent

- provides no clinical advantages over cefuroxime
- cefamandole and cefuroxime are effective against the same bacteria, with cefuroxime having more reliable activity against beta-lactamase–producing *Haemophilus influenzae* (Am Fam Physician 1991;43:937–948)
- cefamandole needs to be dosed Q4–6H, whereas cefuroxime is dosed on a Q8H regimen because of its longer half-life

- cefamandole is usually more expensive than cefuroxime when both are dosed equivalently (cefamandole 1 g IV Q6H versus cefuroxime 750 mg IV Q8H)
- cefamandole has a methylthiotetrazole side chain similar to that found on other antibiotics, which has been associated with bleeding disorders and disulfiram-like reactions

CEFAZOLIN
Bruce Carleton

USA (Ancef, Kefzol, generic)
CANADA (Ancef, Kefzol)

▶ *When Should I Use This Drug?*

check antibiotic susceptibility chart (Table 4–1 in Chapter 4)

Surgical prophylaxis

- cefazolin is the drug of choice for surgical prophylaxis in non–penicillin-allergic patients for noncardiac thoracic, peripheral vascular, gastroduodenal, biliary tract, cesarean section (after clamping the umbilical cord), orthopedic, and gynecological surgeries
- in institutions in which there is a high incidence of infection with coagulase-negative *Staphylococcus* species or methicillin-resistant *Staphylococcus* species, use vancomycin for cardiac, noncardiac thoracic, peripheral vascular, and orthopedic surgeries

Pneumonia

- cefazolin is effective for pneumonias caused by *Streptococcus pneumoniae, Staphylococcus aureus*, and some gram-negative organisms but should be used only if it is less expensive than penicillin (*S. pneumoniae*) or cloxacillin (*S. aureus*)
- cefazolin should not be used if *Haemophilus influenzae* is suspected; use cefuroxime

Upper urinary tract infections

- cefazolin is active against many of the organisms that cause urinary tract infections, but most of these organisms are sensitive to ampicillin (amoxicillin if used orally), and cefazolin should be chosen only if it is less expensive than ampicillin

Cellulitis

- can be used in place of cloxacillin or nafcillin if it is less expensive
- cefazolin has good activity against staphylococcal and streptococcal organisms

▶ *When Should I Not Use This Drug?*

Klebsiella infections

- although many *Klebsiella* organisms are sensitive to cefazolin, *Klebsiella* infections, especially severe infections, do not respond well to first-generation cephalosporins like cefazolin, and other cephalosporins should likely be chosen (cefuroxime, cefoxitin or ceftizoxime, cefotetan, ceftriaxone, cefotaxime)
- in many infections in which *Klebsiella* is suspected, *H. influenzae* is also a potential pathogen, and in these cases, cefazolin is not a useful agent (use cefuroxime, as it has good activity against both *Klebsiella* and *H. influenzae*)

Methicillin-resistant gram-positive bacteria, *Serratia, Pseudomonas, Acinetobacter* and *Bacteroides fragilis* infections

- activity against these organisms is unreliable, and cefazolin should not be used when these organisms are suspected or proven

Surgical prophylaxis when methicillin-resistant staphylococci are a concern

- cephalosporins in general should not be used to treat infections due to methicillin-resistant staphylococci (Antimicrob Agents Chemother 1989;33:407–411)
- controversy exists as to whether cefazolin can be used for surgical prophylaxis when methicillin-resistant staphylococcus is a concern
- whether vancomycin, cefazolin, or a second-generation cephalosporin is used in this situation depends on the frequency with

which methicillin-resistant staphylococcus is cultured in the hospital or ward and the type of surgical procedure involved (Med Lett 1989;31:105–108)

Central nervous system infections

- cefazolin does not penetrate the blood-brain barrier

▶ *What Contraindications Are There to the Use of This Drug?*

Intolerance of or allergic reaction to penicillins or cephalosporins

- if the patient states an allergy to penicillins or cephalosporins, check that the patient has had actual allergic symptoms
- in patients reporting a true allergic reaction to penicillin, cefazolin and all other cephalosporins should not be used
- although experience to date may indicate that many patients who say they are allergic to penicillin do not have problems when they receive a cephalosporin, this is usually because the patient was not truly allergic to penicillins (Rev Infect Dis 1983; 5:S368–S379)
- regardless of when during the course of therapy a drug rash to penicillins or cephalosporins occurred (early or late), these drugs should likely be avoided in the future because there is a good chance that a similar or worse reaction could occur, and this cannot be predicted
- if a penicillin or a cephalosporin needs to be used, the clinician and the patient should be aware of the potential for a more severe reaction and the patient should be told to seek immediate medical attention if symptoms reoccur at any time during treatment

▶ *What Drug Interactions Are Clinically Important?*

- none

▶ *What Route and Dosage Should I Use?*

How to administer

Orally

- not available; however, cephalexin is an oral agent with similar spectrum to that of cefazolin

Parenterally

- cefazolin is available for IV or IM use
- for IV use, give in 100 mL of 5% dextrose in water or normal saline and administer over 30 minutes
- IV use is preferable because most cephalosporins cause pain if given via the IM route
- IM cefazolin is, however, less painful than many other cephalosporins given via the IM route

Surgical prophylaxis

- 1 g IV (2 g IV in knee arthroplasty if a tourniquet is used) 30 minutes prior to surgery and repeated if surgery lasts longer than 4 hours

Pneumonia, upper urinary tract infection, cellulitis

- 1 g IV Q8H for mild to moderate infection
- 2 g IV Q8H for severe infection

Dosage adjustments for renal or hepatic dysfunction

- renally eliminated

Normal Dosing Interval	$C_{cr} > 60$ mL/min or 1 mL/s	C_{cr} 30–60 mL/min or 0.5–1 mL/s	$C_{cr} < 30$ mL/min or 0.5 mL/s
Q8H	no adjustment needed	Q12H	Q24H

▶ *What Should I Monitor with Regard to Efficacy and Toxicity?*

Efficacy

- for antibiotic administration monitoring guidelines, see specific section on drug therapy

Toxicity

Hypersensitivity reactions (anaphylaxis, angioedema, maculopapular rash, urticaria, bronchospasm)

- hypersensitivity reactions occur in 1–5% of cephalosporin-treated patients (Mayo Clin Proc 1987;62:821–834), with maculopapular rash occurring more commonly than anaphylaxis, bronchospasm, and urticaria and usually beginning several days after the onset of therapy (Principles and Practice of Infectious Diseases, 3rd ed 1990:246–257)
- immediate hypersensitivity (anaphylaxis, bronchospasm) or accelerated hypersensitivity (angioedema, urticaria) reactions may occur minutes to hours after administration (Am Fam Physician 1991;43:937–948)

Gastrointestinal

- gastrointestinal symptoms may occur, the most serious of which is diarrhea due to pseudomembranous colitis (see drug-induced diarrhea in Chapter 11)

Pain on injection

- particularly IM injections; therefore, avoid if possible
- if pain occurs after IV injection, ensure that the IV line has not moved into the interstitial space
- if the IV line is properly positioned, slow the infusion rate and consider increasing the volume in which the cefazolin is administered to decrease irritation

Positive Coombs' test result

- frequent occurrence in patients receiving large doses; hemolysis is not usually associated with this but has been reported (Principles and Practice of Infectious Diseases, 3rd ed, 1990:246–257)

▶ *How Long Do I Treat Patients with This Drug?*

Surgical prophylaxis

- for most surgical prophylaxis, 1 g IV 30 minutes prior to surgery is all that is required
- additional doses are necessary only if surgery is longer than 4 hours

Pneumonia

- oral antibiotics should be considered after the patient has clinically improved and has been afebrile for 48 hours

Upper urinary tract infections

- 14 days total IV and PO therapy (e.g., trimethoprim-sulfamethoxazole, amoxicillin)
- consider switching to an oral agent after the patient has become afebrile and has clinically improved for 1–2 days

Cellulitis

- usual duration of therapy is 10 days or 4–5 days after the patient has become afebrile and has clinically improved
- consider switching to oral cephalexin after the patient has become afebrile and has clinically improved for 1–2 days

▶ *How Do I Decrease or Stop the Administration of This Drug?*

- may be stopped abruptly
- cefazolin administration should be discontinued immediately when allergic reactions (particularly anaphylaxis) occur

▶ *What Should I Tell My Patients About This Drug?*

- do you know whether you have ever taken either a penicillin or cephalosporin before? (mention several common names such as penicillin, ampicillin, Keflex, Ceclor)
- have you ever had difficulties or problems taking antibiotics, or medications in general, in the past?
- cefazolin is an antibiotic meant to fight infection and it is similar to penicillins
- cefazolin is normally well tolerated; however, if you notice a rash or have an upset stomach or diarrhea, tell your pharmacist or physician
- complete entire course of therapy prescribed even if you feel better

▶ *Therapeutic Tips*

- never give this medication more frequently than Q8H because the half-life of cefazolin is long enough to prevent the need for more frequent dosing

- for surgical prophylaxis, ensure that therapy is not continued for longer than the appropriate duration (usually 1 dose)

Useful References

Donowitz GR, Mandell GL. Cephalosporins. In: Mandell GL, Douglas RG, Bennett JE, eds. Principles and Practice of Infectious Diseases, 3rd ed. New York: Churchill Livingstone, 1990:246–257

Sussman G, Davis K, Kohler P. Penicillin allergy: A practical approach to management. Can Med Assoc J 1986;134:1353–1356

Thompson RL. Cephalosporin, carbapenem, and monobactam antibiotics. Mayo Clin Proc 1987;62:821–834

Winslade N. Rational use of cephalosporins. On Continuing Practice 1991;18(1):7–10

CEFIXIME

Bruce Carleton

USA (Suprax)
CANADA (Suprax)

▶ When Should I Use This Drug?

check antibiotic susceptibility chart (Table 4–1 in Chapter 4)

Uncomplicated gonorrhea caused by beta-lactamase–producing *Neisseria gonorrhoeae*

- cefixime is the drug of choice because it is a single-dose oral treatment that is as effective as and less expensive than ceftriaxone (J Infect Dis 1992;166:919–922)
- ceftriaxone should be used rather than cefixime in cases of epididymitis owing to a lack of experience with cefixime in this condition
- doxycycline should be added to either cefixime or ceftriaxone because coexisting *Chlamydia trachomatis* is often present

Otitis media

- amoxicillin is the drug of choice for the initial treatment of acute otitis media because it is less expensive than amoxicillin-clavulanate
- use of cefixime is limited by its high cost and its tendency to produce diarrhea
- cefixime or amoxicillin-clavulanate (the decision between these agents should be based on cost and tolerability by the patient) should be chosen after 2–3 treatment failures with amoxicillin or trimethoprim-sulfamethoxazole
- incidence of diarrhea with cefixime is similar to that with amoxicillin-clavulanate in pediatric and adult patients (J Pediatr 1986;109:891–896, Antimicrob Agents Chemother 1986;29:107–111, Antimicrob Agents Chemother 1983;24:716–719, 856–859, Pediatr Infect Dis J 1987;6:976–980)
- erythromycin ethylsuccinate/sulfisoxazole is usually slightly less expensive than cefixime or amoxicillin-clavulanate acid; however, it is likely less well tolerated (abdominal pain)
- although some clinicians suggest that guidelines for antibiotic use be guided by the incidence of beta-lactamase–producing organisms, this information is not readily available because cultures of the middle ear are rarely done

▶ When Should I Not Use This Drug?

Pharyngitis, tonsillitis, acute bronchitis, and urinary tract infections

- amoxicillin is as effective as cefixime in the treatment of these infections (Am J Med 1988;85[suppl 3A]:6–13)

Otitis media caused by *Moraxella (Branhamella) catarrhalis* and beta-lactamase–negative *Haemophilus influenzae*

- amoxicillin is as effective as cefixime in the treatment of these infections (Pediatr Infect Dis J 1987;6:989–991)

Otitis media caused by pneumococci or *Staphylococcus aureus*

- cefixime is less effective than amoxicillin in eradicating these organisms (Pediatr Infect Dis J 1987;6:989–991)

▶ What Contraindications Are There to the Use of This Drug?

see Cefazolin

▶ What Drug Interactions Are Clinically Important?

- none

▶ What Route and Dosage Should I Use?

How to administer

- orally—take with food or milk or on an empty stomach
- parenterally—not available

Uncomplicated gonorrhea caused by beta-lactamase–producing *Neisseria gonorrhoeae*

- 400 mg PO as a single dose

Otitis media

- 400 mg PO daily

Dosage adjustments for renal or hepatic dysfunction

- renal and biliary elimination

Normal Dosing Interval	$C_{cr} > 60$ mL/min or 1 mL/s	C_{cr} 30–60 mL/min or 0.5–1 mL/s	$C_{cr} < 30$ mL/min or 0.5 mL/s
Q24H	no adjustment needed	no adjustment needed	200 mg Q24H

▶ What Should I Monitor with Regard to Efficacy and Toxicity?

Efficacy

- for antibiotic administration monitoring guidelines, see specific section on drug therapy

Toxicity

see Cefazolin

▶ How Long Do I Treat Patients with This Drug?

Uncomplicated gonorrhea caused by beta-lactamase–producing *Neisseria gonorrhoeae*

- single-dose treatment

Otitis media

- 7 days

▶ How Do I Decrease or Stop the Administration of This Drug?

see Cefazolin

▶ What Should I Tell My Patients About This Drug?

see Cefazolin

▶ Therapeutic Tips

- long elimination half-life (~3 hours) allows once- or twice-daily dosing
- peak serum concentrations and the extent of absorption are not affected by food (Pediatr Infect Dis J 1987;6:963–970)
- oral suspension is absorbed more rapidly and completely than the tablets; the manufacturer recommends against using the tablets to treat acute otitis media
- unlike other cephalosporins, cefixime has no activity against staphylococci

Useful References

Plourde PJ, Tyndall M, Agoki E, et al. Single-dose cefixime versus single-dose ceftriaxone in the treatment of antimicrobial-resistant *Neisseria gonorrhoeae* infection. J Infect Dis 1992;166:919–922

Sanders CC. β-Lactamase stability and in vitro activity of oral cephalosporins against strains possessing well-characterized mechanisms of resistance. Antimicrob Agents Chemother 1989;33:1313–1317

Howie VM, Owen MJ. Bacteriologic and clinical efficacy of cefixime compared with amoxicillin in acute otitis media. Pediatr Infect Dis J 1987;6:989–991

CEFONICID

Bruce C. Carleton

USA (Monocid)
CANADA (not available)

▶ *When Should I Use This Drug?*

Consider an alternative agent

- similar spectrum of activity to cefamandole, but not as active against staphylococci (precludes use in surgical prophylaxis)

CEFOPERAZONE

Bruce C. Carleton

USA (Cefobid)
CANADA (Cefobid)

▶ *When Should I Use This Drug?*

Consider an alternative agent

- although cefoperazone has a wide spectrum of activity, including activity against both *Pseudomonas aeruginosa* and *Bacteroides fragilis*, with the availability of ceftazidime and cefoxitin or cefotetan, there are no specific indications for which cefoperazone is considered the antibiotic of choice (Am Fam Physician 1991;43:937–948)
- concerns of bleeding disorders associated with prothrombin deficiency and a disulfiram-like reaction after the ingestion of alcohol (Med Lett 1990;32:107–110) further diminish the usefulness of cefoperazone relative to other available antibiotics

CEFORANIDE

Bruce C. Carleton

USA (Precef)
CANADA (not available)

▶ *When Should I Use This Drug?*

Consider an alternative agent

- ceforanide has less activity against most organisms than does cefuroxime
- there is no reason to use this agent (Med Lett 1984;26:91–92)

CEFOTAXIME

Bruce C. Carleton

USA (Claforan)
CANADA (Claforan)

Cefotaxime and ceftriaxone have equivalent spectrums of activity and are of equal clinical effectiveness • Ceftriaxone causes a slightly higher incidence of diarrhea (3% versus 1%), but the clinical significance of this is unclear • Ceftriaxone may cause pseudolithiasis, frank cholelithiasis, biliary colic, and cholecystitis because of its high degree of biliary excretion (45%) (Antimicrob Agents Chemother 1990;34:1146–1149, Lancet 1988;1:1411–1413) • The clinical significance of this effect is unclear, but cholecystectomy has occurred (MMWR 1993;42:39–42) • Cefotaxime when dosed at 1 or 2 g Q8H is more expensive than ceftriaxone when given at equivalent dosages (1 or 2 g Q24H); however, in patients with poor renal function, cefotaxime can be dosed Q12H and becomes more cost effective than ceftriaxone

▶ *When Should I Use This Drug?*

check antibiotic susceptibility chart (Table 4–1 in Chapter 4)

Spontaneous bacterial peritonitis (in cirrhotics)

- combination of ampicillin and cefotaxime covers enterococci, Enterobacteriaceae, and aerobic streptococci
- ampicillin plus an aminoglycoside may be used; however, some studies suggest an increased incidence of nephrotoxicity in cirrhotic patients receiving aminoglycosides, but this is not yet clearly delineated (Gastroenterology 1982;82:97–105, Hepatology 1985;5:457–462)

Upper urinary tract infection

- useful in patients who are severely ill with contraindications to the use of aminoglycosides (e.g., poor renal function)

Meningitis

- cefotaxime in conjunction with ampicillin is the empirical regimen of choice for meningitis, especially for adults 50 years or older or patients with a history of head injury, concurrent sinusitis, otitis media, pneumonia or epiglottitis, diabetes, alcoholism, or hypogammaglobulinemia, as this combination covers *Streptococcus pneumoniae, Neisseria meningitidis, Listeria monocytogenes, Haemophilus influenzae,* and other gram-negative organisms that may be present in this population (Infect Dis Clin North Am 1990;4:645–659)
- cefotaxime should also be used as empirical therapy if Gram stain of the cerebrospinal fluid (CSF) shows gram-negative organisms and *Pseudomonas* is not suspected
- cefotaxime, ceftriaxone, and ceftazidime are the only cephalosporins that penetrate the CSF in reliable concentrations to treat meningitis

Osteomyelitis, soft tissue infections, pneumonia, sepsis, and other infections

- only when caused, or suspected to be caused, by gram-negative bacteria that are resistant to other less expensive penicillins and cephalosporins, yet sensitive to cefotaxime (including *Serratia* spp., *Klebsiella* spp., *H. influenzae, Proteus* spp., *Enterobacter* spp., and *Escherichia coli*)
- ensure that organisms are resistant to other agents, as many other effective agents are less expensive and should be used

▶ *When Should I Not Use This Drug?*

Infections caused by methicillin-resistant *Staphylococcus aureus* or *epidermidis*, *E. faecalis*, *Pseudomonas* sp., *Bacteroides fragilis*, or *Acinetobacter*

- cefotaxime does not have reliable activity against these organisms (Med Lett 1990;32:107–110)

Mild infections caused by bacteria that are sensitive to other less expensive antibiotics

- cefotaxime should not be used to treat community-acquired pneumonia, uncomplicated urinary tract infections, or other infections caused by bacteria sensitive to less expensive agents

▶ *What Contraindications Are There to the Use of This Drug?*

see Cefazolin

▶ *What Drug Interactions Are Clinically Important?*

- none

▶ *What Route and Dosage Should I Use?*

How to administer

Orally

- not available

Parenterally

- cefotaxime is available only for IV or IM use
- for IV use, give in 100 mL of 5% dextrose in water or normal saline and administer over 30 minutes
- IV use is preferable because most cephalosporins cause pain if given via the IM route

Spontaneous bacterial peritonitis (in cirrhotics), upper urinary tract infection, osteomyelitis, soft tissue infections, pneumonia, sepsis, and other infections

- 2 g IV Q8H for severe infections
- 1 g IV Q8H for less severe infections
- several studies support the use of cefotaxime Q12H in patients with normal renal function who have mild to moderate uncomplicated gram-negative infections (Drugs 1990;40:608–651, Diagn Microbiol Infect Dis 1988;9:97–103)

Meningitis

- 2 g IV Q8H

Dosage adjustments for renal or hepatic dysfunction

- renally eliminated with an active metabolite

Normal Dosing Interval	C$_{cr}$ > 60 mL/min or 1 mL/s	C$_{cr}$ 30–60 mL/min or 0.5–1 mL/s	C$_{cr}$ < 30 mL/min or 0.5 mL/s
Q8H	no adjustment needed	Q12H	Q24H

▶ *What Should I Monitor with Regard to Efficacy and Toxicity?*

Efficacy

- for antibiotic administration monitoring guidelines, see specific section on drug therapy

Toxicity

see Cefazolin

▶ *How Long Do I Treat Patients with This Drug?*

Spontaneous bacterial peritonitis (in cirrhotics)

- treatment should continue for a minimum of 10 days; however, extend treatment if the patient has not been asymptomatic for longer than 72 hours

Upper urinary tract infections

- 14 days of IV and PO therapy
- consider switching to oral therapy with an appropriate oral agent (see antibiotic susceptibility chart [Table 4–1 in Chapter 4]) after the patient has become afebrile and has clinically improved for 1–2 days

Meningitis

- 21 days for meningitis caused by gram-negative organisms

Osteomyelitis, soft tissue infections, pneumonia, sepsis, and other infections

- see specific section on drug therapy

▶ *How Do I Decrease or Stop the Administration of This Drug?*

see Cefazolin

▶ *What Should I Tell My Patients About This Drug?*

see Cefazolin

▶ *Therapeutic Tips*

- when dosed Q8H, it is more expensive than ceftriaxone, but when dosed Q12H (e.g., in patients with poor renal function), it is less expensive than ceftriaxone
- several studies support the use of cefotaxime Q12H in patients with normal renal function who have mild to moderate uncomplicated gram-negative infections (Drugs 1990;40:608–651, Diagn Microbiol Infect Dis 1988;9:97–103)

Useful References

Thompson RL. Cephalosporin, carbapenem, and monobactam antibiotics. Mayo Clin Proc 1987;62:821–834

Neu HC, Carbon C, Pechere JC, eds. Cefotaxime: Proceedings from the 15th International Congress of Chemotherapy. Drugs 1988;35(suppl 2):1–231

Todd PA, Brogden RN. Cefotaxime: An update of its pharmacology and therapeutic use. Drugs 1990;40:608–651

CEFOTETAN

Bruce Carleton

USA (Cefotan)
CANADA (Cefotan)

Cefoxitin, cefotetan, and ceftizoxime have similar spectrums of activity, except cefoxitin has greater activity against certain strains of *Bacteroides* (*distasonis, ovatus, thetaiotaomicron,* and *uniformis*) but lesser activity against enteric bacilli such as *Escherichia coli* and *Klebsiella* (Am J Surg 1988;155:103–107), although the clinical relevance of these findings is questionable • Although few trials have directly compared these drugs, numerous uncontrolled studies have demonstrated virtually identical clinical and bacteriological responses with each agent, including treatment of intraabdominal infections (Am J Surg 1988;155[5A]:61–66) and treatment of pelvic inflammatory disease (Am J Obstet Gynecol 1988;158:736–743) • Cefoxitin when given 1 or 2 g Q6H is more expensive than cefotetan (DICP, Ann Pharmacother 1989;23:1024–1030) or ceftizoxime (Med Lett 1991;33:75–76) when given at equivalent dosages • Cefoxitin, cefotetan, and ceftizoxime have comparable side effect profiles, despite the presence of the methylthiotetrazole side chain on cefotetan (Am J Surg 1988;155[5A]:40–44, 44–46) • The decision among cefoxitin, cefotetan, and ceftizoxime should be based on a cost comparison (including administration costs) of cefoxitin 1 g Q6H, cefotetan 1 g IV Q12H, and ceftizoxime 1 g Q8H

▶ *When Do I Use This Drug?*

check antibiotic susceptibility chart (Table 4–1 in Chapter 4)
see Cefoxitin

▶ *When Should I Not Use This Drug?*

see Cefoxitin

▶ *What Contraindications Are There to the Use of This Drug?*

see Cefazolin

▶ *What Drug Interactions Are Clinically Important?*

- none

▶ *What Route and Dosage Should I Use?*

How to administer

Orally

- not available

Parenterally

- cefotetan is available only for IV or IM use
- for IV use, give in 100 mL of 5% dextrose in water or normal saline and administer over 30 minutes
- IV use is preferable because most cephalosporins cause pain if given via the IM route

Surgical prophylaxis, outpatient treatment of pelvic inflammatory disease

- 2 g IV as a single dose

Intraabdominal infections, pelvic inflammatory disease, cellulitis, *Bacteroides fragilis* infections

- 1 g IV Q12H for mild to moderate infections
- 2 g IV Q12H for severe infections (Am J Surg 1988;155:61–66)

Dosage adjustments for renal or hepatic dysfunction

- renally eliminated

Normal Dosing Interval	C$_{cr}$ > 60 mL/min or 1 mL/s	C$_{cr}$ 30–60 mL/min or 0.5–1 mL/s	C$_{cr}$ < 30 mL/min or 0.5 mL/s
Q12H	no adjustment needed	Q24H	Q24H and reduce dosage by 50%

▶ *What Should I Monitor with Regard to Efficacy and Toxicity?*

Efficacy

- for antibiotic administration monitoring guidelines, see specific section on drug therapy

Toxicity

see Cefazolin

Hematological effects
- cefotetan contains the methylthiotetrazole side chain, which has been associated with bleeding disorders (Rev Infect Dis 1990;12:1109–1120) and disulfiram-like reactions to alcohol
- hypoprothrombinemia and bleeding appear to be no more frequent with cefotetan than with other cephalosporins (Am J Surg 1988;155[5A]:40–44, 44–46)

▶ *How Long Do I Treat Patients with This Drug?*
see Cefoxitin

Surgical prophylaxis
- give as a single dose; a repeated dose is not needed, even if surgery proceeds for longer than 4 hours, because cefotetan has a long half-life

▶ *How Do I Decrease or Stop the Administration of This Drug?*
see Cefazolin

▶ *What Should I Tell My Patients About This Drug?*
see Cefazolin

▶ *Therapeutic Tips*
see Cefoxitin

Useful Reference

Thompson RL. Cephalosporin, carbapenem, and monobactam antibiotics. Mayo Clin Proc 1987;62:821–834

CEFOXITIN
Bruce Carleton

USA (Mefoxin, generics)
CANADA (Mefoxin)
Cefoxitin, cefotetan, and ceftizoxime have similar spectrums of activity, except cefoxitin has greater activity against certain strains of *Bacteroides* (*distasonis, ovatus, thetaiotaomicron,* and *uniformis*) but lesser activity against enteric bacilli such as *Escherichia coli* and *Klebsiella* (Am J Surg 1988;155:103–107), although the clinical relevance of these findings is questionable • Although few trials have directly compared these drugs, numerous uncontrolled studies have demonstrated virtually identical clinical and bacteriological responses with each agent, including treatment of intraabdominal infections (Am J Surg 1988;155[5A]:61–66) and treatment of pelvic inflammatory disease (Am J Obstet Gynecol 1988;158:736–743) • Cefoxitin when given 1 or 2 g Q6H is more expensive than cefotetan (DICP, Ann Pharmacother 1989;23:1024–1030) or ceftizoxime (Med Lett 1991;33:75–76) when given at equivalent dosages • Cefoxitin, cefotetan, and ceftizoxime have comparable side effect profiles, despite the presence of the methylthiotetrazole side chain on cefotetan (Am J Surg 1988;155[5A]:40–44, 44–46) • The decision among cefoxitin, cefotetan, and ceftizoxime should be based on a cost comparison (including administration costs) of cefoxitin 1 g Q6H, cefotetan 1 g IV Q12H, and ceftizoxime 1 g Q8H

▶ *When Should I Use This Drug?*
check antibiotic susceptibility chart (Table 4–1 in Chapter 4)

Surgical prophylaxis
- drug of choice for surgical prophylaxis in non–penicillin-allergic patients for appendectomy, abdominal trauma, emergency colorectal surgery, and lower extremity amputation

Intraabdominal infections
- drug of choice for secondary peritonitis, abdominal trauma, gangrenous or perforated appendix, or cholecystitis or cholangitis if the risk of renal impairment from aminoglycoside is high (elderly patients or those with preexisting renal failure, otic or vestibular dysfunction, or previous aminoglycoside treatment)

Pelvic inflammatory disease
- drug of choice, in combination with either doxycycline or tetracycline

- this combination covers organisms implicated in pelvic inflammatory disease (PID), namely *Chlamydia trachomatis, Neisseria gonorrhoeae,* aerobes (*E. coli,* streptococci) and anaerobes (*Bacteroides* sp.)
- proven efficacy and lower toxicity than clindamycin and gentamicin make it the first choice in mild to moderately ill hospitalized patients with PID
- also useful for outpatient therapy for PID, as a single dose in combination with probenecid and doxycycline, if this combination is less expensive than ceftriaxone and doxycycline (MMWR 1991;40[RR-5]:1–25)

Cellulitis
- useful for high-risk patients if an abscess is present or if anaerobic and gram-negative organisms are suspected (devitalized necrotic foul-smelling tissue or abdominal surgery wound) when aminoglycosides are contraindicated

***Bacteroides fragilis* infections**
- only if the infection is non–life threatening and the patient is unable to tolerate metronidazole
- metronidazole has better activity against *B. fragilis* and is less expensive than cefoxitin, cefotetan, or ceftizoxime

▶ *When Should I Not Use This Drug?*
Routine surgical prophylaxis in obstetrics and gynecology
- includes vaginal and abdominal hysterectomies and cesarean sections
- cefazolin has been shown to provide effective prophylaxis in high-risk patients (Med Lett 1989;31:105–108, DICP, Ann Pharmacother 1990;24:841–846)

***Pseudomonas* species, methicillin-resistant staphylococcus, or *E. faecalis* infections**
- cefoxitin does not have activity against these organisms

Combination with aminoglycosides
- cefoxitin is often used in patients in whom aminoglycosides are contraindicated (i.e., when one would normally use metronidazole or clindamycin plus an aminoglycoside) and so there is no reason to use cefoxitin with an aminoglycoside

Combination with other beta-lactam antibiotics
- cefoxitin can antagonize the activity of other beta-lactam antibiotics (owing to the induction of beta-lactamase production)

▶ *What Contraindications Are There to the Use of This Drug?*
see Cefazolin

▶ *What Drug Interactions Are Clinically Important?*
- none

▶ *What Route and Dosage Should I Use?*
How to administer
Orally
- not available
Parenterally
- cefoxitin is available only for IV or IM use
- for IV use, give in 100 mL of 5% dextrose in water or normal saline and administer over 30 minutes
- IV use is preferable because most cephalosporins cause pain if given via the IM route

Surgical prophylaxis
- 2 g IV as a single dose

Outpatient treatment of pelvic inflammatory disease
- 2 g IV or IM as a single dose combined with probenecid 1 g PO concurrently

Intraabdominal infections, pelvic inflammatory disease, *Bacteroides fragilis* infections
- 1 g IV Q6H for mild to moderate infections
- 2 g IV Q6H for severe infections (Am J Surg 1988;155:61–66)

Dosage adjustments for renal or hepatic dysfunction

- renally eliminated

Normal Dosing Interval	$C_{cr} > 60$ mL/min or 1 mL/s	C_{cr} 30–60 mL/min or 0.5–1 mL/s	$C_{cr} < 30$ mL/min or 0.5 mL/s
Q6H	no adjustment needed	Q8H	Q12H

▶ ### What Should I Monitor with Regard to Efficacy and Toxicity?

Efficacy

- for antibiotic administration monitoring guidelines, see specific section on drug therapy

Toxicity

see Cefazolin

▶ ### How Long Do I Treat Patients with This Drug?

Surgical prophylaxis

- repeated dose is recommended if surgery extends longer than 4 hours

Intraabdominal infection

- treatment should continue for a minimum of 10 days; however, extend treatment if the patient has not been asymptomatic for longer than 72 hours
- oral antibiotics should be considered after the patient has clinically improved and has been afebrile for 48 hours

Pelvic inflammatory disease

- used as a single dose for outpatient treatment of PID
- if PID is being treated on an inpatient basis continue the initial regimen until 48 hours after clinical improvement
- after discharge from the hospital, continue with doxycycline 100 mg PO BID for a total of 10–14 days depending on how quickly patient responds to therapy

Cellulitis

- usual duration is 10 days or 4–5 days after the patient has become afebrile and has clinically improved
- consider switching to oral therapy after the patient has become afebrile and has been clinically improved for 1–2 days

▶ ### How Do I Decrease or Stop the Administration of This Drug?

see Cefazolin

▶ ### What Should I Tell My Patients About This Drug?

see Cefazolin

▶ ### Therapeutic Tips

- most significant problems with cefoxitin are overuse for inappropriate indications (e.g., prophylaxis for obstetrical surgery) and extended use after surgery
- never use in combination with aminoglycosides because cefoxitin is likely indicated only for the treatment of infections in patients in whom aminoglycosides are contraindicated
- cefazolin-metronidazole combination is probably as effective as cefoxitin and, in many areas, is less expensive than cefoxitin (Am J Hosp Pharm 1992;49:1946–1950)

Useful Reference

Thompson RL. Cephalosporin, carbapenem, and monobactam antibiotics. Mayo Clin Proc 1987;62:821–834

CEFTAZIDIME

Bruce Carleton

USA (Fortaz, Ceptaz, Tazicef, Tazidime)
CANADA (Ceptaz, Fortaz)

▶ ### When Should I Use This Drug?

check antibiotic susceptibility chart (Table 4–1 in Chapter 4)

Meningitis, pneumonia, sepsis, osteomyelitis, soft tissue infections, upper urinary tract infections, intraabdominal infections

- only when caused, or suspected to be caused, by *Pseudomonas aeruginosa* or *Acinetobacter* or by other gram-negative organisms proven to be resistant to other less expensive cephalosporins
- ceftazidime is the only cephalosporin with reliable activity against these organisms
- ceftazidime may be used as a single agent to treat the above infections when they are caused by *P. aeruginosa* or polyresistant gram-negative bacteria; however, if the infection is severe (e.g., sepsis, necrotizing pneumonia, and peritonitis) or if the patient is neutropenic, ceftazidime should be used in combination with an aminoglycoside (Med Lett 1990;32:107–110, Hosp Form 1986;21:1130–1139)
- usually chosen over piperacillin and ticarcillin because it is less expensive and dosed less frequently than these agents (Q8H versus Q4H)
- some institutions choose to use aminoglycosides plus piperacillin or ticarcillin instead of third-generation cephalosporins because of the belief that the penicillins are less likely to induce the production of beta-lactamases and thus less likely to cause the development of resistant organisms; however the clinical importance of this is not known (J Infect Dis 1983;147:585–589, J Infect Dis 1986;154:792–800)

Empirical therapy in febrile neutropenic patients

- ceftazidime has also been used as single-agent empirical therapy in febrile neutropenic patients; however, owing to concerns of resistance and its unreliable activity against gram-positive bacteria, if ceftazidime is chosen, it should be combined with an aminoglycoside plus or minus vancomycin in this condition (J Infect Dis 1990;161:381–396)
- if cetazidime is used alone, it should be limited to patients who have had only brief periods of neutropenia and have neutrophil counts of greater than 500 cells/μL (J Infect Dis 1990;161:381–396)
- because the above combination has not been proved to be more effective than the combination of an aminoglycoside plus an antipseudomonal penicillin, consideration should be given to the use of the latter combination (J Infect Dis 1990;161:381–396)

▶ ### When Should I Not Use This Drug?

Staphylococcus aureus or *epidermidis*, *E. faecalis*, *Pseudomonas cepacia*, or *Bacteroides fragilis* infections

- ceftazidime does not have reliable activity against these organisms (Med Lett 1990;32:107–110)

Mild infections caused by bacteria that are sensitive to other less expensive antibiotics

- ceftazidime should not be used to treat community acquired pneumonia or uncomplicated urinary tract infections or other infections caused by bacteria sensitive to less expensive agents

Infections that can be treated with either cefotaxime or ceftriaxone

- ceftazidime is more expensive than these agents

▶ ### What Contraindications Are There to the Use of This Drug?

see Cefazolin

▶ ### What Drug Interactions Are Clinically Important?

- none

▶ ### What Route and Dosage Should I Use?

How to administer

Orally

- not available

Parenterally

- ceftazidime is available only for IV or IM use
- for IV use, give in 100 mL of 5% dextrose in water or normal saline and administer over 30 minutes
- IV use is preferable because most cephalosporins cause pain if given via the IM route

Meningitis

- 2 g IV Q8H

Pneumonia, sepsis, osteomyelitis, soft tissue infections, upper urinary tract infections, intraabdominal infections

- 2 g IV Q8H for severe infections
- 1 g IV Q8H for less severe infections

Dosage adjustments for renal or hepatic dysfunction

- renally eliminated

Normal Dosing Interval	C_{cr} > 60 mL/min or 1 mL/s	C_{cr} 30–60 mL/min or 0.5–1 mL/s	C_{cr} < 30 mL/min or 0.5 mL/s
Q8H	no adjustment needed	Q12H	Q24H

▶ **What Should I Monitor with Regard to Efficacy and Toxicity?**

Efficacy

- for antibiotic administration monitoring guidelines, see specific section on drug therapy

Toxicity

see Cefazolin

▶ **How Long Do I Treat Patients with This Drug?**

Meningitis

- 21 days for meningitis caused by gram-negative organisms

Osteomyelitis, soft tissue infections, pneumonia, sepsis, and other infections

- see specific section on drug therapy

Empirical therapy in febrile neutropenic patients

- if the patient is afebrile for 72 hours, no causative agent is found, and the total granulocyte count is greater than $500/\mu L$, discontinue the antibiotic administration after 7 days of treatment (J Infect Dis 1990;161:381–396)
- if the patient remains neutropenic, continue the antibiotic regimen until the patient is afebrile for 5 days
- if the patient is clinically unwell, continue antibiotic therapy until the granulocyte count is greater than 500 μL (J Infect Dis 1990;161:381–396)

▶ **How Do I Decrease or Stop the Administration of This Drug?**

see Cefazolin

▶ **What Should I Tell My Patients About This Drug?**

see Cefazolin

▶ **Therapeutic Tips**

- use only if organisms are resistant to other less expensive cephalosporins
- do not use in a scattershot fashion because of both expense and concerns for resistance
- ceftazidime should be reserved for the treatment of infections that require an antibiotic with activity against *P. aeruginosa* or polyresistant gram-negative enteric bacteria

Useful References

Thompson RL. Cephalosporin, carbapenem, and monobactam antibiotics. Mayo Clin Proc 1987;62:821–834

EORTC Report. Vancomycin added to empirical combination antibiotic therapy for fever in granulocytopenic cancer patients. J Infect Dis 1991;163:951–958

Hughes WT, Armstrong D, Bodey GP, et al. Infectious Disease Society of America guidelines for the use of antimicrobial agents in neutropenic patients with unexplained fever. J Infect Dis 1990;161:381–396

CEFTIZOXIME

Bruce Carleton

USA (Ceftizox)
CANADA (Ceftizox)

Cefoxitin, cefotetan, and ceftizoxime have similar spectrums of activity, except cefoxitin has greater activity against certain strains of *Bacteroides* (*distasonis, ovatus, thetaiotaomicron,* and *uniformis*) but lesser activity against enteric bacilli such as *Escherichia coli* and *Klebsiella* (Am J Surg 1988;155:103–107), although the clinical relevance of these findings is questionable • Although few trials have directly compared these drugs, numerous uncontrolled studies have demonstrated virtually identical clinical and bacteriological responses with each agent, including treatment of intraabdominal infections (Am J Surg 1988;155[5A]:61–66) and treatment of pelvic inflammatory disease (Am J Obstet Gynecol 1988;158:736–743) • Cefoxitin when given 1 or 2 g Q6H is more expensive than cefotetan (DICP, Ann Pharmacother 1989;23:1024–1030) or ceftizoxime (Med Lett 1991;33:75–76) when given at equivalent dosages • Cefoxitin, cefotetan, and ceftizoxime have comparable side effect profiles, despite the presence of the methylthiotetrazole side chain on cefotetan (Am J Surg 1988;155[5A]:40–44, 44–46) • The decision among cefoxitin, cefotetan, and ceftizoxime should be based on a cost comparison (including administration costs) of cefoxitin 1 g Q6H, cefotetan 1 g IV Q12H, and ceftizoxime 1 g Q8H

▶ **When Do I Use This Drug?**

check antibiotic susceptibility chart (Table 4–1 in Chapter 4)
see Cefoxitin

▶ **When Should I Not Use This Drug?**

see Cefoxitin

▶ **What Contraindications Are There to the Use of This Drug?**

see Cefazolin

▶ **What Drug Interactions Are Clinically Important?**

- none

▶ **What Route and Dosage Should I Use?**

How to administer

Orally

- not available

Parenterally

- ceftizoxime is available only for IV or IM use
- for IV use, give in 100 mL of 5% dextrose in water or normal saline and administer over 30 minutes
- IV use is preferable because most cephalosporins cause pain if given via the IM route

Surgical prophylaxis, outpatient treatment of pelvic inflammatory disease

- 2 g IV as a single dose

Intraabdominal infections, pelvic inflammatory disease, *Bacteroides fragilis* infections

- 1 g IV Q8H for mild to moderate infections
- 2 g IV Q8H for severe infections

Dosage adjustments for renal or hepatic dysfunction

- renally eliminated

Normal Dosing Interval	C_{cr} > 60 mL/min or 1 mL/s	C_{cr} 30–60 mL/min or 0.5–1 mL/s	C_{cr} < 30 mL/min or 0.5 mL/s
Q8H	no adjustment needed	Q12H	Q24H

▶ *What Should I Monitor with Regard to Efficacy and Toxicity?*

Efficacy

- for antibiotic administration monitoring guidelines, see specific section on drug therapy

Toxicity

see Cefazolin

▶ *How Long Do I Treat Patients with This Drug?*

see Cefoxitin

Surgical prophylaxis

- as a single dose; a repeated dose is not needed, even if surgery extends longer than 4 hours, because ceftizoxime has a long half-life

▶ *How Do I Decrease or Stop the Administration of This Drug?*

see Cefazolin

▶ *What Should I Tell My Patients About This Drug?*

see Cefazolin

▶ *Therapeutic Tips*

see Cefoxitin

Useful Reference

Thompson RL. Cephalosporin, carbapenem, and monobactam antibiotics. Mayo Clin Proc 1987;62:821–834

CEFTRIAXONE

Bruce Carleton

USA (Rocephin)
CANADA (Rocephin)

Cefotaxime and ceftriaxone have equivalent spectrums of activity and are of equal clinical effectiveness • Ceftriaxone causes a slightly higher incidence of diarrhea (3% versus 1%), but the clinical significance of this is unclear • Ceftriaxone may cause pseudolithiasis, frank cholelithiasis, biliary colic, and cholecystitis because of its high degree of biliary excretion (45%) (Antimicrob Agents Chemother 1990;34:1146–1149, Lancet 1988;1:1411–1413) • The clinical significance of this effect is unclear, but cholecystectomy has occurred (MMWR 1993;42: 39–42) • Cefotaxime when dosed at 1 or 2 g Q8H is more expensive than ceftriaxone when given at equivalent dosages (1 or 2 g Q24H); however, in patients with poor renal function, cefotaxime can be dosed Q12H and becomes more cost effective than ceftriaxone

▶ *When Should I Use This Drug?*

check antibiotic susceptibility chart (Table 4–1 in Chapter 4)
see Cefotaxime for additional ceftriaxone indications

Uncomplicated gonorrhea caused by beta-lactamase–producing *Neisseria gonorrhoeae*

- cefixime should be chosen over ceftriaxone, as it is a single-dose oral treatment that is as effective as and less expensive than ceftriaxone (J Infect Dis 1992;166:919–922)
- ceftriaxone should be used instead of cefixime in cases of epididymitis owing to a lack of experience with cefixime in this condition
- doxycycline should be added because coexisting *Chlamydia trachomatis* is often present

Pelvic inflammatory disease

- useful for outpatient therapy of pelvic inflammatory disease as a single dose in combination with doxycycline
- use if less expensive than cefoxitin in combination with probenecid and doxycycline (MMWR 1991;40[RR-5]:1–25)

Lyme disease with central nervous system involvement

- drug of choice for meningitis, radiculoneuropathy, peripheral neuropathy, and encephalitis associated with Lyme disease (Ann Intern Med 1991;114:472–481)

Outpatient therapy of infections caused by susceptible organisms

- although less expensive antibiotics may be effective, considerable cost savings and convenience can be achieved by dosing this drug Q24H and treating the patient outside the hospital

▶ *When Should I Not Use This Drug?*

Infections caused by methicillin-resistant *Staphylococcus aureus* or *epidermidis*, *E. faecalis*, *Pseudomonas* sp., *Bacteroides fragilis*, or *Acinetobacter*

- ceftriaxone does not have reliable activity against these organisms (Med Lett 1990;32:107–110)

Mild infections caused by bacteria that are sensitive to other less expensive antibiotics

- ceftriaxone should not be used to treat community-acquired pneumonia or uncomplicated urinary tract infections caused by bacteria sensitive to less expensive agents

Cefotaxime can be given Q12H

- in patients with poor renal function, ceftriaxone becomes more expensive than cefotaxime for the treatment of gram-negative infections
- several studies support the use of cefotaxime Q12H in patients with normal renal function who have mild to moderate uncomplicated gram-negative infections (Drugs 1990;40:608–651, Diagn Microbiol Infect Dis 1988;9:97–103)

▶ *What Contraindications Are There to the Use of This Drug?*

see Cefazolin

▶ *What Drug Interactions Are Clinically Important?*

- none

▶ *What Route and Dosage Should I Use?*

How to administer

Orally

- not available

Parenterally

- ceftriaxone is available only for IV or IM use
- for IV use, give in 100 mL of 5% dextrose in water or normal saline and administer over 30 minutes
- IV use is preferable because most cephalopsorins cause pain if given via the IM route

Spontaneous bacterial peritonitis (in cirrhotics), upper urinary tract infection, osteomyelitis, soft tissue infections, pneumonia, sepsis, and other infections

- 2 g IV Q24H for severe infections
- 1 g IV Q24H for less severe infections

Meningitis

- 2 g IV as a first dose, then 1 g IV Q12H until the patient is stable, then 2 g IV Q24H

Uncomplicated gonorrhea caused by beta-lactamase–producing *Neisseria gonorrhoeae*

- 250 mg IM as a single injection

Pelvic inflammatory disease (ambulatory regimen)

- 250 mg IV or IM as a single dose

Lyme disease with central nervous system involvement

- 2 g IV Q24H

Dosage adjustments for renal or hepatic dysfunction

- renal and biliary elimination
- no dosage adjustments necessary

▶ What Should I Monitor with Regard to Efficacy and Toxicity?

Efficacy

- for antibiotic administration monitoring guidelines, see specific section on drug therapy

Toxicity

see Cefazolin

Gastrointestinal effects

- gastrointestinal symptoms may occur, the most serious of which is diarrhea due to pseudomembranous colitis
- diarrhea is more common with ceftriaxone than with other cephalosporins (Can Med Assoc J 1990;142:450–452) and this is especially true in children
- rarely does this diarrhea necessitate discontinuation of therapy
- see discussion of drug-induced diarrhea in Chapter 11

Pseudocholelithiasis

- ceftriaxone may cause pseudolithiasis, frank cholelithiasis, biliary colic, and cholecystitis because of its high degree of biliary excretion (45%) (Antimicrob Agents Chemother 1990;34:1146–1149, Lancet 1988;1:1411–1413) (precipitation can occur in bile at dosages of >2 g/d) (Gastroenterology 1990;99:454–465, 1772–1778)
- ceftriaxone's effect on the gallbladder appears to occur more commonly in children (than in adults) or in patients with impaired gallbladder emptying (those receiving total parenteral nutrition or not eating well) (Ann Intern Med 1991;115:712–714)
- clinical significance of this effect is unclear, but cholecystectomy has occurred (MMWR 1993;42:39–42)
- symptoms, if they occur, should resolve after ceftriaxone therapy is discontinued

▶ How Long Do I Treat Patients with This Drug?

Uncomplicated gonorrhea caused by beta-lactamase–producing *Neisseria gonorrhoeae*

- single-dose therapy

Pelvic inflammatory disease

- single-dose therapy with ceftriaxone
- continue treatment with doxycycline 100 mg PO BID for a total of 10–14 days

Lyme disease with central nervous system involvement

- 14 days

see Cefotaxime for durations of treatment for other indications

▶ How Do I Decrease or Stop the Administration of This Drug?

see Cefazolin

▶ What Should I Tell My Patients About This Drug?

see Cefazolin

▶ Therapeutic Tips

- ensure that ceftriaxone is being used Q24H and not Q12H for appropriate indications

Useful References

Thompson RL. Cephalosporin, carbapenem, and monobactam antibiotics. Mayo Clin Proc 1987;62:821–834

Hawkins H, et al. Infectious Diseases and Immunization Committee, Canadian Pediatric Society: Ceftriaxone in the treatment of meningitis, gonococcal infections and other serious bacterial infections. Can Med Assoc J 1990;142:450–452

CEFUROXIME, CEFUROXIME AXETIL

Bruce Carleton

USA (Zinacef, Kefurox, Ceftin)
CANADA (Zinacef, Ceftin)

▶ When Should I Use This Drug?

check antibiotic susceptibility chart (Table 4–1 in Chapter 4)

Pneumonia

- cefuroxime has good activity against *Streptococcus pneumoniae,* ampicillin-resistant *Haemophilus influenzae,* and *Klebsiella* and is well tolerated and relatively inexpensive compared with many other parenteral antibiotics
- drug of choice in mild to moderately ill patients when Gram stain shows gram-negative coccobacillus, is not possible or unobtainable, or shows no organisms
- in many areas, ampicillin-resistant *H. influenzae* is too frequent to warrant the empirical use of amoxicillin in patients with a potentially life-threatening infection such as pneumonia
- even in areas with a low incidence of ampicillin-resistant *H. influenzae,* agents with activity against ampicillin-resistant *H. influenzae* should be used until culture and sensitivity testing results are known

Other infections caused by ampicillin-resistant *Haemophilus influenzae* or *Moraxella (Branhamella) catarrhalis*

- only if known to be resistant to ampicillin and sensitive to cefuroxime, as ampicillin is less expensive
- cefuroxime has gram-negative activity similar to cefoxitin, cefotetan, and ceftizoxime and is often less expensive than these agents

▶ When Should I Not Use This Drug?

Meningitis

- cefuroxime should not be used to treat *H. influenzae* meningitis because of a documented delay in sterilization of the cerebrospinal fluid when compared with ampicillin plus chloramphenicol (J Pediatr 1986;109:123–130)
- ceftriaxone or cefotaxime should be used for this indication because they have been shown to be as efficacious as ampicillin plus chloramphenicol (J Pediatr 1985;107:129–133, Lancet 1983;1:1241–1244)

***Serratia, Pseudomonas, Enterobacter, Acinetobacter, Bacteroides fragilis,* or methicillin-resistant staphylococcal infections**

- cefuroxime has poor activity against these organisms and should not be used to treat infections caused by these pathogens

Pneumonias when ampicillin-resistant *Haemophilus influenzae* is not suspected

- less expensive and equally effective agents such as penicillin or ampicillin should be used

Oral administration

- cefuroxime axetil is the ester form of cefuroxime, and it is hydrolyzed rapidly to cefuroxime after oral administration
- spectrum of activity is identical to that of parenterally administered cefuroxime
- although cefuroxime axetil is approved for the treatment of infections caused by susceptible strains of organisms in diseases such as tonsillitis, pharyngitis, lower respiratory tract infections, urinary tract infections, gonorrhea, and skin structure infections, in many instances less expensive oral agents with equivalent therapeutic effectiveness are available (Med Lett 1988;30:57–59)
- cefuroxime axetil is more expensive than oral amoxicillin, trimethoprimsulfamethoxazole, amoxicillin-clavulanate and erythromycin-sulfamethoxazole (Clin Pharm 1990;9:15–34)
- it is comparable in price to cefaclor and cefixime
- lack of an oral suspension form limits its use, particularly in the pediatric patient (the tablets when crushed are bitter and unpalatable)
- attempts to manufacture a palatable suspension have not proved successful

▶ What Contraindications Are There to the Use of This Drug?

see Cefazolin

▶ *What Drug Interactions Are Clinically Important?*

• none

▶ *What Route and Dosage Should I Use?*

How to administer

Orally

• available as cefuroxime axetil
• see discussion of oral administration above

Parenterally

• cefuroxime is available only for IV or IM use
• for IV use, give in 100 mL of 5% dextrose in water or normal saline and administer over 30 minutes
• IV use is preferable because most cephalosporins cause pain if given via the IM route

Pneumonia and other infections

• 1500 mg IV Q8H for severe infections
• 750 mg IV Q8H for mild to moderate infections

Dosage adjustments for renal or hepatic dysfunction

• renally eliminated

Normal Dosing Interval	$C_{cr} > 60$ mL/min or 1 mL/s	C_{cr} 30–60 mL/min or 0.5–1 mL/s	$C_{cr} < 30$ mL/min or 0.5 mL/s
Q8H	no adjustment needed	Q12H	Q24H

▶ *What Should I Monitor with Regard to Efficacy and Toxicity?*

Efficacy

• for antibiotic administration monitoring guidelines, see specific section on drug therapy

▶ *Toxicity*

see Cefazolin

▶ *How Long Do I Treat Patients with This Drug?*

Pneumonia

• usual duration of therapy is 7–10 days or 4–5 days after the patient has become afebrile and clinically improved
• consider switching to oral therapy with an appropriate oral agent (see antibiotic susceptibility chart [Table 4–1 in Chapter 4]) after the patient has become afebrile and has clinically improved for 1–2 days

▶ *How Do I Decrease or Stop the Administration of This Drug?*

see Cefazolin

▶ *What Should I Tell My Patients About This Drug?*

• see Cefazolin

▶ *Therapeutic Tips*

• do not use cefuroxime when beta-lactamase–producing bacteria are not a concern
• dosing should never be more frequent than Q8H and give either 750 mg or 1500 mg, not 1000 mg or 2000 mg, because cefuroxime comes as either a 750 mg or 1500 mg dosage form and it is difficult to prepare odd doses

Useful References

Thompson RL. Cephalosporin, carbapenem, and monobactam antibiotics. Mayo Clin Proc 1987;62:821–834

Marx MA, Fant WK. Cefuroxime axetil. DICP 1988;22:651–658

CEPHALEXIN

Bruce Carleton

USA (Keftab, Ceporex, Keflex)
CANADA (Keflex, Apo-Cephalex, Novolexin, Nu-Cephalex)

▶ *When Should I Use This Drug?*

check antibiotic susceptibility chart (Table 4–1 in Chapter 4)

Cellulitis

• cloxacillin and nafcillin are the drugs of choice if the presence of staphylococcal and streptococcal organisms is suspected or proved or if there are no clues as to what organisms are present
• cephalexin can be used in place of cloxacillin or nafcillin if it is less expensive
• cephalexin has good activity against staphylococcal and streptococcal organisms

▶ *When Should I Not Use This Drug?*

Otitis media

• cephalexin does not have good activity against *Haemophilus influenzae*

Lower urinary tract infections (cystitis)

• although cephalexin is effective, it provides no advantage over amoxicillin or trimethoprim-sulfamethoxazole

▶ *What Contraindications Are There to the Use of This Drug?*

see Cefazolin

▶ *What Drug Interactions Are Clinically Important?*

• none

▶ *What Route and Dosage Should I Use?*

How to administer

• orally—take with food or milk or on an empty stomach
• parenterally—not available

Cellulitis

• 500 mg PO Q6H

Dosage adjustments for renal or hepatic dysfunction

• renal and biliary elimination

Normal Dosing Interval	$C_{cr} > 60$ mL/min or 1 mL/s	C_{cr} 30–60 mL/min or 0.5–1 mL/s	$C_{cr} < 30$ mL/min or 0.5 mL/s
Q6H	no adjustment needed	Q8H	Q12H

▶ *What Should I Monitor with Regard to Efficacy and Toxicity?*

Efficacy

• for antibiotic administration monitoring guidelines, see specific section on drug therapy

Toxicity

see Cefazolin

▶ *How Long Do I Treat Patients with This Drug?*

Cellulitis

• usual duration is 10 days or 4–5 days after the patient has become afebrile and has clinically improved

▶ *How Do I Decrease or Stop the Administration of This Drug?*

see Cefazolin

▶ *What Should I Tell My Patients About This Drug?*

see Cefazolin

▶ *Therapeutic Tips*

• although cephalexin is useful for a number of infections, less expensive, equally effective alternative agents are usually available

Useful References

Thompson RL. Cephalosporin, carbapenem, and monobactam antibiotics. Mayo Clin Proc 1987;62:821–834

Winslade N. Rational use of cephalosporins. On Continuing Practice 1991;18(1):7–10

CEPHRADINE

Bruce Carleton

USA (Anspor, Velosef)
CANADA (Velosef)

▶ *When Should I Use This Drug?*

Consider an alternative agent

- provides no clinical advantages over cephalexin or antistaphylo-coccal penicillins such as cloxacillin
- similar in spectrum of activity to cefazolin
- usually more expensive than cefazolin and cephalexin

CHLORAL HYDRATE

Jonathan Fleming

USA (Noctec)
CANADA (Noctec, Novochlorhydrate)

▶ *When Should I Use This Drug?*

Consider an alternative agent

- there are insufficient data to warrant its preferred use, as a primary hypnotic, over the benzodiazepine hypnotics
- drug interactions and toxicity make it less safe than the benzodiazepines
- tolerance to its hypnotic effect occurs within 2 weeks (Arch Gen Psychiatry 1970;23:226–232)

Useful Reference

Kales A, Allen C, Scharf MB, Kales JD. Hypnotic drugs and their effectiveness. Arch Gen Psychiatry 1970;23:226–232

CHLORAMPHENICOL

George Zhanel and Alfred Gin

USA (Chloromycetin)
CANADA (Chloromycetin, Pentamycetin, Novochlorocap)

▶ *When Should I Use This Drug?*

check antibiotic susceptibility chart (Table 4–1 in Chapter 4)

Brain Abscess

- as alternative to penicillin and metronidazole in patients unable to tolerate penicillin or metronidazole

Meningitis

- drug of choice, as empirical therapy in a patient truly allergic to penicillins and cephalosporins if Gram stain of the cerebrospinal fluid shows gram-positive diplococci or no organisms or if Gram stain not available
- if Gram stain shows gram-negative organisms, chloramphenicol can be used as empirical therapy in the patient who is truly allergic to penicillin or cephalosporin; then desensitize to penicillins and use cefotaxime or ceftriaxone, as chloramphenicol is often not very active against some gram-negative organisms

Rickettsial Infections

- useful for infections caused by *Rickettsia* species if a patient is unable to tolerate tetracyclines or if tetracylines are contraindicated

▶ *When Should I Not Use This Drug?*

Typhoid fever

- ciprofloxacin is now the drug of choice and chloramphenicol should be used only if ciprofloxacin is not available

Intraabdominal abscess

- use only if the patient cannot tolerate metronidazole, clindamycin, cephalosporins, or penicillins

▶ *What Contraindications Are There to the Use of This Drug?*

Intolerance of or allergic reaction to chloramphenicol

- if the patient states an allergy to chloramphenicol, check that the patient has actual allergic symptoms

History of or preexisting bone marrow disease

- risk of additional bone marrow suppression

Concomitant bone marrow suppressive drugs

- risk of additional bone marrow suppression

▶ *What Drug Interactions Are Clinically Important?*

Drugs that may increase the effect of chloramphenicol

MARROW SUPPRESSIVE THERAPY

- concomitant administration of chloramphenicol with marrow suppressive therapy should be avoided, as chloramphenicol may worsen bone marrow suppression

Drugs that may decrease the effect of chloramphenicol

BARBITURATES AND RIFAMPIN

- concurrent administration of these agents with chloramphenicol may reduce the serum concentrations of chloramphenicol

Drugs that may have their effect increased by chloramphenicol

PHENYTOIN

- chloramphenicol may inhibit metabolism of phenytoin and may produce increases in serum phenytoin concentrations
- monitor serum phenytoin measurements weekly until a new steady state is established or if symptoms of toxicity occur and adjust the dosage accordingly

CHLORPROPAMIDE, TOLBUTAMIDE

- chloramphenicol may inhibit the metabolism of these agents
- if chloramphenicol is added to these drugs, treat as if a dosage change of the oral hypoglycemia agent has been made

Drugs that may have their effect decreased by chloramphenicol

- none

▶ *What Route and Dosage Should I Use?*

How to administer

Orally

- give with or without food

Parenterally

- dilute chloramphenicol in 100 mL of 5% dextrose in water or normal saline, infuse over longer than 5 minutes
- IM route is not recommended owing to delayed or incomplete absorption

Brain abcesses, meningitis

- 2 g IV Q6H

Rickettsial infections

- 50 mg/kg/d in 4 divided doses

Dosage adjustments for renal or hepatic dysfunction

- hepatically and renally eliminated
- no adjustment required unless there is combined hepatic and renal dysfunction

▶ *What Should I Monitor with Regard to Efficacy and Toxicity?*

Efficacy

- for antibiotic administration monitoring guidelines, see specific section on drug therapy

Serum concentrations

- to ensure efficacy and minimize toxicity, peak chloramphenicol concentrations should be kept between 10 and 25 mg/L

- monitor peak chloramphenicol serum concentrations (1 hour after the IV dose or 2–3 hours after the oral dose) every 3–4 days

Toxicity

Bone marrow suppression

- 2 types (irreversible and reversible)
- irreversible, rare (1/40,000 patients) idiosyncratic, bone marrow suppression, which may occur after 1 dose or after discontinuation of the drug administration
- reversible, dose-related bone marrow suppression occurs with dosages greater than 4 g/d
- monitor complete blood cell count every 2–3 days; discontinue drug administration if blood dyscrasias are noted
- monitor peak chloramphenicol serum concentrations (1 hour after the IV dose or 2–3 hours after the oral dose) every 3–4 days

Gray baby syndrome

- vomiting, abdominal distention, cyanosis, diarrhea, irregular respiration, and circulatory collapse
- occurs within first week of therapy in children younger than 1 month of age
- owing to high chloramphenicol concentration due to an inability to conjugate chloramphenicol or its metabolite
- discontinue drug administration immediately if these symptoms occur

Optic neuritis

- is rare; occurs in patients receiving high-dose, long-term therapy
- monitor patients receiving long-term therapy for visual disturbances such as loss of visual acuity and scotomas (a small area of abnormally decreased or absent vision)

▶ How Long Do I Treat Patients with This Drug?

Brain abcess, meningitis

- usual duration is 7–14 days or 4–5 days after the patient has become afebrile and has clinically improved
- consider switching to oral chloramphenicol after the patient has become afebrile and has clinically improved for 1–2 days

Rickettsial infections

- 7 days, with a minimum of 48 hours after the patient is afebrile

▶ How Do I Decrease or Stop the Administration of This Drug?

- may be stopped abruptly

▶ What Should I Tell My Patients About This Drug?

- your antibiotic is called chloramphenicol; let your physician or your pharmacist know if you have any sort of adverse reaction (fatigue, tiredness, fever, or sore throat) to this drug
- let your physician or your pharmacist know if you are taking any other medications
- take the medication until it is completed

▶ Therapeutic Tips

- monitor complete blood cell count every 3 days

Useful References

Shalit I, Marks MI. Chloramphenicol in the 1980's. Drugs 1984;29:281–291
Francke El, Neu HC. Chloramphenicol and tetracycline. Med Clin North Am 1987;71:1155–1166
Wilson WR, Cockerill FR III. Tetracyclines, chloramphenicol, erythromycin and clindamycin. Mayo Clin Proc 1987;62:906–915

CHLORDIAZEPOXIDE

Steven Stanislav and Patricia Marken

USA (C-Tran, Libritabs, Librizan, Tropium, Via-Quil)
CANADA (Librium, Apo-Chlordiazepoxide, Novopoxide, Solium, Medilium)

▶ When Should I Use This Drug?

Consider an alternative agent

- there are insufficient data to warrant its preferred use, as a primary hypnotic, antianxiety, or alcohol-withdrawal agent over the other benzodiazepines
- as a primary hypnotic, its long half-life (2–4 days), its production of active metabolites, and its hepatic metabolism (oxidative) make it less desirable than the other benzodiazepine hypnotics

CHLORPROMAZINE

Juan Avila and Patricia Marken

USA (Thorazine, Thoradol, Ormazine, Promaz, Chlorpromazine Intensol)
CANADA (Chlorprom, Novochlorpromazine, Chlorpromanyl, Largactil)

▶ When Should I Use This Drug?

Acute psychosis therapy (if prompt control is required)

- in the acutely psychotic and agitated patient, rapid tranquilization with the goal of quietly calming a dangerous patient
- chlorpromazine is a low-potency antipsychotic with high anticholinergic activity
- chlorpromazine produces more sedation and hypotension than do the medium- or high-potency antipsychotics but produces a low incidence of acute extrapyramidal or dystonic reactions
- drug of choice when sedation is required if it is less expensive than thioridazine
- available in a parenteral form
- when a patient has a previous history of response to this agent

Maintenance psychosis therapy

- to ameliorate the symptoms of psychosis that include hallucinations, delusions, formal thought disorder, bizarre behavior, agitation, and/or hyperactivity
- decision as to when to choose this agent is as above under acute psychosis therapy

Manic phase of bipolar illness

- antipsychotics are often also required for adequate sedation and behavioral control and are usually preferred to benzodiazepines for acutely manic patients with concurrent psychoses; however, there is some evidence that high-dose benzodiazepines may be equally efficacious with less adverse effects (J Clin Psychopharmacol 1985;5:109–113)
- decision as to when to choose this agent is as above under acute psychosis therapy

Migraine treatment

- useful but can cause significant sedation
- most often used in conjunction with ergot alkaloids to decrease nausea

Other uses

- nausea and vomiting, hiccups, intermittent porphyria, tetanus

▶ When Should I Not Use This Drug?

Insomnia

- unless the patient has a concurrent psychosis, antipsychotics should not be used, as they are more toxic and no more effective than benzodiazepines
- for patients who require antipsychotics and who have insomnia as part of their symptom complex, a sedating phenothiazine such as chlorpromazine can be given at night

General anxiety disorder

- unless the patient has a concurrent psychosis, antipsychotics should not be used, as they are more toxic and no more effective than benzodiazepines

Mental retardation

- should be used only if the patient is acutely agitated

- for long-term treatment, use other forms of therapy such as behavioral modification or carbamazepine or lithium administration

▶ *What Contraindications Are There to the Use of This Drug?*

Intolerance of or allergic reaction to chlorpromazine
Comatose or severely depressed states

- because antipsychotics depress the central nervous system (CNS)

Cardiovascular disease

- within 6 weeks of a myocardial infarction
- severe hypotension or conduction disturbances

Bone marrow depression; blood dyscrasias, both endogenous and drug induced

- may cause further bone marrow depression
- can be used in patients recovering from clozapine-induced agranulocytosis (J Clin Psychiatry 1988;49:271–277)

▶ *What Drug Interactions Are Clinically Important?*

Drugs that may increase the effect or toxicity of chlorpromazine
Central nervous system depressants (opiates, barbiturates, general anesthetics, alcohol)

- excessive sedation and CNS depression may occur if these agents are used concomitantly
- start with low doses of both agents to avoid excessive sedation or CNS depression, and adjust dosages on the basis of clinical presentation

Lithium

- most patients who receive lithium and an antipsychotic do not develop unusual adverse effects, but occasionally an acute encephalopathic syndrome has occurred, especially when high serum levels of lithium are present
- this is controversial, as the effect may be no greater than with lithium alone; therefore, observe for clinical signs of this syndrome; but otherwise there is no need to change therapy
- symptoms are manifest as neurological effects
- lithium may also unmask the signs of tardive dyskinesia

Drugs that may decrease the effect of chlorpromazine
PHENOBARBITAL

- has been shown to increase urinary excretion and to decrease plasma concentrations of chlorpromazine
- no empirical dosing changes are recommended, but increase the dosage of chlorpromazine if the patient experiences an exacerbation of the disease state

LITHIUM

- lithium decreases the bioavailability of chlorpromazine (Clin Pharmacol Ther 1978;23:451–455)
- no empirical dosing changes are recommended, but increase the dosage of chlorpromazine if the patient experiences an exacerbation of the disease state

Drugs that may have their effect or toxicity increased by chlorpromazine
PHENYTOIN

- chlorpromazine has been reported to decrease the metabolism of phenytoin if the drugs are used concomitantly
- monitor serum phenytoin measurements weekly until a new steady state is established or if symptoms of toxicity occur, and adjust the dosage accordingly
- if the antipsychotic regimen is stopped, return to the previous dosage

EPINEPHRINE

- acute intravenous infusions of epinephrine have produced hypotension and tachycardia in patients receiving maintenance doses of chlorpromazine
- avoid combination if possible, and if not, monitor blood pressure continuously during epinephrine infusion

Drugs that may have their effect decreased by chlorpromazine
ANTICONVULSANTS (E.G., PHENYTOIN, PHENOBARBITAL, CARBAMAZEPINE)

- chlorpromazine may lower the seizure threshold, and dosage adjustments of anticonvulsants may be necessary when the drugs are used concomitantly, but no adjustments should be made unless seizures develop

PROPRANOLOL

- chlorpromazine increases the oral bioavailability of propranolol by 25–32% because of a decrease in first-pass hepatic metabolism
- both propranolol and chlorpromazine plasma concentrations can be increased; no adjustments are necessary in most cases

▶ *What Route and Dosage Should I Use?*

How to administer

- orally—take with food or milk or on an empty stomach
- parenterally—via the IM route or as an IV infusion (dilute to at least 1 mg/mL and give at a rate of no more than 1 mg/min)

Acute psychosis therapy (if prompt control is required), manic phase of bipolar illness

- 100 mg PO or 25 mg IM (if the patient will not take oral medication) every 30–60 minutes until control is achieved or the patient does not tolerate drug (usually 2–3 doses)
- start a maintenance dose after an adequate response has been seen (see below)
- titrate to sedative effect or cerebellar side effects (ataxia, slurred speech)

Maintenance psychosis therapy

- 150 mg PO BID
- 75 mg PO BID in smaller or elderly patients
- increase the dosage every 2 weeks until an appropriate response has been seen
- typical maintenance dosage is 300–400 mg PO daily given as a single dose
- maximum daily oral dose is 2000 mg

Migraine treatment

- 12.5 mg IV repeated at 20 minute intervals to a total maximum dose of 37.5 mg may be given as required

Dosage adjustments for renal or hepatic dysfunction

- hepatically metabolized
- there are no specific dosage adjustments; just start with a low dose and titrate to effect

▶ *What Should I Monitor with Regard to Efficacy and Toxicity?*

Efficacy

Acute psychosis therapy (if prompt control is desired)

- titrate to decreased agitation, sedative effect, or cerebellar side effects (ataxia, slurred speech)
- initially, monitor a very agitated patient continuously
- monitor vital signs and the degree of agitation hourly
- should see some decrease in agitation within hours and significant improvement within 24–48 hours

Maintenance psychosis therapy

Specific target symptoms of psychosis and thought disorder

- initially, evaluate the patient at least weekly
- agitation and aggression, decreased sleep and appetite, hallucinations, delusions, disorganized thinking, pressured speech, absence of social drive, and restricted or blunted affect
- agitation and sleep improve within days
- hallucinations improve within weeks, and thought disorders within 1–2 months
- negative symptoms such as the absence of social drive and restricted or blunted affect take weeks to months to improve and may not improve at all
- monitor target symptoms at least monthly during maintenance treatment

Signs of decompensation

- after they are stable, patients should be monitored weekly initially for clinical signs of decompensation on an ongoing basis for as long as they are receiving antipsychotic therapy

Manic phase of bipolar illness

Monitor specific target symptoms

- agitation; decreased sleep; rapid, pressured speech with flight of ideas for manic phase; or symptoms of depression
- agitation and sleep disturbances usually resolve within several days to weeks; however, complete mood stabilization (and resolution of thought disorder, if present) may take 6 weeks or longer
- monitor hourly for acute situation and then increase the evaluation frequency to daily and then weekly

Monitor concurrent symptoms of psychoses

- auditory, visual hallucinations, and delusional or disorganized thinking
- symptoms may abate in several days (if related to acute mania), or require 6 weeks or longer for complete resolution

Migraine treatment

Relief of pain and other symptoms such as prodrome, aura, and gastrointestinal complaints

- assess the patient hourly during the early stage of migraine attacks

Toxicity

Anticholinergic effects

- may resolve by lowering the daily dose if the patient is stable
- if not, the following may be done

Dry mouth

- increase fluid intake and/or use sugarless chewing gum or hard candies

Constipation

- increase fluid and fiber in diet, and if needed, use a laxative

Sedation

- may occur, however, and many patients become tolerant of the sedation
- if sedation is a problem, ensure that the drug is given as a nighttime dose

Blurred vision

- tell the patient that tolerance to this adverse effect will likely develop within a few weeks
- if there is no resolution of symptoms, switch to a drug with fewer anticholinergic properties such as a high-potency agent (haloperidol)

Urinary hesitancy or retention

- tell the patient not to ignore the urge to void and recommend frequent voiding
- bethanechol chloride 25 mg PO QID can be used if this becomes an ongoing problem

Orthostatic hypotension

- if hypotension becomes clinically important and does not respond to a dosage reduction, switch to high-potency antipsychotic agents (haloperidol, fluphenazine), as they produce less orthostatic hypotension than do the low-potency agents
- treatment of orthostasis includes rising slowly from supine or sitting positions, wearing support stockings, and ensuring that adequate fluid intake is being maintained

Acute dystonia

- acute dystonic reactions (involuntary muscle contractions of the head and neck) usually occur within hours or days of either starting the administration of or increasing the dosage of an antipsychotic agent
- most often associated with high-potency agents (haloperidol, fluphenazine)

- if an acute dystonic reaction occurs, treat with benztropine 2 mg IM and repeat the dose if a response is not seen within 15 minutes
- if there is still no response, give diphenhydramine 50 mg IM, and repeat the dose if there is not relief within 5 minutes
- after a response has been seen with parenteral therapy, continue oral therapy for 2–3 weeks
- if the patient has a history of acute dystonic reactions, use benztropine or diphenhydramine prophylactically for 2 weeks and then reassess

Parkinsonism

- if pseudoparkinsonism (tremor, rigidity, bradykinesia) occurs, treat by reducing the dosage, changing to an agent less likely to produce extrapyramidal reactions, adding a conventional anticholinergic agent such as benztropine, or adding amantadine (if the patient is intolerant of anticholinergic effects
- if akathisia (jitteriness, restlessness) becomes a problem and does not respond to a decrease in the dosage, beta-blockers (nadolol 20 mg PO daily as an initial dose) have been shown to be of benefit

Tardive dyskinesia

- tardive dyskinesia usually occurs after long-term therapy (longer than 6 months) with antipsychotics (most commonly seen with high-potency agents), occurs in 10–20% of patients, and is unpredictable
- tardive dyskinesia presents as involuntary slow twisting movements of the tongue, lips, or jaws
- problem can be minimized by monitoring regularly and acting early to withdraw medication
- monitoring for tardive dyskinesia should be done at least every 6 months if treatment with antipsychotics continues for several years
- signs of extrapyramidal adverse effects should be monitored using rating scales such as AIMS (abnormal inventory movement scale) or Simpson-Angus scales
- if abnormal movements occur, consider reducing the dosage or stopping administration of the antipsychotic agent (the decision is based on the severity of psychotic illness)
- symptoms may actually worsen initially when the drug therapy is stopped or the dosage is reduced
- if the drug therapy cannot be stopped or the dosage cannot be reduced, justify that the patient is dangerous without antipsychotics and that the risks of no antipsychotic medication outweigh the risk of taking an antipsychotic agent
- some clinicians get the patient to sign a form indicating that the risks of therapy have been discussed with the physician

Neuroleptic malignant syndrome

- most serious adverse effect associated with neuroleptic agents
- more prevalent with the high-potency agents
- presents as fluctuating levels of consciousness, hyperthermia, muscle rigidity, unstable blood pressure (elevated), and dehydration
- neuroleptic regimen must be discontinued immediately and treatment is mainly symptomatic and supportive (cooling, rehydration, and so on)

Cardiac arrhythmias

- pretreatment electrocardiogram (for patients older than 40 years or those with existing cardiovascular disease) is warranted when using this agent but is not routinely done

Increased serum prolactin

- all antipsychotics (primarily the high-potency agents) can increase serum prolactin levels acutely but this usually normalizes
- if amenorrhea, galactorrhea, or gynecomastia (rarely) occurs, rule out pregnancy and pituitary adenoma (serum prolactin level >150 μ/mL)
- if the patient is symptomatic, decrease the dosage, change to a lower potency agent, or add bromocriptine 2.5–5 mg PO BID until symptoms resolve

Central nervous system depression

- patients with early or mild intoxication may experience restlessness, confusion, and excitement and can progress to coma with areflexia in overdoses

Gray skin syndrome

- can occur with any phenothiazine but is most common with chlorpromazine
- risk is increased with higher doses and worsened with exposure to sunlight

▶ How Long Do I Treat Patients with This Drug?

Acute psychosis therapy (if prompt control is desired)

- for acute psychotic episodes that may be drug-induced, related to mania, related to depression, or caused by trauma, antipsychotics are used only as long as the psychosis or thought disorder is present

Maintenance psychosis therapy

- adequate trial period (typically, 4–6 weeks at dosages within the therapeutic range; some patients require up to 8–12 weeks for full response) is necessary to evaluate efficacy
- maintenance treatment may be lifelong and should be implemented if the diagnosis is of a chronic disorder such as schizophrenia or a schizoaffective disorder
- studies indicate that relapses or recurrences occur at a constant rate such that the probability of recurrence increases with the time off medication
- there is a 50% relapse rate at 6 months and 70% at 1 year after antipsychotic drug discontinuation versus only 40% in patients receiving medication (Drugs 1992;44:981–992)
- as a rule, after the first episode, treat for 1 year; after the second episode, treat for at least 3 years; after the third episode, consider at least 5 years of maintenance therapy
- after good control has been achieved, attempt to taper the dosage of the antipsychotic to the lowest effective level
- after the lowest effective dosage has been reached, PRN doses can be made available to patients when they are showing signs of relapse or when stressful events known to worsen symptoms occur or when anticipated
- clinical impressions suggest that elderly chronic schizophrenics need less antipsychotic medication than was needed in the earlier stages of the illness (J Clin Psychiatry 1986;47[suppl 5]:17–22)
- risk of developing tardive dyskinesia increases with the length of therapy and advanced age

Manic phase of bipolar illness

- continue administration of drugs until symptoms have been controlled

Migraine treatment

- for the acute attack, treat until relief of acute headache attacks, development of toxic effects, or maximum daily doses have been achieved

▶ How Do I Decrease or Stop the Administration of This Drug?

- recurrence of symptoms and withdrawal symptoms such as insomnia, headaches, nausea, vomiting, and withdrawal dyskinesias have been reported after rapid withdrawal
- tapering regimen (reduction of the dosage by no more than 10–20% every month) is encouraged when withdrawing drug administration

▶ What Should I Tell My Patient About This Drug?

- you may experience some drowsiness and blurred vision, especially during the first few weeks of therapy; make sure that you know how you react to chlorpromazine before you drive, operate machines, or do other jobs that require you to be alert and see well
- minimize or prevent toxicity by knowing the signs of toxicity and returning for frequent clinical monitoring to enable identification of early signs of toxicity
- dizziness, lightheadedness, or fainting may occur, especially when you get up from a lying or sitting position, and getting up slowly may help, but if the problem continues, check with your physician
- do not stop taking this medication without first consulting your physician
- be aware of the risks of tardive dyskinesia

▶ Therapeutic Tips

- attempt to administer chlorpromazine in a single daily dose, usually at bedtime; or give $^1/_3$ in the morning and $^2/_3$ at bedtime if the patient is bothered by transient side effects
- may take up to 6–12 weeks to see a full response, and complete resolution of all psychotic symptoms may not be possible
- do not use in combination with another antipsychotic, as there is no benefit and increased side effects may occur

Useful References

Black JL, Richelson E, Richardson JW. Antipsychotic agents: A clinical update. Mayo Clin Proc 1985;60:777–789

Kane JM. The current status of neuroleptic therapy. J Clin Psychiatry 1989;50:322–328

CHLORPROPAMIDE

Christy Silvius Scott

USA (Diabinese, Glucamide, generic)
CANADA (Diabinese, Apo-Chlorpropamide, Novopropamide)

▶ When Should I Use This Drug?

Non–insulin-dependent diabetes

- obese (>120% of ideal body weight) and/or older patients (older than 40 years) or those patients not willing to inject insulin and self-monitor blood glucose levels with moderate hyperglycemia and without significant symptoms
- because obese diabetics are in a state of insulin resistance and large doses of insulin may be required and euglycemia may be difficult to achieve (N Engl J Med 1989;321:1231–1245)
- although there are no studies to demonstrate the greater effectiveness of second- over first-generation sulfonylureas (Diabetes Care 1992;15:737–754), most studies suggest that the maximum doses of chlorpropamide, glyburide, and glipizide are equally efficacious and appear superior to tolazamide, acetohexamide, and tolbutamide (N Engl J Med 1989;321:1231–1245)
- is the only truly once a day oral hypoglycemic agent and should be used only in patients who require twice-daily dosing with glyburide, glipizide, or gliclazide (i.e., when higher doses of these agents are used and twice-daily dosing is required), which may cause a compliance problem
- 20% is eliminated unchanged by the kidneys, and therefore, it should not be used in elderly patients or those with renal insufficiency (N Engl J Med 1989;321:1231–1245)
- chlorpropamide causes a relatively high incidence of hypoglycemia, which may be prolonged for several days after, a disulfiram-type reaction with alcohol, and syndrome of inappropriate secretion of antidiuretic hormone, which can produce profound hyponatremia; therefore, it is rarely used (N Engl J Med 1989; 321:1321–1345)

▶ When Should I Not Use This Drug?

see Tolbutamide

Patients at risk for hypoglycemia

- the elderly, malnourished, and/or alcoholic patients and those with renal or hepatic dysfunction or adrenal insufficiency are at increased risk for hypoglycemia
- highest incidence of hypoglycemia occurs with glyburide and chlorpropamide (5 times more than with tolbutamide, 2 times more than with glipizide and gliclazide) (Diabetes Care 1989; 12:203–208, Drugs 1981;22:211–245, N Engl J Med 1989;321: 1231–1245)

Patients with moderate to severe renal dysfunction (creatinine clearance < 50 mL/min)

- chlorpropamide and/or its active metabolite may accumulate
- preferred agents (having no active metabolites) include tolbutamide and glipizide; tolbutamide is probably a better choice because it is shorter acting (N Engl J Med 1989;321:1231–1245)

Patients known to consume alcohol

- these patients may experience chlorpropamide-alcohol flush (disulfiram reaction) (Br Med J 1978;2:1519–1521, Drugs 1981; 22:295–320)

Patients at increased risk for dilutional hyponatremia

- increases the production antidiuretic hormone and may be a problem in patients older than 60 years of age, women, and patients taking thiazide diuretics (N Engl J Med 1989;321: 1231–1245, Diabetes 1983;6:468–471)

▶ *What Contraindications Are There to the Use of This Drug?*

see Tolbutamide

▶ *What Drug Interactions Are Clinically Important?*

see Tolbutamide

▶ *What Route and Dosage Should I Use?*

How to administer

- orally—because chlorpropamide has a long half-life, timing of the dose in relation to meals is probably irrelevant for long-term therapy
- parenterally—not available

Non–insulin-dependent diabetes

- 250 mg PO daily
- increase the dosage every 2 weeks by 100 mg increments to achieve glycemic control or reach a maximum dose of 500 mg PO daily
- average daily dose is 250 mg (N Engl J Med 1989;321:1231–1245)
- all doses should be given once daily

Dosage adjustments for renal or hepatic dysfunction

- 20% eliminated unchanged; metabolized to weakly active compounds, which are retained in renal failure

Normal Dosing Interval	C_{cr} > 60 mL/min or 1 mL/s	C_{cr} 30–60 mL/min or 0.5–1 mL/s	C_{cr} < 30 mL/min or 0.5 mL/s
Q24H	no adjustment needed	not recommended in renal insufficiency	not recommended in renal failure

▶ *What Should I Monitor with Regard to Efficacy and Toxicity?*

Efficacy

see Tolbutamide

Toxicity

see Tolubutamide

Syndrome of inappropriate secretion of antidiuretic hormone

- increases the production of antidiuretic hormone and may be a problem in patients older than 60 years of age, women, and patients taking thiazide diuretics, and therefore, the medication should not be used in these populations (N Engl J Med 1989; 321:1231–1245, Diabetes 1983;6:468–471)
- serum sodium levels may drop without consequence to the patient; if this occurs, therapy may be continued
- if problems such as edema and mental confusion occur, the medication administration should be discontinued and not restarted; another glucose-lowering agent can be tried and syndrome of inappropriate secretion of antidiuretic hormone should not develop

Chlorpropamide-alcohol flush (Eur Pharmacol 1976;35:301, Br Med J 1978;2:1519–1521)

- symptoms are flushing and headache
- may not occur with the first dose; however, occurs after about a week of therapy
- $1/3$ of patients may have this reaction
- patient should be told that this reaction may occur
- if it does occur, the decision should be made with the patient either to avoid alcohol or to change to another glucose-lowering agent

▶ *How Long Do I Treat Patients with This Drug?*

see Tolbutamide

▶ *How Do I Decrease or Stop the Administration of This Drug?*

- may be stopped abruptly
- decrease the dosage by 100 mg every 2 weeks if satisfactory blood glucose control is maintained

▶ *What Should I Tell My Patients About This Drug?*

see Tolbutamide

- there is a risk of chlorpropamide-alcohol flush

▶ *Therapeutic Tips*

- careful patient selection is necessary before using chlorpropamide so that hypoglycemic reactions can be avoided
- because of adverse reactions, this medication should be reserved for the patient who desires or requires once-daily dosing that cannot be achieved with other glucose-lowering agents

see Tolbutamide

Useful References

Gerich JE. Oral hypoglycemic agents. N Engl J Med 1989;321:1231–1245
Groop LC. Sulfonylureas in NIDDM. Diabetes Care 1992;15:737–754
Hansten PD, Horn JR. Drug Interactions and Updates, 7th ed. Philadelphia: Lea & Febiger, 1993
Tatro DS. Drug Interaction Facts. St Louis, MO: Facts and Comparisons, 1995

CHLORTHALIDONE

Ian Petterson

USA (Biogroton, Hygroton, Thalitone)
CANADA (Apo-Chlorthalidone, Hygroton, Novothalidone)

▶ *When Should I Use This Drug?*

Decision among the different thiazide diuretics should be based on cost, as there is little, if any, difference in clinical effect among these agents • Although chlorthalidone has a slightly longer duration of action, this confers no benefit, as thiazide diuretics are all dosed once daily and are well tolerated

see Hydrochlorothiazide

▶ *When Should I Not Use This Drug?*

see Hydrochlorothiazide

▶ *What Contraindications Are There to the Use of This Drug?*

see Hydrochlorothiazide

▶ *What Drug Interactions Are Clinically Important?*

see Hydrochlorothiazide

▶ *What Route and Dosage Should I Use?*

How to administer

- orally—may be given with food or on an empty stomach
- parenterally—not available

Chronic (noncrisis) hypertension

- start with 12.5 mg PO daily
- some clinicians advocate the use of 6.25 mg as a starting dose, but the difficulty in attaining this dose makes it impractical
- dosage may be increased every 2–4 weeks if the current dosage is not adequately controlling blood pressure
- dosage should rarely exceed 25 mg and never exceed 50 mg daily, as there is no greater hypotensive effect with higher dosages and the incidence of adverse effects is increased

Congestive heart failure

- 25 mg PO daily if being used as sole diuretic therapy
- dosage may be increased after 2 weeks to 50 mg PO daily if the current dosage is not adequately controlling the edema
- metabolic effects at dosages greater than 50 mg limit its effectiveness

- in cardiac failure, thiazides are effective in potentiating the action of loop diuretics (furosemide)
- in patients already receiving furosemide, start with low dosages (12.5 mg daily) and be aware of possible profound dehydration and electrolyte disturbances with standard dosages (Ann Intern Med 1991;114:885–894)

Ascites associated with hepatic cirrhosis

- 12.5 mg PO daily
- increase the dosage to 25 mg PO daily in 2 weeks
- if 25 mg PO daily is ineffective, consider switching to furosemide
- in cirrhosis, if an effect is not seen with 50 mg daily, the addition of low-dose spironolactone has an additive effect and reverses hypokalemia

Dosage adjustments for renal or hepatic dysfunction

- renally eliminated
- no adjustment is needed for renal impairment, except avoid in patients with moderate to severe renal function (creatinine clearance < 30 mL/min), as effectiveness is lost

▶ *What Should I Monitor with Regard to Efficacy and Toxicity?*

see Hydrochlorothiazide

▶ *How Long Do I Treat Patients with This Drug?*

see Hydrochlorothiazide

▶ *How Do I Decrease or Stop the Administration of This Drug?*

see Hydrochlorothiazide

▶ *What Should I Tell My Patients About This Drug?*

see Hydrochlorothiazide

▶ *Therapeutic Tips*

see Hydrochlorothiazide

Useful References

Nader C, Thompson JR, Alpern RJ. Complications of diuretic use. Semin Nephrol 1988;8:365–387
Black HR. Metabolic consideration in the choice of therapy for the patient with hypertension. Am Heart J 1991;121:707–715
Freis ED. Critique of the clinical importance of diuretic induced hypokalemia and elevated cholesterol levels. Arch Intern Med 1989;149:2640–2648

CHLORPHENIRAMINE

Penny Miller

USA (Chlor-Trimeton, Aller-chlor, Chlorate, many generics)
CANADA (Chlor-Tripolon, Novopheniram)

▶ *When Should I Use This Drug?*

Seasonal allergic rhinitis, chronic (perennial) rhinitis, chronic dermatological allergies (atopic dermatitis, chronic urticaria, pruritus of unknown cause)

- all antihistamines are considered to have the same efficacy in preventing or treating allergic reactions; however, there is great interpatient variation in the response to a given antihistamine
- selection of any particular antihistamine is based on the degree of sedation and anticholinergic effects, plus the convenience of dosing and cost
- chlorpheniramine is likely the initial drug of choice, as it is much less expensive than the newer agents and is convenient to take because it can be given once daily (Clin Pharmacokinet 1991; 21:372–393)
- chlorpheniramine is rapid acting and causes less sedation and fewer anticholinergic effects than agents such as diphenhydramine and hydroxyzine but more than the newer antihistamines such as astemizole, loratadine, and terfenadine
- if sedation is a problem (seen with 20% of patients), switch to a nonsedating agent such as astemizole, loratadine, or terfenadine, whichever is the least expensive

Acute dermatological allergies (e.g., hives, allergic conjunctivitis caused by allergens or food)

- antihistamines relieve pruritus and prevent further extension of the lesions
- choice of agent to use is as above, except that astemizole is slow acting and should not be used if an acute effect is needed
- if sedation is required (may be desirable for an acute allergic reaction), diphenhydramine or hydroxyzine should be used, as these are effective and very sedating

Common cold

- for the symptoms of sneezing and runny nose, chlorpheniramine has widespread use, proven efficacy most likely because of its anticholinergic effect, a comparatively low incidence of sedation, rapid action, and a lower cost than the newer antihistamines (Health Protection Branch. First Report of the Expert Advisory Committee on Nonprescription Cough and Cold Remedies. Health and Welfare Canada, 1988:6)
- antihistamines do not appear to reduce the symptoms of congestion (J Allergy Clin Immunol 1989;84:845–861)
- newer antihistamines (astemizole, loratadine, terfenadine) do not have the anticholinergic effects likely required to have an effect on symptoms of the common cold

Anaphylaxis and angioedema

- antihistamines prevent further extension of allergic reaction
- drug of choice is usually diphenhydramine, preferably given intravenously, combined with epinephrine
- chewable chlorpheniramine tablets are included in commercial anaphylactic kits

▶ *When Should I Not Use This Drug?*

Sole treatment of anaphylaxis and angioedema

- do not rely solely on any antihistamine to prevent anaphylactic reactions because they can be displaced easily from receptors after a massive release of histamine (On Continuing Practice 1991;18:31–36)

Asthma

- do not use in severe acute asthmatic attacks, as antihistamines have the potential to dry secretions and cause mucous plugs
- evidence is still controversial on the effectiveness of histamine blockade in asthma (Health Protection Branch. First Report of the Expert Advisory Committee on Nonprescription Cough and Cold Remedies. Health and Welfare Canada, 1988:4)

Edema and serum sickness resulting from allergic reactions to drugs

- not relieved by antihistamines (American Hospital Formulary Service, Drug Information, Bethesda, MD, 1992;3)

Vasomotor (nonallergic) rhinitis

- antihistamines are ineffective for this condition

▶ *What Contraindications Are There to the Use of This Drug?*

Intolerance of or allergic reaction to chlorpheniramine

Prostatic hypertrophy, urinary retention, seizure disorders, closed angle glaucoma, asthma

- anticholinergic effects of chlorpheniramine can worsen these disease states
- if an antihistamine is required, use terfenadine, astemizole, or loratadine, as these agents do not have anticholinergic effects

▶ *What Drug Interactions Are Clinically Important?*

Drugs that may increase the effect of chlorpheniramine

ANTICHOLINERGIC DRUGS (E.G., PHENOTHIAZINES, TRICYCLIC ANTIDEPRESSANTS, BELLADONNA ALKALOIDS, MONOAMINE OXIDASE INHIBITORS)

- concomitant use can cause additive effects, which can be detrimental in patients with prostatic hypertrophy, glaucoma, and asthma

- if an antihistamine is required, use terfenadine, astemizole, or loratadine, as these agents do not have anticholinergic effects

CENTRAL NERVOUS SYSTEM DEPRESSANTS (PHENOTHIAZINES, NARCOTICS, BARBITURATES, BENZODIAZEPINES, AND ALCOHOL)

- sedative effects can be additive
- in persons who need to be mentally alert and who work with dangerous machinery where impairment is unacceptable, if an antihistamine is required, use terfenadine, astemizole, or loratadine, as these agents do not cause additive sedative effects

Drugs that may decrease the effect of chlorpheniramine

- none

Drugs that may have their effect increased by chlorpheniramine

CENTRAL NERVOUS SYSTEM DEPRESSANTS

- see above

Drugs that may have their effect decreased by chlorpheniramine

- none

▶ *What Route and Dosage Should I Use?*

How to administer

- orally—take with food or milk or on an empty stomach
- parenterally—not available

Seasonal allergic rhinitis, chronic (perennial) rhinitis, chronic dermatological allergies (atopic dermatitis, chronic urticaria, pruritus of unknown cause)

- 4 mg PO HS
- giving the dose at bedtime can reduce or eliminate the problem of sedation
- increase the dosage by 4 mg PO daily every 2–3 days until an effect is seen, up to a maximum dosage of 24 mg PO daily

Acute dermatological allergies (e.g., hives, allergic conjunctivitis caused by allergens or food), common cold

- 4 mg PO Q6H PRN for symptoms up to a maximum dosage of 24 mg PO daily

Dosage adjustments for renal or hepatic dysfunction

- hepatically metabolized
- no dosage adjustments are required; just titrate the dose up to an effect

▶ *What Should I Monitor with Regard to Efficacy and Toxicity?*

Efficacy

Seasonal allergic rhinitis, chronic (perennial) rhinitis

Improvement of congestion, rhinorrhea, and itching

- effect should be seen within 1–2 hours and partial or complete resolution within 24–48 hours
- if no effect has been seen, increase the dosage
- antihistamines can generally provide a 60% reduction in symptoms (On Continuing Practice 1991;18[2]:31–36)

Chronic dermatological allergies (atopic dermatitis, chronic urticaria, pruritus of unknown cause)

- relief of severe itching within 2–3 days

Acute dermatological allergies

- relief of itching and no more formation of new lesions within 24–48 hours

Common cold

- runny nose and sneezing should be lessened within 2–3 hours

Toxicity

- individual patients vary in their susceptibility to the adverse effects of antihistamines

Sedation

- sedation occurs in approximately 20% of patients (Clin Pharmacokinet 1991;21:372–393) and is a dose-related phenomenon

- sedation should lessen and subside in 3–4 days (On Continuing Practice 1991;18:31–36, American Hospital Formulary Service, Drug Information ASHP, Bethesda, MD, 1993)
- if the drug is being used long term and sedation does not subside, switch to a nonsedating antihistamine (astemizole, terfenadine, loratadine)
- paradoxical excitement, especially in children, is characterized by restlessness, insomnia, euphoria, nervousness, and even seizures

Anticholinergic effects

- in general, if the drug is being used long term and anticholinergic effects do not subside, switch to an antihistamine without anticholinergic effects (astemizole, terfenadine, loratadine)
- some of the anticholinergic effects can be treated as follows

Blurred vision, urinary hesitancy

- switch to a different agent

Dry mouth

- increase fluid intake and/or use sugarless chewing gum or hard candies

Constipation

- increase fluid and fiber in diet, and if needed, use a laxative

Orthostatic hypotension

- treatment of orthostasis includes rising slowly from supine or sitting positions and wearing support stockings

Gastrointestinal effects

- epigastric distress and nausea and vomiting
- can be lessened by taking the drug with food or milk

Blood dyscrasias

- should investigate twice yearly in long-term use, as hemolytic anemia and agranulocytosis have been reported (Postgrad Med 1986;79:75–86)

▶ *How Long Do I Treat Patients with This Drug?*

Seasonal allergic rhinitis, chronic (perennial) rhinitis

- for seasonal rhinitis, treat throughout the season (e.g., 3 weeks to 2 months), beginning early in the season when pollen counts are low
- for chronic rhinitis, this drug may be used continuously but drug-free periods should be tried every 6 months to reassess the diagnosis and the effectiveness of the drug

Chronic dermatological allergies (atopic dermatitis, chronic urticaria, pruritus of unknown cause)

- for acute conditions, treat for 4–7 days
- for chronic conditions, treat intermittently (for years)

Acute dermatological allergies

- treat for 4–7 days, depending on the resolution of symptoms

Common cold

- because the common cold is a self-limited condition lasting no longer than 5–7 days, treatment should not extend beyond this time

▶ *How Do I Decrease or Stop the Administration of This Drug?*

- may be stopped abruptly
- for chronic allergic symptoms, the drug administration should likely be tapered (decrease the dosage by 25% every week)

▶ *What Should I Tell My Patients About This Drug?*

- you may experience sedation for the first few days of use, so be cautious when performing tasks that require mental alertness
- effects of alcohol may be intensified if it is taken together with this agent
- you may experience dry mouth and blurred vision for the first few days of use
- dry mouth can be contolled by sucking on sugarless candy or ice cubes

- contact your physician if you have difficulty in urinating
- if your allergic symptoms are not improving, the dosage may be increased or another antihistamine can be tried

▶ Therapeutic Tips

- there is great interpatient variation in response to antihistamines; therefore, a trial and error approach is required to determine which antihistamine is the most effective for a particular patient
- antihistamines are more effective at preventing allergic reactions from occurring than treating the symptoms after they have occurred
- despite product monograph recommendations, for long-term use, chlorpheniramine can be used once daily
- no reason to use extentabs preparation because chlorpheniramine has a long half-life

Useful References

Sutherland D. Antihistamine agents—New options or just more drugs? On Continuing Practice 1991;18(2):31–36
American Hospital Formulary Service, Drug Information, ASHP. Bethesda, MD, 1993
Report of the Expert Advisory Committee. Nonprescription Cough and Cold Remedies. Ottawa, Ontario, Health and Welfare, Canada, August 1988

CHOLESTYRAMINE

Stephen Shalansky and Robert Dombrowski

USA (Questran, Questran Light, Cholybar)
CANADA (Questran, Questran Light)

▶ When Should I Use This Drug?

Hypercholesterolemia

- bile acid sequestrants are recommended (assuming they are tolerated) if HMG-CoA reductase inhibitors are ineffective or not tolerated as bile acid sequestrants have proven efficacy and safety in the reduction of cardiovascular disease and cardiovascular mortality
- choose the least expensive of either cholestyramine (4 g dose) or colestipol (5 g dose) as these agents are equally effective and equally tolerated
- cholestyramine and colestipol are equally efficacious at lowering total and LDL cholesterol levels, and therefore, the choice is based on cost and convenience of administration

Mixed hyperlipidemias

- bile acid sequestrants raise triglyceride levels and are therefore not particularly useful as a single agent for this indication
- may be used in combination with gemfibrozil or niacin, particularly in patients who experience myositis while receiving the combination of gemfibrozil and lovastatin

▶ When Should I Not Use This Drug?

Hypertriglyceridemia

- bile acid sequestrants may cause a further elevation in triglyceride levels
- niacin or gemfibrozil can be used in these patients

▶ What Contraindications Are There to the Use of This Drug?

Intolerance of or allergic reaction to cholestyramine or aspartame (Questran Light)
Complete biliary obstruction where bile is not excreted into the intestine

- cholestyramine and colestipol are bile acid sequestrants, which work by binding bile acids

▶ What Drug Interactions Are Clinically Important?

Drugs that may increase the effect or toxicity of cholestyramine
- none

Drugs that may decrease the effect of cholestyramine
- none

Drugs that may have their effect or toxicity increased by cholestyramine
- none

Drugs that may have their effect decreased by cholestyramine
WARFARIN, THIAZIDE DIURETICS, BETA-BLOCKERS (ORAL), CORTICOSTEROIDS (ORAL), THYROXINE (ORAL), DIGOXIN (ORAL), GEMFIBROZIL

- bile acid sequestrants can interfere with the absorption of many drugs
- in general, it is advisable to take medications at least 1 hour before or 4 hours after a bile acid sequestrant

▶ What Route and Dosage Should I Use?

How to administer

- orally—give with food, as food stimulates the release of bile
- parenterally—not available

Hypercholesterolemia, mixed hyperlipidemias

- give 2 g ($^1/_2$ packet) PO daily initially, and titrate up every 2–3 days by 2 g PO daily until 4 g PO BID is reached, as this may increase tolerability
- give the 4 g PO BID with breakfast and the evening meal
- increase the dosage to 12 g PO daily (4 g PO in the morning and 8 g with the evening meal) if there is inadequate response in 4 weeks
- continue to increase the dosage by 4 g (1 packet) per week up to a maximum dosage of 24 g/d (12 g in the morning and 12 g with the evening meal); however, be aware that most patients do not tolerate daily dosages greater than 16 g
- remeasure serum lipid levels at 3 months
- if after 3 months, a 15% decrease in LDL or total cholesterol levels is achieved, but the target LDL level is not reached, consider adding another drug (e.g., lovastatin)
- if after 3 months, there is less than a 15% decrease in LDL or total cholesterol or the patient is not tolerating the drug (e.g., because of gastrointestinal side effects), change drugs

Dosage adjustments for renal or hepatic dysfunction

- is not absorbed orally; therefore, no dosage adjustments are required

▶ What Should I Monitor with Regard to Efficacy and Toxicity?

Efficacy
Hypercholesterolemia, mixed hyperlipidemias

Total cholesterol and fractionated lipid profile

- in patients with no coronary heart disease or atherosclerotic disease and with less than 2 CHD risk factors lower total cholesterol below 240 mg/dL (6.2 mmol/L) and LDL cholesterol below 160 mg/dL (4.1 mmol/L)
- in patients with no coronary heart disease or atherosclerotic disease and with 2 or more CHD risk factors lower total cholesterol below 200 mg/dL (5.2 mmol/L) and LDL cholesterol below 130 mg/dL (3.4 mmol/L)
- for patients with coronary heart disease or atherosclerotic disease lower LDL cholesterol to below 100 mg/dL (2.6 mmol/L)
- complete lipid profiles should be measured at 1 and 3 months
- if goals are achieved, check annually

Evidence of coronary heart disease

- myocardial infarction, angina, or coronary bypass grafting

Risk factors

- reduce risk factors such as obesity and smoking
- control risk factors such as diabetes and hypertension

Toxicity
These drugs are not absorbed, and therefore, they lack systemic toxicity
Gastrointestinal effects

- most patients experience tolerance to these side effects within months

Constipation

- increase fluid and fiber intake, increase exercise, and add a stool softener if needed

Bloating

- decrease diluent volume

Epigastric Pain

Nausea

Flatulence

- drink slowly to decrease air swallowing

Hemorrhoids

- can be exacerbated by the gritty texture
- soaking the powder in its diluent for several minutes or overnight can help decrease the grittiness

▶ *How Long Do I Treat Patients with This Drug?*

Hypercholesterolemia, mixed hyperlipidemias

- therapy is long term and may continue for life
- if the patient has achieved and maintained target lipid levels for 2 years, these drugs should be discontinued and a trial of dietary therapy alone should be attempted
- recheck lipid levels at 4–6 weeks and at 3 months after drug administration has been discontinued and restart drug therapy if target levels are not maintained

▶ *How Do I Decrease or Stop the Administration of This Drug?*

- may be stopped abruptly

▶ *What Should I Tell My Patients About This Drug?*

- mix with pulpy fruit (e.g., applesauce), fruit juice, or other liquid of choice to increase palatability
- if using a liquid as a diluent, allow the powder to sit on the surface for 1–2 minutes to avoid lumps when mixed
- stir completely
- rinse the glass and drink the contents to avoid missing the powder that sticks to the sides
- diluted powder can stand in the refrigerator overnight to decrease the grittiness and increase palatability
- always mix thoroughly immediately prior to taking
- store the dry powder in a dry place
- maintaining adequate fiber in the diet significantly reduces constipation associated with the use of cholestyramine or colestipol
- take all other medications at least 1 hour before or 4 hours after a bile acid sequestrant

▶ *Therapeutic Tips*

- Questran and Questran Light powder contain filler: 9 g of Questran powder contains 4 g of cholestyramine, whereas 5 g of Questran Light powder contains 4 g of cholestyramine; doses above refer to grams of cholestyramine
- always order this drug as grams of cholestyramine to avoid confusion between the dose of cholestyramine and grams of the powder preparation (a filler is used)
- one Cholybar contains 4 g of cholestyramine
- palatability of colestipol and cholestyramine is similar; the preference is individual
- may not be a good choice for those who travel extensively, as these are bulky preparations whether they are in the form of powder or bars
- when increasing the dosage, increase slowly to decrease the incidence and intensity of gastrointestinal side effects
- if gastrointestinal side effects are intolerable, a trial of a lower dosage should be used before deciding to discontinue the drug administration
- give patients permission to vary the dosage depending on how they feel because, if patients have flexibility with the dosing regimen, compliance is enhanced

Useful References

Expert Panel on Detection, Evaluation, and Treatment of High Blood Cholesterol in Adults. Summary of the second report of the National Cholesterol Education Program (NCEP) expert panel on detection, evaluation, and treatment of high blood cholesterol in adults. JAMA 1993; 269:3015–3023

Knodel LC, Talbert RL. Adverse effects of hypolipidemic drugs. Med Toxicol 1987;2:10–32
Illingworth DR. Lipid-lowering drugs: An overview of indications and optimum therapeutic use. Drugs 1987;33:259–279
Ast M, Frishman WH. Bile acid sequestrants. J Clin Pharmacol 1990; 30:99–106
LaRosa J. Review of clinical studies of bile acid sequestrants for lowering plasma lipid levels. Cardiology 1989;76(suppl 1):55–64
Lipid Research Clinics Program. The Lipid Research Clinics coronary primary prevention trial results. 1. Reduction in incidence of coronary heart disease. JAMA 1984;251:351–364
Lipid Research Clinics Program. The Lipid Research Clinics coronary primary prevention trial results. 2. The relationship of reduction in incidence of coronary disease to cholesterol lowering. JAMA 1984; 251:365–374
Brensike JF, Levy RI, Kelsey SF, et al. Effects of therapy with cholestyramine on progression of coronary arteriosclerosis: Results of the NHLBI type II coronary intervention study. Circulation 1984;69:313–324
Levy RI, Brensike JF, Epstein SE, et al. The influence of changes in lipid values induced by cholestyramine and diet on progression of coronary artery disease: Results of the NHLBI type II coronary intervention study. Circulation 1984;69:325–337

CHOLINE MAGNESIUM TRISALICYLATE

Kelly Jones

USA (Trilisate)
CANADA (Trilisate)

▶ *When Should I Use This Drug?*

Acute pain, general aches and pain, bone pain

- useful for the acute management of general aches and pains
- only advantage over non–enteric-coated aspirin is that it causes less gastrointestinal intolerance
- decision between this drug and other nonsteroidal antiinflammatory drugs (NSAIDs) should be based on cost

Rheumatoid arthritis

- not considered first line, as this agent is considered less effective than the NSAIDs
- should be used as an alternative for patients with rheumatoid arthritis who cannot tolerate the adverse effects on the gastrointestinal system and kidneys of nonaspirin NSAIDs, as nonacetylated salicylates (salsalate, diflunisal, choline magnesium trisalicylate) are less likely to affect the gastrointestinal tract than is aspirin (Gastroenterology 1990;99:1616–1621)
- can be used as an alternative when platelet function is important, as nonacetylated salicylates have no appreciable effect on platelets (J Am Board Fam Pract 1989;2:257–271)
- decision among nonacetylated salicylates should be based on cost

Osteoarthritis

- if acetaminophen and ibuprofen are not effective
- decision between this drug and other NSAIDs should be based on cost

▶ *When Should I Not Use This Drug?*

see Ibuprofen

▶ *What Contraindications Are There to the Use of This Drug?*

see Aspirin

▶ *What Drug Interactions Are Clinically Important?*

see Ibuprofen

▶ *What Route and Dosage Should I Use?*

How to administer

- orally—take with food or milk
- parenterally—not available

Acute pain, general aches and pain, bone pain

- 500 mg PO Q8–12H PRN

Rheumatoid arthritis

- 1000 mg PO BID and increase to a maximum of 3000 mg PO daily

Osteoarthritis

- 500 mg PO BID

Dosage adjustments for renal or hepatic dysfunction

- hepatically metabolized; therefore, no adjustments needed for renal disease
- reduce dosage 25% in patients with a history of hepatic disease

▶ *What Should I Monitor with Regard to Efficacy and Toxicity?*

see Aspirin

▶ *How Long Do I Treat Patients with This Drug?*

see Aspirin

▶ *How Do I Decrease or Stop the Administration of This Drug?*

- may be stopped abruptly if needed

▶ *What Should I Tell My Patients About This Drug?*

see Aspirin

▶ *Therapeutic Tips*

see Aspirin

Useful References

see Aspirin

CIMETIDINE

James McCormack and Glen Brown

USA (Tagamet)
CANADA (Tagamet, Peptol, Apo-Cimetidine, Novocimetine)

▶ *When Should I Use This Drug?*

Dyspepsia

- drug of choice for empirical therapy of dypepsia not evaluated by endoscopy
- appears to be no better than placebo for nonulcer dyspepsia (Can Fam Physician 1988;34:613–617)

Duodenal or gastric ulcers

- drug of choice for the initial treatment of peptic ulcer disease because it has few adverse effects, can be given once daily, and is less expensive than other treatment modalities such as other H_2 antagonists, sucralfate, and omeprazole
- all H_2 antagonists have equivalent efficacy and toxicity (N Engl J Med 1990;323:1749–1755) and cimetidine is the oral H_2 antagonist of choice, except when the patient is taking drugs that may interact

Prevention of peptic ulcer disease recurrence

- prophylaxis recommended only for patients with more than 2 relapses per year, a history of peptic ulcer disease complications, or severe symptoms
- all antiulcer agents have equivalent efficacy and toxicity in prophylactic dosages and cimetidine is the least expensive (N Engl J Med 1990;323:1749–1755)

Stress ulcer prophylaxis

- for patients with extensive burns, central nervous system injury, prolonged hypotension, sepsis, uncorrectable coagulopathy, acute respiratory failure (undergoing ventilation), or hepatic failure (Am J Gastroenterol 1990;85:95–96) who cannot receive sucralfate by gastric administration
- use the least expensive parenteral H_2 antagonist
- sucralfate is preferred if oral administration is possible because there is less chance of nosocomial infection, it is less expensive

than parenteral H_2 antagonists and does not require pH measurement of gastric contents (Lancet 1989;2:1255–1256)

Gastroesophageal reflux

- only after nondrug therapy has failed
- drug of choice for mild to moderate reflux disease
- effective and less expensive than omeprazole and other H_2 antagonists

Prior to anesthesia for prophylaxis of aspiration pneumonitis

- only patients who are obese, pregnant, or diabetic or who have an incomplete gastrointestinal tract, a history of hiatal hernia, or peptic ulcer disease require prophylaxis
- cimetidine can be used for this indication, even in patients taking interacting drugs, because it is used for only 1–2 doses

▶ *When Should I Not Use This Drug?*

Combination with other antiulcer medications

- no studies to support combination therapy of regularly dosed upper gastrointestinal tract drugs for the treatment of peptic ulcer disease, and combination therapy only increases cost and the chance of adverse effects (Lancet 1988;1:1383–1385, N Engl J Med 1991;325:1017–1025, Am J Gastroenterol 1993;88:675–679)

Stress ulcer prophylaxis in patients not at risk

- after a patient is no longer at risk for gastrointestinal hypoperfusion or is receiving consistent feeding by gastric administration, stress ulcer prophylaxis is not needed

Zollinger-Ellison syndrome

- need large doses of H_2 antagonists at frequent intervals, which can be inconvenient and costly and can potentially cause a higher incidence of adverse effects
- omeprazole is the proven drug of choice (N Engl J Med 1990; 323:1749–1755)

▶ *What Contraindications Are There to the Use of This Drug?*

Intolerance of or allergic reaction to cimetidine

▶ *What Drug Interactions Are Clinically Important?*

Drugs that may increase the effect or toxicity of cimetidine

- none

Drugs that may decrease the effect of cimetidine

ANTACIDS

- antacids decrease absorption of H_2 antagonists; therefore, patients should not take antacids within 1 hour of taking an H_2 antagonist

Drugs that may have their effect or toxicity increased by cimetidine

BENZODIAZEPINES, BETA-BLOCKERS, THEOPHYLLINE, WARFARIN, PHENYTOIN, QUINIDINE, PROCAINAMIDE, NIFEDIPINE

- cimetidine decreases the metabolism of all these drugs to a varying degree owing to the effect on hepatic metabolism
- if the patient is receiving any drugs that can potentially interact with cimetidine, it is best to use an H_2 antagonist (ranitidine, famotidine, nizatidine) that has little, if any, effect on hepatic metabolism
- if cimetidine is being used as only a single 400 mg nighttime dose, the effect is minimal

Drugs that may have their effect decreased by cimetidine

KETOCONAZOLE, IRON

- decreased gastric acidity reduces ketoconazole or iron absorption
- administer ketoconazole or iron at least 2 hours prior to H_2 antagonists, and be aware that absorption of ketoconazole or iron may still be decreased to some extent

▶ *What Route and Dosage Should I Use?*

How to administer

Orally

- can be given with food or on an empty stomach

Parenterally

- dilute to 20 mL and inject over not less than 5 minutes
- dilute to 50 mL and infuse over 15–20 minutes

Dyspepsia or duodenal or gastric ulcers

- 800 mg PO at HS or with the evening meal is as effective as 300 mg PO QID or 400 mg PO BID and more convenient for the patient (Curr Ther Res 1986;40:893–897)
- 400 mg PO BID if the patient has frequent daytime ulcer pain

Prevention of peptic ulcer disease recurrence

- 400 mg PO HS

Stress ulcer prophylaxis

- 300 mg IV Q6H titrated to keep gastric pH greater than 4 at all times
- infusion of drug is not clinically superior (although it does produce better pH control) to intermittent therapy and should be used only if it is more practical or economical than intermittent injections
- analysis of aspirates of gastric fluid should be done Q4H and the dosage increased in 150 mg increments to maintain a gastric pH of greater than 4 at all times

Gastroesophageal reflux

- 400 mg PO BID
- 400 mg PO HS if the patient has only nighttime symptoms

Prior to anesthesia for prophylaxis of aspiration pneumonitis

- 400 mg PO the morning of surgery
- a dose given the evening before surgery is often recommended, but this dose has no effect on gastric acidity in the morning because of cimetidine's short half-life

Dosage adjustments for renal or hepatic dysfunction

- renally eliminated

Normal Dosing Interval	$C_{cr} > 60$ mL/min or 1 mL/s	C_{cr} 30–60 mL/min or 0.5–1 mL/s	$C_{cr} < 30$ mL/min or 0.5 mL/s
Q6H	no adjustment needed	Q8H	Q12H
Q12H	no adjustment needed	Q24H	Q24H and decrease dosage by 50%
Q24H or by infusion	no adjustment needed	decrease dosage by 50%	decrease dosage by 75%

▶ *What Should I Monitor with Regard to Efficacy and Toxicity?*

Efficacy

Dyspepsia

- relief of symptoms such as epigastric pain or discomfort, belching, burning, bloating, fullness, and nausea and vomiting
- if there is no relief of symptoms after 7 days or complete relief of symptoms does not occur after 6 weeks, reevaluate with endoscopy

Duodenal or gastric ulcer

- relief of symptoms such as epigastric pain or discomfort, belching, burning, bloating, fullness, and nausea and vomiting
- if there is no relief after 1 week, endoscopy or reendoscopy is recommended
- for duodenal ulcers, reendoscopy is not needed unless symptoms persist
- for gastric ulcers, reendoscopy is recommended to ensure that complete healing has occurred because loss of symptoms is well described in malignant ulcers

Prevention of peptic ulcer disease recurrence

- recurrence of symptoms as reported by the patient

Acute stress ulcer prophylaxis

- aspirates of gastric fluid Q4H for pH measurements
- if the aspirate contains blood, the need for endoscopy should be considered

Gastroesophageal reflux

- decrease in number and severity of reflux episodes

Prior to anesthesia for prophylaxis of aspiration pneumonitis

- no variables to monitor

Toxicity

Adverse effects are infrequent

- there are a number of unusual adverse effects such as hepatitis, gynecomastia, bradycardia, and rash, but no special monitoring other than symptomatic monitoring is required

Mental confusion

- H_2 antagonists may produce confusion especially in the elderly, patients in an intensive care unit, and patients with poor renal function
- can occur with cimetidine and other H_2 antagonists; however, no studies suggest that cimetidine causes a higher frequency of confusion than the other H_2 antagonists (Arch Intern Med 1991;151:810–815, Ann Intern Med 1991;114:1027–1034)
- if mental confusion occurs, ensure that the dosage is adjusted for patient's renal function
- if the dosage is appropriate and mental confusion is not potentially due to other medications, stop cimetidine administration, reevaluate its need, and if an upper gastrointestinal agent is needed, switch to sucralfate

▶ *How Long Do I Treat Patients with This Drug?*

Dyspepsia or duodenal or gastric ulcers

- 6 weeks
- if satisfactory response occurs, stop drug administration
- if there is an inadequate response after 6 weeks, continue therapy for another 6 weeks
- if there is still no response, consider alternative therapy such as omeprazole

Prevention of peptic ulcer disease recurrence

- indefinitely; however, consideration should be given to a trial off drug therapy in patients who have remained symptom free for longer than 2 years, unless the peptic ulcer disease was associated with complications (bleeding, perforation, and so on)

Stress ulcer prophylaxis

- after a patient is no longer at risk for hypoperfusion or is receiving consistent feeding by gastric administration, stress ulcer prophylaxis is not needed
- in general, if a patient is no longer in an intensive care unit or burn ward and does not have sepsis or central nervous system injury, prophylaxis can be stopped

Gastroesophageal reflux

- initial treatment should be 4 weeks in duration, and if there is no relief, double the dosage of the H_2 antagonist and continue therapy for a total of 8 weeks
- approximately 50% of patients have complete relief with H_2 antagonist therapy
- after symptoms are controlled, reduce the dosage by 50% every few weeks to identify the lowest effective dosage

▶ *How Do I Decrease or Stop the Administration of This Drug?*

- may be stopped abruptly
- if the patient has been receiving the drug for a number of months, it may be best to reduce the dose by 50% every 1–2 weeks

▶ *What Should I Tell My Patients About This Drug?*

- it may take several days for this drug to relieve stomach pain

- if no relief of symptoms is seen in 7 days, contact your physician
- if symptoms are not completely resolved after 3–4 weeks, contact your physician
- this drug interacts with many medications; therefore, check with your physician or your pharmacist before taking other medications
- for peptic ulcer disease, take the drug for the full 6 weeks even if symptoms disappear after 1–2 weeks
- contact your physician if you experience any excessive dizziness or confusion

▶ *Therapeutic Tips*

- ensure that the drug dosage has been adjusted for renal function
- anyone who has been receiving full-dose cimetidine (300 mg QID, 400 mg BID, or 800 mg HS) or any H_2 antagonist for longer than 8 weeks must be evaluated to determine need for continued therapy
- at least 50% of patients taking cimetidine for longer than 8 weeks are receiving it inappropriately (J Am Geriatr Soc 1987; 35:1023–1027, DICP 1987;21:452–458)
- use 400 mg PO at bedtime for the prevention of ulcer recurrence
- do not use cimetidine in patients receiving drugs that may be subject to clinically significant interactions

Useful Reference

Feldman M, Burton ME. Histamine 2–receptor antagonists: Standard therapy for acid-peptic diseases. N Engl J Med 1990;323:1672–1680 (Part 1), 1749–1755 (Part 2)

CIPROFLOXACIN

Peter Jewesson

USA (Cipro)
CANADA (Cipro)

▶ *When Should I Use This Drug?*

check antibiotic susceptibility chart (Table 4–1 in Chapter 4)

Lower urinary tract infections

- ciprofloxacin should be reserved for the treatment of urinary tract infections if patients are known or suspected to be intolerant of trimethoprim-sulfamethoxazole and amoxicillin, or when pathogens associated with the infections are known or suspected to be resistant to trimethoprim-sulfamethoxazole and amoxicillin, because ciprofloxacin is more expensive than these agents and no more effective if the organisms are sensitive
- norfloxacin 400 mg PO Q12H should be used instead of ciprofloxacin 250 mg PO Q12H if it is less expensive or if the patient is taking theophylline (ciprofloxacin interacts with theophylline)

Upper urinary tract infection

- parenteral ciprofloxacin is the drug of choice for severely ill patients who are allergic to penicillins
- also useful as oral step-down therapy after the patient has improved on a regimen of parenteral agents
- oral ciprofloxacin can be used for mildly to moderately ill patients who are allergic to trimethoprim-sulfamethoxazole (this combination is as effective as ciprofloxacin if organisms are sensitive and it is less expensive than ciprofloxacin)

Acute or chronic bacterial prostatitis

- good penetration into the prostate makes ciprofloxacin useful for acute and chronic prostatis
- parenteral ciprofloxacin should be used for patients who are severely ill and allergic to penicillins (ampicillin and gentamicin are the initial drugs of choice)
- oral ciprofloxacin should be used only for mildly to moderately ill patients who are allergic to trimethoprim-sulfamethoxazole (trimethoprim-sulfamethoxazole penetrates the prostate well, provides convenient twice-daily dosing, and is less expensive than the newer agents)

Enteric infections

- ciprofloxacin is at least as active as previously used agents, is usually better tolerated, but is more expensive
- drug of choice for severe shigellosis, traveler's diarrhea, and salmonellosis if it is less expensive than norfloxacin
- use trimethoprim-sulfamethoxazole for mild infections, as it is effective and less expensive

Urethritis or cervicitis

- useful in conjunction with doxycycline in the penicillin-allergic patient if urethral discharge or endocervical discharge shows increased polymorphonuclear neutrophils and gram-negative intracellular diplococci (*Neisseria gonorrhoeae*) or no diagnostic results are available
- ciprofloxacin covers *N. gonorrhoeae* and doxycycline covers *Chlamydia trachomatis*

Mycobacterium avium infection

- ciprofloxacin, in conjunction with a variety of agents (clofazamine, rifampin, ethambutol, and so on) has been a useful regimen (N Engl J Med 1991;324:1332–1338, Ann Intern Med 1990; 113:358–361)

Other systemic infections (including soft tissue infections, osteomyelitis, pneumonias, and so on)

- oral ciprofloxacin can be used as an alternative to parenteral therapy in the treatment of non–life-threatening, non–central nervous system (CNS) infections (ciprofloxacin does not penetrate the CNS) involving susceptible pathogens

Step-down therapy or alternative to aminoglycosides

- oral ciprofloxacin should be used for step-down therapy, after a patient has improved with parenteral therapy, to facilitate early discharge from the hospital
- oral alternative to parenteral aminoglycosides when avoidance of aminoglycosides is desired owing to potential for toxicity and/or the need for hospitalization to administer a parenteral drug

▶ *When Should I Not Use This Drug?*

Urinary tract infections responsive to equally effective and tolerated, less expensive agents

- trimethoprim-sulfamethoxazole and amoxicillin are less expensive
- ciprofloxacin should be used for infections caused by organisms resistant to other antibacterial agents

Treatment of systemic infections involving streptococcal species

- streptoccocal organisms are only moderately susceptible to ciprofloxacin

Treatment of infections involving anaerobic pathogens (e.g., *Clostridium* and *Bacteroides*)

- ciprofloxacin lacks activity against these organisms

Patients with renal failure receiving aluminum products for the intestinal binding of phosphate

- chelation with quinolones may render both treatment courses ineffective

▶ *What Contraindications Are There to the Use of This Drug?*

Intolerance of or allergic reactions to ciprofloxacin

Use in children

- fluoroquinolones have been demonstrated to cause permanent joint damage in juvenile animals
- use in children with cystic fibrosis has not yet been associated with this complication, although arthralgias can develop (Drug Saf 1991;6:8–27)

Pregnancy or lactation

- teratogenic potential of fluoroquinolones not yet determined (nalidixic acid and older quinolones are considered potential teratogens)

▶ *What Drug Interactions Are Clinically Important?*

Drugs that may increase the effect or toxicity of ciprofloxacin

- none

Drugs that may decrease the effect of ciprofloxacin

ANTACIDS, FERROUS SULFATE

- magnesium- or aluminum-containing antacids or ferrous sulfate reduce the absorption of fluoroquinolones
- avoid concomitant use or space doses by 3 hours or longer

SUCRALFATE

- sucralfate contains aluminum salts and has been demonstrated to reduce the bioavailability of fluoroquinolones
- avoid concomitant use or space doses by 3 hours or longer

Drugs that may have their effect or toxicity increased by ciprofloxacin

THEOPHYLLINE

- if ciprofloxacin is to be used for a lower urinary tract infection, use norfloxacin instead
- if ciprofloxacin must be used, empirically decrease the theophylline dosage by 50% and monitor for signs and symptoms of toxicity

WARFARIN

- may reduce the clearance of warfarin
- use alternative agents if possible
- if not, monitor INR every 2 days until the full extent of interaction is seen and adjust the dosage as for a warfarin dosage change
- monitor INR every 2 days when administration of the interacting drug is discontinued and adjust as needed

Drugs that may have their effect decreased by ciprofloxacin

- none

▶ *What Route and Dosage Should I Use?*

How to administer

Orally

- on an empty stomach or with food if gastrointestinal intolerance occurs
- available in 250, 500, and 750 mg tablets only

Parenterally

- give as a 10 mg/mL solution diluted to 1–2 mg/mL with 5% dextrose in water, normal saline, or lactated Ringer's solution and give over 30 minutes
- do not give by rapid injection, and use a large vein if possible to prevent phlebitis

Lower urinary tract infections

- 250 mg PO Q12H

Upper urinary tract infection

- 200 mg IV Q12H for moderate to severe infections and infections in which the oral route must be avoided
- 500 mg PO Q12H for moderate infections
- 750 mg PO Q12H for severe systemic infections

Acute or chronic bacterial prostatitis

- 500 mg PO Q12H for mild to moderate infections
- 200 mg IV Q12H for severe infections

Enteric infections

- 500 mg PO Q12H

***Mycobacterium avium* infection**

- 750 mg PO BID

Other systemic infections (including soft tissue infections, osteomyelitis, pneumonias, and so on)

- 500 mg PO Q12H or 200 mg IV Q12H if parenteral therapy is required
- 750 mg PO Q12H for severe systemic infections or infections involving multiresistant pathogens or difficult to penetrate anatomical sites such as bone
- 400 mg IV is roughly equivalent to 750 mg PO
- 400 mg IV Q8H for serious infections involving *Pseudomonas* species

Normal Dosing Interval	$C_{cr} > 60$ mL/min or 1 mL/s	C_{cr} 30–60 mL/min or 0.5–1 mL/s	$C_{cr} < 30$ mL/min or 0.5 mL/s
Q8H	no adjustment needed	no adjustment needed	Q12H
Q12H	no adjustment needed	no adjustment needed	Q24H

▶ *What Should I Monitor with Regard to Efficacy and Toxicity?*

Efficacy

- for antibiotic administration monitoring guidelines, see specific section on drug therapy

Toxicity

Gastrointestinal

- 2–5% incidence of nausea (with or without vomiting), diarrhea, and upper abdominal discomfort and distention
- take with food if nausea develops
- food delays, but does not reduce, absorption
- if symptoms persist, discontinue use

Central nervous system effects

- 1–4% incidence of dizziness, restlessness, headache, and insomnia
- decrease the dosage or discontinue use if symptoms persist
- seizures have been reported in patients receiving concomitant theophylline, imipenem, and nonsteroidal antiinflammatory drugs and in those with a previous history of seizures (seizures can occur when the patient is receiving standard doses); therefore avoid high doses, as seizures are likely a dose-related effect
- avoid using in these patients if possible

Dermatological effects

- 1–1.5% incidence of maculopapular rash or urticaria
- discontinue use if either occurs
- phototoxic reactions have been reported
- advise the patient to avoid strong sunlight or to use sun-blocking agents while receiving therapy

Renal effects

- a few reports of interstitial nephritis, renal tubular damage, hematuria, and renal insufficiency
- incidence is too low to promote routine screening

Other

- anaphylaxis has rarely been reported

▶ *How Long Do I Treat Patients with This Drug?*

Lower urinary tract infections

- 3 days if uncomplicated

Upper urinary tract infection

- 14 days total (IV and PO)

Acute or chronic bacterial prostatitis

- 30 days for treatment of acute bacterial prostatitis
- for chronic prostatitis: 6 weeks for initial treatment

Enteric infections

- 5 days of treatment are adequate
- empirical therapy of traveler's diarrhea at the onset of diarrheal illness is as effective as prophylaxis, less toxic, and less expensive

***Mycobacterium avium* infection**

- probably life-long, although clinical trials have not addressed this question
- a number of patients, even after 1 year of treatment, can experience recurrent symptoms and mycobacteremia when antimycobacterial medications are stopped

Other systemic infections (including soft tissue infections, osteomyelitis, pneumonias, and so on)

- usual duration of therapy is 10 days or 4–5 days after the patient has become afebrile and has clinically improved

- consider switching to an oral agent after the patient has become afebrile and has clinically improved for 1–2 days
- for osteomyelitis, 4 weeks of parenteral therapy or longer is necessary

▶ How Do I Decrease or Stop the Administration of This Drug?

- may be stopped abruptly

▶ What Should I Tell My Patients About This Drug?

- this agent is an antibacterial, and successful therapy is contingent on good compliance and completion of the full treatment course
- some minor side effects (e.g., gastrointestinal or CNS complaints) can be expected, but these are usually self-limited and therapy should not be stopped
- contact your pharmacist or your physician if side effects are bothersome
- do not take fluoroquinolones with antacids or sucralfate or any other prescription or nonprescription drug products without the knowledge of both your pharmacist and your physician

▶ Therapeutic Tips

- always consider efficacy, toxicity, and cost when determining the role of fluoroquinolones relative to other available agents
- reserve use for difficult to treat infections involving susceptible pathogens
- overuse likely results in the development of resistance over time
- use as a step-down agent to convert parenteral to oral therapy and to facilitate early hospital discharge
- use as a step-down agent after aminoglycosides to decrease the duration of aminoglycoside treatment and associated risk of toxicity

Useful References

LeBel M. Ciprofloxacin: Chemistry, mechanism of action, resistance, antimicrobial spectrum, pharmacokinetics, clinical trials and adverse reactions. Pharmacotherapy 1988;8:3–33

Paton JH, Reeves DS. Clinical features and management of adverse effects of quinolone antibacterials. Drug Saf 1991;6:8–27

Campoli-Richards DM, Monk JP, Price A, et al. Ciprofloxacin: A review of its antibacterial activity, pharmacokinetic properties and therapeutic use. Drugs 1988;35:373–447

CLINDAMYCIN

David Guay and Ann Beardsell

USA (Cleocin, generic)
CANADA (Dalacin C)

▶ When Should I Use This Drug?

check antibiotic susceptibility chart (Table 4–1 in Chapter 4)

Pneumonia

- use if empyema or lung abscess infections due to anaerobic gram-positive organisms are suspected or proved to be resistant to penicillin or if the patient is allergic to penicillins (clindamycin is more expensive and has more toxicities than does penicillin)
- for aspiration pneumonia, use clindamycin if the patient is allergic to penicillin (use clindamycin in conjunction with cefotaxime or ceftriaxone if aspiration pneumonia is hospital acquired or if the patient is very ill, especially if gram-negative organisms are seen on gram stain)

Acute or chronic osteomyelitis

- drug of choice if there is a documented history of penicillin allergy
- although clindamycin has activity against the most common organisms causing acute osteomyelitis (staphylococcal and streptococcal organisms), it is more expensive than cloxacillin or nafcillin and can cause diarrhea and/or pseudomembranous colitis
- combine with gentamicin (or ciprofloxacin if aminoglycosides are contraindicated) for high-risk patients (intravenous drug abusers, hemodialysis patients, and patients with underlying debilitating diseases); patients with peripheral vascular disease (diabetes);

and patients with osteomyelitis if the skull, facial bones, the mandible, the sacrum (especially with decubitus ulcers), the hand (after human bite), or the pelvis (after intraabdominal infections) is involved
- clindamycin with gentamicin has activity against the common organisms causing osteomyelitis in these patients (*Staphylococcus aureus, Klebsiella pneumoniae, Haemophilus influenzae,* and anaerobes)
- clindamycin is useful when both gram-positive and anaerobic organisms are suspected
- if infection is caused by both anaerobic and gram-positive aerobic organisms, consider the merits and costs of clindamycin treatment versus combined therapy with metronidazole and penicillin or cephalosporin or quinolone

Cellulitis

- if the patient is moderately to severely ill with a documented history of penicillin allergy, as clindamycin has better activity against gram-positive organisms than does erythromycin
- if parenteral therapy is required, clindamycin is less expensive than either parenteral erythromycin or vancomycin
- use in combination with gentamicin if patients are at high risk (intravenous drug abusers, hemodialysis patients, and patients with underlying debilitating diseases) or if an abscess is present
- clindamycin has good activity against staphylococcal and streptococcal organisms

Anaerobic sepsis

- use only if the infecting organism is resistant to cephalosporins with anaerobic activity (cefoxitin, ceftizoxime, cefotetan) and metronidazole

Vaginitis

- drug of choice if the patient has bacterial vaginosis (Gram stain of vaginal swab shows gram-positive and/or gram-negative coccobacilli) in patients who cannot take metronidazole

Pelvic inflammatory disease

- drug of choice in combination with an aminoglycoside, if the patient is penicillin allergic
- also useful, in conjunction with an aminoglycoside, if the patient has failed to respond to prior combination therapy of a cephalosporin with anaerobic activity and doxycycline (Am J Obstet Gynecol 1988;158:687–693)

Acne vulgaris

- topical drug of choice

Cerebral toxoplasmosis in patients with acquired immunodeficiency syndrome

- use only if sulfadiazine-pyrimethamine therapy cannot be used (sulfa allergy or intolerance) or this therapy fails, as clindamycin is more expensive than sulfadiazine
- used in combination with pyrimethamine

Intraabdominal infections

- when used with an aminoglycoside, clindamycin is as effective as metronidazole and gentamicin; however, clindamycin is usually more expensive and has more adverse effects than metronidazole (diarrhea and occasionally pseudomembranous colitis)

Surgical prophylaxis

- in conjunction with gentamicin for head and neck surgery
- in conjunction with gentamicin for gastroduodenal, biliary tract, and emergency colorectal surgery; appendectomy; abdominal trauma; lower extremity amputation; and colorectal surgery in patients allergic to penicillin

▶ When Should I Not Use This Drug?

Anaerobic meningitis

- poor central nervous system penetration; therefore, use metronidazole

Combination with erythromycin

- antagonism can occur when these agents are used together

▶ *What Contraindications Are There to the Use of This Drug?*

Intolerance of or allergic reaction to clindamycin
Previous history of pseudomembranous colitis

- increased risk of repeated disease

▶ *What Drug Interactions Are Clinically Important?*

- none

▶ *What Route and Dosage Should I Use?*

How to administer

- orally—can be given with food or on empty stomach
- parenterally—administer in a diluted solution of less than 12 mg/mL over a minimum of 20 minutes
- topically—administer as a thin film to affected areas (gel, lotion, solution)

Pneumonia, cellulitis, acute or chronic osteomyelitis, anaerobic sepsis, intraabdominal infections, pelvic inflammatory disease

- 600 mg IV Q8H if the patient is mildly to moderately ill
- 900 mg IV Q8H if the patient is severely ill
- 300 mg PO Q6H if the patient is moderately ill and the patient is to be treated orally

Vaginitis

- 300 mg PO BID

Acne vulgaris

- apply a thin film BID

Cerebral toxoplasmosis

- 900 mg IV Q6H for 3 weeks until there is marked clinical improvement
- if no clinical improvement, increase dose to 1200 mg IV Q6H
- once marked clinical improvement has occurred, give 300 mg PO QID for 3 more weeks

Surgical prophylaxis

- 600 mg IV as a single dose

Dosage adjustments for renal or hepatic dysfunction

- no adjustment needed for either hepatic or renal impairment

▶ *What Should I Monitor with Regard to Efficacy and Toxicity?*

Efficacy

- for antibiotic administration monitoring guidelines, see specific section on drug therapy

Toxicity

Gastrointestinal effects
- abdominal pain, esophagitis, nausea, vomiting, and diarrhea
- have been seen even with topical formulation
- question the patient, on a daily basis while the patient is in the hospital, about the appearance of these symptoms
- if nausea and vomiting occur, the patient should take clindamycin with food, and if it continues, the patient should stop taking the drug
- if diarrhea occurs and pseudomembranous colitis is suspected (profuse greenish, watery, foul-smelling diarrhea; a fever of 39–41°C (102.2–105.8°F); abdominal tenderness; leukocytosis; and hypoalbuminemia), see drug-induced diarrhea in Chapter 11

Allergic reactions
- skin rash, anaphylaxis, Stevens-Johnson syndrome, and so on
- question the patient, on a daily basis while in the hospital, about the presence of a skin rash

Dermatological effects (topical formulation)
- dryness, dermatitis, and folliculitis

▶ *How Long Do I Treat Patients with This Drug?*

Pneumonia

- oral antibiotics should be considered after the patient has clinically improved and has been afebrile for 48 hours

- if the patient responds rapidly, a 10 day course of therapy is sufficient
- if the patient responds slowly or has a pneumonia caused by gram-negative organisms, *Mycoplasma,* or *Legionella,* a 14 day course of therapy should be given (Clin Chest Med 1991; 12:237–242, Ann Intern Med 1987;106:341–345)

Cellulitis

- usual duration is 10 days or 4–5 days after the patient has become afebrile and has clinically improved
- if using parenteral therapy, consider switching to oral therapy after the patient has become afebrile and has clinically improved for 1–2 days

Acute or chronic osteomyelitis

- treat patients with at least 4 weeks of parenteral antibiotics after debridement surgery (the duration of therapy is based on the patient's clinical response)
- if an amputation is done proximal to the site of the infection, only prophylactic antibiotics are required (Hosp Formul 1993; 28:63–85)
- if the bone is removed and there is still evidence of soft tissue infection, the patient should receive a 2 week course of antibiotics
- for patients with a prosthetic device, treat for 4–6 weeks with parenteral antibiotics followed by 3–6 months of oral antibiotics
- treat patients with peripheral vascular disease with at least 4 weeks of parenteral antibiotics and follow with oral antibiotics until there is no evidence of inflammation (based on clinical or radiological evidence) (Am J Med 1987;83:653–660)
- duration of parenteral antibiotic therapy prior to switching to oral therapy depends on the patient's clinical response

Vaginitis

- 7 days for bacterial vaginosis

Pelvic inflammatory disease

- continue the initial regimen until 48 hours after clinical improvement
- after the patient is discharged from the hospital, continue therapy for a total of 10–14 days, depending on how quickly the patient responds

Acne vulgaris

- may require treatment for several months to years
- continue as long as the response is satisfactory and no intolerable toxicity occurs

Cerebral toxoplasmosis in patients with AIDS

- treat for 6 weeks, at which time there has usually been marked clinical improvement
- lesions that fail to respond to antitoxoplasmosis therapy within 7–14 days should be considered for diagnostic brain biopsy, depending on the general status of the patient
- major symptomatic improvement can be expected to occur within 7–14 days after the initiation of therapy

Intraabdominal infections

- treatment should continue for 10 days; however, extend treatment if the patient has not been asymptomatic for 72 hours

Surgical prophylaxis

- single dose

▶ *How Do I Decrease or Stop the Administration of This Drug?*

- may be stopped abruptly

▶ *What Should I Tell My Patients About This Drug?*

- let your physician know if you have had any sort of reaction to this type of drug in the past (use trade names as a cue)
- contact your physician if symptoms do not improve during the next few days (for systemic therapy) or weeks (for topical treatment)

- if diarrhea develops, contact your physician immediately
- take the medication until it is completely finished

▶ *Therapeutic Tips*

- Q6H IV dosing is not necessary (except for toxoplasmosis)
- oral doses given Q8H may be poorly tolerated, so Q6H oral dosing is usually used
- use metronidazole instead of clindamycin whenever possible
- switch from IV to PO therapy whenever possible

Useful References

Klainer AS. Clindamycin. Med Clin North Am 1987;71:1169–1175
Hammill HA. Metronidazole, clindamycin and quinolones. Obstet Gynecol Clin North Am 1989;16:317–328

CLOFAZIMINE

Ann Beardsell

USA (Lamprene)
CANADA (Lamprene)

▶ *When Should I Use This Drug?*

Mycobacterium avium Infection

- used in conjunction with other antimycobacterial agents owing to the rapid development of resistance when one drug is used alone

Leprosy

- in combination with other antiinfectives (dapsone, rifampin, and possibly ethionamide)

▶ *When Should I Not Use This Drug?*

As a single agent in the treatment of tuberculosis

- must be used in conjunction with other agents to prevent resistance

▶ *What Contraindications Are There to the Use of This Drug?*

- intolerance of or allergic reaction to clofazimine

▶ *What Drug Interactions Are Clinically Important?*

Drugs that may increase the effect of clofazimine

ISONIAZID

- can increase clofazimine concentrations
- no specific guidelines available about dosage adjustment

Drugs that may decrease effect of clofazamine

DAPSONE

- may decrease or nullify some of the antiinflammatory effects of clofazimine when used for leprosy
- monitor the response of inflammation to the drug and add other antiinflammatory drugs or change to another antileprosy agent if required, but this interaction is usually not a problem
- no effect on antimycobacterial activity of either drug

Drugs that may have their effect increased by clofazimine

- none

Drugs that may have their effect decreased by clofazimine

RIFAMPIN

- clofazimine may decrease the rate of absorption of rifampin
- only a consideration if the response to leprosy treatment is poor

▶ *What Route and Dosage Should I Use?*

How to administer

- orally—take with meals to maximize absorption
- parenterally—not available

Mycobacterium avium infection

- 100 mg PO daily with other agents

Leprosy

- 50 mg PO daily and 300 mg PO once a month in combination with other agents

Dosage adjustments for renal or hepatic dysfunction

- eliminated in feces
- no dosage adjustments needed

▶ *What Should I Monitor with Regard to Efficacy and Toxicity?*

Efficacy

Mycobacterium avium infection

Signs and symptoms

- fevers, chills, night sweats, malaise, fatigue, weight loss, abdominal pain, and diarrhea
- there are usually few or no physical signs to follow other than body weight or possibly the presence of a lesion in patients with localized disease (e.g., regional lymphadenopathy)
- patients should also be advised to report new or worsening diarrhea while taking such regimens, because *Clostridium difficile* colitis is a possible complication
- patients should be assessed every 1–2 weeks during the first 1–2 months of treatment

Complete blood count

- monthly or more frequently for severe disease, to detect progressive anemia and cytopenias due to bone marrow involvement, which may persist despite treatment

Blood cultures

- to document reduction or clearance of mycobacteremia, particularly in patients who have persistent symptoms

Leprosy

- tissue stain smears, which should become negative with time
- resolution of skin lesions may take 8–12 weeks, depending on the severity of disease

Toxicity

- generally well tolerated

Discoloration of body tissues

- clofazimine is a bright red dye and crystals accumulate in various body tissues and fluids such as skin (75–100%), eyes (38–57%), gastrointestinal tract, sweat, tears, sputum, urine, feces, nasal secretions, semen, and breast milk

Dermatological effects

- in addition to discoloration, 8–38% of patients experience itching and dry skin, which may be relieved by using oil or an emollient lotion with urea
- pruritus and nonspecific rash (follicular and papular) occur in 1–5%

Ocular effects

- discoloration of conjunctiva, cornea, and lacrimal fluid occurs but does not affect visual acuity
- dryness, burning, itching, irritation, and watering of eyes occur in 2–32%

Gastrointestinal effects

- major dose-limiting adverse effect involving abdominal and epigastric pain, diarrhea, nausea, vomiting, and gastrointestinal intolerance (up to 60%)
- these appear to be dose related and occur more commonly with dosages greater than 100 mg daily
- with usual dosages, these may occur within a few days or weeks after the initiation of therapy as a result of a direct irritant effect on the gut; symptoms generally decrease with decreased dosage
- with higher dosages (300 mg daily or greater), a severe syndrome of crampy or colicky abdominal pain, persistent diarrhea, and weight loss may occur at 3 months or later
- discontinue clofazimine administration; watch for bowel obstruction (hospitalization may be necessary)

▶ *How Long Do I Treat Patients with This Drug?*

Mycobacterium avium infection

- for the lifetime of the patient or as long as the patient tolerates the treatment

Leprosy

- for multibacillary, dapsone-sensitive leprosy, a minimum of 2 years or until skin smears are negative
- for multibacillary, dapsone-resistant leprosy, a minimum of 2 years with rifampin and then as sole therapy until skin smears are negative for 10 years or, depending of the type of leprosy, for life

▶ *How Do I Decrease or Stop the Administration of This Drug?*

- may be stopped abruptly

▶ *What Should I Tell My Patients About This Drug?*

- clofazamine is generally well tolerated
- clofazamine most likely causes a pink to brownish-black discoloration of your skin that gives you a well-tanned appearance, as well as discoloring the conjunctiva, tears, sweat, sputum, urine, feces, nasal secretions, semen, and breast milk, which may take several months or years to disappear after the drug administration has been stopped
- you may experience some gastrointestinal upset when the drug therapy is first started but this should resolve; however, if it persists, contact your physician
- use may result in staining of contact lenses; therefore, wear glasses

▶ *Therapeutic Tips*

- advise the patient to take this medication with meals to improve absorption and to minimize gastrointestinal upset
- spread drugs and/or doses out over the day to reduce the volume of drugs being taken at once, which may improve compliance and tolerance

CLOFIBRATE

Stephen Shalansky and Robert Dombrowski

USA (Atromid-S, generics)
CANADA (Atromid-S, Novofibrate)

▶ *When Should I Use This Drug?*

Consider an alternative agent

- WHO Primary Prevention Trial demonstrated an increased mortality in clofibrate-treated patients compared with those given placebo
- no particular disease accounted for the overall increase in mortality, but causes contributing included an increased incidence of gastrointestinal malignancies and complications from cholecystectomy (Br Heart J 1978;40:1069–1118, Lancet 1980;2:379–385)
- there is an increased incidence of gallstones associated with clofibrate use (Lancet 1980;2:379–385, Br Heart J 1978;40:1069–1118, JAMA 1975;231:360–381)
- Coronary Drug Project trial also showed a significant increase in the incidence of thromboembolism, angina pectoris, intermittent claudication, and cardiac arrhythmias (JAMA 1975;231:360–381)

Useful References

Knodel LC, Talbert RL. Adverse effects of hypolipidemic drugs. Med Toxicol 1987;2:10–32
Illingworth DR. Lipid-lowering drugs: An overview of indications and optimum therapeutic use. Drugs 1987;33:259–279

CLOMIPRAMINE

Lyle K. Laird and Julia Vertrees

USA (Anafranil)
CANADA (Anafranil)

▶ *When Should I Use This Drug?*

Obsessive-compulsive disorders

- first-line therapy as extensive clinical experience and research show greater efficacy than with other tricyclic antidepressants (Pharmacotherapy 1990;10:175–197)

▶ *When Should I Not Use This Drug?*

Major depression, dysthymia, panic disorders, generalized anxiety disorder, chronic pain syndromes

- no more effective than other antidepressants such as imipramine
- more expensive than many other tricyclic antidepressants
- should be used if the patient has depression with obsessional features, as clomipramine is effective for the treatment of obsessive-compulsive disorder
- has been associated with seizures

▶ *What Contraindications Are There to the Use of This Drug?*

see Imipramine

Pregnancy

- adequate human studies have not been performed

▶ *What Drug Interactions Are Clinically Important?*

see Imipramine

▶ *What Route and Dosage Should I Use?*

How to administer

- orally—can be given with food or on an empty stomach
- parenterally—not available

Obsessive-compulsive disorders

- start with 25 mg PO BID
- increase after 3 days to 100 mg PO daily at bedtime
- increase to 150 mg PO daily at bedtime after 1 week and leave at this dosage for 10–14 days
- if target symptoms do not improve by this time, increase the daily dosage weekly by 50 mg until a maximum of 250 mg/d is reached or until target symptoms improve
- in geriatric patients and patients with a seizure history start with 25 mg PO at bedtime, and in general, dosages should be approximately 50% of those used in healthy individuals
- clomipramine has a long duration of action and once-daily dosing is appropriate

Dosage adjustments for renal or hepatic dysfunction

- hepatically metabolized
- start with low doses as for geriatric patients
- decreased renal function does not necessitate dosage adjustments

▶ *What Should I Monitor with Regard to Efficacy and Toxicity?*

Efficacy

Obsessive-compulsive disorders

Target symptoms

- monitor changes in compulsive or ritualistic behavior and obsessional thoughts
- response is slow (3–4 weeks for initial response) and it may take 6–8 weeks to see a 50% decrease in symptoms
- after they are stable, patients should be clinically assessed for target symptoms at least monthly (or weekly if clinical decompensation is suspected)
- patients may need up to 12 weeks of therapy to see an effect

Toxicity

see Imipramine

Sexual dysfunction

- commonly encountered in patients taking clomipramine

▶ How Long Do I Treat Patients with This Drug?

Obsessive-compulsive disorders

- efficacy for longer than 9 months is not established; however, improvement in obsessive-compulsive disorders is maintained as long as drug therapy continues (The American Psychiatric Association Textbook of Psychiatry 1988:443–491)
- because obsessive-compulsive disorders can significantly impair one's ability to function, lifelong therapy may be indicated

▶ How Do I Decrease or Stop the Administration of This Drug?

see Imipramine

▶ What Should I Tell My Patients About This Drug?

see Imipramine

▶ Therapeutic Tips

see Imipramine

Useful References

DeVane CL. Cyclic antidepressants. In: Evans WE, Schentag JJ, Jusko WJ, eds. Applied Pharmacokinetics: Principles of Therapeutic Drug Monitoring. Spokane, WA: Applied Therapeutics, 1987:852–907

McTavish D, Benefield P. Clomipramine: An overview of its pharmacologic properties. Drugs 1990;39:136–153

Hollander E, Liebowitz MR, Gorman JM. Anxiety disorders. In: Talbott JA, Hales RE, Yudofsky SC, eds. The American Psychiatric Association Textbook of Psychiatry. Washington, DC: American Psychiatric Press, 1988:443–491

CLONAZEPAM

Steven Stanislav, Patricia Marken, and William Parker

USA (Klonopin)
CANADA (Rivotril)

▶ When Should I Use This Drug?

Generalized anxiety disorder

- benzodiazepines have been considered first-line therapy due to extensive research and over 30 years' clinical experience
- predictors of response to benzodiazepines are acute symptoms, precipitating stress, high level of psychic and somatic anxiety, absence of or low level of depression, no previous drug treatment, good response in previous therapy, and expectation of recovery or desire for medication
- benzodiazepines have an effect immediately to within several days, whereas buspirone's effect is delayed for 2–4 weeks
- all benzodiazepines are equally effective; therefore, the choice is based on the patient's previous response and cost
- agents with an intermediate duration of action (lorazepam or oxazepam) are preferred because they allow easier dose titration by both the patient and the physician
- clonazepam has an intermediate to long duration of activity (N Engl J Med 1993;328:1398–1405) and no active metabolites

Panic disorder

- clonazepam has been found to be equally efficacious to alprazolam (J Clin Psychiatry 1991;52[2]:69–76)
- clonazepam has a longer duration of action than does alprazolam and can be dosed 2–3 times daily, whereas alprazolam is dosed 3–4 times daily
- some clinicians prefer clonazepam to avoid rebound anxiety that occurs when reducing or stopping alprazolam administration, although this has not been proven in prospective studies
- alprazolam is the only U.S. FDA approved agent for treating panic disorders

Periodic limb movement disorder

- clonazepam, temazepam (Sleep 1986;9:385–392), nitrazepam (Can J Neurol Sci 1986;13:52–54), levodopa (Clin Neuropharmacol 1986;9:456–463), and trazodone (Sleep Res 1988;17:39) have demonstrated efficacy in managing this disorder
- although there are more scientific data for clonazepam and temazepam, on the basis of clinical experience trazodone may have

an advantage over these agents in that patients do not appear to develop tolerance
- with clonazepam being a long-acting agent, it may cause unacceptable daytime sedation or sleepiness in the elderly, who most commonly have periodic limb movement disorders

Rapid eye movement sleep behavior disorder

- although a variety of psychotropic agents have been used to treat this disorder, clonazepam is the preferred benzodiazepine and appears to have specific therapeutic effects in this disorder (JAMA 1987;257:1786–1789)

Generalized seizures (no primary focus)

Absence seizures, myoclonic seizures (including juvenile myoclonic epilepsy)

- clonazepam is an effective alternative drug in treating patients who do not tolerate or respond to first-line drugs
- it is a second-line drug owing to central nervous system and behavioral side effects and the potential for loss of efficacy after several months
- many clinicians prefer clobazam to clonazepam because it has fewer psychomotor side effects

▶ When Should I Not Use This Drug?

Transient and short-term insomnia

- should not be used instead of other benzodiazepines because it produces more hangover effects and daytime sedation is more prominent with this benzodiazepine than with the shorter-acting agents such as triazolam, temazepam, lorazepam, and oxazepam

Multiple types of seizure disorders

- use in patients with multiple types of seizure disorders may increase the frequency of or precipitate tonic-clonic (grand mal) seizures in some patients

Acute manic episode

- although clonazepam may be used (there is a suggestion that it has some specific antimanic properties), it is more expensive than lorazepam and there is little evidence that it is more effective than lorazepam

▶ What Contraindications Are There to the Use of This Drug?

see Lorazepam

▶ What Drug Interactions Are Clinically Important?

see Lorazepam

▶ What Route and Dosage Should I Use?

How to administer

- orally—take with food or milk or on an empty stomach
- parenterally—not available

Generalized anxiety disorder

- start with 0.5 mg PO BID
- if no excessive sedation occurs, increase the dosage by 0.5 mg increments every 3–4 days up to 1 mg PO TID (this dosage provides control for most people) or until symptoms are well under control

Panic disorder

- goal is to prevent attacks and then to decrease the dosage if the drug is tolerated and symptoms are controlled
- 0.5 mg PO TID for 1 week
- advise the patients that this dosage may make them sedated and that they may have to take time off from work or school
- if necessary, titrate the dose up by 0.5 mg increments to 6 mg PO daily on the basis of response and the patient's ability to tolerate sedation
- after symptoms are suppressed, one can attempt to decrease the dosage and to administer twice daily
- 2–3 doses per day are needed to avoid breakthrough anxiety

Periodic limb movement disorder

- 0.25 mg PO HS only, increasing to 0.5 mg if ineffective

Rapid eye movement sleep behavior disorder

- start at 1 mg PO HS, and increase up to 2 mg until the symptoms abate

Generalized seizures (no primary focus)

Absence seizures, myoclonic seizures (including juvenile myoclonic epilepsy)

- start with 0.5 mg PO HS for 7 days, as clonazepam is very sedating
- increase the dosage by 0.5 mg every 3–5 days (given BID) until seizures are controlled or side effects become intolerable or to a maximum daily dosage of 20 mg PO (the usual dosage is 4–6 mg/d)
- largest dose should be given at bedtime if doses are not equally divided

Dosage adjustments for renal or hepatic dysfunction

- hepatically metabolized
- no dosage adjustments for organ dysfunction are recommended; however, always start with the lowest dose and titrate to response

▶ *What Should I Monitor with Regard to Efficacy and Toxicity?*

Efficacy

- see Lorazepam

Panic Disorder

Target symptoms

- monitor changes in shortness of breath, choking or smothering sensations, dizziness, palpitations or chest pain, trembling, nausea, depersonalization, tingling, and fear of impending doom
- should see initial response within several days
- after patients are stable, patients should be clinically assessed for target symptoms at least monthly or weekly if clinical decompensation is suspected

Periodic limb movement disorder, rapid eye movement sleep behavior disorder

Shortening of time taken to fall asleep and improved sleep efficiency

- quantify through the use of a sleep diary and compare with pretreatment sleep performance
- bed partner often reports decreased movements and verbalizations
- patient may report reduced frequency of disturbing dreams and self-injury from striking out or walking during sleep episodes

Improved daytime functioning

- quantify by comparing changes in the symptoms (e.g., anxiety, tension, and fatigue) while receiving treatment with baseline values

Generalized seizures (no primary focus) • Absence seizures, myoclonic seizures (including juvenile myoclonic epilepsy)

Seizure control

- reduction in frequency and severity of seizures
- close attention to changes in seizure frequency is necessary to monitor for therapeutic tolerance
- tolerance to the anticonvulsant effect occurs in up to $^1/_3$ of patients within 3–6 months of starting the drug administration and a dosage increase may restore initial efficacy in some patients

Serum concentrations

- although the accepted anticonvulsant therapeutic range is 20–80 ng/mL (60–250 μmol/L), periodic serum level measurements are of limited or no value because of poor correlation between therapeutic and adverse effects and serum levels

Toxicity

Behavioral disturbances

- irritation, aggressiveness, and loss of self-confidence have been seen
- behavioral disturbances occur most frequently during the initiation of treatment in patients with preexisting brain damage or a history of behavioral or psychiatric disturbances
- best management is starting with low doses, gradually increasing the dosage over 2 weeks, and giving the drug in 3–4 divided daily doses
- if behavioral disturbance occurs, decrease the dosage, and if it is still a problem, stop the drug

Psychomotor impairment and hangover effects

- if this occurs, reduce the dosage, and if this is not effective, switch to another medication
- for rapid eye movement (REM) sleep behavior disorder, other benzodiazepines are not as effective as clonazepam, and it is usually necessary to trade off the daytime impairments for the decrease in self-injurious behavior
- see Lorazepam for other potential adverse effects

▶ *How Long Do I Treat Patients with This Drug?*

see Lorazepam

Periodic limb movement disorder, rapid eye movement sleep behavior disorder

- treatment is indefinite

Generalized seizures (no primary focus)

Absence seizures, myoclonic seizures (including juvenile myoclonic epilepsy)

- 4 year seizure-free period is recommended before attempting to withdraw clonazepam administration
- factors promoting complete withdrawal include a seizure-free period of 2–4 years, complete seizure control within 1 year of onset, an onset of seizures between 2 and 35 years of age, and a normal electroencephalogram
- patients should not drive during withdrawal and for 3–4 months after, and this may make it difficult for some patients to try withdrawal
- prior to withdrawal, patients should be advised that about $^1/_3$ experience relapse, and if this occurs, then the patient and the physician will know that the drug is still necessary
- factors associated with a poor prognosis after stopping the drug administration, despite a seizure-free period, include a history of a high frequency of seizures, repeated episodes of status epilepticus, multiple seizure types, and development of abnormal mental functioning
- drug withdrawal in patients with juvenile myoclonic epilepsy is usually not successful, and therapy probably needs to be lifelong

▶ *How Do I Decrease or Stop the Administration of This Drug?*

see Lorazepam

Generalized seizures (no primary focus)

- sudden withdrawal is to be avoided, especially after long-term, high-dose therapy
- withdrawal is best done over several months
- decrease the dosage by 0.5 mg daily each month until withdrawal is complete
- seizure relapse is most common during withdrawal or the first 3 months after withdrawal
- clinical impression of some neurologists has been that clonazepam is more difficult to withdraw than other antiepileptic drugs, in that withdrawal seizures are more likely to occur
- some patients can continue to withdraw clonazepam administration, despite withdrawal seizures, and then be seizure free thereafter
- if seizures recur, reinstitute treatment with the same drugs used previously
- if multiple anticonvulsant therapy is present, drugs should be withdrawn one at a time

- because of clonazepam's long half-life, withdrawal symptoms may not occur until several days after the drug has been stopped

▶ **What Should I Tell My Patients About This Drug?**

see Lorazepam

▶ **Therapeutic Tips**

- watch for psychomotor impairment
- tolerance to the anticonvulsant effect occurs in up to $1/3$ of patients within 3–6 months of starting the drug therapy and a dosage increase may restore efficacy in some patients
- psychomotor and behavioral problems are frequent at dosages necessary to control seizures; therefore, try clobazam before clonazepam
- this drug is specific treatment for REM sleep behavior disorder
- becoming a drug of choice for panic disorders

Useful References

Teboul E, Chouinard G. A guide to benzodiazepine selection. Part II: Clinical aspects. Can J Psychiatry 1991;36:62–73

Pugh CB, Garnett WR. Current issues in the treatment of epilepsy. Clin Pharm 1991;10:335–358

Parker WA. Epilepsy. In: Herfindal ET, Gourley DR, Hart LL, eds. Clinical Pharmacy and Therapeutics, 4th ed. Baltimore: Williams & Wilkins, 1988:570–592

CLOTRIMAZOLE

Peter Jewesson

USA (Gyne-Lotrimin, Mycelex-G)
CANADA (Canestan, Myclo)

▶ **When Should I Use This Drug?**

Oropharyngeal candidiasis

- topical agents should initially be used because they are often as effective as systemic agents but are associated with less toxicity and less potential for drug interactions
- unfortunately, compliance with these regimens may be poor and this often mandates a change to systemic antifungal therapy such as ketoconazole, fluconazole, or itraconazole (see below under esophageal candidiasis)
- nystatin and cotrimazole are likely equally effective
- clotrimazole is preferred over nystatin as the initial treatment of oropharyngeal candidiasis as it is usually better tolerated; however, clotrimazole is more expensive than nystatin
- patients with severe disease may need to be treated with ketoconazole/fluconazole or itraconazole and those who are unable to swallow will require amphotericin B

Vaginal candidiasis

- topical miconazole/clotrimazole/terconazole are all effective and can be given as a 3 day course of therapy
- choice between these agents should be on the basis of cost and patient tolerance

Vaginal trichomoniasis

- secondary drug to metronidazole, however, considered drug of choice if patient pregnant

▶ **When Should I Not Use This Drug?**

Esophageal candidiasis

- topical agents are usually not effective for esophageal candidiasis and oral agents such as ketoconazole or fluconazole or itraconazole should be used

▶ **What Contraindications Are There to the Use of This Drug?**

- Intolerance or allergic reaction to clotrimazole

▶ **What Drug Interactions Are Clinically Important?**

- none

▶ **What Route and Dosage Should I Use?**

How to administer

- orally—should be dissolved in mouth (for local antifungal effect only)
- vaginally—insert tablet(s) intravaginally at bedtime

Oropharyngeal candidiasis

- 1 vaginal suppository (100 mg) dissolved slowly in the mouth TID
- 1 flavored pastille (100 mg) dissolved slowly in the mouth TID
- 1 troche (100 mg) TID
- choice of the above is dependent on patient preference (none is well tolerated)

Vaginal candidiasis

- 2 × 100 mg vaginal suppository nightly for three nights
- 500 mg × 1 day intravaginal clotrimazole also appears to be effective and could be used if compliance is a potential problem

Vaginal trichomoniasis

- 100 mg vaginal tablet at bedtime for 7 days

▶ **What Should I Monitor with Regard to Efficacy and Toxicity?**

Efficacy

Oropharyngeal candidiasis

- reduction in pain, disappearance of lesions
- assess symptoms daily if in hospital or weekly if outpatient

Vaginal candidiasis, vaginal trichomoniasis

- disappearance of lesions and reduction in pain and itching

Toxicity

Mild localized reactions

- stinging, erythema, urticaria, edema, desquamation, pruritus, and vesication when applied to skin
- mild burning, skin rash, and lower abdominal cramps associated with vaginal application
- discontinue use of drug if symptoms persist or worsen and use alternative (e.g., nystatin)

▶ **How Long Do I Treat Patients with This Drug?**

Oropharyngeal candidiasis

- 1 week and at least 2 days after the symptoms have resolved
- patient should respond within a few days
- continuous therapy may be required in patients with frequent relapses

Vaginal candidiasis

- 3 days

Vaginal trichomoniasis

- 7 days

▶ **How Do I Decrease or Stop the Administration of This Drug?**

- may be stopped abruptly

▶ **What Should I Tell My Patient About This Drug?**

- this agent is an antifungal agent and successful therapy is contingent upon good compliance and completion of the full treatment course
- local side effects (i.e., stinging, erythema, rash) can occur
- if symptoms persist, contact pharmacist or physician

▶ **Therapeutic Tips**

- considered safe in pregnant and breastfeeding women; however, should be avoided in first trimester (as with all drugs) unless deemed essential

References

Bennett JE. Antifungal Agents. In Mandell GL, Douglas RG, Jr, Bennett JE, eds. Principles and Practice of Infectious Diseases, 3rd ed. New York: Churchill Livingstone, 1990; 361–370.

Hoeprich PD, Rinaldi MG. Candidosis. In: Hoeprich PD, Jordan MC. Infectious Diseases, 4th ed. Philadelphia: J.B. Lippincott, 1989;465–481.

CLOXACILLIN

John Rotschafer, Kyle Vance-Bryan, and Rick Zabinski

USA (Cloxapen, Tegopen, parenteral not available)
CANADA (Bactopen, Cloxapen, Novocloxin, Orbenin, Tegopen)

▶ When Should I Use This Drug?

check antibiotic susceptibility chart (Table 4–1 in Chapter 4)

Cellulitis

- drug of choice if staphylococcal and streptococcal organisms are suspected or proved, or if there are no clues as to what organisms are present
- cloxacillin has good activity against staphylococcal and streptococcal organisms and is less expensive than agents such as dicloxacillin and flucloxacillin
- some clinicians suggest adding penicillin to cloxacillin in moderately to severely ill patients; however, this is likely not needed if a high dosage of cloxacillin (2 g IV Q6H) is used
- dicloxacillin produces slightly higher total serum concentrations than does cloxacillin; however, it is more highly protein bound than cloxacillin, and thus at similar dosages, dicloxacillin produces slightly lower free serum concentrations (Br Med J 1970;4:455–460)
- flucloxacillin (not available in USA) produces similar total serum concentrations to dicloxacillin but is less protein bound and produces higher free concentrations than does either cloxacillin or dicloxacillin
- these small differences in pharmacokinetics have never been shown to affect the clinical outcome

Acute or chronic osteomyelitis

- cloxacillin has activity against the most common organisms causing acute or chronic osteomyelitis (staphylococcal and streptococcal organisms)
- is less expensive and less toxic than clindamycin but has to be given more frequently than clindamycin (Q4H versus Q8H)
- combine with gentamicin for high-risk patients (intravenous drug abusers, hemodialysis patients, and patients with underlying debilitating diseases) to cover gram-negative organisms
- combination with metronidazole provides a similar spectrum of activity to clindamycin and can be used if this combination is less expensive than clindamycin

Endocarditis

- drug of choice for endocarditis if caused by methicillin-sensitive *Staphylococcus aureus*
- may actually be superior to vancomycin in terms of outcome and shortened duration of bacteremia

Meningitis

- if infection is proved to be caused by methicillin-sensitive staphylococci

Pneumonia

- if Gram stain shows gram-positive cocci in clusters (*S. aureus*), cloxacillin is the drug of choice for sensitive gram-positive staphylococcal organisms, as it is less expensive than vancomycin and cloxacillin also has good activity against *Streptococcus pneumoniae*, which may be present

▶ When Should I Not Use This Drug?

Empirical treatment of infections proved or presumed to be caused by staphylococci in situations in which the incidence of methicillin-resistant staphylococci is high (>8–10%)

- in these cases, vancomycin should be used as empirical therapy

▶ What Contraindications Are There to the Use of This Drug?

see Penicillin

▶ What Drug Interactions Are Clinically Important?

see Penicillin

▶ What Route and Dosage Should I Use?

How to administer

- orally—take on an empty stomach
- parenterally—administer intravenously in 100 mL of IV fluid (normal saline or 5% dextrose in water) and infuse over 30 minutes

Cellulitis, pneumonia

- 1 g IV Q6H for mild to moderate infections
- 2 g IV Q6H for severe infections
- 250 mg PO Q6H when treating or switching to oral therapy for mild infections
- 500 mg PO Q6H for more serious infections

Endocarditis, meningitis, osteomyelitis

- 2 g IV Q4H

Dosage adjustments for renal or hepatic dysfunction

- renally eliminated and hepatically metabolized, and no dosage adjustments required

▶ What Should I Monitor with Regard to Efficacy and Toxicity?

Efficacy

- for antibiotic administration monitoring guidelines, see specific section on drug therapy

Toxicity

see Ampicillin

▶ How Long Do I Treat Patients with This Drug?

Cellulitis

- usual duration of therapy is 10 days or 4–5 days after the patient has become afebrile and has clinically improved
- consider switching to oral cloxacillin after the patient has become afebrile and has clinically improved for 1–2 days if started on intravenous therapy

Acute or chronic osteomyelitis

- treat patients with at least 4 weeks of parenteral antibiotics after debridement surgery (the duration of therapy is based on the patient's clinical response)
- if an amputation is done proximal to the site of the infection, only prophylactic antibiotics are required (Hosp Formul 1993;28:63–85)
- if the bone is removed and there is still evidence of soft tissue infection, the patient should receive a 2 week course of antibiotics
- treat patients with a prosthetic device for 4–6 weeks with parenteral antibiotics followed by 3–6 months of oral antibiotics
- treat patients with peripheral vascular disease with at least 4 weeks of parenteral antibiotics and follow with oral antibiotics until there is no evidence of inflammation (based on clinical or radiological evidence) (Am J Med 1987;83:653–660)
- duration of parenteral antibiotic therapy prior to switching to oral therapy depends on the patient's clinical response

Endocarditis

- 4 weeks for penicillin-resistant *S. aureus*
- some clinicians suggest that therapy for right-sided *S. aureus* endocarditis be continued for 4 weeks and that left-sided *S. aureus* endocarditis be treated for 4–6 weeks, depending on clinical response (Infect Dis Clin North Am 1993;7:53–68)

Meningitis

- 10 days for shunt infections caused by *S. aureus* or *S. epidermidis* (Infect Dis Clin North Am 1990;4:677–791)

Pneumonia

- oral antibiotics should be considered after the patient has clinically improved and has been afebrile for 48 hours

- if the patient responds rapidly, a 10 day course of therapy is sufficient

▶ How Do I Decrease or Stop the Administration of This Drug?

- may be stopped abruptly

▶ What Should I Tell My Patients About This Drug?

see Penicillin

▶ Therapeutic Tips

- do not use empirically if the probability of methicillin-resistant staphylococcal infection is high (e.g., prosthetic device–related infection, orthopedic surgery, open heart surgery)

see Penicillin

Useful Reference

Wright AJ, Wilkowske CJ. The penicillins. Mayo Clin Proc 1987;62:806–820

CODEINE

Terry Baumann

USA (codeine sulfate and codeine phosphate—various products, combinations: Tylenol with codeine No. 1, No. 2, No. 3, various)
CANADA (codeine sulfate and codeine phosphate—various products, combinations: Tylenol with codeine No. 1, No. 2, No. 3, various)

▶ When Should I Use This Drug?

Acute pain, cancer pain, chronic noncancer pain

- for moderate symptoms if treatment with nonopioid agents (acetaminophen or nonsteroidal antiinflammatory drugs [NSAIDs]) is not effective after titrating rapidly to maximum doses
- use the nonopioid in conjunction with codeine because codeine on its own produces only a weak analgesic effect

Postoperative pain

- after the patient no longer requires regularly dosed medications (e.g., 2–3 days postoperatively), acetaminophen with codeine may be used on an as needed basis or regular basis depending on the patient's need

▶ When Should I Not Use This Drug?

Severe pain

- not very effective for severe pain
- use regularly dosed morphine or other opioid agent for severe pain

Single-therapy or parenteral administration

- codeine on its own is a weak analgesic, and it should be used in combination with aspirin or acetaminophen
- morphine is the opioid of choice for parenteral use

▶ What Contraindications Are There to the Use of This Drug?

Intolerance of or allergic reaction to codeine

- true allergies to codeine are rare
- check that the patient has actual allergic symptoms, and if there is a true allergy, consider meperidine, methadone, or propoxyphene

Severe respiratory depression

- not an absolute contraindication, just start with doses 25% of the normal initial dose and titrate up to an effect while assessing respiratory rate and oxymetry before each dose

▶ What Drug Interactions Are Clinically Important?

see Morphine

▶ What Route and Dosage Should I Use?

How to administer

- orally—may be administered with food or milk or on an empty stomach
- parenterally—not recommended

Acute pain, cancer pain, chronic noncancer pain, postoperative pain

- 30 mg PO Q4H in combination with at least 325 mg of acetaminophen, 300 mg of aspirin, or an NSAID
- use 15 mg of codeine in the elderly
- when using the acetaminophen or aspirin combination for more than 5 days in a round-the-clock fashion be aware of possible acetaminophen or aspirin toxicity

Dosage adjustments for renal or hepatic dysfunction

- hepatically metabolized
- dosage adjustment is usually not required if the dose is titrated properly

▶ What Should I Monitor with Regard to Efficacy and Toxicity?

see Morphine

▶ How Long Do I Treat Patients with This Drug?

see Morphine

- may be used indefinitely on a PRN basis as long as the maximum daily aspirin or acetaminophen dosages are not exceeded

▶ How Do I Decrease or Stop the Administration of This Drug?

see Morphine

▶ What Should I Tell My Patients About This Drug?

see Morphine

▶ Therapeutic Tips

- most effective when used with peripherally acting nonopiate analgesics (acetaminophen or NSAIDs)
- always consider prescribing in conjunction with a laxative and counsel the patient on the appropriate use of fluids and fiber
- do not use parenterally; use morphine
- be aware that, when codeine is used in combination products with acetaminophen or aspirin in a round-the-clock fashion, possible acetaminophen or aspirin toxicity may occur owing to the possible ingestion of large amounts of acetaminophen and/or aspirin

Useful References

see Morphine

COLCHICINE

Wayne Weart

USA (various generic)
CANADA (various generic)

▶ When Should I Use This Drug?

Acute gouty arthritis

- use in patients with a history of heart failure, active peptic ulcer disease, and severe hypertension, as these patients should not take prednisone or nonsteroidal antiinflammatory drugs (NSAIDs)
- indomethacin is the drug of choice for the acute attack, as it is generally better tolerated than colchicine (most patients experience gastrointestinal toxicity when given colchicine) (Aust N Z J Med 1987;17:301–304)
- therapeutic response to colchicine in the absence of synovial fluid examination for sodium urate crystals is suggestive but not necessarily diagnostic of acute gouty arthritis

Prophylaxis of acute gouty arthritis

- low-dose prophylactic therapy should be used in patients with preexisting tophaceous gout, those with a long history of recurrent gouty attacks, or those with significantly elevated serum uric acid levels (>12–13 mg/dL) who are begun on uric acid–lowering therapy to prevent mobilization gout

Prevention of mobilization gout in patients taking allopurinol, probenecid, or sulfinpyrazone

- drug of choice for the prevention of mobilization gout for several months after the initiation of urate-lowering therapy

Familial Mediterranean fever

- is used for both acute abortive and chronic prophylactic therapy of familial Mediterranean fever
- colchicine is the mainstay of therapy in this disease, producing complete remission or a marked reduction in the frequency of attacks in more than 90% of patients (Pharmacotherapy 1991; 11:196–211)

Recurrent pericarditis

- very effective in recurrent steroid- or NSAID-resistant symptomatic pericarditis, regardless of cause (Circulation 1990;82: 117–120)

Cirrhosis of the liver

- improves survival in patients with cirrhosis (N Engl J Med 1988;318:1709–1713)

Other Uses

- Behçet's mucosal ulcers

▶ *When Should I Not Use This Drug?*

Lowering of uric acid levels

- does not lower serum urate levels and should not be used for this purpose

Parenteral use

- parenteral colchicine should not be used owing to its high risk of severe local irritation, central nervous system (CNS) effects, and agranulocytosis

▶ *What Contraindications Are There to the Use of This Drug?*

Intolerance of or allergic reaction to colchicine

Gastrointestinal disease

- patients with preexisting nausea, vomiting, abdominal pain, or diarrhea, as colchicine may worsen these conditions

Renal disease

- avoid long-term use (i.e., longer than for an acute attack) in patients with creatinine clearance less than 60 mL/min or 1 mL/sec

Blood disorders

- avoid in patients with leukopenia, thrombocytopenia, agranulocytosis, or anemia, as colchicine has been reported to cause these conditions rarely

▶ *What Drug Interactions Are Clinically Important?*

Drugs that may increase the effect or toxicity of colchicine

- none

Drugs that may decrease the effect of colchicine

- none

Drugs that may have their effect or toxicity increased by colchicine

CENTRAL NERVOUS SYSTEM DEPRESSANTS

- colchicine may enhance the response to CNS depressants
- may need to decrease dosage of CNS depressants

SYMPATHOMIMETICS

- colchicine may enhance the response to sympathomimetics
- may need to decrease the dosage of sympathomimetic agents

Drugs that may have their effect decreased by colchicine

VITAMIN B$_{12}$

- colchicine may induce reversible malabsorption of vitamin B$_{12}$
- routine monitoring not required
- if signs and symptoms of vitamin B$_{12}$ deficiency develop, assess the vitamin B$_{12}$ level and treat if necessary

▶ *What Route and Dosage Should I Use?*

How to administer

- orally—with food or milk

- parenterally—parenteral colchicine should not be used owing to its high risk of severe local irritation, CNS effects, and agranulocytosis

Acute gouty arthritis

- 1.2 mg PO and repeat every 12 hours until patient gets pain relief, experiences nausea and/or diarrhea, or a total of three 1.2 mg doses have been given
- many clinicans suggest giving 1.2 mg PO followed by 0.6 mg every 1–2 hours until pain relief occurs, gastrointestinal symptoms occur, or a total dose of 7 mg is reached
- however, colchicine does not produce immediate (within 6–12 hours) pain relief and thus all patients will reach, using the every 1–2 hour dosing method, doses at which toxicity will likely occur (Aust NZ J 1987;17:301–304)

Prophylaxis of acute gouty arthritis, prevention of mobilization gout in patients taking allopurinol, probenecid, or sulfinpyrazone

- a dose of 0.6 mg PO daily can be used because of the long duration of activity for colchicine
- if the patient develops symptoms during the prophylactic period while on 0.6 mg PO daily increase the dose to 0.6 mg PO BID

Familial Mediterranean fever

- 0.6 mg PO every hour for 3 doses, followed by 0.6 mg Q2H for 2 doses taken at the onset of symptoms, followed by 0.6 mg PO Q12H for 2 additional days for the acute treatment of Mediterranean fever
- 1–2 mg PO daily (depending on response) for long-term treatment

Recurrent pericarditis

- 1.2 mg PO daily

Cirrhosis of the liver

- 1.2 mg PO daily for 5 d/wk

Dosage adjustments for renal or hepatic dysfunction

- renal and hepatic elimination

Normal Dosing Interval	$C_{cr} > 60$ mL/min or 1 mL/s	C_{cr} 30–60 mL/min or 0.5–1 mL/s	$C_{cr} < 30$ mL/min or 0.5 mL/s
Q24H	no adjustment needed	avoid long-term use	avoid

- decrease the dosage by 50% in patients with hepatic disease

▶ *What Should I Monitor with Regard to Efficacy and Toxicity?*

Efficacy

Acute gouty arthritis

- typically produces symptomatic improvement in acute gouty arthritis within 12–16 hours and complete resolution within 48–72 hours

Prophylaxis of acute gouty arthritis

Number of attacks

- number of acute gouty attacks should decrease

Prevention of mobilization gout in patients taking allopurinol, probenecid, or sulfinpyrazone

- frequency of acute attacks decreased

Familial Mediterranean fever

- acute episodes of familial Mediterranean fever typically respond to colchicine after 4 or 5 doses
- typically produces a marked (90%) reduction in the frequency and severity of familial Mediterranean fever

Recurrent pericarditis

- suppression of symptoms and reduced frequency of recurrence

Cirrhosis of the liver

- signs and symptoms of hepatic cirrhosis

Toxicity

Gastrointestinal symptoms (nausea, vomiting, and/or diarrhea)

- colchicine administration should be discontinued if these symptoms occur and should not be reinstituted for at least 24–48 hours after symptoms disappear

Severe local irritation or thrombophlebitis

- colchicine is irritating to tissues if extravasation occurs
- infuse as a dilute solution over at least 5 minutes

Bone marrow depression

- colchicine may cause agranulocytosis, thrombocytopenia, leukopenia, and/or aplastic anemia with prolonged use of higher doses; therefore, aim for the minimum effective doses that prevent recurrences
- monitor complete blood count at baseline and remeasure if toxicity is suspected

Peripheral neuritis, purpura, hair loss, myopathy, and reversible azoospermia

- drug has been reported to cause these symptoms, but no special monitoring is required

▶ How Long Do I Treat Patients with This Drug?

Acute gouty arthritis

- until symptomatic relief is obtained, gastrointestinal toxicity occurs, or a total of 3.6 mg of oral colchicine is given
- at any of these endpoints, no further colchicine is recommended for the next week

Prophylaxis of acute gouty arthritis

- use colchicine for 12 months if the patient had a uric acid level of 12–13 mg/dL (700 μmol/L) or greater and tophi, and stop after this time if the uric acid level has been decreased and no attacks have occurred
- use colchicine for 3–6 months if the serum uric acid level is less than 12 mg/dL and there are no tophi

Prevention of mobilization gout in patients taking allopurinol, probenecid, or sulfinpyrazone

- discontinue after serum uric acid concentrations have been in the desired range for 3 months

Familial Mediterranean fever

- indefinitely to prevent amyloidosis (N Engl J Med 1986;314: 1001–1005)

Recurrent pericarditis

- present experience is to give for 1–2 years and then to try drug withdrawal
- if recurrence happens, reinstitute therapy

Cirrhosis of the liver

- indefinitely

▶ How Do I Decrease or Stop the Administration of This Drug?

- may be stopped abruptly

▶ What Should I Tell My Patients About This Drug?

- stop taking this medicine as soon as the pain is almost gone or at the first sign of nausea, vomiting, stomach pain, or diarrhea
- do not drink alcoholic beverages while taking this medication
- keep out of the reach of children, as this can be very toxic to young children

▶ Therapeutic Tips

- initial total acute dose should not exceed 3.6 mg to minimize adverse effects
- there is a delay in its effect (12–48 hours), and therefore, do not be impatient and overdose the patient
- this drug has a long duration of action and, for chronic therapy, dosing more frequently than once daily is not required

Useful References

Paulus HE, Schlosstein LH, Godfrey RG, et al. Prophylactic colchicine therapy of intercritical gout. Arthritis Rheum 1974;17:609–614

Wallace SL, Singer JZ. Treatment. In: Primer on Rheumatic Diseases, 9th ed. Atlanta: Arthritis Foundation, 1988:202–206

Wallace SL, Singer ZS. Review: Systemic toxicity associated with the intravenous administration of colchicine—Guidelines for use. J Rheumatol 1988;15:495–499

Levy M, Spino M, Read SE. Colchicine: A state of the art review. Pharmacotherapy 1991;11:196–211

Zemer D, Pras M, Sohar E, et al. Colchicine in the prevention and treatment of the amyloidosis of familial Mediterranean fever. N Engl J Med 1986;314:1001–1005

COLESTIPOL

Stephen Shalansky and Robert Dombrowski

USA (Colestid)
CANADA (Colestid)

▶ When Should I Use This Drug?

Hypercholesterolemia

- bile acid sequestrants are recommended (assuming they are tolerated) if HMG-CoA reductase inhibitors are ineffective or not tolerated as bile acid sequestrants have proven efficacy and safety in the reduction of cardiovascular disease and cardiovascular mortality
- choose the least expensive of either cholestyramine (4 g dose) or colestipol (5 g dose) as these agents are equally effective and equally tolerated
- cholestyramine and colestipol are equally efficacious at lowering total and LDL cholesterol levels, and therefore, the choice is based on cost and convenience of administration

Mixed hyperlipidemias

- bile acid sequestrants raise triglyceride levels and are therefore not particularly useful as a single agent for this indication
- may be used in combination with gemfibrozil or niacin, particularly in patients who experience myositis with the combination of gemfibrozil and lovastatin

▶ When Should I Not Use This Drug?

Hypertriglyceridemia

- bile acid sequestrants may cause a further elevation in triglyceride levels
- niacin or gemfibrozil can be used in these patients

▶ What Contraindications Are There to the Use of This Drug?

- intolerance of or allergic reaction to colestipol

see Cholestyramine

▶ What Drug Interactions Are Clinically Important?

see Cholestyramine

▶ What Route and Dosage Should I Use?

How to administer

- orally—give with food, as food stimulates the release of bile
- parenterally—not available

Hypercholesterolemia, mixed hyperlipidemias

- 2.5 g (^{1}/$_2$ packet) of colestipol PO daily initially and titrate up every 2–3 days by 2.5 g PO daily until 5 g PO BID is reached, as this may increase tolerability
- give the 5 g PO BID with breakfast and the evening meal
- increase the dosage to 15 g PO daily (5 g PO in the morning and 10 g with the evening meal) if inadequate response occurs in 4 weeks
- continue to increase the dosage by 5 g (1 packet) per week up to a maximum dose of 30 g/d (15 g in the morning and 15 g with the evening meal); however, be aware that most patients do not tolerate daily dosages greater than 20 g
- remeasure serum lipid levels at 3 months

- if after 3 months a 15% decrease in LDL or total cholesterol levels is achieved, but the target LDL level is not reached, consider adding another drug (e.g., lovastatin)
- if after 3 months there is less than a 15% decrease in LDL or total cholesterol level or the patient is not tolerating the drug (e.g., because of gastrointestinal side effects), change drugs

Dosage adjustments for renal or hepatic dysfunction

- not absorbed orally; therefore, no dosage adjustments required

▶ *What Should I Monitor with Regard to Efficacy and Toxicity?*

see Cholestyramine

▶ *How Long Do I Treat Patients with This Drug?*

see Cholestyramine

▶ *How Do I Decrease or Stop the Administration of This Drug?*

- may be stopped abruptly

▶ *What Should I Tell My Patients About This Drug?*

see Cholestyramine

▶ *Therapeutic Tips*

see Cholestyramine

Useful References

see Cholestyramine

CROMOLYN

Karen Shalansky and Cindy Reesor Nimmo

USA (Intal)
CANADA (Sodium Cromoglycate, Intal)

▶ *When Should I Use This Drug?*

Chronic asthma

- minimal antiinflammatory activity in comparison with that of high-dose inhaled corticosteroids
- use only in patients taking appropriate doses of beta$_2$-agonist and inhaled corticosteroids who are experiencing major side effects
- in many cases, cromolyn for the treatment of chronic asthma in the adult population is ineffective

Exercise-induced asthma

- use as a prophylactic agent when salbutamol is not effective or well tolerated
- is as effective (for prevention, not acute treatment) as salbutamol but is more expensive

Seasonal asthma

- cromolyn should be tried first in patients with intermittent asthma due to allergen exposure because it is effective and has virtually no side effects

▶ *When Should I Not Use This Drug?*

Acute asthma

- has no value and may exacerbate attack through throat and bronchial irritation

▶ *What Contraindications Are There to the Use of This Drug?*

- intolerance of or allergic reaction to cromolyn

▶ *What Drug Interactions Are Clinically Important?*

- none

▶ *What Route and Dosage Should I Use?*

How to administer

- orally—not useful for asthma

- inhaled—see What Should I Tell My Patients About This Drug? (below)
- parenteral—not available

Chronic asthma

- 2 mg (1 mg per puff of metered-dose inhaler) inhaled QID until the patient is stabilized
- 20 mg of powder (1 capsule in spinhaler) inhaled QID until the patient is stabilized
- choice of inhalers is based on the patient's preference and cost
- 3–6 weeks of therapy are required to achieve maximum effect; however, a significant effect may be seen within 2 weeks
- after adequate response has been obtained it may be possible to reduce the dosage to TID or BID
- 20 mg (1 ampule in a nebulizer) inhaled QID (use only when metered-dose inhaler or spinhaler cannot be used)

Exercise-induced asthma

- inhale 1–2 puffs about 10 minutes prior to exercise

Seasonal asthma

- prophylaxis should be initiated 1 week prior to and continued throughout the anticipated allergen season
- 2 mg inhaled QID via a metered-dose inhaler
- 20 mg inhaled QID via a spinhaler

▶ *What Should I Monitor with Regard to Efficacy and Toxicity?*

Efficacy

see Budesonide

Toxicity

- low incidence of toxicity (approximately 2%)

Irritant bronchospasm

- easily treated with an inhaled beta$_2$-agonist

Rash

- urticaria

▶ *How Long Do I Treat Patients with This Drug?*

Chronic asthma

- therapy may be required indefinitely; however, consider dosage tapering every 6–12 months and possible withdrawal, depending on the severity of the asthma
- long-term treatment is indicated if therapy results in a significant decrease in the severity of the asthma, a reduction or discontinuation of corticosteroid usage, or substitution for another drug with intolerable side effects

Exercise-induced asthma

- use just prior to exercise

Seasonal asthma

- continue therapy for the duration of allergen exposure

▶ *How Do I Decrease or Stop the Administration of This Drug?*

- treatment should not be discontinued abruptly, as a return of symptoms may occur
- dosage should be progressively reduced over a period of 1 week (decrease the daily dose by 1 puff every couple of days)

▶ *What Should I Tell My Patients About This Drug?*

- cromolyn is used to prevent bronchospasm (it does not relieve an attack that has already started and may make the attack worse)
- if you are using a bronchodilator inhaler, use the bronchodilator first
- compliance with regular therapy is essential to maintain control of asthma—use cromolyn exactly as directed
- side effects are uncommon—throat irritation or dryness of the mouth may occur—gargling or rinsing the mouth after each dose may alleviate these side effects

- cough due to throat irritation may be prevented by taking several short breaths rather than one large breath when inhaling the powder form of cromolyn
- notify your physician if you have skin rash, troubled breathing, or dizziness

Spinhaler

1. hold the spinhaler upright with the mouthpiece pointing down—unscrew the body
2. ensure that the propeller is on its spindle—insert a Spincap with the colored end down into the cup of the propeller—screw the body back onto the mouthpiece
3. while still holding the inhaler upright, slide the gray sleeve down as far as it will go and then back up again to pierce the capsule
4. exhale to a normal relaxed expiration, then place the mouthpiece between the teeth and lips
5. tilt your head back and breathe in deeply—hold your breath for 10 seconds—breathe out slowly to a normal relaxed resting position
6. keep repeating the process until the Spincap is empty
7. keep your spinhaler clean—brush off any remaining powder

Metered-dose inhaler

1. place the canister firmly into the outer shell
2. shake well; remove the cap
3. exhale to a normal relaxed expiration
4. place the tip of the mouthpiece—either 2 fingerbreadths in front of widely opened mouth or between the teeth and lips
5. breathe in slowly, and at the same time, press the canister to release 1 puff of the drug
6. continue to inhale as deeply as possible—hold your breath for as long as is comfortable (5–10 seconds)
7. breathe out to a normal relaxed resting position
8. if a second inhalation is prescribed, the same procedure is repeated with the second puff, 30 seconds after the first

▶ Therapeutic Tips

- after long-term therapy, bronchial hyperreactivity is reduced
- drug must be used prophylactically—the best results are obtained if therapy is started 1 week prior to anticipated allergen exposure
- drug deposition in the lungs is dependent on airway patency—concomitant beta$_2$-agonist or corticosteroids may be required prior to achieving a response to cromolyn
- is as efficacious as theophylline but has fewer side effects
- may permit a reduction in corticosteroid dosage in steroid-dependent patients
- in general, this agent is more effective for children than adults

Useful References

Murphy S, Kelly HW. Cromolyn sodium: A review of mechanisms and clinical use in asthma. DICP 1987;21:22–35

Bernstein IL. Cromolyn sodium in the treatment of asthma: Coming of age in the United States. J Allergy Clin Immunol 1985;76:381–388

CYCLOPHOSPHAMIDE

Kelly Jones

USA (Cytoxan, Neosar)
CANADA (Cytoxan, Procytox)

▶ When Should I Use This Drug?

Rheumatoid arthritis

- because of the toxicity associated with cyclophosphamide, this agent should be reserved as a last line for those who have failed to respond to other disease-modifying therapies or those with refractory and progressive disease or patients with serious systemic complications such as rheumatoid vasculitis (Med Clin North Am 1985;69:817–835)

▶ When Should I Not Use This Drug?

Uncomplicated rheumatoid arthritis

- there are other agents available that are effective and less toxic

▶ What Contraindications Are There to the Use of This Drug?

Intolerance of or allergic reaction to cyclophosphamide
Severe bone marrow suppression

- high risk of severe bone marrow toxicity

Patients wishing to become pregnant

- counsel patients about proper contraception (both partners)

▶ What Drug Interactions Are Clinically Important?

- none

▶ What Route and Dosage Should I Use?

How to administer

- orally—best taken on an empty stomach, but if gastrointestinal intolerance occurs, take with meals
- parenterally—available but only for oncological uses

Rheumatoid arthritis

- give 1 mg/kg PO daily and increase to 2 mg/kg PO daily after 6 weeks
- in patients who respond to therapy, decrease the dosage by 25 mg/mo to the lowest effective maintenance level (Clin Pharm 1987;6:475–491)

Dosage adjustments for renal or hepatic dysfunction

- hepatic metabolism

Normal Dosing Interval	C_{cr} > 60 mL/min or 1 mL/s	C_{cr} 30–60 mL/min or 0.5–1 mL/s	C_{cr} < 30 mL/min or 0.5 mL/s
Q24H	no adjustment needed	no dosage adjustment	decrease dosage by 50%

▶ What Should I Monitor with Regard to Efficacy and Toxicity?

Efficacy

Rheumatoid arthritis

Joint tenderness count, sedimentation rate measurements, grip strength, duration of morning stiffness, time to onset of fatigue, and patient's report on specific functions

- patient should be assessed monthly for the first 2 months, and after the symptoms are under control, the patient can be assessed every 3 months for 6 months and then every 6 months
- these variables should be used to guide drug administration initiation and discontinuation
- one study found that clinical and laboratory measures of physical well-being appeared to be unrelated to psychological and social measures of well-being (J Rheumatol 1991;18:650–653)
- it is important to include the patient's self-assessment of the drug's effect on ability to function and well-being

Toxicity

Hemorrhagic cystitis (13–28%)

- presents as dysuria or hematuria
- take the drug in the morning with large amounts of water to stimulate frequent emptying of the bladder throughout the day
- stop drug administration if hematuria or mild dysuria occurs, and it usually resolves spontaneously within a few days
- medical (bladder irrigation) or surgical support may be needed in protracted cases
- urinalysis should be done every 2 weeks during the initial dosing, then every month after the dosage is stable

Hematological effects

- do baseline complete blood count and platelet count initially, then weekly for 2 months, then every 2 weeks for 2 months, and then every month for the duration of treatment
- discontinue the drug administration if the leukocyte count is less than 3500/mm^3, the granulocyte count is less than 1000/mm^3, or the platelet count decreases to less than 100,000/mm^3

Hepatotoxicity

- biliary stasis, jaundice, and portal hypertension
- perform baseline liver enzyme determination and repeat monthly
- discontinue cyclophosphamide administration if levels rise to greater than 3 times baseline

Pulmonary fibrosis

- cyclophosphamide administration should be stopped immediately and the patient treated with supportive care and corticosteroids if a persistent otherwise unexplained nonproductive dry cough occurs
- do yearly chest X-ray (no data on value, but is strongly recommended) (Ann Intern Med 1987;107:358–366)

Alopecia

- reversible after the drug administration is discontinued

Sterility

- drug interferes with oogenesis and spermatogenesis, and sterility may be irreversible (JAMA 1988;259:2446–2449, Clin Pharm 1987;6:475–491)

▶ *How Long Do I Treat Patients with This Drug?*

Rheumatoid arthritis

- stop the drug if there is no response by 4 months
- treatment with this agent is indefinite, but studies show that toxicity is the limiting factor
- treat only if the patient is getting benefit from the drug

▶ *How Do I Decrease or Stop the Administration of This Drug?*

- may be stopped abruptly

▶ *What Should I Tell My Patients About This Drug?*

- use proper contraception (both partners)
- drug is best taken on an empty stomach, but take it with meals if gastrointestinal intolerance occurs
- report any unusual bleeding, headaches, sore throats, unusual lumps or masses, stomach pain, yellow skin, sores in mouth, and darkened urine to your physician
- always make sure to keep follow-up appointments for close monitoring

Useful References

Pugh MC, Pugh CB. Current concepts in clinical therapeutics: Disease-modifying drugs for rheumatoid arthritis. Clin Pharm 1987;6:475–491

Weinblatt ME, Maier AL. Newer immunosuppressive therapies for rheumatoid arthritis. Crit Care Med 1990;18:S126–S131

Wilder RL. Treatment of the patient with rheumatoid arthritis refractory to standard therapy. JAMA 1988;259:2446–2449

CYCLOSPORINE

Nilufar Partovi

USA (Sandimmune)
CANADA (Sandimmune)

▶ *When Should I Use This Drug?*

Transplantation

- cyclosporine has dramatically improved graft and patient survival after organ transplantation (N Engl J Med 1989;321:1725–1738)
- it is used for prophylaxis of rejection either as monotherapy or in combination with 1 or 2 other immunosuppressive agents such as steroids and/or azathioprine
- cyclosporine is also indicated for prophylaxis and treatment of graft versus host disease in bone marrow transplant patients

Rheumatoid arthritis, inflammatory bowel disease

- cyclosporine is nephrotoxic and should be used only when all else fails
- there is little question of its efficacy, but toxicity of the drug (nephrotoxicity) precludes general use (Crit Care Med 1990;18:S126–S131)

Uveitis, Behçet's syndrome, insulin-dependent diabetes mellitus, psoriasis, polymyositis, systemic lupus erythematosus, primary aplastic anemia, idiopathic thrombocytopenia

- cyclosporine use in these autoimmune diseases remains experimental because of its nephrotoxic effects and the relatively immediate relapses that occur after discontinuation of therapy

▶ *When Should I Not Use This Drug?*

Risk of toxicities from cyclosporine outweighs its benefit

- when there is a previous history of intolerance of cyclosporine, the patient has decreased renal function, or the patient is taking other drugs that may increase the risk of cyclosporine toxicities

▶ *What Contraindications Are There to the Use of This Drug?*

Intolerance of or allergic reaction to cyclosporine or polyoxyethylated castor oil

- intravenous formulation of cyclosporine contains Cremophor-EL (polyoxyethylated castor oil)

▶ *What Drug Interactions Are Clinically Important?*

Drugs that may increase the effect or toxicity of cyclosporine

ERYTHROMYCIN, FLUCONAZOLE, KETOCONAZOLE, ITRACONAZOLE, DILTIAZEM, VERAPAMIL, NICARDIPINE, DOXYCYCLINE, MELPHALAN, DANAZOL, METHYLTESTOSTERONE, ORAL CONTRACEPTIVES
(Clin Pharmacokinet 1990;19:319–332, 400–415)

- inhibit hepatic metabolism of cyclosporine
- seen as early as 2 days after the start of the administration of these drugs
- use an alternative if possible (e.g., nifedipine does not interact)
- monitor cyclosporine levels every other day until the full extent of interaction is seen and adjust the dosage accordingly
- may need to decrease the cyclosporine dosage by 30% or more

Drugs that may decrease the effect of cyclosporine

PHENYTOIN, PHENOBARBITAL, CARBAMAZEPINE, PRIMIDONE, RIFAMPIN, ETHAMBUTOL, ISONIAZID

- induce hepatic metabolism of cyclosporine
- cyclosporine levels are markedly reduced; this is usually seen 2–4 days after the start of administration of the interacting drugs
- if possible, use an alternative agent such as valproic acid, as it does not interact with cyclosporine
- monitor cyclosporine levels every other day until the full extent of the interaction is seen and adjust the dosage accordingly
- may need to increase the cyclosporine dosage by 30% or more

SULFAMETHOXAZOLE AND/OR TRIMETHOPRIM (MAINLY WITH PARENTERAL ADMINISTRATION)

- monitor cyclosporine levels twice a week until the full extent of the interaction is seen and adjust the dosage accordingly (Br Med J 1986;292:728–729, Lancet 1983;1:366–367)

Drugs that may have their effect or toxicity increased by cyclosporine
AMINOGLYCOSIDES, AMPHOTERICIN B

- increased risk of nephrotoxicity
- avoid combination if possible
- no change in monitoring frequency of serum creatinine level; just be aware of the potential for toxicity

NONSTEROIDAL ANTIINFLAMMATORY DRUGS

- increased risk of nephrotoxicity
- avoid combination if possible
- monitor serum creatinine levels once weekly until stable

HMG CoA REDUCTASE INHIBITORS

- cyclosporine may decrease the metabolism of these agents
- avoid concurrent use if possible; however, if these agents must be used together, start with a low dose (i.e., ½ of the normal starting dose) and evaluate for effect and toxicities such as myalgias, myopathies, and rhabdomyolysis

DIGOXIN

- cyclosporine can produce an increase in digoxin serum concentrations
- while no empiric changes need to be made, clinicians should be aware of the interaction and if the patient develops signs and symptoms of digoxin toxicity a serum digoxin concentration should be measured and the dose adjusted accordingly

▶ *What Route and Dosage Should I Use?*

How to administer

Orally
- available in liquid form and capsules; the liquid can be mixed in juice or milk

Parenterally
- continuous IV infusion over 24 hours at concentration of 0.5–2.5 mg/mL in 5% dextrose in water or normal saline
- intermittent IV administration over 4 hours (depending on the patient's tolerance, may need to change the rate to 6 hours)
- intermittent IV administration is used when it is not possible to administer the drug as a continuous IV infusion (not enough IV access for all medications or compatibility problems)

Transplantation

Kidney transplant
- starting dose is 3 mg/kg/d IV as a continuous infusion until the patient can take oral medication
- starting oral dose is 10 mg/kg/d
- when the patient is able to take oral medications, switch to the oral form (capsule or solution) at a dosage of 10 mg/kg/d or 3 times the IV dose
- adjust the dosage on the basis of cyclosporine levels (see below)

Liver transplant
- starting dose is 3 mg/kg/d IV as a continuous infusion over 24 hours
- in the initial postoperative period, the absorption of cyclosporine from the intestine is unreliable owing to external bile drainage (i.e., through the T tube)
- keep the patient on IV cyclosporine therapy while there is external bile drainage, and after the external drainage has stopped (i.e., T tube is clamped), switch the patient to oral cyclosporine at a dosage 3 times the IV dose
- adjust the dosage on the basis of cyclosporine levels (see below)

Heart or lung transplant
- starting dosage is 2 mg/kg PO BID initiated on day 4 or 5 after transplantation in patients that are on OKT3
- if patient is not receiving OKT3 then start with 3 mg/kg/d IV as a continuous infusion over 2–4 hours started immediately postoperatively
- the dose is considerably lower in heart or heart-lung transplant patients owing to the high incidence of oliguria and renal failure in the postoperative period
- increase the dosage on the basis of the cyclosporine level
- the goal is to reach the therapeutic range by day 10

Bone marrow transplant
- initial dose is 4 mg/kg/d IV as a continuous infusion over 24 hours
- then titrate the dose to levels of 400–500 μg/L
- because treatment of established acute graft versus host disease is unsatisfactory, most bone marrow transplant centers are aiming for higher levels than for other types of transplants

Rheumatoid arthritis
- start with 5 mg/kg/d PO divided into 2 doses
- decrease the dosage by 50% if hypertension or nephrotoxicity develops
- some patients have been more successfully treated with 3 mg/kg/d (Crit Care Med 1990;18:132–137)

Uveitis
- 8–10 mg/kg/d PO

Psoriasis
- 3 mg/kg/d PO

Behçet's syndrome, insulin-dependent diabetes mellitus, polymyositis, systemic lupus erythematosus, primary aplastic anemia, idiopathic thrombocytopenia
- 4 mg/kg/d PO and increase to higher dosages if required

Dosage adjustments for renal or hepatic dysfunction
- hepatically metabolized
- in severe hepatic dysfunction (e.g., 2–3 times the normal values for liver function test results) start the patients with ½ of the normal dose and adjust the dosage according to level of cyclosporine

▶ *What Should I Monitor with Regard to Efficacy and Toxicity?*

Efficacy

Transplantation

Signs and symptoms of rejection
- rejection is a major cause of morbidity and mortality in solid organ transplant patients
- occurrence of rejection is frequent early after transplantation and diminishes after a year post-transplantation
- there are two types of rejection: acute (onset at 5–7 days) and chronic (ongoing rejection; many years after transplantation)
- signs and symptoms common to all transplant types are fever, malaise, and leukocytosis
- most accurate method of diagnosing rejection is graft biopsy
- refer to the accompanying table for more specific clinical characteristics

Transplant Type	Acute Rejection	Chronic Rejection
kidney	rapid increase in serum creatinine level graft tenderness decreased urine output fluid retention blood in urine renal scan: decreased renal blood flow	gradual increase in serum creatinine level gradual decrease in function
liver	increased aminotransferase, alkaline phosphatase, and bilirubin levels light-colored stools jaundice upper right quadrant pain	intimal proliferation marked fibrosis disappearance of bile ducts
heart	ventricular gallop rhythm electrocardiographic changes arrhythmias congestive heart failure	atherosclerosis or coronary artery disease
lung	chest X-ray changes shortness of breath change in lung function test results	restrictive ventilatory defect
pancreas	change in glucose control change in C peptide levels decrease in amylase concentration	

Cyclosporine levels
- can be measured in serum, plasma, or whole blood
- serum and plasma levels provide a better index of concentration at the site of action; however, concentrations vary depending on temperature, hematocrit, and lipoprotein concentration, and sample preparation is required
- whole blood provides higher concentrations, greater analytical precision, and more metabolites; concentration depends on hematocrit; and less preparation time is required

- several assays are available for measuring cyclosporine: high-performance liquid chromatography (HPLC), radioimmunoassay (RIA), and fluorescence polarization immunoassay (FPIA)
- HPLC is specific to parent cyclosporine, is adaptable to measure metabolites, is sensitive, is expensive, requires extensive sample preparation, and is slow, and other substances interfere
- RIA is simple, fast, and inexpensive, but there is cross-reactivity with metabolites
- RIA analysis can involve either polyclonal or monoclonal antibodies to cyclosporine
- antibodies react to specific sites on the cyclosporine molecule and, depending on the concentration, vary the absorbance (polyclonal method has higher cross-reactivity with cyclosporine metabolites than does monoclonal technique [30% versus <2%])
- FPIA is simple, efficient, and quick; has minimal error; and is reliable, but some cross-reactivity with metabolites occurs (comparable to the case with RIA)

Therapeutic monitoring

- steady state cyclosporine trough levels should be measured every other day for the first 2 weeks after transplantation or until the patient's clinical condition and cyclosporine concentrations are stable
- thereafter, cyclosporine concentrations are generally measured once a week for the first month and then monthly for the first year after transplantation
- steady state levels occur 36–48 hours after starting therapy or after dosage changes
- blood samples for cyclosporine levels should be taken just prior to the morning dose of cyclosporine, and levels should be taken at the same time each day to eliminate variability from the diurnal rhythm of cyclosporine elimination

Desired cyclosporine levels (monoclonal radioimmunoassay whole blood assay)

Kidney transplant

Time Posttransplant (d)	Target Cyclosporine Level (μg/L)
0–28	350–450
28–60	250–350
60–90	150–250
90–180	100–200
>180	75–125

Liver, heart, or lung transplant

Time Posttransplant	Target Cyclosporine Level (μg/L)
14–120 d	350–450
120–180 d	300–350
180–270 d	250–300
270–365 d	200–250
12–18 (mo)	150–200
>18 mo	100–200

Bone marrow transplant

- target cyclosporine level is 400–500 μg/L (depending on the patient's tolerability)
- some patients may not tolerate these levels and the trough may need to be kept at approximately 200 μg/L (Transplantation 1984;38:511–513)

Autoimmune disease

- ranges for cyclosporine have been less clearly defined in autoimmunity and appear to vary according to the nature and activity of disease

Dosage adjustments

- if the level is within 25 μg/L of the target range, do not adjust the dosage and repeat the level in 1 week
- if the level is within 25–50 μg/L of the target range, increase or

decrease the oral dosage by 25 mg/dose, respectively, and recheck the level in 48 hours
- if the level is within 50–100 μg/L of the target range, increase or decrease the oral dosage by 50 mg/dose, respectively, and recheck the level in 48 hours

Rheumatoid arthritis

Joint tenderness count, sedimentation rate measurements, grip strength, duration of morning stiffness, time to onset of fatigue, and patient's report on specific functions

- patient should be assessed monthly for the first 2 months, and after the disease is under control, the patient can be assessed every 3 months for 6 months and then every 6 months
- these variables should be used to guide administration starting and stopping
- one study found that clinical and laboratory measures of physical well-being appeared to be unrelated to psychological and social measures of well-being (J Rheumatol 1991;18:650–653)
- it is important to include the patient's self-assessment of the drug's effect on their function and well-being

Toxicity

Most patients experience one or more cyclosporine toxicities (nephrotoxicity, neurotoxicity, hepatotoxicity) after 1 year of therapy (Crit Care Med 1990;18:S126–S131)

Paresthesias, confusion, hallucinations, and convulsions

- are dose related and usually disappear by lowering the dosage by 25–50 mg and observing for decreased signs of toxicities

Gum hyperplasia

- effects can be minimized by good oral hygiene (frequent cleaning, flossing, gum massage with toothbrush)

Hypertension

- 13–26% occurrence and if it occurs, decrease the dosage (DICP, Ann Pharmacother 1988;22:443–451)
- may necessitate therapy with multiple antihypertensive agents
- calcium channel blockers are considered the drug choice for treatment of cyclosporine-induced hypertension in transplant patients
- nifedipine has been associated with a beneficial effect on cyclosporine nephrotoxicity in both retrospective and prospective studies, and it does not interact with cyclosporine
- beta-blockers or angiotensin converting enzyme inhibitors may also be added if necessary

Nephrotoxicity

- serum creatinine and blood urea nitrogen levels are monitored daily for first 2 weeks after transplantation
- for the next month, the renal function is monitored once to twice weekly, depending on the patient's progress
- it is difficult to differentiate cyclosporine nephrotoxicity from organ rejection in kidney transplant patients, but several clinical criteria can be used
- rejection is suspected if the following are present: sudden increase in serum creatinine level, fever, graft tenderness or swelling, decreased urinary output, renal scan that shows decreased blood flow, biopsy that shows diffuse infiltrate, low cyclosporine level, decreased hematocrit
- cyclosporine nephrotoxicity is suspected if the following are present: a gradual increase in serum creatinine level, absence of fever, nontender graft, normal urinary output, renal scan that shows a normal blood flow, biopsy that shows local infiltrate, high cyclosprorine level, and no change in hematocrit

Hepatotoxicity

- liver function test results should be monitored twice weekly for the first 2 weeks after transplantation and then weekly for the first posttransplant month
- is noted as an increase in both total and direct bilirubin levels
- hepatotoxicity rapidly reverses with dosage reduction
- usually occurs in the first month of therapy

Hypomagnesemia

- monitor magnesium levels twice weekly for the first 2 weeks after transplantation
- add a magnesium supplement if hypomagnesemia develops

Hyperkalemia
- monitor potassium levels 3 times a week for the first 2 weeks after transplantation
- if the serum potassium level is greater than 6 mEq/L, give sodium polystyrene sulfonate 15–30 g with 30 mL of 70% sorbitol

Tremor
- lower the dosage by 25 mg if the patient cannot tolerate tremor, and observe for any changes in tremor

Acne, hirsutism
- is not dose related, and antiacne medications or other cosmetic treatment may be needed
- 30–45% incidence

Leukopenia
- rare
- measure baseline complete blood count and platelet count initially, then weekly for 2 months, then every 2 weeks for 2 months, and then every month for the duration of treatment
- stop cyclosporine administration if the leukocyte count is less than 3500/mm³, the granulocyte count is less than 1000/mm³, or the platelet count decreases to less than 100,000/mm³
- drug therapy can be restarted at 50–75% of the previous dosage after blood counts have recovered (usually 3 weeks) (Clin Pharm 1987;6:475–491)

▶ How Long Do I Treat Patients with This Drug?

Transplantation

Kidney transplant
- for as long as the patient has the transplanted kidney

Liver transplant or heart or lung transplant
- for as long as the patient is alive

Bone marrow transplant
- for 100–180 days after transplantation
- duration of treatment is determined by the degree and severity of graft versus host disease

Rheumatoid arthritis
- treatment is indefinite, but studies show that toxicity is the limiting factor

Uveitis, Behçet's syndrome, insulin-dependent diabetes mellitus, psoriasis, polymyositis, systemic lupus erythematosus, primary aplastic anemia, idiopathic thrombocytopenia
- depending on the disease course and the patient's tolerance

▶ How Do I Decrease or Stop the Administration of This Drug?
- significant disease rebound has occurred on abrupt withdrawal of cyclosporine therapy; therefore, taper the dosage down if toxicity allows
- there are no rules of thumb on how to taper cyclosporine (Crit Care Med 1990;18:S126–S131)

▶ What Should I Tell My Patients About This Drug?

Steps in administering oral cyclosporine solution
- using the supplied measuring pipette, draw up the correct volume of solution by pulling the plunger up to the correct value
- pointing the tip up, remove any excess air from the pipette
- recheck to ensure that the correct amount has been measured
- transfer the solution into a glass half filled with juice or milk at room temperature
- mix and drink immediately
- rinse the glass with more juice or milk and drink (this is to ensure that the full dose is taken)
- dry the outside of the pipette and return it to its protective cover

Points to remember
- always use the same diluent
- do not contaminate the pipette by placing it in the diluting fluid
- do not rinse the pipette
- always use a glass (not plastic or Styrofoam)

- store the solution at room temperature (below 30°C [86°F])
- after the container has been opened, the contents must be used within 2 months
- use proper contraception (both partners)
- when using cyclosporine, do not use oral contraceptives because oral contraceptives can increase the concentration of cyclosporine; use a barrier method

▶ Therapeutic Tips
- cyclosporine capsules contain 12% alcohol, and using concurrent medications known to interact with alcohol (e.g., metronidazole and disulfiram) may cause an adverse reaction
- liquid form is formulated in an olive oil vehicle and must be diluted in either milk or juice before administration
- injectable form is never given via direct IV injection

Useful References

Beveridge T. Pharmacokinetics and metabolism of cyclosporine A. In: White DJG, ed. Cyclosporine A. Oxford: Elsevier Biomedical, 1982:36–44

Buonpane E. Therapeutic drug monitoring of cyclosporine. (Drug information update: Hartford Hospital.) Connecticut Med 1990;54(1):17–19

Burckart GJ, Venkataramanan R, Ptachchinski R. Cyclosporine. In: Taylor WJ, Caviness MHD, eds. A Textbook for the Clinical Application of Therapeutic Drug Monitoring. Irving, TX: Abbott Laboratories, Diagnostics Division, 1986:339–351

Kahan BD, Grevel J. Optimization of cyclosporine therapy in renal transplantion by a pharmacokinetics strategy. Transplantation 1988;46:631–644

Keown PA. Clinical application of therapeutic drug monitoring: Optimizing cyclosporine therapy: Dose, levels, and monitoring. Transplant Proc, 1988;20(suppl 2):382–389

Rodighiero V. Therapeutic drug monitoring of cyclosporine. Clin Pharmacokinet 1989;16:27–37

CYPROHEPTADINE

Jerry Taylor

USA (Periactin)
CANADA (Periactin, Vimicon)

▶ When Should I Use This Drug?
Consider an alternative agent
- cyproheptadine is considered useful in the prophylaxis and treatment of vascular headaches and migraines for children, but troublesome side effects, such as sedation, limit its use in adults
- therapeutic response with this drug is often unpredictable and frequently less than satisfactory (Headache 1977;17:61–63)

DANTHRON

Leslie Mathews

USA (not available)
CANADA (combination: Doss, Regulex-D)

▶ When Should I Use This Drug?
Consider an alternative agent
- danthron was withdrawn in the USA by the manufacturer in 1987 because intestinal and hepatic tumors were found in rats and mice after long-term therapy with high doses (Drug Ther Bull 1988;26:53–56)
- although danthron is not a proven carcinogen in humans, there has been 1 case report of a leiomyosarcoma of the small bowel in an 18-year-old female patient after prolonged use (Postgrad Med J 1989;65:216–217)
- available combination products in Canada contain danthron and docusate sodium
- docusate sodium may increase the absorption of danthron
- chronic hepatitis was reported in 1 patient taking docusate sodium and danthron, but not when either drug was given alone (Ann Intern Med 1976;84:290–292)

Useful References

Tedesco FJ. Laxative use in constipation. Am J Gastroenterol 1985;80:303–309

Laxatives: Replacing danthron. Drug Ther Bull 1988;26:53–56
Patel PM, Selby PJ, Deacon J, et al. Anthraquinone laxatives and human cancer: An association in one case. Postgrad Med J 1989;65:216–217

DAPSONE

Ann Beardsell

USA (Avlosulfon)
CANADA (Avlosulfon)

▶ When Should I Use This Drug?

Pneumocystis carinii pneumonia

- preferred agent in combination with trimethoprim for outpatient treatment of mild to moderate episodes of *P. carinii* pneumonia (PCP) in acquired immunodeficiency syndrome (AIDS), as it is effective and inexpensive
- is also used as a single agent for PCP prophylaxis in patients with AIDS if trimethoprim-sulfamethoxazole cannot be used

Leprosy

- drug of choice for all forms (unless organisms are shown to be resistant) because it is inexpensive, is relatively nontoxic, and has high activity against *Mycobacterium leprae*
- because the incidence of resistant organisms is climbing, combination therapy with other antileprosy drugs is recommended

Dermatitis herpetiformis

- drug of choice

▶ What Contraindications Are There to the Use of This Drug?

Intolerance of or allergic reaction to dapsone

- hypersensitivity reactions are a combination of adverse effects (fever, dermatitis, and eosinophilia) known as the dapsone syndrome
- sulfa cross-reactivity is not a common problem but can occur in some patients (5–10%)

Severe anemia

- dapsone may exacerbate a preexisting anemic state
- use only when absolutely required in patients with glucose-6-phosphate dehydrogenase (G-6-PD) deficiency, methemoglobin reductase deficiency, hemoglobin M, or other conditions associated with hemolysis (e.g., certain infections and diabetic ketoacidosis), as dapsone may precipitate hemolysis
- if it must be used, do weekly monitoring of hemoglobin and reticulocyte counts

▶ What Drug Interactions Are Clinically Important?

Drugs that may increase the effect of dapsone

ZIDOVUDINE

- may cause nonhemolytic anemia in human immunodeficiency virus (HIV)–positive patients and may have additive effects with dapsone
- this is more common when dapsone is used for acute PCP than when it is used for PCP prophylaxis
- monitor hemoglobin and reticulocytes, and if anemia occurs, reduce or stop the administration of zidovudine for the remainder of treatment of acute PCP and resume after treatment is completed and anemia is resolved
- if dapsone is being used for PCP prophylaxis, stop dapsone administration and switch to a different prophylactic agent

PYRIMETHAMINE

- any drug that is capable of causing hemolytic anemia on its own should be used with caution in combination with dapsone
- if used together, weekly monitoring of hematological variables (hemoglobin B level, complete blood count, reticulocyte count) is essential
- if anemia occurs, discontinue administration of the least critical drug

NITRITE, ANILINE, PHENYLHYDRAZINE, NAPHTHALENE, NIRIDAZOLE, NITROFURANTOIN, PRIMAQUINE

- G-6-PD–deficient patients may experience additive effects of dapsone and other drugs or agents, resulting in hemolytic anemia
- if used together, hematological variables (hemoglobin B level, complete blood count, reticulocyte count) should be monitored weekly

Drugs that may decrease the effect of dapsone

CLOFAZIMINE

- some of the antiinflammatory effects of clofazimine may be diminished or nullified with concomitant use of dapsone
- significance of this interaction is unknown and concomitant use for the treatment of leprosy is advised, although higher dosages of clofazimine may be required in some types of leprosy

DIDEOXYINOSINE

- citrate buffer in the powder form of dideoxyinosine (ddI) (when mixed in water) inhibits the absorption of dapsone (the powder form is no longer available but there is still the tablet form)
- avoid simultaneous administration of both drugs; separate by several hours

Drugs that may have their effect increased by dapsone

- none

Drugs that may have their effect decreased by dapsone

- none

▶ What Route and Dosage Should I Use?

How to administer

- orally—take with food or milk
- parenterally—not available

Pneumocystis carinii pneumonia

Mild or moderate disease

- 100 mg PO daily in conjunction with trimethoprim 20 mg/kg daily for treatment of acute PCP

Prophylaxis

- 100 mg PO 3 times weekly

Leprosy

- 1–2 mg/kg daily (50–100 mg PO daily)

Dermatitis herpetiformis

- dose is individually titrated to the response of the lesions
- give 50 mg PO daily initially, increase until full control is achieved, and then reduce as soon as possible to the minimum required dosage for maintenance
- control may necessitate 300 mg or higher
- maintenance dosage ranges from 25 to 400 mg daily
- gluten-free diet may reduce the required maintenance dosage of dapsone

Dosage adjustments for renal or hepatic dysfunction

- 70–80% renally eliminated
- no information on dosage adjustments

▶ What Should I Monitor with Regard to Efficacy and Toxicity?

Efficacy

Pneumocystis carinii pneumonia

- for acute PCP, monitor for improvement in breathing, oxygen saturation, and chest X-ray findings, as well as resolution of fevers, night sweats, and other symptoms
- when using for prophylaxis, monitor the frequency and severity of PCP episodes during prophylaxis
- if episodes are frequent and/or severe, switch to another agent

Leprosy

- tissue stain smears should become negative with time
- resolution of skin lesions

Dermatitis herpetiformis
- resolution of skin lesions

Toxicity

Dose related and uncommon with doses up to 100 mg daily

Hematological effects
- hemolysis and methemoglobinemia are common with dosages greater than 200 mg daily but are seen in HIV-positive patients being treated with dapsone for acute PCP with dosages of 100 mg daily (especially if they are also receiving zidovudine) and in patients with G-6-PD deficiency with dosages greater than 50 mg daily
- monitor hemoglobin B level monthly and discontinue dapsone if it drops by more than 2 g/dL

Gastrointestinal symptoms
- anorexia, nausea, vomiting, and abdominal pain occur
- treat symptomatically

Dermatological effects
- rash and urticaria are common in HIV-positive patients about day 10 of treatment for PCP
- treat symptomatically with diphenhydramine or add prednisone 10 mg daily
- if severe, stop dapsone administration

Neurological effects
- peripheral neuritis is common with high dosages (200–500 mg daily)
- if it develops, stop dapsone administration; symptoms are reversible but resolution may take several months to several years

Hypersensitivity reaction
- also known as dapsone syndrome
- is rare and usually occurs within the first 6 weeks of therapy
- consists of fever; eosinophilia; mononucleosis; lymphadenopathy; leukopenia; jaundice with hepatitis; exanthematous skin eruptions, which may progress to exfoliative dermatitis; toxic epidermal necrolysis; or Stevens-Johnson syndrome
- stop dapsone administration
- some patients respond to desensitization

Hepatic effects
- hepatic impairment may occur shortly after starting therapy
- monitor for elevated levels of alkaline phosphatase, aspartate aminotransferase, bilirubin, and lactate dehydrogenase; lower the dosage if increases are 5 times normal levels and discontinue if the increase is 10 times normal values

▶ How Long Do I Treat Patients with This Drug?

Pneumocystis carinii pneumonia
- acute treatment—14 days
- prophylaxis—indefinite, depending on the patient's tolerance and response

Leprosy
- 6 months to 10 years, depending on the type of leprosy

Dermatitis herpetiformis
- indefinite

▶ How Do I Decrease or Stop the Administration of This Drug?
- may be stopped abruptly

▶ What Should I Tell My Patients About This Drug?
- do not take this drug at the same time as you take ddI (separate doses by several hours)
- this drug may cause anemia in some patients so if you feel excessively fatigued, lightheaded, or short of breath, let your physician know as soon as possible

DESIPRAMINE

Lyle K. Laird and Julia Vertrees

USA (Norpramin, Pertofrane, others)
CANADA (Norpramin, Pertofrane)

▶ When Should I Use This Drug?

Major depression, dysthymia, cyclothymia, panic disorders, generalized anxiety disorders, chronic pain syndromes
- although imipramine is usually chosen for these disorders, desipramine is the least anticholinergic of the tricyclic antidepressants and can be chosen for patients with certain types of glaucoma (e.g., open angle glaucoma), urinary retention, and prostatic hypertrophy (fluoxetine, sertraline, or paroxetine may also be used in patients with glaucoma but they are more expensive); for patients with glaucoma, an ophthalmologist should be consulted
- clinicians often prefer this drug because it is a stimulating tricyclic antidepressant whose efficacy is thought not to decrease at higher dosages
- if desipramine is less expensive than imipramine, desipramine should be chosen because it produces less sedation and fewer anticholinergic effects than does imipramine
- desipramine may also have less cardiovascular effects than does imipramine but nortriptyline hydrochloride is usually chosen, as it produces a lower incidence of orthostatic hypotension in patients with cardiovascular disease

▶ When Should I Not Use This Drug?

see Imipramine

▶ What Contraindications Are There to the Use of This Drug?

see Imipramine

Pregnancy
- adequate human studies have not been performed

▶ What Drug Interactions Are Clinically Important?

see Imipramine

▶ What Route and Dosage Should I Use?

How to administer
- orally—can be given with food or on an empty stomach
- parenterally—not available

Major depression, dysthymia, generalized anxiety disorders
- 50 mg PO daily at bedtime
- increase after 3 days to 100 mg PO daily at bedtime
- increase to 150 mg PO daily at bedtime after 1 week and leave at this dosage for 10–14 days
- if target symptoms are not improving after 3 weeks of therapy, continue to increase the daily dosage by 50 mg at weekly intervals until a response is seen or a dosage of 300 mg PO daily has been reached
- in geriatric patients and patients with a seizure history, start with 25 mg PO at bedtime, and in general, dosages should be approximately 50% of those used in younger patients
- desipramine has a long duration of action; hence, long-acting or sustained-release products are unnecessary and once-daily dosing is appropriate in adults
- after the patient has experienced a therapeutic response, the dosage should be maintained at these levels for 6–9 months because relapses may occur if a dosage reduction is attempted

Panic disorders, chronic pain syndromes
- dosages are often lower than those needed in depressive disorders
- start with 10 mg PO daily, as clinicians have noticed that these patients do not tolerate the adverse effects as well
- for panic disorders, titrate the dose up by 10–25 mg/wk and aim for 150 mg as the total daily dose
- in chronic pain syndromes, the general effective dose range is 25–50 mg PO daily and is generally used as adjuvant therapy

Dosage adjustments for renal or hepatic dysfunction
- hepatically metabolized
- start with low doses as for a geriatric patient

- decreased renal function does not necessitate dosage adjustments

▶ What Should I Monitor with Regard to Efficacy and Toxicity?

Efficacy

see Imipramine

Plasma concentration monitoring

- although routine plasma concentration monitoring is not necessary, a desipramine level in which total desipramine concentrations are 180 ng/mL or greater have been associated with a positive clinical response (Clin Chem 1988;34:863–888); with this in mind, it is generally thought that there is a linear relationship between a response and plasma concentration

Toxicity

see Imipramine

- fewer anticholinergic effects than imipramine

▶ How Long Do I Treat Patients with This Drug?

see Imipramine

▶ How Do I Decrease or Stop the Administration of This Drug?

see Imipramine

▶ What Should I Tell My Patients About This Drug?

see Imipramine

▶ Therapeutic Tips

see Imipramine

DEXAMETHASONE

Karen Shalansky and Cindy Reesor Nimmo

USA (Dalalone, Decadron, Decadron Phosphate Respihaler, Decaject, Dekasol, Dexacen, Dexone, Hexadrol)
CANADA (Decadron, Deronil, Dexasone, Hexadrol, inhaler not available in Canada)

▶ When Should I Use This Drug?

Consider an alternative agent

- intravenous, oral, inhaler
- systemic dexamethasone has a long half-life and duration of action (36–54 hours), which may cause more adrenal suppression than with other corticosteroids, especially if used for prolonged periods (DICP 1991;25:72–78)
- injectable dexamethasone sodium phosphate contains metabisulfites, which can precipitate bronchoconstriction, especially in allergic patients (J Allergy Clin Immunol 1985;76:312–320)
- inhaled dexamethasone could be used in place of other inhaled corticosteroids if it is less expensive (see Budesonide)

DEXTROMETHORPHAN

Penny Miller

USA (Benylin DM, dextromethorphan cough syrup)
CANADA (Benylin DM syrup, Robidex, Balminil D.M., Delsym, Koffex)

▶ When Should I Use This Drug?

Nonproductive coughs

- short-term symptomatic relief of dry nonproductive cough due to the common cold or an unknown cause when repeated bouts of coughing result in interference with performance at work or school, lack of sleep for patients or family members, exhaustion, or emesis
- in other conditions causing a nonproductive cough, in which the underlying disease is unknown, the occasional use of this drug is acceptable, when cough is resulting in emesis, interfering with daily performance or sleep, or causing exhaustion

- is approximately equipotent to codeine on a per milligram basis, but unlike narcotics, it produces no significant analgesia, central nervous system or respiratory depression, constipation, or physical dependence
- dextromethorphan does not inhibit ciliary activity, whereas codeine does (American Hospital Formulary Service, Drug Information, ASHP, Bethesda, MD, 1993; 1669)

▶ When Should I Not Use This Drug?

Coughs associated with infections and fevers

- should be treated with antibiotics

Coughs associated with pathological states such as emphysema, chronic obstructive pulmonary disease, chronic bronchitis, and cystic fibrosis

- in these conditions, the cough reflex is essential to maintain airway patency by cleaning excessive secretions from the tracheobronchial tree
- antitussives are not contraindicated in patients with productive coughs (Health Protection Branch. Second Report of the Expert Advisory Committee on Nonprescription Cough and Cold Remedies. Health and Welfare Canada, 1989: 1–50); however, it should not be used in cases in which cough is important in clearing the bronchial tract

Coughs associated with allergic states such as allergic rhinitis, asthma

- in allergic rhinitis, excess secretions produced by inflamed nasopharyngeal mucosa result in postnasal drip, which causes an irritative cough, which is not reduced by dextromethorphan
- in asthma, the inflammation and bronchospasm are the underlying cause of cough

Chronic coughs in which the cause may be an inhaled foreign body or aspiration of pharyngeal or gastrointestinal content, or a response to chronic irritation from inhaled environmental pollutants such as cigarette smoke

- these coughs should not be suppressed, as treatment should be aimed at the underlying cause

Coughs resulting from any intraluminal or extraluminal mass affecting the trachea or bronchi

- bronchogenic carcinoma necessitates narcotic antitussive agents

Nocturnal coughs associated with congestive heart failure

- treatment should be aimed at relieving the edema

▶ What Contraindications Are There to the Use of This Drug?

- intolerance of or allergic reaction to dextromethorphan

▶ What Drug Interactions Are Clinically Important?

Drugs that may increase the effect of dextromethorphan

- none

Drugs that may decrease the effect of dextromethorphan

- none

Drugs that may have their effect increased by dextromethorphan

MONOAMINE OXIDASE INHIBITORS

- avoid concurrent use or avoid if the patient has taken monoamine oxidase inhibitors in the previous 2 weeks, as there is a single case report of neurological symptoms (Medical Letter Handbook of Adverse Drug Interactions, New York, 1991)

Drugs that may have their effect decreased by dextromethorphan

- none

▶ What Route and Dosage Should I Use?

How to administer

- orally—can be given with food or on an empty stomach

Nonproductive coughs

- 15 mg PO Q4H PRN for symptoms up to a maximum of 120 mg/d

Dosage adjustments for renal or hepatic dysfunction

- hepatically metabolized
- no dosage adjustments are needed, as the drug should be used infrequently for short periods of time

▶ *What Should I Monitor with Regard to Efficacy and Toxicity?*

Efficacy

Nonproductive coughs

- decrease in the severity and/or the frequency of cough

Toxicity

Bronchospasm

- monitor for bronchospasm or other signs of histamine release caused by dextromethorphan in patients with asthma
- if these symptoms occur, stop the drug administration

Central nervous system effects

- monitor for drowsiness, nausea, gastrointestinal upset, and dizziness
- decrease the dosage or discontinue the drug administration if these effects are particularly bothersome
- sedated or debilitated patients or patients confined to a supine position may be at a greater risk for aspirating gastrointestinal or pharyngeal secretions because of the sedating effects of the drug (American Hospital Formulary Service, Drug Information, ASHP, Bethesda, MD, 1993:1669)

▶ *How Long Do I Treat Patients with This Drug?*

Nonproductive coughs

- short-term (1 to 2 weeks) treatment has not been proved harmful

▶ *How Do I Decrease or Stop the Administration of This Drug?*

- may be stopped abruptly

▶ *What Should I Tell My Patients About This Drug?*

- if you have a rash, itching, wheezing, or difficulty with breathing, discontinue the medication regimen and call your physician
- if the cough has not improved in 7 days or if you have a high fever, continuing headache, or large amount of mucus, contact your physician

▶ *Therapeutic Tips*

- ensure that adequate dosages are used
- carefully consider the cause of the cough
- liquid, tablets, or sustained-release liquids are available, and the choice should be up to the patient
- single entity is preferred to allow dosage adjustments
- limit the duration of use to 1–2 weeks

Useful References

USPDI 1993, U.S. Pharmacopeial Convention, Rockville, MD: 1991

American Hospital Formulary Service, Drug Information, ASHP, Bethesda, MD:1993

Health Protection Branch. Second Report of the Expert Advisory Committee on Nonprescription Cough and Cold Remedies. Health and Welfare Canada, 1989: 1–50

Committee on Drugs. American Academy of Pediatrics. Use of codeine and dextromethorphan containing cough syrups in pediatrics. Pediatrics 1978;62:118–122

DIAZEPAM

Steven Stanislav and Patricia Marken

USA (Valium, various generics)

CANADA (Valium, Apo-Diazepam, Diazemuls, Meval, Novodipam, Vivol)

▶ *When Should I Use This Drug?*

Alcohol withdrawal (treatment and prevention of seizures)

- relieves agitation, tremor, and delirium in acute alcohol withdrawal
- both diazepam and lorazepam are effective for preventing alcohol withdrawal seizures
- diazepam has a longer duration of action than does lorazepam and other benzodiazepines, which may be useful when stopping diazepam administration (self-tapering)
- some clinicians prefer lorazepam over diazepam if an intramuscular agent is required (in addition to an oral agent for backup), because intramuscular lorazepam is absorbed more rapidly and completely than intramuscular diazepam

Status epilepticus

- intravenous diazepam is effective for status epilepticus and for acute seizures due to drug overdose or poisoning, although lorazepam is equally effective (JAMA 1983;249:1452–1454)
- lorazepam is the first choice for many clinicians, as it distributes out of the central nervous system (CNS) slower and may work longer, but the clinical significance of this is not known
- diazepam is less expensive than lorazepam

Benzodiazepine withdrawal

- dose of the drug (benzodiazepine) can be titrated down in most patients rather than substituting a cross-tolerant agent
- making a dose-for-dose switch to a longer acting benzodiazepine such as diazepam and then slowly tapering that medication may reduce withdrawal symptoms (J Psychiatr Res 1990;24(suppl 2):81–90)
- clonazepam may also be used but it is more expensive than diazepam (J Psychiatr Res 1990;24(suppl 2):81–90)

Skeletal muscle relaxation

- as adjunct to rest and physical therapy for short-term relief of acute skeletal muscle pain or for long-term therapy for spasticity due to upper motor neuron disorder
- likely all benzodiazepines can be used

Preoperative sedation

- to reduce anxiety and to produce anterograde amnesia prior to endoscopy, cardioversion, and other surgery
- lorazepam is usually preferred because it is shorter acting

▶ *When Should I Not Use This Drug?*

Sleep disorders

- its long half-life (2–4 days), production of active metabolites, and oxidative hepatic metabolism make it less desirable than other benzodiazepine hypnotics

Generalized anxiety disorders

- some clinicians avoid diazepam because they suspect it has a higher abuse potential
- all benzodiazepines are equally effective; therefore, the choice is based on the patient's previous response and cost

Panic disorders

- although limited data suggest that diazepam may be efficacious (J Clin Psychiatry 1986;47:458–460), if cost is a major issue, high-dose lorazepam (shorter acting than diazepam) can be used in place of alprazolam or clonazepam, which are usually the first-line agents
- however, most patients do not tolerate the high doses of diazepam required to prevent panic attacks

▶ *What Contraindications Are There to the Use of This Drug?*

see Lorazepam

▶ *What Drug Interactions Are Clinically Important?*

Drugs that may increase the effect or toxicity of diazepam

ALCOHOL

- about 20% of insomniacs may take alcohol and sleeping pills concurrently to aid sleep (Confin Psychiatr 1977;15:151–172), and these can produce additive sedative effects
- avoid this combination

CENTRAL NERVOUS SYSTEM DEPRESSANTS

- additive, sedative effects are expected when CNS depressants are used
- avoid the combination if possible or minimize by starting with low, divided daily doses and allow tolerance to develop before dosage increases

CIMETIDINE

- cimetidine reduces plasma diazepam clearance and plasma levels may increase, resulting in increased sedation
- if an H₂ antagonist is required, use ranitidine or other H_2 antagonists, which have less of an effect on hepatic enzymes

DISULFIRAM, ISONIAZID, OMEPRAZOLE

- may reduce the clearance of diazepam (Clin Pharmacol Ther 1978;24:583–589)
- if these combinations must be used, be aware of the potential for increased sedation, and if it occurs, reduce the diazepam dosage by 50% and reassess

Drugs that may decrease the effect of diazepam

CARBAMAZEPINE, PHENYTOIN, PHENOBARBITAL, RIFAMPIN

- may increase clearance and reduce serum concentrations of diazepam
- increase the dosage of diazepam if exacerbation of symptoms occur

Drugs that may have their effect or toxicity increased by diazepam

- none

Drugs that may have their effect decreased by diazepam

- none

▶ *What Route and Dosage Should I Use?*

How to administer

Orally
- take with food or on an empty stomach

Parenterally
- can be given as an intravenous push at not faster than 5 mg/min
- do not give intramuscularly, as it is poorly and erratically absorbed (if the intravenous route is not available, use lorazepam intramuscularly)

Alcohol withdrawal (treatment and prevention of seizures)

- give 5 mg IV over 30–60 seconds, and if seizures are not controlled and no cardiorespiratory depression occurs, give another 5 mg in 2–5 minutes
- a further 10 mg IV can be given 10–20 minutes later if tonic-clonic seizures continue
- to prevent alcohol withdrawal seizures, give 10 mg PO Q1H until the patient is sedated and then give 10 mg PO TID
- if symptoms such as tremor and irritability start to occur, increase the dose

Status epilepticus

- give 5 mg IV over 30–60 seconds, and if seizures are not controlled and no cardiorespiratory depression occurs, give another 2 mg in 2–5 minutes
- a further 10 mg IV can be given 10–20 minutes later if tonic-clonic seizures continue (this rarely happens) while phenytoin is being administered

Benzodiazepine withdrawal

- depends on the dosage of the drug that is being stopped
- 5 mg diazepam = 1 mg lorazepam = 15 mg oxazepam = 1 mg clonazepam

Skeletal muscle relaxation

- give 10 mg IV initially and repeat the dose in 3–4 hours if needed

Preoperative sedation

- 10 mg IV 15–20 minutes before surgery

Dosage adjustments for renal or hepatic dysfunction

- hepatically metabolized
- no dosage adjustments for organ dysfunction are recommended; however, always start with the lowest dose and titrate to response
- in patients with severe hepatic disease, use a benzodiazepine metabolized by conjugation such as lorazepam and oxazepam

▶ *What Should I Monitor with Regard to Efficacy and Toxicity?*

Efficacy

Alcohol withdrawal (treatment and prevention of seizures)
- symptoms of withdrawal such as tremor, irritability, and tachycardia

Status epilepticus
- control of seizures

Benzodiazepine withdrawal
- signs and symptoms of withdrawal

Skeletal muscle relaxation
- reduction in severity of symptoms

Preoperative sedation
- memory of events around surgery

Toxicity

see Lorazepam

▶ *How Long Do I Treat Patients with This Drug?*

Alcohol withdrawal (treatment and prevention of seizures)

- continue a maintenance dosage for 2–3 days; then discontinue benzodiazepine administration
- diazepam continues to be effective for 1–2 days after stopping the drug administration owing to its long duration of action
- reinstitute a maintenance dosage if the person starts to exhibit signs and symptoms of withdrawal

Status epilepticus

- until control of seizures is seen

Benzodiazepine withdrawal

- conservative approach is to lower the total daily dose by 10% per week (faster discontinuations may be appropriate for patients receiving lower dosages for shorter periods); if withdrawal symptoms (anxiety, insomnia, malaise, anorexia, diaphoresis, tremor, nausea, vomiting, irritability, and psychoses) or rebound anxiety (similar to previous symptoms, but with increased severity) appears, increase the dosage to the previous week's level, wait for symptoms to abate, and proceed to taper the administration again (only at slower rate)

Skeletal muscle relaxation

- use a 1 week trial and then reevaluate

▶ *How Do I Decrease or Stop the Administration of This Drug?*

see Lorazepam

▶ *What Should I Tell My Patients About This Drug?*

see Lorazepam

▶ *Therapeutic Tips*

- do not use as a stand alone hypnotic
- this drug is not indicated as a hypnotic medicine owing to its long half-life, but its sedative effects can be used to promote sleep through a nocturnal dose schedule in patients receiving daily therapy
- useful when switching patients from short-acting benzodiazepines to allow slow tapering of the daily dosage

Useful References

Uhlenhuth EH, DeWitt H, Balter MD, et al. Risks and benefits of long-term benzodiazepine use. J Clin Psychiatry 1988;8:161–167

Dubovsky SL. Generalized anxiety disorder: New concepts and psychophar-macologic therapies. J Clin Psychiatry 1990;51:3–32

Hayes PE, Dommisse CS. Current concepts in clinical therapeutics: Anxiety disorders I, II. Clin Pharm 1987;6:140–147, 196–215

Noyes R, Garvey MJ, Cook BL, et al. Benzodiazepine withdrawal: A review of the evidence. J Clin Psychiatry 1988;49:382–389

DICLOFENAC

Kelly Jones

USA (Voltaren)
CANADA (Voltaren, Apo-Diclo, Novo-Difenac, Nu-Diclo)

▶ When Should I Use This Drug?

Acute pain, general aches and pain, bone pain

- useful for the short-term management of general aches and pains
- only advantage over non-enteric coated aspirin is that it causes less frequent gastrointestinal intolerance
- decision between this drug and other nonsteroidal antiinflammatory drugs (NSAIDs) should be based on cost

Rheumatoid arthritis

- diclofenac can be used as an alternative for patients who fail to respond to enteric coated aspirin or ibuprofen
- it offers no advantages over enteric coated aspirin or ibuprofen and is more expensive

Osteoarthritis

- if acetaminophen and enteric coated aspirin or ibuprofen are not effective
- decision between this drug and other NSAIDs should be based on cost

▶ When Should I Not Use This Drug?

see Ibuprofen

▶ What Contraindications Are There to the Use of This Drug?

see Ibuprofen

Hepatic disease

- do not use in patients with a history of hepatic disease, as there has been information published on diclofenac-induced hepato-toxicity (JAMA 1990;264:2660–2662)

▶ What Drug Interactions Are Clinically Important?

see Ibuprofen

▶ What Route and Dosage Should I Use?

How to administer

- orally—take with food or milk
- parenterally—not available

Acute pain, general aches and pain, bone pain, dysmenorrhea

- 25–50 mg PO Q12H PRN

Cancer pain

- 50 mg PO Q12H up to a maximum dosage of 200 mg PO daily

Rheumatoid arthritis

- 75 mg PO Q12H up to a maximum dosage of 200 mg PO daily

Osteoarthritis

- 50 mg PO Q12H

Dosage adjustments for renal or hepatic dysfunction

- hepatically metabolized; therefore, no adjustments are needed for renal disease
- reduce the dosage by 25% in patients with a history of hepatic disease

▶ What Should I Monitor with Regard to Efficacy and Toxicity?

see Ibuprofen

▶ How Long Do I Treat Patients with This Drug?

see Ibuprofen

▶ How Do I Decrease or Stop the Administration of This Drug?

- may be stopped abruptly if needed

▶ What Should I Tell My Patients About This Drug?

see Ibuprofen

▶ Therapeutic Tips

see Ibuprofen

Useful References

see Ibuprofen

DICLOXACILLIN

John Rotschafer, Kyle Vance-Bryan, and Rick Zabinski

USA (Dycill, Dynapen, Pathocil, Veracillin)
CANADA (Dynapen)

Consider an alternative agent

- has identical indications to cloxacillin but is more expensive
- dicloxacillin is somewhat better absorbed than cloxacillin but this does not provide dicloxacillin with any clinically significant advantages over oral cloxacillin

DIFLUNISAL

Kelly Jones

USA (Dolobid)
CANADA (Dolobid)

▶ When Should I Use This Drug?

Acute pain, general aches and pain, bone pain

- useful for the short-term management of general aches and pains
- only advantage over non-enteric coated aspirin is that it causes less gastrointestinal intolerance
- decision between this drug and other nonsteroidal antiinflammatory drugs (NSAIDs) should be based on cost

Rheumatoid arthritis

- not considered first line, as this agent is considered less effective than the NSAIDs
- should be used as an alternative for patients with rheumatoid arthritis who cannot tolerate the adverse effects on the gastrointestinal system and kidneys from nonaspirin NSAIDs, as nonacetylated salicylates (salsalate, diflunisal, choline magnesium trisalicylate) are less likely to affect the gastrointestinal tract than is aspirin (Gastroenterology 1990;99:1616–1621)
- can be used as an alternative when platelet function is important, as nonacetylated salicylates have no appreciable effect on platelets (J Am Board Fam Pract 1989;2:257–271)
- decision among nonacetylated salicylates should be based on cost

Osteoarthritis

- if acetaminophen and ibuprofen are not effective
- decision between this drug and other NSAIDs should be based on cost

▶ When Should I Not Use This Drug?

see Ibuprofen

▶ What Contraindications Are There to the Use of This Drug?

see Aspirin

▶ What Drug Interactions Are Clinically Important?

see Ibuprofen

▶ What Route and Dosage Should I Use?

How to administer

- orally—take with food or milk
- parenterally—not available

Acute pain, general aches and pain, bone pain

- 250–500 mg PO Q8–12H PRN

Rheumatoid arthritis

- 500 mg PO BID up to a maximum dosage of 500 mg PO TID

Osteoarthritis

- 250 mg PO BID

Dosage adjustments for renal or hepatic dysfunction

- hepatically metabolized; therefore, no adjustments are needed for renal disease
- reduce the dosage by 25% in patients with a history of hepatic disease

▶ What Should I Monitor with Regard to Efficacy and Toxicity?

see Aspirin

▶ How Long Do I Treat Patients with This Drug?

see Aspirin

▶ How Do I Decrease or Stop the Administration of This Drug?

- may be stopped abruptly if needed

▶ What Should I Tell My Patients About This Drug?

- it is important to be educated about what to expect in terms of the onset of relief
- your pain will not go away with 1 dose or with 2 days of therapy, but by 2 weeks, you should experience significant relief
- avoid concomitant use of other NSAIDs, especially over the counter products containing ibuprofen
- do not crush or chew tablet
- take with food, milk, or antacids if gastrointestinal upset occurs and tell your physician of any gastrointestinal intolerance
- notify your physician of any rash, unusual fever, edema, black stools, or weight gain
- some patients get drowsy with diflunisal; therefore, observe caution when performing tasks requiring alertness

▶ Therapeutic Tips

see Aspirin

Useful References

see Aspirin

DIGOXIN

Jack Onrot

USA (Lanoxin)
CANADA (Lanoxin)

▶ When Should I Use This Drug?

Atrial fibrillation or flutter

- considered the drug of choice for control of ventricular rate, because congestive heart failure is frequently present concurrently with atrial fibrillation or flutter (Drugs 1990;40:841–853, Clin Pharm 1983;2:312–320, Med Lett 1991;33:55–60)
- digoxin can achieve reductions in resting heart rate during chronic atrial fibrillation or flutter; however, digoxin may have relatively little effect on heart rate during exercise in these patients (Ann Intern Med 1991;114:573–575, Drugs 1986;31:185–197)
- digoxin may be ineffective in patients with paroxysmal atrial fibrillation (sinus rhythm punctuated by attacks of fibrillation) (N Engl J Med 1992;326:1264–1271) and less effective in rate control for patients with high catecholamine states (anxiety, exercise)
- although there is some evidence that digoxin may not be effective in paroxysmal atrial fibrillation, it is still considered by some

clinicians the drug of choice (especially because many of these patients have heart failure)

Atrioventricular nodal reentrant tachycardia

Acute episodes

- digoxin should be used in patients who have asthma, who have contraindications to verapamil use, or who are unresponsive to adenosine or verapamil (JAMA 1992;268:2199–2241)

Long-term therapy

- there are no studies comparing the efficacy of agents for the prevention of atrioventricular nodal reentrant tachycardia, but most sources consider digoxin the drug of choice
- therapy may be selected empirically for patients with atrioventricular nodal reentrant tachycardia that is not life threatening and not associated with serious symptoms
- few data exist comparing the efficacy of drugs for the suppression of recurrent episodes of atrioventricular nodal reentrant tachycardia
- because response to intravenous verapamil does not accurately predict long-term response to oral verapamil (Circulation 1980;62:996–1010) and because many of these patients have concomitant left ventricular dysfunction, digoxin is a reasonable choice as a first-line agent

Congestive heart failure

- most patients with severe heart failure need a loop diuretic, angiotensin converting enzyme inhibitors, and digoxin (JAMA 1988;259;539–544)
- triple therapy is warranted for patients who fail to respond to loop diuretic plus angiotensin converting enzyme inhibitors
- because digoxin works by improving contractility, it is useful only for patients with decreased systolic left ventricular function and heart failure (many patients with congestive heart failure have normal systolic left ventricular function but diastolic dysfunction [impedance to filling] because of thickened left ventricle myocardium; this is the situation in hypertensive cardiomyopathy or early hypertensive cardiomyopathy)
- in hypertensive patients with congestive heart failure, assessment of left ventricular function (echo or multigated angiography) is recommended to determine the feasibility of digoxin therapy (i.e., do not use digoxin for solely diastolic dysfunction)
- digoxin should be used in all patients with concomitant atrial fibrillation and may be beneficial in patients with S_3 heart sound (Am J Cardiol 1988;61:371–375)

▶ When Should I Not Use This Drug?

Wolff-Parkinson-White syndrome

- digoxin should not be administered to patients with atrial fibrillation who are known to have Wolff-Parkinson-White syndrome or other syndromes characterized by ventricular preexcitation, as it may paradoxically increase the ventricular rate (Circulation 1977;56:260–267)

Hypertrophic cardiomyopathy

- postive inotropic effect may enhance cardiac outflow obstruction

Congestive heart failure in patients with sinus rhythm and normal left ventricular function

- because digoxin works by improving contractility, it is useful only in patients with decreased systolic left ventricular function and heart failure

▶ What Contraindications Are There to the Use of This Drug?

Intolerance of or allergic reaction to digoxin
Sinus bradycardia, second- or third-degree heart block, or sick sinus syndrome in the absence of a functioning pacemaker

- digoxin can worsen these conditions

Severe hypokalemia (potassium level <3 mmol/L)

- correct potassium levels before using digoxin

▶ *What Drug Interactions Are Clinically Important?*

Drugs that may increase the effect or toxicity of digoxin

QUINIDINE

- quinidine therapy has been reported to result in 2- to 3-fold elevations in serum digoxin concentrations, which may occur as early as several hours after the initiation of quinidine therapy (N Engl J Med 1979;301:400–404, Int J Cardiol 1981;1:109–116)
- when quinidine therapy is added in patients receiving digoxin, decrease the digoxin dosage by 50% when starting these agents and make further dosage changes on the basis of clinical response

VERAPAMIL, AMIODARONE

- digoxin concentrations may increase by 50–75% during the first week of verapamil therapy and may be more substantial in patients with underlying hepatic disease
- may raise digoxin levels (by inhibition of renal clearance)
- decrease the digoxin dosage by 50% when adding verapamil and make further dosage changes on the basis of clinical response (efficacy and toxicity)

Drugs that may decrease the effect of digoxin

CHOLESYTRAMINE, COLESTIPOL

- binds to digoxin and may reduce absorption
- in general, it is advisable to take medications at least 1 hour before or 4 hours after a bile acid sequestrant

Drugs that may have their effect or toxicity increased by digoxin

- none

Drugs that may have their effect decreased by digoxin

- none

▶ *What Route and Dosage Should I Use?*

How to administer

- orally—can be administered with or without food
- parenterally—can be given undiluted as a bolus or may be diluted in sterile water, 5% dextrose in water, or normal saline

Atrial fibrillation or flutter, atrioventricular nodal reentrant tachycardia, congestive heart failure

Loading dose

- digoxin is rarely given as an intravenous loading dose for the treatment of heart failure (except for patients with acute pulmonary edema) and is used more frequently for rate control in atrial fibrillation
- 0.013 mg/kg (Ann Intern Med 1968;69:703–717) rounded to the closest 0.25 mg dose is the initial loading dose given over the first 24 hours
- if the total loading dose is 0.75 mg or greater, administer an initial dose of 0.5 mg IV
- if the total loading dose is less than 0.75 mg, administer an initial dose of 0.25 mg IV
- remainder of calculated loading dose should be administered orally or IV (if patient cannot tolerate oral medications) in 0.25 mg increments every 6 hours
- give $2/3$ of a loading dose to patients with renal impairment (estimated creatinine clearance <20 mL/min)

Maintenance dose

- 0.25 mg PO daily
- 0.125 mg daily in patients older than the age of 65 years or patients taking drugs that may interact with digoxin to elevate serum digoxin concentrations

Dosage adjustments for renal or hepatic dysfunction

- approximately 85% renally eliminated

Normal Dosing Interval	C_{cr} > 60 mL/min or 1 mL/s	C_{cr} 30–60 mL/min or 0.5–1 mL/s	C_{cr} < 30 mL/min or 0.5 mL/s
Q24H	no adjustment needed	decrease dosage by 50%	decrease dosage by 75%

▶ *What Should I Monitor with Regard to Efficacy and Toxicity?*

Efficacy

Atrial fibrillation or flutter

Control of ventricular rate

Vital signs

- check vital signs every 15 minutes until the patient is stable, then every 4 hours for 24 hours
- resting apical ventricular rate of 60–80 bpm is a reasonable target, although 90–100 bpm may be acceptable if the patient is asymptomatic at this heart rate
- presence or absence of symptoms related to arrhythmia (palpitations, shortness of breath, dizziness, and angina)

Digoxin serum concentrations

- need not be determined unless signs or symptoms of digoxin toxicity are suspected
- if the ventricular rate is within the desired range and there is no evidence of digoxin toxicity, the digoxin dosage should be considered appropriate

Atrioventricular nodal reentrant tachycardia

Acute episodes

Electrocardiogram

- electrocardiogram (ECG) should be monitored continuously until the arrhythmia has stopped

Vital signs

- should be assessed every 5 minutes during drug administration
- presence or absence of symptoms related to arrhythmia (palpitations, shortness of breath, dizziness, and angina)

Long-term therapy

- frequency or duration of episodes (may be evaluated by ambulatory ECG or by patients' reports of the frequency of symptoms)
- patients should be assessed every few weeks during the first few months of therapy and every few months thereafter

Congestive heart failure

Signs and symptoms

- monitoring the response to digoxin is often difficult because the patient with congestive heart failure is undergoing concomitant adjustments in the dosage of diuretics and angiotension converting enzyme inhibitors; thus, it is difficult to titrate digoxin dose to efficacy
- dyspnea, orthopnea, paroxysmal nocturnal dyspnea, fatigue, ankle swelling, fine crackles on chest auscultation, weight, liver size, and absence of S_3 heart sound
- jugular venous pressure should be normal to slightly increased
- for patients with acute symptoms, assess patients at least twice daily while they are in the hospital
- after the patient is discharged, assess within a week of discharge
- after the patient is stabilized, decrease the frequency of evaluation
- for patients with mild symptoms, assess weekly until symptoms are controlled

Digoxin serum concentration

- digoxin serum concentration measurement is not required unless one is assessing compliance, absorption, or possible toxicity
- other clinical monitoring variables are more beneficial in assessing efficacy or toxicity

Toxicity

Cardiovascular effects

- electrocardiographic monitoring is required to detect cardiovascular toxicities
- ECG may show digoxin effect (ST depression, ''Salvadore Dali moustache,'' or ''coving'' and T wave flattening); however, this is nonspecific for toxicity and can be seen with other conditions
- atrioventricular nodal blocks, sinoatrial blocks to a lesser degree, bradycardia, accelerated junctional rhythm, and paroxysmal

atrial tachycardia with atrioventricular block are more specific for digoxin toxicity

Gastrointestinal effects

- anorexia, nausea, vomiting, abdominal pain, and diarrhea may occur
- these symptoms are important because a fall in intake leads to prerenal failure, leading to reduced digoxin clearance and further elevation of toxic levels (a vicious cycle)

Central nervous system effects

- confusion, headache, and fatigue can occur, especially in elderly patients who are digoxin toxic
- blurred vision, "frosting" or "halo," and disturbed color vision may occur (the well-known yellow vision along with the other visual disturbances is uncommon)

Digoxin serum concentration measurement

- not useful, unless toxicity is suspected
- digoxin may result in toxicities over a wide range of serum concentrations, including concentrations required for therapeutic benefit; therefore, a concentration measurement adds little to the clinical assessment of toxicities but may be useful in patients with potential toxicity as a guide to diagnosis ("therapeutic range" of 0.5–2 ng/mL)
- serum measurement may be useful in determining digoxin antibody (digoxin immune Fab [Digibind]) dose in severe chronic toxicity
- in an acute ingestion, the antibody dose can also be determined from the amount of drug ingested (if known)
- when toxicity is suspected, digoxin should be withheld

▶ How Long Do I Treat Patients with This Drug?

Atrial fibrillation or flutter

- unless factors stimulating arrhythmia can be eliminated, digoxin therapy should be continued indefinitely

Atrioventricular nodal reentrant tachycardia

- unless factors stimulating arrhythmia can be eliminated, digoxin therapy should be continued indefinitely

Congestive heart failure

- if the initial indication for digoxin was appropriate (see above under When Should I Use This Drug) then lifelong treatment is probably necessary
- if precipitating factors can be reversed, then a trial of digoxin withdrawal would be warranted

▶ How Do I Decrease or Stop the Administration of This Drug?

- may be stopped abruptly

▶ What Should I Tell My Patients About This Drug?

- be alert to side effects, especially gastrointestinal effects, palpitations, and lightheadedness, which may indicate dysrrhythmias
- prolonged periods of negative fluid balance might precipitate toxicity
- monitoring and follow-up are necessary

▶ Therapeutic Tips

- in atrial fibrillation, titrate the dose to heart rate
- avoid hypokalemia
- young patients (younger than 50 years) are usually placed on 0.25 mg daily, whereas the elderly (older than 60 years) are given 0.125 mg daily as a rule
- smaller patients and those with any degree of renal impairment or those taking interacting agents need smaller dosages
- if serum digoxin concentrations are measured, they should be obtained at least 8 hours after a dose (to allow complete distribution)

DIHYDROERGOTAMINE

Jerry Taylor

USA (DHE 45)
CANADA (Dihydroergotamine-Sandoz)

▶ When Should I Use This Drug?

Migraine treatment

- is as effective and better tolerated (less nausea) than ergotamine but is available only parenterally
- parenteral DHE plus metoclopramide is an effective treatment for moderate to severe migraine and is less expensive than parenteral sumatriptan
- DHE can be used at home if the patient is taught how to use a subcutaneous injection
- dihydroergotamine has diminished oxytocic and vasodilator effects compared with those with ergotamine

▶ When Should I Not Use This Drug?

Delayed therapy and well-established pain

- dihydroergotamine is not as effective when therapy has been delayed and the pain has become well established
- may be risky in patients with prolonged prodromes (complicated migraine) and may lead to irreversible sequelae in these circumstances
- avoid use in patients with signs of chronic ergotism or rebound headache

Daily administration

- to prevent rebound headache and subsequent dependency problems, the drug must never be used on a daily basis

▶ What Contraindications Are There to the Use of This Drug?

see Ergotamine

▶ What Drug Interactions Are Clinically Important?

see Ergotamine

▶ What Route and Dosage Should I Use?

How to administer

- orally—not available
- parenterally—direct intravenous injection into catheters containing 5% dextrose in water or normal saline

Migraine treatment

- 0.5 mg IV or subcutaneously (1 mg in large patients) and repeat dose at 1 hour intervals as needed
- maximum dose should not exceed 3 mg/24 h or 6 mg/wk
- can be given subcutaneously by the patient at home if needed

Dosage adjustments for renal or hepatic dysfunction

- extensively metabolized and eliminated by biliary excretion, necessitating dosage reductions in hepatic disease
- dihydroergotamine is probably best avoided in patients with renal or hepatic disease
- specific recomendations in hepatic disease are not available

▶ What Should I Monitor with Regard to Efficacy and Toxicity?

see Ergotamine

▶ How Long Do I Treat Patients with This Drug?

see Ergotamine

▶ How Do I Decrease or Stop the Administration of This Drug?

see Ergotamine

▶ What Should I Tell My Patients About This Drug?

- proper timing of dose administration and appropriate use of the dosage form prescribed is most important
- take medication early, after the onset of prodromal symptoms or headache in those without aura, to be most effective
- total daily and weekly dose limitations are important
- you and family members should watch for signs of confusion and other signs of possible acute ergot toxicity

▶ *Therapeutic Tips*

- is better tolerated; therefore, should be used instead of ergotamine
- prochlorperazine should be used prior to the use of dihydroergotamine to decrease the occurrence of nausea
- can be used at home if the patient is taught how to use a subcutaneous injection
- repeated dosing over an extended time may reduce effectiveness by allowing the establishment of vasodilatation
- total dose requirement can be given early as a single dose, at the onset of headache, to abort attack

Useful References

Raskin NH. Repetitive intravenous dihydroergotamine as therapy for intractable migraine. Neurology 1986;36:995–997

Callaham M, Raskin N. A controlled study of dihydroergotamine in the treatment of acute migraine headache. Headache 1986;26:168–171

DILTIAZEM

Stephen F. Hamilton, Stan Horton, and Udho Thadani
USA (Cardizem, Cardizem CD, Cardizem SR)
CANADA (Apo-Diltiaz, Cardizem, Novo-Diltiazem, Nu-Diltiaz, Syn-Diltiazem, Cardizem CD, Cardizem SR)

▶ *When Should I Use This Drug?*

Chronic stable angina

- in patients with no concomitant disease states, calcium channel blockers are useful for patients who do not tolerate or do not have complete control with nitrates and beta-blockers
- beta-blockers should be chosen instead of calcium channel blockers for new-onset angina or chronic stable angina because there is more cumulative information about the overall value of beta-blockers in these patients and they are less expensive than calcium antagonists
- calcium antagonists can be used as monotherapy when contraindications to the use of beta-blockers and nitrates are present and can be added when optimum 2 drug therapy (nitrates and beta-blockers) is not adequate for symptom control (Am Heart J 1989;118:1093–1097)
- triple-drug therapy (maximum therapy) has not had advantages over optimized therapy with nitrates and beta-blockers and should be reserved for those patients who are symptomatic with double-drug (nitrates and beta-blockers) therapy (J Am Coll Cardiol 1984;3:1051–1057)
- in patients with concomitant hypertension, calcium channel blockers should be chosen in patients unable to take beta-blockers
- in patients with concomitant diabetes or chronic obstructive pulmonary disease or asthma, calcium channel blockers should be chosen in patients who cannot tolerate nitrates or in whom nitrates are ineffective
- all calcium channel blockers are equally effective; however, diltiazem is usually the best tolerated calcium channel blocker and should be chosen instead of other agents unless there are significant price differences
- calcium channel blocking agents are considered the drugs of choice for the management of Prinzmetal's variant angina

Chronic (noncrisis) hypertension

- use in only patients who do not tolerate, do not respond to, or have contraindications to thiazide diuretics and beta-blockers because thiazide diuretics and beta-blockers have proven long-term benefit and are generally less expensive than calcium channel blockers
- calcium channel blockers are useful for hypertension in patients with ischemic heart disease if beta-blockers are not effective or tolerated and in patients with asthma, diabetes, or moderate to severe hyperlipidemias, as they have no effect on these disease states
- all calcium channel blockers are equally effective; however, diltiazem is usually the best tolerated calcium channel blocker and should be chosen instead of other agents unless there are significant price differences

Atrial fibrillation or flutter, atrioventricular nodal reentrant tachycardia

- diltiazem is an alternative to parenteral verapamil if the negative inotropic effects of verapamil would be detrimental to the patient (likely neither verapamil nor diltiazem should be used long term if the patient has left ventricular dysfunction)

Raynaud's syndrome

- diltiazem has been effective but has not been as extensively studied as nifedipine (Hypertension 1991;17:593–602)
- nifedipine has proven efficacy in the treatment of Raynaud's syndrome and should be chosen if the patient can tolerate the drug

▶ *When Should I Not Use This Drug?*

Post–myocardial infarction patients

- addition of a calcium antagonist is indicated only if optimum (beta-blocker and nitrate) therapy does not control anginal symptoms
- data for empirical use of calcium antagonists after myocardial infarction have not shown a decrease in mortality

Acute (crisis) hypertension

- no evidence of the use of verapamil in this condition

▶ *What Contraindications Are There to the Use of This Drug?*

Intolerance of or allergic reaction to diltiazem

Severe left ventricular dysfunction (ejection fraction < 20–30%)

- diltiazem can depress left ventricular function and should be avoided

Ventricular dysfunction and atrioventricular conduction abnormalities if the patient is receiving a beta-adrenergic blocking agent

- these 2 agents can produce an additive effect on blocking the atrioventricular node, which can progress to second- or third-degree heart block

Severe hypotension (systolic blood pressure < 90 mmHg)

- lowers blood pressure and/or blocks an appropriate rise in heart rate

Cardiogenic shock

- decreases contractility and further decreases cardiac output and counteracts appropriate vasoconstriction

Second- or third-degree atrioventricular block or sick sinus syndrome (unless a functioning ventricular pacemaker is in place)

- worsens heart block

Wolff-Parkinson-White syndrome

- atrioventricular node blocking activity with no increased conduction in accessory atrioventricular pathways and therefore possible increased ventricular response in patients with WPW

Wide-complex ventricular tachycardia

- may decrease blood pressure and is not effective

▶ *What Drug Interactions Are Clinically Important?*

Drugs that may increase the effect or toxicity of diltiazem

BETA-ADRENERGIC BLOCKING AGENTS

- when used concomitantly with diltiazem, this increases the incidence of congestive heart failure, arrhythmia, and severe hypotension
- these agents should be used together only when anginal symptoms fail to be controlled by other drug therapy or either agent alone

Drugs that may decrease the effect of diltiazem

CALCIUM

- calcium therapy may result in antagonism of the beneficial effects and unwanted effects of calcium channel blocking agents, and therefore concomitant use is not recommended
- therapy to maintain eucalcemia is not a problem

CAFFEINE, EPINEPHRINE, ISOPROTERENOL, THEOPHYLLINE

- drugs that increase cyclic adenosine monophosphate inhibit the calcium channel blocking activity and patients should be observed for alterations in response
- if episodic hypertension is suspected because of these agents, an ambulatory blood pressure monitor may be useful

Drugs that may have their effect or toxicity increased by diltiazem

PROPRANOLOL

- is a lipophilic beta-adrenergic blocker
- bioavailability is increased 50% by diltiazem therapy
- choose another beta-blocker

DIGOXIN

- conflicting reports about the effect of diltiazem on digoxin
- if diltiazem is being added to digoxin, be aware of the potential for an interaction and adjust the dosage on the basis of clinical signs and symptoms of toxicity

CARBAMAZEPINE

- hepatic metabolism is inhibited by diltiazem via the cytochrome P-450 microsomal enzyme system, which may result in increased plasma carbamazepine concentrations and subsequent toxicity
- 40–50% reduction in carbamazepine dosage may be necessary during concomitant therapy
- use nifedipine in place of diltiazem if possible
- if diltiazem must be added for longer than 3 days, obtain a baseline serum carbamazepine concentration prior to adding inhibitor, recheck the concentration in 1 week, and reduce the dosage proportionately if the concentration is greater than 12 mg/L
- monitor for symptoms of toxicity, and if they occur, stop the drug administration, get a repeat concentration, and adjust the dosage accordingly
- if a concentration not available within 24 hours, restart the carbamazepine regimen at 50% of the previous dosage as long as toxicity is not present
- if no toxicity occurs, measure concentrations weekly until a new steady state has been reached
- if diltiazem administration is stopped, increase the carbamazepine dosage to preinhibitor levels

CYCLOSPORINE

- diltiazem inhibits hepatic metabolism of cyclosporine
- seen as early as 2 days after the start of these drugs
- use an alternative if possible (e.g., nifedipine does not interact)
- monitor cyclosporine levels every other day until the full extent of the interaction is seen and adjust the dosage accordingly
- may need to decrease the cyclosporine dosage by 30% or more

Drugs that may have their effect decreased by diltiazem

- none

▶ What Route and Dosage Should I Use?

How to administer

Orally
- diltiazem should be taken before meals and at bedtime

Parenterally
- not available in Canada
- diltiazem is physically compatible with 5% dextrose in water injection and normal saline injection
- diltiazem bolus injection should be given as a slow intravenous push, over 2 minutes
- maintenance intravenous infusion can be initiated after bolus injection for continued reduction of the heart rate

Chronic stable angina

- 60 mg of diltiazem SR (a twice-daily product) PO BID, increasing the dosage by 60 mg/d at weekly intervals until symptoms are controlled or a maximum dosage of 300 mg/d is reached
- 180 mg of diltiazem CD (a once-daily product) PO daily, increasing the dosage by 60 mg/d at weekly intervals until symptoms are controlled or a maximum dosage of 300 mg/d is reached

- sustained-release preparations are recommended, as they are more convenient and usually not much different in price from the regular-release products (unless generic regular-release forms are available)
- regular-release form is started at 30 mg PO Q6H, increasing the dosage weekly by 30 mg PO Q6H until symptoms are controlled or a maximum dosage of 360 mg/d is reached

Chronic (noncrisis) hypertension

- 60 mg of diltiazem SR (a twice-daily product) PO BID, increasing the dosage every 4 weeks by 60 mg/d until an effect is seen or a maximum dosage of 300 mg/d is reached
- 180 mg of diltiazem CD (a once-daily product) PO daily, increasing the dosage every 4 weeks by 60 mg/d until an effect is seen or a maximum dosage of 300 mg/d is reached
- sustained-release preparations are recommended, as they are more convenient and usually not much different in price from the regular-release products (unless generic regular-release forms are available)
- regular-release form is started at 30 mg PO Q6H, increasing the dosage every 4 weeks by 30 mg PO Q6H until an effect is seen or a maximum dosage of 360 mg/d is reached

Atrial fibrillation or flutter, atrioventricular nodal reentrant tachycardia

- 0.25 mg/kg IV bolus administered over 2 minutes
- second dose of 0.35 mg/kg may be administered after 15 minutes if the response is inadequate
- continuous IV infusion of 10 mg/h may be initiated immediately after the last IV bolus
- infusion rate may be increased to 15 mg/h after 1 hour if a further reduction in heart rate is required
- oral doses as above

Raynaud's syndrome

- 30 mg PO just prior to cold exposure or at the onset of an attack
- 30 mg PO Q8H for long-term prevention

Dosage adjustments for renal or hepatic dysfunction

- hepatically metabolized
- specific diltiazem dosage recommendations for patients with impaired renal or hepatic function are not available
- start with a low dose and titrate to effect

▶ What Should I Monitor with Regard to Efficacy and Toxicity?

Efficacy

Chronic stable angina
- relief of chest pain and decreased frequency of chest pain
- reduction in the use of nitroglycerin tablets
- resolution of ST segment depression or decreased amount of total daily ischemia on Holter monitoring
- patient should be evaluated every time the dosage of an agent needs to be increased
- patients should be reevaluated with treadmill exercise tests when symptoms change or at least every 3 years

Chronic (noncrisis) hypertension

Blood pressure
- patients with diastolic blood pressures greater than 115 mmHg or with symptoms should be evaluated again within 48 hours to ensure that at least a 5–10 mmHg drop in blood pressure has occurred
- for patients with diastolic blood pressures less than 115 mmHg, follow-up blood pressure measurements should be done within a couple of weeks
- at each visit, do 2 blood pressure measurements, supine or sitting, after the patient has been resting without conversation for 5–10 minutes
- continue to do this every 4 weeks to assess the effect of each new drug or dosage until control is achieved
- for most patients with mild hypertension, after blood pressure is controlled, blood pressure measurements 2–4 times per year are sufficient

Evidence of end-organ damage

- if blood pressure is well controlled and no other disease states exist (e.g., diabetes), measure baseline serum creatinine, blood glucose, and serum cholesterol levels and perform urinalysis and repeat every 5 years
- repeat every year if other disease states are present

Atrial fibrillation or flutter

Control of ventricular rate

Electrocardiogram

- during acute loading, the patient's electrocardiogram (ECG) should be monitored every 8 hours

Vital signs

- every 15 minutes until the patient is stable, then every 4 hours for 24 hours
- resting apical ventricular rate of 60–80 bpm is a reasonable target, although 90–100 bpm may be acceptable if the patient is asymptomatic at this heart rate
- presence or absence of symptoms related to arrhythmia (palpitations, shortness of breath, dizziness, and angina)

Atrioventricular nodal reentrant tachycardia

Acute episodes

Electrocardiogram

- ECG should be monitored continuously until the arrhythmia has stopped

Vital signs

- should be assessed every 5 minutes during drug administration
- presence or absence of symptoms related to arrhythmia (palpitations, shortness of breath, dizziness, and angina)

Long-term therapy

- frequency or duration of episodes (may be evaluated by ambulatory ECG)
- patients should be assessed every few weeks during the first few months of therapy and every few months thereafter

Raynaud's syndrome

Acute treatment or prophylaxis

- reduction in the severity and duration of attack

Long-term prevention

- subjective improvement seen as a reduction in the frequency, severity, or duration of attacks best determined by diary records

Toxicity

Hypotension

- all calcium channel blockers can cause hypotension and it is dose related
- if systolic pressures become less than 90 mmHg, stop the drug administration, and if the drug is still needed, reinstitute at 50% of the dosage after the blood pressure has improved

Bradycardia

- is most common with verapamil but can occur with diltiazem
- if symptomatic bradycardia occurs, stop the drug administration, and if the drug is still needed, reinstitute at 50% of the dosage after bradycardia has resolved

Dizziness or lightheadedness

- all calcium channel blockers can cause this; however, nifedipine is likely the worst

Exacerbation of congestive heart failure

- all calcium antagonists have the potential to depress left ventricular function and cause exacerbation of symptoms of congestive heart failure in some patients with ejection fractions of less than 30%
- verapamil and diltiazem can both depress left ventricular function and should not be used in patients with congestive heart failure
- peripheral vasodilatation seen with nifedipine may offset its negative inotropic effect; however, nifedipine can still worsen congestive heart failure in some patients

- if congestive heart failure symptoms occur, consider alternative therapy

Constipation

- all calcium channel blockers can cause constipation, with verapamil likely being the worst offender
- increase fluid and fiber in the diet, and if needed, use a laxative

Peripheral edema

- peripheral edema (ankle edema) occurs in 5–10% of patients receiving calcium channel blockers
- if this occurs, ensure that this is not an exacerbation of congestive heart failure (see above)
- try a dosage reduction, or low-dose diuretics may be effective at reducing peripheral edema if the dosage cannot be reduced or the drug administration cannot be stopped

▶ *How Long Do I Treat Patients with This Drug?*

Chronic stable angina

- maintenance drug therapy should likely be continued indefinitely; however, a change in lifestyle and the natural history of the disease should suggest continual reevaluation for the lowest effective dosage, replacement with a better or less expensive agent, or even discontinuation of drug
- patients should be reevaluated with treadmill exercise tests when symptoms change or at least every 3 years

Chronic (noncrisis) hypertension

Stepped-down therapy, in general, should be considered in patients whose blood pressures during the previous few visits have been well controlled

- approximately 50% of patients with well-controlled disease successfully undergo either dosage or drug reduction and remain so for a period of time, but unfortunately, this period varies from patient to patient and consistent reevaluation is necessary
- this may be explained by reversal of cardiac and vascular changes that may occur after prolonged treatment with drug therapy and may be a means of "setting back the clock" of primary hypertension evolution
- as with every treatment, not everyone has their blood pressure successfully respond to drug discontinuation or drug dosage reduction
- patients most likely to have a successful reduction or discontinuation of therapy may be predicted by a low pretreatment blood pressure (mild hypertension with diastolic pressure <100 mmHg), no evidence of target organ damage, requirement of only monotherapy for blood pressure control, and weight loss, salt restriction, increased exercise, and a decrease in alcohol intake
- drug administration discontinuation in patients with severe to malignant hypertension or target organ damage (e.g., myocardial infarction, congestive heart failure, stroke, and renal failure) is not advised
- reassessment allows a reevaluation of the efficacy of nondrug measures in the treatment of hypertension such as reducing weight and reducing salt and alcohol intake
- reassessment allows hypertension to be treated with the least number of drugs at the lowest dosage, which reduces the incidence of adverse effects, reduces the frequency of drug administration, and is more cost effective

Atrial fibrillation or flutter

- patients with acute atrial fibrillation or flutter for which an underlying cause can be identified require rate control therapy until the underlying cause can be corrected
- patients with chronic or paroxysmal atrial fibrillation or flutter require rate control therapy indefinitely
- patients with paroxysmal atrial fibrillation or flutter require therapy for the maintenance of sinus rhythm indefinitely

Atrioventricular nodal reentrant tachycardia

Acute episodes

- therapy should be continued until arrhythmia is terminated

Long-term oral therapy

- unless nonpharmacological arrhythmia cure (such as radiofrequency ablation or surgery) is attempted and achieved, therapy is required indefinitely

Raynaud's syndrome

- treatment with diltiazem can be continued as long as symptoms recur during drug-free periods

▶ *How Do I Decrease or Stop the Administration of This Drug?*

- should be tapered in hypertension or angina unless other antianginal or antihypertensive agents are added concurrently
- in patients with disease controlled with single-drug therapy, the dosage should be reduced by 50% with reassessment of blood pressure at 2 weeks
- if blood pressure is still normotensive, reduce the dosage by another 50% (i.e., to 25% of the initial dose) and recheck blood pressure in another 2 weeks
- if the blood pressure is still well controlled, stop the medication administration and recheck the blood pressure in 2 weeks
- so-called rebound hypertension does not occur if the dosage is gradually tapered, with dosage reductions of no more than 50% at 2–4 week intervals
- final dose before full drug discontinuation should be less than $^1/_4$ the dose of the initial therapy

▶ *What Should I Tell My Patients About This Drug?*

- diltiazem should be taken on an empty stomach
- excessive caffeine consumption (>5 cups per day) should be avoided, as this may inhibit the action of calcium channel blocking agents
- high-fiber diets are helpful in maintaining normal bowel habits

▶ *Therapeutic Tips*

- patients are usually more compliant with extended-release products, which are usually less expensive when the cost of daily therapy is considered

Useful References

Follath F. The role of calcium antagonists in the treatment of myocardial ischemia. Am Heart J 1989;118:1093–1097

Tolins M, Weir EK, Chesler E, Pierpont GL. "Maximal" drug therapy is not necessarily optimal in chronic angina pectoris. J Am Coll Cardiol 1984;3:1051–1057

DIMENHYDRINATE

Lynne Nakashima

USA (Dramamine, Dymenate, Dinate, Dommanate, Dramocen, Dramoject)
CANADA (Gravol, Nauseatol, Travel Aids, Travel-Eze)

▶ *When Should I Use This Drug?*

Motion sickness

- for mild to moderate road, air, or sea travel, especially if sedation is desired
- decision between dimenhydrinate and promethazine should be based on cost

General nausea and vomiting, postoperative nausea and vomiting

- if sedation is desired, dimenhydrinate should be chosen instead of agents such as prochlorperazine, perphenazine, or thiethylperazine

▶ *When Should I Not Use This Drug?*

Chemotherapy-induced nausea and vomiting

- dimenhydrinate is not usually used in chemotherapy-induced nausea and vomiting because it is generally considered no more effective than placebo (Drugs 1992;43:295–315)

▶ *What Contraindications Are There to the Use of This Drug?*

Intolerance of or allergic reaction to dimenhydrinate
Bladder neck or urethral obstruction

- may precipitate or aggravate urinary retention

Angle closure glaucoma

- may cause increased intraocular pressure, leading to an acute attack of glaucoma

▶ *What Drug Interactions Are Clinically Important?*

Drugs that may increase the effect or toxicity of dimenhydrinate

OTHER ANTICHOLINERGICS (E.G., ATROPINE, ANTIDEPRESSANTS, ANTIPSYCHOTICS)

- may cause additive anticholinergic effects
- use the lowest effective dosage of all agents

OTHER CENTRAL NERVOUS SYSTEM DEPRESSANTS (E.G., NARCOTIC ANALGESICS, HYPNOTICS, ALCOHOL)

- additive sedative effects are expected when other central nervous system depressants are used
- avoid combinations if possible, or use the lowest effective dosages of all agents

Drugs that may decrease the effect of dimenhydrinate

- none

Drugs that may have their effect or toxicity increased by dimenhydrinate

OTOTOXIC MEDICATIONS (E.G., AMINOGLYCOSIDES, AMPHOTERICIN B, SALICYLATES, CISPLATIN)

- dimenhydrinate may mask the symptoms of ototoxicity, such as tinnitus, dizziness, and vertigo
- avoid combination if possible

Drugs that may have their effect decreased by dimenhydrinate

- none

▶ *What Route and Dosage Should I Use?*

How to administer

- orally—take with food or milk or on an empty stomach
- parenterally—dilute 50 mg in 10 mL of normal saline or 5% dextrose in water and inject slowly over 2 minutes; may also dilute 50 mg in 50 mL of normal saline or 5% dextrose in water and administer over 15 to 30 minutes
- also available as rectal suppositories in Canada

Motion sickness

- 50 mg PO BID starting 1–2 hours before the trip

Postoperative nausea and vomiting

- 50 mg IV or IM every 3 hours when needed
- 25 mg PO every 3 hours may be used if the patient can tolerate sips of fluid

Dosage adjustments for renal or hepatic dysfunction

- no dosage adjustments are currently recommended; little information is available on the metabolism of dimenhydrinate

▶ *What Should I Monitor with Regard to Efficacy and Toxicity?*

Efficacy

Number and severity of vomiting episodes

- determine time of day, force, description of vomitus, and associated symptoms

Toxicity

Anticholinergic effects

- effects include dry mouth and blurred vision
- if dry mouth occurs, try increasing fluid intake or try sugarless gum to keep the mouth moist
- if blurred vision occurs, try using comfort drops and avoid the use of contact lenses

Sedation

- can be quite sedating

- tell patients to avoid activities that require mental alertness until they see the extent of sedation
- if sedation becomes a problem, reduce the dosage by 50%
- avoid other sedating medications if possible

▶ *How Long Do I Treat Patients with This Drug?*

Motion sickness

- treatment should continue for the duration of susceptibility to motion sickness

Postoperative nausea and vomiting

- may continue for 24 hours after surgery as needed

▶ *How Do I Decrease or Stop the Administration of This Drug?*

- may be stopped abruptly

▶ *What Should I Tell My Patients About This Drug?*

- for the prevention of motion sickness, take the first dose 1–2 hours before a trip
- it may cause drowsiness; therefore, avoid activities requiring you to be mentally alert
- drowsiness may also be increased if you are taking other medications that cause drowsiness

Useful Reference

Wood CD. Antimotion sickness and antiemetic drugs. Drugs 1979;17: 471–479

DIPHENHYDRAMINE

Penny Miller

USA (Benadryl, many generics)
CANADA (Benadryl, many generics)

▶ *When Should I Use This Drug?*

Nonproductive coughs

- only antihistamine with proven efficacy as an antitussive in the treatment of coughs caused by the common cold or irritants
- unless sedation is also desired, dextromethorphan should be chosen instead of diphenhydramine, as it is effective and causes much less sedation

Nausea and vomiting

- can be used for the prevention and treatment of nausea and vomiting associated with motion sickness, but unless sedation is desired, dimenhydrinate should be chosen instead of diphenhydramine, as it is more effective and produces less sedation (Drug Evaluations 1986)

Transient situational insomnia, short-term insomnia (of up to 3 weeks' duration)

- antihistamines are available in many over the counter sleep preparations, and although these agents promote sleep, they are not as effective or as safe as benzodiazepines, they have more side effects, and compounds with long half-lives are not recommended because they may cause hangover effects
- if prescription sleep agents are not available, diphenhydramine may be useful, as it causes a high level of sedation

Drug-induced extrapyramidal reaction

- can be useful for dystonic reactions but use instead of benztropine or trihexyphenidyl only if these agents are ineffective or unavailable

Anaphylaxis and angioedema

- antihistamines prevent further extension of allergic reaction
- drug of choice is usually diphenhydramine, preferably intravenous, combined with epinephrine

Parkinson's disease

- when patients do not respond to less sedating agents such as benztropine, trihexyphenidyl, and procyclidine

Acute dermatological allergies (e.g., hives and allergic conjunctivitis caused by allergens or food)

- antihistamines relieve pruritus and prevent further extension of the lesions
- if sedation is required (may be a desirable property in an acute allergic reaction), diphenhydramine is useful; if not, use chlorpheniramine

▶ *When Should I Not Use This Drug?*

Seasonal allergic rhinitis, chronic (perennial) rhinitis, chronic dermatological allergies (atopic dermatitis, chronic urticaria, and pruritus of unknown cause)

- diphenhydramine causes a high incidence of sedation and must be given 3–4 times daily and therefore provides no advantages over other antihistamines (e.g., chlorpheniramine, terfenadine, and loratidine) unless sedation is desirable

▶ *What Contraindications Are There to the Use of This Drug?*

see Chlorpheniramine

▶ *What Drug Interactions Are Clinically Important?*

see Chlorpheniramine

▶ *What Route and Dosage Should I Use?*

How to administer

Orally
- take on an empty stomach or with food or milk

Parenterally
- can be given intramuscularly and by intravenous push over 1 minute
- do not give subcutaneous injection because it is irritating

Nonproductive coughs

- 25 mg PO Q4H up to 150 mg PO daily as needed to control symptoms

Nausea and vomiting

- 25–50 mg PO or IM Q4H

Transient situational insomnia, short-term insomnia (of up to 3 weeks' duration)

- 25 mg PO 40 minutes before retiring
- if after 1–2 nights of therapy this dose is not effective, increase the dose to 50 mg

Drug-induced extrapyramidal reaction

- 50 mg IM or IV

Anaphylaxis and angioedema

- 50 mg IV over 5 minutes or IM if there is no IV access

Parkinson's disease

- 25 mg PO TID up to 50 mg PO QID

Acute dermatological allergies (e.g., hives and allergic conjunctivitis caused by allergens or food)

- 50 mg PO Q4H up to 300 mg PO daily as needed to control symptoms

▶ *What Should I Monitor with Regard to Efficacy and Toxicity?*

Efficacy

Nonproductive coughs
- monitor for relief or a reasonable degree of reduction of cough, runny nose, and sneezing

Nausea and vomiting
- monitor for relief within 15–45 minutes of parenteral administration and 30–60 minutes of oral ingestion

Transient situational insomnia, short-term insomnia (of up to 3 weeks' duration)

Shortening of the time taken to fall asleep and improved sleep efficiency

- quantify through the use of a sleep diary and compare with pretreatment sleep performance

Improved daytime functioning

- quantify by comparing changes in the symptoms (e.g., anxiety, tension, and fatigue) with treatment with baseline values

Drug-induced extrapyramidal reaction

- dystonic reactions should be relieved within 10–30 mintues after injection

Anaphylaxis and angioedema

- laryngeal edema, bronchial obstruction, and prevention of progression to respiratory and cardiovascular collapse

Parkinson's disease

- assess signs and symptoms weekly during the titration period, using one of several available evaluation scores
- evaluate for improvement or worsening of symptoms
- after the patient has been stabilized, assess the patient every 3 months
- see Chapter 6 for signs and symptoms of Parkinson's disease

Acute dermatological allergies (e.g., hives and allergic conjunctivitis caused by allergens or food)

- relief of itching and no more formation of new lesions within 24–48 hours

▶ *How Long Do I Treat Patients with This Drug?*

Nonproductive coughs

- some coughs may persist longer than a week, and these should be evaluated

Nausea and vomiting

- therapy should be continued until vomiting is controlled and the underlying pathophysiological changes are treated

Transient situational insomnia, short-term insomnia (of up to 3 weeks' duration)

- 1–4 days when a recurrent stressor is causing sleep disruption with impairment in awake functioning

Drug-induced extrapyramidal reaction

- after acute dystonic reactions have been relieved with a parenteral dose, oral therapy should be continued for 3 days

Anaphylaxis and angioedema

- use for 1–6 weeks after the acute phase has resolved

Parkinson's disease

- therapy for Parkinson's disease is lifelong
- in the majority of cases, anticholinergic drugs can be discontinued, as symptoms deteriorate when another drug class is instituted

Acute dermatological allergies (e.g., hives and allergic conjunctivitis caused by allergens or food)

- treat for 4–7 days depending on the resolution of symptoms

▶ *How Do I Decrease or Stop the Administration of This Drug?*

- may be stopped abruptly

▶ *What Should I Tell My Patients About This Drug?*

see Chlorpheniramine

▶ *Therapeutic Tips*

- diphenhydramine is a drug that abusers seek; therefore, control the quantities prescribed
- diphenhydramine is extremely sedating and the combination of alcohol or other central nervous system depressants with this drug is dangerous

Useful References

Sutherland D. Antihistamine agents—New options or just more drugs? On Continuing Practice 1991;18:31–36

American Hospital Formulary Service, Drug Information ASHP. Bethesda, MD:1993

Health Protection Branch. First Report of the Expert Advisory Committee on Nonprescription Cough and Cold Remedies. Health and Welfare Canada, 1988

Health Protection Branch. Second Report of the Expert Advisory Committee on Nonprescription Cough and Cold Remedies. Health and Welfare Canada, 1989

American Medical Association. Drug Evaluations, 6th ed. Philadelphia: Saunders, 1986

DIPYRIDAMOLE

J. Chris Bradberry

USA (Persantine)
CANADA (Apo-Dipyridamole, Persantine)

▶ *When Should I Use This Drug?*

Prevention of cardiogenic cerebral embolism in patients with mechanical prosthetic valves

- although some studies have shown no benefit, this agent should be used if the patient has systemic embolism and warfarin and aspirin are not allowed

▶ *When Should I Not Use This Drug?*

Transient ischemic attack, completed stroke, angina

- there is no evidence to support the use of dipyridamole in these conditions (Stroke 1985;16:406–415)

▶ *What Contraindications Are There to the Use of This Drug?*

Intolerance of or allergic reaction to dipyridamole

Unstable angina

- increases the risk of ischemia due to a coronary steal mechanism, and worsening of angina may occur

▶ *What Drug Interactions Are Clinically Important?*

Drugs that may increase the effect or toxicity of dipyridamole

ASPIRIN, NONSTEROIDAL ANTIINFLAMMATORY DRUGS, SULFINPYRAZONE

- concurrent use with agents that inhibit platelet aggregation may increase the risk of bleeding
- do not use dipyridamole in conjunction with these agents

Drugs that may decrease the effect of dipyridamole

- none

Drugs that may have their effect or toxicity increased by dipyridamole

- none

Drugs that may have their effect decreased by dipyridamole

- none

▶ *What Route and Dosage Should I Use?*

How to administer

- orally—take with food or milk to minimize gastrointestinal discomfort
- parenterally—not available

Prevention of cardiogenic cerebral embolism in patients with mechanical prosthetic valves

- 100 mg PO Q6H

Dosage adjustments for renal or hepatic dysfunction

- hepatically metabolized

Normal Dosing Interval	C_{cr} > 60 mL/min or 1 mL/s	C_{cr} 30–60 mL/min or 0.5–1 mL/s	C_{cr} < 30 mL/min or 0.5 mL/s
Q6H	no adjustment needed	no adjustment needed	no adjustment needed

▶ *What Should I Monitor with Regard to Efficacy and Toxicity?*

Efficacy

Prevention of cardiogenic cerebral embolism

Evidence of cerebral embolism

- transient ischemic attacks or strokes

Toxicity

- dizziness, weakness, syncope, and myocardial ischemia occur rarely

▶ *How Long Do I Treat Patients with This Drug?*

Prevention of cardiogenic cerebral embolism in patients with mechanical prosthetic valves

- mechanical valves necessitate treatment indefinitely (J Am Coll Cardiol 1986;8:41B–56B)

▶ *How Do I Decrease or Stop This Drug?*

- may be stopped abruptly

▶ *What Should I Tell My Patients About This Drug?*

- because of its effect on platelets, you should report any abnormal bleeding or bruising
- if you experience stomach upset or diarrhea, remember to take this drug with food and this should help
- if stomach upset or diarrhea continues or you develop a rash, contact your physician

Useful Reference

The American-Canadian Cooperative Study Groups. Persantine aspirin trial in cerebral ischemia. Part II. Endpoint results. Stroke 1985;16:406–415.

DISOPYRAMIDE

James Tisdale

USA (Norpace, Norpace CR, generic)
CANADA (Norpace, Norpace CR, Rythmodan, Rythmodan-LA, generic)

▶ *When Should I Use This Drug?*

Disopyramide should not be used without consulting a cardiologist or a cardiac electrophysiologist

Atrial fibrillation or flutter

- maintenance of sinus rhythm in patients with paroxysmal atrial fibrillation or flutter in whom quinidine, procainamide, and flecainide have been proven ineffective and/or not well-tolerated

Ventricular tachycardia

- disopyramide should be used in patients who are unable to tolerate therapy with quinidine or procainamide and in whom procainamide has been shown to suppress ventricular tachycardia during electrophysiological study or on Holter monitoring

Wolff-Parkinson-White syndrome

- disopyramide should be used in patients with supraventricular tachycardia due to Wolff-Parkinson-White syndrome who have no history of left ventricular dysfunction, in whom the syndrome is not cured by nonpharmacological techniques such as radioablation and surgery, and in whom disopyramide has been shown to be effective during electrophysiological testing

Syncope

- disopyramide should be used for the management of vasovagal syncope in patients in whom disopyramide prevents the provocation of syncope during upright tilt-table testing (Am J Cardiol 1990;65:1339–1344)

▶ *When Should I Not Use This Drug?*

Asymptomatic ventricular arrhythmias

- treatment of asymptomatic ventricular arrhythmias with antiarrhythmic drugs has not been shown to be of benefit

▶ *What Contraindications Are There to the Use of This Drug?*

Intolerance of or allergic reaction to disopyramide
Congestive heart failure

- disopyramide has profound negative inotropic effects and may cause cardiovascular collapse and death in patients with congestive heart failure (N Engl J Med 1980;302:614–617)
- disopyramide should not be used in any patient with clinical congestive heart failure, a history of congestive heart failure, or known left ventricular dysfunction (left ventricular ejection fraction < 40%)

Prostatic hypertrophy or urinary retention

- disopyramide has potent anticholinergic effects and may cause or aggravate urinary retention

Long QT interval syndrome or history of torsades de pointes

- disopyramide may prolong QT intervals on surface electrocardiogram and provoke torsades de pointes in susceptible patients

Myasthenia gravis or glaucoma

- anticholinergic properties may aggravate this condition

Second- or third-degree atrioventricular nodal block

- may be aggravated by disopyramide, and therefore, the drug should not be used in such patients unless a functioning ventricular pacemaker is present

▶ *What Drug Interactions Are Clinically Important?*

Drugs that may increase the effect or toxicity of disopyramide

- none

Drugs that may decrease the effect or toxicity of disopyramide
PHENYTOIN, PHENOBARBITAL, RIFAMPIN

- induce the hepatic metabolism of disopyramide
- if therapy with any of these agents is initiated for a patient with disopyramide, a serum disopyramide concentration should be determined 1 week after the initiation of therapy, and the dose adjusted if necessary

Drugs that may have their effect or toxicity increased by disopyramide

- none

Drugs that may have their effect or toxicity decreased by disopyramide

- none

▶ *What Route and Dosage Should I Use?*

How to administer

- orally—administer with or without food
- parenterally—not available in USA

Atrial fibrillation or flutter, ventricular tachycardia, Wolff-Parkinson-White syndrome, syncope

- initial dosage is 150 mg PO Q6H
- increase in 48 hours to 200 mg PO Q6H if arrhythmia is not controlled
- do not change to a sustained-release preparation until arrhythmias are controlled
- do not use sustained-release disopyramide in patients with renal insufficiency

Dosage adjustments for renal or hepatic dysfunction

- hepatically metabolized and renally eliminated

Normal Dosing Interval	$C_{cr} > 60$ mL/min or 1 mL/s	C_{cr} 30–60 mL/min or 0.5–1 mL/s	$C_{cr} < 30$ mL/min or 0.5 mL/s
Q6H	no adjustment needed	Q12H	Q24H

▶ What Should I Monitor with Regard to Efficacy and Toxicity?

Efficacy

see Quinidine

Serum concentrations

- therapeutic range of disopyramide levels is usually quoted as 2–5 µg/mL
- range of serum disopyramide concentrations necessary for efficacy varies widely among patients, and therefore, the therapeutic range is of relatively little use in monitoring the efficacy of disopyramide
- if therapeutic monitoring is performed, use the method of monitoring target serum disopyramide concentrations (see Quinidine) (Clin Pharmacokinet 1991;20:151–166)

Toxicity

Adverse effects necessitating discontinuation of therapy occur in 10–20% of patients

Anticholinergic effects

Dry mouth

- increase fluids and/or use sugarless chewing gum or hard candies

Constipation

- increase fluid and fiber in the diet, and if needed, use a laxative

Sedation

- may occur; however, many patients become tolerant of the sedation

Orthostatic hypotension

- treatment of orthostatic hypotension includes having the patient rise slowly from supine or sitting positions and wear support stockings

Blurred vision

- dosage reduction may alleviate this effect, but antiarrhythmic effect must be ensured

Urinary hesitancy

- anticholinergic effects may be alleviated or attenuated with sustained-release pyridostigmine bromide

Congestive heart failure

- evaluate the patient within 72 hours for signs or symptoms of congestive heart failure
- if this occurs, stop the drug administration immediately

Electrocardiogram

- repeat electrocardiogram within 1 week for prolongation of QT interval greater than 25%
- if this occurs, the dosage should be reduced

▶ How Long Do I Treat Patients with This Drug?

Atrial fibrillation or flutter, ventricular tachycardia, Wolff-Parkinson-White syndrome, syncope

- patients treated for atrial fibrillation or flutter, ventricular tachycardia, Wolff-Parkinson-White syndrome, or syncope may require therapy indefinitely if contributing factors cannot be reversed

▶ How Do I Decrease or Stop the Administration of This Drug?

- disopyramide therapy should not be discontinued without consulting a cardiologist or a cardiac electrophysiologist
- may be stopped abruptly if ineffective or poorly tolerated

▶ What Should I Tell My Patients About This Drug?

- consult your physician if you experience dry mouth, blurred vision, difficulty with urinating, shortness of breath, or palpitations

- do not change your dosage or discontinue therapy without consulting your physician

▶ Therapeutic Tips

- range of serum disopyramide concentrations required for efficacy varies widely among patients, and therefore, the therapeutic range is of relatively little use in monitoring the efficacy of disopyramide

Useful References

Willis PW. The clinical scope of disopyramide 7 years after introduction: An overview. Angiology 1987;38:165–173

Podrid PJ, Schoeneberger A, Lown B. Congestive heart failure caused by oral disopyramide. N Engl J Med 1980;302:614–617

Brogden LM, Todd PA. Focus on disopyramide. Drugs 1987;34:151–187

DOCUSATE

Leslie Mathews

USA (Colace, Doxinate, Surfak, Dialose, Kasof; combination: Feen-a-Mint, Disolan, Phillips' LaxCaps, Gentlax, Senokot-S, Modane Plus, Correctol)
CANADA (Colace, Regulex, sodium docusate, Surfak; combination: Senokot-S, Correctol, Peri-Colace, Calcium Docuphen, Dulcodos)

▶ When Should I Use This Drug?

Fecal impaction

- docusate enemas are useful for impaction when sodium phosphate enemas are contraindicated, not effective, or not recommended (e.g., patients who are sensitive to fluid and electrolyte changes or who have renal disease, hypocalcemia, abnormal colonic mucosa, or congestive heart failure)
- also useful for softening hard stools prior to manual disimpaction
- decision between this agent and mineral oil enemas should be based on availability, cost, and the patient's preference

Chronic constipation

- when bulk-forming laxatives or lactulose are ineffective, are contraindicated, or are poorly tolerated
- suitable for short-term use only (7 days)
- is effective at producing soft stools, which are easy to pass, without a great increase in bulk and is therefore useful for constipation associated with hard, dry stools, or conditions in which straining should be avoided (e.g., anorectal disorders, hernias, recovery from myocardial infarction, and cerebrovascular accident)
- use for hard, dry stools only if lactulose is ineffective or not tolerated

▶ When Should I Not Use This Drug?

Acute constipation

- with recommended dosage, docusate exerts little or no laxative effect (Gastroenterology 1985;89:489–493)
- ineffective when used alone on a regular basis (J Chronic Dis 1976;29:59–63, Med Clinics North Am 1989;73:1502–1509)

▶ What Contraindications Are There to the Use of This Drug?

Intolerance of or allergic reaction to docusate
Symptoms of acute abdomen

- undiagnosed abdominal pain, nausea, and vomiting

▶ What Drug Interactions Are Clinically Important?

- none

▶ What Route and Dosage Should I Use?

How to administer

- orally—with a glass of water or juice
- parenterally—not available

Chronic constipation

- there is little therapeutic difference among the various docusate salts

- 100 mg PO BID of docusate sodium or potassium (or 240 mg PO daily of docusate calcium)
- assess effectiveness after 3 days and increase as needed to a maximum of 500 mg PO daily of docusate sodium or 300 mg PO daily of docusate potassium
- can be used as a retention enema to soften stool with fecal impaction (50 mg [5 mL of drops] added to 90 mL of enema fluid) or as a flushing enema (10 mg [1 mL of drops] added to 100 mL of enema fluid)

Dosage adjustments for renal or hepatic dysfunction

- absorbed orally and appears in bile in significant concentrations
- extent of absorption after rectal administration is unknown
- no dosage adjustments for renal dysfunction
- do not use in patients with hepatic dysfunction

▶ *What Should I Monitor with Regard to Efficacy and Toxicity?*

Efficacy

Fecal impaction, chronic constipation

- softens stool within 1–3 days if given orally
- question the patient about the consistency of stool and the ease of passage after 3 days of regular use, and adjust the dosage up or down as needed

Toxicity

Gastrointestinal symptoms

- abdominal cramping, nausea, and diarrhea
- decrease or discontinue administration of the drug if symptoms are significant or prolonged
- nausea occurs with liquid preparation; use capsules instead

Hepatotoxicity

- clinical and laboratory evidence suggests that docusate can be hepatotoxic and may increase absorption of other hepatobiliary toxins (Med Clin North Am 1989;73:1502–1509)
- avoid regular use for longer than 7 days, monitor liver enzyme test results when used for longer than 7 days and when used in conjunction with other potentially hepatoxic drugs

▶ *How Long Do I Treat Patients with This Drug?*

Chronic constipation

- use for 3–7 days and then substitute lactulose for patients unable to tolerate regular bulk-forming laxatives

▶ *How Do I Decrease or Stop the Administration of These Drugs?*

- may be stopped abruptly

▶ *What Should I Tell My Patients About This Drug?*

- it may take 3 days to see full softening effect
- to be used on a short-term basis only (1 week) unless directed otherwise by your physician
- do not take with mineral oil
- cramping can occur; in the event of persistent abdominal pain, stop administration of the drug and see your physician
- liquid preparations can cause nausea
- add syrup to juice or pop to mask the bitter taste

▶ *Therapeutic Tips*

- always use in conjunction with laxatives and/or dietary fiber
- ineffective if used alone to prevent or treat constipation
- combination products are not recommended and there are no controlled studies supporting added efficacy, the dose of each component drug is usually inadequate, and there is increased risk of hepatotoxicity
- it is common for patients to require the maximum dosage
- appears to be little therapeutic difference among the activities of the sodium, calcium, or potassium salts
- consider using the calcium or potassium salt for patients with sodium restrictions

Useful References

Tedesco FJ. Laxative use in constipation. Am J Gastroenterol 1985; 80:303–309

Elliot DL, Watts WJ, Girard DE. Constipation—mechanisms and management of a common clinical problem. Postgrad Med 1983;73:143–149
Goodman J, Pang J, Bessman AN. Dioctyl sodium sulfosuccinate—An ineffective prophylactic laxative. J Chronic Dis 1976;29:59–63

DOXEPIN

Lyle K. Laird and Julia Vertrees

USA (Adapin, Sinequan, others)
CANADA (Sinequan, Triadapin)

▶ *When Should I Use This Drug?*

Consider an alternative agent

- doxepin is no more effective than other antidepressants and is associated with a high incidence of adverse effects similar to those with amitriptyline
- doxepin has been touted as having fewer cardiovascular adverse effects (specifically, decreasing intracardiac conduction) than the other tricyclic antidepressants; however, the main study supporting this conclusion was methodologically flawed in that it compared subtherapeutic doxepin doses to therapeutic doses for the comparison drug, nortriptyline (Prog Neuropsychopharmacol 1977;1:371–375)
- is very sedating and is therefore used as a sleeping aid in the elderly but it has no special advantages over other agents

Useful References

Bryant SG, Brown CS. Major depressive disorders. In: Young LY, Koda-Kimble MA, eds. Applied Therapeutics: The Clinical Use of Drugs, 4th ed. Vancouver, WA: Applied Therapeutics, 1988:1231–1253
Wells BG, Hayes PE. Depressive illness. In: DiPiro JT, Talbert RL, Hayes PE, et al, eds. Pharmacotherapy: A Pathophysiologic Approach. New York: Elsevier, 1989:748–764

DOMPERIDONE

Lynne Nakashima

USA (Motilium)
CANADA (Motilium)

▶ *When Should I Use This Drug?*

Nausea and vomiting associated with gastric stasis

- domperidone increases lower esophageal sphincter tone and improves gastric emptying
- metoclopramide and domperidone have similar activity and are likely equally effective
- domperidone causes less frequent sedation and a lower incidence of anticholinergic and extrapyramidal adverse effects than does metoclopramide
- if the oral route can be used, choose domperidone over metoclopramide, as it produces fewer adverse effects; the cost difference may be significant and affect this decision

Reflux esophagitis

- effective agent for mild esophagitis; however, it is no more effective than the H_2 antagonists, which are usually less expensive and dosed less frequently
- effective in combination with H_2 blockers (when therapy with H_2 blockers fails); however, this dual therapy provides no advantage over omeprazole (combination therapy may be more expensive and domperidone is usually dosed QID versus daily or BID dosing for omeprazole)
- domperidone should initially be chosen over cisapride, as it is less expensive and is well tolerated by the majority of patients (no comparative trials of cisapride and domperidone are available)
- omeprazole is the drug of choice for severe reflux esophagitis

▶ *When Should I Not Use This Drug?*

Chemotherapy-induced nausea and vomiting

- not much information about this agent in the treatment of chemotherapy-induced nausea and vomiting
- for this reason, metoclopramide is more widely used

Nausea and vomiting caused by motion sickness and vestibular conditions

- does not appear to be useful (Drugs 1992;43:295–315)

▶ *What Contraindications Are There to the Use of This Drug?*

Intolerance of or allergic reaction to domperidone

Parkinsonism

- may exacerbate parkinsonian symptoms

Gastrointestinal hemorrhage, mechanical obstruction, and perforation

- stimulation of gastrointestinal motility may exacerbate symptoms or worsen the disease state

▶ *What Drug Interactions Are Clinically Important?*

Drugs that may increase the effect or toxicity of domperidone

- none

Drugs that may decrease the effect of domperidone

ANTACIDS OR H₂ ANTAGONISTS

- may inhibit absorption because gastric acidity is needed for the absorption of domperidone
- space doses at least 2 hours apart

OMEPRAZOLE

- may inhibit absorption because gastric acidity is needed for the absorption of domperidone
- as omeprazole produces relative achlorhydria, this combination should be avoided
- metoclopramide could be used as an alternative to domperidone

Drugs that may have their effect or toxicity increased by domperidone

- none

Drugs that may have their effect decreased by domperidone

- none

▶ *What Route and Dosage Should I Use?*

How to administer

- orally—take with food or milk or on an empty stomach
- parenterally—not available

Nausea and vomiting, reflux esophagitis

- 10 mg Q6H may be increased to a maximum of 20 mg PO Q6H if needed (Drugs 1982;24:360–400)

Dosage adjustments for renal or hepatic dysfunction

- hepatically metabolized
- no dosage adjustments required in renal disease
- start with a low dose and titrate up to effect in patients with hepatic disease

▶ *What Should I Monitor with Regard to Efficacy and Toxicity?*

Efficacy

Nausea and vomiting • Frequency of assessment depends on the severity and frequency of nausea and vomiting

Number and severity of vomiting episodes

- determine time of day, force, description of vomitus, and associated symptoms

Fluid balance

- only needed if vomiting occurs for a prolonged period
- assess jugular venous pressure and orthostatic changes in blood pressure and heart rate; any decrease in upright diastolic pressure plus a rise in heart rate of 20 bpm or greater is abnormal
- oliguria
- weight
- rising values of hematocrit and creatinine, urea, sodium, and bicarbonate levels plus decreasing levels of potassium and chloride are an indication of dehydration

Reflux esophagitis

Signs and symptoms

- decrease in heartburn, pain on swallowing, and sour or bitter taste in mouth

- aim is to be virtually symptom free
- initially assess the patient every month and then every 3–6 months after symptoms are under control to encourage lifestyle changes (losing weight, and so on)

Toxicity

Anticholinergic effects

- incidence of less than 7% with domperidone versus 20% with metoclopramide (Can Med Assoc J 1986;135:457–461)
- effects include dry mouth (2%), headache (1.2%), and transient rash or itching (Drugs 1982;24:360–400)
- reduce the dosage or discontinue the administration of domperidone if side effects are severe and intolerable

Extrapyramidal effects

- occasionally may occur; frequency appears to be less than that seen with metoclopramide (Drugs 1982;24:360–400)
- can usually be prevented with diphenhydramine 25 mg PO Q6H or, if severe, 25 mg IV
- discontinue domperidone administration if these effects occur

Sedation

- incidence of sedation is 4.6% with domperidone versus up to 80% with metoclopramide (Am J Med Sci 1987;293:34–44)

▶ *How Long Do I Treat Patients with This Drug?*

Nausea and vomiting associated with gastric stasis

- assess the efficacy of treatment within 72 hours and continue if symptoms persist

Reflux esophagitis

Mild to moderate cases

- approximately 80% of patients experience relapse within a year after discontinuation of short-term treatment
- patients with frequent relapse should be considered for long-term prophylaxis
- prophylaxis usually necessitates dosages equivalent to those for treatment; however, after symptoms are controlled, cut back the dose by 50% every few weeks to identify the lowest effective dosage

Severe cases

- continued treatment with a successful drug regimen is recommended

▶ *How Do I Decrease or Stop the Administration of This Drug?*

- may be stopped abruptly

▶ *What Should I Tell My Patients About This Drug?*

- domperidone can be taken with food or on an empty stomach
- it will take ½–1 hour to become fully effective
- side effects include restlessness or muscle spasms, which may be controlled by diphenhydramine 25 mg every 6 hours; however, if severe facial or neck muscle spasms occur (uncommon), stop taking domperidone and go to nearest emergency department
- drowsiness should decrease after 1–2 days; however, it may be increased if you are taking other medication that causes drowsiness (e.g., narcotic painkillers, alcohol, and some cough remedies)

▶ *Therapeutic Tips*

- domperidone does not cross the blood-brain barrier and therefore less central nervous system toxicity is seen with this agent when compared to metoclopramide

Useful References

Brogden RN, Carmine AA, Heel RC, et al. Domperidone. A review of its pharmacological activity, pharmacokinetics and therapeutic efficacy in the symptomatic treatment of chronic dyspepsia and as an antiemetic. Drugs 1982;24:360–400

Champion MC, Hartnett M, Yen M. Domperidone, a new dopamine antagonist. Can Med Assoc J 1986;135:457–461

DOXYCYCLINE

Alfred Gin and George Zhanel

USA (Doxy Caps, Doxychel Hyclate, Vibramycin, Vibra-Tabs)
CANADA (Apo-Doxy, Doxycin, Novo-doxylin, Vibramycin)

▶ When Should I Use This Drug?

Both tetracycline and doxycycline are equally effective • Doxycycline has the advantages of less frequent dosing (BID for doxycycline versus QID for tetracycline), can be used in patients with decreased renal function, and may be taken with food and should be recommended unless tetracycline is less expensive • Parenteral tetracycline is no longer available
check antibiotic susceptibility chart 1 (Table 4–1 in Chapter 4)

Urethritis

- doxycycline as sole therapy can be used if urethral discharge shows increased polymorphonuclear neutrophils (PMNs) and no diplococci (no *Neisseria gonorrhoeae*), as doxycycline is effective against *Chlamydia trachomatis*
- doxycycline should be used in combination with cefixime if urethral discharge or endocervical disharge shows increased PMNs and gram-negative intracellular diplococci or if no results are available, as this combination covers both gonorrhea and chlamydial infection

Cervicitis

- regardless of cervical stain results, doxycycline in combination with cefixime is the regimen of choice, as this combination covers both gonorrhea organisms and *Chlamydia*, which are usually present

Genital ulcers

- drug of choice in penicillin-allergic patients, if there is clinical suspicion and lesions suggestive (usually painless) of syphilis and/or if dark-field microscopy shows corkscrew spirochetes

Pelvic inflammatory disease

- use in combination with cefoxitin, cefotetan, or ceftizoxime for the inpatient treatment of pelvic inflammatory disease, as doxycycline provides good coverage against *Chlamydia*
- for outpatient treatment, doxycycline can be combined with ceftriaxone or ciprofloxacin if the patient is penicillin allergic

Lyme disease

- drug of choice for the treatment of early stage of disease, but ceftriaxone is recommended in late disease, especially in patients with neurological disease

Rickettsial infection

- doxycycline is the drug of choice for Rocky Mountain spotted fever, Q fever, typhus fever, and tick bite fever

Vibrio infections

- doxycycline is the drug of choice for *Vibrio cholerae*

Prevention of postoperative infections

- prophylactic agent of choice for hysterectomy when the patient is allergic to penicillin

Pneumonia

- useful in patients with proven atypical pneumonias (*Mycoplasma, Legionella*) who cannot tolerate erythromycin

Animal bites

- useful if the patient is penicillin allergic
- although clindamycin or erythromycin may be useful, they have limited activity against *Pasteurella multocida*

▶ When Should I Not Use This Drug?

Gram-negative infections

- many gram-negative organisms are resistant to the tetracyclines

▶ What Contraindications Are There to the Use of This Drug?

see Tetracycline

▶ What Drug Interactions Are Clinically Important?

see Tetracyline

▶ What Route and Dosage Should I Use?

How to administer

- orally—take with a full glass of water 1 hour before or 2 hours after meals, but can take with food (not milk) to decrease gastrointestinal irritation
- parenterally—dilute doxycycline in 100 mL of 5% dextrose in water or normal saline when given intravenously

Urethritis, cervicitis, endocervicitis, genital ulcers, animal bites

- 100 mg PO BID

Pelvic inflammatory disease

- 100 mg PO Q12H
- 100 mg IV Q12H for severely ill patients

Lyme disease, rickettsial infection, Vibrio infections

- 100 mg PO Q12H
- 100 mg IV Q12H for severely ill patients

Prevention of postoperative infections

- 200 mg IV as a single dose

Pneumonia

- 100 mg of PO Q12H for moderately ill patients
- 100 mg IV Q12H for severely ill patients

Dosage adjustments for renal or hepatic dysfunction

- renally eliminated

Normal Dosing Interval	$C_{cr} > 60$ mL/min or 1 mL/s	C_{cr} 30–60 mL/min or 0.5–1 mL/s	$C_{cr} < 30$ mL/min or 0.5 mL/s
Q12H	no adjustment needed	Q24H	Q24H and reduce dosage by 50%

▶ What Should I Monitor with Regard to Efficacy and Toxicity?

see Tetracycline

▶ How Long Do I Treat Patients with This Drug?

see Tetracycline

▶ How Do I Decrease or Stop the Administration of This Drug?

- may be stopped abruptly

▶ What Should I Tell My Patients About This Drug?

- doxycycline may cause your skin to be more sensitive to sunlight; therefore, avoid sun exposure or protect yourself with clothing or sunscreen (need a product that protects against both ultraviolet B and A rays)
- avoid taking doxycycline with antacids or milk products (e.g., take 1 hour before or 2 hours after these products)
- take the medication until it is completed
- take with a full glass of water

▶ Therapeutic Tips

see Tetracycline

Useful References

Franke EL, Neu AC. Chloramphenicol and tetracycline. Med Clin North Am 1987;71:1155–1166
Wilson WR, Cockerill FR III. Tetracycline, chloramphenicol, erythromycin, and clindamycin. Mayo Clin Proc 1987;62:906–915

DRONABINOL

Lynne Nakashima

USA (Marinol)
CANADA (Marinol)

▶ *When Should I Use This Drug?*

see Nabilone

- use only if less expensive than nabilone, as there are insufficient data to select dronabinol over nabilone
- nabilone may be associated with fewer central nervous system euphoric effects than is dronabinol (Drugs 1983;25[suppl 1]: 52–62, Pharmacotherapy 1990;10:129–145)

▶ *When Should I Not Use This Drug?*

see Nabilone

▶ *What Contraindications Are There to the Use of This Drug?*

see Nabilone

▶ *What Drug Interactions Are Clinically Important?*

see Nabilone

▶ *What Route and Dosage Should I Use?*

How to administer

- orally—take with or without food
- parenterally—not available

Chemotherapy-induced nausea and vomiting, intractable nausea and vomiting in acquired immunodeficiency syndrome

- 5 mg/m^2 1 hour prechemotherapy followed by 5 mg/m^2 Q4H (doses must be rounded off to the nearest 2.5 mg)
- if ineffective, increase in 2.5 mg/m^2 increments to a maximum of 10 mg/m^2

Dosage adjustments for renal or hepatic dysfunction

- hepatically metabolized to active metabolites
- avoid in patients with severe hepatic dysfunction

▶ *What Should I Monitor with Regard to Efficacy and Toxicity?*

see Nabilone

▶ *How Long Do I Treat Patients with This Drug?*

see Nabilone

▶ *How Do I Decrease or Stop the Administration of This Drug?*

see Nabilone

▶ *What Should I Tell My Patients About This Drug?*

see Nabilone

Useful References

Cocchetto DM, Cook LF, Cato AE. A critical review of the safety and antiemetic efficacy of delta-9-tetrahydrocannabinol. DICP 1981;15: 867–875

Anderson PO, McGuire GG. Delta-9-tetrahydrocannabinol as an antiemetic. Am J Hosp Pharm 1981;38:646–649

DROPERIDOL

Lynne Nakashima

USA (Inapsine)
CANADA (Inapsine)

▶ *When Should I Use This Drug?*

Postoperative nausea and vomiting

- considered antiemetic of choice to control postoperative vomiting prophylactically owing to its effectiveness and long duration of action (Can Anaesth Soc J 1979;26:125–127, Drugs 1992;

43:443–463, Anesth Analg 1974;53:361–364, Anesth Analg 1977; 56:674–677)

- only drug that appears truly to prevent nausea and vomiting; however, it produces dysphoria in some patients, delays awakening, and prolongs the time to discharge from the postanesthetic care unit
- routine prophylaxis after surgery is discouraged (Drugs 1981;22:246–253) because nausea and vomiting necessitating treatment is seen in only about 5% of patients postoperatively (Can Anaesth Soc J 1986;33:22–31)
- patients at high risk for aspiration (e.g., patients who have their jaws occluded by wires after oral surgery or patients with a history of moderate to severe postoperative vomiting) should receive prophylactic therapy

▶ *When Should I Not Use This Drug?*

Pregnancy

- safety of droperidol in pregnancy has not been established

▶ *What Contraindications Are There to the Use of This Drug?*

Intolerance of or allergic reaction to droperidol
Epilepsy

- may precipitate seizures

▶ *What Drug Interactions Are Clinically Important?*

Drugs that may increase the effect or toxicity of droperidol
OTHER CENTRAL NERVOUS SYSTEM DEPRESSANTS (E.G., NARCOTIC ANALGESICS, HYPNOTICS, ALCOHOL)

- additive sedative effects are to be expected when other central nervous system depressants are used
- avoid combinations if possible, or use the lowest effective dosages of all agents

Drugs that may decrease the effect of droperidol

- none

Drugs that may have their effect or toxicity increased by droperidol
NARCOTIC ANALGESICS

- when droperidol is used in combination with narcotic analgesics, additive respiratory depression, apnea, and muscle rigidity may occur
- use the lowest effective dosages of both agents
- monitor the patient for signs of decreased respiration and use naloxone to reverse the effects of the narcotic analgesic if necessary

Drugs that may have their effect decreased by droperidol

- none

▶ *What Route and Dosage Should I Use?*

How to administer

- orally—not available
- parenterally—may be given intramuscularly; may be given intravenously undiluted at a rate of 10 mg/min or can be diluted in 5% dextrose in water or normal saline

Postoperative nausea and vomiting

- 0.0175 mg/kg IV or IM, as a single dose at the end of surgery

Dosage adjustments for renal or hepatic dysfunction

- hepatically metabolized
- dosage adjustments are not currently available for patients with hepatic failure but are not required if it is being used as a single dose

▶ *What Should I Monitor with Regard to Efficacy and Toxicity?*

Efficacy

Postoperative nausea and vomiting • Number and severity of vomiting episodes

- determine time of day, force, description of vomitus, and associated symptoms

Toxicity

Extrapyramidal reactions

- dystonic reactions, tetanus, restlessness, facial spasms, involuntary movement, torticollis, and muscular twitching can occur
- if an acute dystonic reaction occurs, treat with benztropine 2 mg IM and repeat the dose if a response is not seen within 15 minutes
- if there is still no response, give diphenhydramine 50 mg IM and repeat the dose if there is no relief within 5 minutes

Sedation

- avoid other sedating medications if possible

Hypotension

- usually transient and of mild to moderate severity
- may occur immediately after droperidol, especially after rapid intravenous, administration
- if hypotension persists, this may suggest hypovolemia
- administer while the patient is recumbent
- tell the patient to avoid rising quickly
- ensure that the patient is well hydrated

Hypertension

- has occurred after the use of droperidol combined with fentanyl or other parenteral analgesics

▶ *How Long Do I Treat Patients with This Drug?*

Postoperative nausea and vomiting

- single prophylactic dose has a duration of action of up to 24 hours (Can Anaesth Soc J 1984;31:407–415)

▶ *How Do I Decrease or Stop the Administration of This Drug?*

- may be stopped abruptly

▶ *What Should I Tell My Patients About This Drug?*

- it may cause drowsiness; therefore, avoid activities requiring you to be mentally alert
- drowsiness may also be increased if you are taking other medications that cause drowsiness
- avoid rising quickly to prevent hypotension

Useful Reference

Palazzo MGA, Strunin L. Anaesthesia and emesis II: Prevention and management. Can Anaesth Soc J 1984;31:407–415

DYPHYLLINE

Karen Shalansky and Cindy Reesor Nimmo

USA (Dyflex, Lufyllin, Neothylline)
CANADA (Protophylline)

▶ *When Should I Use This Drug?*

Consider an alternative agent

- contains 70% theophylline and offers no advantage over other theophylline preparations unless it is less expensive

ENALAPRIL

Jack Onrot and James McCormack

USA (Vasotec)
CANADA (Vasotec)

▶ *When Should I Use This Drug?*

All angiotensin converting enzyme (ACE) inhibitors are likely equally effective and the decision about which agent to use should be based on convenience of administration and cost • Captopril has a relatively short half-life and should be dosed twice daily for hypertension • Enalapril and lisinopril can both be dosed once daily • Only captopril and enalapril have been shown to provide survival benefit • Although ramipril, quin-april, benazepril, and fosinopril can also be dosed once daily (for most patients), they offer no advantages over other more extensively used ACE inhibitors (Med Lett 1991;33:83–84, Med Lett 1992;34:27–28) and should likely be chosen only if they are significantly less expensive (Drug Ther Perspect 1993; 1[9]:4–7) • Captopril has a faster onset of action (30 minutes; peak effect, 60–90 minutes) than the other available ACE inhibitors (onset, 1–2 hours; peak effect, 2–6 hours) and should be chosen instead of these other agents if a fast onset is desired (acute hypertension or titration in the initial treatment of congestive heart failure) • The duration of action for captopril is shorter (6–12 hours) than that for other agents (12–24 hours), and this allows easier titration, and if side effects occur, they are less prolonged than those seen with the other agents • Captopril and enalapril have caused taste disturbances, but this adverse effect has not been reported with other ACE inhibitors

Congestive heart failure

Acute pulmonary edema

- captopril is chosen in the acute setting, instead of other ACE inhibitors, because its onset of action is faster (30 minutes versus 2–4 hours) and its duration of action is shorter and this allows easier titration, and if side effects occur, they are less prolonged
- after the patient has been stabilized, the ACE inhibitors for long-term therapy should be chosen on the basis of cost and frequency of administration

Mild to moderate heart failure

- ACE inhibitors have proven beneficial effects on survival (N Engl J Med 1987;316:1429–1435, N Engl J Med 1991;325:293–302, 303–310)
- all ACE inhibitors are likely equally effective, and the decision about which agent to use should be based on convenience (all but captopril can be given once daily) and cost
- best used in conjunction with furosemide (Ann Intern Med 1984;100:777–782)
- no evidence yet exists to support the use of ACE inhibitors alone in heart failure

Chronic (noncrisis) hypertension

- ACE inhibitors are drugs of choice in patients with preexisting congestive heart failure because both conditions can be treated by the single agent
- selection of a specific ACE inhibitor should be based on cost and convenience
- use only in patients who do not tolerate, do not respond to, or have contraindications to thiazide diuretics and beta-blockers because thiazide diuretics and beta-blockers have proven long-term benefit and are generally less expensive than ACE inhibitors
- if compliance is a potential problem, a once-daily ACE inhibitor (whichever is the least expensive) should be chosen

Other Uses

- diabetic nephropathy, rheumatoid arthritis

▶ *When Should I Not Use This Drug?*

Acute (crisis) hypertension

- onset of action for ACE inhibitors other than captopril is likely too slow to be used in this condition

see Captopril

▶ *What Contraindications Are There to the Use of This Drug?*

see Captopril

▶ *What Drug Interactions Are Clinically Important?*

see Captopril

▶ *What Route and Dosage Should I Use?*

How to administer

- orally—can be administered with or without food
- parenterally—available as enalaprilat—can be administered undiluted over at least 5 minutes or given diluted in up to 50 mL of 5% dextrose in water normal saline, or lactated Ringer's solution

Congestive heart failure

- 2.5 mg PO daily
- rapidity of dosage escalation depends on the severity of symptoms
- in general, increase dosages weekly, however, dosages may be increased daily
- no value in exceeding a total daily dose of 40 mg

Chronic (noncrisis) hypertension

- 2.5 mg PO daily
- increase the dosage by 2.5 mg PO daily every 4 weeks until adequate blood pressure is achieved or a daily dosage of 20 mg is reached (dosages as high as 40 mg PO daily have been used)
- BID dosing with this agent is not necessary unless side effects preclude once-daily dosing
- intravenous dose is 1.25 mg Q6H; however, patients who are volume depleted should receive a test dose of 0.625 mg and be evaluated for an hour after the dose for excessive hypotension

Dosage adjustments for renal or hepatic dysfunction

- renally eliminated
- titrate the dose to clinical response and not concurrent renal or hepatic function

▶ *What Should I Monitor with Regard to Efficacy and Toxicity?*

see Captopril

▶ *How Long Do I Treat Patients with This Drug?*

see Captopril

▶ *How Do I Decrease or Stop the Administration of This Drug?*

see Captopril

▶ *What Should I Tell My Patients About This Drug?*

see Captopril

▶ *Therapeutic Tips*

see Captopril

EPHEDRINE

Karen Shalansky and Cindy Reesor Nimmo

USA (combination: Bronkolixir, Bronkotabs, Mudrane GG, Primatene P formula, Quibron Plus, Tedral)
CANADA (combination: Tedral)

▶ *When Should I Use This Drug?*

Consider an alternative agent

- ephedrine stimulates beta$_1$-, beta$_2$-, and alpha-receptors and therefore causes more frequent and numerous side effects than do more selective beta-agonists
- ephedrine produces bronchodilation, cardiac stimulation, and increased blood pressure when administered orally, parenterally, or topically

Useful References

Kelly HW. New beta$_2$-adrenergic agonist aerosols. Clin Pharm 1985;4: 393–403
McFadden ER. Clinical use of beta-adrenergic agonists. J Allergy Clin Immunol 1985;76:352–356

EPINEPHRINE

Karen Shalansky and Cindy Reesor Nimmo

USA (Adrenalin, Ana-Guard Epinephrine, AsthmaHaler, Bronitin Mist, Bronkaid Mist, Epinephrine Mist, EpiPen, Sus-Phrine, Medihaler-Epi, Primatene Mist)

CANADA (Adrenalin, Bronkaid Mistometer, EpiPen, Medihaler-Epi, Vaponefrin)

▶ *When Should I Use This Drug?*

Anaphylaxis (bites, insect stings, drugs, and so on)

- for use by patients with an emergency allergic reaction (anaphylaxis)

Acute asthma unresponsive to other agents

- subcutaneous injection or intravenous infusion for the emergency treatment of acute asthma only after failure from inhaled beta$_2$-agonists, ipratropium bromide, systemic corticosteroids, and theophylline (if intravenous salbutamol is available, it is preferred over epinephrine)

Croup (laryngotracheobronchitis)

- racemic epinephrine is useful owing to its vasoconstrictive properties in the upper airways

Cardiac arrest

- part of advanced cardiac life support protocol
- for asystole or ventricular fibrillation unresponsive to electrical cardioversion

▶ *When Should I Not Use This Drug?*

Acute or chronic asthma

- subcutaneous epinephrine for the initial emergency treatment of acute asthma has not been shown to be superior to inhaled beta$_2$-agonists (Am Rev Respir Dis 1980;122:365–371, J Pediatr 1983;102:465–469)
- inhaled form is not recommended because it stimulates alpha-, beta$_1$-, and beta$_2$-receptors (beta$_1$ > beta$_2$ > alpha) and there are selective beta$_2$-agonists available (e.g., salbutamol and terbutaline), which produce fewer side effects
- shorter acting and less effective than selective beta$_2$-agonists (Med Lett 1991;33:9–12)

▶ *What Contraindications Are There to the Use of This Drug?*

Intolerance of or allergic reaction to epinephrine
Cardiac tachyarrhythmias

- epinephrine may produce serious cardiac arrhythmias

▶ *What Drug Interactions Are Clinically Important?*

Drugs that may increase the effect or toxicity of epinephrine
NONSELECTIVE BETA-BLOCKERS (E.G., PROPRANOLOL, NADOLOL, TIMOLOL, SOTALOL)

- hypertension followed by bradycardia may occur owing to unopposed alpha effects and reflex stimulation of baroreceptors; it is best to avoid this combination or discontinue the beta-blocker 3 days prior to use of epinephrine

TRICYCLIC ANTIDEPRESSANTS

- potentiation of pressor effects of epinephrine (e.g., dysrhythmias and hypertension) may occur owing to inhibition of re-uptake of epinephrine by the tricyclic antidepressants; epinephrine dosage reduction is necessary with this combination (i.e., start with $^1/_{10}$ of the usual dose and titrate upward)

Drugs that may decrease the effect of epinephrine

- none

Drugs that may have their effect increased by epinephrine

- none

Drugs that may have their effect decreased by epinephrine

- none

▶ *What Route and Dosage Should I Use?*

How to administer

- parenterally—for infusion, dilute 2 mg (2 mL of 1:1000 solution) in 250 mL of 5% dextrose in water or normal saline to provide a concentration of 8 μg/mL

- subcutaneously
- intramuscularly
- inhaled—dilute to 4 mL with normal saline and nebulize for 10–15 minutes

Anaphylaxis (bites, insect stings, drugs, and so on)

- (1:1000 solution) 0.5 mL subcutaneously every 5–10 minutes as necessary to maintain blood pressure or patent airway
- 0.3 mg IM; may repeat every 5–20 minutes (EpiPen delivers 0.3 mg per intramuscular autoinjection)
- for nonresponding, severe, or prolonged hypotension, give 0.5 mg (5 mL of 1:10,000 solution) IV and may repeat every 5–20 minutes

Acute asthma, croup (laryngotracheobronchitis)

- 0.3–0.5 mg subcutaneously every 20 minutes for 3 doses
- initiate intravenous infusion at 1 μg/min (0.015 μg/kg/min) and taper according to response
- racemic epinephrine 2.25%—0.5 mL (0.05 mL/kg to maximum of 0.5 mL) inhaled every 1–2 hours (Can J Hosp Pharm 1988;41:216)

Cardiac arrest

- 0.5–1 mg (5–10 mL of 1:10,000 solution) IV or endotracheally every 5 minutes

▶ What Should I Monitor with Regard to Efficacy and Toxicity?

Efficacy

Anaphylaxis (bites, insect stings, drugs, and so on)

Vital signs

- monitor blood pressure, heart rate and rhythm, and signs of respiratory compromise continuously

Acute asthma • For severe acute asthma, assess the patient after each dose and until improvement is seen

Heart rate, degree of respiratory distress, and presence of cyanosis
Pulmonary function tests
Peak expiratory flow rate

- should be measured before treatment if possible
- measured after treatment to assess the effect of treatment
- patients with an acute attack should be given a peak flow gauge and should record peak expiratory flow rate (PEFR) at least twice daily

Forced expiratory volume in 1 second

- assess once to determine the reversibility of bronchoconstriction
- reversibility is indicated by an increase of 15–20% in forced expiratory volume in 1 second after bronchodilator administration

Arterial blood gases

- if the patient has a PEFR less than 40% of predicted values or is not responding to treatment
- repeat within 24 hours if blood carbon dioxide level is elevated or the patient is fatiguing

Croup (laryngotracheobronchitis)

- decrease in intensity of inspiratory stridor

Cardiac arrest

Vital signs

- monitor blood pressure, heart rate and rhythm, and signs of respiratory compromise continuously

Toxicity

Side effects are generally dose related and occur more frequently with systemic formulations
Tachycardia (common), palpitations, arrhythmias

- due to beta$_1$ and beta$_2$ effects

Hypertension

- due to alpha effects

Tremor (up to 20% of patients)

- due to beta$_2$ effects
- may improve with continued use

Gluconeogenesis, hypokalemia (more prominent with parenteral use)

- due to beta$_2$ effects
- hospitalized patients should have electrolytes determined at least twice weekly if receiving intravenous epinephrine

Respiratory effects

- may reduce bronchial secretions, resulting in thick mucus

▶ How Long Do I Treat Patients with This Drug?

Anaphylaxis (bites, insect stings, drugs, and so on)

- until vital signs have stabilized and there is no evidence of cardiac or respiratory compromise
- after mild symptoms responding quickly to treatment and involving a known causative agent that is metabolized or excreted rapidly, continue monitoring in a supervised setting for a minimum of 2 hours after complete resolution of symptoms
- when anaphylaxis is caused by a long-acting drug, the patient should be monitored in a supervised setting for 24 hours

Acute asthma, croup

- should be used only until the patient is stabilized
- patients should be continued on selective beta$_2$-agonist therapy for prolonged use

Cardiac arrest

- for duration of resuscitation

▶ How Do I Decrease or Stop the Administration of This Drug?

- may be stopped abruptly

▶ What Should I Tell My Patients About This Drug?

- should not be prescribed on an outpatient basis for the treatment of asthma

EpiPen

- read the package insert for proper directions for use
- do not use if you are allergic to sulfites, as this product contains sulfites
- check the expiration date regularly and replace prior to expiration
- if an allergic reaction occurs, use EpiPen immediately as follows:
  1. remove the safety cap
  2. place the black tip on the anterolateral aspect of the thigh at right angles to the leg
  3. press hard on the thigh until the autoinjector functions; hold in place for several seconds
  4. remove and discard the autoinjector after the injection is completed
  5. massage the injection area for 10 seconds

▶ Therapeutic Tips

- do not use this drug via the inhalation route for asthma except in emergency use when no other drugs are available (e.g., salbutamol)
- use frequent and high doses of other bronchodilators before using epinephrine parenterally; use parenteral salbutamol if available

Useful Reference

Drugs for ambulatory asthma. Med Lett Drug Ther 1991;33:9–12

ERGOTAMINE TARTRATE

Jerry Taylor

USA (Ergostat, Wigrettes)
USA or CANADA (Ergomar, Gynergen, Medihaler Ergotomine)
CANADA (Gravergol, Megral)

▶ When Should I Use This Drug?

Migraine treatment

- should be given to the patient who has failed to respond to simple analgesics or who has moderate to severe symptoms

- dihydroergotamine is as effective and better tolerated (less nausea) and has only modest arterial effects when compared with ergotamine, but is available only parenterally (Headache 1990;8:857–865)
- advantageous over dihydroergotamine because it is available as in oral, rectal, sublingual, and inhalation dosage forms
- oral and sublingual forms are erratically absorbed (J Neurol 1991;238:S28–S35)
- ergotamine is most effective if used during the prodromal phase of the headache

▶ *When Should I Not Use This Drug?*

Delayed therapy and well-established pain

- ergotamines are not as effective when therapy has been delayed and the pain has become well established
- ergotamines may be risky in patients with prolonged prodromes (complicated migraine) and may lead to irreversible sequelae in these circumstances
- avoid use in patients with signs of chronic ergotism or rebound headache

Daily administration

- to prevent rebound phenomena and subsequent dependency problems, the drug must never be used on a daily basis

▶ *What Contraindications Are There to the Use of This Drug?*

Intolerance of or allergic reaction to ergotamine

Peripheral vascular disease

- these patients are particularly susceptible to the vasoconstrictive complications

Severe hypertension, coronary disease, hepatic and renal failure, and pregnancy

- because of the vasoconstrictor effects seen with this drug

▶ *What Drug Interactions Are Clinically Important?*

Drugs that may increase the effect or toxicity of ergotamine

METHYSERGIDE

- risk of arterial occlusion exists when given with methysergide; therefore, avoid this combination

BETA-BLOCKERS

- although many patients can take propranolol and ergots without ill effects, one must monitor for signs and symptoms of peripheral vascular insufficiency such as ergotism, peripheral ischemia, and gangrene

DOPAMINE AND OTHER VASOCONSTRICTIVE THERAPY

- should be undertaken only if constant monitoring of potentially excessive peripheral vasoconstriction such as ergotism, peripheral ischemia, and gangrene is done

Drugs that may decrease the effect of ergotamine

- none

Drugs that may have their effect increased by ergotamine

- none

Drugs that may have their effect decreased by ergotamine

NITRATES

- ergotamine may precipitate angina and may counteract the antianginal effects of nitroglycerin
- if worsening of angina occurs, immediate discontinuation and avoidance of further treatment with vasoconstrictor agents is required

▶ *What Route and Dosage Should I Use?*

How to administer

- orally—take with food or milk

- rectally—if vomiting
- parenterally—not available
- inhaled

Migraine treatment

- ergotamine inhalation is preferred for its rapid onset of action
- one inhalation repeated in 10 minutes as needed to a maximum of 6 inhalations per 24 hours or 15 inhalations per week
- 2 mg PO, rectally, or sublingually (all routes are equally effective, the choice is based on the status of the gastrointestinal tract) initially, then 1–2 mg repeated at 30 minute intervals, up to 6 mg per attack with the maximum dose not exceeding more than 10 mg of ergotamine per week

Dosage adjustments for renal or hepatic dysfunction

- no dosage adjustments, as its use is contraindicated in patients with renal or hepatic dysfunction

▶ *What Should I Monitor with Regard to Efficacy and Toxicity?*

Efficacy

Migraine treatment

Relief of pain and other symptoms such as prodromal, aural, and gastrointestinal complaints

- assess the patient hourly during the early stage of migraine attacks

Toxicity

Nausea and vomiting

- mild symptoms are noted in about 45% of patients

Ergotism

- nausea, diarrhea, thirst, pruritus, vertigo, muscle cramps, paresthesias, cold skin, or decreased pulses
- occurs more often in predisposed patients (i.e., patients with hepatic, renal, or cardiovascular disorders), when ergotamine is taken concurrently with sympathomimetic agents, and when high doses are used
- use the lowest effective dose, employ agents lacking vasoconstrictive properties in those at risk, and use prophylactic agents when appropriate
- stop drug administration if these occur

Rebound headache and subsequent dependency problems

- may be common in those patients who take ergot medications several times a week

▶ *How Long Do I Treat Patients with This Drug?*

Migraine treatment

- should be limited to maximum allowable dosages
- reducing dosing to 4 d/wk decreases the risk of developing a pattern of cyclic headaches, and if a patient is not responsive to ergot drugs, nonsteroidal antiinflammatory drugs (NSAIDs) can be tried

▶ *How Do I Decrease or Stop the Administration of This Drug?*

- in the patient with dependency problems, detoxification should be undertaken in an inpatient setting
- ergotamines should be discontinued and pain relief can be provided by the administration of an NSAID
- should an NSAID be ineffective in providing relief, a rapidly tapering course of prednisone with chlorpromazine may offer benefit for severe withdrawal headache

▶ *What Should I Tell My Patients About This Drug?*

- use proper timing of dose administration and appropriate use of the dosage form prescribed
- take medication early, after the onset of prodromal symptoms or headache, in those without aura, to be most effective
- total daily and weekly dose limitations are important

- you and your family members should watch for signs of confusion and other signs of possible acute ergot toxicity

▶ Therapeutic Tips

- ergotamine dosage requirements should be titrated for each patient until the appropriate dose is determined for subsequent attacks
- prochlorperazine should be used prior to the use of ergotamine to decrease the occurrence of nausea with these agents
- patients should be given ergotamine to treat future attacks at home at the earliest stages of the migraine attack to lessen its intensity and shorten its duration
- repeated dosing over an extended time may be less efficacious by allowing establishment of vasodilatation
- this medicine is best given in the period preceding the headache or in the initial hours of headache onset (i.e., before first 2 hours of headache pain)
- total dose requirements determined from previous use can be given early as a single dose, at the onset of headache, to abort attacks
- oral and sublingual ergotamine bioavailability is poor in comparison with that from inhalation, which allows rapid absorption
- detoxification of patients is necessary for those with rebound or withdrawal headaches
- maximum effectiveness of prophylactic medications does not occur until excessive habit-forming medications have been withdrawn

Useful Reference

Perrin VL. Clinical pharmacokinetics of ergotamine in migraine and cluster headache. Clin Pharmacokinet 1985;10:334–352

ERYTHROMYCIN

Alfred Gin and George Zhanel

USA (ERYC, Ilosone, various)
CANADA (ERYC, Ilosone, various)

▶ When Should I Use This Drug?

check antibiotic susceptibility chart (Table 4–1 in Chapter 4)

Upper respiratory tract infections

- if caused by streptococcal species in penicillin-allergic patients
- erythromycin causes frequent gastrointestinal discomfort and is more expensive than penicillin

Pneumonia

- erythromycin covers the main organisms responsible for community-acquired pneumonia (*Streptococcus pneumoniae* and *Mycoplasma pneumoniae*), whereas penicillin does not cover *Mycoplasma*
- drug of choice in community-acquired pneumonia in mild to moderately ill patients with no underlying disease states when Gram stain is not possible or is unobtainable or Gram stain shows no organisms
- also useful if Gram stain shows gram-positive diplococci (*S. pneumoniae*) and the patient is allergic to penicillin and sulfa drugs
- should also be used in patients who do not have abrupt onset of fever, chills, and pleuritic pain, which are classic signs and symptoms of bacterial pneumonia, as these patients may have atypical pneumonia (*M. pneumoniae, Legionella pneumophila* or *Chlamydia pneumoniae*) (Clin Chest Med 1987;8:441–453)
- drug of choice for proven atypical pneumonias (*Mycoplasma, Legionella*)
- useful in combination with ciprofloxacin in mild to moderately ill patients with underlying disease states such as alcoholism and chronic obstructive pulmonary disease (these patients have a high incidence of infections caused by gram-negative organisms) when Gram stain is not possible or is unobtainable or Gram stain shows either gram-negative coccobacilli or no organisms

Cellulitis

- useful in mildly to moderately ill patients with a documented history of penicillin allergy in whom oral therapy can be used

(if the patient is severely ill, clindamycin should be chosen instead of erythromycin, as it has better activity against gram-positive organisms than does erythromycin)
- erythromycin has activity against staphylococcal and streptococcal organisms and is less expensive than oral clindamycin

Erysipelas

- useful for patients with documented history of penicillin allergy

Urethritis, cervicitis

- erythromycin is useful if a patient is unable to tolerate a tetracycline or if use of a tetracycline is contraindicated in patients with urethritis if urethral discharge shows increased polymorphonuclear neutrophils and no diplococci, as it has good activity against *Chlamydia trachomatis*
- useful in conjunction with cefixime (for gonorrhea coverage) for cervicitis, if the patient is unable to tolerate doxycycline

Genital ulcers

- drug of choice in a penicillin-allergic patient if there is clinical suspicion and lesions suggestive of chancroid and dark-field microscopy does not show corkscrew spirochetes (syphilis) in a penicillin-allergic patient

Bacterial endocarditis prophylaxis

- for dental, oral, or respiratory tract procedures as an alternative to amoxicillin in penicillin-allergic patients (JAMA 1990;264:2919–2922)

Prevention of postoperative infections

- for colorectal surgery, as an oral agent, in conjunction with neomycin on the day prior to surgery followed by either cefoxitin, ceftizoxime, or cefotetan or clindamycin and gentamicin if the patient is penicillin allergic

▶ When Should I Not Use This Drug?

Urinary tract infections

- other agents are available at less cost and are more efficacious against urinary pathogens

Infections caused by Enterobacteriaceae, *Pseudomonas,* and *Bacteroides fragilis*

- erythromycin is inactive against many strains of these organisms

▶ What Contraindications Are There to the Use of This Drug?

- Intolerance of or allergic reaction to erythromycin

▶ What Drug Interactions Are Clinically Important?

Drugs that may increase the effect of erythromycin

- none

Drugs that may decrease the effect of erythromycin

- none

Drugs that may have their effect increased by erythromycin

THEOPHYLLINE

- theophylline levels may increase 20–40% in patients taking erythromycin, with onset after 3–5 days of concomitant therapy
- toxicity due to increased theophylline levels can be life threatening
- use an alternative antibiotic if possible; if not, and the combination will be used for longer than 3 days, measure theophylline level every 2 days until the extent of interaction is known

CARBAMAZEPINE

- use alternative antibiotics to erythromycin if possible, as it inhibits the metabolism of carbamazepine
- if erythromycin must be added for longer than 3 days, obtain baseline serum carbamazepine concentrations prior to adding erythromycin, recheck the concentration in 1 week, and reduce

the dosage proportionately if the concentration is greater than 12 mg/L

- monitor for symptoms of toxicity, and if they occur, stop carbamazepine administration, get a repeated concentration, and adjust the dosage accordingly
- if the concentration is not available within 24 hours, restart carbamazepine therapy at 50% of the previous dose as long as toxicity is not present
- if no toxicity occurs, measure concentrations weekly until a new steady state has been reached
- when erythromycin administration is stopped, increase the dosage back to preinhibitor levels

CYCLOSPORINE

- empirically decrease the cyclosporine dosage by 30%, especially in patients with cyclosporine concentrations in the higher end of the therapeutic range, and monitor cyclosporine levels every other day until the full extent of interaction is seen and adjust the dosage accordingly

WARFARIN

- may reduce the clearance of warfarin
- use alternative agents if possible
- if not, monitor INR every 2 days until the full extent of interaction is seen and adjust the dosage as for a warfarin dosage change
- monitor INR every 2 days when the interacting drug is discontinued and adjust dosage to obtain desired degree of anticoagulation

Drugs that may have their effect decreased by erythromycin

- none

▶ *What Route and Dosage Should I Use?*

How to administer

- orally—take with food or milk to decrease the amount of gastrointestinal upset
- parenterally—when given intravenously, dilute erythromycin in 5% dextrose in water to a concentration of no less than 1 mg/mL

Many dosage forms (enteric-coated, suspension, and microencapsulated) and salt forms (base, ethylsuccinate, estolate, or stearate) are available

- clinically important differences in bioavailability do not exist among the various salt forms
- erythromycin base, estolate, and ethylsuccinate products may be given with or without food, whereas food decreases the absorption of erythromycin stearate
- erythromycin base is the least expensive and selection of an erythromycin product should be based on the patient's tolerance of the erythromycin base
- all erythromycin products cause gastrointestinal upset, and this appears to be greater with the erythromycin base than the ethylsuccinate and stearate salts (taking these agents with food reduces the incidence of gastrointestinal adverse effects) (DICP 1987;21:734–738)

Upper respiratory tract infections

- 500 mg PO Q6H

Pneumonia

- 500 mg PO Q6H for moderate illness
- 500 mg IV Q6H for severe illness
- 1 g IV Q6H if *Legionella* is suspected

Cellulitis, erysipelas

- 500 mg PO Q6H

Urethritis, cervicitis

- 500 mg PO Q6H

Genital ulcers

- 500 mg PO Q6H

Endocarditis prophylaxis

- 1 g PO 2 hours before the procedure and 500 mg PO 6 hours after first dose

Prevention of postoperative infections

- 1 g PO in combination with neomycin at 1 PM, 2 PM, 11 PM, on the day prior to surgery

Dosage adjustments for renal or hepatic dysfunction

- hepatically eliminated
- no adjustments required, except in end-stage renal failure (maximum dose, 2 g/d)

▶ *What Should I Monitor with Regard to Efficacy and Toxicity?*

Efficacy

- for antibiotic administration monitoring guidelines, see specific section on drug therapy

Toxicity

Gastrointestinal symptoms

- nausea, vomiting, diarrhea, and cramps occur in 30–40% of patients
- erythromycin should be taken with food, which may decrease the effects
- caused by direct effect of erythromycin on gastrointestinal motility
- central effect may also be present because gastrointestinal symptoms also occur when the drug is given parenterally
- all erythromycin products cause gastrointestinal symptoms, which may be minimized if erythromycin is taken with food or the dosage is reduced
- selection of an erythromycin product should be based on the patient's tolerance of the erythromycin base
- use of erythromycin stearate or ethylsuccinate in adults or the estolate in children may be useful

Thrombophlebitis

- occurs with parenteral administration
- dilute erythromycin in large volume of diluent to a concentration of 5 mg/mL less

Ototoxicity

- is usually reversible; occurs in patients with severe renal impairment receiving high-dose erythromycin (4 g/d or greater)
- patients with severe renal function should be questioned about hearing loss every 1–2 days
- reduce the dosage or discontinue the drug administration on occurrence

Hepatotoxity

- hepatic dysfunction with or without jaundice may occur rarely; cholestatic jaundice associated with erythromycin estolate is reported mainly in adults
- risk of hepatotoxicity likely does not differ from salt to salt (Lancet 1988;1:1104)
- monitor liver enzymes and bilirubin levels every 2–3 days in patients with preexisting hepatic impairment
- discontinue the drug administration on occurrence

▶ *How Long Do I Treat Patients with This Drug?*

Upper respiratory tract infections

- usual duration is 10 days or 4–5 days after the patient has become afebrile and has clinically improved

Pneumonias

- consider switching to oral erythromycin (500 mg PO Q6H) after the patient has become afebrile and has clinically improved for 1–2 days
- if the patient responds slowly or has a pneumonia caused by *Mycoplasma* or *Legionella*, a 14 day course of therapy should be given (Clin Chest Med 1991;12:237–242, Ann Intern Med 1987;106:341–345)
- *Legionella* may necessitate 3 weeks of treatment if the patient responds slowly

Cellulitis, erysipelas

- usual duration is 10 days or 4–5 days after the patient has become afebrile and has clinically improved
- if using the parenteral form, consider switching to oral erythromycin (500 mg PO Q6H) after the patient has become afebrile and has clinically improved for 1–2 days

Urethritis, cervicitis

- 7 days

Genital ulcers

- 7 days

Endocarditis prophylaxis

- 2 doses

Prevention of postoperative infections

- 3 doses preoperatively

▶ How Do I Decrease or Stop the Administration of This Drug?

- may be stopped abruptly

▶ What Should I Tell My Patients About This Drug?

- your antibiotic is called erythromycin; let me know if you have any sort of adverse reaction (decreased hearing or irritation of your veins) to this drug
- erythromycin may cause diarrhea or cramping; minimize by taking with food or a glass of milk, contact your physician if symptoms are severe
- let me know if you are taking any other medications such as carbamazepine, theophylline, cyclosporine, and warfarin
- take the medication until it is completed

▶ Therapeutic Tips

- reduce the dosage in patients with severe renal impairment (e.g., for end-stage renal diseases, use a maximum of 2 g/d)
- convert to oral erythromycin as soon as possible to minimize thrombophlebitis associated with intravenous administration
- take erythromycin with food to decrease the incidence of gastrointestinal adverse effects

Useful References

Washington JA, Wilson WR. Erythromycin: Antimicrobial and clinical perspective after 30 years of use (part 1). Mayo Clin Proc 1985;60:189–203

Washington JA, Wilson WR. Erythromycin: Antimicrobial and clinical perspective after 30 years of use (part 2). Mayo Clin Proc 1985;60:271–278

Wilson WR, Cockerill FR III. Tetracyclines, chloramphenicol, erythromycin and clindamycin. Mayo Clin Proc 1987;62:906–915

Brittain DC. Erythromycin. Med Clin North Am 1987;71:1147–1154

ESMOLOL

Robert Rangno and James McCormack

USA (Brevibloc)
CANADA (Brevibloc)

Esmolol is a parenteral beta-receptor antagonist with a short half-life (approximately 10 minutes) for use in hospitalized patients

▶ When Should I Use This Drug?

Any situation in which rapid onset, very short duration beta-blockade is required (e.g., patients with potential contraindications to beta-blockade such as patients with severe left ventricular dysfunction or asthma)

- preferred to longer-acting beta-receptor antagonists when it is desired to produce a rapid onset and offset of action in critically ill patients
- in contrast to the case with propranolol, esmolol-induced cardiovascular effects disappear within 30 minutes after discontinuation of the drug administration
- esmolol's effect on heart rate is proportional to its blood concentration (Drugs 1987;33:392–412)
- esmolol's unique pharmacological properties suggest that it may be useful in perioperative situations, especially in the presence

of tachycardia, hypertension, and arrhythmias, particularly in high-risk patients (patients with poor ventricular function)

Atrioventricular nodal reentrant tachycardia

- for acute episodes if parenteral adenosine and verapamil are ineffective or contraindicated, esmolol may be used (except in patients with severe left ventricular dysfunction or contraindications to beta-blockade)

Perioperative management of hemodynamic effects

- during general anesthesia, certain surgical procedures cause reflex sympathetic activity with profound hemodynamic effects
- laryngoscopy and endotracheal intubation cause transient hypertension and tachycardia associated with an increase in myocardial oxygen demand
- in patients with preexisting hypertension or coronary artery disease, this autonomic response may pose a potential danger and esmolol may be useful in the treatment of these patients

▶ When Should I Not Use This Drug?

Long-term control of arrhythmias or tachycardia

- esmolol is available only for parenteral administration and has a short duration of activity so other beta-adrenergic antagonists should be used for long-term treatment

▶ What Contraindications Are There to the Use of This Drug?

- intolerance of or allergic reaction to esmolol

Although esmolol potentially has the same contraindications as other beta-blockers, the main reason for its use is to see if beta-blockade is tolerated by patients with potential contraindications to beta-blocker therapy

▶ What Drug Interactions Are Clinically Important?

- none

▶ What Route and Dosage Should I Use?

How to administer

Orally

- not available

Parenterally

- esmolol should not be injected at a concentration exceeding 10 mg/mL to minimize the possibility of phlebitis
- at this concentration, it is stable for 24 hours at a controlled room temperature or under refrigeration
- esmolol is not compatible with 5% sodium bicarbonate solution (Clin Pharm 1986;5:288–303)
- esmolol is compatible with 5% dextrose injection, 5% dextrose in lactated Ringer's solution, 5% dextrose in Ringer's injection, 5% dextrose and normal or half-normal saline injection, or normal or half-normal saline injection

Any situation in which rapid onset, very short duration beta-blockade is required, atrioventricular nodal reentrant tachycardia

- 500 μg/kg bolus over 1 minute followed by 50 μg/kg/min infusion for 4 minutes
- if there is inadequate response, give another 500 μg/kg bolus and increase the infusion to 100 μg/kg/min for 4 minutes
- if there is inadequate response, give another 500 μg/kg bolus and increase the infusion to 150 μg/kg/min for 4 minutes
- if there is inadequate response, give another 500 μg/kg bolus and increase the infusion to 200 μg/kg/min for 4 minutes
- dosages greater than 200 μg/kg/min are not recommended
- as desired heart rate is approached, the incremental dosage for maintenance may be reduced from 50 to 25 μg/kg/min while the interval titration steps are increased from 4 to 10 minutes

Dosage adjustment for renal or hepatic dysfunction

- renally eliminated

- in general, even in patients with renal dysfunction, start with a low dose and titrate up to an effect

Normal Dosing Interval	$C_{cr} > 60$ mL/min or 1 mL/s	C_{cr} 30–60 mL/min or 0.5–1 mL/s	$C_{cr} < 30$ mL/min or 0.5 mL/s
infusion	no adjustment needed	decrease dosage by 50%	decrease dosage by 75%

▶ *What Should I Monitor with Regard to Efficacy and Toxicity?*

Efficacy

Atrioventricular nodal reentrant tachycardia

Electrocardiogram

- electrocardiogram should be monitored continuously until the arrhythmia has stopped

Vital signs

- should be assessed every 5 minutes during drug administration
- presence or absence of symptoms related to arrhythmia (palpitations, shortness of breath, dizziness, angina)

Perioperative management of hemodynamic effects

Heart rate, blood pressure

- heart rate and blood pressure should decrease almost immediately
- monitor continuously while the patient is receiving esmolol

Toxicity

see Nadolol

Severe bradycardia, congestive heart failure, hypotension, heart block, and asthma

- if these occur, stop the infusion

▶ *How Long Do I Treat Patients with This Drug?*

Any situation in which rapid onset, very short duration beta-blockade is required atrioventricular nodal reentrant tachycardia

- esmolol is primarily used for short-term control of heart rate in tachyarrhythmias, and information on administration for longer than 24 hours is scarce
- after achieving adequate hemodynamic control, it is advisable to transfer to a long-acting agent depending on the condition being treated

Perioperative management of hemodynamic effects

- as long as blood pressure and heart rate control is required

▶ *How Do I Decrease or Stop the Administration of This Drug?*

- dosage of esmolol should be reduced as follows: 30 minutes after the first dose of the alternative agent, reduce esmolol infusion by 50%
- after the second dose of the alternative agent (or 4–6 hours after administration of the agent if it is dosed daily), if satisfactory control is maintained for the first hour, discontinue the esmolol infusion

▶ *What Should I Tell My Patients About This Drug?*

- esmolol is a short-acting drug that can only be given intravenously; some irritation of the injection site occurs in some patients but is resolved by changing the injection site

Useful References

Benfield P, Sorkin EM. Esmolol. A preliminary review of its pharmacodynamic and pharmacokinetic properties, and therapeutic efficacy. Drugs 1987;33:392–412

Reves JG, Flezzani P. Perioperative use of esmolol. Am J Cardiol 1985;56:57F–62F

Angaran DM, Schultz NJ, Tschida VH. Esmolol hydrochloride, an ultra-short-acting beta-adrenergic blocking agent. Clin Pharm 1986;5:288–303

ESTROGENS (estradiol, estrone, ethinyl estradiol, mestranol, estropipate, conjugated equine estrogens)

Deborah Stier Carson

USA (Premarin, Ogen, Estrace, Estratab, Estraderm, Menest, Orthoest)

CANADA (Neo-estrone, Estinyl, Estrace, Estraderm, Ogen)

Also many birth control pills (in combination with progestins)

▶ *When Should I Use This Drug?*

Menopausal symptoms

- estrogens are effective in reducing flushing, night sweats, outer genital and vaginal irritation, insomnia, and other symptoms of menopause
- all women with the above symptoms should be given the option of using estrogen to eliminate or decrease these symptoms unless it is contraindicated

Prevention of osteoporosis or bone loss, treatment of osteoporosis (low bone mass and fractures)

- estrogen prevents osteoporosis, decreases incidence of vertebral and other fractures, and prevents further loss of height (JAMA 1984;252:799–802, N Engl J Med 1987;817:1169–1174); however, the major effect is seen in the first 10–15 years after menopause
- estrogens are the only treatment that prevents menopausal symptoms and decreases cardiovascular risk (N Engl J Med 1991;325:756–762)
- oral and transdermal estrogen appear to be equally effective, and the decision should be based on the patient's preference
- transdermal estrogen is more expensive than oral therapy
- transdermal estrogen may be safer if the patient has a history of clotting disorders (in general, estrogen therapy is not recommended for patients with active disease) or hypertension, as nonoral administration avoids the first-pass hepatic effects, thereby possibly avoiding alterations in renin substrate and coagulation factors
- recent data show some benefit on lipid levels from transdermal administration of estrogen (Obstet Gynecol 1994;84:222–226)

Hormonal contraception

see Chapter 7 for discussion of birth control

Dysmenorrhea

- oral contraceptives are the drugs of choice for the treatment of dysmenorrhea in women who desire contraception as well
- see Chapter 7 for discussion of birth control
- nonsteroidal antiinflammatory drugs are drugs of choice if hormonal therapy is not wanted

Other Uses

- dysfunctional uterine bleeding, endometriosis, benign breast disease, functional ovarian cysts

▶ *What Contraindications Are There to the Use of This Drug?*

Intolerance of or allergic reaction to estrogens

Absolute contraindications

- known or suspected pregnancy
- known or suspected cancer of the breast
- known or suspected estrogen-dependent neoplasia or a history thereof
- undiagnosed abnormal genital bleeding
- active thrombophlebitis or thromboembolic disorders
- cerebrovascular accident or a history thereof
- benign or malignant liver tumor or a history thereof
- impaired hepatic function

Strong relative contraindications (can be used if no useful alternatives)

- severe headaches that start after the initiation of estrogen therapy

- history of migraines; however, some patients get better and some patients get worse
- hypertension
- immobility
- major injury to lower leg
- older than 35 years and currently a heavy smoker (more for oral contraception than estrogen replacement)
- abnormal bleeding
- previous cholestasis during pregnancy

▶ What Drug Interactions Are Clinically Important?

Drugs that may increase the effect or toxicity of estrogens

- none

Drugs that may decrease the effect of estrogens

ANTIBIOTICS

- may reduce the effectiveness of oral contraceptives, and although the clinical significance of this has been questioned, it is prudent to recommend additional methods of birth control to women while they are taking the combination of low-dose oral contraceptives and antibiotics
- no changes required when using estrogen as replacement therapy

PHENOBARBITAL, RIFAMPIN, PHENYTOIN, CABAMAZEPINE, AND OTHER DRUGS THAT MAY BE EXPECTED TO INDUCE HEPATIC MICROSOMAL ENZYMES

- with concomitant use, these agents may produce lower estrogen levels than expected by increasing the metabolism of estrogen to a less active form
- patients taking oral contraceptives should be started on a high-estrogen product
- although higher-dose estrogens can decrease spotting in patients taking interacting drugs, the efficacy may be decreased but is likely still greater than with any other single form of birth control

Drugs that may have their effect or toxicity increased by estrogens

TRICYCLIC ANTIDEPRESSANTS

- effects of these agents may be altered by estrogens; the effects of this interaction may depend on the dose of the estrogen, and an increased incidence of side effects from the tricyclic antidepressant may occur
- empirically reduce the dosage of the tricyclic antidepressant by $1/3$ or use another method of birth control

Drugs that may have their effect decreased by estrogens

WARFARIN

- estrogens may theoretically reduce the effects of anticoagulants
- with nonoral routes of administration, which do not alter production of antithrombin III, this interaction may not be clinically relevant
- if estrogen is added to the regimen of a patient receiving warfarin, treat it as if there was a warfarin dosage change
- generally, the concomitant use of these drugs is contraindicated because estrogen can worsen thromboembolic disease

▶ What Route and Dosage Should I Use?

How to administer

Orally

- bedtime doses help to circumvent some side effects (e.g., nausea, breast tenderness, and chloasma)

Topically

- patch is applied to a clean, dry, nonhairy area of the trunk
- buttock area may be best
- should not be applied to breast
- patch site should be rotated

Preparations available for estrogen replacement

Active Ingredient	Brand Name	Maximum Daily Dose to Prevent Bone Loss	Dosage Form	Onset (h)	Duration of Action (h)
estradiol-17β	Estrace	1 mg	oral tablet	0.5–1	12–24
	Estrace		vaginal cream	0.5–1	12–24
	Estraderm	0.05 mg/d	transdermal	0.5–1	72–96
	Estrogel (not in USA)	1.5 mg (estimate)	percutaneous	0.5–1	24
estradiol valerate	generic		intramuscular		14–21 days
estradiol cypionate	generic		intramuscular		14–28 days
estropipate	Ogen	0.625 mg	oral tablet	0.5–1	12–24
	Ogen		vaginal cream	0.5–1	12–24
estrone	generic		intramuscular		
conjugated estrogens	Premarin, Estratab, Menest	0.625 mg	oral	3	24
	Premarin	0.625 mg	vaginal cream	3	24
synthetic ethinyl estradiol	Estinyl	0.02 mg	oral	0.5–1	12–24

Menopausal symptoms, prevention of osteoporosis or bone loss, treatment of osteoporosis (low bone mass and fractures)

Oral

- product selection should be based on cost
- 0.625 mg of conjugated equine estrogen or the equivalent PO daily in patients with or without an intact uterus
- if breast tenderness develops, give estrogen for just the first 25 days of each month
- any estrogen dose less than or equivalent to 0.625 mg of conjugated equine estrogen may not be sufficient to prevent bone loss (data suggest that doses < 0.625 mg are effective if elemental calcium intake is > 1700 mg/day)
- if the woman is close to the perimenopausal period and retains some ability to produce estradiol, 0.625 mg of conjugated equine estrogen may not be tolerated
- a lower dose (0.325 mg) may be necessary initially, but an attempt to increase to 0.625 mg/d of conjugated equine estrogen should be tried within 3 to 6 months

Transdermal

- 0.05 mg/24 hours (Estraderm 50) transdermal patch applied twice weekly; if breast tenderness develops, give for only 3 weeks each month
- change the patch on same days of the week (e.g., every 3–4 days)

Topical

- useful if the patient has dermatological problems
- 2–4 gm of conjugated equine estrogen

Hormonal contraception, dysmenorrhea

see Chapter 7 for discussion of birth control

Dosage adjustments for renal or hepatic dysfunction

- hepatically metabolized
- no dosage adjustments for renal dysfunction
- avoid in patients with active hepatic disease or history of hepatitis B

▶ What Should I Monitor with Regard to Efficacy and Toxicity?

Efficacy

Menopausal symptoms

- suppression of all menopausal syndrome symptoms

Prevention of osteoporosis or bone loss, treatment of osteoporosis (low bone mass and fractures)

Breast and pelvic examination

- yearly examination with mammogram at least every 2–3 years

Incidence of fractures or pain

- assess at each follow-up

Bone density

- not recommended for everyone because of expense
- recommended for early menopause (medical or surgical) or a history of osteoporosis

Serum calcium concentrations

- not recommended, as the serum calcium level is usually normal and routine measurement is not recommended for hormone therapy or calcium replacement

Hormonal contraception, dysmenorrhea
see Chapter 7 for discussion of birth control

Toxicity

Most of the serious side effects relating to estrogen therapy can be discovered early if the patient is monitored properly

Initial assessment

- needed for all patients prior to prescribing estrogens
- do a complete medical, social, and family history to identify possible contraindications
- predisposing risk factors to cardiovascular, thromboembolic, and metabolic diseases (including, but not limited to, hypercholesterolemia, diabetes, hypertension, obesity, smoking, positive family history of cardiovascular disease, and diabetes) should be carefully assessed

Hypertension

- measure blood pressure prior to the initiation of estrogen therapy and reevaluate at 3 months
- if unchanged at 3 months, yearly measurements are sufficient

Lipid changes

- measure lipid levels prior to the initiation of estrogen therapy and reevaluate at 3 months
- if unchanged at 3 months, yearly measurements are sufficient

Endometrial hyperplasia and carcinoma

- more commonly occurs in women receiving unopposed large doses of estrogen
- progestin component of oral contraceptives and the addition of medroxyprogesterone during the last days of each month of estrogen replacement reduces the risk of endometrial hyperplasia and endometrial cancer
- do Papanicoloau's (Pap) test and pelvic examination prior to estrogen therapy
- reevaluate at 3 months and then annually

Breast cancer

- there is little evidence that estrogens given to women increase the risk of breast cancer, although metaanalysis in postmenopausal women again raised this possibility (JAMA 1991;265:1985–1990)
- because of this and animal data, estrogen replacement in women who have a strong family history of breast cancer or who have breast nodules, fibrocystic disease, or abnormal mammograms should be done only with biannual mammograms and regular self-examination
- although there is some controversy about the effectiveness, regular breast self-examinations are recommended
- annual mammograms are indicated for all women older than 40 years of age, regardless of their estrogen use

Thromboembolism

- patients should be alerted to the early danger signs of thromboembolism, such as severe abdominal pain; severe chest pain, cough, or shortness of breath; severe headache; dizziness, weakness, or numbness; eye or speech problems; and severe leg pain

Uterine bleeding

- any abnormal or undiagnosed bleeding must be investigated
- if breakthrough bleeding (2 episodes or more) occurs or the bleeding is heavier than premenstrual bleeding, an endometrial biopsy is indicated to rule out endometrial hyperplasia or cancer
- if regular withdrawal bleeding occurs about days 7–9 of medroxyprogesterone administration or if the onset of bleeding has varied

by 5–6 days, increase the medroxyprogesterone dose if it is presently at 5 mg or less
- if the dose is greater than 5 mg, a biopsy should be done

Nausea

- usually disappears and can be diminished if estrogen is taken at bedtime or with food; transdermal route may be tried

▶ How Long Do I Treat Patients with This Drug?

Menopausal symptoms

- treat for 3–6 months, then taper and see if symptoms return

Prevention of osteoporosis or bone loss, treatment of osteoporosis (low bone mass and fractures)

- best duration of hormonal therapy or calcium replacement is unknown, but with available data, 10 years seems reasonable
- because bone loss resumes immediately after discontinuation of therapy, patients who have tolerated therapy and who are willing to continue treatment can continue therapy indefinitely
- may be continued indefinitely unless contraindications are present

Hormonal contraception, dysmenorrhea

- see Chapter 7 for discussion of birth control

▶ How Do I Decrease or Stop the Administration of This Drug?

- estrogens do not need to be tapered if the decision is made to discontinue their use; however, if estrogens are being used for menopausal syndrome, symptoms may recur or have exaggerated rebound
- depending on the status of the endometrium, uterine bleeding may be experienced at irregular times after estrogen therapy is stopped

▶ What Should I Tell My Patients About This Drug?

- estrogens must be dispensed with patient package inserts, as they provide balanced information regarding benefits and risks of estrogen therapy
- review all of the information in these inserts, at least briefly, with your physician or pharmacist
- you are encouraged to ask questions at return visits
- it may take up to 3 months for the uterine bleeding patterns to become established after adding or changing estrogen therapy
- alert your physician if you experience depression, jaundice, or a breast lump

Useful References

Dickey RP. Managing Contraceptive Pill Patients, 7th ed. Durant, OK: CIP, 1993
Sitruk-Ware R. Estrogen therapy during menopause. Drugs 1990;39:203–217

ETHAMBUTOL
Ann Beardsell

USA (Myambutol, Etibi)
CANADA (Myambutol, Etibi)

▶ When Should I Use This Drug?

Mycobacterium avium infection

- used in conjunction with other antimycobacterial agents owing to the rapid development of resistance when only one drug is used alone

Tuberculosis

- used in conjunction with other antituberculosis agents owing to the rapid development for resistance when only one drug is used alone

▶ When Should I Not Use This Drug?

Single agent in the treatment of tuberculosis

- must be used in conjunction with other agents to prevent resistance

► *What Contraindications Are There to the Use of This Drug?*

Intolerance of or allergic reaction to ethambutol

Optic neuritis

- as ethambutol may cause optic neuritis, it is contraindicated in patients with preexisting optic neuritis unless it is absolutely required

► *What Drug Interactions Are Clinically Important?*

- none

► *What Route and Dosage Should I Use?*

How to administer

- orally—with food or milk
- parenterally—not available

***Mycobacterium avium* infection**

- 15 mg/kg PO daily

Tuberculosis

- 15 mg/kg PO daily for initial treatment
- 25 mg/kg PO daily for 60 days, then reduce to 15 mg/kg PO daily if retreating after primary treatment fails

Dosage adjustments for renal or hepatic dysfunction

- renally eliminated

Normal Dosing Interval	$C_{cr} > 60$ mL/min or 1 mL/s	C_{cr} 30–60 mL/min or 0.5–1 mL/s	$C_{cr} < 30$ mL/min or 0.5 mL/s
Q24H	no adjustment needed	decrease dosage by 50%	decrease dosage by 75%

► *What Should I Monitor with Regard to Efficacy and Toxicity?*

Efficacy

Mycobacterium avium infection

Signs and symptoms

- fevers, chills, night sweats, malaise, fatigue, weight loss, abdominal pain, and diarrhea
- there are usually few or no physical signs to follow other than body weight or possibly the presence of a lesion in patients with localized disease (e.g., regional lymphadenopathy)
- patients should also be advised to report new or worsening diarrhea while taking such regimens, because *Clostridium difficile* colitis is a possible complication
- patients should be assessed every 1–2 weeks during the first 1–2 months of treatment

Complete blood count

- monthly or more frequently if there is severe disease, to detect progressive anemia and cytopenias due to bone marrow involvement, which may persist despite treatment

Blood cultures

- to document reduction or clearance of mycobacteremia, particularly in patients who have persistent symptoms

Tuberculosis

- disease improvement or resolution of symptoms such as fevers, sweats, and weight loss

Toxicity

Ocular effects

- ethambutol can cause retrobulbar (ocular) neuritis, which results in a reduction in visual acuity, constriction of visual field, central or peripheral scotoma, and red-green color blindness
- may occur in one or both eyes

- degree of impairment appears to be dose and duration dependent and can occur after many months of therapy
- visual acuity testing should precede treatment and be repeated regularly monthly while the patient is receiving ethambutal, with discontinuation of the medication if changes occur
- changes are reversible, usually within a few weeks or months, unless the impairment is severe, in which case recovery may be years, if at all

Gastrointestinal symptoms

- nausea, vomiting, and diarrhea may occur initially but usually resolves within 2–4 weeks
- treat symptomatically

Other effects

- rash, itchiness, and dizziness may occur but can be managed symptomatically
- increased uric acid serum levels and possibly gout, as ethambutol may inhibit the excretion of uric acid
- if symptoms of gout occur, check serum uric acid concentration and start uricosuric agents if appropriate

► *How Long Do I Treat Patients with This Drug?*

***Mycobacterium avium* infection**

- lifelong or as long as the patient tolerates the drug

Tuberculosis

- 6 or 9 months, depending on the regimen

► *How Do I Decrease or Stop the Administration of This Drug?*

- may be stopped abruptly

► *What Should I Tell My Patients About This Drug?*

- this medication may be taken with food
- ethambutol should always be taken with other prescribed medications
- do not stop taking this or any other antituberculosis medications without your physician's approval
- if you miss a dose, take it as soon as you remember; however, if it is time for your next dose, skip the missed dose and continue on your regular schedule
- contact your physician immediately if you have blurred vision, eye pain, red-green color blindness, or any loss of vision
- this medication may cause dizziness; therefore, use caution driving or operating machinery until you know how you are going to react to this medication
- if you have pain and/or swelling in your joints, especially the big toe, contact your physician

► *Therapeutic Tips*

- if gastrointestinal upset occurs in patients taking numerous antimycobacterial agents, stop the administration of all drugs and restart with just 1–2 drugs and slowly add back the rest
- if gastrointestinal upset reappears, stop administration of the last drug added

ETHOSUXIMIDE

William Parker

USA (Zarontin)
CANADA (Zarontin)

► *When Should I Use This Drug?*

Absence seizures

- ethosuximide is as effective as valproic acid
- ethosuximide is preferred because of the risk of serious hepatotoxicity and pancreatitis with valproic acid (valproic acid hepatotoxicity is much lower in adults than in children)

► *When Should I Not Use This Drug?*

Seizures other than absence seizures

- ineffective against other generalized and partial seizures

- when used alone in mixed seizures, ethosuximide may increase the frequency of tonic-clonic seizures

▶ *What Contraindications Are There to the Use of This Drug?*

- intolerance of or allergic reaction to ethosuximide

▶ *What Drug Interactions Are Clinically Important?*

Drugs that may increase the effect or toxicity of ethosuximide

CENTRAL NERVOUS SYSTEM DEPRESSANTS (ALCOHOL, BENZODIAZEPINES, ANTIDEPRESSANTS, ANTIPSYCHOTICS, AND SO ON)

- if used concomitantly, there is increased potential for excessive sedation
- give the largest doses of CNS depressants at bedtime and/or reduce drug dosage if possible

VALPROIC ACID

- may produce a modest increase in ethosuximide levels, but no dosage reduction is necessary unless gastrointestinal or central nervous system (CNS) side effects occur

Drugs that may decrease the effect of ethosuximide

CARBAMAZEPINE

- may produce a modest decrease in ethosuximide levels
- ethosuximide dosage can be increased if seizure frequency is increased

Drugs that may have their effect or toxicity increased by ethosuximide

- none

Drugs that may have their effect decreased by ethosuximide

- none

▶ *What Route and Dosage Should I Use?*

How to administer

- orally—take with food or milk
- parenterally—not available

Absence seizures

- loading dose is not appropriate
- initial dose is 250 mg BID
- data suggest that patients can be successfully managed on once-daily therapy, but gastrointestinal distress appears to be dose related and most patients better tolerate a BID regimen
- maintenance dosage is 20 mg/kg/d; achieve by increasing the daily dosage by 250 mg every 5 days until seizure control is achieved or side effects become intolerable

Dosage adjustments for renal or hepatic dysfunction

- hepatically metabolized
- no dosage adjustment is needed
- just titrate the dose upward on the basis of efficacy or adverse effects

▶ *What Should I Monitor with Regard to Efficacy and Toxicity?*

Efficacy

Absence seizures

Seizure frequency

- reduction in the frequency and severity of seizures

Serum concentrations

- accepted therapeutic range is 40–100 μg/mL (280–370 μmol/L))
- many patients respond with levels at the low end, whereas many patients require and tolerate concentrations up to 150 μg/mL (550 μmol/L) without adverse effects
- measurement of trough levels is preferred
- steady state is reached in 7–10 days after the maintenance dosage is attained

- patients initiated on therapy and growing children with changing body weight and metabolism should have their serum drug concentrations checked at least monthly initially until a pattern stabilization is established
- patients with good therapeutic response who are not experiencing rapid changes in body weight or passing through puberty should have their serum drug concentrations checked every 6 months

Toxicity

- ethosuximide is a relatively benign anticonvulsant
- there is no obvious correlation between ethosuximide serum concentrations and clinical side effects

Gastrointestinal effects

- up to 40% of patients experience nausea, vomiting, and anorexia; minimize by giving smaller doses in a divided regimen and by giving with food

Central nervous system effects

- drowsiness, fatigue, and dizziness are also common, especially in the first few days
- these effects frequently decrease or disappear during continued therapy
- minimize by avoiding concomitant administration of CNS depressants and by starting with low doses, gradually increasing the dosage and giving in 2–3 divided daily doses
- if CNS effects persist, decrease the dosage gradually

Hematological effects

- blood dyscrasias occur rarely and appear to be a hypersensitivity reaction; leukopenia occurs in about 7% of patients and may be transient
- patients should be generally monitored for unexplained bruising, infection, and fever, but periodic complete blood counts are of questionable efficacy, given the unpredictability and suddenness of the reaction
- if leukopenia occurs, stop the drug administration
- reintroduction of the drug may be attempted after the leukopenia resolves if a suitable alternative drug is unavailable

▶ *How Long Do I Treat Patients with This Drug?*

Absence seizures

- ethosuximide therapy is long-term therapy for a minimum of 2 years
- drug-free periods (''drug holidays'') are not indicated
- withdrawal is not recommended for absence seizures with tonic-clonic seizures
- a 2-year seizure-free period is recommended for withdrawing ethosuximide in absence seizures, and 4 years for absence seizures associated with tonic-clonic seizures
- factors promoting complete withdrawal include a seizure-free period of 2–4 years, complete seizure control within 1 year of onset, an onset of seizures between 2 and 35 years of age, and a normal electrocardiogram
- factors associated with a poor prognosis in stopping drug administration despite a seizure-free period include a history of a high frequency of seizures, repeated episodes of status epilepticus, multiple seizure types, and the development of abnormal mental functioning

▶ *How Do I Decrease or Stop the Administration of This Drug?*

- sudden withdrawal is to be avoided, especially during long-term, high-dose therapy
- withdrawal is best done over 6 months
- seizure relapse is more common if the drug is withdrawn over 1–3 months
- if seizures recur, reinstitute treatment with the same drugs used previously
- if multiple-anticonvulsant therapy is present, drugs should be withdrawn one at a time
- absence seizures necessitating ethosuximide therapy frequently cease by the age of 20 years, although occasionally they are then replaced by other forms of generalized seizures

▶ *What Should I Tell My Patients About This Drug?*

- using ethosuximide with alcohol or other CNS depressants may cause excessive drowsiness
- initially, ethosuximide may make some patients drowsy, so take in small doses and do not undertake activities requiring mental alertness or physical coordination until you know how you will react to ethosuximide
- this effect should lessen with time
- using ethosuximide may cause nausea, vomiting, or loss of appetite, so take in small doses with food
- abrupt stoppage of therapy may result in the precipitation of seizures, so do not stop taking ethosuximide or reduce the dosage without prior advice from your physician
- patients should be advised to avoid situations that could be dangerous or life threatening if further seizures should occur

▶ *Therapeutic Tips*

- syrup and capsule forms are equally bioavailable, but the rate of absorption of the syrup is faster; however, this does not appear to be clinically important

Useful References

Pugh CB, Garnett WR. Current issues in the treatment of epilepsy. Clin Pharm 1991;10:335–358

Parker WA. Epilepsy. In: Herfindal ET, Gourley DR, Hart LL, eds. Clinical Pharmacy and Therapeutics, 4th ed. Baltimore: Williams & Wilkins, 1988:570–592

Levy RH, Wilensky AJ, Friel PN. Other antiepileptic drugs. In: Evans WE, Schentag JJ, Jusko WJ, eds. Applied Pharmacokinetics. Principles of Therapeutic Drug Monitoring, 2nd ed. Spokane WA: Applied Therapeutics, 1986:540–569

ETODOLAC

Kelly Jones

USA (Lodine)
CANADA (not available)

▶ *When Should I Use This Drug?*

Acute pain, general aches and pain, bone pain, dysmenorrhea

- useful for the acute management of general aches and pains
- only advantage over non-enteric coated aspirin is that it causes less frequent gastrointestinal intolerance
- decision between this drug and other nonsteroidal antiinflammatory drugs should be based on cost

Rheumatoid arthritis

- has no approved indication but could be used as an alternative for patients who fail to respond to enteric coated aspirin or ibuprofen
- it offers no advantages over enteric coated aspirin or ibuprofen and is more expensive

Osteoarthritis

- if acetaminophen has not been effective and the patient does not tolerate enteric coated aspirin or ibuprofen
- etodolac does have a good safety profile and may become the agent of choice in patients with a history of gastrointestinal bleeds or renal insufficiency, as microbleed studies suggest a reduction in mean gastrointestinal blood loss for etodolac as compared with ibuprofen, indomethacin, and naproxen, and long-term therapy may not adversely affect renal function (J Clin Pharmacol 1986;26:269–274)
- at present, the drug is expensive

▶ *When Should I Not Use This Drug?*

see Ibuprofen

▶ *What Contraindications Are There to the Use of This Drug?*

see Aspirin

▶ *What Drug Interactions Are Clinically Important?*

see Ibuprofen

▶ *What Route and Dosage Should I Use?*

How to administer

- orally—take with food or milk
- parenterally—not available

Acute pain, general aches and pain, bone pain, dysmenorrhea

- 200–400 mg PO Q6H PRN up to a maximum dosage of 1200 mg PO daily

Rheumatoid arthritis

- 400 mg PO BID up to maximum dosage of 1200 mg PO daily

Osteoarthritis

- 200 mg PO BID up to maximum dosage of 1200 mg PO daily

Dosage adjustments for renal or hepatic dysfunction

- hepatically metabolized; therefore, no adjustments needed for renal disease
- reduce the dosage by 25% in patients with a history of hepatic disease

▶ *What Should I Monitor with Regard to Efficacy and Toxicity?*

see Aspirin

▶ *How Long Do I Treat Patients with This Drug?*

see Aspirin

▶ *How Do I Decrease or Stop the Administration of This Drug?*

- may be stopped abruptly if needed

▶ *What Should I Tell My Patients About This Drug?*

see Aspirin

▶ *Therapeutic Tips*

see Aspirin

Useful References

see Aspirin

FAMOTIDINE

James McCormack and Glen Brown

USA (Pepcid)
CANADA (Pepcid)

▶ *When Should I Use This Drug?*

All H_2 antagonists have equivalent efficacy and toxicity (N Engl J Med 1990;323:1749–1755) • The decision among these agents should be based on cost
see Ranitidine

▶ *When Should I Not Use This Drug?*

see Ranitidine

▶ *What Contraindications Are There to the Use of This Drug?*

- intolerance of or allergic reaction to famotidine

▶ *What Drug Interactions Are Clinically Important?*

see Ranitidine

▶ *What Route and Dosage Should I Use?*

How to administer

Orally

- may be given with food or on an empty stomach

Parenterally

- dilute to 5–10 mL and inject over not less than 2 minutes
- dilute to 100 mL and infuse over 15–20 minutes

Dyspepsia or duodenal or gastic ulcers

- 40 mg PO at bedtime or with the evening meal
- 20 mg PO BID if the patient has frequent daytime ulcer pain

Prevention of peptic ulcer disease recurrence

- 20 mg PO at bedtime

Gastroesophageal reflux

- 20 mg PO BID
- 20 mg PO at bedtime if the patient has only nighttime symptoms

Stress ulcer prophylaxis

- 20 mg IV Q8H
- infusion is not clinically superior (although it does produce better pH control) to intermittent therapy and should be used only if it is more practical or economical than intermittent injections
- analysis of aspirates of gastric fluid should be done Q4H and the dosage increased in 10 mg increments to maintain gastric pH of greater than 4 at all times

Dosage adjustments for renal or hepatic dysfunction

- renally eliminated

Normal Dosing Interval	$C_{cr} > 60$ mL/min or 1 mL/s	C_{cr} 30–60 mL/min or 0.5–1 mL/s	$C_{cr} < 30$ mL/min or 0.5 mL/s
Q8H	no adjustment needed	Q12H	Q24H
Q12H	no adjustment needed	Q24H	Q24H and decrease dosage by 50%
Q24H or by infusion	no adjustment needed	decrease dosage by 50%	decrease dosage by 75%

▶ *What Should I Monitor with Regard to Efficacy and Toxicity?*

see Cimetidine

▶ *How Long Do I Treat Patients with This Drug?*

see Cimetidine

▶ *How Do I Decrease or Stop the Administration of This Drug?*

see Cimetidine

▶ *What Should I Tell My Patients About This Drug?*

see Ranitidine

▶ *Therapeutic Tips*

see Ranitidine

FENOFIBRATE

Stephen Shalansky and Robert Dombrowski

USA (not available)
CANADA (Lipidil)

▶ *When Should I Use This Drug?*

Hypercholesterolemia

- fibric acid derivatives generally decrease low density lipoprotein (LDL) cholesterol less than bile acid sequestrants, niacin, or HMG-CoA reductase inhibitors do and in some cases may increase LDL cholesterol
- should be considered only if all other agents have failed
- unless there is significant cost advantage, gemfibrozil should be used instead of fenofibrate, as there are no long-term studies evaluating fenofibrate's effect on cardiovascular morbidity and mortality

Hypertriglyceridemia

- consider drug therapy only in patients with symptomatic (pancreatitis, xanthomas) hypertriglyceridemia, as there is no evidence yet to support or screen patients with asymptomatic elevated triglyceride levels (Br Med J 1992;304:394–396)
- unless there is significant cost advantage, gemfibrozil should be used instead of fenofibrate, as there are no long-term studies evaluating fenofibrate's effect on cardiovascular morbidity and mortality

Mixed hyperlipidemia

- should be used after niacin and when the HMG-CoA reductase inhibitors have failed

▶ *When Should I Not Use This Drug?*

First-line agent for hyperlipidemias

- do not use as a first-line agent, as there are no studies evaluating its effect on cardiovascular morbidity or mortality

▶ *What Contraindications Are There to the Use of This Drug?*

- intolerance of or allergic reaction to fenofibrate

see Gemfibrozil

▶ *What Drug Interactions Are Clinically Important?*

Few reported drug interactions so far but one should assume that fenofibrate exhibits the same drug interactions as gemfibrozil

see Gemfibrozil

▶ *What Route and Dosage Should I Use?*

How to administer

- orally—give with meals
- parenterally—not available

Hypercholesterolemia, hypertriglyceridemia, mixed hyperlipidemias

- 100 mg PO TID
- if at 3 months the drug is tolerated and there has been at least a 15% decrease in lipid level but not to the desired level, continue the drug administration and add second-line agent
- if adding another drug, monitor as if initiating therapy
- if the drug is not tolerated or there is less than a 15% decrease in total cholesterol level after 3 months of therapy, stop the fenofibrate administration and start a different drug

Dosage adjustments for renal or hepatic dysfunction

- hepatically metabolized
- decrease daily dose to 100 mg PO daily if creatinine clearance is less than 15 mL/min
- do not use in severe renal or hepatic failure

▶ *What Should I Monitor with Regard to Efficacy and Toxicity?*

Efficacy

see Gemfibrozil

Toxicity

Gastrointestinal symptoms

- constipation and diarrhea in 3–5% of patients

Gallstones

- clofibrate, another fibric acid derivative, has been linked to gallstone formation (JAMA 1975;231:360–381)
- although fenofibrate increases cholesterol saturation in the bile, it does not appear to increase the incidence of gallstones (Drugs 1990;40:260–290)

Hepatic toxicity

- mild elevations in aminotransferase levels are common
- there are several reports of hepatitis associated with fenofibrate

- serum aminotransferases should be monitored after 6 months of treatment and yearly thereafter
- if serum aminotransferase levels are substantially elevated (>3 times normal), fenofibrate should be discontinued

Dermatological reactions

- erythema, pruritus, urticaria
- 0.3–8.4% (Cardiology 1989;76:169–179)

Myalgia

- up to 3%
- may be associated with elevated creatinine phosphokinase levels

Uric acid and alkaline phosphatase levels

- may be mildly decreased

▶ *How Long Do I Treat Patients with This Drug?*

see Gemfibrozil

▶ *How Do I Decrease or Stop the Administration of This Drug?*

- may be stopped abruptly

▶ *What Should I Tell My Patients About This Drug?*

see Gemfibrozil

▶ *Therapeutic Tips*

- do not use as a first-line agent for hypercholesterolemia

Useful References

Balfour JA, McTavish D, Heel RC. Fenofibrate: A review of its pharmacodynamic and pharmacokinetic properties and therapeutic use in dyslipidemia. Drugs 1990;40:260–290

Brown WV, ed. Fenofibrate, a third-generation fibric acid derivative. Am J Med 1987;83(suppl 5B):1–89

FENOPROFEN

Kelly Jones

USA (Nalfon, various generic)
CANADA (Nalfon)

▶ *When Should I Use This Drug?*

Consider an alternative agent

- there is no reason to use this agent for the treatment of rheumatoid arthritis because fenoprofen is too toxic and not well tolerated when compared with other NSAIDs
- 15% incidence of headache
- this agent is the most renally toxic agent in this class
- accounts for 50% of the reports on nephrotic syndrome, 30% with acute tubular necrosis, 28% with acute interstitial nephritis (J Am Board Fam Pract 1989;2:257–271)

FENOTEROL

Karen Shalansky and Cindy Reesor Nimmo

USA (Berotec)
CANADA (Berotec)

▶ *When Should I Use This Drug?*

Consider an alternative agent

- on a per milligram basis, fenoterol has been shown to be equipotent to salbutamol; with a 200 μg/puff inhaler, a higher incidence of side effects, including hypokalemia and cardiac toxicity, has been reported (Lancet 1990;336:1396–1399, Chest 1978;73:348–351, Am Rev Respir Dis 1989;139:176–180)
- possible increase in asthmatic deaths with regular use of fenoterol (200 μg/puff) has been reported (Lancet 1989;1:917–922, Lancet 1990;336:1391–1396, N Engl J Med 1992;326:501–506)

Useful Reference

Woolcock AJ. Beta-agonists and asthma mortality. What have we learned, what questions remain? Drugs 1990;40:653–656

FENTANYL

Terry Baumann

USA (fentanyl, Sublimaze, Duragesic)
CANADA (fentanyl, Sublimaze, Duragesic)

▶ *When Should I Use This Drug?*

Anesthesia

- most often as an adjunct to general anesthesia

Postoperative pain

- seldom used for postoperative pain via the intramuscular or the intravenous route because of its short duration of action
- opioid of choice for epidural administration because it has a faster onset of action and is easier to titrate than epidural morphine because of its lipid solubility
- epidural fentanyl also produces less frequent and severe respiratory depression, nausea and vomiting, and itch than does epidural morphine (epidural morphine also produces a greater incidence of later respiratory depression)
- after epidural fentanyl administration has been stopped, patients need to be monitored (for toxicity) only for 4 hours, whereas toxicity from epidural morphine can cause adverse effects for up to 24 hours

Cancer pain

- a patch may be useful after the patient is controlled on a regular-release oral opioid
- fentanyl patch may be as effective as sustained-release morphine but is more difficult to titrate
- a patch allows a convenient Q72H dosing schedule

▶ *When Should I Not Use This Drug?*

Mild to moderate pain (acute or chronic)

- unless drugs such as acetaminophen, acetaminophen-codeine, nonsteroidal antiinflammatory drugs (NSAIDs), and morphine have been used on a regularly scheduled basis (not PRN) and are shown to be ineffective

Postoperative pain (patch)

- fentanyl patch should not be used for postoperative pain because it is difficult to titrate the dose acutely, which is necessary for many patients postoperatively

▶ *What Contraindications Are There to the Use of This Drug?*

Intolerance of or allergic reaction to fentanyl

- true allergies to fentanyl are rare
- check whether the patient has actual allergic symptoms, and if there is a true allergy, consider giving morphine

Severe respiratory depression

- not an absolute contraindication, just start with doses 25% of the normal initial dose and titrate up to an effect, assessing respiratory rate and oxymetry before each dose

▶ *What Drug Interactions Are Clinically Important?*

see Morphine

MONOAMINE OXIDASE INHIBITORS

- combination of fentanyl and monoamine oxidase inhibitors has caused coma, severe respiratory depression, and extreme central nervous system stimulation
- do not use in combination or if patient has received monoamine oxidase inhibitors during the previous 14 days

▶ *What Route and Dosage Should I Use?*

How to administer

- transdermal—see below
- parenterally—can be administered intramuscularly, intravenously, or epidurally

Anesthesia

- 1–20 μg/kg IV, most often as an adjunct to general anesthesia

Postoperative pain

- initial epidural dose of 50–100 μg may be given with a 20 μg/h infusion
- this route should be used only by anesthetists skilled in this technique

Cancer pain

- transdermal patch should be used only after good pain control has been achieved with other opioids such as morphine and nonopioids such as NSAIDs and patient wants to switch to a more convenient dosage form
- a fentanyl patch may be as effective as sustained-release morphine but is more difficult to titrate
- has the advantage of requiring only Q27H dosing
- dosage is determined by the daily morphine requirements
- fentanyl patches come in only strengths of 25, 50, 75, and 100 μg/h
- for initial dosing, start with 25 μg/h patch if patient is receiving 45–134 mg of morphine/day; 50 μg/h patch if patient is receiving 135–224 mg of morphine/day; 75 μg/h patch if patient is receiving 225–314 mg of morphine/day; and the 100 μg/h patch if the patient is receiving 215–404 mg of morphine/day
- always use transdermal fentanyl with an order for PRN rapid-release morphine for breakthrough pain
- do not adjust the fentanyl dosage upward for inadequate analgesia until the initial 72 hour period has been reached
- further fentanyl dosage adjustments should be made no more frequently than every 6 days
- fentanyl dosage adjustments should be based on the daily dose of supplementary opioids required
- if the patient does not tolerate the fentanyl patch, it may be removed and the patient converted to another narcotic
- it usually takes 17 hours or longer for the fentanyl serum concentration to decline by 50%; therefore, for the first 12–18 hours after the patch is removed, half the equianalgesic dose of narcotic should be administered; then titrate to the patient's need

Dosage adjustments for renal or hepatic dysfunction

- hepatically metabolized
- dosage adjustment is usually not required if the dose is titrated properly

▶ What Should I Monitor with Regard to Efficacy and Toxicity?

see Morphine

▶ How Long Do I Treat Patients with This Drug?

see Morphine

▶ How Do I Decrease or Stop the Administration of This Drug?

see Morphine

▶ What Should I Tell My Patients About This Drug?

see Morphine

- fentanyl should not be used in patients who have received monoamine oxidase inhibitors within 14 days
- the patch should be applied to dry, nonirritated, flat surfaces of the upper torso by firmly pressing it for 10–20 seconds
- when a patch is to be replaced, a new site on the upper torso should be chosen
- hair at the site of application may be clipped but not shaved (this may cause irritation and changes the absorption characteristics of the transdermal system)
- clean the area of application with water only
- flush any unused portion down the toilet
- if the gel from the patch accidentally contacts the skin, the area should be washed with water only

▶ Therapeutic Tips

see Morphine

- do not use the fentanyl patch for the initial titration
- always give intravenous or subcutaneous morphine for severe unrelieved pain in cancer patients

- morphine may then be changed to the patch after the pain is under control
- most effective when used with peripheral acting nonopiate analgesics (acetaminophen, aspirin, or NSAIDs)
- in patients who will be given regularly dosed narcotics for longer than 3–4 days, always prescribe narcotics in conjunction with a laxative and counsel the patient on the appropriate use of fluids and fiber

Useful References

see Morphine

FLECAINIDE

James Tisdale

USA (Tambocor)
CANADA (Tambocor)

▶ When Should I Use This Drug?

Flecainide should not be used without consulting a cardiologist or a cardiac electrophysiologist

Life-threatening ventricular arrhythmias

- flecainide should be used for the prevention of life-threatening ventricular arrhythmias in patients without a history of congestive heart failure, acute myocardial infarction, or ischemic heart disease who have failed to respond to therapy with class IA drugs such as quinidine and procainamide, class IB drugs such as mexiletine and tocainide, and/or the combination of class IA and IB antiarrhythmic drugs during serial drug testing in the electrophysiology (EP) laboratory and in whom flecainide is shown to suppress inducible ventricular arrhythmias during EP testing or on Holter monitoring

Atrioventricular nodal reentrant tachycardia

- flecainide should be used for the long-term prevention of atrioventricular (AV) nodal reentrant tachycardia in patients without a history of congestive heart failure, myocardial infarction, or ischemic heart disease in whom empirical therapy with oral digoxin alone and in combination with a beta-blocker has been unsuccessful, and in patients with contraindications to beta-blocker therapy in whom digoxin therapy has been unsuccessful (Circulation 1991;83:119–125)

Atrial fibrillation or flutter

- flecainide should be used for the prevention of episodes of paroxysmal atrial fibrillation or flutter in patients with no history of congestive heart failure, myocardial infarction, or ischemic heart disease in whom therapy with quinidine has been unsuccessful or poorly tolerated (Am J Cardiol 1991;67:713–717)

Wolff-Parkinson-White syndrome

- flecainide should be used in patients with supraventricular tachycardia due to Wolff-Parkinson-White syndrome who have no history of left ventricular dysfunction or ischemic heart disease in whom Wolff-Parkinson-White syndrome is not cured by nonpharmacological techniques such as radioablation or surgery, and in whom flecainide has been shown to be effective during electrophysiological testing

▶ When Should I Not Use This Drug?

Asymptomatic ventricular arrhythmias

- treatment of asymptomatic arrhythmias with antiarrhythmic drugs has not been shown to be of benefit, and flecainide has adversely influenced mortality in post–myocardial infarction patients with asymptomatic ventricular arrhythmias (N Engl J Med 1989;321:406–412)

▶ What Contraindications Are There to the Use of This Drug?

Intolerance of or allergic reaction to flecainide
History of myocardial infarction

- flecainide should not be used in any patient who has a history of myocardial infarction, as the drug has adversely influenced mortality in this population (N Engl J Med 1989;321:406–412)

Congestive heart failure

- flecainide should not be used in any patient with a history of congestive heart failure, as the drug has negative inotropic activity and may aggravate congestive heart failure

Atrioventricular block

- flecainide impairs the conduction of electrical impulses through the AV node and therefore should not be used in patients with second- or third-degree AV block in the absence of a functioning ventricular pacemaker
- flecainide may be used in patients with first-degree AV block, but the electrocardiogram (ECG) should be monitored closely for progression of heart block

Bundle branch blocks

- flecainide slows conduction through the His-Purkinje system and therefore should not be used in patients with bifascicular or trifascicular bundle branch blocks unless a functioning pacemaker is present

Pacemakers

- flecainide has been reported to increase the threshold for pacemaker impulse capture and therefore should be used with caution in patients with temporary or permanent pacemakers
- if flecainide therapy is initiated in a patient with a pacemaker, the device should be programmed to stimulus strengths 3 times higher than threshold levels (rather than the usual 2 times threshold values), and pacing thresholds should be determined when serum flecainide concentrations reach steady state (PACE 1983;6:892–899)

▶ *What Drug Interactions Are Clinically Important?*

Drugs that may increase the effect or toxicity of flecainide

AMIODARONE

- concomitant amiodarone therapy has resulted in elevated serum flecainide concentrations
- if amiodarone therapy is initiated in patients receiving flecainide, the flecainide dosage should be decreased by 50% and the patient should be monitored for adverse effects

CIMETIDINE

- concomitant cimetidine therapy may result in elevations in serum flecainide concentrations of 10–30%
- switch to ranitidine or other H_2 antagonist if a combination must be used, as these agents have less of an effect on metabolism

BETA-BLOCKERS, VERAPAMIL, DILTIAZEM

- flecainide impairs conduction of impulses through the AV node, and this effect may be additive when flecainide is used in combination with agents with similar properties
- in patients receiving flecainide in combination with one of the above agents, the ECG should be monitored for prolongation of the PR interval to longer than 0.2 second monthly for the first 3 months of therapy and every 6 months thereafter

Drugs that may decrease the effect or toxicity of flecainide

- none

Drugs that may have their effect or toxicity increased by flecainide

DIGOXIN

- concomitant flecainide therapy may result in elevations of serum digoxin concentrations (approximately 25%)
- if flecainide therapy is initiated in patients receiving digoxin, patients should be monitored for signs or symptoms of digoxin toxicity

Drugs that may have their effect or toxicity decreased by flecainide

- none

▶ *What Route and Dosage Should I Use?*

How to administer

- orally—administer with or without food
- parenterally—unavailable

Life-threatening ventricular arrhythmias, atrioventricular nodal reentrant tachycardia, atrial fibrillation or flutter, Wolff-Parkinson-White syndrome

- start with 100 mg PO Q12H
- if there is an inadequate response, the dosage may be increased by 50 mg Q12H every 4 days until a response is achieved, or a maximum dosage of 200 mg Q12H is reached
- some patients have adverse effects with Q12H dosing (if these develop, smaller doses administered Q8H may alleviate adverse effects)

Dosage adjustments for renal or hepatic dysfunction

- 25% renal elimination, 75% hepatic elimination

Normal Dosing Interval	$C_{cr} > 60$ mL/min or 1 mL/s	C_{cr} 30–60 mL/min or 0.5–1 mL/s	$C_{cr} < 30$ mL/min or 0.5 mL/s
Q12H	no adjustment needed	no adjustment needed	initial dose 50 PO Q12H maximum dosage, 100 mg PO Q12H

▶ *What Should I Monitor with Regard to Efficacy and Toxicity?*

Efficacy

Life-threatening ventricular arrhythmias, atrioventricular nodal reentrant tachycardia, atrial fibrillation or flutter, Wolff-Parkinson-White syndrome

- continuous ECG monitoring daily during initiation and stabilization, then ECG's every 3–6 months to detect the presence or absence of arrhythmia or reduced frequency of arrhythmia episodes
- symptoms associated with arrhythmia (palpitations, shortness of breath, chest pain, and syncope) should resolve

Serum concentrations

- therapeutic range of flecainide is usually quoted as 0.2–1 μg/mL
- range of serum flecainide concentrations required for efficacy varies widely among patients, and therefore, the therapeutic range is of relatively little use in monitoring the efficacy of flecainide
- if therapeutic monitoring is performed, use the method of monitoring target serum flecainide concentrations (see Quinidine) (Clin Pharmacokinet 1991; 20:151–166)

Toxicity

Adverse effects necessitating discontinuation of therapy occur in approximately 5–10% of patients
Blurred vision, difficulty in accomodation, lightheadedness, dizziness, ataxia, parasthesias

- blurred vision and difficulty in accomodation are dose related and occur in approximately 30% of patients taking 400 mg daily
- dizziness, ataxia, and paresthesias may also occur
- flecainide dosage should be reduced in patients who experience intolerable blurred vision, difficulty in accommodation, lightheadedness, or dizziness (after it has been confirmed that lightheadedness or dizziness is not the result of arrhythmia recurrence)
- dosage may be reduced by 50 mg Q12H with reevaluation of adverse effects
- if the dosage is reduced, patients should be instructed to report changes in symptoms or pulse rate

Congestive heart failure

- rare in patients with no history of congestive heart failure
- flecainide therapy should be discontinued abruptly in patients who have signs or symptoms of congestive heart failure

Electrocardiogram

- repeat ECG at 1 week to monitor for prolonged PR interval (>0.2 second), prolonged duration of QRS complex (>25% increase compared with baseline measurement), and initiation of new arrhythmia or worsening of clinical arrhythmia

- flecainide therapy should be discontinued abruptly in patients who experience new cardiac arrhythmias or worsening of their clinical arrhythmia in association with flecainide therapy

▶ How Long Do I Treat Patients with This Drug?

Life-threatening ventricular arrhythmias, atrioventricular nodal reentrant tachycardia, atrial fibrillation or flutter, Wolff-Parkinson-White syndrome

- patients treated for life-threatening ventricular arrhythmias, atrioventricular nodal reentrant tachycardia, or atrial fibrillation or flutter may require therapy indefinitely if contributing factors cannot be reversed

▶ How Do I Decrease or Stop the Administration of This Drug?

- flecainide therapy should not be discontinued or dosage reduction performed without consulting a cardiologist or an electrophysiologist
- may be stopped abruptly if ineffective or poorly tolerated

▶ What Should I Tell My Patients About This Drug?

- notify your physician if you have any disturbances in vision, nausea, vomiting, tingling in hands or feet, shortness of breath, palpitations, chest pain, dizziness, or lightheadedness
- do not discontinue flecainide therapy without consulting your physician

▶ Therapeutic Tips

- range of serum flecainide concentrations required for efficacy varies widely among patients, and therefore, the therapeutic range is of relatively little use in monitoring the efficacy of flecainide

Useful References

Flecainide Ventricular Tachycardia Study Group. Treatment of resistant ventricular tachycardia with flecainide acetate. Am J Cardiol 1986; 57:1299–1304

Anderson JL, Gilbert EM, Alpert BL, et al. Prevention of symptomatic recurrences of paroxysmal atrial fibrillation in patients initially tolerating antiarrhythmic therapy. A multicenter, double-blind, crossover study of flecainide and placebo with transtelephonic monitoring. Circulation 1989;80:1557–1570

Cockrell JL, Scheinman MM, Titus C, et al. Safety and efficacy of oral flecainide therapy in patients with atrioventricular re-entrant tachycardia. Ann Intern Med 1991;114:189–194

Anderson JL, Jolivette DM, Fredell PA. Summary of efficacy and safety of flecainide for supraventricular arrhythmias. Am J Cardiol 1988; 62:62D–66D

FLUCLOXACILLIN

John Rotschafer, Kyle Vance-Bryan, and Rick Zabinski

USA (not available)
CANADA (Fluclox)

▶ When Should I Use This Drug?

Consider an alternative agent

- identical indications to those for cloxacillin but is more expensive
- flucloxacillin reaches somewhat higher peak free serum concentrations than does cloxacillin, but this does not offer any clinically significant advantages over oral cloxacillin

FLUCONAZOLE

Peter Jewesson

USA (Diflucan)
CANADA (Diflucan)

▶ When Should I Use This Drug?

Cryptococcal meningitis

- fluconazole as initial therapy can be considered in mild disease without poor prognostic factors (i.e., abnormal mental status or both cryptococcal antigen titer > 1:1024 and CSF white blood count <20 per mm³) (N Engl J Med 1992;326:83)

- fluconazole 200 mg PO daily for prevention of relapse (suppressive therapy) is the preferred approach (N Engl J Med 1992;326:793–798, N Engl J Med 1991;324:580–584) despite its cost and potential drug interactions, because it has greater efficacy, convenience (once daily oral dosing), and tolerance compared to amphotericin B

Oropharyngeal and esophageal candidiasis

- use if failure to achieve some symptomatic improvement after 5–7 days with ketoconazole or initially where a drug interaction may be more likely to result in failed therapy with ketoconazole (e.g., rifampin, H_2 blockers, omeprazole)
- more expensive than ketoconazole

Systemic candidiasis

- alternative to amphotericin B
- direct comparative trials are in progress but good data still lacking
- choose amphotericin B over fluconazole in patients who are immunocompromised or who are severely ill
- reserve fluconazole for patients who have contraindications to amphotericin B

Vaginal candidiasis

- use when topical therapy is unsuccessful and where ketoconazole is not tolerated
- a 1 day course of fluconazole appears to be equivalent to a 3 day course of ketoconazole
- more expensive yet better tolerated than systemic ketoconazole

▶ When Should I Not Use This Drug?

Treatment of fungal infection involving pathogens resistant to fluconazole

- fluconazole is ineffective against aspergillosis

Bowel sterilization (selective decontamination) for immunocompromised patients

- antifungal prophylaxis with fluconazole may reduce the incidence of mucosal candidiasis; it does not reduce the frequency of deep invasive candidiasis (Clin Infectious Dis 1993;17(suppl 2):S468–S480)

▶ What Contraindications Are There to the Use of This Drug?

- intolerance or allergic reaction to fluconazole

▶ What Drug Interactions Are Clinically Important?

Drugs that may increase the effect or toxicity of fluconazole

- none

Drugs that may decrease the effect of fluconazole

RIFAMPIN

- rifampin decreases fluconazole serum concentrations by stimulating hepatic metabolism
- if existing dose ineffective, consider increasing dose to a maximum of 400 mg daily

Drugs that may have their effect or toxicity increased by fluconazole

THEOPHYLLINE

- fluconazole inhibits cytochrome P450 enzyme systems, resulting in reduced theophylline clearance
- avoid concomitant use; however, if used together, monitor serum theophylline concentrations weekly and evaluate for clinical signs of theophylline toxicity
- reassess again upon discontinuation of fluconazole if changes occur while on combination

WARFARIN

- fluconazole inhibits cytochrome P450 enzyme systems, resulting in reduced warfarin clearance
- avoid concomitant use of fluconazole and warfarin
- if used together, monitor INR every 2 days and adjust warfarin dose to maintain therapeutic values
- reassess again upon discontinuation of fluconazole

CYCLOSPORINE

- inhibits hepatic metabolism of cyclosporine
- seen as early as 2 days after the start of these drugs
- monitor cyclosporine levels every other day until full extent of interaction is seen, and adjust dose accordingly
- may need to decrease the cyclosporine dose by 30% or more

PHENYTOIN

- inhibits metabolism of phenytoin and may produce increases in serum phenytoin concentrations
- monitor serum phenytoin measurements weekly until a new steady-state is established or symptoms of toxicity occur, and adjust dose accordingly
- return to previous dose upon discontinuation of fluconazole

TOLBUTAMIDE

- fluconazole inhibits cytochrome P450 enzyme systems resulting in interference with tolbutamide clearance
- if fluconazole is added to tolbutamide therapy, monitor blood glucose daily for first 3–4 days and adjust dose of tolbutamide accordingly
- reassess after discontinuation of fluconazole

Drugs that may have their effect decreased by fluconazole

- none

▶ What Route and Dosage Should I Use?

How to administer

- orally—take oral preparation on empty stomach or with food if intolerance occurs
- parenterally—administer IV preparation in normal saline solution at a maximum rate of 200 mg/h (400 mg/h via central line)
- daily doses for oral and parenteral therapy are equivalent

Cryptococcal meningitis

- 400 mg PO daily
- 200 mg PO daily for prophylaxis

Oropharyngeal candidiasis, esophageal candidiasis

- 200 mg followed by 100 mg PO once daily

Systemic candidiasis

- start with 400 mg IV at onset of treatment and consider stepping down to oral therapy once the clinical condition stabilizes

Vaginal candidiasis

- 150 mg × 1 dose

Dosage adjustments for renal or hepatic liver dysfunction

- eliminated by renal, hepatic pathways
- fluconazole is removed by hemodialysis; give the usual dose once after each dialysis
- no adjustment for liver disease

Normal Dosing Interval	$C_{cr} > 60$ mL/min or 1.0 mL/s	C_{cr} 30–60 mL/min or 0.5–1.0 mL/s	$C_{cr} < 30$ mL/min or 0.5 mL/s
Q24H	no adjustment needed	decrease dosage by 50%	decrease dosage by 75%

▶ What Should I Monitor with Regard to Efficacy and Toxicity?

Efficacy

Cryptococcal meningitis

- relief of headache, neurologic signs and fever
- assess daily until clinical response, then 1–2 × a week until completed 10 weeks of treatment

Oropharyngeal candidiasis

- reduction in pain, disappearance of lesions
- assess symptoms daily if in hospital or weekly as an outpatient

Esophageal candidiasis

- relief of dysphagia
- assess symptoms daily if in hospital or weekly as an outpatient

Systemic candidiasis

see Amphotericin B

Vaginal candidiasis

- disappearance of lesions and reduction in pain and itching

Toxicity

- considered minor compared to amphotericin B

Gastrointestinal

- 9% incidence of nausea and vomiting
- take with food if nausea develops; if symptoms persist, discontinue use
- food delays but does not reduce absorption

Dermatologic

- 4% incidence of rash

Hepatic

- approximately 1% of patients will develop reversible elevation of liver enzymes; rare reports of hepatotoxicity (lower incidence than ketoconazole)
- monitor liver enzymes at baseline and once weekly

▶ How Long Do I Treat Patients with This Drug?

Cryptococcal meningitis

- indefinitely with suppressive therapy

Oropharyngeal candidiasis

- 1 week and at least 2 days after the symptoms have resolved
- patient should respond within a few days

Esophageal candidiasis

- treat for at least 2–3 weeks and 1 week following resolution of symptoms

Systemic candidiasis

- a minimum of 4 weeks and at least 2 weeks following resolution of symptoms

Vaginal candidiasis

- 1 day

▶ How Do I Decrease or Stop Administration of This Drug?

- may be stopped abruptly

▶ What Should I Tell My Patient About This Drug?

- this agent is a newer antifungal agent and successful therapy is contingent upon good compliance and completion of the full treatment course
- some minor side effects (i.e., gastrointestinal or reversible liver changes) can be expected but these are usually self-limiting and therapy should not be stopped
- contact pharmacist or physician if any new symptoms arise

▶ Therapeutic Tips

- always consider efficacy, toxicity, and cost when determining the role of fluconazole relative to other available agents

Useful Reference

Bennett JE. Antifungal agents. In: Mandell GL, Douglas RG Jr., Bennett JE, eds., Principles and Practice of Infectious Diseases, 3rd ed. New York: Churchill Livingstone, 1990:361–370.

FLUCYTOSINE (5-FC, 5-fluorocytosine)

Peter Jewesson

USA (Ancobon)
CANADA (Ancotil)

▶ When Should I Use This Drug?

Disseminated or severe candidiasis

- add to amphotericin therapy when fungal resistance suspected or infection is considered severe enough to warrant combination therapy
- considered additive or slightly synergistic against *Candida* and additive effects may allow amphotericin B to be given in lower doses

Cryptococcal meningitis

- amphotericin in combination with flucytosine has been shown to be the treatment of choice in non-AIDS patients (N Engl J Med 1979;301:126) but it is unclear whether it is more effective than amphotericin B alone in AIDS patients (Ann Intern Med 1990;113:183,N Engl J Med 1992;326:83–89)
- add flucytosine to amphotericin B unless there are significant cytopenias or renal impairment

Chromomycosis

- drug of choice, as single therapy, because it is as effective as amphotericin and less toxic

▶ *When Should I Not Use This Drug?*

As single agent

- clinical efficacy, except for treatment of chromomycosis, is inferior to amphotericin B
- secondary drug resistance is common when used as monotherapy

▶ *What Contraindications Are There to the Use of This Drug?*

- intolerance or allergic reaction to flucytosine

▶ *What Drug Interactions Are Clinically Important?*

Drugs that may increase effect/toxicity of flucytosine

Concomitant nephrotoxic drugs (e.g., amphotericin B)

- can reduce the clearance of flucytosine
- monitor serum creatinine every 2 days and adjust dose based on renal function estimates
- if parameters continue to be stable, reduce frequency of serum creatinine monitoring to three times weekly

Drugs that may decrease effect of flucytosine

- none

Drugs that may have effect/toxicity increased by flucytosine

- concomitant bone marrow suppressing drugs
- when this combination is used in AIDS patients, profound cytopenias may develop

Drugs that may have effect decreased by flucytosine

- none

▶ *What Route and Dosage Should I Use?*

How to administer

- orally—on an empty stomach, or with food if gastrointestinal intolerance occurs

Disseminated or severe candidiasis, Cryptococcal meningitis, Chromomycosis

Moderately severe infections

- 25 mg/kg PO Q6H (rounded to nearest 500 mg as only available in 500 mg tablets)

Severe infections

- 37.5 mg/kg PO Q6H (rounded to nearest 500 mg)

Dosage adjustment for renal/hepatic dysfunction

- renally eliminated

Normal Dosing Interval	$C_{cr} > 60$ mL/min or 1.0 mL/sec	C_{cr} 30–60 mL/min or 0.5–1.0 mL/sec	$C_{cr} < 30$ mL/min or 0.5 mL/sec
Q6H	no adjustment needed	Q8H	Q12H

▶ *What Should I Monitor with Regard to Efficacy and Toxicity?*

Efficacy

see Amphotericin

Toxicity

- when used on its own, flucytosine rarely causes serious toxicities

Gastrointestinal

- nausea and vomiting common and in part due to large number of capsules administered for each dose
- administration of capsules at 5 minute intervals may be helpful

Severe enterocolitis

- monitor daily for loose stools or dull abdominal pain

Hematological

- leukopenia, thrombocytopenia, aplastic anemia have been reported and are potentially lethal
- monitor blood counts at baseline and at least twice weekly
- bone marrow suppression may be more pronounced in AIDS patients receiving AZT

Renal

- not nephrotoxic but routinely administered with amphotericin B
- monitor serum creatinine a minimum of every 2 days when receiving with amphotericin
- adjust dose empirically according to estimated creatinine clearance and/or according to serum concentrations (see below)

Hepatic

- 5% incidence of asymptomatic, reversible liver function tests
- evaluate liver enzymes at baseline and once weekly
- reduce dose or discontinue drug if elevated greater than 2 times baseline

Serum concentration monitoring

- 5-flucytosine is converted to 5-fluorouracil in vivo and this appears responsible for hematological and gastrointestinal tract toxicities
- hematological and gastrointestinal tract toxicities appear more common when serum concentrations exceed 100 mg/mL
- 5-flucytosine serum concentration monitoring is still considered experimental
- if used, predose serum concentrations should be kept greater than 25 mg/L and postdose levels at less than 100 mg/L

▶ *How Long Do I Treat Patients with This Drug?*

Disseminated or severe candidiasis, cryptococcal meningitis

- total amount of 5-flucytosine needed to treat any fungal infection is not known
- response to therapy varies according to nature of infection and immune status of host
- 5-flucytosine should be discontinued when amphotericin B is discontinued

Chromomycosis

- 2–3 months

▶ *How Do I Decrease or Stop the Administration of This Drug?*

- may be stopped abruptly

▶ *What Should I Tell My Patients About This Drug?*

- this agent is an antifungal agent and successful therapy is contingent upon good compliance and completion of the full treatment course
- some side effects (i.e., gastrointestinal or reversible bone marrow suppression) can be expected but these can be monitored for and therapy stopped if necessary
- contact pharmacist or physician if diarrhea, dull abdominal pain, or mouth sores develop

▶ *Therapeutic Tips*

- with availability of newer azoles, use of this drug is generally restricted to combination therapy with amphotericin B
- expect amphotericin B–related nephrotoxicity and plan to alter 5-flucytosine doses accordingly

Useful Reference

Bennett JE. Antifunal agents. In: Mandell GL, Douglas RG Jr., Bennett JE, eds. Principles and Practice of Infectious Diseases, 3rd ed. New York: Churchill Livingstone, 1990; 361–370.

FLUNISOLIDE

Karen Shalansky and Cindy Reesor Nimmo

USA (AeroBid)
CANADA (Bronalide)

▶ When Should I Use This Drug?

Consider an alternative agent

- flunisolide provides no advantages over the other inhaled corticosteroids
- flunisolide has a potential disadvantage, in that it has a disagreeable taste, which may interfere with patient compliance

FLUOXETINE

Lyle K. Laird and Julia Vertrees

USA (Prozac)
CANADA (Prozac)

▶ When Should I Use This Drug?

Major depression

- as effective as other antidepressants for the treatment of major depression
- although imipramine is usually chosen for these disorders, if cost is not a factor, fluoxetine may be chosen instead of imipramine, as it is generally better tolerated (no anticholinergic effects, not usually sedating)
- fluoxetine has less potential to cause orthostatic hypotension than do other antidepressants and can be chosen in those patients for whom orthostasis may be a significant concern, such as the elderly; however, if cost is an issue, nortriptyline can be used, as it also causes a low incidence of adverse effects and is less expensive than fluoxetine
- other antidepressants can lower the seizure threshold, and fluoxetine appears to have a lower propensity to cause seizures than do other tricyclic antidepressants
- fluoxetine appears to cause few cardiovascular effects and can be chosen in patients with certain types of heart block (first and second degree)

Obsessive-compulsive disorders

- fluoxetine should be chosen in patients with inadequate response to clomipramine, hypersensitivity to clomipramine, significant cardiovascular disease (e.g., bundle branch block), or a history of past response to fluoxetine

Dysthymia, panic disorders, bulimia, obesity

- fluoxetine has been investigated in these conditions and may be considered alternative drug therapy when more traditional therapy fails

▶ When Should I Not Use This Drug?

see Imipramine

▶ What Contraindications Are There to the Use of This Drug?

Intolerance of or allergic reaction to fluoxetine

Currently, there are no known absolute contraindications to the use of fluoxetine

Pregnancy

- human studies have not been done; however, animal studies have not shown fluoxetine to cause adverse effects on the fetus

Breast-feeding

- not known whether fluoxetine is excreted into breast milk
- problems in humans not reported

▶ What Drug Interactions Are Clinically Important?

Drugs that may increase the effect or toxicity of fluoxetine

CENTRAL NERVOUS SYSTEM DEPRESSANTS

- central nervous system (CNS) depressant effects are enhanced; therefore, avoid use with other CNS depressants

MONOAMINE OXIDASE INHIBITORS

- concurrent administration or administration of a monoamine oxidase inhibitor shortly after stopping fluoxetine administration may lead to serotonin syndrome, which includes CNS irritability, increased muscle tone, shivering, myoclonus, and altered consciousness (Lancet 1988;2:850–851)
- manufacturer recommends a 5 week interval between stopping fluoxetine and beginning monoamine oxidase inhibitor therapy

LITHIUM

- several reports exist of a serotoninergic hyperarousal syndrome with concurrent use of fluoxetine and lithium (Am J Psychiatry 1989;146:278, 1515, Am J Psychiatry 1991;148:146–147)
- alternatively, there have been a number of reports of safe concurrent use (J Clin Psychiatry 1992;53:28–29, Biol Psychiatry 1991;29:946–948, Can J Psychiatry 1991;36:154–155, Acta Psychiatr Scand 1991;83:188–192, Am J Psychiatry 1988;145:1292–1294)
- monitor for toxicity during concurrent administration and discontinue administration of one or both medications if symptoms of CNS hyperarousal occur

Drugs that may decrease the effect of fluoxetine

- none

Drugs that may have their effect or toxicity increased by fluoxetine

TRICYCLIC ANTIDEPRESSANTS

- fluoxetine is a hepatic enzyme inhibitor and can lead to increased levels of other hepatically eliminated drugs
- elevated tricyclic blood levels and adverse effects, including drowsiness, lethargy, psychomotor retardation, depressed mood, dry mouth, and confusion, have been reported during concurrent use with tricyclic antidepressants
- these effects have developed over periods ranging from 5 days to 5 weeks, in spite of lowering the antidepressant dosage, and may persist for several weeks after stopping fluoxetine therapy
- monitor for signs of toxicity and adjust the tricyclic dosage if necessary

CARBAMAZEPINE

- there have been 2 reports of increased carbamazepine concentrations in patients receiving carbamazepine and fluoxetine (J Clin Psychiatry 1990;51:126–127)
- if fluoxetine is added, obtain a baseline serum carbamazepine concentration prior to adding inhibitor, recheck the concentration in 1 week, and reduce the dosage proportionately if the concentration is greater than 12 mg/L
- monitor for symptoms of toxicity, and if they occur, stop the drug administration, get a repeated concentration, and adjust the dosage accordingly
- if the concentration is not available within 24 hours, restart carbamazepine therapy at 50% of the previous dose as long as toxicity is not present
- if no toxicity occurs, measure concentrations weekly until a new steady state has been reached
- if fluoxetine stopped, increase the dosage back to the preinhibitor level

TRYPTOPHAN

- concurrent administration of these agents may lead to symptoms of CNS toxicity (e.g., agitation, aggressiveness, and worsening of obsessive-compulsive symptoms) and peripheral toxicity (e.g., nausea and vomiting) (Biol Psychiatry 1986;21:1067–1071)
- concurrent use should be avoided
- if concurrent use is necessary, monitor for toxic reactions and discontinue the tryptophan regimen if symptoms occur

WARFARIN

- interferes with warfarin metabolism and can increase INR
- use alternative agents if possible
- if not, monitor INR every 2 days until the extent of the interaction is seen and adjust warfarin dosage as needed
- monitor INR every 2 days when interacting drug therapy is discontinued and adjust warfarin dosage as needed to attain desired INR

Drugs that may have their effect decreased by fluoxetine

BUSPIRONE

- fluoxetine is a selective inhibitor of serotonin neuronal reuptake and may block serotoninergic activity of other serotoninergic drugs and, therefore, the pharmacological effect of buspirone may be decreased (J Clin Psychopharmacol 1989;9:150)
- consider avoiding the concurrent use of these agents (only a single case report of the interaction exists in the literature at this time)

▶ What Route and Dosage Should I Use?

How to administer

- orally—can be given with food or on an empty stomach
- parenterally—not available

Major depression, dysthmia, panic disorders, generalized anxiety disorder, chronic pain syndromes, obsessive-compulsive disorders

- 10 mg PO daily for 2 weeks, and if there is some improvement, maintain this dosage; if not, increase to 20 mg PO daily and reevaluate in another 2 weeks
- if there is minimal to no change in symptoms after this time, increase the dosage to 40 mg PO daily
- if there is some response with 40 mg after another 2 weeks but not complete effect, increase the dosage to 60 mg PO daily
- if the desired effect is still not seen after another 2 weeks, consider increasing the dosage to 80 mg PO daily
- maximum adult dosage is 80 mg/d (60 mg/d in geriatric patients), but studies have shown that few patients need greater than 20 mg/d and that side effects increase with 60 mg/d or greater (Psychopharmacol Bull 1987;23:164–168)
- manufacturer recommends that dosages larger than 20 mg be taken in 2 divided doses, in the morning and at noon, but this is not necessary, and even high dosages can be given as a single morning dose
- some patients respond to 5–10 mg/d (Psychopharmacol Bull 1988; 24:183–188) and these lower dosages decrease cost

Dosage adjustments for renal or hepatic dysfunction

- hepatically metabolized
- no dosage adjustment guidelines are available
- in patients with renal or hepatic dysfunction, start with the lowest available dosage and titrate the dose on the basis of efficacy and toxicity

▶ What Should I Monitor with Regard to Efficacy and Toxicity?

Efficacy

see Imipramine
Plasma concentrations
- therapeutic range has not been established

Toxicity

Fluoxetine is generally better tolerated than other antidepressants
Central nervous system effects
- anxiety, nervousness, and insomnia; drowsiness and fatigue; tremor; sweating; dizziness or lightheadedness; headache
- if intolerable, lower the dosage
Gastrointestinal effects
- anorexia, nausea, diarrhea
- approximately 9% of patients experienced anorexia in premarketing trials
- significant weight loss is possible, especially in underweight and depressed individuals; however, fluoxetine therapy has been discontinued only rarely because of weight loss
- if intolerable, lower the dosage
Suicide
- several reports suggest that suicidal preoccupation may be increased by serotoninergic antidepressants, specifically fluoxetine; while receiving much lay press coverage, this reaction has by no means been established and remains highly controversial (at this time there is no reason to avoid the use of fluoxetine in any

known group of individuals on the basis of current information; however, be aware that as with any antidepressant, as patients begin to have more energy, yet may remain suicidal, they may be better able to act on suicidal impulses (Am J Psychiatry 1990;147:207–210, 1380–1381, 1570–1572, 1691–1693, N Engl J Med 1991;324:420, J Clin Psychiatry 1991;52:108–111, Am J Psychiatry 1991;148:543)

▶ How Long Do I Treat Patients with This Drug?

see Imipramine

▶ How Do I Decrease or Stop the Administration of This Drug?

- fluoxetine, because of its extremely long half-life (3–4 days) and its active metabolite's half-life of 7 days, is considered self-tapering and may be abruptly discontinued

▶ What Should I Tell My Patients About This Drug?

see Imipramine
- there is controversy about suicide reports (see above)

▶ Therapeutic Tips

- although fluoxetine is generally thought to be activating and therefore dosed in the morning, significant numbers of patients experience drowsiness and it may be dosed at night with no effect on efficacy (J Clin Psychiatry 1991;52:134–136)
- because fluoxetine is generally activating, it may be a good choice for patients with psychomotor retardation and hypersomnolence
- useful in patients intolerant of anticholinergic effects of the other antidepressants
- for patients prone to overdose, fluoxetine may be safer than tricyclic antidepressants, as there have been no reported deaths with fluoxetine despite large overdoses (60 tablets)

Useful References

USP Dispensing Information. Rockville, MD: United States Pharmacopeial Convention, 1991
Olin BR, ed. Drug Interaction Facts. St Louis: Facts and Comparisons, 1994
Facts and Comparisons. St Louis: Facts and Comparisons, 1994
Young LY, Koda-Kimble MA, eds. Applied Therapeutics. The Clinical Use of Drugs, 5th ed. Vancouver WA: Applied Therapeutics, 1992

FLUPHENAZINE

Juan Avila and Patricia Marken

USA (Prolixin, Permitil, Prolixin decanoate)
CANADA (Moditen, Apo-Fluphenazine, Modecate, Permitil)

▶ When Should I Use This Drug?

Acute psychosis therapy (if prompt control is required)

- in the acutely psychotic and agitated patient, rapid tranquilization with the goal of quietly calming a dangerous patient
- fluphenazine is a high-potency antipsychotic with low anticholinergic activity
- fluphenazine produces a lower incidence of sedation and orthostatic hypotension than the low potency antipsychotics (chlorpromazine) but produces a high incidence of acute, extrapyramidal or dystonic reactions
- drug of choice if patients are elderly or cardiovascular or seizure disorders are present and if it is less expensive than haloperidol
- is available in a parenteral form and a depot preparation
- when a patient has a previous history of response to this agent

Maintenance psychosis therapy

- to ameliorate the symptoms of psychosis that include hallucinations, delusions, formal thought disorder, bizarre behavior, agitation, and/or hyperactivity
- drug of choice if the patient is not compliant, because a depot form is available
- must be dosed every 2–3 weeks in comparison with every 4 weeks for the haloperidol depot form

Manic phase of bipolar illness

- antipsychotics are often also required for adequate sedation and behavioral control and are usually preferred to benzodiazepines for acutely manic patients with concurrent psychoses; however, there is some evidence that high-dose benzodiazepines may be equally efficacious with fewer adverse effects (J Clin Psychopharmacol 1985;5:109–113)
- decision as to when to choose this agent is as above under acute psychosis therapy

▶ *When Should I Not Use This Drug?*

see Chlorpromazine

▶ *What Contraindications Are There to the Use of This Drug?*

see Chlorpromazine

▶ *What Drug Interactions Are Clinically Important?*

Drugs that may increase the effect or toxicity of fluphenazine

CENTRAL NERVOUS SYSTEM DEPRESSANTS (OPIATES, BARBITURATES, GENERAL ANESTHETICS, ALCOHOL)

- excessive sedation and central nervous system (CNS) depression may occur if used concomitantly
- start with low doses of both agents to avoid excessive sedation or CNS depression, and adjust the dosages on the basis of clinical presentation

LITHIUM

- concurrent administration of fluphenazine and lithium has produced hypothalamic extrapyramidal syndromes that have been difficult to distinguish from a neuroleptic malignant syndrome
- observe for any clinical signs of this syndrome or neuroleptic malignant syndrome and stop fluphenazine administration if signs appear

Drugs that may decrease the effect of fluphenazine

- none

Drugs that may have their effect or toxicity increased by fluphenazine

- none

Drugs that may have their effect decreased by fluphenazine

ANTICONVULSANTS (PHENYTOIN, PHENOBARBITAL)

- fluphenazine may lower the seizure threshold and dosage adjustments of anticonvulsants may be necessary when the drugs are used concomitantly, but no adjustments should be made unless seizures develop

▶ *What Route and Dosage Should I Use?*

How to administer

- orally—take with food or milk or on an empty stomach
- parenterally—IM or subcutaneously

Acute psychosis therapy (if prompt control is required), manic phase of bipolar illness

- 5–10 mg PO or 2.5–5 mg IM (if the patient will not take oral medication) every 30–60 minutes until control is achieved or the patient does not tolerate the drug (usually 2–3 doses)
- start a maintenance dosage after an adequate response has been seen (see below)
- some clinicians suggest that after 20 mg IM has been administered, higher dosages may not work but the risk of adverse effects increases
- after a dosage of 20 mg has been reached, consider increasing the benzodiazepine dosage or switching to a different antipsychotic

Maintenance psychosis therapy

- 5 mg PO BID
- 2.5 mg PO BID in smaller or elderly patients

- increase the dosage every 2 weeks until an appropriate response has been seen
- typical maintenance dosage is 15 mg PO daily given as a single daily dose
- maximum daily oral dosage is 60 mg
- to convert to a depot preparation, start with a dose of 12.5 mg IM of fluphenazine decanoate for every 10 mg of daily oral fluphenazine required
- supplement initial IM dose with PRN doses of oral fluphenazine for breakthrough symptoms that may occur between injections
- repeat injection in 2–3 weeks, increasing the IM dose by 12.5 mg, if the patient became symptomatic between injections
- IM doses can be increased up to 100 mg; however, experience is limited with doses greater than 75 mg/2 weeks

Dosage adjustments for renal or hepatic dysfunction

- hepatically metabolized
- no specific dosage adjustments, just start with a low dose and titrate to effect

▶ *What Should I Monitor with Regard to Efficacy and Toxicity?*

see Chlorpromazine

▶ *How Long Do I Treat Patients with This Drug?*

see Chlorpromazine

▶ *How Do I Decrease or Stop the Administration of This Drug?*

see Chlorpromazine

▶ *What Should I Tell My Patients About This Drug?*

see Chlorpromazine

▶ *Therapeutic Tips*

see Chlorpromazine

Useful References

Kane JM. The current status of neuroleptic therapy. J Clin Psychiatry 1989;50:322–328

Black JL, Richelson E, Richardson JW. Antipsychotic agents: A clinical update. Mayo Clinic Proc 1985;60:777–789

Alexander B. Antipsychotics: How strict the formulary? DICP 1988; 22:324–326

FLURBIPROFEN

Kelly Jones

USA (Ansaid)
CANADA (Ansaid, Froben)

▶ *When Should I Use This Drug?*

Acute pain, general aches and pain, bone pain, dysmenorrhea

- useful for the acute management of general aches and pains
- only advantage over non-enteric coated aspirin is that it causes less gastrointestinal intolerance
- decision between this drug and other nonsteroidal antiinflammatory drugs (NSAIDs) should be based on cost

Rheumatoid arthritis

- flurbiprofen can be used as an alternative for patients who fail to respond to enteric coated aspirin or ibuprofen; however, it offers no advantages over enteric coated aspirin or ibuprofen and it is more expensive

Osteoarthritis

- if acetaminophen and enteric coated aspirin or ibuprofen are not effective
- decision between this drug and other NSAIDs should be based on cost

▶ *When Should I Not Use This Drug?*

see Ibuprofen

▶ *What Contraindications Are There to the Use of This Drug?*

see Ibuprofen

▶ *What Drug Interactions Are Clinically Important?*

see Ibuprofen

▶ *What Route and Dosage Should I Use?*

How to administer

- orally—take with food or milk
- parenterally—not available

Acute pain, general aches and pain, bone pain, dysmenorrhea

- 50–100 mg PO Q8–12H PRN

Cancer pain

- 50 mg PO Q12H up to a maximum dosage of 300 mg PO daily

Rheumatoid arthritis

- 100 mg PO Q12H up to a maximum dosage of 300 mg PO daily

Osteoarthritis

- 50 mg PO Q12H

Dosage adjustments for renal or hepatic dysfunction

- hepatically metabolized; therefore, no adjustments needed for renal disease
- reduce dosage 25% in patients with a history of hepatic disease

▶ *What Should I Monitor with Respect to Efficacy and Toxicity?*

see Ibuprofen

▶ *How Long Do I Treat Patients with This Drug?*

see Ibuprofen

▶ *How Do I Decrease or Stop the Administration of This Drug?*

- may be stopped abruptly if needed

▶ *What Should I Tell My Patients About This Drug?*

see Ibuprofen

▶ *Therapeutic Tips*

see Ibuprofen

Useful References

see Ibuprofen

FOLIC ACID
Eric M. Yoshida and Angela Kim-Sing

USA (Folvite)
CANADA (Apo-Folic, Folvite)

▶ *When Should I Use This Drug?*

Prevention of folic acid depletion

- recommended during pregnancy, lactation, questionable nutritional intake (e.g., "skid row" alcoholics), malabsorptive syndromes (e.g., celiac sprue), and increased utilization (e.g., hemolytic anemia, conditions of bone marrow recovery)

Treatment of folic acid deficiency

- macrocytic anemia (exclude other causes of macrocytosis, especially vitamin B_{12} deficiency), pancytopenia due to folic acid deficiency

Primary prevention of neural tube defects

- it is recommended that women who have given birth to offspring with neural tube defects receive folate supplementation even with normal red blood cell folate levels

- it is speculated that the neural tube defects are secondary to a metabolic block in folic acid metabolism

▶ *When Should I Not Use This Drug?*

Anemia not secondary to folic acid deficiency

Macrocytosis associated with folic acid antagonists (e.g., methotrexate, trimethoprim, pyrimethamine)

- folinic acid (calcium leucovorin), not folic acid, should be used in "rescue"

Empiric treatment of macrocytic anemia

- folic acid may mask vitamin B_{12} deficiency; progressive neurologic impairment may result (subacute spinal cord degeneration, dementia)

▶ *What Contraindications Are There to the Use of This Drug?*

- none

▶ *What Drug Interactions Are Clinically Important?*

Drugs that may increase effect/toxicity of folic acid

- none

Drugs that may decrease effect of folic acid

PHENYTOIN

- patients receiving phenytoin should be observed for symptoms of folic acid deficiency and, if necessary, folic acid 1 mg/day may be added as supplemental therapy
- pregnant epileptics on anticonvulsants may be at greater risk for early folate deficiency and therefore these individuals should receive folic acid supplementation, and hemoglobin, and mean cell volume (MCV) should be measured every 1–2 months and the dose of folic acid should be adjusted on the basis of these lab results

PYRIMETHAMINE, SULFASALAZINE, TRIMETHOPRIM

- monitor hemoglobin, WBC, and platelets in patients receiving these drugs for longer than 14 days, especially when these drugs are used in high doses
- these lab values should be measured every 1–2 months and the use and dose of folic acid should be based on the basis of these lab results

METHOTREXATE

- folic acid deficiency is associated with high doses, underlying renal disease, and infection
- get baseline CBC and platelets after 14 days of treatment, then every 4 weeks once dose is stable
- discontinue methotrexate if neutrophil count decreases less than $2,000/mm^3$ or platelets decrease less than $150,000/mm^3$

ALCOHOL, ORAL CONTRACEPTIVES

- while these agents may produce folic acid deficiency, routine monitoring is likely not required
- patients receiving these agents should be observed for symptoms of folic acid deficiency and, if necessary, folic acid 1 mg/day may be added as supplemental therapy

Drugs that may have effect/toxicity increased by folic acid

- none

Drugs that may have effect decreased by folic acid

PHENYTOIN

- folate can increase the metabolism of phenytoin
- at the RDA the interaction is not clinically significant; however, supplementation in excess of the RDA may result in lower serum phenytoin concentrations and loss of seizure control
- measure a baseline and initially measure monthly phenytoin concentrations until the extent of the interaction is seen and adjust the dose based on serum concentrations

▶ What Route and Dosage Should I Use?

How to administer

- orally—take with food or milk or on an empty stomach
- commercially available as 5 mg tablet; dose will vary in multivitamin preparations
- parenterally—may be given IM, SQ, or IV as a bolus or infusion in D_5W or NS

Prevention of folic acid depletion

- RDA for men is 200 μg/day
- RDA for women is 180 μg/day
- RDA 400 μg PO daily during pregnancy; decreased to 280 μg (first 6 months) and 260 μg PO daily (for second 6 months) while breastfeeding

Treatment of folic acid deficiency

- treatment dose will vary between 500 and 1000 μg daily
- folic acid is found in many multivitamin preparations
- as a single entity product most dosage forms in the USA contain 5 mg and in Canada they contain 1 mg
- doses of 1–5 mg PO daily will provide enough folic acid even in patients with intestinal malabsorption
- in patients with ongoing folic acid losses (e.g., sprue, chronic hemodialysis, chronic hemolytic anemia, etc.), maintenance dose ranging from 200–500 μg/day is given indefinitely

Prevention of neural tube defects in pregnancy

- a minimum dose of 0.8 mg PO daily should be used to decrease the incidence of neural tube defects
- women who have had a previous baby with neural tube defects should use 4 or 5 mg PO daily

▶ What Should I Monitor for with Regard to Efficacy and Toxicity?

Efficacy

Prevention of folic acid depletion

- in patients at risk of folic acid deficiency (i.e., pregnancy), initially measure hemoglobin and MCV every 1–2 months and adjust dose based on response
- if MCV increased (> 100 fL) measure red cell folate, which is a more reliable indicator of recent folate deficiency

Treatment of folic acid deficiency

- measure hemoglobin and reticulocytes weekly until improvement seen
- reticulocytosis generally begins within 2–5 days following initiation of folic acid therapy
- hemoglobin should increase by 10 g/L per week until within normal range
- if no improvement in reticulocytosis within the first week, evaluate compliance and confirm diagnosis of folate deficiency

Signs and symptoms of deficiency

- nonspecific symptoms of anemia (gastrointestinal symptoms, stomatitis, glossitis, weight loss, etc.) or complications of pancytopenia

Toxicity

- no toxicities occur since this is a water-soluble vitamin and excess is excreted in the urine

▶ How Long Do I Treat Patients with This Drug?

Prevention of folic acid depletion

- for duration of underlying disorder or condition

Treatment of folic acid deficiency

- continue until hemoglobin is normalized

Primary prevention of neural tube defects

- administer during the periconceptual period and for duration of pregnancy
- folic acid should be continued while breastfeeding; however, lower doses can be used (see above under prevention)

▶ How Do I Decrease or Stop This Drug?

- may discontinue abruptly

▶ What Should I Tell My Patients About This Drug?

- dietary folate present in green leafy vegetables and fruits

▶ Therapeutic Tips

- red blood cell folate levels should be measured during investigation of macrocytosis as serum folate levels reflect acute nutritional intake

Useful References

Kones R. Folic acid, 1991. An update, with new recommended daily allowances. South Med J 1990;83:1454–1458

MacCosbe PE, Toomey K. Interaction of phenytoin and folic acid. Clin Pharm 1983;2:362–369

Colon-Otero G, Menke D, Hook CC. A practical approach to the differential diagnosis and evaluation of the adult patient with macrocytic anemia. Med Clin North Am 1992;76:581–597

Van Allen MI, Fraser FC, Dallaire L, et al. Recommendations on the use of folic acid supplementation to prevent the recurrence of neural tube defects. Clinical Teratology Committee, Canadian College of Medical Geneticists. Can Med Assoc J 1993;149:1239–1243

FOSINOPRIL

Jack Onrot and James McCormack

USA (Monopril)
CANADA (Monopril)

▶ When Should I Use This Drug?

see Enalapril

▶ When Should I Not Use This Drug?

see Enalapril

▶ What Contraindications Are There to the Use of This Drug?

see Captopril

▶ What Drug Interactions Are Clinically Important?

see Captopril

▶ What Route and Dosage Should I Use?

How to administer

- orally—should be administered on an empty stomach
- parenterally—not available

Congestive heart failure

- 5 mg PO daily
- rapidity of dosage escalation depends on the severity of symptoms
- dosage may be increased daily if necessary
- no value in exceeding a total daily dose of 40 mg

Chronic (noncrisis) hypertension

- 5 mg PO daily
- increase the dosage by 5 mg PO daily every 4 weeks until adequate blood pressure is achieved or a daily dosage of 20 mg is reached
- limited value in exceeding a total daily dose of 20 mg (dosages as high as 40 mg PO daily have been used)
- for some patients, the antihypertensive effect may be diminished before 24 hours and twice-daily dosing may be required

Dosage adjustments for renal or hepatic dysfunction

- renal and biliary elimination
- titrate the dose to clinical response and not concurrent renal or hepatic function

▶ What Should I Monitor with Regard to Efficacy and Toxicity?

see Captopril

▶ How Long Do I Treat Patients with This Drug?

see Captopril

▶ *How Do I Decrease or Stop the Administration of This Drug?*

see Captopril

▶ *What Should I Tell My Patients About This Drug?*

see Captopril

▶ *Therapeutic Tips*

see Captopril

FUROSEMIDE

Ian Petterson

USA (Lasix, Furomide)
CANADA (Lasix, Apo-Furosemide, Novo-semide)

▶ *When Should I Use This Drug?*

Congestive heart failure

Acute pulmonary edema

- furosemide mobilizes interstitial lung fluid and promotes rapid diuresis
- avoid aggressive diuresis if the patient is intravascularly depleted (e.g., low jugular venous pressure [JVP]), as this may lead to further hypovolemia, which may reduce the cardiac output and blood pressure

Mild to moderate heart failure

- oral furosemide should be the initial drug therapy selected, based on consistent beneficial effects and synergistic effects seen with subsequent additional therapy
- furosemide should be chosen instead of thiazide diuretics because it is more effective, has a faster onset, provides more diuresis, and causes fewer metabolic changes than do thiazides when used in equivalent natriuretic dosages
- angiotensin converting enzyme (ACE) inhibitors, in the absence of furosemide, may be ineffective (Lancet 1987;2:709–711)

Ascites associated with hepatic cirrhosis

- considered secondary therapy if spironolactone has failed to control edema (Gastroenterology 1983;84:961–968)
- too rapid or marked diuresis in a patient with ascites can cause serious acid-base, fluid, and electrolyte imbalances and can precipitate hepatic encephalopathy

Acute renal failure

- perception is that converting nonoliguric to oliguric renal failure allows easier patient management, but there is no evidence that furosemide or other diuretics alter the associated high morbidity and mortality
- probably useful in prophylaxis against acute tubular necrosis induced by surgery in jaundiced patients, rapid intravascular hemolysis, rhabdomyolysis, radiocontrast dyes, cisplatin, and acute hyperuricemia

Hypercalcemia

- used in cases of severe hypercalcemia (>13 mg/dL or >3.3 mmol/L)
- most patients with severe hypercalcemia also have a depletion of extracellular fluid
- high-rate saline infusions should be the initial therapy, and furosemide should be reserved for those patients whose fluid balance becomes positive
- for those patients unable to tolerate the fluid or for those without an extracellular depletion, furosemide should be given initially and saline infusions used to prevent hypovolemia
- major hypocalcemic effect is seen early and therapy for longer than 1–2 days causes little further decrease in calcium levels

▶ *When Should I Not Use This Drug?*

Chronic (noncrisis) hypertension

- use only in patients with renal failure and/or concomitant volume overload
- for furosemide to be effective as an antihypertensive agent, it must be given 3–4 times daily, which makes furosemide undesirable compared with other diuretics
- there is evidence that furosemide is inferior to thiazides or other agents in the management of uncomplicated mild to moderate hypertension
- in patients unresponsive to thiazide therapy, furosemide alone does not produce an adequate response

▶ *What Contraindications Are There to the Use of This Drug?*

Intolerance of or allergic reaction to furosemide

Systemic lupus erythematosus

- may activate or exacerbate this condition; therefore, use the drug only if other alternatives are not possible

Patients who are intravascularly volume depleted

- may potentially cause severe hypovolemia if overdiuresis occurs
- furosemide should be withheld if JVP is low and/or the urea creatinine level is rising

▶ *What Drug Interactions Are Clinically Important?*

Drugs that may increase the effect or toxicity of furosemide

AMINOGLYCOSIDES (GENTAMICIN, TOBRAMYCIN, AMIKACIN)

- increased irreversible hearing loss associated with concomitant use
- more likely with large doses, intravenous administration, and renal failure
- avoid combination, and be aware of the increased risk, but no extra monitoring is required

OTHER DIURETICS

- other diuretics, especially metolazone and hydrochlorothiazide, may increase the risk of hypokalemia, hypomagnesemia, hypotension, and prerenal failure
- avoid combination if possible; if not, ensure the lowest effective dose of each agent is used

DIGOXIN

- furosemide's hypokalemic and hypomagnesemic effects may predispose the patient to arryhthmias
- supplement magnesium as necessary, and maintain potassium serum levels at greater than 4 mEq/L

ANGIOTENSIN CONVERTING ENZYME INHIBITORS

- overdiuresis can exaggerate the rise in urea and creatinine levels and cause reversible renal insufficiency
- if this occurs, withhold diuretics and ACE inhibitors and monitor the patient's volume status and renal function
- start with low dosage of ACE inhibitors whenever adding to the regimen of patients already receiving furosemide

Drugs that may decrease the effect of furosemide

NONSTEROIDAL ANTIINFLAMMATORY DRUGS

- nonsteroidal antiinflammatory drugs may oppose diuresis and natriuresis and concomitant use may blunt the furosemide response and higher doses of furosemide may be required
- especially in the context of overdiuresis and hypovolemia, these agents, by interfering with renal prostaglandins, can exaggerate the rise in urea and creatinine levels
- avoid combination if at all possible
- in patients who must use NSAIDs, ensure the lowest effective dose is being used

Drugs that may have their effect or toxicity increased by furosemide

- none

Drugs that may have their effect decreased by furosemide

- none

▶ *What Route and Dosage Should I Use?*

How to administer

Orally

- can be given with food or on an empty stomach

Parenterally

- when administering IV doses, toxicity is rate related, and therefore, maximum rates are 20 mg/min if the dose is less than 100 mg or 4 mg/min if the dose is greater than 100 mg (mix in 50–100 mL IV fluid)
- when converting from PO to IV or IM administration, reduce the dosage by 50%

Congestive heart failure

Acute pulmonary edema

- 20 mg IV if the patient is furosemide naive, and if there is no response in 30 minutes, double the dose (40 mg IV), and if there is still no response after another 30 minutes, give 80 mg IV
- for patients already receiving furosemide, begin with an IV dose equal to the previous PO maintenance dose and then double every 30 minutes until a response is seen
- after symptoms begin to resolve and edema begins to clear, therapy can be switched to oral by doubling the effective daily IV dosage and giving it once daily
- although furosemide exhibits an almost limitless dose-response curve, single doses greater than 160 mg IV (320 mg PO) are rarely required in patients without renal impairment
- if a greater response is desired, give the dose more frequently during the day (e.g., 360 mg PO once daily is not equivalent in terms of response to 120 mg PO TID)

Mild to moderate heart failure

- 20 mg PO daily
- double the dosage every 3–4 days until the desired effect is seen
- too low a dosage is characterized by worsening symptoms, high JVP, edema, crackles, S_3 heart sound, and weight gain
- too high a dosage is indicated by a low JVP, rising urea or creatinine levels, weight loss, and orthostatic hypotension
- divide the dose if the patient has paroxysmal nocturnal dyspnea (give the dose before dinner, not at bedtime)

Ascites associated with hepatic cirrhosis

- if initial spironolactone therapy is ineffective (or creatinine clearance < 30 mL/min), start with 40 mg PO daily and titrate every 2 days for response (use in addition to the spironolactone)
- if a more rapid diuresis is desired, the IV route may be preferable because of delayed absorption (Clin Pharm Ther 1991;49: 241–247)

Acute renal failure

- usually large dosages are required regardless of renal function
- start with 40 mg IV and increase at 6 hour intervals until response or 120 mg is reached
- edema associated with decreased renal function may cause an erratic and delayed absorption of the drug; therefore, for acute renal failure, parenteral dosing should always be used (Kidney Int 1984;26:183–189)
- increase the dosage until urine output is maintained at 40 mL/h (realize that this goal may not be possible if patients have preexisting renal impairment [e.g., acute renal failure superimposed on chronic failure])
- as usual concentrations of drug reach the nephrons, doses greater than 120 mg IV do not give added diuresis
- in severely refractory patients or in patients with preexisting renal impairment, the addition of a low-dose thiazide (metolazone 2.5 mg) 1 hour before the furosemide administration may improve the diuretic response (Curr Ther Res 1977;22:686–691)

Hypercalcemia

- after rehydration is accomplished (normal saline at 200–300 mL/ h), 40 mg IV every 2–4 hours to maintain a urine output of 250–300 mL/h is effective in reducing the serum calcium level
- monitor serum potassium and magnesium levels and replace as necessary

- continue for a maximum of 48 hours, because after that furosemide does not exhibit any additive hypocalcemic effect

Dosage adjustments for renal or hepatic dysfunction

- renally eliminated
- no dosage adjustments are required
- titrate to effect and realize that higher than normal dosages may be required in patients with poor renal function

▶ *What Should I Monitor with Regard to Efficacy and Toxicity?*

Efficacy

Acute pulmonary edema

Pulmonary signs and symptoms

- for a parenteral furosemide dose, the onset of diuresis is 15–30 minutes (peak effect, approximately 1 hour) and the duration of effect is 3–4 hours, but resolution of pulmonary edema occurs within 15 minutes
- for an oral dose, the onset of diuresis is 30–60 minutes (peak, 1–2 hours) and the duration of effect is 4–6 hours
- patient should initially be assessed after each dose of furosemide
- do arterial blood gas determinations initially if the patient is distressed and repeat hourly until patient is stable
- look for relief of dyspnea, orthopnea, paroxysmal nocturnal dyspnea, and distribution of crackles
- after the patient is stable, monitor the patient daily while receiving intravenous furosemide

Other signs and symptoms

- assess JVP, the presence of peripheral edema, and liver size after each dose of furosemide
- JVP should be normal to slightly increased (be aware that right-sided filling pressures do not always accurately reflect left-sided pressure)
- after some of the acute symptoms have decreased, assess the patient at least twice daily
- initially assess weight daily

Urea, creatinine, and sodium levels

- may improve if cardiac output is improved, and in patients who are hyponatremic, the serum sodium level may normalize
- in overdiuresis, levels of urea increase out of proportion to creatinine increase
- monitor daily in patients with acute disease undergoing rapid diuresis
- in patients with severe chronic congestive heart failure, accept modest urea and creatinine level increases above baseline values if this is needed to maintain optimum symptom control

Mild to moderate heart failure

Signs and symptoms

- dyspnea, orthopnea, paroxysmal nocturnal dyspnea, fatigue, ankle swelling, fine crackles on chest auscultation, weight, liver size, and absence of S_3 heart sound
- JVP should be normal to slightly increased
- for patients with acute symptoms assess patients at least twice daily while they are in the hospital
- after the patient is discharged, assess within a week of discharge
- after the patient is stabilized, decrease the frequency of evaluation
- for patients with mild symptoms, assess weekly until symptoms are controlled

Ascites associated with hepatic cirrhosis

- treatment needs to proceed slowly to prevent acid-base, fluid, and electrolyte imbalances, which can precipitate hepatic encephalopathy
- three primary goals of therapy are weight loss of 0.3–1 kg/d, urine output of 300–1000 mL/d over daily input, and patient comfort

Acute renal failure

- increase the dosage until urine output is maintained at 40 mL/h

Hypercalcemia

- hydration and furosemide decrease serum calcium levels by 2–3 mg/dL (0.5–0.7 mmol/L) in 24–48 hours
- serum calcium levels (ionized calcium if possible) should be monitored twice daily for the first 48 hours, then daily thereafter until the calcium level is normalized

Toxicity

Ototoxicity (manifested by tinnitus or deafness)

- less ototoxic than ethacrynic acid
- incidence of 3–6%
- occurrence associated with large doses (e.g., > 200 mg IV [400 mg PO]) or rapid intravenous rates, renal failure, or concomitant administration of ototoxic drugs
- generally reversible

Hypokalemia

- causes less hypokalemia than do thiazides (e.g., 40 mg PO daily of furosemide produces less hypokalemia than 50 mg PO daily of hydrochlorothiazide) (Arch Intern Med 1983;143:1694–1699) because of furosemide's relatively short duration of action (4–6 hours) compared with that seen with hydrochlorothiazide (18–24 hours)
- monitor the potassium levels at 2 weeks and at the end of 1 month (measure twice weekly if using high and frequent doses [e.g., more than once per day] of furosemide)
- after the patient is stable, repeat measurement only if the dosage or the disease state changes occur
- if serum potassium levels decrease to less than 3.5 mEq/L (or < 4 mEq/L while the patient is receiving digoxin), supplement by increasing dietary potassium and restricting sodium intake

Renal function

- increased serum urea and creatinine levels may occasionally be seen but are likely not indicative of nephrotoxity but due to hypovolemia and decreased glomerular filtration rate, possibly indicating excess diuresis
- monitor baseline urea and creatinine levels every 3–4 months thereafter for patients with initially diminished function

Rash

- furosemide can cause photosensitivity
- tell patients that the sun may burn them more easily and they should see how they react
- if patients are more sensitive, a sunscreen should be used

Hyponatremia

- especially if heart failure is due to saluresis and failure to clear free water because of excess antidiuretic hormone release

Hypomagnesemia

- parallels potassium loss
- as serum magnesium levels do not correlate with cellular levels, all patients requiring large intravenous doses for acute congestive heart failure should receive magnesium supplements

▶ *How Long Do I Treat Patients with This Drug?*

Congestive heart failure

Acute pulmonary edema, mild to moderate heart failure

- seek the lowest dose of furosemide compatible with maximum symptom relief
- usually need less diuretic when stable and free from acute precipitants that may have brought the patient to medical attention
- trial of a decreased dosage is warranted after the patient has been stabilized for 2–3 months; however, one can rarely withdraw diuretics completely

Ascites associated with hepatic cirrhosis

- treat until the cause of exacerbation of ascites is gone
- treatment may be lifelong if ascites is due to alcoholic cirrhosis; however, always reevaluate for the lowest effective dosage

Acute renal failure

- treat as long as required to maintain urine output or treat until such time that the failure is no longer reversible

Hypercalcemia

- continue for a maximum of 48 hours, because after that furosemide does not exhibit any additive hypocalcemic effect

▶ *How Do I Decrease or Stop the Administration of This Drug?*

- tapering of the drug is not necessary

▶ *What Should I Tell My Patients About This Drug?*

- this drug works on your kidney to help it eliminate excess salt and water from your body
- limiting your salt ingestion helps this drug to work
- if you notice your feet or any other part of your body becoming puffy, this may indicate that the current dosage of furosemide is no longer effective or your salt intake is excessive and you should contact your physician
- once-daily doses should be taken in the morning
- if you take furosemide twice daily, make sure that you take the second dose in the afternoon to avoid having to go the bathroom in the middle of the night
- if you begin to feel weak, dizzy, or lightheaded, you should contact your physician as this may indicate an electrolye abnormality or low blood pressure
- report any unusual ringing in your ears or unsteadiness on your feet
- diuresis may be abrupt and voluminous; therefore, initially have close access to a bathroom until the effect of the drug has been seen
- increase potassium and magnesium intake through dietary means

▶ *Therapeutic Tips*

- not a useful agent for uncomplicated mild to moderate hypertension
- if patients receiving furosemide become unresponsive to therapy, the addition of a low-dose thiazide often restores effectiveness
- effective diuretic even in patients with poor renal function
- avoiding rapid administration of large intravenous doses, especially if using concomitant aminoglycosides, may reduce the incidence of ototoxicity
- always titrate the dose to effect
- increase the dosage as renal function decreases
- monitor JVP as a bioassay
- administer other diuretics concurrently in low doses because they may magnify the potential for side effects (Ann Intern Med 1991;114:886–894)
- when treating any edematous state that requires rapid diuresis, intravenous dosing is preferable to oral doses because of delayed and erratic absorption associated with these disease states
- patients must maintain a sodium-restricted diet, as a high-sodium diet overcomes the diuretic effect and worsens hypokalemia
- additive diuresis is achieved by the administration of metolazone 1 hour before the furosemide
- furosemide does not adversely affect lithium levels as seen with thiazides or potassium-sparing diuretics

Useful References

Ellison DH. The physiologic basis of diuretic synergism: Its role in treating diuretic resistance. Ann Intern Med 1991;114:886–894

Brater DC. Use of diuretics in chronic renal insufficiency and nephrotic syndrome. Semin Nephrol 1988;8:333–341

Nader PC, Thompson JR, Alpern RJ. Complications of diuretic use. Semin Nephrol 1988;8:365–387

GANCICLOVIR

Ann Beardsell

USA (Cytovene)
CANADA (Cytovene)

▶ *When Should I Use This Drug?*

Cytomegalovirus infection

Chorioretinitis

- drug of choice in the treatment of cytomegalovirus (CMV) retinitis in immunocompromised patients

- unless there is no useful vision in the involved eye, chorioretinitis should be treated promptly after the detection of characteristic retinal lesions

Gastrointestinal disease or disease at other sites

- drug of choice for the treatment of symptomatic CMV disease in the gut, lungs, esophagus, and nervous system (polyradiculopathy)

▶ *When Should I Not Use This Drug?*

Infections in immunocompetent patients

- is not recommended for use in immunocompetent patients because of the high risk of toxicity

▶ *What Contraindications Are There to the Use of This Drug?*

Intolerance of or allergic reaction to ganciclovir

Neutropenia

- is not recommended if the patient is neutropenic (neutrophil count < 500/mm^3) or thrombocytopenic (platelet count < 25,000/mm^3), as ganciclovir may further potentiate these conditions

▶ *What Drug Interactions Are Clinically Important?*

Drugs that may increase the effect or toxicity of ganciclovir

ZIDOVUDINE

- both ganciclovir and zidovudine alone may cause myelosuppression and concomitant use may result in additive or synergistic effects on the bone marrow
- stop zidovudine administration during ganciclovir induction
- if both are used together, monitor leukocyte and erythrocyte counts every 2 days initially and then weekly
- discontinue zidovudine therapy if neutrophil counts decline by greater than 50% from baseline levels or are less than 500/mm^3

AZATHIOPRINE, CYCLOSPORINE, CORTICOSTEROIDS

- concomitant use of these agents with ganciclovir may result in excessive suppression of the bone marrow or immune system
- monitor complete blood count (CBC), and if excessive suppression of the immune system occurs, decrease the dosage or discontinue the administration of these agents temporarily until ganciclovir treatment is completed
- foscarnet could be used as an alternative to ganciclovir

DAPSONE, PENTAMIDINE, PYRIMETHAMINE, FLUCYTOSINE, TRIMETHOPRIM-SULFAMETHOXAZOLE, VINCRISTINE, VINBLASTINE, DOXORUBICIN, AMPHOTERICIN B

- these drugs inhibit the replication of rapidly dividing cells, and concomitant use with ganciclovir may produce additive effects
- if used concomitantly, monitor CBC weekly

IMIPENEM-CILASTATIN

- concomitant use with ganciclovir has resulted in seizures in several reports
- alternatives to imipenem-cilastatin should be used with ganciclovir if possible; otherwise, ensure that the lowest effective dosages of both agents are being used and have been adjusted for hepatic or renal dysfunction

Drugs that may decrease the effect of ganciclovir

- none

Drugs that may have their effect increased by ganciclovir

- none

Drugs that may have their effect decreased by ganciclovir

- none

▶ *What Route and Dosage Should I Use?*

How to administer

- orally—not available

- parenterally—administer over 1 hour diluted in 5% dextrose in water to a maximum concentration of 10 mg/mL

Cytomegalovirus infection

Chorioretinitis

- 5 mg/kg IV Q12H for 14 days (21 days if patient responds slowly) followed by a maintenance dosage of 5 mg/kg IV daily, or 6 mg/kg IV daily 5 d/wk

Gastrointestinal disease

- 5 mg/kg IV Q12H for 14 days (21 days if patient responds slowly)
- role of maintenance therapy is unclear in gastrointestinal disease; some clinicians reserve maintenance therapy for patients having frequent recurrences

Dosage adjustments for renal or hepatic dysfunction

- renally eliminated

Normal Dosing Interval	C$_{cr}$ > 60 mL/min or 1 mL/s	C$_{cr}$ 30–60 mL/min or 0.5–1 mL/s	C$_{cr}$ < 30 mL/min or 0.5 mL/s
Q12H	no adjustment needed	Q24H	Q24H and decrease dosage by 50%

▶ *What Should I Monitor with Regard to Efficacy and Toxicity?*

Efficacy

Chorioretinitis

- ophthalmological assessment for evidence of progression
- these patients should be assessed every 1–2 weeks until retinitis is inactive, then monthly, by an experienced ophthalmologist

Gastrointestinal disease

- relief of diarrhea, abdominal discomfort, and fever
- assess clinical changes in symptoms daily initially and then 2–3 times a week

Toxicity

- adverse reactions to ganciclovir are common and can be severe
- drug toxicity is complicated by the complex disease states in which CMV infections become symptomatic enough to necessitate treatment (acquired immunodeficiency syndrome [AIDS], organ and bone marrow transplants)

Hematological effects

- neutropenia and thrombocytopenia are the 2 most common hematological problems and appear to be a dose-related direct effect on the bone marrow
- neutropenia is more common in patients with AIDS than in other immunocompromised patients and usually occurs within the first 2 weeks of induction therapy but can occur at any time and, in 1 study, resulted in discontinuation of the drug in 20% of patients
- thrombocytopenia is more common in patients with other causes of immunosuppression than human immunodeficiency virus (HIV) infection or AIDS but may occur in 20% of patients
- monitor CBC and differential leukocyte count every 3–4 days during induction and reduce the dosage if the neutrophil count decreases to less than 1000/mm^3 or 50% of baseline values and/or the platelet count decreases below 50,000/mm^3
- if neutrophils are less than 500/mm^3 and/or platelets are less than 25,000/mm^3, discontinue ganciclovir administration until counts improve (usually within 3–7 days), then restart at a reduced dosage (50%)
- in cases in which neutrophil counts remain low and continued ganciclovir treatment is necessary, the addition of granulocyte-macrophage colony-stimulating factor may maintain higher neutrophil counts during ganciclovir administration
- other less frequent effects are anemia and eosinophilia (<2%)

Ocular effects

- retinal detachment has developed in ganciclovir-treated CMV retinitis that has responded to treatment (more common in AIDS patients)

Neurological effects

- confusion, headaches, and behavioral changes (ranging from mood swings to psychosis) have been reported
- for mild cases, treat symptomatically, but for more severe symptoms (e.g., psychosis and hallucinations), reduction or discontinuation of the drug may be required

Gastrointestinal effects

- nausea and vomiting are the most common gastrointestinal effects (2%)
- treat symptomatically

Hepatic effects

- elevated liver enzyme levels may occur with ganciclovir
- monitor alanine aminotransferase, aspartate aminotransferase, alkaline phosphatase, and gamma-glutamyltransferase and reduce or discontinue the drug administration if marked elevations occur (>5 times normal values)

Other reactions

- fever and rash have occurred in 2% of patients
- treat symptomatically and reduce or discontinue the drug administration if fever and rash persist or are severe

▶ *How Long Do I Treat Patients with This Drug?*

Chorioretinitis

- administer ganciclovir as long as the patient retains sight and tolerates the drug
- in cases in which the eyesight continues to deteriorate, consider using an alternative investigational drug, foscarnet, or repeating the induction dosage

Gastrointestinal disease

- some authorities (Ann Intern Med 1992;116:63–77) recommend maintenance therapy; however, some clinicians reserve maintenance therapy for patients with frequent recurrences
- treat as long as the drug is tolerable

▶ *How Do I Decrease or Stop the Administration of This Drug?*

- may be stopped abruptly

▶ *What Should I Tell My Patients About This Drug?*

- this drug is administered intravenously, usually in a hospital daycare setting, 5 or 7 d/wk
- this drug has the potential to decrease the production of some components of blood; it is important to have your blood drawn for laboratory studies as instructed by your physician on a regular basis
- any fevers, chills, or infections should be reported to your physician immediately
- any unusual or prolonged bleeding should be reported to your physician immediately
- if you are being treated for CMV retinitis, it is important to have regular eye examinations
- report any eye pain to your physician immediately

▶ *Therapeutic Tips*

- monitor CBC and differential leukocyte count weekly and initiate dosage changes early to prevent infection resulting from neutropenia
- ensure that the patient has frequent eye examinations to monitor for retinal progression of CMV or retinal detachment

GEMFIBROZIL

Stephen Shalansky and Robert Dombrowski

USA (Lopid)
CANADA (Lopid)

▶ *When Should I Use This Drug?*

Hypercholesterolemia

- fibric acid derivatives generally decrease low density lipoprotein (LDL) cholesterol less than bile acid sequestrants, niacin, or HMG-CoA reductase inhibitors do and, in some cases, may increase LDL cholesterol
- should be considered only if all other agents have failed
- this is true even after the results of the Helsinki Trial were published showing gemfibrozil to be safe and effective in treating hyperlipidemias (N Engl J Med 1987;317:1237–1245)
- there was an apparent inconsistency in gemfibrozil's effects, which may be related to triglyceride levels
- Helsinki Trial results showed that gemfibrozil can actually increase LDL cholesterol in patients with very elevated triglyceride levels (>500 mg/dL, or >5.6 mmol/L), while decreasing LDL in patients with normal or moderately elevated triglyceride levels
- unless there is significant cost advantage, gemfibrozil should be used instead of fenofibrate, as there are no long-term studies evaluating fenofibrate's effect on cardiovascular morbidity and mortality

Hypertriglyceridemia

- consider drug therapy only in patients with symptomatic (pancreatitis, xanthomas) hypertriglyceridemia, as there is no evidence yet to support the treatment of or screening of patients with asymptomatic elevated triglyceride levels (Br Med J 1992; 304:394–396)
- unless there is significant cost advantage, gemfibrozil should be used instead of fenofibrate, as there are no long-term studies evaluating fenofibrate's effect on cardiovascular morbidity and mortality

Mixed hyperlipidemia

- should be used after niacin and HMG-CoA reductase inhibitors have failed
- gemfibrozil has mainly a triglyceride-lowering effect with a variable effect on LDL cholesterol and mild HDL-elevating effects

▶ *When Should I Not Use This Drug?*

First-line agent for hypercholesterolemia

- gemfibrozil has its main effect on triglycerides and therefore is not useful in patients whose primary lipid disorder is hypercholesterolemia

▶ *What Contraindications Are There to the Use of This Drug?*

Intolerance of or allergic reaction to gemfibrozil

Preexisting gallbladder disease and primary biliary cirrhosis

- alters the lithogenic index of bile, which may predispose these patients to the formation of gallstones

Severe hepatic failure

- rarely gemfibrozil can induce hepatic toxicity

▶ *What Drug Interactions Are Clinically Important?*

Drugs that may increase the effect or toxicity of gemfibrozil

LOVASTATIN

- incidence of myopathy is increased to about 5% (N Engl J Med 1988;318:48)
- can be used together but be aware of the increased risk and monitor creatine kinase levels if the patient reports muscle aches and pains

Drugs that may decrease the effect of gemfibrozil

BILE ACID SEQUESTRANTS (CHOLESTYRAMINE AND COLESTIPOL)

- decrease gemfibrozil absorption by up to 50%; therefore, give 1 hour before or 4 hours after cholestyramine or colestipol

Drugs that may have their effect or toxicity increased by gemfibrozil

WARFARIN

- gemfibrozil may enhance the effects of anticoagulants
- monitor INR every 2 days until the full extent of interaction is seen and adjust the dosage as for a warfarin dosage change
- monitor INR every 2 days when administration of the interacting drug is discontinued and adjust as for a warfarin dosage change

Drugs that may have their effect decreased by gemfibrozil

- none

▶ What Route and Dosage Should I Use?

How to administer

- orally—give 30 minutes before meals
- parenterally—not available

Hypercholesterolemia, hypertriglyceridemia, mixed hyperlipidemias

- 600 mg PO BID
- if at 3 months the drug is tolerated and there has been at least a 15% decrease in lipid levels but not to the desired level, continue gemfibrozil and add a second agent
- if adding another drug, monitor as if initiating therapy
- if the drug is not tolerated or there is less than a 15% decrease in total cholesterol levels, after 3 months of therapy stop gemfibrozil administration and start therapy with a different drug

Dosage adjustments for renal or hepatic dysfunction

- hepatically metabolized
- no dosage adjustment necessary in renal failure (J Clin Pharmacol 1987;27:994–1000)
- do not use in severe hepatic failure, because although rare, gemfibrozil can induce hepatic toxicity

▶ What Should I Monitor with Regard to Efficacy and Toxicity?

Efficacy

Hypercholesterolemia, hypertriglyceridemia, mixed hyperlipidemias

Total cholesterol and fractionated lipid profile

- initially, measure baseline lipid levels (cholesterol, fractionated lipid profile) when deciding on initiating drug therapy for hyperlipidemias
- in patients with no coronary heart disease or atherosclerotic disease and with less than 2 CHD risk factors lower total cholesterol below 240 mg/dL (6.2 mmol/L) and LDL cholesterol below 160 mg/dL (4.1 mmol/L)
- in patients with no coronary heart disease or atherosclerotic disease and with 2 or more CHD risk factors lower total cholesterol below 200 mg/dL (5.2 mmol/L) and LDL cholesterol below 130 mg/dL (3.4 mmol/L)
- for patients with coronary heart disease or atherosclerotic disease lower LDL cholesterol to below 100 mg/dL (2.6 mmol/L)
- complete lipid profiles should be measured at 1 and 3 months

Evidence of coronary heart disease

- myocardial infarction, angina, and coronary bypass grafting

Risk factors

- reduce risk factors such as obesity and smoking
- control risk factors such as diabetes and hypertension

Toxicity

Generally well tolerated

- no patients in clinical trials have required hospitalization for side effects (Drugs 1988;36:314–339)

Gastrointestinal symptoms

- gastrointestinal symptoms (abdominal pain, diarrhea, nausea, vomiting, epigastric pain, and flatulence)
- 2–11% incidence, depending on the study
- patient may develop tolerance to these side effects within the first year of therapy

Rash

- approximately a 2% incidence

Hepatic toxicity

- hepatic toxicity has occurred in animals administered very high dosages of gemfibrozil
- increases in hepatic enzyme levels are rarely seen in humans

- liver function tests should be performed before starting gemfibrozil administration (baseline), after 6 months of therapy, and every year thereafter
- if substantially elevated (aminotransferase levels > 3 times normal values), gemfibrozil administration should be discontinued

Gallstones

- clofibrate, another fibric acid derivative, has been linked to gallstone formation (JAMA 1975;231:360–381)
- gemfibrozil does not appear to increase the incidence of gallstones (N Engl J Med 1987;317:1237–1245, Drugs 1988;36:314–339)

▶ How Long Do I Treat Patients with This Drug?

Hypercholesterolemia, hypertriglyceridemia, mixed hyperlipidemias

- therapy is long term and may continue for life
- if the patient has achieved and maintained target lipid levels for 2 years, gemfibrozil administration should be discontinued and a retrial on dietary therapy alone should be tried
- recheck lipid levels at 4–6 weeks and at 3 months after the drug administration has been discontinued, and restart drug therapy if target levels are not maintained

▶ How Do I Decrease or Stop the Administration of This Drug?

- may be stopped abruptly

▶ What Should I Tell My Patients About This Drug?

- take this medication 30 minutes before meals (usually before breakfast and dinner)
- you may experience some gastrointestinal side effects (nausea, constipation, diarrhea, and abdominal pain) or a rash, and most patients develop tolerance to these side effects within the first few months

▶ Therapeutic Tips

- do not use as a first-line agent for hypercholesterolemia

Useful References

Expert Panel on Detection, Evaluation, and Treatment of High Blood Cholesterol in Adults. Summary of the second report of the National Cholesterol Education Program (NCEP) expert panel on detection, evaluation, and treatment of high blood cholesterol in adults. JAMA 1993;269:3015–3023

Knodel LC, Talbert RL. Adverse effects of hypolipidemic drugs. Med Toxicol 1987;2:10–32

Illingworth DR. Lipid-lowering drugs: An overview of indications and optimum therapeutic use. Drugs 1987;33:259–279

Todd PA, Ward A. Gemfibrozil: A review of its pharmacodynamic and pharmacokinetic properties, and therapeutic use in dyslipidemia. Drugs 1988;36:314–339

Frick MH, Elo O, Haapa K, et al. Helsinki Heart Study: Primary-prevention trial with gemfibrozil in middle-aged men with dyslipidemia. N Engl J Med 1987;317:1237–1245

Manninen V, Elo O, Frick MH, et al. Lipid alteration and decline in the incidence of coronary heart disease in the Helsinki Heart Study. JAMA 1988;260:645–651

GENTAMICIN

David Guay

USA (Garamycin, Gentafair, generics)
CANADA (Cidomycin, Garamycin, generics)

▶ When Should I Use This Drug?

check antibiotic susceptibility chart (Table 4–1 in Chapter 4)
Gentamicin is the aminoglycoside of choice for the following infections caused by sensitive organisms, with the exception of *Pseudomonas aeruginosa* (use tobramycin), as it is equally effective and toxic and less expensive than other aminoglycosides

Upper urinary tract infection (pyelonephritis), acute or chronic bacterial prostatitis

- in combination with ampicillin as empirical therapy for moderately to severely ill patients (signs of sepsis) until culture and sensitivity testing results are known

- ampicillin and gentamicin have activity against organisms that commonly cause urinary tract infection: *Escherichia coli, Proteus* sp., *Klebsiella-Enterobacter* sp., *P. aeruginosa*, and enterococcus

Pneumonias

- for nosocomial respiratory tract infections due to gram-negative aerobic organisms known or suspected to be resistant to penicillins or cephalosporins

Intraabdominal infections

- use in combination with antianaerobic agents such as metronidazole and clindamycin with or without ampicillin for enterococci
- ampicillin plus an aminoglycoside may be used for spontaneous bacterial peritonitis; however, some studies suggest an increased incidence of nephrotoxicity in cirrhotic patients receiving aminoglycosides, but this is not yet clearly delineated (Gastroenterology 1982;82:97–105, Hepatology 1985;5:457–462)
- cefotaxime or ceftriaxone in conjunction with ampicillin is likely preferable for spontaneous bacterial peritonitis in cirrhotic patients

Endocarditis

In conjunction with penicillin for the following:

- penicillin-sensitive streptococci (minimum inhibitory concentration [MIC] < 0.1 mg/L) if the patient is younger than 65 years and has no renal or auditory impairment
- intermediate-sensitive streptococci (MIC 0.1–1.0 mg/L)
- penicillin-sensitive enterococci
- penicillin-sensitive diphtheroids (JK diphtheroids, a frequent cause of endocarditis, are often penicillin-resistant and necessitate vancomycin)
- negative culture
- native valve endocarditis if the patient is acutely ill with cardiovascular or neurological complications

In conjunction with vancomycin for the following:

- methicillin-resistant *Staphylococcus aureus* with a prosthetic valve
- penicillinase-producing enterococcus
- if the patient has a history of an immediate-type hypersensitivity to penicillin and has penicillin-sensitive streptococci (MIC < 0.1 mg/L) and if the patient is younger than 65 years and has no renal or auditory impairment
- penicillin-resistant streptococci (MIC ≥ 2.0 mg/L)
- gentamicin-sensitive diphtheroids
- for new valvular insufficiency or suspected intravenous drug abuse if the patient is acutely ill or has cardiovascular or neurological complications

In conjunction with vancomycin and rifampin for the following:

- methicillin-resistant *S. aureus* or *S. epidermidis* if the patient does not respond to vancomycin and gentamicin
- if staphylococci are resistant to gentamicin, use another aminoglycoside, and if they are resistant to all aminoglycosides, omit aminoglycosides (JAMA 1989;261:1471–1477)

Bacterial endocarditis prophylaxis

- in conjunction with ampicillin (vancomycin if the patient is penicillin allergic) for all genitourinary or gastrointestinal procedures

Cellulitis

- useful in conjunction with cloxacillin or nafcillin (or vancomycin or clindamycin if the patient is penicillin allergic) for high-risk patients (intravenous drug abusers, patients undergoing hemodialysis, and patients with underlying debilitating diseases) and/or patients in whom both gram-positive and gram-negative organisms are suspected or proven pathogens (gram-negative cellulitis most commonly presents in patients with diabetes, ischemia, trauma, or surgery of the abdomen or perineum)

Acute or chronic osteomyelitis

- useful in conjunction with cloxacillin or nafcillin for high-risk patients (intravenous drug abusers, patients undergoing hemodialysis, and patients with underlying debilitating diseases)

- cloxacillin or nafcillin with gentamicin has activity against the common organisms causing acute osteomyelitis in these patients (*S. aureus, E. coli, Klebsiella pneumoniae*, and *Haemophilus influenzae*)
- if anaerobes are suspected, add metronidazole or use clindamycin with gentamicin (the decision is based on cost)

Meningitis

- rarely used for gram-negative meningitis
- use in combination with a third-generation cephalosporin with good central nervous system penetration (e.g., cefotaxime, ceftriaxone, and ceftazidime) when the patient is severely ill or the organism (gram negative) has become resistant to third-generation cephalosporins
- if the patient fails to respond to initial parenteral antibiotics, administer aminoglycoside intrathecally or intraventricularly in addition to parenterally
- parenteral aminoglycoside therapy is mainly for the extracerebral manifestations because aminoglycosides penetrate poorly into the cerebrospinal fluid

Prevention of postoperative infections

- in conjunction with vancomycin for neurosurgery
- in conjunction with clindamycin for head and neck surgery
- in conjunction with clindamycin for gastroduodenal or biliary tract surgery, emergency colorectal surgery, appendectomy, abdominal trauma, lower extremity amputation, and colorectal surgery when the patient is allergic to penicillins

Gram-negative shock

- in conjunction with a beta-lactam that has gram-negative activity

Febrile neutropenia

- can be used in combination with a beta-lactam antibiotic that has activity against *Pseudomonas* species (ceftazidime, piperacillin, and ticarcillin-clavulanate)
- tobramycin should likely be chosen instead of gentamicin if *Pseudomonas* is proven or suspected, as tobramycin has better activity against *Pseudomonas* (J Infect Dis 1976;134[suppl]:S3–S19)

▶ *When Should I Not Use This Drug?*

Streptococcal infections caused by organisms other than enterococci

- aminoglycosides are not active against these organisms (except for synergy in endocarditis)

Staphylococcal infections

- use antistaphylococcal penicillins or vancomycin, as the latter is more effective (especially against methicillin-resistant strains) and less toxic (except for synergy in endocarditis)

Uncomplicated urinary tract infections

- less toxic antibiotics are just as effective

Community-acquired respiratory tract infections

- less toxic antibiotics are just as effective

Skin or skin structure infections

- unless gram-negative organisms are proved to be resistant to beta-lactams or quinolones

Any infections

- if less toxic antimicrobials (e.g., beta-lactams, trimethoprim-sulfamethoxazole, and fluoroquinolones) can be used

Single therapy

- there are likely no indications to use gentamicin as sole parenteral therapy for the treatment of any systemic infections
- always combine with another agent such as a penicillin and cephalosporin, which allows the use of lower dosages and a shorter duration of therapy with aminoglycosides

▶ *What Contraindications Are There to the Use of This Drug?*

Intolerance of or allergic reaction to gentamicin

- true allergy to aminoglycosides is extremely rare

Relative contraindications

- aminoglycosides should be used only if no other alternatives are available for patients with these risk factors, as these patients are at greatest risk for toxicity
  - existing renal dysfunction (creatinine clearance < 0.8 mL/s)
  - advanced age (older than 60 years)
  - existing hearing or balance impairment
  - previous aminoglycoside therapy within the last 2–3 months or more than 2 previous courses of an aminoglycoside

▶ What Drug Interactions Are Clinically Important?

Drugs that may increase the effect or toxicity of gentamicin

DIURETICS, AMPHOTERICIN B, VANCOMYCIN, CISPLATIN

- increased chance of nephrotoxicity and ototoxicity
- no change in monitoring frequency; just be aware of the potential for toxicity

Drugs that may decrease the effect of gentamicin

ANTIPSEUDOMONAL PENICILLINS (CARBENICILLIN, TICARCILLIN, PIPERACILLIN, MEZLOCILLIN, AZLOCILLIN)

- inactivation of aminoglycoside on admixture in same intravenous bottle or minibag, in the infusion port, or into the peritoneal cavity
- avoid admixture and infuse via separate intravenous catheters if possible

Drugs that may have their effect increased by gentamicin

- none

Drugs that may have their effect decreased by gentamicin

- none

▶ What Route and Dosage Should I Use?

How to administer

- orally—not absorbed
- parenterally—dilute in 100 mL of saline or 5% dextrose in water and infuse over 30 minutes
- can be given intramuscularly if the intravenous route is not available

Dosages depend on the patient's size, severity of illness, and renal function • Round the dosage up to nearest 20 mg (i.e., the 60, 80, 100, 120, 140, and 160 mg) to allow ease of administration

Upper urinary tract infection (pyelonephritis), acute or chronic bacterial prostatitis, pneumonias, cellulitis, acute or chronic osteomyelitis, intraabdominal infections

- 1.5 mg/kg IV Q8H for mild to moderate illness
- 2 mg/kg IV Q8H for severe illness

Endocarditis

- 1 mg/kg IV Q8H
- only low dosages are required because using only for synergy with beta-lactams or vancomycin against enterococci or staphylococci
- low dosages should also be used because an aminoglycoside may be needed for up to 2–4 weeks, and it is best to use a low dosage to minimize toxicity

Bacterial endocarditis prophylaxis

- 1.5 mg/kg (maximum, 80 mg) IV or IM 30 minutes before the procedure

Meningitis

- 2 mg/kg IV Q8H plus 7.5 mg intrathecally or intraventricularly Q24H if the patient fails to respond to IV therapy

Prevention of postoperative infections

- 2 mg/kg IV

Gram-negative shock

- 2.5 mg/kg IV Q8H

Febrile neutropenia

- 2 mg/kg IV Q8H

Dosage adjustments for renal or hepatic dysfunction

- renally eliminated

Normal Dosing Interval	C_{cr} > 60 mL/min or 1 mL/s	C_{cr} 30–60 mL/min or 0.5–1 mL/s	C_{cr} < 30 mL/min or 0.5 mL/s
Q8H	no adjustment needed	Q12H	Q24H

▶ What Should I Monitor with Regard to Efficacy and Toxicity?

Efficacy

- for antibiotic administration monitoring guidelines, see specific section on drug therapy

Nephrotoxicity

- monitor serum creatinine levels every 3 days during therapy
- if the serum creatinine level rises more than 25% over baseline values, no dosage changes are needed, but be on the alert for further increases
- if there is an increase in the serum creatinine level of 50% over baseline values, the need for continued aminoglycoside therapy should be reassessed and discontinuation of aminoglycoside therapy and the use of an alternative nonnephrotoxic agent (e.g., cephalosporins and quinolones) to complete the treatment course is advised
- if aminoglycoside therapy is to be continued, serum aminoglycoside concentrations should be determined and dosage regimens adjusted to maintain adequate levels (see below)

Ototoxicity

- aminoglycoside-related ototoxicity is usually irreversible and can have a significant impact on the future lifestyle of the patient
- decrease the risk by limiting total aminoglycoside therapy to a maximum of 7–10 days (in some cases, such as endocarditis and osteomyelitis, therapy may need to be continued after 7–10 days)
- stop aminoglycoside therapy when the patient has improved or change to an oral agent (e.g., quinolone)
- for patients anticipated to require more than 5 days of aminoglycoside therapy, inform them of the potential toxicities and question them daily about the presence of the following symptoms: tinnitus, loss of hearing, fullness in their ears, headache, nausea and vomiting, giddiness, lightheadedness, vertigo, nystagmus, and ataxia
- if these symptoms develop and no other causes can be ascertained, aminoglycoside therapy should be stopped and alternative agents initiated
- patients requiring longer than 14 days of aminoglycoside therapy (e.g., patients with osteomyelitis or febrile neutropenia) should have baseline and weekly auditory and vestibular function tests

Serum concentrations

Desired serum concentrations

- 1–2 mg/L (predose) and 4–10 mg/L (postdose) for most infections (3 mg/L postdose for gram-positive endocarditis)
- remember that these ranges are guidelines, and patients may require higher or lower concentrations depending on the clinical course and toxicity
- prior to ordering any serum concentrations, ensure that patients are receiving an appropriate dosage for their age, weight, renal function, and disease state

If the empirical dosage is appropriate, concentrations are not required

- patients anticipated to require less than 5–7 days of therapy
- patients receiving aminoglycosides for the treatment of lower urinary tract infections or mild infections

- immunocompetent patients receiving aminoglycoside therapy for moderate infections who lack physiological conditions (e.g., burn patients, hyperdynamic critically ill patients, cystic fibrotis patients), which may significantly alter drug disposition
- immunocompetent patients receiving aminoglycoside therapy for moderate infections who are receiving concomitant broad-spectrum antibiotics (Clin Infect Dis 1992;14:320–339)

Concentrations should be done after the third dose and then weekly

- patients with life-threatening infections, particularly immuno-suppressed patients
- patients anticipated to require extended (longer than 7 days) aminoglycoside therapy
- patients who are not responding to treatment after 48 hours
- patients in whom aminoglycoside-related toxicity is suspected if the continuation of therapy is needed

▶ *How Long Do I Treat Patients with This Drug?*

Upper urinary tract infections (pyelonephritis)

- 14 days total intravenous and oral therapy (e.g., trimethoprim-sulfamethoxazole and amoxicillin)
- consider switching from an aminoglycoside to an oral agent after the patient has become afebrile and has clinically improved for 1–2 days

Acute or chronic bacterial prostatitis

- for acute disease, treat for a total of 30 days (Med Clin North Am 1991;75:405–424)
- for chronic disease, treat for a total of 6 weeks
- symptoms usually resolve during 7 days, but a prolonged treatment course is mandatory for eradication
- consider switching to an oral agent after patient has become afebrile and has clinically improved for 1–2 days

Pneumonias

- usual duration of therapy is 10 days or 4–5 days after the patient has become afebrile and has clinically improved
- consider switching to an oral agent after the patient has become afebrile and has clinically improved for 1–2 days
- if the patient has a pneumonia caused by gram-negative organisms, a 14 day course of therapy should be given (Clin Chest Med 1991;12:237–242, Ann Intern Med 1987;106:341–345)

Intraabdominal infections

- treatment should continue for 10 days; however, extend treatment if the patient has not been asymptomatic for 72 hours

Cellulitis

- usual duration is 10 days or 4–5 days after the patient has become afebrile and has clinically improved
- consider switching to oral therapy after patient has become afebrile and has clinically improved for 1–2 days

Acute or chronic osteomyelitis

- treat patients with at least 4 weeks of parenteral antibiotics after debridement surgery (the duration of therapy is based on the patient's clinical response)
- if an amputation is done proximal to the site of the infection, only prophylactic antibiotics are required (Hosp Formul 1993; 28:63–85)
- if the bone is removed and there is still evidence of soft tissue infection, the patient should receive a 2 week course of antibiotics
- treat patients with a prosthetic device for 4–6 weeks with parenteral antibiotics followed by 3–6 months of oral antibiotic treatment
- treat patients with peripheral vascular disease with at least 4 weeks of parenteral antibiotics and follow with oral antibiotics until there is no evidence of inflammation (on the basis of clinical or radiological evidence) (Am J Med 1987;83:653–660)
- duration of parenteral antibiotic therapy prior to switching to oral therapy depends on the patient's clinical response
- in patients receiving aminoglycosides as part of their parenteral regimen, consideration should be given to switching to cefotax-

ime, ceftriaxone, or a quinolone after 10–14 days of aminoglycoside therapy to decrease the chance of serious ototoxicity

Meningitis

- 21 days if meningitis is caused by gram-negative organisms

Endocarditis

- gentamicin is usually continued for 2 weeks (4 weeks for penicillinase-producing enterococcus, intermediate-sensitive or penicillin-resistant streptococci, enterococci, penicillin-sensitive diphtheroids, or culture-negative endocarditis)
- depending on the site and the organism, other antibiotics that are being used in conjunction with the aminoglycoside may need to be continued for longer than the aminoglycoside

Bacterial endocarditis prophylaxis

- single dose

Prevention of postoperative infections

- single dose

Gram-negative shock

- for 4–5 days after the patient has become afebrile and clinically improved

Febrile neutropenia

- if the patient is afebrile for 72 hours, no causative agent is found, and the total granulocyte count is greater than $500/\mu L$, discontinue antibiotic treatment after 7 days (J Infect Dis 1990;161: 381–396)
- if patient remains neutropenic, continue the antibiotic regimen until the patient is afebrile for 5 days
- if the patient is clinically unwell, continue antibiotic therapy until the granulocyte count is greater than $500/\mu L$ (J Infect Dis 1990;161:381–396)

▶ *How Do I Decrease or Stop the Administration of This Drug?*

- may be stopped abruptly

▶ *What Should I Tell My Patients About This Drug?*

- if you have dizziness, vertigo, ringing in the ears, roaring sensation in the ears, loss of balance, or hearing loss, tell your physician

▶ *Therapeutic Tips*

- ensure that the dosing interval is adjusted for renal function, especially in the elderly and patients with prior renal impairment
- if the expected duration of therapy is 5–7 days or less, avoid blood concentration monitoring unless the patient is renally impaired
- switch to an alternative less toxic agent as soon as possible (base the decision on culture and sensitivity testing results)
- decrease the risk of toxicity by limiting therapy to 7–10 days and switch to oral therapy as soon as possible
- a number of clinicians are now recommending once-daily dosing of aminoglycosides (a useful regimen is 5 or 6 mg/kg IV Q24H and extending the interval to Q36H in patients with estimated creatinine clearance <1 mL/s)
- serum concentrations with once-daily dosing are not presently recommended, as there is no evidence of a relation between concentrations and efficacy or toxicity

Useful References

Pancoast SJ. Aminoglycoside antibiotics in clinical use. Med Clin North Am 1988;72:581–612

Chan GL. Alternative dosing strategy for aminoglycosides: Impact of efficacy, nephrotoxicity, and ototoxicity. DICP 1989;23:788–794

Mattie H. Determinants of efficacy and toxicity of aminoglycosides. J Antimicrob Chemother 1989;24:281–293

Garrison MW, Zaske DE, Rotschafer JC. Aminoglycosides: Another perspective. DICP 1990;24:267–272

Gruninger RP, Tsukayama DT, Wicklund B. Antibiotic-impregnated PMMA beads in bone and prosthetic joint infections. In: Gustilo RB, Gruninger

RP, Tsukayama DT, eds. Orthopedic Infection. Diagnosis and Treatment. Philadelphia: WB Saunders, 1989:66–74

GLICLAZIDE

Christy Silvius Scott

USA (not available)
CANADA (Diamicron)

▶ When Should I Use This Drug?

Non–insulin-dependent diabetes

- obese (>120% of ideal body weight) and/or older patients (older than 40 years) with moderate hyperglycemia and without significant symptoms
- because obese diabetics are in a state of insulin resistance and large dosages of insulin may be required and euglycemia may be difficult to achieve (N Engl J Med 1989;321:1231–1245)
- similar potency and duration of action to those of glyburide
- metabolized to less than 20% active metabolites; however, they may be retained in renal failure (Can Med Assoc J 1992;124:1571–1581, Clin Pharmacokinet 1981;6:215–241)
- also reduced platelet adhesiveness and impairs aggregation, enhances fibrinolytic activity, possesses antithrombotic activity, and is a free radical scavenger; however, the extent to which these effects alter the microvascular long-term complications in patients with diabetes is unknown (Metabolism 1992;41:33–39, 40–45, JAMA 1991;90[suppl 6A]:50S–54S)
- cost is much higher than with glyburide or tolbutamide
- future role of gliclazide depends on its ability to decrease the long-term microvascular complications of diabetes

▶ When Should I Not Use This Drug?

see Tolbutamide

▶ What Contraindications Are There to the Use of This Drug?

see Tolbutamide

▶ What Drug Interactions Are Clinically Important?

see Tolbutamide

▶ What Route and Dosage Should I Use?

How to administer

- orally—the timing of the dose in relation to meals appears to be irrelevant with long-term therapy (Eur J Clin Pharmacol 1990;38:465–467)
- parenterally—not available

Non–insulin-dependent diabetes

- 40 mg PO daily
- timing of the dose in relation to meals appears to be irrelevant with long-term therapy (Eur J Clin Pharmacol 1990;38:465–467)
- increase the dosage weekly by 40 mg increments until glycemic control or a maximum daily dosage of 320 mg is reached
- daily dosages greater than 160 mg should be divided BID because patients requiring high dosages likely need a split dose to ensure adequate effective concentrations throughout the day

Dosage adjustments for renal or hepatic dysfunction

- 20% metabolized to active metabolites, which are retained in renal failure

Normal Dosing Interval	C_{cr} > 60 mL/min or 1 mL/s	C_{cr} 30–60 mL/min or 0.5–1 mL/s	C_{cr} < 30 mL/min or 0.5 mL/s
Q12H	no adjustment needed	Q24H	not recommended in renal failure
Q24H	no adjustment needed	decrease dosage by 50%	not recommended in renal failure

▶ What Should I Monitor with Regard to Efficacy and Toxicity?

see Tolbutamide

▶ How Long Do I Treat Patients with This Drug?

see Tolbutamide

▶ How Do I Decrease or Stop the Administration of This Drug?

- may be stopped abruptly, if necessary
- if satisfactory blood glucose control is maintained for 6 months, decrease the dosage by 40 mg every 2 weeks

▶ What Should I Tell My Patients About This Drug?

see Tolbutamide

▶ Therapeutic Tips

see Tolbutamide

Useful References

Groop LC. Sulfonylureas in NIDDM. Diabetes Care 1992;15:737–754
Rodger W. Non–insulin-dependent (type II) diabetes mellitus. Can Med Assoc J 1991;145:1571–1581

GLIPIZIDE

Christy Silvius Scott

USA (Glucotrol)
CANADA (not available)

▶ When Should I Use This Drug?

Non–insulin-dependent diabetes

- obese (>120% of ideal body weight) and/or older patients (older than 40 years); patients with moderate hyperglycemia and without significant symptoms
- obese diabetics are in a state of insulin resistance; therefore, large dosages of insulin may be required and euglycemia may be difficult to achieve with insulin (N Engl J Med 1989;321:1231–1245)
- although there are no studies demonstrating the greater effectiveness of second- over first-generation sulfonlyureas (Diabetes Care 1992;15:737–754), most studies suggest that maximum dosages of chlorpropamide, glyburide, and glipizide are equally efficacious and appear superior to tolazamide, acetohexamide, and tolbutamide (N Engl J Med 1989;321:1231–1245)
- similar potency and duration of action to those of glyburide
- more expensive than glyburide
- causes a lower incidence (approximately 50% less) of hypoglycemia in comparison with glyburide (Drugs 1981;22:211–245)
- metabolized to inactive compounds
- therefore, reserve for patients with renal insufficiency who desire once-daily dosing and are willing to pay more for the convenience
- tolbutamide is probably a better choice for patients older than 60 years because of decreased potency and duration of action (Drug Ther Bull 1987;25:13–16)

▶ When Should I Not Use This Drug?

see Tolbutamide

▶ What Contraindications Are There to the Use of This Drug?

see Tolbutamide

▶ What Drug Interactions Are Clinically Important?

see Tolbutamide

▶ What Route and Dosage Should I Use?

How to administer

- orally—food delays the absorption of glipizide; however, with long-term therapy, this delay is not clinically important and administration before meals is not necessary (Diabetes Care 1990;3[suppl 3]:26–31)
- parenterally—not available

Non–insulin-dependent diabetes

- 5 mg PO daily
- increase the dosage weekly by 2.5 mg increments until glycemic control or a maximum daily dosage of 40 mg is reached
- average daily dosage is 10 mg (N Engl J Med 1989;321:1231–1245)

• daily dosages greater than 15 mg PO should be divided BID because patients requiring high doses likely need a split dose to ensure adequate effective concentrations throughout the 24 hour period

Dosage adjustments for renal or hepatic dysfunction

• 90% metabolized to inactive compounds; however, renal excretion of the parent compound is reduced in severe failure and the parent compound may accumulate

Normal Dosing Interval	C_{cr} > 60 mL/min or 1 mL/s	C_{cr} 30–60 mL/min or 0.5–1 mL/s	C_{cr} < 30 mL/min or 0.5 mL/s
Q12H	no adjustment needed	no adjustment needed	Q24H
Q24H	no adjustment needed	no adjustment needed	decrease dosage by 50%

▶ What Should I Monitor with Regard to Efficacy and Toxicity?

see Tolbutamide

▶ How Long Do I Treat Patients with This Drug?

see Tolbutamide

▶ How Do I Decrease or Stop the Administration of This Drug?

• drug administration may be abruptly stopped, if necessary
• if satisfactory blood glucose control is maintained for 6 months, decrease the dosage by 2.5 mg every 2 weeks

▶ What Should I Tell My Patients About This Drug?

see Tolbutamide

▶ Therapeutic Tips

see Tolbutamide

Useful References

Gerich JE. Oral hypoglycemic agents. N Engl J Med 1989;321:1231–1245
Groop LC. Sulfonylureas in NIDDM. Diabetes Care 1992;15:737–754
Hansten PD, Horn JR. Drug Interactions and Updates, 7th ed. Philadelphia: Lea & Febiger, 1991
Tatro DS. Drug Interaction Facts. St Louis: Facts and Comparisons, 1995

GLYBURIDE (GLIBENCLAMIDE)

Christy Silvius Scott
USA (DiaBeta, Micronase)
CANADA (Diabeta, Euglucon)

▶ When Should I Use This Drug?

Non–insulin-dependent diabetes

• obese (>120% of ideal body weight) and/or older patients (older than 40 years) with moderate hyperglycemia and without significant symptoms
• obese diabetics are in a state of insulin resistance; therefore, large dosages of insulin may be required and euglycemia may be difficult to achieve (N Engl J Med 1989;321:1231–1245)
• although there are no studies demonstrating the greater effectiveness of second- over first-generation sulfonylureas (Diabetes Care 1992;15:737–754), most studies suggest that maximum dosages of chlorpropamide, glyburide, and glipizide are equally efficacious and appear superior to tolazamide, acetohexamide, and tolbutamide (N Engl J Med 1989;321:1231–1245)
• glyburide is as effective as other oral hypoglycemics and can be given less frequently than tolbutamide
• highest incidence of hypoglycemia occurs with glyburide and chlorpropamide (5 times more frequently than with tolbutamide, 2 times more often than with glipizide and gliclazide) (Diabetes Care 1989;12:203–208, Drugs 1981;22:211–245, N Engl J Med 1989;321:1231–1245)
• some studies suggest that glyburide causes the highest incidence of hypoglycemia (Diabetes Care 1989;12:203–208, Br Med J 1988;296:949–950)

• is a reasonable starting medication for younger patients (40–60 years) with good renal function who desire less frequent dosing schedules and who are not at risk for hypoglycemia
• careful patient selection is required before using this medication because glyburide causes more hypoglycemia than does any other glucose-lowering agent (Diabetes Res Clin Pract 1991;14:139–148, Br Med J 1988;296:949–950)
• for patients who are at risk for hypoglycemia (patients older than 60 years, malnourished or alcoholic patients, or patients with renal or hepatic dysfunction or adrenal insufficiency), it is best to avoid glyburide (N Engl J Med 1989;321:1231–1245)

▶ When Should I Not Use This Drug?

see Tolbutamide

▶ What Contraindications Are There to the Use of This Drug?

see Tolbutamide

Patients with moderate or severe renal dysfunction (creatinine clearance < 30–50 mL/min)

• glyburide and/or its active metabolites may accumulate
• preferred agents (having no active metabolites) include tolbutamide and glipizide; tolbutamide is probably a better choice because it is shorter acting and less potent (N Engl J Med 1989;321:1231–1245)

▶ What Drug Interactions Are Clinically Important?

see Tolbutamide

▶ What Route and Dosage Should I Use?

How to administer

• orally—the timing of the dose in relation to meals appears to be irrelevant with long-term therapy (Diabetes Care 1990;13[suppl 3]:26–31)
• parenterally—not available

Non–insulin-dependent diabetes

• 2.5 mg PO daily
• increase the dosage weekly by 2.5 mg increments until glycemic control or a maximum daily dosage of 20 mg is reached
• average daily dosage is 7.5 mg (N Engl J Med 1989;321: 1231–1245)
• daily dosages greater than 10 mg should be divided BID because patients requiring high dosages likely need a split dose to ensure adequate effective concentrations throughout the day

Dosage adjustments for renal or hepatic dysfunction

• active metabolites renally eliminated

Normal Dosing Interval	C_{cr} > 60 mL/min or 1 mL/s	C_{cr} 30–60 mL/min or 0.5–1 mL/s	C_{cr} < 30 mL/min or 0.5 mL/s
Q12H	no adjustment needed	avoid because of increased risk of hypoglycemia	do not use
Q24H	no adjustment needed	avoid because of increased risk of hypoglycemia	do not use

▶ What Should I Monitor with Regard to Efficacy and Toxicity?

see Tolbutamide

▶ How Long Do I Treat Patients with This Drug?

see Tolbutamide

▶ How Do I Decrease or Stop the Administration of This Drug?

• may be stopped abruptly, if necessary
• if satisfactory blood glucose control is maintained for 6 months, decrease by 2.5 mg every 2 weeks

► *What Should I Tell My Patients About This Drug?*

see Tolbutamide

► *Therapeutic Tips*

- careful patient selection is necessary before using glyburide so that hypoglycemic reactions can be avoided

see Tolbutamide

Useful References

Gerich JE. Oral hypoglycemic agents. N Engl J Med 1989;321:1231–1245

Groop LC. Sulfonylureas in NIDDM. Diabetes Care 1992;15:737–754

Hansten PD, Horn JR. Drug Interactions and Updates. Philadelphia: Lea & Febiger, 1991

Tatro DS. Drug Interaction Facts. St Louis: Facts and Comparisons, 1995

GLYCERIN

Leslie Mathews

USA (Glycerin)
CANADA (Glycerin)

► *When Should I Use This Drug?*

Acute constipation

- for occasional use to evacuate the lower bowel when oral laxatives are ineffective
- glycerin suppositories are safe to use, require less nursing time, and are aesthetically more acceptable to patients than enemas

Chronic constipation

- useful for patients with atonic or severe idiopathic constipation
- glycerin is necessary in these conditions in which the rectum is filled but the defecation reflex is not triggered, or intestinal transit time is severely delayed, because it stimulates the rectal mucosa
- glycerin is sometimes referred to as a stimulant laxative but is generally classified as an osmotic laxative
- is less likely to produce anorectal irritation and is less expensive than bisacodyl suppository
- suitable for occasional use if bulk-forming laxatives, lactulose, and other laxatives are ineffective alone

► *When Should I Not Use This Drug?*

Stool is hard and dry

- if stool is hard and dry, glycerin may be ineffective (Pharm Bull 1987;21:1–7)

Oral laxatives are effective

- oral laxatives are easier to administer

Regular use for long periods or routine use without indication

- anorectal irritation can occur with persistent use

► *What Contraindications Are There to the Use of This Drug?*

Intolerance of or allergic reaction to glycerin
Symptoms of acute abdomen

- undiagnosed abdominal pain, nausea, vomiting

Anal or rectal fissures, ulcerated hemorrhoids

- glycerin can cause irritation and worsen fissures

► *What Drug Interactions Are Clinically Important?*

- none

► *What Route and Dosage Should I Use?*

How to administer

- orally—not useful for constipation because it is absorbed, leaving an insufficient amount to exert activity by the time it reaches the colon
- parenterally—not available
- rectally—inserted rectally 30 minutes after breakfast or dinner

Acute constipation, chronic constipation

- one 3 g suppository rectally administered 30 minutes after breakfast or dinner to take full advantage of the gastrocolic reflex
- should be retained for at least 15 minutes

Dosage adjustments for renal or hepatic dysfunction

- dosage adjustments are not required for rectal administration, as it is poorly absorbed

► *What Should I Monitor with Regard to Efficacy and Toxicity?*

Efficacy

Prevention of fecal impaction, acute constipation, chronic constipation

- initiates a bowel movement within 15–60 minutes of administration

Toxicity

Anorectal irritation

- anal inflammation and fissures can occur with continued use
- if they occur, discontinue use and try a different laxative

► *How Long Do I Treat Patients with This Drug?*

Acute constipation

- give 1 dose only

Chronic constipation

- to help reestablish bowel habits, give daily as needed, preferably for no longer than 10 days
- may be used on a regular or intermittent basis (e.g., every 3–4 days) in bedridden, institutionalized, or chronically constipated patients

► *How Do I Decrease or Stop the Administration of This Drug?*

- may be stopped abruptly

► *What Should I Tell My Patients About This Drug?*

- drugs usually work within 15–60 minutes
- stay close to a bathroom
- to use, allow the suppository to stand at room temperature
- remove the wrapper and insert the tapered end into the rectum
- remain lying down for a few minutes after insertion
- use after a meal or before a short walk to be most effective
- drug may produce anal or rectal irritation or burning or abdominal cramping
- discontinue use if marked swelling of the anus, bleeding, or discharge of mucus occurs

► *Therapeutic Tips*

- suppositories are most effective if inserted against the wall of the rectum rather than directly into stool
- glycerin is ineffective orally because it is well absorbed, leaving little active drug left to work at rectal site

Useful Reference

Yakabowich M. Prescribe with care: The role of laxatives in the treatment of constipation. Gerontol Nurs 1990;16:4–11

GOLD COMPLEXES

Kelly Jones

Aurothioglucose Injection (Oil Based)

USA (Solganal)
CANADA (Solganal)

Gold Sodium Thiomalate Injection (Water Based)

USA (Myochrysine)
CANADA (Myochrysine)

Auranofin Capsules

USA (Ridaura)
CANADA (Ridaura)

▶ When Should I Use This Drug?

Rheumatoid arthritis

- gold complexes are considered by many rheumatologists as the second-line drugs of choice for treating rheumatoid arthritis
- injectable gold is by far the most effective in treating rheumatoid arthritis as compared with the oral gold formulation (auranofin)
- some clinicians consider oral gold a good agent to treat mild rheumatoid arthritis when the patient has no effect from hydroxychloroquine or cannot tolerate the side effects
- injectable gold is considered by most clinicians to be the second-line agent of choice in progressive disease, and the decision becomes choosing between injectable gold and methotrexate
- most rheumatologists choose gold simply based on experience using these compounds
- for patients who dislike injections, oral methotrexate may be the agent of choice
- use oral gold in mild disease, as it is much less toxic; use injectable gold for progressive disease
- aurothioglucose (Solganal) is considered the injectable agent of choice because the injection is an oil-based product (sesame oil), which allows slower absorption and less chance for the nitritoid reaction (this reaction consists of flushing, weakness, dizziness, syncope, and hypotension and is related to the rate of absorption)
- gold sodium thiomalate (Myochrysine) still has a place in therapy in patients allergic to the oil component

▶ When Should I Not Use This Drug?

Progressive rheumatoid arthritis

- do not use oral gold, even though it is less toxic, because it is also less effective than injectable gold

Unreliable patients who will not have regular follow-ups

- in the United Kingdom, gold complexes were one of the major causes of drug-induced death, and follow-up is essential (Paulus HE, Furst DR, Dromgate SH, eds. Drugs for Rheumatic Disease. New York: Churchill Livingstone, 1987:49–83)

▶ What Contraindications Are There to the Use of This Drug?

Intolerance of or allergic reaction to gold
Patients with the HLA-DR locus histocompatability antigen DR3

- these patients appear to be genetically predisposed to adverse effects from gold complexes (proteinuria), and there is evidence that the gold-induced adverse effects may be immunologically mediated

Dermatitis

- check the patient's history of dermatitis (e.g., eczema, urticaria, and exfoliative dermatitis) because these patients may be more sensitive to the dermatological adverse effects of gold complexes

Hematological abnormalities

- patients should have baseline hematological workup to rule out any possible blood dyscrasias

▶ What Drug Interactions Are Clinically Important?

Drugs that may increase the effect or toxicity of gold

- none

Drugs that may decrease the effect of gold

- none

Drugs that may have their effect or toxicity increased by gold
PHENYTOIN

- one report of a possible interaction with auranofin and phenytoin, whereby the serum level of phenytoin was raised with concurrent administration
- be aware of the interaction, but it should not warrant a change of therapy

Drugs that may have their effect or toxicity decreased by gold

- none

▶ What Route and Dosage Should I Use?

How to administer

- orally—take with food or milk or on an empty stomach
- parenterally—the drug should be administered by deep intramuscular injection, preferably intragluteally

Rheumatoid arthritis
Oral

- 6 mg PO daily as a single dose or in divided doses twice daily
- splitting the dose may help the patient to tolerate the gastrointestinal side effects
- if there is no response in 6 months, increase the dosage to 9 mg daily (3 mg PO TID) for 3 months
- if the patient does not respond to 3 months of 9 mg daily, discontinue the drug

Intramuscular

- give a 10 mg IM test dose of the drug and observe for anaphylaxis, shock, syncope, bradycardia, thickening of the tongue, dysphagia, and dyspnea
- patient should remain still for 10 minutes after the injection
- after the test dose, give doses weekly
- increase second and third doses to 25 mg IM
- continue therapy with 50 mg IM doses weekly until a total of 1 g has been given
- if the patient has responded to therapy at 1 g, then the injections can be given every 2–3 weeks for 3 months, then monthly as long as the patient tolerates the drug
- if the patient does not respond at 1 g cumulative dose, increase the dosage by 10 mg/wk every 2–4 weeks until a maximum of 100 mg/wk is reached, until the wanted response is achieved, or until the patient cannot tolerate the drug

Dosage adjustments for renal or hepatic dysfunction

- renally eliminated

Normal Dosing Interval	$C_{cr} > 60$ mL/min or 1 mL/s	C_{cr} 30–60 mL/min or 0.5–1 mL/s	$C_{cr} < 30$ mL/min or 0.5 mL/s
Q24H	no adjustment needed	avoid	avoid

▶ What Should I Monitor with Regard to Efficacy and Toxicity?

Efficacy

Severe rheumatoid arthritis

Joint tenderness count, sedimentation rate measurements, grip strength, and a physician's assessment

- has been shown to be adequate in evaluating the disease activity (Arthritis Rheum 1989;32:1093–1099)
- patient should be assessed monthly for the first 2 months, and after the disease is under control, the patient can be assessed every 3 months for 6 months, and then every 6 months
- these variables should be used to guide drug starting and stopping
- one study found that clinical and laboratory measures of physical well-being appeared to be unrelated to psychological and social measures of well-being (J Rheumatol 1991;18:650–653)
- it is important to include patients' self-assessment of the drug's effect on their function and well-being
- evidence from radiographic studies suggests that parenteral gold may slow or arrest the progression of joint space narrowing and bone erosion but it does not reverse damage already done to the joint and surrounding tissues

Toxicity

Toxicity is common with gold therapy • A metaanalysis found that injectable gold had higher toxicity rates and higher total dropout rates than did any of the other second-line drugs (methotrexate, penicillamine, sulfasalazine, antimalarials, and auranofin), and this study revealed injectable gold as the drug with the highest toxicity and auranofin as the agent with the least toxicity (Arthritis Rheum 1990;33:1449–1461)

Hematological effects

- do baseline and monthly (prior to each injection if intramuscular) complete blood count with differential leukocyte count and platelet counts
- order the laboratory tests less often (e.g., after every second injection), depending on the patient's history of tolerability
- discontinue the drug administration if white blood cell counts are less than 3500/mm^3, if there is a rapid decrease in hemoglobin concentration from previous measurements, or platelet counts are less than 100,000/mm^3
- dimercaprol therapy has been used as a chelator in patients with toxicity, but the efficacy is questionable
- suggested protocol for thrombocytopenia is 100 mg of dimercaprol IM twice daily for 2 weeks

Liver toxicity

- baseline liver enzyme levels and every 6 months
- if liver enzyme levels are 3 times baseline values, discontinue the drug administration

Renal toxicity

- proteinuria results from gold complexes depositing in the kidney
- baseline and monthly urinalysis or dipstick tests for protein (prior to each injection if intramuscular)
- order the laboratory test less often (e.g., after every second injection), depending on the patient's history of tolerability
- discontinue the drug administration if proteinuria is greater than 1 g/d

Gastrointestinal effects

- diarrhea can occur in 50% of patients taking oral gold
- diarrhea can be minimized by starting with 3 mg PO daily and titrating up to 6 mg/d after several weeks and splitting higher doses BID
- bulk-forming laxatives BID or other fiber-providing products may help to decrease the diarrhea

Dermatological effects

- mucocutaneous reactions are the most common problems, and skin reactions can range from simple erythema to a severe exfoliative dermatitis
- pruritus is often a warning sign that a cutaneous reaction is going to occur and the drug administration should be stopped for assessment
- often, the nonspecific rash goes away in 2–4 weeks and the drug administration can be reinstituted at a lower dosage (50% of the initial dosage)
- for minor dermatitis, topical corticosteroids may help; however, if dermatitis is severe, 40 mg PO daily of prednisone should be used
- if the patient experiences an exfoliative dermatitis, reinstitution of gold therapy is not warranted
- dimercaprol therapy has been used as a chelator in patients with toxicity, but the efficacy is questionable (a suggested protocol is 2.5 mg/kg IM every 4 hours for 2 days, then twice daily for a week)

Metallic taste

- stomatitis is often preceded by a metallic taste and is a warning of probable toxicity

Nephrotic syndrome, hypersensitivity pneumonitis, and agranulocytosis

- all occur in less than 1% of patients receiving injectable gold and rarely in patients receiving oral gold

Necrotizing enterocolitis, peripheral neuropathy, exfoliative dermatitis, and bone marrow aplasia

- occur rarely with either the injectable or the oral agent

▶ How Long Do I Treat Patients with This Drug?

Severe rheumatoid arthritis

- gold therapy should be given at least a 6 month trial before switching to another therapy

- it is important to try to give the patient a 1 g cumulative trial dose before stopping
- gold administration can be continued in a patient indefinitely if tolerated but many patients fail therapy owing to side effects (35%)

▶ How Do I Decrease or Stop the Administration of This Drug?

- may be stopped abruptly

▶ What Should I Tell My Patients About This Drug?

- it is important to be compliant with physician visits
- watch for the warning signs of toxicity: pruritus and metallic taste
- effectiveness is slow and expect relief in 3–6 months, not within days

▶ Therapeutic Tips

- do not interchange oral gold for injectable gold in patients who have had potentially life-threatening adverse effects (proteinuria, hematological reactions) from the injectable gold; however, many clinicians administer oral gold cautiously in a patient who has had a mild adverse effect (e.g., mucocutaneous reaction) from injectable gold
- injectable gold is more efficacious, but more toxic, than oral gold
- injectable gold takes away the problems of compliance but necessitates close follow-up on the part of the physician
- aurothioglucose (Solganal) injection is an oil-based product that should be used first in patients not allergic to sesame oil because this product is less likely to cause the nitritoid reaction than is the water-based product (gold sodium thiomalate)
- injectable gold should be used in patients with progressive disease, and oral gold should be used in patients with mild disease unresponsive to hydroxychloroquine
- it is important to dose gold therapy appropriately and give an adequate trial of the drug (6 months)
- 35% of patients fail gold therapy owing to adverse effects, and it is important to monitor for these effects

Useful References

Clair WE, Poisson RP. Therapeutic approaches to the treatment of rheumatoid arthritis. Med Clin North Am 1986;70:285–304

Delafuente JC, Osborn TG. Review of auranofin, an oral chrysotherapeutic agent. Clin Pharm 1984;3:121–127

Blocka K, Paulus HE. The clinical pharmacology of the gold compounds. In: Paulus HE, Furst DR, Dromgate SH, eds. Drugs for Rheumatic Disease. New York: Churchill Livingstone 1987;49–83

GUAIFENESIN

Penny Miller

USA (Breonesin, Humibid, Hytuss, Robitussin)
CANADA (Robitussin, Balminil expectorant, Benylin E, Resyl)

▶ When Should I Use This Drug?

Productive coughs

- coughs associated with the common cold, laryngitis, bronchitis, pharyngitis, pertussis, influenza, and measles and coughs provoked by chronic paranasal sinusitis in patients not responsive to increased fluid intake
- guaifenesin reduces the viscosity of tenacious secretions by increasing the volume of respiratory tract fluid
- is the only expectorant that has some scientific evidence to support its efficacy in decreasing sputum thickness (Federal Register 1989;54:8507)
- efficacy of an expectorant is difficult to demonstrate because there are no generally accepted standard techniques of study in humans (Health Protection Branch. Second Report of the Expert Advisory Committee on Nonprescription Cough and Cold Remedies. Health and Welfare Canada, 1989)

▶ When Should I Not Use This Drug?

Nonproductive coughs

- it is a misconception to believe that guaifenesin is useful in nonproductive coughs by supposedly relieving irritated membranes in the respiratory passageways by preventing dryness through increased mucous flow (Federal Register 1989;54: 8494–8509)

Persistent or chronic cough occurring with smoking, asthma, chronic bronchitis, or emphysema

- this may indicate a serious development such as worsening of the patient's condition or an infection (American Hospital Formulary Service, Drug Information, ASHP, Bethesda, Md: 1993:1675)

▶ **What Contraindications Are There to the Use of This Drug?**

- intolerance of or allergic reaction to guaifenesin

▶ **What Drug Interactions Are Clinically Important?**

Drugs that may increase the effect of guaifenesin

- none

Drugs that may decrease the effect of guaifenesin

ANTIHISTAMINES, DEXTROMETHORPHAN, CODEINE, AND OTHER NARCOTIC ANTITUSSIVES

- avoid concomitant use because antihistamines dry secretions and dextromethorphan or codeine prevents the expectoration by suppressing the cough

Drugs that may have their effect increased by guaifenesin

- none

Drugs that may have their effect decreased by guaifenesin

- none

▶ **What Route and Dosage Should I Use?**

How to administer

- orally—can be given with food or on an empty stomach

Productive coughs

- 200 mg PO Q6H PRN for symptoms up to a maximum of 2400 mg PO daily

Dosage adjustments for renal or hepatic dysfunction

- hepatically metabolized
- no dosage adjustments are needed, as the drug should be used infrequently for short periods

▶ **What Should I Monitor with Regard to Efficacy and Toxicity?**

Efficacy

Productive coughs

- sputum should be more fluid (i.e., loose and thin) and easier to cough up

Toxicity

Nausea and gastrointestinal upset

- infrequent and usually dose related
- high doses can cause vomiting

▶ **How Long Do I Treat Patients with This Drug?**

Productive coughs

- for the duration of the common cold up to 7 days
- intermittently for chronic bronchitis while under the supervision of a physician (e.g., regularly dosed for 1–2 weeks at a time)

▶ **How Do I Decrease or Stop the Administration of This Drug?**

- may be stopped abruptly at any time

▶ **What Should I Tell My Patients About This Drug?**

- it has a bitter taste but rarely causes gastrointestinal upset
- use adequate dosages and always take with plenty of fluids

- if there is any change in the nature of sputum (e.g., changes in color and blood-tinged sputum) contact your physician

▶ **Therapeutic Tips**

- ensure that adequate dosages are used
- encourage increased fluid intake for expectoration to occur
- liquid, tablets, or sustained-release liquids are available and are a personal preference
- single entity is preferred to allow dosage adjustments
- some clinicians suggest that proper hydration (6–8 cups of water per day) is likely as effective an expectorant as guaifenesin

Useful References

American Hospital Formulary Service. Drug Information, ASHP. Bethesda, MD: 1993.
Health Protection Branch, Second Report of the Expert Advisory Committee on Nonprescription Cough and Cold Remedies. Health and Welfare Canada, 1989:1–50.

HALOPERIDOL

Juan Avila and Patricia Marken

USA (Haldol, Haloperon, Haldol Decanoate)
CANADA (Haldol, Novoperidol, Apo-Haloperidol, PMS Haloperidol, Peridol, Haldol LA)

▶ **When Should I Use This Drug?**

Acute psychosis therapy (if prompt control is required)

- in the acutely psychotic and agitated patient, rapid tranquilization with the goal of quietly calming a dangerous patient
- haloperidol is a high-potency antipsychotic with low anticholinergic activity
- haloperidol produces a lower incidence of sedation and orthostatic hypotension than the low potency antipsychotics (chlorpromazine) but produces a higher incidence of acute, extrapyramidal or dystonic reactions
- drug of choice if the patient is elderly or cardiovascular or seizure disorders are present and if it is less expensive than fluphenazine
- is available in a parenteral form and as a depot preparation
- when a patient has a previous history of response to this agent

Maintenance psychosis therapy

- to ameliorate the symptoms of psychosis that include hallucinations, delusions, formal thought disorder, bizarre behavior, agitation, and/or hyperactivity
- drug of choice if the patient is not compliant because a depot form is available (dosed every 4 weeks in comparison with the fluphenazine depot form, which is given every 2–3 weeks)

Manic phase of bipolar illness

- antipsychotics are often also required for adequate sedation and behavioral control and are usually preferred to benzodiazepines for acutely manic patients with concurrent psychoses; however, there is some evidence that high-dose benzodiazepines may be equally efficacious with fewer adverse effects (J Clin Psychopharmacol 1985;5:109–113)
- decision as to when to choose this agent is as above under acute psychosis therapy

Other uses

- nausea and vomiting, Tourette's disorder

▶ **When Should I Not Use This Drug?**

see Chlorpromazine

▶ **What Contraindications Are There to the Use of This Drug?**

see Chlorpromazine

▶ **What Drug Interactions Are Clinically Important?**

Drugs that may increase the effect or toxicity of haloperidol

CENTRAL NERVOUS SYSTEM DEPRESSANTS (OPIATES, BARBITURATES, GENERAL ANESTHETICS, ALCOHOL)

- excessive sedation and central nervous system (CNS) depression may occur if used concomitantly

- start with low dosages of both agents to avoid excessive sedation or CNS depression, and adjust dosages on the basis of clinical presentation

LITHIUM

- most patients who receive lithium and an antipsychotic agent do not have unusual adverse effects, but occasionally, an acute encephalopathic syndrome has occurred, especially when high serum levels of lithium are present
- this is controversial, as the effect may be no greater than with lithium alone; therefore, observe for clinical signs of this syndrome, but otherwise there is no need to change therapy
- symptoms manifest as neurologic effects
- lithium may also unmask the signs of tardive dyskinesia, which may lead to the discontinuation of haloperidol therapy if tardive dyskinesia develops

Drugs that may decrease the effect of haloperidol

- none

Drugs that may have their effect or toxicity increased by haloperidol

METHYLDOPA

- dementia has been reported in patients using haloperidol concurrently with methyldopa; if this is noted, stop the concomitant use

Drugs that may have their effect decreased by haloperidol

- none

▶ *What Route and Dosage Should I Use?*

How to administer

- orally—take with food or milk or on an empty stomach
- parenterally—intramuscularly only

Acute psychosis therapy (if prompt control is required), manic phase of bipolar illness

- 5–10 mg PO or 2.5–5 mg IM (if the patient will not take oral medication) every 30–60 minutes until control is achieved or the patient does not tolerate the drug (usually 2–3 doses)
- start a maintenance dosage after an adequate response has been seen (see below)
- some clinicians suggest that, after 20 mg IM has been administered, higher dosages may not work but the risk of adverse effects increases
- after 20 mg has been reached, consider increasing the benzodiazepine dosage or switching to a different antipsychotic agent

Maintenance psychosis therapy

- 5 mg PO BID
- 2.5 mg PO BID in smaller or elderly patients
- increase the dosage every 2 weeks until an appropriate response has been seen
- typical maintenance dosage is 15 mg PO daily given as a single daily dose
- maximum daily oral dosage is 100 mg
- to convert to a depot preparation, start with an intramuscular dose of haloperidol decanoate 10–20 times the daily oral dose
- supplement the initial intramuscular dose with an oral dose ($^1/_2$ of the previous oral dose for the first month, then $^1/_4$ of the previous oral dose for the second month) of haloperidol for breakthrough symptoms that may occur
- after the patient is stable, PRN doses may be stopped
- repeat the injection in 4 weeks, increasing the intramuscular dose if the patient became symptomatic between injections
- intramuscular doses can be increased up to 500 mg; however, experience is limited with doses greater than 300 mg/mo

Dosage adjustments for renal or hepatic dysfunction

- hepatically metabolized
- no specific dosage adjustments; just start with a low dose and titrate to effect

▶ *What Should I Monitor with Regard to Efficacy and Toxicity?*

see Chlorpromazine

▶ *How Long Do I Treat Patients with This Drug?*

see Chlorpromazine

▶ *How Do I Decrease or Stop the Administration of This Drug?*

see Chlorpromazine

▶ *What Should I Tell My Patients About This Drug?*

see Chlorpromazine

▶ *Therapeutic Tips*

see Chlorpromazine

Useful References

Kane JM. The current status of neuroleptic therapy. J Clin Psychiatry 1989;50:322–328

Hemstrom CA, Evans RL, Lobeck FG. Haloperidol decanoate: A depot antipsychotic. DICP 1988;22:290–295

Coryell W, Kelly M, Perry PJ, Miller DD. Haloperidol plasma levels and acute clinical change in schizophrenia. J Clin Psychopharmacol 1990; 10:397–402

Alexander B. Antipsychotics: How strict the formulary? DICP 1988;22: 324–326

HEPARIN

Frances Chow

USA (sodium salt: Liquaemin Sodium, Hep-Lock; calcium salt: Calciparine)
CANADA (sodium salt: Hepalean, Heparin Leo; calcium salt: Calciparine subcutaneous, Calcilean)

▶ *When Should I Use This Drug?*

Deep vein thrombosis or pulmonary embolism

- heparin acts immediately to inhibit the clotting cascade and speeds the resolution of symptoms
- if the patient is pregnant, use heparin only until postpartum, then institute warfarin therapy
- heparin is the anticoagulant of choice in pregnancy because it does not cross the placenta (N Engl J Med 1991;324:1565–1574, Chest 1992;102:385S–390S)

Venous thromboembolism prevention

Bedridden patients with one or more of the following risk factors should receive prophylaxis

- advanced age (older than 40 years)
- prolonged immobility or paralysis
- prior venous thromboembolism
- cancer
- surgical operations (particularly those involving the lower extremities or pelvis)
- obesity
- varicose veins
- CHF
- oral contraceptive use
- patients with known hypercoagulable states

Drug therapy is not required for low-risk general surgery patients without any of the above risk factors

Progressing stroke

- anticoagulation for this condition is controversial and the use of heparin is anecdotal
- anticoagulation should be used only in cases of progressing stroke in which hemorrhage has been ruled out by computed tomographic scan and there are major progressing neurological deficits; otherwise, do not anticoagulate

Prevention of cardiogenic cerebral embolism

Mechanical prosthetic valves, bioprosthetic mitral valves

- anticoagulation with warfarin is required
- heparin would be needed only if the patient could not take warfarin

Myocardial infarction

- all patients with a myocardial infarction (MI) should receive heparin to prevent thromboembolism, further coronary artery thrombosis, mural thrombus, and systemic embolism (Chest 1992;102[suppl]:456S–481S)

- heparin therapy should be instituted, even in patients who do not receive thrombolytic therapy
- heparin should be used to prevent coronary reocclusion with tissue plasminogen activator and should be started concomitantly with tissue plasminogen activator to help decrease the risk of reocclusion
- American College of Chest Physicians offers a Grade C (their weakest) recommendation for the use of heparin after thrombolysis with streptokinase (Chest 1992;102:4565–4815), which have not been strengthened by the results of the GUSTO trial (N Engl J Med 1993;329:673–682)
- heparin therapy should be used for high-risk patients to prevent deep vein thrombosis
- high-risk patients are those older than 70 years, with a history of previous MI, large anterior MI, heart failure, or shock
- preventive subcutaneous regimen should be considered in patients who are immobilized for longer than 3 days, are obese, or have signs of chronic venous insufficiency

▶ When Should I Not Use This Drug?

Maintaining patency of indwelling venipuncture device

- normal saline is as effective, less expensive, and less toxic (DICP 1991;25:399–406)

Transient ischemic attacks

- potential side effects are greater than the benefit, and aspirin is the drug of choice

Disseminated intravascular coagulation

- clotting mechanisms already impaired
- however, in cases of promyelocytic leukemia and disseminated intravascular coagulation (DIC) complicated by thrombosis, heparin can be used

▶ What Contraindications Are There to the Use of This Drug?

Intolerance of or allergic reaction to heparin
Uncontrolled bleeding

- arterial bleeding or presently active bleeding can be worsened with heparin

Hemorrhagic blood dyscrasias (hemophilia, vascular purpuras, thrombocytopenia)

- heparin makes these conditions worse

Dissecting aneurysm, or eye, brain, or spinal cord surgery

- risk of hemorrhage is high

▶ What Drug Interactions Are Clinically Important?

Drugs that may increase the effect or toxicity of heparin
ASPIRIN, NONSTEROIDAL ANTIINFLAMMATORY DRUG, DIPYRIDAMOLE

- these drugs affect platelet function and can increase the risk of hemorrhage
- use acetaminophen or narcotic analgesics
- in the case of post–MI patients, low-dose aspirin therapy should be used in combination, as the benefit outweighs the risk
- in patients who require high-dose aspirin or nonsteroidal antiinflammatory drugs to control adequately a life-altering disease (e.g., rheumatoid arthritis), the combination can be used; however, keep partial thromboplastin time (PTT) at the lower limit of desired values and make the patient aware of the potential for bleeding

Drugs that may decrease the effect of heparin
PROTAMINE

- used for severe hemorrhage or heparin overdose (with clinical evidence of bleeding)

Drugs that may have their effect or toxicity increased by heparin

- none

Drugs that may have their effect decreased by heparin

- none

▶ What Route and Dosage Should I Use?

How to administer

- parenterally—25,000 units in 500 mL of dextrose or saline solutions

Deep vein thrombosis or pulmonary embolism

- 100 units/kg (either 5000 units, 7500 units, or 10,000 units) IV bolus followed by a continuous infusion of 1250 units/h
- measure PTT 6 hours after the initiation of infusion and 6 hours after every dosage change
- adjust the dosage to prolong PTT to 1.5–2 times normal values (normal, 25–35 seconds)

PTT Results	Dosage Adjustment	Time of Repeated PTT
<50	give 5000 unit bolus and increase infusion by 100 units/h	repeat in 6 hours
50–59	increase infusion by 100 units/h	repeat in 6 hours
60–85	no change	repeat next morning
86–95	decrease infusion by 100 units/h	repeat next morning
96–120	stop infusion for 30 minutes and decrease infusion by 100 units/h	repeat in 6 hours
>120	stop infusion for 60 minutes and decrease infusion rate by 200 units/h	repeat in 6 hours

Venous thromboembolism prevention
High-risk patients with low bleeding risk

- 5000 units subcutaneously 2 hours prior to surgery and 5000 units subcutaneously Q8H
- PTT measurements are not required

Moderate-risk patients with low bleeding risk

- 5000 units subcutaneously 2 hours prior to surgery and 5000 units subcutaneously Q12H
- PTT measurements are not required

Progressing stroke

- 100 units/kg (either 5000 units, 7500 units, or 10,000 units) IV bolus followed by a continuous infusion of 1250 units/h started after hemorrhagic stroke has been ruled out
- adjust the dosage to prolong PTT to 1.5–2 times normal values (normal, 25–35 seconds)

Prevention of cardiogenic cerebral embolism

- 100 units/kg (either 5000 units, 7500 units, or 10,000 units) IV bolus followed by a continuous infusion of 1250 units/h started 6 hours after valve replacement or concomitantly with tissue type plasminogen activator and 1–3 hours after the start of streptokinase administration to help to decrease the risk of reocclusion in MI patients (Chest 1992;102[suppl]:456S–481S)

Dosage adjustments for renal or hepatic dysfunction

- hepatically eliminated
- no dosage adjustments for renal failure
- adjust dosage on the basis of PTT in patients with hepatic dysfunction

▶ What Should I Monitor with Regard to Efficacy and Toxicity?

Efficacy
Deep vein thrombosis or pulmonary embolism
Vein thrombosis
Limb circumference, swelling, tenderness, perfusion

- assess the patient daily

Partial thromboplastin time

- measure PTT every 6 hours until therapeutic and then monitor daily

Pulmonary embolism
Apprehension, cough, tachycardia, hypotension, pleuritic chest pain, hemoptysis
- assess the patient daily

Partial thromboplastin time
- measure PTT every 6 hours until therapeutic and then monitor daily

Venous thromboembolism prevention
Clinical signs
- monitor daily for signs of venous thromboembolism, such as changes in limb circumference, swelling, tenderness, and perfusion

Partial thromboplastin time
- no need to monitor PTT in otherwise healthy patients
- if patients are malnourished, have prior coagulation problems, or are receiving broad-spectrum antibiotics, do baseline PTT and repeat in 3 days to evaluate the effect of heparin

Progressing stroke
Stroke stabilization
- assess whether the stoke is stabilizing

Partial thromboplastin time
- measure PTT every 6 hours until therapeutic and then monitor daily

Prevention of cardiogenic cerebral embolism
Evidence of cerebral embolism
- transient ischemic attacks or strokes

Partial thromboplastin time
- measure PTT every 6 hours until therapeutic and then monitor daily

Toxicity
Symptoms of bleeding
- check daily for epistaxis, bleeding gums, hemoptysis, orthostatic hypotension, melena or bright red stools, blood in urine, increased bruising, local irritation, erythema, and hematomas
- if minor hemorrhage occurs, check PTT and decrease heparin administration if PTT is elevated
- if severe hemorrhage occurs, stop heparin administration and give protamine and/or blood transfusion
- administer protamine sulfate IV only if necessary (e.g., patient is bleeding and still has enough heparin in circulation to have problems potentially)
- protamine is more likely useful if the patient is being given subcutaneous heparin, as the heparin is released over an extended period
- calculate the amount of heparin still in the circulation (assume heparin has a half-life of $1^1/_2$ hours)
- for every $1^1/_2$ hours, the amount of heparin present is reduced by 50% (e.g., if 10,000 units are given by accident, 3 hours later only 2500 units of heparin are still in circulation)
- 1 mg of protamine neutralizes 100 units of heparin

Thrombocytopenia
- occurs in 5% of patients and is usually only a small change and is reversible
- monitor platelet count after 5 days of heparin therapy and weekly thereafter
- stop heparin administration if the platelet count falls below $100,000/mm^3$ because a severe heparin-induced thrombosis-thrombocytopenia syndrome may occur

Osteoporosis and spontaneous fractures
- can occur if the patient receives greater than 10,000 units/d for 3 months but is rare

▶ How Long Do I Treat Patients with This Drug?
Deep vein thrombosis or pulmonary embolism
- heparin should be given for a minimum of 5 days but should be continued until warfarin therapy has yielded an international

normalized ratio (INR) of 2–3 (a PT ratio of 1.3–1.5 times control values) (Chest 1992;102:408S–425S, N Engl J Med 1991;324: 1565–1574)
- in pregnancy, heparin should be given in full intravenous dosages for 7–10 days followed by subcutaneous injections given Q12H to prolong the 6 hour postinjection PTT to 1.5–2 times control values until delivery

Venous thromboembolism prevention
- should be continued until the patient is ambulatory (i.e., no longer confined to bed)
- patients with recurrent vein thrombosis or with a continuing risk factor such as antithrombin III deficiency, protein C or S deficiency, and malignancy should be treated indefinitely (Chest 1992;102:408S–425S)

Progressing stroke
- continue anticoagulation until the patient has stabilized (typically used for 3–5 days) (Chest 1992;102:529S–537S)
- if the stroke has not stabilized after 48 hours of therapy, stop the anticoagulation and be sure that worsening of the clinical condition is not due to hemorrhagic stroke or another medical condition

Prevention of cardiogenic cerebral embolism
- heparin should be given for a minimum of 5 days but should not be discontinued before warfarin therapy has yielded a therapeutic INR (Chest 1989;95:37S–51S, N Engl J Med 1991;324:1565–1574)

▶ How Do I Decrease or Stop the Administration of This Drug?
- may be stopped abruptly

▶ What Should I Tell My Patients About This Drug?
- this drug reduces the risk of your developing another blood clot in your legs or lungs
- it may cause you to bleed a little longer if you cut yourself but you should still stop bleeding spontaneously or by applying slight pressure to the site
- if it does not or the cut is deep, go to the emergency department
- if a simple analgesic is required, use acetaminophen

▶ Therapeutic Tips
- start warfarin administration simultaneously with heparin when treating deep vein thrombosis or pulmonary embolism to decrease the time required to get the patient anticoagulated with warfarin and to decrease the length of hospital stay
- risk of bleeding is not closely correlated with a particular PTT but rather the amount and duration of heparin therapy
- major risk in the first 24 hours with heparin therapy is underdosing not overdosing; therefore, do not titrate the dose slowly upward over 48–72 hours
- rebolusing and quick titration is important to prevent recurrence of deep vein thromboses
- avoid IM injections, if possible, to prevent the risk of hematomas while patient is on heparin

Useful References
Third ACCP Consensus Conference on Antithrombotic Therapy Chest 1992;102:303S–550S
Hirsh J. Heparin. N Engl J Med 1991;324:1565–1574
Cruickshank MK, Levine MN, Hirsh J, et al. A standard heparin nomogram for the management of heparin therapy. Arch Intern Med 1991; 151:333–337

HYDROCHLOROTHIAZIDE
Ian Petterson

USA (Aquazide H, Diaqua, Esidrix, Hydro-D, HydroDIURIL, Ezide, Oretic)
CANADA (Apo-Hydro, HydroDIURIL)

▶ When Should I Use This Drug?
Decision among the different thiazide diuretics should be based on cost, as there is little, if any, difference in clinical effect

among these agents • Although chlorthalidone has a slightly longer duration of activity, this confers no benefit, as thiazide diuretics are all dosed once daily and are well tolerated

Chronic (noncrisis) hypertension

- drug of choice for initial management of mild to moderate hypertension in patients with no other disease states, and in patients with congestive heart failure, chronic obstructive pulmonary disease, or asthma
- is as effective as any of the other antihypertensive agents, allows once-a-day dosing, and is inexpensive
- low-dose therapy is associated with few adverse effects and has proven effectiveness in reducing mortality and morbidity due to strokes, myocardial infarction (JAMA 1991;265:3255–3264), and cardiac and renal failure
- also useful for the treatment of hypertension in patients with insulin-dependent diabetes because, when used in low doses, there is little if any effect on glucose control; however, in patients with non–insulin-dependent diabetes, other agents should be chosen, as thiazide diuretics, mainly in high doses, can cause an increase in blood glucose concentrations
- also useful for the treatment of hypertension in patients with mild hyperlipidemia, as the lipid changes are usually slight, are short lived, and have no proven consequence
- complications due to atherosclerosis are decreased with these agents (e.g., a reduction in myocardial infarctions has been seen in elderly patients when treated with thiazide diuretics) (Br Med J 1992;304:412–416)
- drug of choice for hypertension in patients with recurrent urinary calcium calculi, as the urine calcium level is decreased and the serum calcium level is increased
- has additive hypotensive effects with most other antihypertensives and is especially useful in combination with beta-blockers and angiotensin converting enzyme (ACE) inhibitors (Arch Intern Med 1990;150:1175–1183)
- drug of choice in elderly patients with either diastolic or isolated systolic hypertension because of unquestionable effectiveness (JAMA 1991;265:3255–3264) plus decreased osteoporosis (Lancet 1989;1:687–690, N Engl J Med 1990;322:286–290, JAMA 1991;265:370–373)

Congestive heart failure

- is the diuretic of choice for the management of symptoms associated with mild congestive heart failure in patients with preexisting hypertension
- effective for both hypertension and mild congestive heart failure and less expensive than ACE inhibitors
- in mild failure without hypertension, or in severe congestive heart failure or congestive heart failure with renal insufficiency, use furosemide because it is a more effective diuretic and causes less severe metabolic changes than do thiazide diuretics when used in equivalent saluretic dosages
- diuretic effect (versus the antihypertensive effect) of hydrochlorothiazide is not always maintained for an extended period

Ascites associated with hepatic cirrhosis

- in cirrhosis with ascites and edema, thiazide diuretics are useful in low-dose combination with spironolactone
- spironolactone is considered the diuretic of choice because of increased production and decreased metabolism of aldosterone in patients with ascites
- furosemide should be considered before thiazide diuretics, as it is a more effective diuretic

Other uses

- diabetes insipidus

▶ When Should I Not Use This Drug?

Acute (crisis) hypertension

- thiazide diuretics have not been evaluated in this condition but can be started along with other therapy if thiazide diuretics would be considered appropriate long-term therapy

Edema associated with more severe cardiac or renal failure

- furosemide is a more effective and reliable diuretic agent

Edema due to nephrotic syndrome

- this is frequently thiazide resistant; therefore, furosemide should be used as first-line therapy

▶ What Contraindications Are There to the Use of This Drug?

Intolerance of or allergic reaction to hydrochlorothiazide

Moderate to severe renal insufficiency (creatinine clearance < 30 mL/min)

- drug is ineffective

Hyperparathyroidism or vitamin D toxicity

- thiazides decrease calciuresis and increase serum calcium levels and may lead to severe hypercalemia

Severe hyperlipidemia or hypercholesterolemia

- low doses of thiazides for hypertension do not cause alterations in lipid levels or acceleration of atherosclerosis
- however thiazide diuretics should likely not be used in patients with severe hyperlipidemia necessitating drug therapy

Hypovolemia or volume depletion

- may cause further volume depletion and lead to serious hyponatremia

▶ What Drug Interactions Are Clinically Important?

Drugs that may increase the effect or toxicity of hydrochlorothiazide

OTHER DIURETICS

- other diuretics, especially furosemide, may increase the risk of hypokalemia, hypomagnesemia, hypotension, and prerenal failure
- avoid combination if possible; if not, ensure the lowest effective dose of each agent is used

Drugs that may decrease the effect of hydrochlorothiazide

NONSTEROIDAL ANTIINFLAMMATORY DRUGS

- combination increases risk of renal failure and may reverse antihypertensive effect
- avoid combination if possible; and if not, monitor serum creatinine and potassium levels and weight at baseline and every 4 days for 2–3 weeks, then every 2 weeks for 8 weeks, then every month for 3 months, and then as needed (J Musculoskel Med 1991;8[8]:31–46)
- in patients who must use NSAIDs, ensure the lowest effective dose is being used

Drugs that may have their effect or toxicity increased by hydrochlorothiazide

LITHIUM

- decreases renal lithium clearance and increases serum lithium levels
- if possible, use alternative agent such as spironolactone and furosemide
- toxicity due to increased lithium levels can be life-threatening
- monitor lithium level as for a dosage change of lithium (after 5 days) after initiating thiazide therapy or earlier if symptoms of toxicity are seen
- adjust lithium dosage on the basis of lithium levels
- new steady state should be achieved in 5–7 days
- if the dosage is already at upper end of lithium's therapeutic range, empirically decrease the lithium dosage by 30%

Drugs that may have their effect decreased by hydrochlorothiazide

ORAL HYPOGLYCEMICS

- is dose related and is most likely with thiazide diuretics, chlorthalidone, metolazone; less likely with furosemide; much less likely with bumetanide and ethacrynic acid; and least likely with amiloride, spironolactone, and triameterene
- while clinicians must be aware that hydrochlorothiazide, especially in high doses, can worsen glycemic control in some patients, data suggest that diuretics, when used long term, prevent the onset of microalbuminuria in non–insulin-dependent diabet-

ics and do not worsen glycemic control (Hypertension 1993; 21:786–794)

▶ *What Route and Dosage Should I Use?*

How to administer

- orally—may be given with food or on an empty stomach
- parenterally—not available

Chronic (noncrisis) hypertension

- start with 12.5 mg PO daily
- some clinicians advocate the use of 6.25 mg as a starting dose, but the difficulty in attaining this dose makes it impractical
- dosage may be increased every 2–4 weeks if the current dosage is not adequately controlling blood pressure
- dosage should rarely exceed 25 mg and never exceed 50 mg daily, as there is no greater hypotensive effect with higher dosages and an increased incidence of adverse reactions occurs

Congestive heart failure

- 25 mg PO daily if being used as sole diuretic therapy
- dosage may be increased after 2 weeks to 50 mg PO daily if the current dosage is not adequately controlling the edema
- adverse metabolic effects at dosages greater than 50 mg limit effectiveness; however, dosages up to 100 mg PO daily can be tried in patients unresponsive to 50 mg PO daily
- in cardiac failure, thiazide diuretics are effective in potentiating the action of loop diuretics (furosemide) especially in resistant heart failure
- for patients already receiving furosemide, start with low dosages (12.5 mg daily) and be aware of possible profound volume depletion and electrolyte disturbances with standard dosages (Ann Intern Med 1991;114:886–894)

Ascites associated with hepatic cirrhosis

- 12.5 mg PO daily
- increase the dosage to 25 mg PO daily in 2 weeks
- if 25 mg PO daily is ineffective, consider switching to furosemide
- in cirrhosis, if an effect is not seen with 50 mg daily, the addition of low-dose spironolactone has an additive effect and reverses hypokalemia

Dosage adjustments for renal or hepatic dysfunction

- renally eliminated
- no adjustment is needed for renal impairment, except avoid use in patients with moderate to severe renal function (creatinine clearance < 30 mL/min), as effectiveness is lost

▶ *What Should I Monitor with Regard to Efficacy and Toxicity?*

Efficacy

Chronic (noncrisis) hypertension

Blood pressure

- patients with diastolic blood pressures greater than 115 mmHg or with symptoms should be evaluated again within 48 hours to ensure that at least a 5–10 mmHg drop in blood pressure has occurred
- for patients with diastolic blood pressures less than 115 mmHg, follow-up blood pressures should be done within a couple of weeks
- at each visit, do 2 blood pressure measurements, supine or sitting, after the patient has been resting without conversation for 5–10 minutes
- continue to do this every 4 weeks to assess the effect of each new drug or dosage until control is achieved
- for most patients with mild hypertension, after blood pressure is controlled, blood pressure measurement 2–4 times per year is sufficient

Evidence of end-organ damage

- if blood pressure is well controlled and no other disease states exist (e.g., diabetes), measure baseline serum creatinine, blood glucose, serum cholesterol levels and perform urinalysis and repeat every 5 years
- repeat every year if other disease states are present

Congestive heart failure

Signs and symptoms of mild to moderate heart failure

- dyspnea, orthopnea, paroxysmal nocturnal dyspnea, fatigue, ankle swelling, fine crackles on chest auscultation, weight, liver size, and absence of S_3 heart sound
- jugular venous pressure should be normal to slightly increased
- for patients with acute symptoms, assess at least twice daily while the patient is in the hospital
- after the patient is discharged, assess within a week of discharge
- after the patient is stabilized, decrease the frequency of evaluation
- for patients with mild symptoms, assess weekly until symptoms are controlled

Ascites associated with hepatic cirrhosis

- treatment needs to proceed slowly to prevent acid-base, fluid, and electrolyte imbalances, which can precipitate hepatic encephalopathy
- 3 primary goals of therapy are weight loss of 0.3–1 kg/d, urine output of 300–1000 mL/d over daily input, and the patient's comfort

Toxicity

Hypokalemia

- dose dependent but the incidence and the magnitude are low on dosages of 12.5–25 mg PO daily, with the maximum hypokalemic effect seen in the first month
- effect is variable, the drop ranges from 0.1 to 0.6 mEq/L within the first week
- monitor the potassium levels at 2 weeks and at the end of 1 month
- after the patient is stable, repeat measurement only if dosage or disease state changes occur
- if serum potassium levels decrease to less than 3.5 mEq/L (or <4 mEq/L while receiving digoxin), supplement by increasing dietary potassium and restricting sodium intake
- if this is not effective, add amiloride 2.5 mg PO daily (if treating hypertension, there is an additive hypotensive effect) or spironolactone 25 mg PO daily (if treating edema)
- potassium supplements are routinely not effective; large dosages (>40 mEq/d) are required, and these are often inconvenient and not well tolerated

Hyponatremia

- rare and unpredictable but worse in dehydrated and elderly patients
- measure sodium levels daily in patients with acute congestive heart failure

Hypomagnesemia

- incidence less than with loop diuretics and rare with dosages less than 50 mg PO daily
- routine serum magnesium levels are not recommended, as they are not a good indication of total body magnesium concentrations

Hyperuricemia

- only a concern if the patient has a personal or family history of gout; routine monitoring of uric acid levels is unnecessary (Am J Med 1987;82:421–426)
- if the patient has a history of gout and hydrochlorothiazide is to be started, tell the patient to let you know if an attack occurs and measure uric acid level at the time of the attack
- uricosuric agents or allopurinol can be used without compromising diuretic activity or efficacy

Hypercalcemia

- rare in a patient who is previously normocalcemic
- expect a rise in serum calcium level of approximately 0.2 mg/dL (0.05 mmol/L) within the first month
- may be a useful effect in preventing osteoporosis and fractures in elderly patients (Lancet 1989;1:687–690, N Engl J Med 1990;322:286–290, JAMA 1991;265:370–373)
- effect probably useful only with pure thiazide use, as the effect is not seen in combination products
- 30% reduction in recurrent calcium urinary tract calculi

Hyperlipidemia

- expect an occasional, transient, small rise in total serum cholesterol, LDL, and triglyceride levels, with HDL levels usually not affected
- effect on cholesterol is no different from that with most other antihypertensives and placebo and does not persist at 1 year (N Engl J Med 1993;328:914–921)
- clinical significance of this is not known, and there is no evidence of enhanced atheroslerosis and in fact, atherosclerotic associated target organ events are reduced

Hyperglycemia

- thiazide diuretics cause impairment of glucose tolerance, decrease insulin sensitivity, increase hemoglobin A_{1c} levels, and cause worsening of glucose control, but this effect is small and uncommon with low dosages (Ann Intern Med 1992;118:273–278)
- high dosages have been associated with the precipitation of diabetes mellitus and the development of hyperosmolar, nonketotic diabetic coma in the elderly
- when used in low dosages in patients with insulin-dependent diabetes, there is little if any effect on glucose control
- data suggest that diuretics, when used long term, prevent the onset of microalbuminuria in non–insulin-dependent diabetes and do not worsen glycemic control (Hypertension 1993;21: 786–794)
- diuretics need not be avoided in patients with non–insulin-dependent diabetes

Renal function

- increased serum urea and creatinine level may occasionally be seen but is likely not indicative of nephrotoxity but due to hypovolemia and decreased glomerular filtration rate, indicating excess diuretic use
- monitor baseline urea and creatinine levels every 3–4 months thereafter for patients with initial diminished function

▶ How Long Do I Treat Patients with This Drug?

Chronic (noncrisis) hypertension

Stepped-down therapy, in general, should be considered in patients whose blood pressures during the previous few visits have been well controlled

- approximately 50% of patients with well-controlled disease successfully undergo either dosage or drug reduction and the disease remains controlled for a time, but unfortunately, this time period varies from patient to patient and consistent reevaluation is necessary
- this may be explained by reversal of cardiac and vascular changes that may occur after prolonged treatment with drug therapy and may be a means of "setting back the clock" of primary hypertension evolution
- as with every treatment, not everyone has blood pressure successfully respond to drug discontinuation or drug dosage reduction
- patients most likely to have a successful reduction or discontinuation of therapy may be predicted by a low pretreatment blood pressure (mild hypertension with diastolic pressure < 100 mmHg), no evidence of target organ damage, requirement of only monotherapy for blood pressure control, and weight loss, salt restriction, increased exercise, and a decrease in alcohol intake
- reassessment allows a reevaluation of the efficacy of nondrug measures in the treatment of hypertension such as reducing weight and reducing salt and alcohol intake

Congestive heart failure

- seek the lowest dosage of diuretic compatible with maximum symptom relief
- usually need less diuretic when the patient is stable and free from acute precipitants that may have brought the patient to medical attention
- trial of decreased dosage is warranted after the patient has been stabilized for 2–3 months; however, one can rarely withdraw diuretics completely

Ascites associated with hepatic cirrhosis

- treat until the cause of exacerbation of ascites is gone
- treatment may be lifelong if ascites is due to alcoholic cirrhosis; however, always reevaluate for the lowest effective dosage

▶ How Do I Decrease or Stop the Administration of This Drug?

Chronic (noncrisis) hypertension

- gradual dosage or drug reduction along with a precise discussion of why the reduction is being done and what the goals of therapy are avoids most of the patient's psychological dependence
- in patients controlled with single-drug therapy, the dosage should be reduced by 50% with reassessment of blood pressure at 2 weeks
- if the patient is still normotensive, reduce the dosage by another 50% (i.e., to 25% of the initial dose) and recheck blood pressure in another 2 weeks
- if the blood pressure is still well controlled, discontinue the drug and recheck the blood pressure in 2 weeks
- so-called rebound hypertension does not occur if the dosage is gradually tapered, with dosage reductions of no more than 50% at 2–4 week intervals
- final dose before full drug discontinuation should be less than ¼ the dose of the initial therapy

Congestive heart failure, ascites associated with cirrhosis

- tapering of the drug is wise because rebound salt and water retention over 1–2 weeks occurs unpredictably and can be prevented by slow withdrawal over 2–4 weeks (as above)

▶ What Should I Tell My Patients About This Drug?

- this drug works on your kidney to eliminate excess salt and water from your body and/or to decrease your blood pressure
- if you notice your feet or any other part of your body becoming puffy, this may indicate that your salt consumption is excessive or the current dosage is no longer effective, and you should consult your physician
- if you begin to feel weak, dizzy, or lightheaded, you should contact your physician, as this may indicate an electrolyte abnormality
- take this drug in the morning, and it may be taken with food or on an empty stomach, but try to take it the same way every day

▶ Therapeutic Tips

- drug is ineffective in moderate to severe renal failure (creatinine clearance < 30 mL/min)
- always start with a low dose and titrate slowly upward as needed
- start with 12.5 mg/d and do not exceed 50 mg/d, except in patients with severe unresponsive congestive heart failure
- drug effectiveness is enhanced and hypokalemia minimized by a sodium-restricted diet
- 60% of patients receiving 50 mg/d can have the dosage effectively decreased to 25 mg/d or less without loss of efficacy, and this is usually associated with lower side effects (Arch Intern Med 1990;150:1009–1011)
- never start with a combination product (e.g., hydrochlorothiazide plus amiloride) and always titrate each drug individually and use a combination product only if dosages are correct for the individual patient
- thiazide diuretics may reduce osteoporosis and fractures in the elderly
- addition of small doses of hydrochlorothiazide to patients with furosemide-resistant heart failure markedly potentiates diuresis

Useful References

Nader C, Thompson JR, Alpern RJ. Complications of diuretic use. Semin Nephrol 1988;8:365–387

Black HR. Metabolic considerations in the choice of therapy for the patient with hypertension. Am Heart J 1991;121:707–715

Freis ED. Critique of the clinical importance of diuretic induced hypokalemia and elevated cholesterol levels. Arch Intern Med 1989;149:2640–2648

HYDROCORTISONE SODIUM SUCCINATE

Karen Shalansky and Cindy Reesor Nimmo

USA (Cortef, Solu-Cortef, generics)
CANADA (Cortef, Solu-Cortef)

▶ *When Should I Use This Drug?*

Acute asthma or bronchitis, prevention of adrenal insufficiency, rheumatoid arthritis, migraine, acquired immunodeficiency syndrome (AIDS) with *Pneumocystis carinii* pneumonia, ulcerative colitis, skin disorders, organ transplant, collagen disease

- hydrocortisone is the parenteral corticosteroid of choice in patients unable to take oral prednisone who require short-term therapy (shorter than 3 days)
- hydrocortisone has significant mineralocorticoid activity and high dosages for prolonged periods may cause significant fluid and electrolyte abnormalities and hypertension
- if high-dose parenteral steroids are required for longer than 3 days, use methylprednisolone instead of hydrocortisone because methylprednisolone has less mineralocorticoid activity (20 mg of hydrocortisone is equivalent to 4 mg of methylprednisolone)

▶ *When Should I Not Use This Drug?*

When oral corticosteroids can be used

- oral corticosteroids are as effective as parenteral steroids for the treatment of acute asthma

As oral therapy

- hydrocortisone has a short half-life and may not provide relief throughout the day
- use prednisone as an alternative

▶ *What Contraindications Are There to the Use of This Drug?*

Intolerance of or allergic reaction to hydrocortisone

Patients with coexisting heart failure or hypertension

- hydrocortisone displays significant mineralocorticoid activity, and high dosages for prolonged periods may aggravate these conditions
- use methylprednisolone if parenteral corticosteroid therapy is required

Viral, fungal, or active or quiescent tuberculosis infections

- corticosteroids depress the body's immune system and its ability to fight infections and should not be used unless absolutely required

Vaccinations

- poor response due to lack of antibody production and possible neurological complications
- avoid live viral vaccines (e.g., varicella vaccine)

Osteoporosis, psychoses, diabetes mellitus, or glaucoma

- corticosteroids may potentiate these conditions; therefore, use in the lowest possible dosages

▶ *What Drug Interactions Are Clinically Important?*

see Prednisone

▶ *What Route and Dosage Should I Use?*

How to administer

- orally—do not use; use prednisone
- parenterally—for hydrocortisone sodium succinate, dilute in either 2 mL of bacteriostatic water or normal saline and infuse over 30–60 seconds; may also be diluted in a further 100 mL (for a 100 mg dose) or 250 mL (250 mg dose) of 5% dextrose in water or normal saline

Acute asthma, bronchitis, rheumatoid arthritis

- 250 mg IV Q6H for 24–48 hours, then taper (25% of dose every 1–2 days as tolerated) or convert to oral prednisone if oral therapy is tolerated

- although a conversion of 20 mg of hydrocortisone to 5 mg of prednisone can be used, most clinicians use a maximum of 60 mg of prednisone daily

Prevention of adrenal insufficiency

- 100 mg IV the night before surgery, then 100 mg every 6 hours for 72 hours for major surgery
- 100 mg IV every 6 hours for 24 hours for minor or short procedures
- 100 mg IV prior to the procedure for short surgical or stressful diagnostic procedures

Migraine

- 250 mg IV Q6H for 24–48 hours or until the patient can take oral prednisone

AIDS with *Pneumocystis carinii* pneumonia

- 250 mg IV Q6H for 24–48 hours or until the patient can take oral prednisone

Ulcerative colitis

- 100 mg IV Q8H for 24–48 hours or until the patient can take oral prednisone

Dosage adjusments for renal or hepatic dysfunction

- hepatically metabolized
- no adjustments required; just titrate dosage to effect and toxicity

▶ *What Should I Monitor with Regard to Efficacy and Toxicity?*

see Prednisone

▶ *How Long Do I Treat Patients with This Drug?*

see Prednisone

▶ *How Do I Decrease or Stop the Administration of This Drug?*

see Prednisone

▶ *What Should I Tell My Patients About This Drug?*

see Prednisone

Useful References

Kelly HW, Murphy S. Corticosteroids for acute, severe asthma. DICP 1991;25:72–79

Siegel SC. Overview of corticosteroid therapy. J Allergy Clin Immunol 1985;76:312–320

HYDROMORPHONE

Terry Baumann

USA (Dilaudid, various)
CANADA (Dilaudid, various)

▶ *When Should I Use This Drug?*

Acute pain, cancer pain, chronic noncancer pain

- there are no apparent clinical differences between hydromorphone and morphine
- hydromorphone has an advantage over morphine when used parenterally in that it can be administered in smaller volumes of fluid, because of its higher potency, which may be useful for subcutaneous infusions or epidural administration when extremely high doses and small volumes are needed

Postoperative pain

- other than a slightly more rapid onset of analgesic effect after oral dosing (AHFS Drug Information 1994:1296), hydromorphone has no advantages over morphine (similar side effects and analgesic effect)

▶ *When Should I Not Use This Drug?*

Mild to moderate pain (acute or chronic)

- unless drugs such as acetaminophen, acetaminophen-codeine (or nonsteroidal antiinflammatory drugs (NSAIDs)) have been used on a regularly scheduled basis (not PRN) and are shown to be ineffective

▶ What Contraindications Are There to the Use of This Drug?

Intolerance of or allergic reaction to hydromorphone

- true allergies to hydromorphone are rare
- check that the patient has actual allergic symptoms, and if there is a true allergy, consider meperidine, anileridine (N/A USA) methadone, or fentanyl

Severe respiratory depression

- not an absolute contraindication, just start with dosages of 25% of the normal initial dose and titrate up to an effect while assessing respiratory rate and oximetry before each dose

▶ What Drug Interactions Are Clinically Important?

see Morphine

▶ What Route and Dosage Should I Use?

How to administer

- orally—may be administered with food or milk or on an empty stomach
- parenterally—may be administered intramuscularly, intravenously (dilute IV hydromorphone in 10 mL of normal saline and give over at least 2 minutes), subcutaneously, and epidurally

Acute pain

- 4 mg PO Q4H (not PRN) or 2 mg PO Q4H (not PRN) for elderly patients because of concerns about sedation and respiratory depression
- consider giving oral hydromorphone if the patient is able to tolerate oral medications because it is less expensive than the parenteral route and has high patient and nurse acceptability; but be aware that the oral route has a slightly slower onset (15–60 minutes) than does the intramuscular route (15–30 minutes)
- 1 mg IM or SC Q4H (not PRN) or 0.5 mg IM or SC Q4H (not PRN) for elderly patients because of concerns about sedation and respiratory depression
- question patients frequently about the degree of pain they are having (ideally within at most 1–2 hours after the first dose if the drug was administered via the PO or IM route)
- if pain is unrelieved by this time, and there are no signs of sedation or respiratory depression, give another dose 50% higher than the first dose
- continue this approach until pain is 75% relieved and then maintain at this dosage for 12 hours before further adjustments are made
- normal dose increments are 1, 2, and 4 mg
- if an immediate response (within 1–5 minutes) for severe pain is needed, use intravenously as recommended for postoperative pain

Chronic cancer pain, chronic noncancer pain

Patient who has received only weak opioids in the past

- 2 mg PO Q4H (not PRN) or 1 mg PO Q4H for elderly patients because of concerns about sedation and respiratory depression
- almost always give by mouth unless the patient has uncontrollable nausea or vomiting
- oral route is inexpensive and has high patient and nurse acceptability

Patient being switched from another opioid

- determine the average daily requirements for the previous opioids and determine the 24 hour morphine equivalent
- 24 hour requirements for hydromophone should be divided by 6 and given every 4 hours
- if the previous opioid has not been effective, the total daily dose of hydromorphone should be increased by 25–50%
- adjust as above for acute pain
- attempt to get pain at least 90% controlled
- after pain has been controlled, always order PRN doses at 25–50% of the maintenance dosage for breakthrough pain in addition to the regular dose

Continuous infusion intravenously and subcutaneously

- initial infusion rate should be based on the previous 24 hour opioid requirements
- 0.5–1 mg bolus may be administered hourly on a PRN basis with a subsequent 10–20% increase in the hourly rate
- additional 0.5–1 mg bolus doses may be given on a PRN basis without a subsequent increase in the hourly rate when patients are subjected to or perform exceptionally painful activities

Postoperative pain

In the postanesthetic care unit

- 0.5 mg IV repeated every 5 minutes PRN
- adjust the dosage on the basis of response to each dose and titrate to pain control and desired level of sedation or respiratory rate

On the ward

Intermittent therapy

- as above for acute pain
- use the parenteral route initially, but switch to the oral route as soon as the patient is able to take agents orally (usually 24–36 hours postoperatively)
- question the patient frequently and increase the dosage on the basis of pain relief and level of sedation (as above for acute pain)

Patient-controlled analgesia

- 0.1 mg/bolus with a lockout of 6 minutes
- some clinicians believe that 0.1–0.3 mg/h as an infusion with patient-controlled analgesia enables patients to sleep through the night; however, evidence suggests that using a bolus with a baseline infusion may increase the amount of narcotic used and side effects, without improving efficacy (Anaesth Intensive Care 1991;19:555–560, Anesthesiology 1992;76:362–367)
- question the patient frequently hours about his or her degree of pain
- if pain is not controlled with bolus doses, increase the bolus dose by 25–50%
- if pain relief from a bolus is adequate but the duration of pain relief is too short, decrease the lockout period

Epidural or intrathecal use

- can be used as an alternative to parenteral routes, but these routes should be used only by anesthetists skilled in this technique
- 1 mg epidurally as a single dose, with breakthrough pain treated as above with oral or parenteral opioids

Dosage adjustments for renal or hepatic dysfunction

- hepatically metabolized
- dosage adjustment is usually not required if the dose is titrated properly

Normal Dosing Interval	C_{cr} > 60 mL/min or 1 mL/s	C_{cr} 30–60 mL/min or 0.5–1 mL/s	C_{cr} < 30 mL/min or 0.5 mL/s
Q4H	adjust dose on basis of response	adjust dose on basis of response	adjust dose on basis of response

▶ What Should I Monitor with Regard to Efficacy and Toxicity?

see Morphine

▶ How Long Do I Treat Patients with This Drug?

see Morphine

▶ How Do I Decrease or Stop the Administration of This Drug?

see Morphine

▶ What Should I Tell My Patients About This Drug?

see Morphine

▶ Therapeutic Tips

- always prescribe hydromorphone doses at regularly scheduled intervals (e.g., Q4H, never PRN)

- always give intravenous or subcutaneous hydromorphone for severe unrelieved pain in patients with cancer and change to oral therapy after pain is controlled
- in patients who will be taking regularly dosed narcotics for longer than 3–4 days, always consider prescribing narcotics in conjunction with a laxative and counsel the patient on the appropriate use of fluids and fiber
- oral route is preferred because of better patient acceptance and decreased cost
- NSAIDs may be useful in conjunction with hydromorphone, especially when pain is due to bone metastases
- there is no theoretical upper limit to the dose of hydromorphone
- hydromorphone is much more soluble than morphine and can be used when high concentrations of drug are needed in a relatively small volume (e.g., subcutaneous infusion)

Useful References

see Morphine

HYDROXYCHLOROQUINE

Kelly Jones
USA (Plaquenil)
CANADA (Plaquenil)

▶ When Should I Use This Drug?

Mild rheumatoid arthritis

- is effective for mild disease and is well tolerated
- not as effective as gold, but better tolerated
- if there is uncertainty between the diagnoses of rheumatoid arthritis and systemic lupus erythematosus, hydroxychloroquine could be used to treat either condition (Postgrad Med 1990;87:79–92)

Systemic lupus and chronic discoid lupus erythematosus

- considered as adjunctive therapy to topical corticosteroids for discoid lupus erythematosus and to systemic corticosteroids and/or salicylates for systemic lupus erythematosus
- consider hydroxychloroquine in those who have an arthritis component

▶ When Should I Not Use This Drug?

Severe rheumatoid arthritis

- if the disease progression is determined as severe, then agents such as gold and methotrexate should be considered
- hydroxychloroquine is considered slow in onset, with 40–60% of patients responding within 3–6 months and some patients needing 9–12 months for an adequate trial

▶ What Contraindications Are There to the Use of This Drug?

Intolerance of or allergic reaction to hydroxychloroquine

Pregnancy

- this agent is a known teratogen in animal models but an unknown potential risk to the human fetus

▶ What Drug Interactions Are Clinically Important?

- none

▶ What Route and Dosage Should I Use?

How to administer

- orally—give with food
- parenterally—not available

Mild to moderate rheumatoid arthritis, systemic lupus and chronic discoid lupus erythematosus

- give 6 mg/kg PO daily up to a maximum of 400 mg/d, and assess effectiveness in 12 weeks
- if patients have intolerable gastrointestinal side effects, the dose can be split BID
- if therapy is not adequate after 12 weeks for patients receiving less than 400 mg PO daily, increase to 400 mg PO daily

- continue therapy for at least 6 months before discontinuing the drug administration, and some patients may take 9–12 months before efficacy is noted

Dosage adjustments for renal or hepatic dysfunction

- hepatically metabolized to active metabolites

Normal Dosing Interval	$C_{cr} > 60$ mL/min or 1 mL/s	C_{cr} 30–60 mL/min or 0.5–1 mL/s	$C_{cr} < 30$ mL/min or 0.5 mL/s
Q24H	no dosage adjustment needed	no dosage adjustment needed	decrease dosage by 50%

▶ What Should I Monitor with Regard to Efficacy and Toxicity?

Efficacy

Rheumatoid arthritis

Joint tenderness count, sedimentation rate measurements, grip strength, duration of morning stiffness, time to onset of fatigue, and patient's report of specific symptoms

- patient's symptoms and X-rays should be assessed monthly for the first 2 months, and after the disease is under control, the patient can be assessed every 3 months for 6 months and then every 6 months
- these variables should be used to guide drug initiation and discontinuation
- one study found that clinical and laboratory measures of physical well-being appeared to be unrelated to psychological and social measures of well-being (J Rheumatol 1991;18:650–653)
- it is important to include the patient's self-assessment of the drug's effect on the patient's ability to function and well-being

Toxicity

Ocular toxicity

- can cause 3 types of toxicity to the eye but the incidence is low when the drug therapy is monitored appropriately
- risk factors include dosage and duration (≥400 mg/d for 2 years) and age

Ciliary body effects

- disturbance of accommodation with blurred vision occurs and is dose related and reversible on discontinuation of the drug

Corneal deposits

- edema, opacities, blurred vision, halos, and/or photophobia can occur as soon as 3 weeks after the onset of therapy, but are reversible when the drug is discontinued

Retinopathy

- 0.45–5% incidence (Clin Pharm 1987;6:475–491)
- most worrisome toxicity occurring in the eye
- patients have edema, atrophy, abnormal pigmentation of the retina, and retinopathy, causing difficulty in seeing and reading
- can also get a loss of peripheral vision and photophobia
- retinopathy can continue despite discontinuation of the drug and is not readily reversible; therefore, monitoring is important when using hydroxychloroquine
- slit lamp examination and funduscopic examination and visual field tests should be done at baseline and every 6 months and the drug should be discontinued if there is any indication of abnormalities in visual acuity or visual field, pigmentary changes in the macular area, and other visual symptoms such as flashing lights and streaks

Gastrointestinal intolerance

- 5% of patients have nausea, vomiting, or abdominal cramps
- give the daily dose with meals to minimize these effects and splitting the dose BID may also help patients unable to tolerate the gastrointestinal effects

Hematological problems (leukopenia, thrombocytopenia, aplastic anemia)

- can occur, but are not common

- do baseline complete blood count and platelet count and repeat every 3 months

Psoriasis

- hydroxychloroquine can precipitate or exacerbate a flare of psoriasis, and patients should be monitored for a flare-up of their disease

▶ *How Long Do I Treat Patients with This Drug?*

Moderate rheumatoid arthritis

- continue therapy for at least 6 months before discontinuing the drug administration, and some patients may take 9–12 months before efficacy is noted
- if the patient can tolerate the trial, continue for 9 months
- if a good clinical effect is seen, decrease the dosage to the minimum effective dosage to decrease the incidence of side effects, as this drug is typically used long term
- reduce the dosage by 50%, usually to 200 mg daily and monitor for exacerbation of the disease

▶ *How Do I Decrease or Stop the Administration of This Drug?*

- drug may be stopped abruptly

▶ *What Should I Tell My Patients About This Drug?*

- take this medication with meals, which should help reduce possible gastrointestinal side effects
- be compliant with follow-up visits for laboratory work
- eye toxicities are possible, ophthalmological examinations are important, and you should contact your physician if you experience any changes with your eyes

▶ *Therapeutic Tips*

- keep the dosage of hydroxychloroquine at 400 mg/d or less to prevent ocular toxicity
- lower dosages are associated with less toxicity overall
- after a response has been seen, titrate to the lowest effective dosage (usually 200 mg PO daily or every other day)
- do not stop the nonsteroidal antiinflammatory drug and nonpharmacological approaches, rather add this drug to the ongoing therapy
- if tolerated, use for at least a 6–9 month trial

Useful Reference

Clair WE, Poisson RP. Therapeutic approaches to the treatment of rheumatoid arthritis. Med Clin North Am 1986;70:286–304

IBUPROFEN

Kelly Jones, Terry Baumann, and Jerry Taylor

USA (Motrin, Rufen, various generic and over the counter brands)
CANADA (Advil, Motrin, various generic and over the counter brands)

▶ *When Should I Use This Drug?*

Acute pain, general aches and pain, bone pain, dysmenorrhea

- is useful for the acute management of general aches and pains and should be used when inflammation is thought to play a role (pulled muscles, toothaches, and so on) because ibuprofen has an antiinflammatory effect, whereas acetaminophen does not
- for cancer pain, a nonsteroidal antiinflammatory drug (NSAID) should always be added if bone pain is present and the patient can tolerate an NSAID
- ibuprofen causes less gastric distress than does non–enteric-coated aspirin, and although aspirin is usually slightly less expensive, the difference is marginal
- causes more gastric distress than does acetaminophen

Cancer pain

- ibuprofen is useful, in conjunction with codeine, for moderate symptoms if treatment with nonopioid agents are ineffective after titrating rapidly to maximum doses
- NSAID should always be added if bone pain is involved

Rheumatoid arthritis

- good first-line drug for the treatment of rheumatoid arthritis in patients with gastrointestinal disease, as it seems, along with enteric-coated aspirin, to have the least gastrointestinal toxicity and it is inexpensive (J Am Board Fam Pract 1989;2:257–271, Clin Pharm 1992;11:690–713)
- other NSAIDs such as indomethacin and tolmetin may have an advantage over ibuprofen in the treatment of ankylosing spondylitis

Osteoarthritis

- all NSAIDs, including aspirin, are effective for osteoarthritis and should be considered if maximal doses (4 g/d) of acetaminophen are ineffective
- decision among NSAIDs should be based on cost because no predictive measures are available to determine which agent will work

Migraine treatment

- for mild symptoms, ibuprofen is effective and safe
- decision among NSAIDs for the treatment of migraine should be based on cost because no predictive measures are available to determine which agent will work

Migraine prophylaxis

- NSAIDs should be tried in patients not responding to or not able to tolerate beta-blockers, antidepressants, and calcium channel blockers
- NSAIDs are drugs of choice for prophylaxis in patients with menstrual migraine
- at present, there are no predictive measures for deciding which NSAID a patient will respond to
- aspirin is considered the first-line drug of choice because it is as effective as other NSAIDS and is the least expensive agent
- if the patient is at risk for gastrointestinal intolerance or does not tolerate aspirin, ibuprofen is effective, causes less gastrointestinal tolerance than does aspirin, but is more expensive than aspirin

▶ *When Should I Not Use This Drug?*

Combination with other NSAIDs

- combinations of NSAIDs provide no increase in effectiveness compared with maximum doses of single agents and significantly increase the risk of adverse effects

▶ *What Contraindications Are There to the Use of This Drug?*

Intolerance of or allergic reaction to ibuprofen

- allergic reactions occur with NSAIDs as a class and NSAIDs are cross-reactive with aspirin
- patients who are allergic to aspirin or have the classic triad of rhinosinusitis, nasal polyps, and asthma symptoms should avoid the use of ibuprofen and other NSAIDs
- hypersensitivity reactions can range from fever, rash, headache, abdominal pain, and nausea and vomiting to hepatic damage and aseptic meningitis (may occur within 48 hours)

Systemic lupus erythematosus

- should not take ibuprofen owing to the association of hypersensitivity reactions with ibuprofen (J Am Board Fam Pract 1989; 2:257–271, Clin Pharm 1982;1:561–565)

▶ *What Drug Interactions Are Clinically Important?*

Drugs that may increase the effect or toxicity of ibuprofen
DIURETICS

- diuretics plus NSAIDs increase risk of renal failure
- avoid this combination if possible; if not, monitor serum creatinine and potassium levels and weight at baseline and every 4 days for 2–3 weeks, then every 2 weeks for 8 weeks, then every month for 3 months, and then as needed (J Musculoskel Med 1991;8[8]:31–46)

PROBENECID

- decreases renal clearance of NSAIDs; therefore, reduce dosages of NSAID and monitor as for a dosage change

Drugs that may decrease the effect of ibuprofen

CHOLESTYRAMINE

- binds NSAIDs and decreases absorption; therefore, separate the time of administration by 4 hours

Drugs that may have their effect or toxicity increased by ibuprofen

LITHIUM

- causes a decrease in lithium clearance; therefore, use either sulindac or aspirin

POTASSIUM-SPARING DIURETICS

- avoid the combination if possible, and if not, monitor serum creatinine and potassium levels and weight at baseline and every 4 days for 2–3 weeks, then every 2 weeks for 8 weeks, then every month for 3 months, and then as needed (J Musculoskel Med 1991;8[8]:31–46)

METHOTREXATE

- NSAIDs decrease the clearance of methotrexate and increase the risk of toxicity
- no problem if using dosages for rheumatoid arthritis but the combination must not be used when high dosages (for chemotherapy) of methotrexate are being used
- it is important when patients begin methotrexate therapy that their NSAID therapy not be stopped and started (i.e., be consistent) owing to the potential of this drug interaction

Drugs that may have their effect decreased by ibuprofen

ANTIHYPERTENSIVES

- NSAIDs can reduce the hypotensive effect by causing salt and water retention
- among NSAIDs, aspirin and sulindac appear to have the least hypertensive effect (Ann Intern Med 1994;121:289–300) however, all NSAIDs likely have the potential to worsen blood pressure control and blood pressure should be measured at every follow-up visit for patients who are hypertensive or borderline hypertensive
- avoid NSAIDs, if possible, in patients with hypertension
- in patients who must use NSAIDs ensure the lowest effective dose is being used

DIURETICS

- NSAIDs may oppose the diuretic and natriuretic effects of diuretics, and increased doses of diuretics may be required
- avoid combination if at all possible
- in patients who must use NSAIDs, ensure the lowest effective dose is being used

▶ *What Route and Dosage Should I Use?*

How to administer

- orally—take with food or milk
- parenterally—not available

Acute pain, general aches and pain, bone pain, dysmenorrhea

- 200–400 mg PO Q4–6H PRN

Cancer pain

- 400 mg PO Q8H up to a maximum of 3200 mg PO daily

Rheumatoid arthritis

- 800 mg PO Q8H up to a maximum dosage of 3200 mg PO daily

Osteoarthritis

- 400 mg PO Q8H

Migraine treatment

- 800 mg PO Q4H PRN up to a maximum of 3200 mg PO daily

Migraine prophylaxis

- 400 mg PO Q8H

Dosage adjustments for renal or hepatic dysfunction

- hepatically metabolized; therefore, no adjustments are needed for renal disease
- reduce dosage by 25% in patients with a history of hepatic disease

▶ *What Should I Monitor with Regard to Efficacy and Toxicity?*

Efficacy

Acute pain, general aches and pain, bone pain, dysmenorrhea, cancer pain

- key to achieving effective pain control is to question patients frequently about the degree of pain they are having
- frequency of pain evaluation should be based on the knowledge of how quickly the drug should work

Rheumatoid arthritis

- patient's self-assessment is important in making a clinical decision on whether to try another NSAID
- pain and the ability to conduct normal daily activities are important variables to follow when assessing NSAID efficacy

Osteoarthritis

- pain and the ability to conduct normal daily activities are important variables to follow when assessing NSAID efficacy

Migraine treatment

- relief or decrease in the amount of pain within 1–2 hours

Migraine prophylaxis

- frequency and severity of headache can be evaluated for response to medication
- patients with frequent migraine may need evaluation at 2–4 week intervals during the initial dose titration, then the time between visits may be extended in patients showing response to treatment

Toxicity

Gastrointestinal effects

- nausea, vomiting, epigastric discomfort, dyspepsia, diarrhea, and constipation
- gastritis, ulceration, perforation, and occult bleeding
- consider prophylactic therapy with misoprostol in patients taking NSAIDs who are older than 60 years of age, have a past history of peptic ulcer, are also receiving corticosteroids or anticoagulants, or would be a poor surgical risk if ulcer complications occur (Mayo Clin Proc 1992;67:354–364)
- if clinician is solely concerned about reactivation of a duodenal ulcer, an H_2 antagonist could be used (Clin Pharm 1992;11:690–704)

Prevention of NSAID-induced gastropathy

- not required for all patients receiving NSAIDs
- patients at risk (see above) should have an adequate trial of acetaminophen and/or nonacetylated salicylates before NSAID therapy is initiated
- use the lowest dosage of the NSAID for the shortest time possible
- if patients are at risk, use misoprostol 100 μg PO QID
- misoprostol has been effective in preventing NSAID-induced ulceration (Lancet 1988;2:1277–1280), and other agents have generally been no better than placebo (Mayo Clin Proc 1992;67:354–364)
- there is no evidence that misoprostol prevents ulcer complications and death (Am J Gastroenterol 1991;86:264–266)

Treatment of NSAID-induced gastropathy

- stop the drug administration if possible and analyze the need for continued therapy
- consider other agents such as acetaminophen (4 g/d—1000 mg Q6H) and the nonacetylated salicylates (salsalate, diflunisal, choline salicylate); although nonacetylated agents are not as effective as NSAIDs, they do not disrupt gastroprotective mechanisms as do NSAIDs
- give an 8 week course of an H_2 antagonist; however, if administration of NSAIDs must be continued, misoprostol is needed for prophylaxis

- small gastric lesions may heal spontaneously despite continued NSAID therapy (Dig Dis Sci 1982;27:976–980)

Hepatotoxicity (hepatocellular or cholestatic)

- obtain baseline liver enzyme determinations and repeat at 8 weeks for patients at high risk for hepatic disease (e.g., heavy alcohol abusers, patients with a medical history of liver disease, and patients taking hepatotoxic agents concomitantly)
- common in patients with systemic lupus erythematosus, juvenile rheumatoid arthritis, and mixed connective tissue disorders
- liver enzyme levels greater than 3 times normal values should constitute a reason for discontinuation of the drug administration
- if 1 NSAID from a particular class causes a rise in liver function test results, it does not mean that an NSAID from another class would do the same
- for slight elevations in liver enzyme levels, monitor every month

Renal toxicity

- NSAIDs may result in acute renal failure in patients with mild chronic renal failure (Arch Intern Med 1990;112:568–576)
- elderly patients (older than 60 years), patients taking diuretics, and patients with hypovolemia, gout history, or congestive heart failure are at greatest risk for NSAID-induced renal dysfunction
- NSAIDs have caused a wide range of renal toxicities, such as elevations in serum creatinine levels, sodium and water retention, hyperkalemia, papillary necrosis, interstitial nephritis, proteinuria, and acute renal failure
- sulindac is generally believed to have the least adverse effect on the kidney; however, all NSAIDs have the potential to cause adverse renal effects (N Engl J Med 1991;324:1716–1725)
- approximate order of nephrotoxicity: fenoprofen > indomethacin > ibuprofen = flurbiprofen = mefenamic acid = naproxen = diclofenac > tolmentin = piroxicam > sulindac (DICP 1989;23:76–85)
- in patients at risk, monitor serum creatinine and potassium levels and weight at baseline and every 4 days for 2–3 weeks, then every 2 weeks for 8 weeks, and then every month for 3 months

Dermatitis or maculopapular rash

- not that common with aspirin but common with other NSAIDs
- reactions are generally mild and settle with drug administration discontinuation
- Stevens-Johnson syndrome and toxic epidermal necrolysis have been reported with NSAIDs, and if rash is severe, drug therapy should be stopped

Blood pressure

- blood pressure should be measured at every follow-up visit in patients who are hypertensive or borderline hypertensive
- if patients are hypertensive and are concomitantly taking an NSAID, consider the NSAID as the culprit for lack of control
- discontinue the NSAID and get the blood pressure under control before starting another NSAID
- among NSAIDs, aspirin and sulindac appear to have the least hypertensive effect (Ann Intern Med 1994;121:289–300)
- consider use of acetaminophen for pain relief

▶ How Long Do I Treat Patients with This Drug?

Acute pain, general aches and pain, bone pain, dysmenorrhea, cancer pain

- use on a regular basis for the duration of the pain
- acute pain should subside within days after the offending event; if this has not occurred within 1 week, further investigate the cause of the pain

Rheumatoid arthritis

- if the initial dosage does not work within 7 days after starting the drug administration, increase to the maximum dosage
- if maximum dosages have not worked within another 7 days, a change in therapy to another NSAID is appropriate
- give the drug a total of 14 days to work
- treatment of rheumatoid arthritis with ibuprofen or any other NSAID is indefinite
- try to decrease the dosage to the lowest effective level, and the dosage can be decreased during times of disease inactivity to the lowest possible amount to maintain control

- administration of NSAIDs should not be stopped when other second- or third-line agents are added to the treatment of rheumatoid arthritis

Osteoarthritis

- therapy should be continued as long as the drug is effective
- use on a regular basis when pain affects the quality of life
- after pain control is achieved, decrease the daily dosage by 25% every 1–2 weeks until the minimum effective dosage is identified

Migraine treatment

- initial therapy with ibuprofen should prevent or provide pain relief within a couple of hours
- if headaches are persistent after 1–2 hours, alternative therapy should be instituted

Migraine prophylaxis

- prophylactic agents often necessitate adjustment in dosage and may need to be given for several weeks to provide maximum benefit
- if tolerated, each drug should be tried for 4–6 weeks before alternative agents are tried
- if the patient achieves a headache-free state, therapy should be reduced or withdrawn after 6 months to assess continued requirements

▶ How Do I Decrease or Stop the Administration of This Drug?

- may be stopped abruptly if needed

▶ What Should I Tell My Patients About This Drug?

- it is important to be educated about what to expect in terms of the onset of relief
- your pain (rheumatoid arthritis) will not go away with 1 dose or with 2 days of therapy, but by 2 weeks, you should be experiencing significant relief
- avoid concomitant use of other NSAIDs, especially over the counter products containing ibuprofen or aspirin
- take with food, milk, or antacids if gastrointestinal upset occurs, and tell your physician of any gastrointestinal intolerance
- notify your physician of any rash, unusual fever, edema, black stools, or weight gain
- some patients get drowsy with ibuprofen therapy

▶ Therapeutic Tips

- for rheumatoid arthritis, use higher dosages initially and decrease to the lowest effective level
- give a 14 day trial at maximum dosages before changing agents
- there is little support in selecting an NSAID from another chemical class when switching agents
- concurrent administration of acetaminophen (4 g/d) augments the analgesic effects of ibuprofen without increasing toxicity
- do not use 2 NSAIDs concomitantly because this may increase toxicity
- most effective in cancer pain when used with opioids and given on a regular basis

Useful References

Levy RA, Smith DL. Clinical differences among nonsteroidal antiinflammatory drugs: Implications for therapeutic substitution in ambulatory patients. DICP, Ann Pharmacother 1989;23:76–85

Miller LG, Prichard JG. Selecting nonsteroidal anti-inflammatory drugs: pharmacologic and clinical considerations. J Am Board Fam Pract 1989;2:257–271

Roth SH, Bennett RE. Nonsteroidal anti-inflammatory drug gastropathy. Arch Intern Med 1987;147:2093–2099

IMIPENEM-CILASTATIN

James McCormack

USA (Primaxin)
CANADA (Primaxin)

▶ When Should I Use This Drug?

check antibiotic susceptibility chart (Table 4–1 in Chapter 4)

Pneumonia, sepsis, osteomyelitis, cellulitis, urinary tract infections, intraabdominal infections, pelvic inflammatory disease

- for these infections if they are presumed or proved to be caused by organisms resistant to less expensive agents
- imipenem has a broad spectrum of activity; however, it is expensive and should be reserved for infections caused by organisms resistant to less expensive agents
- imipenem may be useful for these infections, if they are caused by multiple organisms and if imipenem is less expensive than combinations of antibiotics

▶ *When Should I Not Use This Drug?*

For infection caused by *Streptococcus faecium*, methicillin-resistant staphylococci, *Pseudomonas* species other than *P. aeruginosa*, *Mycoplasma*, and *Chlamydia*

- imipenem is not active against these organisms

▶ *What Contraindications Are There to the Use of This Drug?*

Intolerance of or allergic reaction to imipenem or penicillins

- patients allergic to penicillins may also be allergic to imipenem, and its use in these patients should be restricted to those patients in whom no other drugs can be used

▶ *What Drug Interactions Are Clinically Important?*

Drugs that may increase the effect or toxicity of imipenem

PROBENECID

- when used with high dosages of imipenem, this may precipitate seizures
- do not use together

GANCICLOVIR

- may increase the risk of seizures
- no extra monitoring is required

Drugs that may decrease the effect of imipenem

- none

Drugs that may have their effect or toxicity increased by imipenem

- none

Drugs that may have their effect decreased by imipenem

- none

▶ *What Route and Dosage Should I Use?*

How to administer

Orally

- not available

Parenterally

- reconstitute with 100–200 mL of either sterile water or normal saline to provide a concentration not greater than 5 mg/mL
- each 250 or 500 mg dose should be infused over 30 minutes, and 1 g doses should be given over 60 minutes

Pneumonia, sepsis, osteomyelitis, cellulitis, urinary tract infections, intraabdominal infections, pelvic inflammatory disease

- 500 mg IV Q6H for mildly or moderately ill patients
- 1000 mg IV Q6H for severely ill patients

Dosage adjustments for renal or hepatic dysfunction

- renally eliminated

Normal Dosing Interval	$C_{cr} > 60$ mL/min or 1 mL/s	C_{cr} 30–60 mL/min or 0.5–1 mL/s	$C_{cr} < 30$ mL/min or 0.5 mL/s
Q6H	no adjustment needed	Q8H	Q12H

▶ *What Should I Monitor with Regard to Efficacy and Toxicity?*

Efficacy

- for antibiotic administration guidelines, see specific section on drug therapy

Toxicity

Allergic reactions (rash, angioedema, anaphylaxis)

- morbilliform rash (5–10%); fatal anaphylactic reaction (1/50,000)
- question the patient about the appearance of these symptoms on a daily basis while the patient is in the hospital

Gastrointestinal symptoms

- question the patient about the appearance of diarrhea, abdominal pain, and cramping
- question the patient about these symptoms on a daily basis while the patient is in the hospital
- for specific treatment, see discussion of drug-induced diarrhea in Chapter 11

Seizures

- occur in 1.5% of patients and are seen in patients receiving high dosages of imipenem and in patients with decreased renal function; therefore, ensure that the dosage is adjusted for the patient's renal function
- seen more frequently in patients with central nervous system disorders
- if they occur and the patient still requires the drug, decrease the dosage

Dizziness

- may occur and is usually due to too rapid an infusion rate
- if this occurs, decrease the infusion rate

Hematological effects

- eosinophilia occurs in 4% and a positive Coombs' test result occurs in 2% of patients
- no routine monitoring is required

Nephrotoxicity

- may cause increased serum creatinine concentrations in 2% of patients
- no specific monitoring is required unless this drug is being used in conjunction with aminoglycosides

▶ *How Long Do I Treat Patients with This Drug?*

- for antibiotic administration duration, see specific section on drug therapy

▶ *How Do I Decrease or Stop the Administration of This Drug?*

- may be stopped abruptly

▶ *What Should I Tell My Patients About This Drug?*

- this agent is related to penicillins and cephalosporins
- have you ever had an allergic reaction to a penicillin? if so, describe the reaction and how long ago it happened
- if you develop a rash, itching, wheezing, or difficulty with breathing, please notify a nurse or physician
- imipenem can cause diarrhea, and if the diarrhea is severe, tell your physician

▶ *Therapeutic Tips*

- for *Pseudomonas* infections, use imipenem in conjunction with an aminoglycoside
- cilastatin sodium is added to imipenem to decrease the renal metabolism of imipenem and increase concentrations in the urinary tract
- ensure that the dosage is appropriate for the patient's renal function

Useful Reference

Wright AJ, Wilkowske CJ. The penicillins. Mayo Clin Proc 1987;62:806–820

IMIPRAMINE

Lyle K. Laird and Julia Vertrees

USA (Tofranil, Janimine, Tipramine, others)
CANADA (Impril, Novo-Pramine, Tofranil, others)

▶ *When Should I Use This Drug?*

Major depression

- imipramine is the initial drug of choice in patients without concomitant disease states because it is as effective as and less expensive than other tricyclic antidepressants
- although imipramine can cause more adverse effects than many of the newer agents, many patients experience tolerance of these adverse effects, and many patients may be effectively treated with this inexpensive drug

Dysthymia

- is formally known as depressive neurosis or as a personality disorder and is now recognized as a depressive disorder that tends to run a more chronic course and is possibly a more heterogeneous entity than major depression
- although previously thought to be refractory to pharmacotherapy, current literature supports the efficacy of tricyclic antidepressants and monoamine oxidase inhibitors; however, the response is often less robust than in major depression (J Clin Psychopharmacol 1991;11:83–92, J Clin Psychiatry 1992;10:15–23)

Panic disorders

- extensive research supports the use of imipramine for panic attacks, and imipramine has been superior to placebo and chlordiazepoxide (J Psychiatr Res 1988;22:7–31)
- alprazolam is the only approved agent for treating panic disorders; however, other benzodiazepines may have efficacy for panic disorders
- comparative studies between alprazolam and imipramine, desipramine, or phenelzine are lacking; the superiority of one agent over another is unknown
- imipramine has minimum effects on anticipatory anxiety; therefore, use benzodiazepines if symptoms are predominantly of the anticipatory type
- antidepressants may be useful in patients who are drug abusers (alcohol, etc.) because these patients are less likely to become dependent on antidepressants than on benzodiazepines
- if an antidepressant is used as initial therapy, concurrent benzodiazepine therapy may be necessary for the first 2–4 weeks (owing to a lag time for response to antidepressants)

Generalized anxiety disorders

- although it is not typically a first-line agent, use in the presence of coexisting depression and dysthymia, a history of substance abuse, or a history of past response to antidepressants in treating similar symptoms

Chronic pain syndromes

- in patients with neuropathic pain that does not respond to narcotics, consider adding imipramine

▶ *When Should I Not Use This Drug?*

Bipolar disorder, depressed

- patients who have this illness (also known as manic depression) may experience an exacerbation of the manic phase of the illness if given imipramine (Arch Gen Psychiatry 1979;36:555–559)

Depression after a bereavement

- in cases of depressed mood that does not meet the definition of clinical depression (e.g., an otherwise depressed feeling that follows a normal periodic fluctuation in mood or a depression that is due to bereavement and lasts shorter than 2 weeks)

Depression with psychotic features

- patient with psychotic features, including delusions and hallucinations, are generally not thought to respond well to tricyclic antidepressants alone (Arch Gen Psychiatry 1976;33:1479–1489)

Insomnia

- tricyclic antidepressants are not appropriate for insomnia not related to or accompanied by depression, as they cause a higher incidence of adverse effects than do benzodiazepines or other appropriate hypnotics

Cyclothymia

- for these patients who chronically experience periods of depression alternating with periods of near mania (hypomania), treatment with imipramine may speed up the cycling pattern and thereby worsen the condition

Obsessive-compulsive disorders

- imipramine does not appear to be as effective for the treatment of obsessive-compulsive disorders as are other agents

Migraine prophylaxis

- imipramine does not appear to be as effective as amitriptyline

▶ *What Contraindications Are There to the Use of This Drug?*

Intolerance of or allergic reaction to imipramine

Acute (first 6 weeks) period after myocardial infarction

- increased risk of arrhythmia, conduction problems, and congestive heart failure

Glaucoma

- closed angle glaucoma is an absolute contraindication to the use of any antidepressant with anticholinergic properties
- if a tricyclic agent must be used, use desipramine
- if a tricyclic agent is not needed, use fluoxetine, sertraline, or paroxetine

Heart block

- in patients with second- or third-degree atrioventricular blocks or left bundle branch disease
- increased risk of arrhythmia and conduction problems

Pregnancy

- adequate studies have not been performed; there are case reports of fetal abnormalities associated with imipramine use; however, animal studies have been inconclusive

Just prior to delivery

- there have been reports of respiratory distress and cardiac problems in infants of mothers given imipramine (USP Dispensing Information 1991:353)
- stop the drug administration at labor or 24 hours before delivery

▶ *What Drug Interactions Are Clinically Important?*

Drugs that may increase the effect or toxicity of imipramine

CENTRAL NERVOUS SYSTEM DEPRESSANTS

- central nervous system (CNS) depressant effects are enhanced; therefore, avoid use with other CNS depressants
- if possible, use bedtime dosing to minimize daytime sedation

MONOAMINE OXIDASE INHIBITORS

- results in gastrointestinal complaints; symptoms of CNS excitability; hyperthermia; cardiovascular events, including dysrhythmia; seizures; and coma
- most likely to occur if the imipramine is added to a monoamine oxidase (MAO) inhibitor regimen
- combination may be used if both imipramine and the MAO inhibitor are started together or if the MAO inhibitor is added to an imipramine regimen
- if the patient is taking MAO inhibitor and imipramine is to be added, the patient should be MAO inhibitor free for at least 2 weeks prior to starting the new combination regimen (J Clin Psychopharmacol 1981;1:264–282) to allow time for new enzyme synthesis

CIMETIDINE

- inhibits hepatic microsomal enzymes, which metabolize imipramine
- significant decrease in imipramine clearance with side effects and toxicity is possible
- if an H_2 antagonist is necessary, prescribe an alternative H_2 antagonist, which does not interact (e.g., ranitidine and famotidine)

ANTIPSYCHOTIC DRUGS

- significant increases in imipramine blood levels may occur owing to competition for hepatic metabolic enzyme systems
- monitor the patient for adverse drug effects if a combination of imipramine and an antipsychotic is indicated and adjust the imipramine dosage on the basis of the development of adverse effects

FLUOXETINE

- significant increases (2-fold) in imipramine blood levels due to competitive inhibition in oxidative metabolism
- avoid the combination of imipramine and fluoxetine, except in patients in whom depression has been difficult to treat and the combination needs to be used

LEVOTHYROXINE

- both therapeutic and toxic effects can be increased for both drugs
- mechanism not known but thought to be result of thyroid hormone correcting subclinical hypothyroidism or augmenting norepinephrine receptor sensitivity in the CNS
- monitor patients for cardiovascular effects (e.g., blood pressure elevation and tachycardia) and CNS excitatory symptoms (e.g., agitation)
- combination may be useful when the patient is deemed refractory to an adequate trial of antidepressant medication alone (J Clin Psychiatry 1991;52[suppl 5]:21–27)

ALPRAZOLAM, BASIC pH (SODIUM BICARBONATE), BETA-BLOCKERS, CHLORAMPHENICOL, DISULFIRAM, ERYTHROMYCIN, ESTROGENS, FENFLURAMINE, ISONIAZID, METHYLPHENIDATE, PERPHENAZINE, THIORIDAZINE
(Neuropsychobiology 1982;8:73–85)

- these drugs have the potential to increase serum imipramine steady state concentrations
- monitor for adverse reactions and any changes should be maximum by 1–2 weeks
- when discontinuing 1 of these agents in patients stabilized on both, loss of efficacy may be due to a decline in serum concentration, which may require an increase in dosage

Drugs that may decrease the effect of imipramine

ACID pH (AMMONIUM CHLORIDE), BARBITURATES, CARBAMAZEPINE, CHLORAL HYDRATE, DOXYCYCLINE, GLUTETHIMIDE, PRIMIDONE, TRIHEXYPHENIDYL
(Neuropsychobiology 1982;8:73–85)

- these drugs have the potential to decrease imipramine steady state serum concentrations
- when adding one of these agents to the regimen of a patient stabilized on imipramine a decline in imipramine concentration may occur and should be maximum by 3–4 weeks
- any loss of efficacy within 1–2 weeks of the change may reflect a need to increase the imipramine dosage
- when discontinuing administration of one of these drugs in patients stabilized on both, an increase in imipramine steady state serum concentrations may occur and be near maximum by 4 weeks
- monitor for the development of adverse effects and adjust the dosage accordingly

Drugs that may have their effect or toxicity increased by imipramine

DIRECT-ACTING SYMPATHOMIMETICS (EPINEPHRINE, NOREPINEPHRINE, PHENYLEPHRINE)

- vasopressor response of these agents may be enhanced by as much as 8-fold
- mechanism thought to be imipramine's interference with neurotransmitter reuptake at the synapse
- avoid this combination

WARFARIN

- hypoprothrombinemic effect of warfarin (and other oral anticoagulants) can be increased
- mechanism not fully understood; it may result from enhanced warfarin absorption due to imipramine or imipramine inhibition of hepatic enzymes
- monitor INR every 2 days until the full extent of the interaction is seen, and adjust the dosage as for a warfarin dose change if needed
- monitor INR every 2 days when administration of the interacting drug is discontinued and adjust as required

Drugs that may have their effect decreased by imipramine

METHYLDOPA, CLONIDINE

- reversal of antihypertensive effect
- mechanism is probably due to imipramine's blocking neurotransmitter reuptake or desensitizing the presynaptic alpha-receptor
- suggest use of an alternative antihypertensive drug if imipramine use is indicated (e.g., diuretics, beta-blocker, and so on)

▶ *What Route and Dosage Should I Use?*

How to administer

- orally—can be given with food or on an empty stomach
- parenterally—intramuscular form is available, but its administration is painful and it has not been shown to work faster

Major depression, dysthymia, generalized anxiety disorders

- 50 mg PO daily at bedtime
- increase after 3 days to 100 mg PO daily at bedtime
- increase to 150 mg PO daily at bedtime after 1 week and leave at this dosage for 10–14 days
- if target symptoms are not improving after 3 weeks of therapy, continue to increase the daily dosage by 50 mg at weekly intervals until a response is seen or a dosage of 300 mg PO daily has been reached
- in geriatric patients and patients with a seizure history, start with 25 mg PO at bedtime, and in general, dosages should be approximately 50% of those used in younger patients
- imipramine has a long duration of action; hence, long-acting or sustained-release products are unnecessary and once-daily dosing is appropriate in adults
- after the patient has experienced a therapeutic response, the dosage should be maintained at these levels for 6–9 months because relapses may occur if a dosage reduction is attempted

Panic disorders

- dosages are often lower than those needed in depressive disorders
- start with 10 mg PO daily for a couple of days, as clinicians have noticed that these patients do not tolerate the adverse effects as well
- for panic disorders, titrate the dose up by 10–25 every 3–5 days and aim for 150 mg as the total daily dose

Chronic pain syndromes

- dosages are often lower than those needed in depressive disorders
- start with 10 mg PO daily
- the general effective dosage range is 25–50 mg PO daily and is generally used as adjuvant therapy

Dosage adjustments for renal or hepatic dysfunction

- hepatically metabolized
- start with low doses as for geriatric patients
- decreased renal function does not necessitate dosage adjustments

▶ *What Should I Monitor with Regard to Efficacy and Toxicity?*

Efficacy

Major depression, dysthymia

Sleep disturbances

- first symptom to improve (after 10–14 days) and should be assessed weekly

Nervousness, somatic complaints, appetite, feelings of helplessness and hopelessness, depressed mood

- tend to improve more slowly over 2–3 weeks
- close friends or relatives notice signs of improvement before the patient is aware of changes
- adequate clinical response should not be expected for at least 4 weeks
- after patients are stable, patients should be clinically assessed for target symptoms at least monthly (or weekly if clinical decompensation is suspected)

Plasma concentrations

- although routine plasma concentration monitoring is not necessary, an imipramine concentration of total imipramine plus its metabolite desipramine of 180 ng/mL or more has been associated with a positive clinical response (Clin Chem 1988;34: 863–888)
- if a patient has had a positive therapeutic response (efficacy and toxicity) from normal dosages, routine measurement of serum concentrations is not needed
- when available, plasma concentrations are useful to assess for compliance, adjust the maintenance dosage into the therapeutic range in patients who do not respond to normal dosage titration, patients with adverse effects or toxicity at low to therapeutic dosages, cases in which the maximum dosage of 300 mg/d is going to be exceeded, overdose, or investigations for research purposes
- plasma concentration sampling should be obtained just prior to the dose

Panic disorders

Target symptoms

- monitor changes in shortness of breath, choking or smothering sensations, dizziness, palpitations or chest pain, trembling, nausea, depersonalization, tingling, and fear of impending doom
- should see initial response within 3–4 weeks with antidepressants
- after they are stable, patients should be clinically assessed for target symptoms at least monthly (or weekly if clinical decompensation is suspected)

Generalized Anxiety Disorders

Target symptoms

- monitor changes in increased motor or muscle tension, restlessness, autonomic hyperactivity (shortness of breath, palpitations, dry mouth, nausea, vomiting, and so on), and hypervigilance
- monitor at least weekly
- after they are stable, patients should be clinically assessed for target symptoms at least monthly (or weekly if clinical decompensation is suspected)

Chronic pain syndromes

- may take several weeks to see a measurable decrease in pain

Toxicity

Anticholinergic effects

Dry mouth

- increase fluid intake and/or use sugarless chewing gum or hard candies

Constipation

- increase fluid and fiber in diet, and if needed, use a laxative

Sedation

- may occur, however, and many patients become tolerant of the sedation
- if sedation is a problem, ensure that the drug is given as a nighttime dose

Blurred vision

- tell the patient that tolerance of this adverse effect will likely develop within a few weeks
- if there is no resolution of symptoms, switch to a drug with fewer anticholinergic properties

Urinary hesitancy

- tell the patient not to ignore the urge to void and recommend frequent voiding
- if there is no resolution of symptoms, switch to drug with fewer anticholinergic properties
- for severe depression that has responded to imipramine, small dosages of the cholinergic drug bethanechol chloride may be effective

Allergic reactions (skin rash, itching, swelling of face or tongue)
(Drugs 1981;21:201–219)

- photosensitivity, urticaria, and cutaneous vasculitis; generally considered benign and not necessarily a reason to discontinue therapy
- often occur within the first few months of treatment
- rashes are often mild and settle on their own
- if hives occur, stop the drug administration and can rechallenge later if there are no systemic symptoms

Hematological effects

- agranulocytosis is rare but is considered fatal in 10–20% of cases
- drug administration discontinuation is recommended
- monitor white blood cell count if signs and symptoms of agranulocytosis (fever, infections, and so on) occur
- eosinophilia is frequently seen in the initial weeks of treatment but is often transient
- drug administration discontinuation is usually not necessary

Hepatic effects

- jaundice has been reported
- aminotransferase and alkaline phosphatase level elevations are commonly seen with tricyclic antidepressants, and drug administration discontinuation is recommended
- hepatic necrosis has occurred and is potentially fatal
- measure liver enzyme levels if signs and symptoms of hepatic dysfunction are present

Cardiovascular effects

- orthostatic hypotension is the most common cardiovascular effect and is found even with therapeutic dosages
- treatment of orthostatic hypotension includes having the patient rise slowly from supine or sitting positions and wear support stockings, ensuring that adequate fluid intake is being maintained, sleep with the head of the bed elevated 6 inches, or switching to nortriptyline or one of the newer antidepressants such as fluoxetine or bupropion
- imipramine is currently believed to worsen left ventricular function when used in therapeutic dosages (JAMA 1986;256:3253–3257)
- for patients with prolonged PR intervals and first-degree atrioventricular block, tricyclic antidepressants can be used up to maximum dosages but only if regular electrocardiographic monitoring is performed
- overdose situations can result in life-threatening arrhythmias, severe hypotension, cardiac failure, shock, and seizures

Switch from depression to a manic phase

- rare but can occur

▶ *How Long Do I Treat Patients with This Drug?*

Major depression, dysthymia, generalized anxiety disorders

- after target symptoms have been controlled and the depression has lifted, the medication administration should be continued for 6–9 months to ensure that the episode has run its course
- after this time, the antidepressant regimen should be tapered to avoid possible withdrawal reactions such as cholinergic rebound with the tricyclic antidepressants
- in patients with a history of repeated and perhaps increasingly frequent episodes, long-term treatment should be considered

Panic disorders

- no long-term follow-up studies longer than 6 months exist, and the efficacy of drug therapy after 6 months is unknown but patients receiving long-term therapy do experience relapse when administration of drugs is discontinued

- some clinicians recommend at least a 6–12 month symptom-free period prior to attempting discontinuation (J Clin Psychiatry 1990;51:11–15) and then taper the drug regimen over several months to prevent rebound symptoms
- concurrent behavioral or desensitization therapy after drug administration discontinuation may decrease the risk of relapse

Chronic pain syndromes

- may be required indefinitely

▶ *How Do I Stop or Decrease the Administration of This Drug?*

- should be gradually tapered over 3–4 weeks (likely over 2–3 months for panic disorders)
- dosage should be reduced at 50 mg/wk for outpatients; inpatients may be tapered more quickly at 50 mg/d every 2 days if needed
- monitor for withdrawal effects (consisting of influenza-like symptoms, nausea and vomiting, and diarrhea); such effects are from cholinergic rebound and are best treated by slowing the withdrawal protocol, adding some imipramine back, or giving 25–50 mg of diphenhydramine TID PRN for symptoms
- in cases of emergency (e.g., toxicity), imipramine administration should be stopped abruptly

▶ *What Should I Tell My Patients About This Drug?*

- alcohol may increase the sedative effect of this drug
- occasional social drink is alright; however, the first drink taken in this situation should be done in a controlled environment (i.e., one that does not potentially require alertness)
- imipramine can interact with several types of medications, including over the counter products and alcohol; inform your physician and pharmacist of all medications that you are taking
- discuss common adverse effects and how to treat them
- imipramine may be taken on an empty stomach
- it can take several weeks before the depression begins to lift
- if you are receiving this drug for depression, it is likely best if you stay at home until full dosages have been achieved and potential adverse effects have been seen (1 week)
- keep this medication out of the reach of children
- do not stop taking this medication without first consulting your physician or pharmacist

▶ *Therapeutic Tips*

- for adults, once-daily dosing is effective and enhances compliance, and bedtime dosing is recommended
- routine plasma concentration monitoring is not necessary but may help in specific situations
- maximum effect may not be seen for up to 4 weeks, assuming adequate dosage
- serious toxicity can occur with doses greater than 1.2 g and doses of greater than 2.5 g are often fatal
- consider dispensing only up to 1 week's worth at a time when the patient is considered at high risk for suicide
- have some family member obtain and supervise medication administration if possible

Useful References

Bryant SG, Brown CS. Major depressive disorders. In: Young LY, Koda-Kimble MA, eds. Applied Therapeutics: The Clinical Use of Drugs, 4th ed. Vancouver, WA: Applied Therapeutics, 1988:1231–1253

Wells BG, Hayes PE. Depressive illness. In: DiPiro JT, Talbert RL, Hayes PE, et al, eds. Pharmacotherapy: A Pathophysiologic Approach. New York: Elsevier, 1989:748–764

USP Dispensing Information. Rockville, MD: United States Pharmacopeial Convention, 1991:335

INDAPAMIDE

Ian Petterson

USA (Lozol)
CANADA (Lozide)

▶ *When Should I Use This Drug?*

Consider an alternative agent

- there is no reason to use this drug instead of other thiazide diuretics because its effects are identical and indapamide is considerably more expensive

- indapamide has similar metabolic adverse effects on potassium and uric acid levels as hydrochlorothiazide
- although there is a suggestion that indapamide might have fewer effects on serum levels of lipids and glucose, comparison studies using comparable antihypertensive dosages have not been done
- even if there were small differences, the clinical significance of these differences is likely unimportant
- indapamide has been shown to produce alterations in glucose metabolism (Arch Intern Med 1986;146:1973–1977)

INDOMETHACIN

Wayne Weart

USA (Indocin, Indocin SR, various generics)
CANADA (Indocid, Indocid SR, Apo-Indomethacin, Novomethacin)

▶ *When Should I Use This Drug?*

Acute attack of gout

- initial drug of choice for the acute attack, as it is generally better tolerated than colchicine because most patients experience gastrointestinal toxicity when given colchicine (Aust N Z J Med 1987;17:301–304)
- some patients get more effect from indomethacin than colchicine especially when treating a patient whose symptoms have been present for ≥24 hours (Primary Care 1984;11:283–294)
- other nonsteroidal antiinflammatory drugs (NSAIDs) have been used (e.g., naproxen and ibuprofen) with apparent similar efficacy, but experience is much less extensive to date, and additional fast-acting NSAIDs should be tried if the patient cannot tolerate indomethacin

Rheumatoid arthritis

- do not use this drug as first-line therapy because indomethacin has more side effects than do most NSAIDs
- indomethacin is considered toxic to the kidneys, as is fenoprofen (J Am Board Fam Pract 1989;2:257–271)
- indomethacin is considered harsh on the gastrointestinal tract; has a number of central nervous system adverse effects such as headaches, psychotic reactions, and depression; and is potentially toxic to the liver
- indomethacin should be reserved for patients who have failed to respond to trials of other NSAIDs
- indomethacin affects platelets for a shorter duration than aspirin
- the time required to return to normal platelet function following cessation of indomethacin is 18–32 hours, whereas it is 7–12 days for aspirin, 2 weeks for piroxicam, and 24 hours for ibuprofen (J Am Board Fam Pract 1989;2:257–271)
- indomethacin may be important for patients who experience a flare of their disease, and some clinicians use the drug initially to gain control of the flare and change to another NSAID for long-term control

▶ *When Should I Not Use This Drug?*

Acute pain, general aches and pain, bone pain, dysmenorrhea, cancer pain, osteoarthritis

- do not use this drug for these indications because indomethacin has more side effects than do most NSAIDs

Combination with other nonsteroidal antiinflammatory drugs

- combinations of NSAIDs provide no increase in effectiveness compared with maximum dosages of single agents and significantly increase the risk of adverse effects

▶ *What Contraindications Are There to the Use of This Drug?*

see Ibuprofen

▶ *What Drug Interactions Are Clinically Important?*

see Ibuprofen

▶ *What Route and Dosage Should I Use?*

How to administer

- orally—take with food or milk
- parenterally—available but not recommended for use

Acute attack of gout

- give 50 mg PO TID until a significant response occurs, then reduce the dosage to 25 mg PO TID until the attack has fully resolved

Rheumatoid arthritis

- 25 mg PO Q8H up to a maximum dosage of 200 mg PO daily

Dosage adjustments for renal or hepatic dysfunction

- hepatically metabolized; therefore, no adjustments are needed for renal disease
- reduce dosage by 25% in patients with a history of hepatic disease

▶ *What Should I Monitor with Regard to Efficacy and Toxicity?*

Efficacy

Acute attack of gout

- reduction in pain and swelling typically occurs within 12–48 hours for agents used for acute treatment; however, if the attack is already established (e.g., 48 hours), response to treatment is slower

Rheumatoid arthritis

- patient's self-assessment is important in making a clinical decision on whether to try another NSAID
- pain and the ability to conduct normal daily activities are important variables to follow when assessing NSAID efficacy

Toxicity

Central nervous system effects

- indomethacin causes depression, psychotic reactions, and headaches
- if these side effects occur, discontinue indomethacin administration and use an alternative agent

see Ibuprofen

▶ *How Long Do I Treat Patients with This Drug?*

Acute attack of gout

- give full dosages until a significant response occurs (typically, 2–3 days) and then reduce the dosage and continue administration until the attack is fully resolved (typically, 7–10 days)

Rheumatoid arthritis

- if the initial dosage does not work within 7 days after starting the drug increase to the maximum dosage
- if maximum dosages have not worked within another 7 days, a change in therapy to another NSAID is appropriate
- give the drug a total of 14 days to work
- indomethacin may best be used by giving temporarily to gain initial control and then switching to another better tolerated NSAID, such as ibuprofen, diclofenac, and naproxen
- treatment of rheumatoid arthritis with indomethacin or any other NSAID is indefinite
- try to decrease the dosage to the lowest effective level, and the dosage can be decreased during times of disease inactivity to the lowest possible amount to maintain control
- NSAIDs should not be stopped when other second- or third-line agents are added to the treatment of rheumatoid arthritis

▶ *How Do I Decrease or Stop the Administration of This Drug?*

- may be stopped abruptly if needed

▶ *What Should I Tell My Patients About This Drug?*

see Ibuprofen

▶ *Therapeutic Tips*

- do not use sustained-release indomethacin for acute pain or initial therapy, as it is difficult to titrate
- for rheumatoid arthritis, use higher dosages initially and decrease to the lowest effective level

see Ibuprofen

Useful References

see Ibuprofen

INSULIN

Christy Silvius Scott

USA (Humulin, Lente, NPH, Regular, Semilente, Ultralente, Insulatard)
CANADA (Humulin, Lente, NPH, Regular, Semilente, Ultralente, Novolin, Insulatard)

▶ *When Should I Use This Drug?*

Long-term uses

Insulin-dependent diabetes mellitus

- all patients require insulin for treatment because they are unable to produce insulin

Non–insulin-dependent diabetes mellitus

Nonobese (within 120% of ideal body weight) and young (younger than 40 years old) patients willing to inject insulin and self-monitor blood glucose levels and patients with severe, symptomatic hyperglycemia

- these patients are generally started on insulin injections, especially if they are symptomatic and have urinary ketones because they rarely respond to oral agents (Can Med Assoc J 1991;145: 1571–1581, Diabetes Care 1990;13:1240–1262)

Patients who fail to respond to oral hypoglycemic agents

- if metformin is not available, insulin therapy must be initiated in patients whose diabetes control is unsatisfactory with a sulfonylurea
- if metformin is available, it should be added to therapy before the initiation of insulin therapy
- with failure to respond to a sulfonylurea, switching to insulin therapy alone (although somewhat controversial) is preferable to adding insulin therapy (Can Med Assoc J 1992;147:697–712, Diabetes Care 1990;13:1240–1262, N Engl J Med 1989;321: 1231–1245)

Temporary uses

Non–insulin-dependent diabetes mellitus

Pregnancy

- insulin is required to produce good control of diabetes during pregnancy if diet and exercise alone are not successful (Clin Obstet Gynecol 1981;8:353–382, The Management of Diabetes Mellitus 1990:29); there is a risk to the fetus if oral agents are used during pregnancy; therefore, as insulin is a naturally occurring hormone it is the drug of choice for control of diabetes during pregnancy (Drugs in Pregnancy and Lactation, 4th ed, 1994)

Breast-feeding

- if glucose-lowering medications are required, insulin should be used, as it does not appear in breast milk and oral medications are contraindicated (Drugs in Pregnancy and Lactation, 4th ed, 1994)

Perioperative use

- surgery produces a stress state, resulting in increased blood glucose levels and a catabolic state (Diabetes: Theory and Practice, 4th ed, 1990:626–633)
- insulin is required perioperatively in the non–insulin-dependent diabetic to control the metabolic response to surgery

Periods of significant stress

- patients who are experiencing significant stress, such as infection, trauma, surgery, myocardial infarction and other serious illness, require insulin for adequate control

Gestational diabetes

- diagnosis depends on a 100 mg oral glucose tolerance test with 2 or more of the following results: fasting levels of less than 105 mg/dL (5.8 mmol/L), 1 hour post–glucose load level of

190 mg/dL (10.6 mmol/L), 2 hour post–glucose load level of greater than 165 mg/dL (9.2 mmol/L), and 3 hour post–glucose load level of greater than 145 mg/dL (8.1 mmol/L) (Diabetes Care 1993;16[suppl 2]:5)

- as most women with gestational diabetes are overweight, a diet consisting of 25 cal/kg of prepregnancy body weight should be instituted along with appropriate exercise (The Management of Diabetes Mellitus 1990:29)
- if dietary measures do not maintain fasting plasma glucose levels of 105 mg/dL (5.8 mmol/L) or less and/or 2 hour post–glucose load levels of 120 mg/dL (6.9 mmol/L) or less, insulin administration should be instituted; oral hypoglycemic agents are contraindicated (The Management of Diabetes Mellitus 1990:29, Diabetes Care 1993;16[suppl 2]:5)

Diabetic ketoacidosis or hyperglycemic hyperosmolar coma

- use intravenous regular insulin infusions in normal saline

Severe hyperkalemia

- potassium level greater than 8 mmol/L or greater than 6.5 mmol/L with clinical symptoms or electrocardiographic changes
- although glucose alone may promote redistribution of potassium from extracellular to intracellular spaces, insulin is usually administered concomitantly (Clinical Physiology of Acid-Base and Electrolyte Disorders 1989:757)

▶ *When Should I Not Use This Drug?*

Noncompliant patients

- do not use insulin in non–insulin-dependent diabetic patients unwilling or unable to self-administer insulin and/or self-monitor blood glucose levels

Non–insulin-dependent diabetes mellitus

- when a program of diet, exercise, and oral agents alone would produce adequate control (N Engl J Med 1989;321:1231–1245)
- if insulin requirements are 20 units/d or less, a trial with a sulfonylurea alone is warranted (Diabetes Care 1990;13:1240–1262)
- definite indications for insulin withdrawal are sustained excellent control and suspected hypoglycemia (Br Med J 1981;283:1386–1388, Diabetes Care 1990;13:1240–1262)

▶ *What Contraindications Are There to the Use of This Drug?*

Intolerance of or allergic reaction to insulin

- patients with insulin-dependent diabetes who must inject insulin require desensitization or a change to human insulin
- for a detailed protocol, consult the following reference: Galloway JA, deShazo RD. The clinical use of insulin and the complications of insulin therapy. In: Ellenberg M, Rifkin H, eds. Diabetes Mellitus: Theory and Practice, 3rd ed. Philadelphia: Medical Examination Publishing, 1983

▶ *What Drug Interactions Are Clinically Important?*

Drugs that may increase the effect or toxicity of insulin

BETA-ADRENERGIC BLOCKERS

- may lengthen hypoglycemic episodes in experimentally induced hypoglycemia, however, the clinical importance of this, particularly with selective beta-blockers, is not well described
- may block insulin secretion (owing to inhibition of beta$_2$-receptors), occasionally causing hyperglycemia; however, this is not usually clinically relevant
- in general, cardioselective beta-blockers can be used in patients with diabetes because CNS symptoms are usually unaltered and sweating is enhanced; however, symptoms such as palpitations and tremor are decreased or diminished
- nonselective beta-blockers should be avoided in diabetic patients
- if a beta-blocker must be used, choose a cardioselective agent (atenolol, metoprolol, or acebutolol) in a low dosage to maintain its cardioselectivity
- particularly when the benefits outweigh the risks (e.g., postmyocardial infarction) beta-blockers should not be avoided in diabetic

patients (Diabetes Care 1983;6:285–290, Eur HJ 1989; 10:423–428)

CLOFIBRATE

- patients with non–insulin-dependent diabetes may be at risk for hypoglycemia if clofibrate is added to insulin therapy
- mechanism of this drug interaction is unknown
- if clofibrate is added, monitor blood glucose levels twice daily for 1 week; if blood glucose levels fall to low levels or signs and symptoms of hypoglycemia are present, reduce the insulin dosage

ETHANOL

- inhibits hepatic gluconeogenesis, causing hypoglycemia when gluconeogenesis is required to maintain normal glucose blood levels (e.g., during fasting or decreased food intake)
- avoid the use of glyburide (and all long-acting sulfonylureas) in alcoholic patients; tolbutamide may be a more useful medication
- patients should limit their consumption of alcohol to an occasional 1 drink per day with food while receiving this medication

FENFLURAMINE

- enhances insulin action at the receptor site, producing increased glucose uptake and/or decreased hepatic gluconeogenesis
- monitor blood glucose levels more closely than usual for 2 weeks, and if blood glucose levels fall to low levels or signs and symptoms of hypoglycemia are present, reduce the insulin dosage

MONOAMINE OXIDASE INHIBITORS

- inhibit gluconeogenesis and, in non–insulin-dependent diabetic patients, stimulate endogenous insulin secretion
- monitor blood glucose levels more closely than usual for 2 weeks, and if blood glucose levels fall to low levels or signs and symptoms of hypoglycemia are present, reduce the insulin dosage

SALICYLATES

- sodium salicylate and aspirin used in high dosages by non–insulin-dependent diabetic patients may cause hypoglycemia by increasing insulin secretion
- in many patients, long-term use of salicylates has reduced the dosage or the need for insulin therapy
- patients should monitor blood glucose levels twice daily for 1 month and monitor closely for signs and symptoms of hypoglycemia
- insulin dosage should be reduced if blood glucose levels fall to low levels or signs and symptoms of hypoglycemia are present

Drugs that may decrease the effect of insulin

CORTICOSTEROIDS

- increase hepatic gluconeogenesis and decrease tissue responsiveness to insulin
- ensure that the use of oral corticosteroids is essential and use the lowest possible dose of corticosteroid
- monitor blood glucose levels more closely for 2 weeks in all patients with diabetes, and if blood glucose levels are not controlled and signs and symptoms of hyperglycemia occur, increase the dosage of insulin

Drugs that may have their effect or toxicity increased by insulin

- none

Drugs that may have their effect decreased by insulin

- none

▶ *What Route and Dosage Should I Use?*

How to administer

- orally—not available
- intravenously—insulin in normal saline is given for the treatment of diabetic ketoacidosis; insulin in dextrose solution is given for perioperative management and acute severe hyperkalemia; intravenous regular insulin may bind to polyvinyl chloride tubing and decrease the bioavailability of insulin; some authors suggest using albumin in the insulin solution; however, this practice is expensive; the amount absorbed may be decreased by running 50 mL of insulin infusion containing greater than 5 units/100

50 mL of insulin infusion containing greater than 5 units/100 mL prior to administering the solution to the patient (Diabetes 1976;25:72–75)

- intramuscularly—may be used for diabetic ketoacidosis, but generally the intravenous route is preferred because it is more easily titrated
- subcutaneously—for routine, daily treatment of diabetes

Available products

Human, beef, pork, beef-pork

- most clinicians recommend initiating human insulin treatment to minimize the potential for immunological complications, which may result from use of the more antigenic beef-pork mixed-species insulins; however, the evidence to support this practice is not conclusive (Diabetes Care 1989;12:641–648)
- there is no clinical difference between biosynthetic and semisynthetic human insulins (Diabetes Care 1989;12:641–648)
- patients who require insulin on only an intermittent or short-term basis (e.g., because of surgery, infection, total parenteral nutrition supplementation, and gestational diabetes) should use human insulin to decrease the possibility of immunological complications with future uses of insulin
- patients who are stabilized on beef-pork insulins (less expensive than human insulins) and who are experiencing no adverse effects do not need to be switched to human insulin
- there appears to be an increased risk of severe hypoglycemia when patients are transferred from animal source insulins to human insulins (Br Med J 1991;303:617–621)
- there are 3 different formulations of insulin, and they vary with respect to time of onset, time to peak effect, and duration of effect

Short acting (onset, ½–1 hour; peak, 2–4 hours; duration, 5–7 hours)

Regular insulin (crystalline zinc insulin)—available as human or animal species insulin

- is the preferred subcutaneous rapid-acting insulin and is the only agent that can be used intravenously

Semilente

- should not be used instead of regular insulin because its onset of action is less prompt and its duration is more prolonged

Intermediate acting (onset, 1–3 hours; peak, 6–12 hours; duration, approximately 24 hours)

NPH and Lente insulin—available as human or animal species insulin

- are widely used and can be considered interchangeable
- NPH may be mixed with regular insulin in the same syringe; Lente may not, as the extra zinc binds with the regular insulin, changing it to intermediate acting

Long acting (onset, 6 hours; peak, 18–24 hours [10–14 hours for human]; duration, 36 hours [16–18 hours for human])

Ultralente insulin—available as human or beef insulin

- is the preferred type in this class

Protamine zinc insulin suspension

- no longer available

Premixed fixed ratios of regular and NPH insulin (USA: 85/15, 70/30, 50/50; Canada 90/10, 85/15, 80/20, 70/30, 50/50)

- are generally recommended for convenience in selected patients who have previously been stabilized on mixed-dose regimens and should not be used for initiating insulin therapy

Long-term uses

Insulin-dependent diabetes mellitus (numbers in parentheses are dosages for a 60 kg patient)

- 0.5 unit/kg/d (30 units)
- insulin can be initiated in either a BID (before breakfast and dinner) or a TID regimen (before breakfast and dinner and at bedtime)

BID regimen

- more convenient than the TID regimen; however, the patient must eat a bedtime snack before retiring to avoid a hypoglycemic reaction in early morning (2–4 AM) when the NPH insulin peaks
- suggested starting regimen: give ⅔ of the total daily dose (20 units) before breakfast, with ⅔ of the morning dose (14 units) given as an intermediate-acting insulin and ⅓ (6 units) given as a short-acting insulin; give ⅓ of the total daily dose (10 units) before dinner, with ½ (5 units) given as an intermediate-acting insulin and ½ (5 units) given as a short-acting insulin
- short-acting insulins provide coverage for breakfast and dinner; the intermediate-acting insulin provides coverage for lunch and bedtime snack and basal amounts throughout the day and night
- evening dose of intermediate-acting insulin may have to be given at bedtime (TID regimen) rather than before dinner in patients who experience 3 AM hypoglycemia followed by fasting 7 AM hyperglycemia owing to a peak effect of insulin occurring during early morning hours followed by counterregulatory hormones causing increased glucose production and hyperglycemia (Somogyi effect) (Diabetes Mellitus: Theory and Practice, 4th ed 1990:526–546)
- insufficient duration of action of the intermediate-acting insulin administered before dinner may also cause 7 AM fasting hyperglycemia; increasing the dose of NPH at dinner or administering the NPH at bedtime may be required
- to determine which of the above is the cause of 7 AM fasting hyperglycemia, blood glucose levels should be measured between 2 and 4 AM (in addition to HS levels)

TID regimen

- allows more flexibility than the BID regimen and can be more readily adjusted (time and amount)
- give a mixed dose (as above for the BID regimen) before breakfast and split the dinner dose by giving ⅙ of the daily dose (5 units) of short-acting insulin before dinner and ⅙ of the daily dose (5 units) of intermediate-acting insulin at bedtime

Intensive insulin regimen

- used in patients who are extremely compliant and willing and able to self-monitor blood glucose levels and change insulin dosages on the basis of these results
- patient must have thorough understanding of the actions of insulin, the effects of diet and exercise, and insulin dosage adjustments on the basis of blood glucose levels
- generally, patients require 3–4 injections per day for maximum control
- suggested regimens include regular insulin prior to each meal with intermediate or long-acting insulins given once to twice a day
- example for starting: ¼ of the daily insulin dosage given as regular insulin prior to breakfast, lunch, and dinner and ¼ of the daily insulin dosage as NPH at bedtime
- example for starting: ⅕ of the daily insulin dosage given as regular insulin prior to breakfast, lunch, and dinner and ⅕ of the day insulin dosage as Ultralente given at breakfast and dinner
- other examples include using standard BID or TID regimens with supplemental dosages of regular insulin as needed for hyperglycemia
- patient would administer 1–2 units of regular insulin before meals for each 50 mg/dL (2.8 mmol/L) above the goal; if blood glucose level prior to a meal is less than 70 mg/dL (3.9 mmol/L), give 1–2 units less of regular insulin (Diabetes Care 1990;13:1265–1283, Applied Therapeutics: The Clinical Use of Drugs, 5th ed 1993; Chap. 72, pp 1–53)

Further insulin dosage adjustments should be based on blood glucose measurements

- gradually increase or decrease the daily dosage by 1–2 units/d as needed to achieve desired glycemic control
- in general, dosage changes of greater than 10% should not be done except in the acute care setting
- early in the course of insulin-dependent diabetes, a period of relative remission ("honeymoon period") may occur and insulin requirements may fall to as low as 0.2 unit/kg/d; insulin therapy must not be interrupted, despite very low requirements because

of the concern about future immunological reactions (Diabetes Care 1987;10:164–168)

- aggressive therapy is recommended for most young, otherwise healthy, patients to normalize blood glucose levels and thereby potentially to minimize the incidence and severity of long-term complications
- consider a less aggressive approach for elderly patients in whom long-term complications are absent and/or unlikely to occur during their expected lifetime (Diabetes Care 1990;13:1011–1019, Clin Diabetes 1985;3:73–90)
- do not attempt to achieve a degree of blood glucose control tighter than that which can be attained safely without frequent and/or severe hypoglycemic episodes
- accept higher plasma glucose values in patients who are predisposed to hypoglycemia and/or unaware of the signs and symptoms and/or likely unable to recover
- dosage adjustments should not be made more frequently than every 3 days (so that a pattern may be established)

Non–insulin-dependent diabetes mellitus

- 0.2–0.5 unit/kg (of actual body weight) of intermediate-acting insulin (NPH or Lente) given once daily before breakfast is the most common starting dosage (Diabetes Care 1990;13:1240–1262, Can Med Assoc J 1991;145:1571–1581)
- alternatively, long-acting pork or mixed beef-pork Ultralente may be given once daily in the evening to supply 24 hour basal insulin levels (long-acting human Ultralente insulin must be given twice daily) (Diabetes Care 1990;13:1240–1262)
- if the patient is in the hospital and has urinary ketones, 4–6 units of regular insulin subcutaneously every 6 hours should be administered until ketosis is resolved (Diabetes Care 1990;13:1240–1262)
- for patients in the hospital, dosages may be increased by 20–40% daily, with close monitoring, to pursue more efficient and cost-effective therapy (Diabetes Care 1990;13:1240–1262)
- for outpatients, dosage increases of 2–5 units/d may be made every 3 days (Can Med Assoc J 1991;145:1571–1581)
- if the NPH dose in the morning reaches 60–80 units without achieving desirable 7 AM fasting blood glucose levels, a second dose of NPH should be added at bedtime (Diabetes Care 1990;13:1240–1262) so that 50–70% of the daily dose is administered before breakfast and 30–50% of the daily dose is administered before dinner (Can Med Assoc J 1991;145:1571–1581); more insulin is usually required during daytime hours
- owing to inherent insulin resistance, daily doses may exceed 1 unit/kg to achieve euglycemia (Can Med Assoc J 1991;145:1571–1581)
- after euglycemia is achieved, dosage decreases may be necessary because insulin sensitivity improves with control of blood glucose levels (Can Med Assoc J 1991;145:1571–1581, Diabetes Care 1990;13:1240–1262)

Temporary uses

- use human insulin to decrease the risk of antibody production and immunological reactions with subsequent uses of insulin

Non–insulin-dependent diabetes mellitus

Pregnancy

- treat as non–insulin-dependent diabetes mellitus as outlined above

Periods of significant stress

- 32 units of regular insulin and 20 mmol of potassium chloride in 1000 mL of dextrose 10% administered at 100 ml/h (3.2 units/h or approximately 0.05 unit/kg/h)
- if blood glucose levels are less than 80 mg/dL (4.4 mmol/L), decrease the rate to 2.4 units/h; 80–120 mg/dL (4.4–6.6 mmol/L), decrease the rate to 2.8 units/h; 120–180 mg/dL (6.6–10 mmol/L), maintain current regimen; greater than 180–270 mg/dL (10–15 mmol/L), increase the rate to 3.6 units/h; greater than 270 mg/dL (15 mmol/L), increase the rate to 4 units/h (Diabetes Theory and Practice, 4th ed 1990:626–633)

Perioperative use

- initiate intravenous insulin regimen 12–24 hours prior to surgery

- begin infusion of dextrose 5% in half-normal saline with potassium 20 mEq/L at 100 mL/h
- insulin infusion is separate so it can easily be titrated
- insulin 50 units in 500 mL of normal saline to infuse initially at 1.5 units/h (15 mL/h) to maintain blood glucose levels of 120–180 mg/dL (6.5–10 mmol/L)
- rate is adjusted according to frequent blood glucose concentrations and is as follows: if less than 80–120 mg/dL (4.5–6.5 mmol/L), decrease the rate by 0.5 unit/h and if less than 80 mg/dL (4.5 mmol/dL), administer 12.5 g of dextrose IV; if blood glucose levels are 180–240 mg/dL (10–13.5 mmol/L) or greater, increase rate by 0.5 unit/h, and if greater than 240 mg/dL (13.5 mmol/L), give additional 8 units of regular insulin as an IV bolus (Applied Therapeutics: The Clinical Use of Drugs, 5th ed 1993; Chap. 72, pp 1–53)

Gestational diabetes

- treat as non–insulin-dependent diabetes mellitus as outlined above

Diabetic ketoacidosis or hyperglycemic hyperosmolar nonketotic syndrome

- regular insulin 0.1 unit/kg IV bolus, followed initially by 0.1 unit/kg/h continuous infusion; mix 50 units of regular insulin in 500 mL of normal saline and run an infusion rate equal to patient's weight (Applied Therapeutics: The Clinical Use of Drugs, 5th ed 1993; Chap. 72, pp 1–53, The Management of Diabetes Mellitus 1990:24–25)
- if glucose concentrations remain unchanged after 2 hours, increase the infusion to 0.2 unit/kg/h
- when glucose concentrations fall to 250–300 mg/dL (14–16.5 mmol/L), decrease the infusion rate to 0.05 unit/kg/h and add dextrose 5% in half-normal saline infusion to prevent hypoglycemia

Severe hyperkalemia

- administer insulin with glucose to prevent hypoglycemia
- if the patient is hyperglycemic, glucose should not be administered with insulin
- regular insulin 20 units in 1000 mL of dextrose 10% administered intravenously over 1–2 hours
- serum postassium levels should decrease within 30 minutes and continue to remain lowered for 2–6 hours
- insulin (and glucose) only shifts potassium stores and does not remove total body stores of potassium; removal of total body stores is also required (Pharmacotherapy: A Pathophysiological Approach 1989:1490–1492)

Dosage adjustments for renal or hepatic dysfunction

- insulin is metabolized by the liver and metabolized and excreted by the kidney
- standard dosages should be used initially and adjusted according to blood glucose levels

▶ *What Should I Monitor with Regard to Efficacy and Toxicity*

Efficacy

Long-term uses

- frequency of assessment of an individual patient depends on the type, severity, and complications of diabetes; the difficulty experienced in controlling blood glucose levels; changes in therapy; and other medical conditions (Diabetes Care 1993;16[suppl 2]:4–13)
- all patients should be referred to a diabetes education center after diagnosis and attend periodically for refresher courses (Diabetes Care 1993;16[suppl 2]:4–13)

Insulin-dependent and non–insulin-dependent diabetes mellitus (Diabetes Care 1993;16[suppl 2]:4–13)

- daily contact may be required during the initiation of insulin therapy or after any major change in insulin regimen and should continue until satisfactory control is achieved, the risk of hypoglycemia is low, and the patient demonstrates competence in insulin administration and monitoring

- after a major change in insulin therapy, contact with the patient should be made within at least 1 week
- in general, regular office visitis are scheduled every 3 months for patients receiving insulin
- children and adolescents should be managed in consultation with persons who have expertise in treating diabetes in this age group
- all insulin-treated patients should be taught self-monitoring of blood glucose levels
- in patients with insulin-dependent diabetes receiving intensive therapy (3–4 injections a day) and requiring insulin dosage that is based on the interpretation of blood glucose results, testing should initially be done as frequently as 4 to 8 times daily (before and 2 hours after meals, at bedtime, and between 2 and 4 AM)
- this intensive schedule need not be done every day during stable periods (e.g., only 3 d/wk) or can be staggered (e.g., before breakfast and lunch 1 day and before dinner and at bedtime on the following day)
- patients receiving minimum insulin therapy (e.g, those with non–insulin-dependent diabetes) may be required to test only once or twice daily (e.g., before breakfast and/or supper) and, during stable periods, only 3 or 4 times per week (Can Med Assoc J 1992;147:697–712)
- frequency and scheduling of blood glucose testing must be individualized according to the type of diabetes, the goals and the agents used for treatment, the extent of blood glucose fluctuation, and the patient's willingness to self-monitor
- every 4–6 months, a blood glucose level obtained by the patient should be compared simultaneously with a laboratory-measured level to verify the patient's self-monitoring technique (Can Med Assoc J 1992;147:697–712)

Self-monitoring of preprandial blood glucose levels (N Engl J Med 1989;321:1231–1245, Can Med Assoc J 1992;147:697–712)

- 80–120 mg/dL (4.4–6.7 mmol/L) is considered good or optimum control
- 120–140 mg/dL (6.7–7.8 mmol/L) is considered acceptable control
- 140–180 mg/dL (7.8–10 mmol/L) is considered fair control
- greater than 180 mg/dL (greater than 10 mmol/L) is considered poor control
- patients should strive for levels in the optimum range, unless they are elderly, and then fair control is acceptable
- all patients must be carefully taught by a qualified trainer how to use the individual testing devices, to try to avoid errors (Diabetes Care 1993;16:60–65)
- in the elderly, it may be best to use devices that do not require wiping blood from sticks or pressing buttons to start the timer (Br Med J 1992;305:1171–1172)

Urine glucose testing (Diabetes Care 1993;16[suppl 2]:39)

- patients should monitor blood glucose, not urine glucose, levels
- normal renal threshold for glucose is 180 mg/dL (10 mmol/L)
- renal threshold may be increased in patients with diabetes of long duration or may be decreased in children and pregnant women
- urine concentration may affect the results
- reflects only an average level of blood glucose since last voiding
- hypoglycemia cannot be detected
- color tests used for urine testing are not very accurate

Glycosylated hemoglobin (e.g., HbA$_{1c}$) (N Engl J Med 1989;321:1231–1245, Can Med Assoc J 1992;147:697–712)

- HbA$_{1c}$ should be determined in all diabetics at least every 6 months, but preferably every 3 months in insulin-treated patients and non-insulin-treated patients with poor glycemic control
- HbA$_{1c}$ values of 6–8% suggest good glucose control
- HbA$_{1c}$ values of 8–11% suggest fair glucose control
- HbA$_{1c}$ values of 11–13% suggest poor glucose control
- upper limit of normal varies from laboratory to laboratory: in general, a HbA$_{1c}$ within 1% of the upper limit reflects good control, within 1–3% indicates acceptable control, and less than 3% above normal values reflects poor control
- the goal of therapy is to have HbA$_{1c}$ values suggesting good control

- glycosylated hemoglobin is expressed as a percentage of total hemoglobin
- hemoglobin is slowly and irreversibly glycosylated throughout the life of the red blood cell; the amount that is glycosylated depends on blood glucose concentrations
- because the life of a red blood cell is approximately 120 days, measuring HbA$_{1c}$ more frequently than 4 times per year is not beneficial
- is the best index of glycemic control because it reflects the mean blood glucose values over the preceding 6–10 weeks

Urinary ketones (Diabetes Care 1993;16[suppl 2]:4–13)

- indicative of impending keotacidosis
- patient with insulin-dependent diabetes should test urine for ketones during periods of stress or acute illness and when blood glucose levels consistently exceed 240 mg/dL (13.4 mmol/L) or symptoms of diabetic ketoacidosis are present (nausea, vomiting, and abdominal pain)
- if ketones are present, medical advice should be sought, as this is a serious danger sign

Eye examination (Diabetes Care 1993;16[suppl 2]:16–18, Can Med Assoc J 1992;147:697–712)

- retinal examination by an ophthalmologist should be performed at least once annually in all patients with a 5 year history of insulin-dependent diabetes
- patients with non–insulin-dependent diabetes should have a complete eye examination at the time of diagnosis and then yearly
- pregnant women with preexisting diabetes should have a complete eye examination during the first trimester and be followed closely throughout the remaining months

Lipid profile (Diabetes Care 1993;16[suppl 2]:4–13, 106–112, Can Med Assoc J 1992;147:697–712)

- in adults, monitor fasting serum triglyceride and total, high density lipoprotein, and calculated low density lipoprotein (LDL) cholesterol once yearly
- if abnormalities exist, complete the above testing every 4 months
- in children, complete testing as for an adult at time of diagnosis; if any abnormality exists, complete testing annually; if no abnormality exists, complete testing every 2 years
- high triglyceride and LDL cholesterol levels may be associated with poor glycemic control
- dyslipidemia should first be treated by weight reduction (if necessary), decreased saturated fat and cholesterol intake, and increased exercise
- if the response is not adequate with nonpharmacological treatment in 4 months, lipid-lowering drug therapy should be considered

Blood pressure (Diabetes Care 1993;16[suppl 2]:4–13)

- measure blood pressure at regular office visits
- results do not affect diabetic therapy but may suggest the need for further diet consultation or antihypertensive drug therapy
- because hypertension contributes to the risk and progression of diabetic complications, increased blood pressure should be treated aggressively

Renal profile (Diabetes Care 1993;16[suppl 2]:4–13, Can Med Assoc J 1992;147:697–712)

- at diagnosis and once yearly, a routine urinalysis and serum creatinine level should be completed
- in patients past puberty or younger patients with a 5 year history of diabetes, total urinary protein excretion should be determined yearly (if possible, by a microalbuminuria method)
- if abnormalities are present, the above testing should be done during all regular office visits
- if declining renal function or persistent proteinuria is confirmed, the patient should be referred to a nephrologist specializing in diabetic renal disease

Neurological profile (Diabetes Care 1993;16[suppl 2]:4–13, Can Med Assoc J 1992;147:697–712)

- sensory, motor, and autonomic nervous systems may be affected by diabetes

- complete neurological examination should be performed at the time of diagnosis and at least annually

Foot care (Diabetes Care 1993;16[suppl 2]:4–13, Can Med Assoc J 1992;147:697–712)

- complete foot and leg examination should be completed at the time of diagnosis and at regular office visits
- patients should routinely inspect their feet for any abnormality each evening

Symptoms

- reduction in symptoms such as polyuria, polydipsia

Temporary uses

Non–insulin-dependent diabetes mellitus

Pregnancy

- optimum control of diabetes is important prior to conception
- optimum target values for blood glucose are: 7AM fasting: 60–90 mg/dL (3.3–5 mmol/L); 2 hours after meals: less 120 mg/dL (6.6 mmol/L); and before meals and bedtime snack and 2–6 AM: 60–90 mg/dL (3.3–5 mmol/L) (The Management of Diabetes Mellitus 1990:29)

Periods of Significant Stress

- monitor blood glucose concentrations every 2 hours and adjust the insulin dosage as outlined above
- monitor potassium levels every 6 hours during this time
- when the patient is more stable and blood glucose levels have remained in the normal range for 12 hours, monitor blood glucose levels every 4 hours (Diabetes Theory and Practice, 4th ed 1990:626–633)
- after the patient is stable and oral intake has resumed, the patient's regular monitoring schedule should be resumed

Perioperative Use

- as for periods of significant stress (see above)

Gestational Diabetes

- as for pregnancy in non–insulin-dependent diabetes (see above)

Diabetic Ketoacidosis or Hyperglycemic Hyperosmolar Nonketotic Syndrome

- rate of fall of blood glucose levels should be 10% per hour (The Management of Diabetes Mellitus 1990:24–25)
- monitor serum glucose concentrations every hour until concentrations reach 250–300 mg/dL (14–16.5 mmol/L) and then every 4–6 hours until subcutaneous injections are initiated

Severe Hyperkalemia

- monitor plasma potassium concentrations every 4 hours until levels are within the normal range
- then monitor concentrations every 6–24 hours, depending on the cause and acuity of increased potassium levels

Toxicity

Long-term uses

Dermatological effects

- patient should rotate the injection site within an anatomical area to decrease the risk of lipoatrophy and lipohypertrophy
- dermatological reactions are rare with purified pork and human insulin products

Hypoglycemia

- patient, family, and friends need to be aware of the signs and symptoms of hypoglycemia
- ask whether the patient has experienced any symptoms of hypoglycemia: sweaty palms, generalized sweating, tremors, palpitations, anxiety, irritability, hunger, restlessness, loss of concentration, confusion, visual disorders, headache, night sweats, restless sleep, nightmares, and difficulty rising in the morning
- if these symptoms occur, the patient should be instructed to take in simple carbohydrates: 1/2 cup of orange juice or nondiet soda, 2 sugar cubes, 6 Life-Savers, or 2 glucose tablets
- if the patient becomes unconscious, glucagon 1 mg SC or IM (or IV if the patient is in the emergency department or the hospital) should be given

- unconscious patient in the hospital or emergency department may be given glucose 25–50 g IV
- investigate the reason for hypoglycemia: fasting or decreased food intake, vomiting, excessive exercise, or alcohol consumption; and educate the patient about the causes of hypoglycemia
- if the patient has 3 hypoglycemic reactions in less than 6 months, insulin dosages should be adjusted by 1–2 units on the basis of premeal blood glucose levels and the type of insulin administered (see below)
- if the fasting 7 AM blood glucose level is not in the range desired, adjust predinner or bedtime intermediate- or long-acting insulin administration
- if the prelunch blood glucose level is not in the range desired, adjust prebreakfast regular insulin dosage
- if the predinner blood glucose level is not in the range desired, adjust prebreakfast intermediate-acting or prelunch regular insulin dosage
- if the bedtime blood glucose level is not in the range desired, adjust the predinner regular insulin dosage
- if 2–4 AM blood glucose concentration is not in the range desired, adjust predinner intermediate-acting insulin dosage
- if the patient is receiving an intensive schedule of insulin, regular insulin dosages should be decreased by 1 unit if the blood glucose level is 50 to less than 80 mg/dL (2.8–4.4 mmol/L) and by 2 units if the blood glucose level is 50 mg/dL (2.8 mmol/L)

Temporary uses

Hypoglycemia

- see above under efficacy, which includes complete monitoring for both hypoglycemia and hyperglycemia

▶ *How Long Do I Treat Patients with This Drug?*

Long-term uses

Insulin-dependent diabetes mellitus

- patients require insulin treatment continuously for the rest of their lives
- early in the course of insulin-dependent diabetes, during a period of relative remission ("honeymoon period"), insulin requirements may fall to as low as 0.2 unit/kg/d; insulin therapy must not be interrupted despite very low requirements because of the concern for future immunological reactions (Diabetes Care 1987; 10:164–168)

Non–insulin-dependent diabetes mellitus

- each patient should be viewed as a candidate for insulin withdrawal
- if insulin requirements are 20 units/d or less, a trial with a sulfonylurea alone is warranted (Diabetes Care 1990;13:1240–1262)
- definite indications for insulin withdrawal are sustained excellent control and suspected hypoglycemia (Br Med J 1981;283: 1386–1388, Diabetes Care 1990;13:1240–1262)
- patients require insulin treatment continuously for the rest of their lives

Temporary uses

Non–insulin-dependent diabetes mellitus

Pregnancy

- if pregnancy induced diabetes, continue insulin administration until delivery and then discontinue; glucose-lowering agents should not be required after this time
- if diabetes existed prior to pregnancy, insulin should be used because oral glucose-lowering agents are contraindicated

Perioperative use

- continue with the regimen until patient's oral intake has stabilized and previous glucose-lowering therapy has been reinstituted

Periods of significant stress

- many patients with non–insulin-dependent diabetes receive insulin treatment for specific periods of instability
- after metabolic control has been reestablished, withdrawal of insulin therapy should be attempted, usually when the patient has resumed normal oral intake

Gestational diabetes

- at delivery, insulin therapy is discontinued and a normal diet is resumed (The Management of Diabetes Mellitus 1990:29)
- patients should be followed post partum with an oral glucose tolerance test to detect non–insulin-dependent diabetes early (Diabetes Care 1993;16[suppl 2]:5–6)

Diabetic ketoacidosis or hyperglycemic hyperosmolar nonketotic syndrome

- continue intravenous insulin in normal saline for diabetic ketoacidosis until ketosis is resolved, the glucose level is controlled, and the patient can resume eating and giving subcutaneous injections
- when the plasma glucose level declines to 14–16.5 mmol/L, continue intravenous insulin for resolution of ketosis but ensure that 5% dextrose is infused to avoid hypoglycemia
- for hyperglycemic hyperosmolar nonketotic syndrome, continue intravenous insulin until the glucose level is adequately controlled and the patient can receive other therapy as required

Severe hyperkalemia

- continue therapy until potassium levels are less than 6 mmol/L and clinical signs and symptoms are relieved
- repeated administration may be necessary after 2–6 hours unless total body stores of potassium are decreased

▶ *How Do I Decrease or Stop the Administration of This Drug?*

- if necessary, insulin may be stopped abruptly

▶ *What Should I Tell My Patients About Insulin?*

Product-related advice

- know your insulin product by name, species source, and manufacturer
- always check the expiration date printed on the insulin box and vial or cartridge, which indicates the expiration date if the insulin is kept refrigerated
- never use a vial of regular insulin that is cloudy, discolored, or unusually thick
- all other insulins are suspensions, which should be cloudy; however, do not use vials that contain clumps of insulin, insulin caked at the bottom, or a frosting of crystals on the walls of the vial
- store unopened vials in the refrigerator
- store in-use vials at room temperature for up to 1 month
- avoid direct sunlight and hot temperatures
- discard insulin that has been frozen because the insulin can aggregate
- when traveling, carry insulins with you and avoid storage in the glove compartments in cars or in the luggage compartments on airplanes; in hot climates, carry an insulated container for insulin storage

Dosage administration

- gently disperse all insulin suspensions just prior to use (avoid shaking and bubbles)
- inject air equal to the amount of insulin that will be withdrawn prior to trying to withdraw insulin and then withdraw the proper dose
- when combining 2 insulins in 1 syringe:
  1. inject the proper amount of air into the NPH vial
  2. withdraw the regular insulin
  3. withdraw the longer-acting insulin in the same syringe
- this process avoids contamination of the regular insulin vial, which may delay the prompt action of the regular insulin
- inject insulin within the same area at all times (e.g., abdomen, thigh, and arm) to allow more consistent absorption
- rotate injection sites within the same anatomical area to avoid local dermatological complications
- be consistent with the administration times of insulin from day to day
- injections of rapid-acting insulin should be followed by ingestion of food (complex carbohydrates such as milk, sandwiches, crackers, etc.) within 30–60 minutes

Hypoglycemia

- you should be familiar with the signs and symptoms of low blood glucose levels
- have you experienced any symptoms of hypoglycemia such as sweating, tremor, palpitations, anxiety, irritability, hunger, restlessness, loss of concentration, confusion, visual disorders, and nightmares?
- family members should be aware of hypoglycemic symptoms
- common causes of low blood glucose levels are missed meals, poor eating habits, excessive exercise, and alcohol consumption
- if these symptoms occur and are mild, you should take in simple carbohydrates: 1/2 cup of orange juice or nondiet soda, 2 sugar cubes, 6 Life-Savers, or 2 glucose tablets followed by a longer acting carbohydrate (e.g., milk or a sandwich) to replete glycogen stores and decrease the risk of a hypoglycemic reaction
- for severe cases and occasions when loss of consciousness occurs or is likely, you or your family or friends should obtain emergency medical assistance
- friends or relatives can inject glucagon 1 unit subcutaneously when professional assistance is unavailable
- if you check home blood glucose levels, hypoglycemia should be confirmed

Hyperglycemia

- be familiar with the signs and symptoms of high blood glucose, including increased urination, unusual thirst, dry mouth, drowsiness, flushed, dry skin, fruit-like breath odor, loss of appetite, and troubled breathing
- have guidelines regarding blood glucose testing, including injection of supplemental rapid-acting insulin and instructions for seeking medical assistance and urine ketone testing

Diet and exercise

- appreciate the significance of the size, composition, and timing of meals and snacks and adhere to the devised meal plan
- establish an exercise plan that provides a guide for the type, extent, and timing of your physical activities

Useful References

Banting and Best Diabetes Centre. The Management of Diabetes Mellitus. Toronto: University of Toronto, 1990

Rifkin H, Porte D, eds. Diabetes Mellitus: Theory and Practice, 4th ed. New York: Elsevier, 1990

Briggs GG, Freeman RD, Yaffe SL, eds. Drugs in Pregnancy and Lactation, 3rd ed. Baltimore: Williams & Wilkins, 1994

Hanslen PD, Horn JR, eds. Drug Interactions and Updates. Philadelphia: Lea & Febiger, 1993

Tatro DS, ed. Drug Interaction Facts. St. Louis: Facts and Comparisons, 1995

Koda-Kimble MA. Diabetes mellitus. In: Koda-Kimble MA, Young LY, eds. Applied Therapeutics: The Clinical Use of Drugs, 5th ed. Vancouver, WA: Applied Therapeutics, 1993: Chap. 72, pp 1–53

IPRATROPIUM

Karen Shalansky and Cindy Reesor Nimmo

USA (Atrovent)
CANADA (Atrovent)

▶ *When Should I Use This Drug?*

Acute asthma or acute exacerbation of chronic obstructive pulmonary disease

- adjunct to beta₂-agonist therapy in patients with severe obstruction (less than 35% of predicted peak expiratory flow rate, forced expiratory volume in 1 second ≤1 L) (DICP 1990;24:409–416, Lung 1990;suppl:295–303)
- ipratropium may provide additional bronchodilation and may be initiated with the first dose of the beta₂-agonist
- ipratropium, although giving an additional small increment in expiratory flow rates when used with submaximum dosages of beta-agonists, has never been shown to reduce other variables such as the need for admission to a hospital or shortened duration of hospital stay
- use for severe asthma, but do not use for the routine treatment of less severe asthma

- ipratropium should never be used before beta-agonists owing to concern about ipratropium initially causing bronchoconstriction (Postgrad Med J 1991;67:1–3)

Chronic asthma or chronic obstructive pulmonary disease

- only after appropriate doses of beta$_2$-agonists, corticosteroids, and cromolyn have been tried in asthmatic patients
- ipratropium appears to be more effective in COPD than in asthma (Arch Intern Med 1989;149:544–547) and has been recommended as first-line therapy for COPD before beta$_2$-agonists by some authors (N Engl J Med 1993;328:1017–1022)

▶ When Should I Not Use This Drug?

Alone for the treatment of acute asthma

- nebulized ipratropium may cause paradoxical bronchoconstriction (J Allergy Clin Immunol 1990;85:1098–1111, N Engl J Med 1989;321:1517–1527)

▶ What Contraindications Are There to the Use of This Drug?

- intolerance of or allergic reaction to ipratropium or atropine

▶ What Drug Interactions Are Clinically Important?

- none

▶ What Route and Dosage Should I Use?

How to administer

Inhaled

- dilute each nebulized dose to 4 mL with normal saline (water, half-normal saline, or hypertonic saline may be used), place in the nebulizer, and use an airflow rate of 6–8 L/min (compatible with salbutamol [albuterol]) if mixed together and nebulized
- for a metered-dose inhaler, see below

Acute asthma or acute exacerbation of chronic obstructive pulmonary disease

- 0.5 mg with the first dose of nebulized salbutamol then Q4H
- 4 puffs via a metered-dose inhaler with the first dose of salbutamol, then Q4H

Chronic asthma or chronic obstructive pulmonary disease

- 2 puffs inhaled QID; may double the dosage if there is inadequate response (Chest 1990;97[suppl 27]:19S–23S, N Engl J Med 1993;328:1017–1022)

▶ What Should I Monitor With Regard to Efficacy and Toxicity?

Efficacy

see Salbutamol

Toxicity

Dry mouth, cough, metallic taste

- rinse mouth with warm water after each use

Blurred vision

- if sprayed into the eyes, prolonged pupillary dilatation may result

▶ How Long Do I Treat Patients with This Drug?

Acute asthma or acute exacerbation of chronic obstructive pulmonary disease

- continue frequent dosing of bronchodilators until pulmonary function returns to normal or the best result achievable is obtained
- after full control has been achieved (absence of night and morning symptoms, normalization or maximization of pulmonary function or peak flow readings), the dosage should be reduced to the minimum necessary (PRN) to maintain control
- ipratropium has not been proved to offer any benefit in combination with a beta-agonist after 24 hours of initial therapy (Chest 1990;98:295–297)

Chronic asthma or chronic obstructive pulmonary disease

- after control or the best possible result is achieved and the lowest level of effective treatment is established, the patient should

be reassessed every 1–6 months, depending on the severity of disease
- administer indefinitely as long as the patient continues to obtain benefit from the drug with minimum toxicity

▶ How Do I Decrease or Stop the Administration of This Drug?

- may be discontinued abruptly; however, tapering is rational and may prevent psychological rebound
- recurrence of symptoms is not rebound, rather verification of usefulness

▶ What Should I Tell My Patients About This Drug?

- do not exceed the dosage recommended by your physician
- dry mouth may be relieved by rinsing with warm water after you use the inhaler
- you may experience a short cough after use of the inhaler; if this becomes bothersome, contact your physician
- rinse the outer shell of the metered-dose inhaler with warm water at least every 2 weeks
- if combination inhalers are used, use ipratropium after the beta$_2$-agonist

Metered-dose inhaler

1. place the canister firmly into the outer shell
2. shake well and remove the cap
3. exhale to a normal relaxed expiration
4. place the tip of the mouthpiece—either 2 fingerbreadths in front of widely opened mouth (preferable) or between the teeth and lips
5. breathe in slowly, and at the same time, press the canister to release 1 puff of the drug
6. continue to inhale as deeply as possible—hold breath for as long as is comfortable (5–10 seconds)
7. breathe out to a normal relaxed resting position
8. if a second inhalation is prescribed, the same procedure is repeated with the second puff, 30 seconds after the first

Extension device (for use with metered-dose inhalers)

1. remove the mouthpiece covers from the inhaler and the extension device
2. shake the inhaler well and insert into the appropriate opening on the extension device
3. exhale to a normal relaxed expiration, then place the mouthpiece of the extension device between the teeth and lips—do not cover the small holes on either side of the mouthpiece
4. activate the metered-dose inhaler into the extension device
5. breathe in slowly and deeply—hold your breath for 5–10 seconds—breathe out slowly to a normal relaxed resting position
6. if you are unable to take a deep breath, breathe in and out normally for 3 or 4 breaths
7. if a second inhalation is prescribed, the same procedure is repeated with the second puff, at least 30 seconds after the first

▶ Therapeutic Tips

- if ipratropium is ineffective, ensure that proper technique is being used
- ensure that the patient does not spray into the eyes
- never use ipratropium before beta-agonists in the treatment of acute asthma because of the concerns about bronchoconstriction

Useful References

Kelly HW, Murphy S. Should anticholinergic be used in acute severe asthma? DICP 1990;24:409–416

Chapman KR. The role of anticholinergic bronchodilators in adult asthma and chronic obstructive pulmonary disease. Lung 1990;suppl:295–303

Gross NJ. Ipratropium bromide. N Engl J Med 1988;319:486–494

IRON

Eric M. Yoshida and Angela Kim-Sing

USA (Ferrous fumarate: Span-FF, Feostat, Femiron, Fumasorb, Hemocyte, Difuleron, Ferro-DSS, Ferrous-DSS, Ferro sequels)

(Ferrous gluconate: Simron, Fergon) (Ferrous sulfate: Fer-in-Sol, Feosol, Fer-Gen-Sol, Mol-iron, Ferrous sulfate enseals, Ferogradumet, Fermalox, Ferralyn, Slow FE, Hytinic, Niferex, Nu-Iron) (Iron dextran injection: Imferon)
CANADA (Ferrous fumarate: Palafer) (Ferrous gluconate: Fergon) (Ferrous sulfate: Apo-ferrous sulfate, Fer-In-Sol, Slow Fe) (Ferrous sucinnate: Cerevon) (Iron dextran injection: Imferon) (Iron sorbitol injection: Jectofer)

▶ When Should I Use This Drug?

Prevention of iron depletion

- iron supplementation should be considered during pregnancy, in menstruating women with suspected inadequate dietary intake (e.g., vegetarians, adolescents with poor dietary habits), and the elderly "tea and toaster" in whom dietary consumption is poor
- in chronic renal failure patients receiving erythropoietin, in whom iron stores are inadequate as indicated by decreased serum iron indices (serum iron, fractional saturation, ferritin)

Treatment of iron deficiency

- microcytic anemia (low MCV, ferritin, serum iron, total iron binding capacity, and increased transferrin) secondary to decreased dietary intake (rare—always rule out blood loss, which may be occult), chronic blood loss (e.g., inadequately compensated menstrual losses, gastrointestinal lesions), or malabsorption syndromes

▶ When Should I Not Use This Drug?

Anemia not due to iron deficiency

- do not supplement iron in patients with thalassemia (often have a low MCV) as these patients have increased iron absorption and can develop iron overload
- in patients with normocytic anemias (e.g., anemia of chronic disease, hemolytic anemia, etc.) as iron is ineffective and the underlying disease process must be treated

▶ What Contraindications Are There to the Use of This Drug?

Intolerance or allergic reaction to iron preparations
Hemosiderosis, hemochromatosis, thalassemia

- these conditions may predispose patient to excessive iron accumulation and multiorgan iron overload

▶ What Drug Interactions Are Clinically Important?

Drugs that may increase effect/toxicity of iron

- none

Drugs that may decrease effect of iron
Phosphate binders (antacids, sucralfate)

- decreases oral iron absorption
- separate oral administration of these agents by at least 2 hours

Drugs that may have effect/toxicity increased by iron

- none

Drugs that may have effect decreased by iron
Floroquinolone antibiotics (e.g., ciprofloxacin), tetracycline, penicillamine, levodopa

- oral iron interferes with the absorption of these drugs; dosing of these agents should be separated by at least 2 hours

▶ What Route and Dosage Should I Use?

How to administer

Orally

- it is preferable to give iron an hour before meals or 2 hours after
- iron may be taken with meals or food if patient is unable to tolerate, but absorption will be decreased by as much as 50%

Oral forms available

- when using oral iron, use a non–enteric-coated, prompted-release (standard) ferrous salt preparation

- ferrous salts are inexpensive and have improved absorption over other iron preparations
- slow release preparations offer no advantage over standard preparations as maximal iron absorption occurs in the duodenum and proximal jejunum
- use least expensive agent listed below that patient is able to tolerate:
  Ferric pyrophosphate contains 12% elemental iron
  Ferrous gluconate contains 12% elemental iron
  Ferrous sulfate contains 20% elemental iron
  Ferrous sulfate, dried, contains 30% elemental iron
  Ferrous fumarate contains 33% elemental iron ferrous carbonate, anhydrous contains 48% elemental iron

Parenteral

- parenteral therapy should be reserved for patients with increased iron requirements and cannot be met with oral supplementation, patients noncompliant or intolerant of oral preparations or with decreased absorption of iron secondary to diseases of the small intestine (e.g., Crohn's disease, celiac sprue)
- a test dose of iron dextran should be administered prior to initiating therapy as both intramuscular and intravenous routes can be complicated by anaphylaxis
- epinephrine and other support measures should be readily available

Intramuscular guidelines

- may use iron sorbitol or iron dextran product with or without phenol
- administer test dose of iron dextran product
- use separate needle to draw up dose
- use Z-track technique, 19–20 gauge needle to inject deeply into muscle; preferably inject into upper outer quadrant of buttock
- painful and inconvenient route of administration as repeated intramuscular injections into both buttocks are required
- if using iron sorbitol, the recommended daily dose in adults is 1.5 mg iron/kg body weight (single daily dose not to exceed 100 mg iron)

Intravenous guidelines

- do *not* use iron dextran product containing phenol for IV administration
- if given "push," the iron dextran should not be administered at a rate greater than 50 mg/min
- extravasation into subcutaneous tissue may cause staining on skin
- if given as a total dose infusion (use is not currently included in FDA approved labeling) dilute in ≥250 ml NS (higher incidence of local pain and phlebitis with D_5W); infuse at 5 mg/min for 10 minutes, and if this is well tolerated the rate may be increased
- flush line with NS after administration to avoid staining skin

Prevention of iron depletion

- 30 mg elemental iron PO daily for prophylaxis in pregnant women
- 65 mg elemental iron PO TID for prophylaxis in chronic renal failure patients on erythropoietin

Treatment of iron deficiency

- 50 mg elemental iron PO TID for the first 3 days, then increase to 100 mg of elemental iron PO TID
- upward dose titration every 3 days may improve gastrointestinal tolerance and compliance
- use oral route unless patient is intolerant to the oral route or has poor absorption secondary to disease
- if oral route not possible, calculate total dose of parenteral iron required to restore hemoglobin concentration to normal using product-specific monograph guidelines
- dilute 100 mg dose to 10 mg/mL with 8 mL NS
- give 25 mg (2.5 mL) over 1–2 minutes and if no reaction occurs after 1 hour, remainder of dose may be given at a rate not exceeding 50 mg/min
- if no reactions have occurred after 2 doses, the total dose may be given at a rate not exceeding 50 mg/min

▶ *What Should I Monitor for with Regard to Efficacy and Toxicity?*

Efficacy

Prevention of iron depletion

- hemoglobin concentration should be assessed monthly during pregnancy to ensure normal value
- if hemoglobin is low, consider causes other than inadequate iron intake
- if inadequate iron intake is the cause, increase dosage by 30 mg elemental iron per day

Treatment of iron deficiency

Hemoglobin

- should increase by week 2–4 at a rate of 10–20 g/L every week until within normal range; rate of regeneration will be proportional to the severity of the anemia

Toxicity

Gastrointestinal

- may cause gastrointestinal irritation, anorexia, nausea, vomiting, diarrhea or constipation, dark stools
- for gastrointestinal upset, increase dose slowly or administer with food

Pain

- repeated intramuscular injections can be painful and should not be used if alternate route of administration available

Staining of the skin

- can occur with parenteral route of administration; advisable to administer IM route to unexposed areas and to flush line with NS following total dose infusions

Anaphylaxis

- can occur with parenteral route of administration; advisable to administer iron test dose with epinephrine, diphenhydramine, and other support measures readily available

Delayed reactions

- arthralgias, myalgia, nausea, vomiting, fever, backache may occur within 24–48 hours following IV or IM administration
- effects generally subside within 3–7 days
- patients with inflammatory diseases may be predisposed to delayed reactions although exact etiology is unknown and in these patients reducing the dose or increasing the interval between doses may reduce the frequency and severity of adverse effects

▶ *How Long Do I Treat Patients with This Drug?*

Prevention of iron depletion

- for duration of pregnancy or until causes are reversed

Treatment of iron deficiency

- continue therapy until hemoglobin maintained at desired level (130–170 g/L for men, 120–160 g/L for women) for 3 months
- 6–12 months of iron therapy may be necessary to replete stores if severe deficiency
- if there is less than a 20 g/L increase in the hemoglobin by week 4, reevaluate diagnosis and/or reassess dose
- for parenteral administration, continue therapy until total calculated dose administered

▶ *How Do I Decrease or Stop This Drug?*

- may be stopped abruptly

▶ *What Should I Tell My Patients About This Drug?*

- oral liquid iron preparations should be diluted and taken through a straw to prevent staining of the teeth
- iron should be taken on an empty stomach if possible; however, if GI intolerance, iron may be taken with meals although absorption will be decreased
- may cause constipation, diarrhea, or dark stools

▶ *Therapeutic Tips*

- only use in patients with documented risk factors or clinical evidence of iron deficiency anemia
- if hemoglobin has not changed after 2–3 weeks of treatment, reconsider diagnosis
- supplemental oral iron intake may interfere with stool guaiac test
- usefulness of concurrent ascorbic acid to increase iron absorption is controversial and not likely to be advantageous as large doses of ascorbic acid are needed to increase iron absorption by only 20–30%

Useful References

Eschback JW, Adamson JW. Hematologic consequences of renal failure. In: Brenner BM, Rector FC, eds. The Kidney. Philadelphia: WB Saunders Co., 1991:2019–2035

Massey AC. Microcytic anemia. Med Clin North Am 1992;76:549–66

Olin BR, ed. Drug Facts and Comparisons. St. Louis, J.B. Lippincott Co., 1992

Kumpf VJ, Holland EG. Parenteral iron dextran therapy. DICP 1990; 24:162–166

Solomons MW. Iron. In: Baumgartner TG, ed. Clinical Guide to Parenteral Micronutrition. Melrose Park, IL: Educational Publications, 1984: 103–114

ISOCARBOXAZID

Lyle K. Laird and Julia Vertrees

USA (Marplan)
CANADA (Marplan)

▶ *When Should I Use This Drug?*

Consider an alternative agent

- provides no advantages over other presently available antidepressants

ISOMETHEPTENE MUCATE

Jerry W. Taylor

Multiingredient preparation (isometheptene mucate 65 mg, dichloralphenazone 100 mg, and acetaminophen 325 mg)

USA (Midrin, Migralam)
CANADA (not available)

▶ *When Should I Use This Drug?*

Consider an alternative agent

- although considered a secondary agent for the acute management of migraine, it is not as effective as ergotamine and, although safe, it is unnecessary with the availability of agents such as sumatriptan or dihydroergotamine

ISONIAZID

Ann Beardsell

USA (Nydrazid, Laniazid)
CANADA (Isotamine, PMS Isoniazid)

▶ *When Should I Use This Drug?*

Mycobacterium avium infection

- isoniazid was used in a variety of protocols to treat this human immunodeficiency virus (HIV)–related infection and was used in combination with other antimycobacterial agents to prevent resistance but is now not commonly used
- *M. avium* infection is less sensitive and responsive to these agents, including isoniazid, and response may be slow

Tuberculosis

- is a major agent in the treatment of pulmonary and extrapulmonary tuberculosis and is always used in initial treatment unless the organism is resistent or izoniazid is contraindicated
- isoniazid is used in combination with other drugs (rifampin, ethambutol, cycloserine, pyrazinamide, streptomycin), depending on the type and sensitivity of the organism and the protocol being used to prevent the development of resistance to any one of the drugs
- isoniazid is the drug of choice for prophylaxis in high-risk individuals and is generally used alone

Other mycobacterial infections (*M. kansasii, M. marinum, M. scrofulaceum, M. xenopi*)

- isoniazid is used in combination with other antituberculous agents according to sensitivities and protocols for each organism

▶ *When Should I Not Use This Drug?*

Resistant organism

- if cultures show that the identified organism is resistant to the drug

Single agent in the treatment of tuberculosis

- as a single agent for the treatment of active or clinical disease, as resistance rapidly develops and the infectious period is prolonged

▶ *What Contraindications Are There to the Use of This Drug?*

Intolerance of or allergic reaction to isoniazid
Hepatic disease

- acute hepatic disease or a previous history of isoniazid-associated hepatic injury

▶ *What Drug Interactions Are Clinically Important?*

Drugs that may increase the effect of isoniazid

ANTITUBERCULOUS DRUGS (CYCLOSERINE, ETHIONAMIDE)

- adverse neurological effects of cycloserine, ethionamide, and isoniazid may be additive

Drugs that may decrease the effect of isoniazid

ALUMINUM HYDROXIDE

- decreases gastrointestinal absorption of isoniazid; therefore, antacids should be administered at least 1 hour after isoniazid is taken

Drugs that may have their effect increased by isoniazid

PHENYTOIN

- isoniazid inhibits the hepatic metabolism of phenytoin, resulting in increased serum levels of phenytoin
- monitor serum phenytoin measurements weekly until a new steady state is established or if symptoms of toxicity occur and adjust the dosage accordingly
- if administration of the inhibitor is stopped, return to the previous dosage of phenytoin

CARBAMAZEPINE

- isoniazid inhibits the hepatic metabolism of carbamazepine, resulting in increased serum levels of carbamazepine
- if the inhibitor must be added for longer than 3 days, obtain a baseline serum carbamazepine concentration prior to adding inhibitor, recheck the concentration in 1 week, and reduce the dosage proportionately if concentrations are greater than 12 mg/L
- monitor for symptoms of toxicity, and if they occur, stop the drug administration, get a repeated concentration, and adjust the dosage accordingly

PRIMIDONE, ETHOSUXIMIDE

- their concurrent use need not be avoided; however, patients should be monitored to ensure effective anticonvulsant control and to avoid possible phenobarbital toxicity (primidone is metabolized to phenobarbital)

Drugs that may have their effect decreased by isoniazid

BCG VACCINE

- isoniazid inhibits the replication of BCG; therefore, the vaccine is ineffective if administered while isoniazid is being administered

▶ *What Route and Dosage Should I Use?*

How to administer

- orally—take on an empty stomach
- parenterally—IM available

Mycobacterium avium infection

300 mg PO daily

Tuberculosis

- 5 mg/kg PO once daily to a maximum of 300 mg PO daily for treatment
- 300 mg PO daily for prophylaxis

Dosage adjustments for renal or hepatic dysfunction

- metabolized in the liver with some renal elimination

Normal Dosing Interval	$C_{cr} > 60$ mL/min or 1 mL/s	C_{cr} 30–60 mL/min or 0.5–1 mL/s	$C_{cr} < 30$ mL/min or 0.5 mL/s
Q24H	no adjustment needed	no dosage adjustment needed	decrease dosage by 50%

▶ *What Should I Monitor with Regard to Efficacy and Toxicity?*

Efficacy

Mycobacterium avium infection

Signs and symptoms

- fevers, chills, night sweats, malaise, fatigue, weight loss, abdominal pain, and diarrhea
- there are few or no physical signs to follow other than body weight or possibly the presence of a lesion in patients with localized disease (e.g., regional lymphadenopathy)
- patients should also be advised to report new or worsening diarrhea while taking such regimens, because *Clostridium difficile* colitis is a possible complication
- patients should be assessed every 1–2 weeks during the first 1–2 months of treatment but more often for severe cases

Complete blood count

- monthly or more frequently for severe disease, to detect progressive anemia and cytopenias due to bone marrow involvement, which may persist despite treatment

Blood cultures

- to document reduction or clearance of mycobacteremia, particularly in patients who have persistent symptoms

Tuberculosis

- disease improvement or resolution of symptoms such as fevers, sweats, and weight loss

Toxicity

Low incidence of adverse effects, especially with lower dosages (< 10 mg/kg)

Neurological effects

- peripheral neuropathy, including numbness, tingling, burning, and pain, may occur if pyridoxine is not concurrently administered
- should always be administered with pyridoxine (50 mg PO daily) to prevent neurotoxicity associated with isoniazid
- headache and fatigue may occur with initial therapy but are usually transient and treatable with common analgesics

Hepatic effects

- transient, mild elevations of liver enzyme levels (aspartate aminotransferase, alanine aminotransferase, and bilirubin) occur in the first 4–6 months of treatment in 10–20% of patients but usually return to baseline levels despite continued treatment
- severe progressive hepatic disease has been seen in a small number of patients, primarily older than 35 years of age who concurrently drink alcohol; therefore, monitor liver enzyme levels on a monthly basis and discontinue isoniazid administration if doubling of values occurs each months for 3 consecutive months

Hypersensitivity reactions

- most commonly occur during the first 2 months of therapy and include fever, rashes, lymphadenopathy, and vasculitis

- if symptoms of a hypersensitivity reaction occur, isoniazid administration should be discontinued immediately and then, after all symptoms are resolved, restarted in small increasing dosages, stopping immediately if symptoms recur

Hematological effects

- agranulocytosis; hemolytic, sideroblastic, or aplastic anemia; thrombocytopenia, and eosinophilia have occurred, especially in patients with HIV infection
- monitor complete blood count on a regular monthly basis

Gastrointestinal symptoms

- anorexia, nausea, vomiting, dry mouth, and epigastric distress may occur, usually with initial therapy, but are transient and can be treated symptomatically

▶ *How Long Do I Treat Patients with This Drug?*

Mycobacterium avium infection

- treatment length is indefinite

Tuberculosis

- for treatment, 6–9 months, depending on the regimen
- for prophylaxis, 12 months

▶ *How Do I Decrease or Stop the Administration of This Drug?*

- may be stopped abruptly

▶ *What Should I Tell My Patients About This Drug?*

- preferably, take this drug on an empty stomach, but it can be taken with meals if it upsets your stomach
- adverse effects are not common, especially if you take pyridoxine regularly
- if adverse effects, such as headache, nausea, and vomiting, occur, it is usually at the beginning of therapy and these effects go away with time
- if persistent nausea and vomiting, upper abdominal pain, or yellowing of the skin and eyes occur, contact your physician or pharmacist as soon as possible

ISOPROTERENOL

Karen Shalansky and Cindy Reesor Nimmo

USA (Norisodrine Aerotrol, Isuprel Mistometer, Vapo-Iso)
CANADA (Isuprel; combination: Aerolone compound, Duo-Medihaler, Isuprel-Neo Mistometer)

▶ *When Should I Use This Drug?*

Consider an alternative agent

- isoproterenol stimulates both beta$_1$- and beta$_2$-receptors equally; it has a higher propensity to produce myocardial infarction and excessive tachycardia compared with selective beta$_2$-agonists (The Pharmacological Approach to the Critically Ill Patient, 2nd ed 1988:591–592)
- the main effects from isoproterenol include bronchodilation, cardiac stimulation, and peripheral vasodilation

Useful References

Kelly HW. New beta$_2$-adrenergic agonist aerosols. Clin Pharm 1985;4: 393–403
McFadden ER. Clinical use of beta-adrenergic agonists. J Allergy Clin Immunol 1985;76:352–356
Zaritsky AL, Chernow B. Catecholamines and other inotropes. In: Chernow B, ed. The Pharmacological Approach to the Critically Ill Patient, 2nd ed. Baltimore: Williams & Wilkins, 1988:584–602

KETOCONAZOLE

Peter Jewesson

USA (Nizoral)
CANADA (Nizoral)

▶ *When Should I Use This Drug?*

Oropharyngeal candidiasis

- drug of choice in patients who do not respond to topical therapy

Esophageal candidiasis

- ketoconazole is the preferred agent for the initial treatment of esophageal candidiasis as it is less expensive than fluconazole and itraconazole
- not tolerated as well and somewhat less effective compared to fluconazole (Ann Intern Med 1992;117:655)

Vaginal candidiasis

- use when topical therapy is unsuccessful
- a 3 day course of ketoconazole appears to be equivalent to a 1 day course of fluconazole
- fluconazole is more expensive yet better tolerated than systemic ketoconazole

Histoplasmosis, paracoccidiodomycosis

- drug of choice in less severe infections
- use amphotericin B in patients who are immunocompromised or who are severely ill

Coccidioidomycosis

- limited in treatment of disseminated disease but useful alternative to amphotericin B in progressive pulmonary coccidioidomycosis

▶ *When Should I Not Use This Drug?*

Chromomycosis, cryptococcosis, mucormycosis, aspergillosis

- ketoconazole not effective against these organisms

▶ *What Contraindications Are There to the Use of This Drug?*

- intolerance or allergic reaction to ketoconazole
- not to be used during pregnancy or lactation

▶ *What Drug Interactions Are Clinically Important?*

Drugs that may increase the effect or toxicity of ketoconazole

- none

Drugs that may decrease the effect of ketoconazole

ANTACIDS, ANTICHOLINERGICS, H$_2$ BLOCKERS, OMEPRAZOLE

- decreased gastric acidity reduces ketoconazole absorption (Clin Pharmacol 1988;14:13–34)
- administer ketoconazole at least 2 hours prior to these agents
- as omeprazole virtually produces achlorhydria these agents should not be used together and if omeprazole is required fluconazole should be used in place of ketoconazole

RIFAMPIN AND ISONIAZID

- rifampin and isoniazid decrease ketoconazole serum concentrations by stimulating hepatic metabolism
- if existing dose ineffective, consider increasing dose to 400 mg/day

Drugs that may have their effect or toxicity increased by ketoconazole

WARFARIN

- interferes with warfarin metabolism and can increase INR
- use alternative agents if possible
- if not, monitor INR every 2 days until full extent of interaction is seen and adjust dose to maintain therapeutic values
- monitor INR every 2 days when interacting drug is discontinued and adjust as normal

CYCLOSPORINE

- inhibits hepatic metabolism of cyclosporine
- seen as early as 2 days after the start of these drugs
- monitor cyclosporine levels every other day until full extent of interaction is seen and adjust dose accordingly
- may need to decrease the cyclosporine dose by 30% or more

PHENYTOIN

- inhibits metabolism of phenytoin and may produce increases in serum phenytoin concentrations

- monitor serum phenytoin measurements weekly until a new steady-state is established or if symptoms of toxicity occur and adjust dose accordingly
- if the inhibitor is stopped return to previous dose

TOLBUTAMIDE

- ketoconazole inhibits cytochrome P450 enzyme systems resulting in interference with tolbutamide clearance
- if ketoconazole is added to tolbutamide therapy, monitor blood glucose daily for first 3–4 days and adjust dose of tolbutamide accordingly

Drugs that may have their effect decreased by ketoconazole

- none

▶ What Route and Dosage Should I Use?

How to administer

- orally—take oral preparation with food to improve bioavailability and patient tolerance

Oropharyngeal candidiasis

- 200 mg PO daily and increase to 400 mg PO daily if unresponsive after 5–7 days

Esophageal candidiasis

- 400 mg PO daily

Vaginal candidiasis

- 200 mg PO daily

Histoplasmosis, paracoccidioidomycosis, coccidioidomycosis

- 400 mg PO daily

Dosage adjustment for renal or hepatic dysfunction

- eliminated by hepatic pathway
- no adjustment for renal insufficiency; however, consider lowest possible dose or avoid ketoconazole if an alternative antifungal agent can be used

▶ What Should I Monitor with Regard to Efficacy and Toxicity?

Efficacy

Oropharyngeal candidiasis

- reduction in pain, disappearance of lesions
- assess symptoms daily if in hospital or weekly if outpatient

Esophageal candidiasis

- relief of dysphagia
- assess symptoms daily if in hospital or weekly if outpatient

Vaginal candidiasis

- disappearance of lesions and reduction in pain and itching

Histoplasmosis, paracoccidioidomycosis, coccidioidomycosis

- see Amphotericin

Toxicity

Gastrointestinal

- 9% incidence of nausea and vomiting
- take with food or at bedtime if nausea develops
- food will reduce absorption
- if symptoms persist, discontinue use

Dermatological

- itching and rash
- discontinue if persists

Hepatic

- 2–5% incidence reversible elevation of liver function tests, reversible (non–dose-related) hepatitis has been observed in 1/10,000 cases (especially in children)
- monitor liver enzymes at baseline and once weekly (critical if on other potentially hepatotoxic drugs)

- discontinue if abnormalities persist or symptoms associated with hepatic dysfunction appear

Adrenal suppression/gynecomastia

- inhibition of steroid synthesis
- if prolonged therapy anticipated, monitor testosterone and cortisol concentrations at week 1 and monthly
- discontinue if abnormalities develop or symptoms appear

▶ How Long Do I Treat Patients with This Drug?

Oropharyngeal candidiasis

- 1 week and at least 2 days after the symptoms have resolved
- patient should respond within a few days

Esophageal candidiasis

- treat for at least 2–3 weeks and 1 week following resolution of symptoms

Vaginal candidiasis

- 3 days

Histoplasmosis, paracoccidioidomycosis, coccidioidomycosis

- 6–12 months

▶ How Do I Decrease or Stop the Administration of This Drug?

- may be stopped abruptly

▶ What Should I Tell My Patients About This Drug?

- this agent is a new antifungal agent and successful therapy is contingent upon good compliance and completion of the full treatment course
- some minor side effects (i.e., gastrointestinal or reversible liver enzyme changes) can be expected but these are usually self-limiting and therapy should not be stopped
- contact pharmacist or physician if anorexia, abdominal pain, jaundice, or increased nausea arise

▶ Therapeutic Tips

- always consider efficacy, toxicity, and cost when determining the role of ketoconazole relative to other available agents
- achlorhydria or concurrent administration of agents that reduce gastric acidity will significantly decrease absorption of ketoconazole and lead to therapeutic failure (use fluconazole in these patients)

Useful Reference

Bennett JE. Antifungal agents. In: Mandell GL, Douglas RG Jr, Bennett JE, eds. Principles and Practice of Infectious Diseases, 3rd ed. New York: Churchill Livingstone, 1990;361–370

KETOPROFEN

Kelly Jones
USA (Orudis)
CANADA (Orudis, Rhodis)

▶ When Should I Use This Drug?

Acute pain, general aches and pain, bone pain

- useful for the acute management of general aches and pains
- only advantage over non–enteric-coated aspirin is that it causes less gastrointestinal intolerance
- decision between this drug and other nonsteroidal antiinflammatory drugs (NSAIDs) should be based on cost

Rheumatoid arthritis

- ketoprofen can be used as an alternative for patients who fail to respond to enteric coated aspirin or ibuprofen
- it offers no advantages over enteric coated aspirin or ibuprofen and is more expensive

Osteoarthritis

- if acetaminophen and enteric coated aspirin or ibuprofen are not effective

- decision between this drug and other NSAIDs should be based on cost

▶ **When Should I Not Use This Drug?**

Combination with other nonsteroidal antiinflammatory drugs

- combinations of NSAIDs provide no increase in effectiveness compared with maximum dosages of single agents and significantly increase the risk of adverse effects

▶ **What Contraindications Are There to the Use of This Drug?**

see Ibuprofen

▶ **What Drug Interactions Are Clinically Important?**

see Ibuprofen

▶ **What Route and Dosage Should I Use?**

How to administer

- orally—take with food or milk
- parenterally—not available

Acute pain, general aches and pain, bone pain, dysmenorrhea

- 25–50 mg PO Q6–8H PRN

Cancer pain

- 50 mg PO Q8H up to a maximum of 300 mg PO daily

Rheumatoid arthritis

- 75 mg PO Q8H up to a maximum dosage of 300 mg PO daily

Osteoarthritis

- 50 mg PO Q8H

Dosage adjustments for renal or hepatic dysfunction

- hepatically metabolized; reduce dosage by 25% in patients with a history of hepatic disease; no adjustments needed for renal disease

▶ **What Should I Monitor with Regard to Efficacy and Toxicity?**

see Ibuprofen

▶ **How Long Do I Treat Patients with This Drug?**

see Ibuprofen

▶ **How Do I Decrease or Stop the Administration of This Drug?**

- may be stopped abruptly if needed

▶ **What Should I Tell My Patients About This Drug?**

see Ibuprofen

▶ **Therapeutic Tips**

see Ibuprofen

Useful References

see Ibuprofen

KETOROLAC

Kelly Jones
USA (Toradol)
CANADA (Toradol)

▶ **When Should I Use This Drug?**

Acute pain

- because of ketorolac's expense, this drug should be reserved for the treatment of acute pain that would normally be treated with narcotics in patients who cannot or should not receive narcotics (e.g., postoperative pain in patients at risk for narcotic-induced respiratory depression and acute pain control in drug addicts seeking narcotics)
- can be used to decrease the amount of opioids required (useful in patients who do not like the sensation associated with opioid use)
- can also be used in conjunction with opioids in patients who do not get adequate pain control with appropriately titrated narcotics

Rheumatoid arthritis

- ketorolac is the first injectable (intramuscular) nonsteroidal antiinflammatory drug (NSAID) but should be used in rheumatoid arthritis only in patients who cannot take medications by mouth
- oral ketorolac offers no advantages over other NSAIDs and is more expensive

▶ **When Should I Not Use This Drug?**

Oral use

- oral ketorolac offers no advantages over other NSAIDs, as it is expensive, and it is recommended that it be given 4 times daily

Combination with other NSAIDs

- combinations of NSAIDs provide no increase in effectiveness compared with maximum dosages of single agents and significantly increase the risk of adverse effects

▶ **What Contraindications Are There to the Use of This Drug?**

see Aspirin

▶ **What Drug Interactions Are Clinically Important?**

see Ibuprofen

▶ **What Route and Dosage Should I Use?**

How to administer

- orally—not recommended
- parenterally—give via the intramuscular route

Acute pain

- 30 mg IM or IV Q6H PRN
- 15 mg IM or IV Q6H PRN in the elderly

Rheumatoid arthritis

- 60 mg IM followed by 30 mg IM Q6H
- in patients with reduced renal function or those older than 65 years, load with 30 mg IM and dose 15 mg IM Q6H

Dosage adjustments for renal or hepatic dysfunction

- hepatically metabolized; reduce the dosage by 25% in patients with a history of hepatic disease; no adjustments are needed for renal disease

▶ **What Should I Monitor with Regard to Efficacy and Toxicity?**

see Ibuprofen

▶ **How Long Do I Treat Patients with This Drug?**

Acute pain

- until oral medications can be used

Rheumatoid arthritis

- until oral medications can be used

▶ **How Do I Decrease or Stop the Administration of This Drug?**

- may be stopped abruptly if needed

▶ **What Should I Tell My Patients About This Drug?**

- it is important to be educated about what to expect in terms of onset of relief
- notify your physician of any rash, unusual fever, edema, black stools, or weight gain

▶ *Therapeutic Tips*

- do not use 2 NSAIDs concomitantly because this may increase toxicity

Useful References

see Ibuprofen

KETOTIFEN

Karen Shalansky and Cindy Reesor Nimmo

USA (not available)
CANADA (Zaditen)

▶ *When Should I Use This Drug?*

Chronic asthma

- prophylactic add-on therapy to reduce the frequency and severity of asthmatic symptoms after failure from appropriate doses of inhaled beta$_2$-agonists, inhaled corticosteroids, and cromolyn
- appears to be clinically equivalent to cromolyn in terms of reduction of asthmatic symptoms and drug requirements (Drugs 1990;40:412–448)
- role not well established but may be beneficial if patients have asthma, allergic rhinitis, and dermatitis or when oral therapy is preferred (e.g., young children with poor inhaler technique)

▶ *When Should I Not Use This Drug?*

Acute asthmatic attacks

- of no value in acute attacks
- use a beta$_2$-agonist with or without ipratropium bromide and, if required, systemic corticosteroids

Exercise-induced asthma

- unlike inhaled cromolyn, it does not appear to provide protection against exercise-induced asthma after short-term therapy
- long-term therapy may provide protection (Allergy 1987;42: 315–317)

▶ *What Contraindications Are There to the Use of This Drug?*

intolerance of or allergic reaction to ketotifen

▶ *What Drug Interactions Are Clinically Important?*

Drugs that may increase the effect or toxicity of ketotifen

CENTRAL NERVOUS SYSTEM DEPRESSANTS

- potentiation of sedation
- avoid or warn the patient of the potential for sedation

Drugs that may decrease the effect of ketotifen

- none

Drugs that may have their effect or toxicity increased by ketotifen

- none

Drugs that may have their effect decreased by ketotifen

- none

▶ *What Route and Dosage Should I Use?*

How to administer

- orally—with food or milk
- parenterally—not available

Chronic asthma

- 1 mg PO BID taken with meals, increasing to a maximum of 2 mg PO BID after 6–12 weeks if the patient is still symptomatic
- 6–12 weeks of therapy are required before a response is seen
- in seasonal allergic asthma, initiate therapy 6–8 weeks prior to peak pollen season

Dosage adjustments for renal or hepatic dysfunction

- hepatically metabolized

- little information on dosage adjustments in renal or hepatic dysfunction; therefore, titrate the dose on the basis of efficacy and toxicity

▶ *What Should I Monitor with Regard to Efficacy and Toxicity?*

Efficacy

Chronic asthma

Clinical improvement

- change in frequency and severity of attacks
- effect is delayed for 6–12 weeks
- responding patients may continue to improve for up to 6 months with continuous therapy

Ability to discontinue or reduce concomitant asthmatic therapy

- pulmonary function test results unlikely to improve; however, they will remain stable as bronchodilator administration is withdrawn

Toxicity

- generally well tolerated

Sedation

- is the most frequent side effect and occurs in 10–20% of patients
- sedation decreases after 1–2 weeks of use
- to minimize sedation, therapy may be initiated at $\frac{1}{2}$ the daily dosage (e.g., 0.5 mg BID), or alternatively, administer a single dose of the drug at bedtime (e.g., 1 mg HS)
- dosage should be increased after a period of 5 days to 2 mg/d (1 mg PO BID)

Headache, dizziness, nausea, and dry mouth

- occur in 1–2% of patients on initiation of therapy
- these side effects usually do not persist with long-term therapy

Weight gain

- associated with long-term therapy
- average of 1 kg over 1 year in adults

▶ *How Long Do I Treat Patients with This Drug?*

Chronic asthma

- therapy may be required indefinitely; however, consider dosage tapering every 6–12 months and possible withdrawal, depending on severity
- long-term therapy is justified if therapy results in a significant decrease in the severity of the asthma, a reduction or discontinuation of bronchodilator or corticosteroid use, or substitution for another drug with intolerable side effects

▶ *How Do I Decrease or Stop the Administration of This Drug?*

- may be stopped abruptly

▶ *What Should I Tell My Patients About This Drug?*

- ketotifen is used to prevent bronchospasm—it does not relieve an attack that has already started
- compliance with regular therapy is essential to maintain control of asthma—use ketotifen exactly as directed
- sedation is the most common side effect
- use caution when operating a car or dangerous machinery
- concomitant use of other central nervous system depressants increases sedation

▶ *Therapeutic Tips*

- drug must be used prophylactically—response may not been seen for 6–12 weeks
- with long-term use (minimum, 6–12 weeks), a reduction or discontinuation of therapy with beta$_2$-agonists, theophylline, or corticosteroids may be possible in some patients
- antiasthmatic and antiinflammatory effects last at least 1 month after discontinuation of the drug

Useful References

Grant SM, Goa KL, Fitton A, Sorkin EM. Ketotifen. A review of its pharmacodynamic and pharmacokinetic properties, and therapeutic use in asthma and allergic disorders. Drugs 1990;40:412–448

Tan WC, Lim TK. Double-blind comparison of the protective effect of sodium cromoglycate and ketotifen on exercise-induced asthma in adults. Allergy 1987;42:315–317

LABETALOL

Robert Rangno and James McCormack

USA (Normodyne)
CANADA (Trandate)

Labetalol is a racemic mixture of compounds that together have the capacity to block both beta- and alpha-adrenergic receptors • Labetalol should be viewed as a fixed dose combination tablet of a beta-adrenergic antagonist combined with an alpha$_1$-selective antagonist in a ratio of 4:1 (this ratio may vary from patient to patient)

▶ When Should I Use This Drug?

Acute (crisis) hypertension

- in these patients, typically the choice of drug has been based on predictable route of administration (intravenous) and titratability; however, oral routes can be used for crisis hypertension (Br J Clin Pharmacol 1986;21:377–383) and oral routes are useful in patients when intravenous access is not possible or feasible
- labetalol provides rapid onset with sustained effect, causes no rebound tachycardia, and has no central nervous system effects
- compared with diazoxide, labetalol causes a decrease in heart rate
- alternative to diazoxide or hydralazine in the emergency treatment of hypertension in pregnancy (Aust N Z J of Obstet Gynaecol 1986;26:26–29)
- labetalol is often a rationale addition (with vasodilators) to avoid or reverse reflex tachycardia and to decrease shear force
- in hypertension-tachycardia syndrome after severe trauma to the head or chest, labetolol may be preferable to nitroprusside because, in contrast to nitroprusside, it results in a decrease in cerebral blood flow (Crit Care Med 1988;16:765–768, 1159–1160)

Deliberate induction of hypotension during anesthesia

- can be used in patients who are undergoing procedures in which a relative hypotension is desirable (intracranial aneurysm clipping), but nitroprusside, nitroglycerin, or deepening of anesthesia can also be used alternatively

▶ When Should I Not Use This Drug?

Chronic (noncrisis) hypertension

- substantially greater incidence of symptomatic orthostatic hypotension and impotence in male patients than with other beta-blockers
- is expensive and must be given more often than once daily
- complete tachyphylaxis to alpha-blockade after 6 months of long-term use (Clin Pharm Ther 1983;33:278–282)
- unlike other beta-blockers, labetalol has been associated with hepatotoxicity and hepatic necrosis with deaths (Ann Intern Med 1990;113:210–213)

Chronic stable angina

- no advantages over other beta-blockers

Clonidine withdrawal hypertension

- this adverse severe hypertensive reaction to abrupt withdrawal of clonidine is characterized by excessive sympathetic nervous system activity, and blockade of both alpha- and beta-adrenergic receptors is a reasonable method of treating this uncommon problem; however, it is best to just restart clonidine administration and then withdraw clonidine slowly

Pheochromocytoma

- unpredictable balance between alpha- and beta-adrenergic receptor blockade and labetalol may not provide enough alpha-antagonism

▶ What Contraindications Are There to the Use of This Drug?

see Nadolol

Postural hypotension

- may be worsened by alpha-receptor blockade

▶ What Drug Interactions Are Clinically Important?

Drugs that may increase the effect of labetalol

CIMETIDINE

- if the patient is already receiving cimetidine then there is no problem; however, if not, do not use cimetidine, use ranitidine instead

HALOGENATED HYDROCARBONS AND HALOTHANE IN HIGH CONCENTRATIONS

- significant reductions in cardiac output, stroke volume, and blood pressure can occur when these agents are used together
- halothane concentration should not exceed 1–1.5% (Drugs 1989;37:583–627)

NITROGLYCERIN

- blunts reflex tachycardia induced by nitroglycerin and may potentiate its hypotensive effect
- titrate doses of each agent on the basis of blood pressure response

Drugs that may decrease the effect of labetalol

- none

Drugs that may have their effect increased by labetalol

- none

Drugs that may have their effect decreased by labetalol

- none

▶ What Route and Dosage Should I Use?

How to administer

Orally

- use other oral beta-blockers

Parenterally

- as an IV bolus over 2 minutes
- for infusion, dilute 200 mg (40 mL) of labetolol in 160 mL of normal saline and dextrose or 5% dextrose in water

Acute (crisis) hypertension

- administration by infusion provides a smoother, less precipitous fall in blood pressure compared with that with intermittent bolus injections (Br J Clin Pharmacol 1982;13[suppl 1]:97s–99s)
- start with 20 mg/h and double the dosage every 30 minutes until a satisfactory response is obtained or a maximum dosage of 160 mg/h is reached
- in hypertension complicating acute myocardial infarction, start the infusion at 15 mg/h and increase gradually to a maximum of 120 mg/h, depending on blood pressure response

Deliberate induction of hypotension during anesthesia

- give 2.5 mg as a bolus and follow with 2.5 mg every 5–10 minutes until a response is seen (seldom need more than 10 mg)

▶ What Should I Monitor with Regard to Efficacy and Toxicity?

Efficacy

see Nadolol

Deliberate induction of hypotension during anesthesia

- measure blood pressure continuously (a mean arterial pressure of 50–60 mmHg is the goal)

Toxicity

see Nadolol

Hepatotoxicity

- elevations in aminotransferase levels have been reported to occur in 8% of patients (Ann Intern Med 1991;114:341)
- do not use as long-term therapy

Postural hypotension, retrograde ejaculation

- is seen with high dosages and is due to the alpha-blockade
- do not use for long-term therapy

▶ *How Long Do I Treat Patients with This Drug?*

see Nadolol

▶ *How Do I Decrease or Stop the Administration of This Drug?*

see Nadolol

▶ *What Should I Tell My Patients About This Drug?*

see Nadolol

- do not stand up suddenly, especially early in treatment, as postural hypotension due to alpha- and beta-adrenergic receptor blockade may occur, particularly in the elderly

Useful References

Townsend RR, DiPette DJ, Goodman R, et al. Combined alpha/beta-blockade versus beta₁-selective blockade in essential hypertension in black and white patients. Clin Pharmacol Ther 1990;48:665–675

Smith WB, Clifton GG, O'Neill WM Jr, Wallin JD. Antihypertensive effectiveness of intravenous labetalol in accelerated hypertension. Hypertension 1983;5:579–583

Dal Palu C, Pessina AC, Semplicini A, et al. Intravenous labetalol in severe hypertension. Br J Clin Pharmacol 1982;13(suppl 1):97s–99s

Michael CA: Intravenous labetalol and intravenous dioxide in severe hypertension complicating pregnancy. Aust N Z J Obstet Gynaecol 1986; 26:26–29

Harnier HD. Use of labetalol in trauma. Crit Care Med 1988;16:1159–1160

Orlowski JP, Shiesley D, Vidt DG, et al. Labetalol to control blood pressure after cerebrovascular surgery. Crit Care Med 1988;16:765–768

Scott DB, Buckley FP, Littlewood DG, et al. Circulating effect of labetalol during halothane anesthesia. Anaesthesia 1978;34:145

Goa KL, Benfield P, Sorkin EM. Labetalol. A reappraisal of its pharmacology, pharmacokinetics and therapeutic use in hypertension and ischaemic heart disease. Drugs 1989;37:583–627

LACTULOSE

Leslie Mathews

USA (Chronulac, Cephulac, Duphalac)
CANADA (Chronulac, Lactulax, Laxilose, Comalose-R)

▶ *When Should I Use This Drug?*

Fecal impaction

- other laxative therapy (senna, cascara, bisacodyl, lactulose, bulk-forming laxatives) is likely required after the colon has been emptied to prevent further impactions
- decision among these agents is based on the reason for constipation, side effects, duration of therapy, and cost
- oral osmotic agents (magnesium) and the oral stimulant laxatives are usually well tolerated and are less expensive than lactulose

Acute constipation

- if a rapid response is needed and if stimulant laxatives or magnesium are ineffective or not tolerated, oral lactulose can be tried, as it is effective and most patients prefer this to an enema or suppository
- more expensive than stimulant laxatives or magnesium hydroxide but can be used long term
- also useful when constipation is associated with hard, dry stools, or conditions in which straining should be avoided (e.g., anorectal disorders, hernias, recovery from myocardial infarction, and cerebrovascular accident), as lactulose softens stools by retaining water in the lumen of the bowel and should be chosen if bulk-forming laxatives are ineffective or not tolerated
- for occasional use when bulk-forming laxatives, magnesium hydroxide, and the stimulant laxatives are contraindicated, ineffective, or poorly tolerated
- for postoperative management of hemorrhoidectomy, as it relieves pain by facilitating easy passage of stool (Br J Clin Pract 1975;29:235–236)

Chronic constipation

- use only when bulk-forming laxatives are ineffective, contraindicated, or poorly tolerated because lactulose is expensive
- also particularly useful for constipation in bed-bound patients, neurogenic constipation, and constipation in debilitated or terminally ill patients as it softens stool and prevents impaction and is likely a better choice than bulk-forming laxatives (these patients may also require regular stimulation of the rectal mucosa with suppositories or enemas) (Postgrad Med 1988;83:339–349, Med Clin North Am 1989;73:1502–1509)
- use in conjunction with bulk-forming laxatives to wean off stimulant laxatives
- chosen instead of magnesium hydroxide, stimulant laxatives, and docusate, as these agents should not be used long term

Hepatic encephalopathy

- enhances the removal of nitrogenous waste products

▶ *When Should I Not Use This Drug?*

Bulk-forming agents or occasional use of osmotic or stimulant laxatives are effective

- avoid the use of this drug because of its high cost when these other agents are effective

▶ *What Contraindications Are There to the Use of This Drug?*

Intolerance of or allergic reaction to lactulose

Symptoms of acute abdomen

- undiagnosed abdominal pain, nausea, and vomiting

Low-galactose diet

- lactulose contains galactose (<2.2 g of galactose per 15 mL)

▶ *What Drug Interactions Are Clinically Important?*

- none

▶ *What Route and Dosage Should I Use?*

How to administer

- orally—take with 250 mL of fluid (water, juice, or milk)
- parenterally—not available
- rectally—200 g mixed in 700 mL of water

Fecal impaction, acute constipation, chronic constipation

- 15 mL PO BID (can be given as a single dose but this may cause increased nausea and vomiting) and increase the dosage after 24–48 hours, if there is no response, to a total daily maximum of 60 mL
- higher dosages are less likely to be tolerated and are more likely to produce fluid and electrolyte problems

Hepatic encephalopathy

- start with 30 mL (20 g) PO TID
- adjust the dosage every 1–2 days as needed
- retention enema can be used when patient is comatose, is restricted to nothing by mouth, or is unable to tolerate oral lactulose
- 300 mL of lactulose (200 g) mixed in 700 mL of water or saline given rectally and repeated Q4H PRN for 3 doses
- should be retained for 30–60 minutes; if not, repeat the dose promptly

Dosage adjustments for renal or hepatic dysfunction

- absorbed to only a small degree; therefore, no dosage adjustments are required

▶ *What Should I Monitor with Regard to Efficacy and Toxicity?*

Efficacy

Fecal impaction, acute constipation, chronic constipation

- produces a soft or semifluid stool in 6–24 hours
- full effects generally occur within 24–48 hours
- question the patient and/or consult the stool chart regarding the frequency and consistency of stool

- reports suggest that tolerance may develop with continued use (this finding is controversial) (J Clin Invest 1985;75:608–613, Br Med J 1989;298:188)

Hepatic encephalopathy

- monitor the frequency of stools, with the goal being 2–3 soft stools per day with a pH of 5–5.5
- level of consciousness, mental state, and so on should improve within 1–3 days
- when lactulose is used rectally, reversal of hepatic coma may occur within 2 hours of the first enema (AHFS Drug Information 1994:1649–1651)
- asterixis decreases or disappears

Toxicity

Gastrointestinal symptoms

- lactulose frequently produces flatulence, bloating, abdominal cramps, diarrhea, nausea, and vomiting
- monitor for these symptoms, particularly when therapy is first started and with higher dosages
- is often transient and usually subsides with continued therapy, but if not, decrease the dosage
- nausea and vomiting occur owing to the sweet taste; minimize this by diluting syrup with water, juice, or milk to taste

Fluid and electrolyte imbalance

- hypernatremia may occur with high dosages used to treat hepatic encephalopathy (DICP 1984;18:70–71)
- hypokalemia and dehydration may occur with diarrhea, higher dosages (40–60 mL) and long-term therapy
- assess the hydration status and measure serum electrolyte levels if diarrhea is acute or prolonged
- decrease or discontinue the drug administration; replace fluid and electrolytes
- measure the serum electrolyte levels of patients receiving the drug for longer than 6 months

Nontoxic megacolon

- X-rays are indicated for patients with severe diarrhea, severe abdominal pain, and distention
- discontinue lactulose administration; give broad-spectrum antibiotics (Gastrointest Endosc 1988;34:489–490)

▶ How Long Do I Treat Patients with This Drug?

Fecal impaction

- prevent further impaction with drug therapy until predisposing factors are eliminated (e.g., immobility, low-residue diet, and anorectal injury)
- substitute a bulk-forming laxative (if possible) as soon as possible to prevent constipation

Acute constipation

- may be used long term but best to avoid use for longer than 7 days
- if needed for longer than this, consider increasing the bulk in the patient's diet and/or using bulk-forming laxatives

Chronic constipation

- while bulk-forming laxatives can be continued indefinitely, if needed it is best to limit the use of other laxatives to 7 days when possible

Hepatic encephalopathy

- if necessary, may need to use indefinitely

▶ How Do I Decrease or Stop the Administration of This Drug?

- may be stopped abruptly

▶ What Should I Tell My Patients About This Drug?

- may cause flatulence, abdominal cramping, and bloating, but these symptoms are often transient; if not, decrease the dosage
- decrease the dosage or stop the drug administration if diarrhea occurs

- chilling and/or adding lactulose to water or juice improves the taste and reduces nausea
- take each dose with 250 mL (8 ounces) of fluid to prevent dehydration and enhance effect

▶ Therapeutic Tips

- owing to its expense, reserve its use for chronic constipation when bulk-forming laxatives are ineffective, contraindicated, or poorly tolerated
- encourage fluid intake to prevent any possible net loss of body water
- diabetic patients must consider calorie intake with daily dosing (e.g., 30 mL of Chronulac contains about 110 cal)
- absorption is reportedly minimal (Drugdex Information System, Micromedex, Inc., Denver, Colorado)

Useful References

Rousseau P. Treatment of constipation in the elderly. Postgrad Med 1988;83:339–349
Lactulose (Chronulac) for constipation. Med Lett 1980;22:2–4
Lederle FA, Busch DL, Mattox KM, et al. Cost-effective treatment of constipation in the elderly: A randomized double-blind comparison of sorbitol and lactulose. Am J Med 1990;89:597–601
AHFS Drug Information. Bethesda, MD: American Society of Hospital Pharmacists, 1992:1497
McEvoy GK, Litvak K, Welsh OH, et al, eds. AHFS 94 Drug Information, American Society of Hospital Pharmacists, Inc., Bethesda, MD, 1995:1649–1651

LEVODOPA-BENSERAZIDE

Ruby Grymonpre

USA (not available)
CANADA (Prolopa)

▶ When Should I Use This Drug?

see Levodopa-carbidopa

▶ When Should I Not Use This Drug?

see Levodopa-carbidopa

▶ What Contraindications Are There to the Use of This Drug?

see Levodopa-carbidopa

▶ What Drug Interactions Are Clinically Important?

see Levodopa-carbidopa

▶ What Route and Dosage Should I Use?

How to administer

- orally—absorption of levodopa is reduced and delayed when taken with food; however, gastrointestinal side effects and dose-response fluctuations are minimized—take it in similar fashion each time
- parenterally—not available

Parkinson's disease

- one 50 mg/12.5 mg capsule PO QID
- increase the dosage by one 50 mg/12.5 mg capsule at weekly intervals until improvement or toxicities are seen
- total daily doses of benserazide greater than 200 mg are not required as 200 mg will provide adequate decarboxylase inhibition
- unfortunately, this preparation does not come as a 10:1 formulation

Dosage adjustments for renal or hepatic dysfunction

- peripheral metabolism
- no dosage adjustment is required; just start with low dose and titrate up to effect or toxicity

▶ What Should I Monitor with Regard to Efficacy and Toxicity?

see Levodopa-carbidopa

▶ How Long Do I Treat Patients with This Drug?

see Levodopa-carbidopa

▶ *How Do I Decrease or Stop the Administration of This Drug?*

see Levodopa-carbidopa

▶ *What Should I Tell My Patients About This Drug?*

see Levodopa-carbidopa

▶ *Therapeutic Tips*

see Levodopa-carbidopa

LEVODOPA-CARBIDOPA

Ruby Grymonpre

USA (Sinemet)
CANADA (Sinemet, Sinemet CR)

▶ *When Should I Use This Drug?*

Parkinson's disease

- levodopa therapy should be initiated early in Parkinson's disease when symptoms interfere with the patient's social, emotional, or work life
- levodopa is the initial drug of choice and is used in conjunction with anticholinergics when tremor is a problem
- addition of a peripheral decarboxylase inhibitor (carbidopa or benserazide) allows a 60–80% reduction in the oral dosage of levodopa required for therapeutic effect and reduces nausea and other peripheral effects (NY State J Med 1987;87:147–153)
- there is clinically no difference between levodopa-carbidopa or levodopa-benserazide, and the decision about which agent to use should be based on cost and dosage flexibility (Drugs 1984;28:236–262)
- levodopa-carbidopa is available in more useful dosages and dosage forms, and in practice, most patients take this combination
- levodopa-benserazide capsules can be opened and may be useful in patients having difficulty with swallowing tablets or capsules
- regular levodopa-carbidopa tablets (not the sustained-release products) can be crushed and administered in a fruit-based liquid or soft food but must be used immediately after disruption of the dosage form

▶ *When Should I Not Use This Drug?*

Parkinson's disease

Early, mild symptoms causing no disability (clumsiness of the hands, fatigue, sensory discomfort)

- treatment not warranted

▶ *What Contraindications Are There to the Use of This Drug?*

Intolerance of or allergic reaction to levodopa-carbidopa

History of melanoma or undiagnosed pigmented lesions

- alternative dopaminergic therapy should be prescribed
- levodopa is a metabolic precursor of skin melanin, and although the risk is small, levodopa may enhance the growth rate of a melanoma

▶ *What Drug Interactions Are Clinically Important?*

Drugs that may increase the effect or toxicity of levodopa-carbidopa

METHYLDOPA

- acts as a decarboxylase inhibitor and a false neurotransmitter and causes a variable therapeutic response to levodopa, and this combination should be avoided.

Drugs that may decrease the effect of levodopa-carbidopa

ANTICHOLINERGICS

- by inhibiting gastrointestinal motility, anticholinergics and other drugs with anticholinergic effects such as phenothiazines, amantadine, meperidine, tricyclic antidepressants, quinidine, disopyramide, or some antihistamines can decrease the extent of levodopa absorption

- when anticholinergic therapy is discontinued, patients should be monitored for levodopa toxicity

PHENOTHIAZINES, BUTYROPHENONES, THIOXANTHINES

- these drugs block dopamine receptors, but if they are needed clinically and alternative agents are not available, they can be used together

RESERPINE, METHYLDOPA, METOCLOPRAMIDE

- these drugs reduce dopamine receptor stimulation, and these combinations should not be used
- alternative agents should be used

Drugs that may have their effect or toxicity increased by levodopa-carbidopa

ANTIHYPERTENSIVE AGENTS

- may have an additive hypotensive effect
- dosage of antihypertensive agents may need to be adjusted when these agents are used concomitantly
- treat as for a dosage change in antihypertensive therapy (e.g., assess the effect after 1–2 weeks of the combination)

GENERAL ANESTHETICS (e.g., HALOTHANE, CYCLOPROPANE)

- arrhythmias can occur
- levodopa can be stopped before surgery if there is a concern about arrhythmia (usually not a problem)

MONOAMINE OXIDASE INHIBITORS

- combination can cause hypertensive crisis; therefore, discontinue monoamine oxidase inhibitor therapy 2 weeks, or preferably 1 month, before starting levodopa

Drugs that may have their effect decreased by levodopa-carbidopa

- none

▶ *What Route and Dosage Should I Use?*

How to administer

- orally—absorption of levodopa is reduced and delayed when taken with food; however, gastrointestinal side effects and dose-response fluctuations are minimized
- take levodopa in similar fashion each time
- parenterally—not available

Parkinson's disease

- $1/2$ of a scored levodopa-carbidopa 100 mg/25 mg tablet PO QID
- increase the dosage by $1/2$ of a 100 mg/25 mg tablet at weekly intervals until improvement or toxicities are seen
- after the total daily dose exceeds 200 mg of carbidopa (2 100 mg/25 mg tablets PO QID), switch to a 10:1 formulation, as only 75 mg is needed to block fully the peripheral dopa decarboxylase enzyme
- increase the dosage until a maximum of 300 mg (levodopa) PO QID is reached
- patients who have not responded to 300 mg of levodopa (with carbidopa) PO QID are not likely to respond to higher dosages
- if the patient reaches a daily dose of 1200 mg of levodopa (combined with at least 75 mg of carbidopa) with no response, reevaluate the diagnosis of Parkinson's disease
- patients requiring more than 700 mg of levodopa (with carbidopa) should be initiated on adjunctive therapy (usually selegiline)
- in patients who find the QID dosing regimen inconvenient, a sustained-release formulation (Sinemet CR) is available and allows fewer daily doses and reduced dose-response fluctuations
- do not start the sustained-release preparation until the patient is stabilized on the regular-release formulation because dose adjustments are more difficult with the sustained-release formulation
- owing to a reduced bioavailability of Sinemet CR relative to Sinemet (levodopa: 0.71; carbidopa: 0.58), the daily dosage may need to beincreased when switching from regular Sinemet (Neurology 1989;39[suppl]:25–38)
- Sinemet CR has a delayed onset of activity, which is problematic for the initial morning dose when the patient's level of function

is usually at its worst; it may be useful early in therapy before morning symptoms are a major problem
- a dose of regular Sinemet tablets has a more rapid absorption rate and is recommended for the morning dose

Dosage adjustments for renal or hepatic dysfunction
- hepatically metabolized
- no dosage adjustment is required; just start with low dose and titrate up to effect or toxicity

▶ *What Should I Monitor with Regard to Efficacy and Toxicity?*

Efficacy
Signs and symptoms
- assess symptoms weekly during the titration period
- after the patient has been stabilized, assess the patient every 3 months

Toxicity
Cardiovascular side effects
- orthostatic hypotension is seen especially when initiating therapy but usually decreases with continued therapy
- advise the patient to rise slowly from supine position
- if symptoms are severe and the patient needs to wear elastic stockings (e.g., thromboembolic stockings) and increase sodium in the diet, suspect Shy-Drager syndrome

Central nervous system effects
- confusion, agitation, hallucinations, delusions, sleep disturbances, and abnormal involuntary movements, including orofacial dyskinesias, facial grimacing, and choreic movements of trunk and limbs
- some degree of symptoms affect 80% of patients after 3 years of therapy
- symptoms are dose related and can be minimized with dosage reduction
- must titrate dose to minimize abnormal involuntary movements while maintaining optimum control of Parkinson's symptoms
- if the patient has a psychiatric illness, monitor for a recurrence of psychiatric episodes (including dementia, depression, and psychosis)

Gastrointestinal side effects
- nausea and vomiting can occur especially when initiating therapy but usually decreases with continued therapy
- less problematic when levodopa is combined with carbidopa
- increase the dosage of levodopa gradually to allow tolerance of the gastrointestinal side effects
- ensure that the patient receives at least 75 mg of carbidopa per day
- take each dose with food
- if nausea and vomiting is a problem, domperidone may be used
- if the patient has had a recent gastrointestinal bleed or peptic ulcer disease, monitor for symptoms of gastrointestinal bleeding (coffee ground emesis, black tarry stools, decreased hematocrit or hemoglobin count, occult blood in stool, gastric pain) annually

Dyskinesia
- occurs in more than 80% of patients treated for longer than 5 years
- characterized by chorea (orofacial chewing movements, ballistic flinging movements of the limbs) and dystonia (prolonged and often painful spasm, frequently in the foot) and occurs most commonly at the time of the drug's peak action
- may also occur throughout the dosing interval, especially when the patient is excited or is concentrating, or as the effect of the drug begins to wane (end of dose)

End-of-dose effect
- transition between normal mobility to severe parkinsonism occurring toward the end of the dosing interval
- usually responds to a shortened dosing interval
- bromocriptine may help to alleviate symptoms

Akinesia paradoxica
- "on-off" or freezing effect
- abrupt, unpredictable fluctuations in drug response that tend to be resistant to any form of therapy

Glaucoma
- monitor intraocular pressure annually, and ask the patient to report any visual disturbances and/or eye pain

Hemolytic anemia and glucose-6-phosphate dehydrogenase deficiency
- monitor hemoglobin count, hematocrit, red blood cell count, reticulocyte count, and peripheral blood smear annually
- especially important after surgery and/or bleeding episodes

▶ *How Long Do I Treat Patients with This Drug?*
Parkinson's disease
- although levodopa's efficacy deteriorates after 3–5 years of treatment, long-term therapy is recommended
- there is no role for drug-free periods ("drug holidays"), as any benefit derived from drug holidays (withdrawal of antiparkinsonian therapy for 3–14 days) is usually short lived and risks include immobility and subsequent thromboembolism, aspiration and pneumonia, and severe depression

▶ *How Do I Decrease or Stop the Administration of This Drug?*
- do not stop abruptly, as parkinsonian crisis and the neuromuscular malignant syndrome have been associated with the abrupt discontinuation of levodopa therapy
- decrease the daily levodopa dosage by 50% every 3 days

▶ *What Should I Tell My Patients About This Drug?*
- levodopa may cause dark discoloration of urine, sweat, and saliva
- taking this drug with food reduces any nausea or vomiting you may be experiencing
- you may experience dizziness when getting up suddenly from a lying or sitting position to a standing position, and if this occurs, rise slowly
- you may experience confusion and mild hallucinations; call your physician if this occurs
- long-term complications may occur as treatment continues and the disease progresses; this can be helped by adjusting dosage schedules and adding other drugs
- treatment is symptomatic only and does not cure Parkinson's disease, and as the disease progresses, symptoms may worsen
- the sustained-release tablet can be split in half; however, the tablets should not be chewed or crushed
- the regular levodopa-carbidopa tablets (not the sustained-release products) can be crushed and administered in a fruit-based liquid or soft food but must be used immediately after disruption of the dosage form

▶ *Therapeutic Tips*
- unless the patient is incontinent during the night, it is best to avoid bedtime doses of levodopa because a drug-free interval may be beneficial and levodopa may be disruptive to sleep (sleep movements and vivid dreams)
- be aware of false elevations with certain laboratory procedures; levodopa may cause asymptomatic and clinically insignificant elevations in uric acid, blood urea nitrogen, alanine aminotransferase, aspartate aminotransferase, lactate dehydrogenase, bilirubin, and alkaline phosphatase levels
- also be aware of false-positive results for urine glucose using Clinitest, false-positive results for urine ketones using Ketostix and Labstix, and false-negative glucosuria using Clinistix and Tes-Tape
- patients who are restricted to nothing by mouth near the time of surgery and cannot take levodopa may be treated with injectable benztropine if symptoms are a problem, although patients can stop receiving levodopa for several days before symptoms worsen

- controlled-release Sinemet CR (200 mg/50 mg) PO BID can be tried in new patients who do not have trouble with symptoms in the morning; however, later on in the disease, they may require TID dosing and eventually regular levodopa in the morning or may need a complete change to regular levodopa
- sustained-release preparations can be helpful to use at nighttime for patients who have difficulty getting up and going to the bathroom
- food increases the absorption of the sustained-release preparation (Sinemet CR)

LEVORPHANOL

Terry Baumann

USA (Levo-Dromoran)
CANADA (Levo-Dromoran)

▶ When Should I Use This Drug?

Consider an alternative agent

- this drug offers no advantages over sustained-release morphine

LEVOTHYROXINE

Ruby Grymonpre

USA (Levothroid, Levoxine, Synthroid)
CANADA (Eltroxin, Synthroid)

▶ When Should I Use This Drug?

Hypothyroidism

Patients with signs and symptoms of hypothyroidism and thyrotropin level greater than 15 mU/L and thyroxine level below normal

- signs and symptoms of hypothyroidism can be treated effectively with thyroid hormone replacement

Patients with mild or no symptoms of hypothyroidism and moderately elevated thyrotropin level (6–15 mU/L) and thyroxine level within normal limits

- approximately 80% of patients in this category ultimately have overt hypothyroidism and early rather than late treatment in this group with subclinical disease is appropriate (South Med J 1989;82:681–685)

▶ When Should I Not Use This Drug?

Nonspecific signs and symptoms of hypothyroidism

- patients with fatigue, difficulty in losing weight, and irregular menstruation should not receive levothyroxine without a proper workup and diagnosis of hypothyroidism (Postgrad Med 1989; 86:67–74)

Thyrotropin level within normal limits (0.5–6 mU/L) and low or low normal thyroxine levels

- thyroid hormone replacement is not required

▶ What Contraindications Are There to the Use of This Drug?

- intolerance of or allergic reaction to levothyroxine

▶ What Drug Interactions Are Clinically Important?

Drugs that may increase the effect or toxicity of levothyroxine

- none

Drugs that may decrease the effect of levothyroxine

CHOLESTYRAMINE OR COLESTIPOL

- absorption of levothyroxine is reduced by 30% up to 5 hours after cholestyramine or cholestipol administration
- if patients must use these 2 agents together, administer levothyroxine at least 6 hours after the administration of cholestyramine or cholestipol

- because the extent of this interaction is unknown, identify the effect of the interaction by measuring thyrotropin levels a couple of weeks after the start of this combination of agents and adjust levothyroxine dosages on the basis of these results

Drugs that may have their effect or toxicity increased by levothyroxine

WARFARIN

- levothyroxine may increase the anticoagulant effect of warfarin, probably owing to increased clearance of vitamin K–dependent clotting factors in the euthyroid patient
- addition of levothyroxine therapy to warfarin treatment necessitates weekly monitoring of INR until it is stabilized (for a minimum of 30 days)

Drugs that may have their effect decreased by levothyroxine

THEOPHYLLINE

- levothyroxine may decrease the activity of theophylline as a result of increased hepatic metabolism
- monitor the clinical effect of theophylline, and if a clinical deterioration occurs, measure a serum theophylline concentration and increase the dosage as needed

DIGOXIN

- pharmacodynamics of digoxin may be decreased by concurrent levo-thyroxine therapy by an unknown mechanism
- assess the effects of digoxin monthly and increase the dosage of digoxin if clinical deterioration occurs

▶ What Route and Dosage Should I Use?

How to administer

- orally—administer in the morning with or without food
- parenterally—give IV push at a rate not exceeding 100 μg/min

Hypothyroidism

- therapy that is initiated too aggressively may lead to thyroid hormone toxicity, including chest pain, increased pulse rate, palpitations, excessive sweating, headache, heat intolerance, and nervousness
- 0.1 mg PO daily for young, otherwise healthy patients
- 0.05 mg PO daily for patients older than 45 years of age with no cardiac disease
- 0.025 mg PO daily for elderly patients and patients with cardiac disease or long-standing hypothyroidism
- increase the dosage by 0.025 mg increments every 4 weeks until thyrotropin levels are within normal limits
- some patients (elderly, those with cardiac disease) are able to tolerate a maximum dose of only 0.05–0.075 mg of levothyroxine
- half-life of levothyroxine is approximately 7 days, and therefore, thyrotropin measurements and subsequent dosage adjustments should be made no more frequently than every 4 weeks

Switching patients from liothyronine to levothyroxine

- daily dosage of levothyroxine can be estimated by multiplying the daily liothyronine dose by 2.5
- liothyronine can be discontinued when levothyroxine administration is started
- to avoid overdosing, levothyroxine administration should be initiated at a dosage lower than the estimated daily dosage and titrated upward

Switching patients from desiccated thyroid to levothyroxine

- daily dosage of levothyroxine in micrograms is approximately equal to the daily dosage of desiccated thyroid in milligrams

Dosage adjustments for renal or hepatic dysfunction

- levothyroxine is primarily metabolized by the liver
- dosing adjustments should be based on serum thyrotropin concentrations
- if hepatic failure develops during stabilized levothyroxine therapy, measurement of serum thyrotropin levels guides dosing reductions

▶ What Should I Monitor with Regard to Efficacy and Toxicity?

Efficacy

Hypothyroidism

Thyrotropin and thyroxine

- optimal replacement is achieved when thyrotropin and thyroxine (T_4) levels are normal
- measure thyrotropin and T_4 levels every 4 weeks until within normal limits
- serum T_4 may occasionally be above normal values when a normal thyrotropin level is maintained; however, this is rare
- after an optimum levothyroxine dosage has been established, evaluate thyrotropin levels annually
- in patients known to be compliant, thyrotropin can be monitored every 4–5 years to ensure that T_4 requirements are not decreasing with age

Free thyroxine index

- this test is redundant and an excessive use of laboratory resources

Triiodothyronine

- T_3 level is often within normal limits in early or mild hypothyroidism and is an insensitive indicator of hypothyroidism (Can Med Assoc J 1981;124:1181–1183)
- is usually not readily available

Thyrotropin-releasing hormone

- thyrotropin response to thyrotropin-releasing hormone has been used to fine-tune the optimum levothyroxine dose; however, this is not clinically practical

Signs and symptoms of hypothyroidism

- assess symptoms every 4 weeks until the dosage is stabilized
- some reversal of hypothyroid symptoms (such as reduced skin temperature and physical activity) occurs within 2–3 weeks of therapy; however, maximum effects are not noticed until 4–6 weeks, and certain symptoms (e.g., anemia and hair or skin changes) do not respond until several months of replacement therapy

Toxicity

Signs and symptoms of hyperthyroxinemia

- palpitations, diarrhea, nervousness, intolerance of heat, and weight loss
- in elderly patients and patients with cardiac disease, monitor cardiovascular effects such as congestive heart failure, angina, tachycardia, and myocardial infarction
- if toxicity occurs, stop the drug until symptoms resolve (3–7 days) and restart the drug regimen at a dosage 25% lower than the previous level

▶ How Long Do I Treat Patients with This Drug?

Hypothyroidism

- therapy with levothyroxine is usually lifelong
- transient forms of hypothyroidism (subacute thyroiditis, postpartum thyroiditis) do not usually necessitate lifelong thyroid hormone replacement therapy

▶ How Do I Decrease or Stop the Administration of This Drug?

- may be stopped abruptly

▶ What Should I Tell My Patients About This Drug?

- medication is to replace a hormone produced by the thyroid gland
- medication must be taken daily, preferably in the morning, and may be taken with or without food
- if you forget to take your medication, but remember later in the day, take the usual dosage of medication at that time
- if you forget until the next day, do not double the dosage, but instead continue with your usual daily dosage
- symptoms that you have because of lack of this hormone will gradually disappear over 2–4 weeks

- contact your physician if any signs of excessive thyroid hormone occur (e.g., chest pain, rapid heart rate, palpitations, and excessive nervousness)
- you may notice a slight weight loss, increase in bowel movement frequency, and increased appetite, but these require no action unless they are persistent or severe

▶ Therapeutic Tips

- in 1982, the content of levothyroxine in Synthroid was increased from 78% to 100%
- patients stabilized on 1 brand of levothyroxine should not be changed to any other brand owing to differences in bioequivalence among products
- it is likely that many persons currently prescribed thyroid hormone replacement are, for various reasons, not hypothyroid and this is especially true for elderly persons
- in cases in which the need for thyroid hormone is not documented or is questionable, a single thyrotropin test drawn 8 weeks after thyroid hormone administration withdrawal determines whether a patient is hypothyroid or euthyroid (J Clin Epidemiol 1989; 42:417–420)
- long half-life (7 days) of levothyroxine makes parenteral administration rarely indicated, unless prolonged restriction of oral administration occurs
- instability of the parenteral product and its high cost (approximately $65/d) encourages oral administration if at all possible

LIDOCAINE

James E. Tisdale

USA (lidocaine hydrochloride, LidoPen, Xylocaine)
CANADA (Lidocaine, Xylocard)

▶ When Should I Use This Drug?

Ventricular tachycardia

- lidocaine should be used for the short-term treatment of sustained, symptomatic, hemodynamically stable ventricular tachycardia and for the short-term prevention of recurrent episodes of ventricular tachycardia

Ventricular fibrillation

- lidocaine should be used for the short-term treatment of ventricular fibrillation and for the short-term prevention of recurrent episodes of ventricular fibrillation after an initially successful defibrillation attempt

Prophylaxis of primary ventricular fibrillation in acute myocardial infarction

- defibrillation should be used to treat ventricular fibrillation and cardioversion should be used to treat unstable symptomatic ventricular tachycardia; the routine prophylactic use of lidocaine to prevent ventricular fibrillation is not recommended
- lidocaine has been shown to reduce the incidence of primary ventricular fibrillation after acute myocardial infarction (MI), but has not been shown to influence mortality positively, and evidence suggests that routine prophylaxis may increase mortality (Arch Intern Med 1989;149:2694–2698)
- American Heart Association and the American College of Cardiology recommend the prophylactic administration of lidocaine for 12–24 hours to patients with suspected acute MI who experience frequent (>6/min) ventricular premature beats (VPBs), closely coupled (R-on-T) VPBs, multiform VPBs, or VPBs that occur in short bursts of 3 or more in succession (Circulation 1990;82:664–707)

Diagnosis or management of wide QRS complex tachycardia of uncertain origin

- lidocaine is the drug of choice for this indication (JAMA 1992; 268:2199–2241) because 80–85% of wide QRS complex tachycardias are ventricular tachycardia

▶ When Should I Not Use This Drug?

Asymptomatic ventricular arrhythmias

- lidocaine should not be used for the treatment of asymptomatic arrhythmias, unless they occur in association with acute MI as described above

Supraventricular arrhythmias

- lidocaine is not effective for the management of supraventricular arrhythmias

▶ *What Contraindications Are There to the Use of This Drug?*

Intolerance of or allergic reaction to lidocaine

- lidocaine is contraindicated in patients with known hypersensitivity to lidocaine or to amide-type local anesthetics (bupivicaine, dibucaine, etidocaine, mepivacaine, prilocaine)

Sick sinus syndrome

- lidocaine has been reported to cause sinus bradycardia, sinus arrest, and asystole and should not be used in patients with sick sinus syndrome in the absence of a pacemaker

Atrioventricular block

- lidocaine has been reported to cause atrioventricular (AV) conduction disturbances and should not be used in patients with Mobitz type II second-degree heart block or complete (third-degree) heart block in the absence of a pacemaker; lidocaine should be used with caution in patients with Mobitz type I second-degree heart block (Wenckebach) or first-degree heart block

▶ *What Drug Interactions Are Clinically Important?*

Drugs that may increase the effect or toxicity of lidocaine

BETA-BLOCKERS

- concomitant administration of propranolol or metoprolol with lidocaine may result in elevations in plasma lidocaine concentrations by reducing the clearance of lidocaine, probably as a result of decreasing cardiac output and hepatic blood flow and hepatic enzyme inhibition
- if therapy with one of these drugs is initiated in a patient receiving lidocaine, the rate of infusion should be decreased by $1/3$, and the patient should be monitored for arrhythmia recurrence and signs or symptoms of lidocaine toxicity
- although it has not been studied, it should be assumed that other beta-blockers also interact with lidocaine

CIMETIDINE

- concomitant administration of lidocaine and cimetidine may result in elevations in plasma lidocaine concentrations
- switch to ranitidine or other H_2 antagonist if the combination must be used, as these agents have less of an effect on metabolism
- if cimetidine must be used, decrease lidocaine infusion by $1/3$ and monitor for arrhythmia recurrence and signs or symptoms of lidocaine toxicity

Drugs that may decrease the effect or toxicity of lidocaine

- none

Drugs that may have their effect or toxicity increased by lidocaine

- none

Drugs that may have their effect or toxicity decreased by lidocaine

- none

▶ *What Route and Dosage Should I Use?*

How to administer

- orally—significant first-pass metabolism makes oral administration potentially toxic owing to high concentrations of active metabolites
- intravenously—as a bolus or continuous infusion in dextrose or saline solutions

Ventricular tachycardia, ventricular fibrillation, prophylaxis of primary ventricular fibrillation in acute myocardial infarction

Loading dose

- 1.5 mg/kg IV (usually 100 mg) over 1–2 minutes as an initial loading dose
- 5–10 minutes later, administer a second loading dose of 0.75 mg/kg IV over 1–2 minutes

- maximum loading dose is 3 mg/kg (JAMA 1992;268:2199–2241)
- if arrhythmia suppression occurs, follow the loading dose with a maintenance infusion
- breakthrough ventricular arrhythmias are managed by giving additional boluses of 0.5 mg/kg and increasing the maintenance infusion by 1 mg/min up to a maximum of 4 mg/min

Maintenance dosage

- maintenance dosage of 3 mg/min in patients younger than 65 years without acute MI, congestive heart failure, or chronic hepatic disease
- 2 mg/min in patients older than 65 years of age, those with acute MI, and those receiving concomitant beta-adrenergic receptor blocking agent therapy
- 1.5 mg/min in patients with chronic hepatic disease or both acute MI and congestive heart failure
- 1 mg/min in patients with congestive heart failure and those older than 65 years of age with chronic hepatic disease

Dosage adjustments for renal or hepatic dysfunction

- hepatically metabolized
- lidocaine dosages do not need adjustment in patients with renal dysfunction
- although 1 of the metabolites of lidocaine may accumulate in patients with renal dysfunction, this metabolite is not believed to be responsible for significant toxicity
- for patients with chronic hepatic disease, use a maintenance dosage of 1.5 mg/min

▶ *What Should I Monitor with Regard to Efficacy and Toxicity?*

Efficacy

Ventricular tachycardia, ventricular fibrillation

Vital signs

- heart rate, blood pressure, and respiratory rate should be assessed continuously until arrhythmia is under control
- presence or absence of symptoms related to arrhythmia (palpitations, shortness of breath, dizziness, angina, or syncope)

Electrocardiogram

- frequency of ventricular ectopic activity and rate and duration of episodes of ventricular tachycardia should be assessed continuously until arrhythmia is under control

Serum lidocaine concentrations

- if the patient's ventricular arrhythmia is under control and no toxicities are present, the lidocaine dosage should be considered appropriate and no measurement of concentration is required
- if signs or symptoms of lidocaine toxicity are present, or if an inadequate response is achieved with the current dosage, serum lidocaine concentrations should be obtained
- serum concentrations should also be monitored within 24 hours in patients with congestive heart failure and hepatic dysfunction (repeated serum concentrations are not needed unless dosage changes are made)
- if arrhythmia recurs, obtain a serum concentration and increase the dosage by 0.5–1 mg/min pending the results of the concentration (if the concentration is between 2 and 6 mg/L, change to a different drug)
- lidocaine therapy should be discontinued abruptly in patients with plasma concentrations greater than 6 mg/L (restart at $2/3$ of the original dosage if concentrations are between 6 and 8 mg/L)

Prophylaxis of primary ventricular fibrillation in acute myocardial infarction

- as above, except lidocaine concentrations are not required

Toxicity

Intermittent electrocardiographic assessment

- for AV block, sinus bradycardia, sinus arrest, and asystole
- if this occurs, stop the drug administration and give atropine

Dizziness; drowsiness; confusion; numbness of the face, extremities, or whole body; dysarthria; double vision; euphoria; tremors; twitching; hypotension; new cardiac arrhythmias; seizures

- should be assessed every 12 hours
- lidocaine therapy should be abruptly discontinued if any of the adverse effects of lidocaine develops
- if the patient has seizures, new cardiac arrhythmias, sinus arrest, second- or third-degree heart block, or asystole, the drug administration should not be restarted
- if the patient has one of the other adverse effects of lidocaine, the drug regimen may be restarted at 50% of the original dosage in 2 hours in patients with normal hepatic and cardiac function; in 4 hours, in patients with congestive heart failure; and in 6 hours, in patients with hepatic disease
- lidocaine therapy should be discontinued abruptly in patients with plasma concentrations greater than 6 mg/L (restart at ²/₃ of the original dose if concentrations are between 6 and 8 mg/L, and at 50% of the original dose if concentrations > 8 mg/L)

▶ *How Long Do I Treat Patients with This Drug?*

Ventricular tachycardia, ventricular fibrillation

- lidocaine therapy should be continued until the underlying cause of the arrhythmia may be identified and corrected
- if no correctable underlying cause is identified, lidocaine therapy should be continued until ventricular tachycardia is terminated and for 24 hours after termination, after which the patient should be referred to a cardiac electrophysiologist for assessment of the need for long-term oral antiarrhythmic drug therapy

Prophylaxis of primary ventricular fibrillation in acute myocardial infarction

- continue lidocaine therapy for 12–24 hours after MI

▶ *How Do I Decrease or Stop the Administration of This Drug?*

- lidocaine infusion rates do not have to be decreased in a tapering fashion prior to discontinuation
- when therapy is no longer indicated, lidocaine infusions may be discontinued abruptly

▶ *What Should I Tell My Patients About This Drug?*

- you are receiving an intravenous drug to control your irregular heartbeat and you should inform your nurse or physician if you have palpitations, shortness of breath, chest pain, dizziness, drowsiness, twitching, tremors, double vision, or numbness of any part of the body

▶ *Therapeutic Tips*

- lidocaine accumulates in patients with an acute MI who receive the drug for longer than 24–36 hours (if prolonged infusions are necessary in this population, a plasma lidocaine concentration is recommended at 36–48 hours to prevent toxicity)

Useful References

Tisdale JE. Lidocaine prophylaxis in acute myocardial infarction. Henry Ford Hosp Med J 1991;39:217–225

Pieper JA, Johnson KE. Lidocaine. In: Evans WE, Schentag JJ, Jusko WJ, eds. Applied Pharmacokinetics. Principles of Therapeutic Drug Monitoring, 3rd ed. Spokane, WA: Applied Therapeutics, 1992:21-1–21-37

Collingsworth KA, Kalman SM, Harrison DC. The clinical pharmacology of lidocaine as an antiarrhythmic drug. Circulation 1974;50:1217–1230

LISINOPRIL

Jack Onrot and James McCormack

USA (Prinivil, Zestril)
CANADA (Prinivil, Zestril)

▶ *When Should I Use This Drug?*

see Enalapril

▶ *When Should I Not Use This Drug?*

see Enalapril

▶ *What Contraindications Are There to the Use of This Drug?*

see Captopril

▶ *What Drug Interactions Are Clinically Important?*

see Captopril

▶ *What Route and Dosage Should I Use?*

How to administer

- orally—can be administered with or without food
- parenterally—not commercially available

Congestive heart failure

- 2.5 mg PO daily
- rapidity of the dosage escalation depends on the severity of symptoms
- in general, increase dosages weekly; however, dosages may be increased daily
- no value in exceeding a total daily dose of 40 mg

Chronic (noncrisis) hypertension

- 2.5 mg PO daily
- increase the dosage by 2.5 mg PO daily every 4 weeks until adequate blood pressure is acheived or a daily dosage of 20 mg is reached
- limited value in exceeding a total daily dosage of 20 mg (dosages as high as 40 mg PO daily have been used)

Dosage adjustments for renal or hepatic dysfunction

- renally eliminated
- titrate dose to clinical response and not concurrent renal or hepatic function

▶ *What Should I Monitor with Regard to Efficacy and Toxicity?*

see Captopril

▶ *How Long Do I Treat Patients with This Drug?*

see Captopril

▶ *How Do I Decrease or Stop the Administration of This Drug?*

see Captopril

▶ *What Should I Tell My Patients About this Drug?*

see Captopril

▶ *Therapeutic Tips*

see Captopril

LITHIUM

Steven Stanislav and Patricia Marken

Lithium Carbonate

USA (Eskalith, Eskalith CR, Lithane, Lithobid, Lithotabs)
CANADA (Lithane, Duralith)

Lithium Citrate

USA (Cibalith-S)
CANADA (not available)

▶ *When Should I Use This Drug?*

Prophylactic therapy for bipolar disorder (started in conjunction with acute therapy)

- is the drug of choice because of extensive clinical experience and more controlled studies compared with the case for alternative agents and should be started as soon as the acutely manic patient is willing or able to take oral agents (within 24 hours)

- drug of choice for the prevention or the attenuation of recurrent bipolar episodes, although approximately 20–40% of lithium-treated patients experience relapse (Am J Psychiatry 1990;147:431–434)

Depression

- patients with bipolar depression who may not be good candidates for tricyclic antidepressants or fluoxetine and possibly other antidepressants, as these medications can cause a switch to a manic phase (Biol Psychiatry 1982;17:271–274)
- may also be used as augmentation therapy to conventional antidepressants in partial responders (J Clin Psychopharmacol 1982;3:303–307)

Aggression

- treatment option in episodic aggressive behavior (Am J Psychiatry 1976;133:1409–1413)
- one of the first-line agents in chronic, impulsive, nonpsychotic patients (e.g., mentally retarded patients)

▶ *When Should I Not Use This Drug?*

Organic cause of mania is known

- drug-induced mania, hyperthyroidism, severe metabolic abnormalities, tumor, etc.

Mild, behavioral dyscontrol or psychotic agitation

- may respond equally well to temporary therapy with other agents (e.g., antipsychotics and sedative-hypnotics)

Prophylactic therapy after a single manic episode in patients without a prior psychiatric history

- use prophylactic or maintenance therapy only after at least 2 well-documented episodes within 5 years (or after the first episode if the occurrence of a second episode is potentially life threatening) (Handbook of Biological Psychiatry, Part IV 1981:225–242)

▶ *What Contraindications Are There to the Use of This Drug?*

Intolerance of or allergic reaction to lithium

Severe dehydration

- rehydrate the patient before giving lithium because of the increased risk of adverse effects

Patients with renal dysfunction (< 50% normal renal function)

- lithium is renally eliminated and it is best to use an alternative agent such as carbamazepine or valproic acid
- in patients with stable chronic renal failure, lithium may be used, but serum concentrations must be monitored

Patients in congestive heart failure or sick sinus syndrome

- may impair conduction (Hosp Formul 1985;20:726–735)
- use an alternative agent such as carbamazepine and valproic acid

▶ *What Drug Interactions Are Clinically Important?*

Drugs that may increase the effect of lithium

CHLOROTHIAZIDE, HYDROCHLOROTHIAZIDE

- decreases renal lithium clearance and increases serum lithium levels
- if possible, use an alternative agent such as spironolactone and furosemide
- toxicity due to increased lithium levels can be life threatening
- monitor lithium level several days after initiating thiazide therapy or earlier if symptoms of toxicity are seen
- adjust the dosage on the basis of lithium levels
- if the dosage is already at upper end of lithium's therapeutic range, decrease the lithium dosage by 20–40%

NONSTEROIDAL ANTIINFLAMMATORY DRUGS

- increase renal tubular reabsorption of sodium and increase serum lithium levels
- use acetaminophen and aspirin when possible owing to their minimum effects on lithium concentration

- as needed use of nonsteroidal antiinflammatory drugs (NSAIDs) is probably not significant
- if the patient is receiving regularly dosed NSAIDs, monitor the lithium level 1 week after initiating NSAID therapy or earlier if symptoms of toxicity are seen

Drugs that may decrease the effect of lithium

THEOPHYLLINE

- increases renal clearance of lithium
- upward adjustment in lithium dosages should be guided by the lithium level obtained after reaching new steady state in approximately 5 days

Drugs that may have their effect increased by lithium

- none

Drugs that may have their effect decreased by lithium

- none

▶ *What Route and Dosage Should I Use?*

How to administer

- orally—with food or milk or on an empty stomach
- parenterally—not available

Prophylactic therapy for bipolar disorder, depression, aggression

- 300 mg PO TID is the starting dosage in normal, healthy adults with good renal function
- check level in 3–4 days and, if the serum concentration is not in the therapeutic range, increase the dose to 600 mg PO BID
- start with 300 mg PO BID in patients with estimated creatinine clearance less than 80 mL/min, those with a low serum sodium level, or patients receiving diuretics
- 300 mg PO BID in elderly patients
- because there is much interpatient variability in response to dosages, serum concentration monitoring, rather than dosage, is the most important monitoring variable to ensure therapeutic levels
- sustained-release products are more expensive and offer no advantage over conventional dosing forms; however, consider using sustained-release products when patients are intolerant to conventional formulations (J Clin Psychopharmacol 1981;1:406–408)

Dosage adjustments for renal or hepatic dysfunction

- renally eliminated
- in patients with renal dysfunction start with 300–600 mg/d and obtain weekly serum concentrations until steady state is achieved
- once steady state is achieved, obtain monthly serum concentrations and serum creatinine (ensure stable sodium and fluid intake)

▶ *What Should I Monitor with Regard to Efficacy and Toxicity?*

Efficacy

Bipolar disorder

Specific target symptoms

- agitation; decreased sleep; rapid, pressured speech with flight of ideas for manic phase; or symptoms of depression
- agitation and sleep disturbances usually resolve within several days to weeks; however, complete mood stabilization (and resolution of thought disorder, if present) may necessitate 6 weeks or longer

Concurrent symptoms of psychoses

- auditory, visual hallucinations, and delusional or disorganized thinking
- symptoms may abate in several days (if related to acute mania) or necessitate 6 weeks or longer for complete resolution

Lithium concentrations

- therapeutic lithium levels have been delineated in the treatment of bipolar disorder; however, it is unclear whether the same therapeutic range exists for other psychiatric disorders treated with lithium

- similar steady state levels are attained with different dosage forms (e.g., carbonate, citrate, sustained-release); once-daily dosing may result in higher 12 hour lithium levels (Acta Psychiatr Scand 1981;64:281–294)
- initial serum concentration should be determined after 5 days with the initial dosage
- obtain all serum levels 12 hours after the dose is given
- obtain further lithium level 5 days after each dosing increase and monthly thereafter
- attempt to achieve levels of 0.8–1.2 mEq/L, which are often required in therapy for acute mania; however, the dosage should be maintained at lowest possible level to decrease the incidence of dose-related side effects
- typically dosage increases of 300 mg result in an increase in lithium levels by approximately 0.2–0.3 mEq/L
- studies suggest that relapse rates may increase as lithium levels decrease; however, therapy must be individualized for each patient (J Clin Psychiatry 1989;50:17–22)

Depression

Sleep disturbance

- is the first symptom to improve (after 7–14 days) and should be assessed weekly

Nervousness, somatic complaints, appetite, mood

- tend to improve more slowly over 2–3 weeks
- close friends or relatives notice signs of improvement before the patient is aware of changes
- adequate clinical response may take at least 4 weeks
- after they are stable, patients should be clinically assessed for target symptoms at least monthly (or weekly if clinical decompensation is suspected)

Aggression

- look for less frequent or less severe aggressive outbursts
- may take up to 3 months for patients to respond

Toxicity

Clinical monitoring is the most effective means of detecting early signs of toxicity

Worsening tremor, severe nausea, vomiting, or persistent diarrhea, and neurological toxicity suggested by weakness, ataxia, confusion, or slurred speech

- lithium toxicity is potentially fatal
- discontinue lithium administration at the first signs of possible toxicity and draw blood for a serum lithium concentration
- withold lithium if dehydration is suspected
- fine hand tremor, polyuria, and mild nausea often occur with dosages within the therapeutic range and do not always suggest toxicity

Gastrointestinal effects

- intolerance often resolves after several weeks of therapy, by changing salt or formulation (regular to sustained release or vice versa) or by dividing doses

Tremor

- often resolved by lowering the total daily dose by 150–300 mg (provided it is not at the low end of the therapeutic range)

Polyuria (impaired renal concentrating ability)

- if patients report polyuria (>3 L/d), the dosage should be reduced by 25%, and if this does not resolve the problem, lithium discontinuation should be considered because patients with an impaired renal concentrating ability may be at increased risk for renal toxicity from this agent

Renal function

- measure blood urea and serum creatinine at least every 6 months
- if there is evidence of renal dysfunction, reassess the lithium dosage (via serum concentrations)

Thyroid function

- many patients become hypothyroid when taking lithium
- obtain baseline and every 6 month thyroid function tests

▶ How Long Do I Treat Patients with This Drug?

Bipolar disorder, depression

- duration of therapy is not well defined
- at the minimum, treatment should continue until symptoms resolve, the patient is euthymic, and sleep normalizes (some clinicians recommend continuing therapy for several months after symptoms resolve)
- prophylactic or maintenance therapy should be continued in rapid cyclers (>4 episodes per year), and probably in patients with a history of recurrent bipolar disorder (at least 1 episode per year) with marked severity and substantial disruption of functioning
- after they are stable, patients receiving maintenance or prophylactic therapy should be clinically assessed at least monthly (or weekly at the first signs of clinical decompensation) and serum levels measured every 3 months and then every 6 months when the patient has been stable for at least 1 year
- reassess the need for prophylactic therapy in patients with no signs of mania or depression for 5 years

▶ How Do I Decrease or Stop the Administration of This Drug?

- most patients do not experience a withdrawal syndrome or rebound phenomenon on abrupt discontinuation; however, certain individuals may have increased risks of recurrence of symptoms after discontinuation (Br J Psychiatry 1986;149:498–501)
- if tapering is warranted decrease the daily dosage by 300 mg every week and monitor the patient weekly for the first few weeks (monitoring for early relapse) and then monthly after that (monitoring for late relapse)

▶ What Should I Tell My Patients About This Drug?

- you may experience mild hand tremor, diarrhea, and/or increased urination while taking this drug—do not be alarmed, these are common side effects; however, inform your physician immediately if the intensity of these side effects increases
- recognize early symptoms of toxicity
- it is important to maintain adequate fluid intake and not to change your diet without your physician's knowledge
- contact your physician if you notice extreme sedation, confusion, incoordination or shakiness on your feet, or difficulty with talking
- do not take any other medications (including nonprescription or over the counter medicines) without your physician's knowledge

▶ Therapeutic Tips

- obtain all lithium levels as close to 12 hours after a dose as possible to ensure standardization when interpreting subsequent levels
- 12 hour lithium levels may be slightly higher with a sustained-release formulation compared with a carbonate form
- sustained-release products are more expensive and offer no advantage over conventional dosing forms (J Clin Psychopharmacol 1981;1:406–408)

Useful References

Schou M. Lithium prophylaxis: Myths and realities. Am J Psychiatry 1989;146:573–576

Jefferson JW, Greist JH, Ackerman DL, Carroll JA. Lithium Encyclopedia for Clinical Practice, 2nd ed. Washington, DC: American Psychiatric Press, 1989

Angst J. Bipolar disorder. In: van Praag H, Lader M, Rafaelson OJ, Sachar ER. Handbook of Biological Psychiatry, Part IV. New York: Dekker, 1981:225–242

LORATADINE

Penny Miller

USA (not available)
CANADA (Claritin)

▶ When Should I Use This Drug?

Seasonal allergic rhinitis, chronic (perennial) rhinitis, chronic dermatological allergies (atopic dermatitis, chronic urticaria, pruritus of unknown cause)

- all antihistamines are considered to have relatively the same efficacy in preventing or treating allergic reactions; however, there is great interpatient variation in the response to a given antihistamine

- selection of any particular antihistamine is based on the degree of sedation and anticholinergic effects, plus the convenience of dosing and cost
- loratadine is useful if the patient has sedative effects or would be sensitive to the sedative effects from less expensive antihistamines such as chlorpheniramine
- choice among astemizole, terfenadine, and loratadine should be based on cost and the onset of action (astemizole has a slow onset of action)
- does not impair psychomotor activity or potentiate ethanol's central nervous system effects such as sedation, decreased visual discrimination, and slowed reaction times
- it does not lower the seizure threshold (unlike diphenhydramine and chlorpheniramine)
- demonstrates few or no anticholinergic side effects (antihistamine effects are responsible for the relief of allergic symptoms)

Acute dermatological allergies (e.g., hives and allergic conjunctivitis caused by allergens or food)

- antihistamines relieve pruritus and prevent further extension of the lesions
- if sedation from an antihistamine would be a problem, choose either loratadine or terfenadine, whichever is the least expensive
- if mild sedation would not be a problem, use chlorpheniramine, which is less expensive than loratadine

▶ When Should I Not Use This Drug?

Common cold

- for the symptoms of sneezing and runny nose, loratadine is not effective because it has little or no anticholinergic effects

▶ What Contraindications Are There to the Use of This Drug?

- intolerance of or allergic reaction to loratadine

▶ What Drug Interactions Are Clinically Important?

- none

▶ What Route and Dosage Should I Use?

How to administer

- orally—take on an empty stomach or with food or milk
- parenterally—not available

Seasonal allergic rhinitis, chronic (perennial) rhinitis, chronic dermatological allergies (atopic dermatitis, chronic urticaria, pruritus of unknown cause), acute dermatological allergies (e.g., hives and allergic conjunctivitis caused by allergens or food)

- 10 mg PO daily up to a maximum dosage of 40 mg PO daily

Dosage adjustments for renal or hepatic dysfunction

- hepatically metabolized
- no dosage adjustments are required, titrate the dose up to an effect

▶ What Should I Monitor with Regard to Efficacy and Toxicity?

Efficacy

see Chlorpheniramine

Toxicity

Mild fatigue, headache, dry mouth, and sedation

- can occur, but less often than with chlorpheniramine, and is likely not clinically significant

Cardiac toxicity

- no reported cases of arrhythmias or electrocardiographic alterations

▶ How Long Do I Treat Patients with This Drug?

see Chlorpheniramine

▶ How Do I Decrease or Stop the Administration of This Drug?

- may be stopped abruptly
- for chronic allergic symptoms, the drug administration should likely be tapered (decrease the dosage by 25% every week)

▶ What Should I Tell My Patients About This Drug?

- do not exceed maximum daily dosages

▶ Therapeutic Tips

- adverse cardiac effects reported for other nonsedating antihistamines (astemizole and terfenadine) have not occurred to date with loratadine; however, experience with loratadine is still limited (HPB, Health and Welfare Canada, Dear Doctor #42 (letter), re terfenadine and astemizole, August 28, 1992)

Useful References

Mann KV, Crowe JP, Tietze KJ. Drug reviews. Non-sedating histamine H_1 receptor antagonists. Clin Pharm 1989;8:331–344

Sutherland D. Antihistamine agents—New options or just more drugs? On Continuing Practice 1991;18:31–36

Estelle F, Simmons R, Simons KJ. Pharmacokinetic optimization of histamine H_1-receptor antagonist therapy. Clin Pharmacokinet 1991;21:372–393

LORAZEPAM

Steven Stanislav, Patricia Marken, William Parker, and Jonathan Fleming

USA (Ativan)

CANADA (Ativan, Apo-Lorazepam, Novolorazepam, PMS Lorazepam, Nu-Loraz)

▶ When Should I Use This Drug?

Generalized anxiety disorder

- benzodiazepines have been considered first-line therapy due to extensive research and more than 30 years' clinical experience
- all benzodiazepines are equally effective (N Engl J Med 1993;328:1398–1405); therefore, the choice is based on the patient's previous response and cost
- agents with an intermediate duration of action (lorazepam or oxazepam) are preferred because they allow easier dose titration by both the patient and the physician
- onset of action of lorazepam is a little faster (15–45 minutes versus 45–90 minutes) than that of oxazepam (likely because it is absorbed faster), but this difference is probably not important when these agents are dosed long term
- predictors of response to benzodiazepines are acute symptoms, a precipitating stressful event, high level of psychic and somatic anxiety, absence of or low level of depression, no previous drug treatment, good response to previous therapy, and expectation of recovery or desire for medication
- benzodiazepines have an effect immediately to within several days, whereas buspirone's effect is delayed for 2–4 weeks

Panic disorder

- limited data suggest that lorazepam and diazepam may be efficacious (J Clin Psychiatry 1986;47:458–460)
- if cost is a major issue, high-dose lorazepam can be used in place of alprazolam or clonazepam, which are usually the first-line agents

Transient situational insomnia, short-term insomnia (of up to 3 weeks' duration)

- all of the marketed benzodiazepines have sedative properties and can be used as hypnotics
- they differ in their pharmacokinetics, side effect profile, capacity to cause discontinuation syndromes (e.g., rebound insomnia), and cost
- lorazepam, oxazepam, and temazepam are equally effective, although there are fewer data on the use of lorazepam and oxazepam as hypnotics
- lorazepam, as with other high-potency, short-acting benzodiazepines, is associated with worse rebound effects than less potent

or longer-acting compounds (this is not important if it is being used for just a few nights)
- decision should also include cost (lorazepam and oxazepam are available as generics and are usually less expensive)

Long-term treatment of insomnia
- effective in the intermittent treatment of long-term insomnia if alternative, behavioral techniques for controlling insomnia are ineffective
- although studies on the efficacy of long-term use of hypnotics are scant and many sleep laboratory studies show a loss of hypnotic effect (tolerance) by the fourth week of continuous use, about 10% of patients benefit from continuous or intermittent use of hypnotics, and long-term users often report high satisfaction with their sleep and few adverse effects (Age Ageing 1984;13:335–343)
- continued, intermittent medication use (provided there is demonstrable benefit) may be the most sensible approach
- lorazepam, as with other high potency, short-acting benzodiazepines, may be associated with worse rebound effects than less potent or longer-acting compounds, although this is disputed by some clinicians (N Engl J Med 1993;328:1398–1405)

Acute psychosis
- short-term therapy with benzodiazepines can be used to control initial agitation and decrease the need for initial high dosages of antipsychotics
- can be given parenterally, which may be useful in patients unwilling to take oral medications

Bipolar disorder
- for short-term therapy in the initial stages of an acute manic episode, lorazepam should be used, as it is available in both oral and parenteral forms and may decrease the amount of antipsychotic needed
- although clonazepam may be used (there is a suggestion that it has some specific antimanic properties), it is more expensive than lorazepam and there is little evidence that it is more effective than lorazepam

Preoperative sedation
- drug of choice, as it is effective, is rapidly absorbed, and is available as a parenteral agent

Status epilepticus
- is the first choice for many clinicians, as it distributes out of the central nervous system (CNS) more slowly and may work longer than diazepam (even though it has a shorter half-life than does diazepam), but the clinical significance of this is not known
- diazepam is as effective as and less expensive than lorazepam

Alcohol withdrawal (treatment and prevention of seizures)
- as under status epilepticus
- many clinicians prefer lorazepam for the treatment of seizures due to alcohol withdrawal
- both diazepam and lorazepam are effective for preventing alcohol withdrawal seizures
- diazepam has a longer duration of action than does lorazepam and other benzodiazepines, which may be useful when stopping diazepam (self-tapering)
- some clinicians prefer lorazepam to diazepam because, if an intramuscular agent is required (in addition to an oral agent for backup), intramuscular lorazepam is absorbed more rapidly and completely than intramuscular diazepam

▶ When Should I Not Use This Drug?

Transient and short-term insomnia when it is important to avoid daytime sedation or effects on psychomotor performance, such as for the management of jet lag
- lorazepam has a moderately long half-life; therefore, use triazolam, which has less severe hangover effects

▶ What Contraindications Are There to the Use of This Drug?

Intolerance of or allergic reaction to lorazepam

Patients with chronic obstructive pulmonary disease and sleep-related breathing disorders (particularly obstructive sleep apnea)
- these conditions are worsened by the use of benzodiazepines

Pregnant or lactating women
- because effects are unknown

Patients with a history of abusing benzodiazepines or alcohol
- concurrent alcohol use increases amnestic effects (JAMA 1987; 258:945–946)

▶ What Drug Interactions Are Clinically Important?

Drugs that may increase the effect or toxicity of lorazepam

ALCOHOL
- about 20% of insomniacs may take alcohol and sleeping pills concurrently to aid sleep (Confin Psychiatry 1977;15:151–172), and this can produce additive sedative effects
- avoid the combination if possible

CENTRAL NERVOUS SYSTEM DEPRESSANTS
- additive, sedative effects are expected when CNS depressants are given concomitantly
- avoid the combination if possible or minimize the effects by starting with low, divided daily doses and allowing tolerance to develop before dosage increases

Drugs that may decrease the effect of lorazepam
- none

Drugs that may have their effect or toxicity increased by lorazepam
- none

Drugs that may have their effect decreased by lorazepam
- none

▶ What Route and Dosage Should I Use?

How to administer

Orally
- take with food or milk or on an empty stomach

Parenterally
- for IV administration, dilute in an equal volume of sterile water, normal saline, or 5% dextrose in water immediately prior to use
- can be given as an IV bolus or into the tubing of an existing IV infusion at a rate of less than 2 mg/min
- can also be given IM

Generalized anxiety disorder
- start with 0.5 mg PO BID
- if no excessive sedation occurs, increase the dosage by 0.5 mg increments every 3–4 days up to 1 mg PO TID (this dosage affords control for most people) or until symptoms are well under control

Panic disorder
- goal is to prevent attacks and then to decrease the dosage if the drug is tolerated and symptoms are controlled
- 0.5 mg PO TID for 1 week
- advise the patient that this dosage may make him or her sedated and that he or she may have to take time off work or school
- if necessary, titrate the dose up by 0.5 mg increments to 6 mg PO daily on the basis of the response and the patient's ability to tolerate sedation
- patients usually require higher doses than those needed for anxiety
- after symptoms are suppressed, one can attempt to decrease the dosage and administer twice daily
- 2–3 doses per day are needed to avoid breakthough anxiety

Transient situational insomnia, short-term insomnia, long-term treatment of insomnia
- 0.5 mg PO taken 40 minutes before retiring
- sublingual form, which has a more rapid onset of action but, as a hypnotic, has no particular advantages over the standard oral form
- use the 0.5 mg dose for 1–2 nights' therapy, and if this low dosage is not effective, the dosage should be doubled

Acute psychosis, bipolar disorder (if acutely agitated)

- 2 mg PO or IM (if the patient will not take oral medication) Q1H until the patient is settled (usually ≤4 mg)
- some clinicians recommend a maximum of 10 mg/d, but there is no specific reason not to give higher dosages in the absence of side effects
- at dosages greater than 8 mg/24 h, disinhibition and ataxia (especially in the elderly) can occur
- goal of therapy is to treat acute agitation only, not core symptoms of psychosis or bipolar disorder

Preoperative sedation

- 0.05 mg/kg IM up to a maximum of 4 mg given at least 2 hours before surgery
- if given IV, give 15–20 minutes before surgery

Status epilepticus, alcohol withdrawal (treatment and prevention of seizures)

- 2 mg IV over 30–60 seconds, and if seizures are not controlled and no cardiorespiratory depression occurs, give another 2 mg in 2–5 minutes
- further 2 mg IV can be given 10–20 minutes later if tonic-clonic seizures continue (this rarely happens) while phenytoin is being administered
- to prevent alcohol withdrawal seizures, give 2 mg PO TID for 2 days, 2 mg PO BID for 2 days, 2 mg PO daily for 1 day, and then stop
- if symptoms of withdrawal, such as tremor and irritability occur, increase the dosage

Dosage adjustments, for renal or hepatic dysfunction

- hepatically metabolized
- no dosage adjustments for organ dysfunction are recommended; however, always start with the lowest dose and titrate to response

▶ *What Should I Monitor with Regard to Efficacy and Toxicity?*

Efficacy

Generalized anxiety disorder

Target symptoms

- monitor changes in increased motor or muscle tension, restlessness, autonomic hyperactivity (shortness of breath, palpitations, dry mouth, nausea, vomiting and so on), and hypervigilance
- monitor initially every 2–3 days for benzodiazepines and weekly for buspirone
- after they are stable, patients should be clinically assessed for target symptoms at least monthly (or weekly if clinical decompensation is suspected)

Panic disorder

Target symptoms

- monitor changes in shortness of breath, choking or smothering sensations, dizziness, palpitations or chest pain, trembling, nausea, depersonalization, tingling, and fear of impending doom
- should see initial response within several days
- after they are stable, patients should be clinically assessed for target symptoms at least monthly (or weekly if clinical decompensation is suspected)

Transient situational insomnia, short-term insomnia, long-term treatment of insomnia

Shortening of the time taken to fall asleep and improved sleep efficiency

- quantify through the use of a sleep diary and compare with pretreatment sleep performance

Improved daytime functioning

- quantify by comparing changes in the symptoms (e.g., anxiety, tension, and fatigue) with treatment with baseline values

Acute psychosis

- titrate dose to decrease agitation, sedative effect, or cerebellar side effects (ataxia, slurred speech)
- initially, monitor very agitated patients continuously
- monitor vital signs and degree of agitation hourly
- should see some decrease in agitation within hours and significant improvement within 24–48 hours

Bipolar disorders

Target symptoms

- agitation; decreased sleep; rapid, pressured speech with flight of ideas for manic phase; or symptoms of depression
- agitation and sleep disturbances usually resolve within several days to weeks; however, complete mood stabilization (and resolution of thought disorder if present) may require 6 weeks or longer
- monitor hourly for acute situation, then increase evaluation to daily and then weekly

Preoperative sedation

- memory of events near the time of surgery

Status epilepticus

- cessation of seizures

Alcohol withdrawal (treatment and prevention of seizures)

- prevention or reduction of symptoms of withdrawal such as tremor, irritability, and tachycardia

Toxicity

Confusion or memory impairment, sedation

- may or may not indicate toxicity
- common early in therapy or after a dosage increase
- suspect toxicity if symptoms persist for longer than 5–7 days after dosage stabilization and decrease the dosage if sedation or memory impairment continues
- tolerance of the sedative effects occurs

Ataxia, hyperreflexia, and slurred speech

- these often suggest toxicity, and the dosage should be reduced if they occur

Addiction

- both psychological and physical dependence can occur
- physical dependence is more likely with continuous use for longer than 3 months
- all benzodiazepines, whether they are short or long acting, likely cause a similar frequency of physical dependence (N Engl J Med 1993;328:1398–1405)
- may occur, especially in alcoholic patients and those known to be dependent on other drugs
- withdrawal syndrome (with abrupt discontinuation or rapid taper) rises to 10% in patients receiving continuous therapy for more than 1 year and consists of tremor, insomnia, palpitations, sweating, and excessive sensitivity to sight and sound

Hangover effects in the morning (when used as a hypnotic)

- hangover effects are therapeutic effects (sedation) carried over into the daytime, and usually the patient accommodates to this effect within 2–3 days
- if accommodation does not occur or impairments are unacceptable, reduce the dosage or switch to a shorter-acting agent such as triazolam or zopiclone
- tell the patient about hangover effects, and if the patient is noticeably impaired, he or she should avoid driving or other tasks requiring coordination and attention

Psychomotor impairment

- rebound insomnia and rebound anxiety may be apparent on discontinuation of therapy
- may be associated with anterograde amnesia and is related to the potency of the agent

▶ How Long Do I Treat Patients with This Drug?

Generalized anxiety disorder

- chronic, yet fluctuating, clinical course of anxiety disorder raises difficult issues regarding long-term drug management
- use the lowest effective dosage for the shortest period of time; attempt periodic discontinuation of therapy
- several well-designed studies describe general anxiety disorder as a chronic illness with fluctuating levels of symptom severity, yet few long-term efficacy studies (longer than 6 months) exist and the efficacy of drug therapy after 6 months is unknown
- clinical experience shows no tolerance of anxiolytic effect with prolonged therapy, but tolerance of sedation occurs (Neurosci Biobehav 1985;9:13–21)
- because of the waxing and waning nature of generalized anxiety disorder, attempt drug discontinuation every 6–12 months if the patients is symptom free (if the patient has a well-documented history of recurrent relapses after previous drug discontinuation, indefinite therapy may be needed)

Panic disorder

- as is the case for generalized anxiety disorders, studies suggest that panic disorders are a chronic illness with waxing and waning symptoms
- no long-term follow-up studies for longer than 6 months exist, and the efficacy of drug therapy after 6 months is unknown
- some clinicians recommend at least a 6–12 month symptom-free period prior to attempting discontinuation (J Clin Psychiatry 1990;51:11–15)
- concurrent behavioral or desensitization therapy after drug discontinuation may decrease the risk of relapse

Transient situational insomnia, short-term insomnia

- as briefly as possible and less than 1 month of continuous use

Long-term treatment of insomnia

- although studies on the efficacy of long-term use of hypnotics are scant and many sleep laboratory studies show a loss of hypnotic effect (tolerance) by the fourth week of continuous use, about 10% of patients benefit from continuous or intermittent use of hypnotics and long-term users often report high satisfaction with their sleep and few adverse effects (Age Ageing 1984;13:335–343)
- continued, intermittent medication use (provided there is demonstrable benefit) may be the most sensible approach

Acute psychosis

- benzodiazepines are used to treat agitation but are used only as short-term therapy (1–2 weeks), although low-dose PRN benzodiazepines may be needed for periods of agitation

Bipolar disorder

- used as short-term therapy until full antimanic effects of the primary drug are obtained (usually 1–2 weeks but may be up to 6 weeks)

Preoperative sedation

- single dose

Status epilepticus

- continue to administer drug therapy until the seizure has stopped and then decide (as above) about the need for long-term therapy

Alcohol withdrawal (treatment and prevention of seizures)

- continue a maintenance dosage for 2–3 days, then discontinue benzodiazepine administration
- reinstitute a maintenance dosage if the person starts to exhibit signs and symptoms of withdrawal

▶ How Do I Decrease or Stop the Administration of This Drug?

Use for only a few days

- abrupt cessation is possible, although patients should be forewarned that the sleep on the first few nights off the medication may be less sound

- advise the patient to keep a regulated sleep-wake schedule
- partial sleep restriction (e.g., delaying the retiring time and advancing the arising time by 30 minutes) during the withdrawal period may help to consolidate sleep

Patient has been taking the drug for a long time (longer than a month) or at high dosages

- conservative approach is to lower the total daily dose by 10% per week (faster discontinuations [25% per week] may be appropriate in patients receiving lower doses for shorter periods of time); if withdrawal symptoms (anxiety, insomnia, malaise, anorexia, diaphoresis, tremor, nausea, vomiting, irritability, and psychoses) or rebound anxiety (similar to previous symptoms, but with increased severity) appears, increase the dosage to the previous week's level, wait for symptoms to abate, and proceed to taper again (only at a slower rate)
- discontinuation syndromes are usually not problematic when therapy is shorter than 2 weeks
- making a dose for dose switch to a longer-acting, cross-tolerant benzodiazepine such as diazepam and then slowly tapering that medication may reduce withdrawal symptoms in patients who experience difficulty discontinuing lorazepam (J Psychiatr Res 1990;24[suppl 2]:81–90) and patients with marked psychological dependence on the benzodiazepine likely do better with a cross-tolerant substitution (see Diazepam)
- shorter acting benzodiazepines must be tapered and discontinued much slower than longer-acting benzodiazepines such as diazepam

▶ What Should I Tell My Patients About This Drug?

- never abruptly discontinue this medication for any reason without your physician's knowledge
- this is a potent drug so avoid alcohol consumption while taking this medication
- you may experience mild to moderate drowsiness and/or mild irritability early in therapy, or after each dosage increase; these drug effects usually decrease and go away after about a week
- tell your physician if you notice difficulty in talking, walking, concentrating, or remembering things
- do not take any other medications (including nonprescription or over the counter medicines) without your physician's knowledge
- psychomotor impairment and hangover effects may occur
- rebound insomnia may occur, so transitory sleep disturbance on withdrawal is not an indication to restart the medication administration
- report any adverse effects as soon as they occur
- medication administration should be discussed with your doctor if you are planning to become pregnant
- disturbances in memory may occur
- sedative properties are additive; if used with over the counter antihistamines, increased sedation may occur

▶ Therapeutic Tips

- use in short courses for sleep disturbance; however, panic disorder is a chronic disorder and usually courses are 6–9 months
- do not use one type of benzodiazepine during the day and a different one at night; just adjust the doses of one benzodiazepine to achieve the desired effect
- rearrange dosing times to cover periods when anxiety is excessive

Useful References

McClure DJ, Walsh J, Chang H, et al. Comparison of lorazepam and flurazepam as hypnotic agents in chronic insomniacs. J Clin Pharmacol 1988;28:52–63

Sanders LD, Yeomans WA, Rees J, et al. A double-blind comparison between nitrazepam, lorazepam, lormetazepam and placebo as preoperative night sedatives. Eur J Anaesthesiol 1988;5:377–383

LOVASTATIN

Stephen Shalansky and Robert Dombrowski

USA (Mevacor)
CANADA (Mevacor)

► When Should I Use This Drug?

Hypercholesterolemia

- HMG-CoA reductase inhibitors are recommended as first-line agents because they have proven efficacy in the reduction of cardiovascular mortality and morbidity (Lancet 1994;344: 1383–1389) and they are better tolerated than niacin or the bile acid sequestrants
- choose the least expensive of either lovastatin, pravastatin, simvastatin, or fluvastatin as these agents are likely equally effective and equally well tolerated

Mixed hyperlipidemias

- choose for patients who cannot take or tolerate niacin
- choose the least expensive of lovastatin, pravastatin, simvastatin, or fluvastatin as these agents are equally effective and equally well tolerated

► When Should I Not Use This Drug?

Hypertriglyceridemia

- primary effect of HMG-CoA reductase inhibitors is on LDL cholesterol not triglycerides and therefore they should not be used in patients with increased triglyceride levels as their only lipid abnormality

► What Contraindications Are There to the Use of This Drug?

Intolerance of or allergic reaction to lovastatin

Active hepatic disease or persistent serum aminotransferase elevations

- see under Toxicity

► What Drug Interactions Are Clinically Important?

Drugs that may increase the effect or toxicity of lovastatin

The following drugs can be used in combination with lovastatin, but should be discontinued immediately if myopathy occurs

CYCLOSPORINE WITH OTHER IMMUNOSUPPRESSIVES

- incidence of myopathy is about 30% (N Engl J Med 1988;318: 46–48)

GEMFIBROZIL

- incidence of myopathy is increased to about 5% (N Engl J Med 1988;318:46–48)
- can be used together and just be aware of the increased risk and monitor creatine kinase (CK) levels if the patient reports muscle aches and pains

NIACIN

- incidence of myopathy is increased to about 2% (Am J Cardiol 1988;62:28–34)

ERYTHROMYCIN

- several cases of rhabdomyolysis have been reported (West J Med 1991;154:213–215)

Drugs that may decrease the effect of lovastatin

- none

Drugs that may have their effect or toxicity increased by lovastatin

WARFARIN

- several cases of substantial increases in effect have been reported (Arch Intern Med 1990;150:2407)
- monitor INR every 2 days until the full extent of interaction is seen and adjust the dosage of warfarin based on the result

Drugs that may have their effect decreased by lovastatin

- none

► What Route and Dosage Should I Use?

How to administer

- orally—can be given with food to enhance bioavailability
- parenterally—not available

Hypercholesterolemia, mixed hyperlipidemias

- start with 10 mg PO daily given with the evening meal
- increase the dosage to 20 mg PO daily if there is inadequate response after 4 weeks
- dosage range is 20–80 mg daily; however, little added benefit is achieved at dosages greater than 40 mg
- dosages greater than 20 mg/d are more effective when given twice daily (JAMA 1986;256:2829–2834)
- lovastatin may be given once daily to enhance compliance
- if at 3 months of optimum therapy, there is at least a 15% decrease in LDL or total cholesterol level, but the target level is not reached, continue lovastatin therapy and add a second drug
- if at 3 months of optimum therapy, there is less than a 15% decrease in LDL or total cholesterol level, consider switching to or adding another agent
- if the patient is not tolerating lovastatin, change to another drug

Dosage adjustments for renal or hepatic dysfunction

- hepatically metabolized
- do not use in severe hepatic dysfunction
- no dosage adjustments are needed for renal dysfunction

► What Should I Monitor with Regard to Efficacy and Toxicity?

Efficacy

Hypercholesterolemia, mixed hyperlipidemias

Total cholesterol and fractionated lipid profile

- in patients with no coronary heart disease or atherosclerotic disease and with less than 2 CHD risk factors, lower total cholesterol below 240 mg/dL (6.2 mmol/L) and LDL cholesterol below 160 mg/dL (4.1 mmol/L)
- in patients with no coronary heart disease or atherosclerotic disease and with 2 or more CHD risk factors, lower total cholesterol below 200 mg/dL (5.2 mmol/L) and LDL cholesterol below 130 mg/dL (3.4 mmol/L)
- for patients with coronary heart disease or atherosclerotic disease, lower LDL cholesterol to below 100 mg/dL (2.6 mmol/L)

Evidence of coronary heart disease

- myocardial infarction, angina, and coronary bypass grafting

Risk factors

- reduce risk factors such as obesity and smoking
- control risk factors such as diabetes mellitis and hypertension

Toxicity

Hepatotoxicity

- persistent elevations of serum aminotransferase levels greater than 3 times the upper limit of normal values (measured on at least 2 occasions) occurred in 0.1% of patients taking 20 mg of lovastatin a day, occurred in 0.9% of patients taking 40 mg of lovastatin a day, and increased to 1.5% in patients taking 80 mg of lovastatin per day (Arch Intern Med 1991;151:43–49)
- serum aminotransferase determinations should be performed after 4–6 weeks of therapy and, if normal, at 6 months and then yearly
- stop lovastatin administration if serum aminotransferase levels are greater than 3 times the upper limit of normal values

Musculoskeletal effects

- incidence of muscle symptoms combined with CK elevations greater than 10 times the normal limit occurred in 0.3% of the patients receiving 40–80 mg of lovastatin daily (Arch Intern Med 1991;151:43–49)
- if patients report muscle pain or weakness, discontinue administration of the drug and measure the CK level
- if the CK level is elevated, stop lovastatin and monitor until it returns to normal then, if the patient is asymptomatic, rechallenge the patient with lovastatin and see whether the CK level increases and monitor for signs and symptoms of myopathy
- remember that, at any given time, 20–30% of the population have elevated CK levels because of bruising, trauma, exercise, and so on

Lens opacities

- after 48 weeks of therapy, lovastatin was found to have no effect on human crystalline lens (Am J Cardiol 1991;67:447–453)
- at present, no data substantiate an increased incidence of lens opacity; therefore, routine slit lamp examinations are not recommended

Constipation

- treat with diet and/or lifestyle changes

Rash

- discontinue administration of the drug

Headache and dizziness

- decision to continue therapy depends on the severity of the side effect and the willingness of the patient to comply with continued therapy

▶ *How Long Do I Treat Patients with This Drug?*

Hypercholesterolemia, mixed hyperlipidemias

- therapy is long term and may continue for life
- if the patient has achieved and maintained target lipid levels for 2 years, lovastatin should be discontinued and a retrial on dietary therapy alone should be begun
- recheck lipid levels at 4–6 weeks and at 3 months after drug administration has been discontinued and restart drug therapy if target levels are not maintained

▶ *How Do I Decrease or Stop the Administration of This Drug?*

- may be stopped abruptly

▶ *What Should I Tell My Patients About This Drug?*

- taking with food enhances absorption and decreases gastrointestinal side effects
- you will have liver function assessed at frequent intervals during the first year
- report symptoms of muscle pain, fever, tenderness, and malaise (myositis)
- expense of the drug is a consideration

▶ *Therapeutic Tips*

- drug is more effective if given twice daily compared with once daily in the evening, but patients may be more compliant on once-daily dosing
- doses given once daily are more effective if given in the evening instead of the morning (Clin Pharmacol Ther 1986;40:338–343)
- maximum response-cost benefit occurs at a dosage of approximately 40 mg PO daily, and if further lowering of LDL cholesterol levels is required, it is more cost-effective to add a second agent
- one can sometimes get a good response with 10 mg PO daily, and if a desired lipid effect has been seen with a 20 mg dosage, a trial on 10 mg should be considered

Useful References

Scandinavian Simvastatin Study Group. Randomized trial of cholesterol lowering in 4444 patients with coronary heart disease: The Scandinavian Simvastin survival study (4S). Lancet 1994;344:1383–1389

Expert Panel on Detection, Evaluation, and Treatment of High Blood Cholesterol in Adults. Summary of the second report of the National Cholesterol Education Program (NCEP) expert panel on detection, evaluation, and treatment of high blood cholesterol in adults. JAMA 1993;269: 3015–3023

McKenney JM. Lovastatin: A new cholesterol lowering agent. Clin Pharm 1988;7:21–36

Bradford RH, Shear CL, Chremos AN, et al. Expanded clinical evaluation of lovastatin (EXCEL) study results. Arch Intern Med 1991;151:43–49

Tolbert JA. Efficacy and long-term adverse effect pattern of lovastatin. Am J Cardiol 1988;62:28J–34J

Grundy SM. HMG-CoA reductase inhibitors for treatment of hypercholesterolemia. N Engl J Med 1988;319:24–33

LOXAPINE

Juan Avila and Patricia Marken

USA (Loxitane, generics)
CANADA (Loxapac)

▶ *When Should I Use This Drug?*

Acute psychosis therapy (if prompt control is required)

- in the acutely psychotic and agitated patient, rapid tranquilization with the goal of calming a dangerous patient
- loxapine is a medium-potency antipsychotic with moderate anticholinergic activity
- loxapine produces a moderate amount of sedation and orthostatic hypotension (less than that seen with chlorpromazine) and a medium incidence of acute extrapyramidal or dystonic reactions
- while loxapine is not commonly used, loxapine is a good choice in a young, otherwise healthy patient
- is available in a parenteral form
- when a patient has a previous history of response to this agent
- although, for most antipsychotic agents, after control has been achieved, once-daily dosing is possible, loxapine (half-life of approximately 6–12 hours, which is shorter than that of other antipsychotic agents) may need to be given more frequently than once daily (a once-daily dose may be tried; however, if the patient reports symptoms near the end of the dosing interval, give loxapine twice daily)

Maintenance psychosis therapy

- to ameliorate the symptoms of psychosis that include hallucinations, delusions, formal thought disorder, bizarre behavior, agitation, and/or hyperactivity
- drug of choice in the young, otherwise healthy, patient if it is less expensive than thiothixene
- one disadvantage, in contrast to the case with other antipsychotic agents, is that it must be given more frequently than once daily

Manic phase of bipolar illness

- antipsychotics are often also required for adequate sedation and behavioral control and are usually preferred to benzodiazepines for acutely manic patients with concurrent psychoses; however, there is some evidence that high-dose benzodiazepines may be equally efficacious with fewer adverse effects (J Clin Psychopharmacol 1985;5:109–113)
- decision as to when to choose this agent is as above for acute psychosis therapy

▶ *When Should I Not Use This Drug?*

see Chlorpromazine

▶ *What Contraindications Are There to the Use of This Drug?*

see Chlorpromazine

▶ *What Drug Interactions Are Clinically Important?*

Drugs that may increase the effect or toxicity of loxapine

CENTRAL NERVOUS SYSTEM DEPRESSANTS (OPIATES, BARBITURATES, GENERAL ANESTHETICS, ALCOHOL)

- excessive sedation and central nervous system (CNS) depression may occur if used concomitantly
- start with low dosages of both agents to avoid excessive sedation or CNS depression, and adjust dosages on the basis of clinical presentation

Drugs that may decrease the effect of loxapine

- none

Drugs that may have their effect or toxicity increased by loxapine

- none

Drugs that may have their effect decreased by loxapine

ANTICONVULSANTS (PHENYTOIN, PHENOBARBITAL)

- loxapine may lower the seizure threshold, and dosage adjustments of anticonvulsants may be necessary when the drugs are used concomitantly, but no adjustments should be made unless seizures develop

EPINEPHRINE

- epinephrine should not be used in conjunction with loxapine, as loxapine inhibits the vasopressor effect of epinephrine

▶ *What Route and Dosage Should I Use?*

How to administer

- orally—take with food or milk or on an empty stomach
- parenterally—IM only

Acute psychosis therapy (if prompt control required), manic phase of bipolar illness

- 50 mg PO or 25 mg IM (if the patient will not take oral medication) every 30–60 minutes until control is achieved or the patient does not tolerate the drug (usually 2–3 doses)
- start a maintenance dosage after an adequate response has been seen (see below)

Maintenance psychosis therapy

- 25 mg PO BID
- 10 mg PO BID in smaller or elderly patients
- increase the dosage every 2 weeks until an appropriate response has been seen
- typical maintenance dosage is 100 mg PO daily divided into 2 doses
- maximum daily oral dosage is 150 mg

Dosage adjustments for renal or hepatic dysfunction

- hepatically metabolized
- no specific dosage adjustments; just start with a low dose and titrate to effect

▶ *What Should I Monitor with Regard to Efficacy and Toxicity?*

see Chlorpromazine

▶ *How Long Do I Treat Patients with This Drug?*

see Chlorpromazine

▶ *How Do I Decrease or Stop the Administration of This Drug?*

see Chlorpromazine

▶ *What Should I Tell My Patients About This Drug?*

see Chlorpromazine

▶ *Therapeutic Tips*

see Chlorpromazine

Useful References

Black JL, Richelson E, Richardson JW. Antipsychotic agents: A clinical update. Mayo Clinic Proc 1985;60:777–789
Kane JM. The current status of neuroleptic therapy. J Clin Psychiatry 1989;50(9):322–328
Alexander B. Antipsychotics: How strict the formulary? DICP 1988;22:324–326

MAGNESIUM

Leslie Mathews, James McCormack, and Glenda Meneilly

Magnesium Hydroxide

USA (milk of magnesia, Phillips' Milk of Magnesia; combination: Haley's M-O, Alma-Mag No. 4, Aludrox)
CANADA (milk of magnesia, Phillips' magnesia tablets; combination: Haley's M-O, Magnolax)

Magnesium Citrate

USA (citrate of magnesia, Citroma, Citro-Nesia; combination: Citralax, Evac-Q-Kwik)
CANADA (Citro-Mag; combination: Citrocarbonate, Osmopak-Plus, Royvac kit)

Magnesium sulfate

USA (magnesium sulfate)
CANADA (magnesium sulphate, Epsom salts)

Magnesium Glucoheptonate

USA (not available)
CANADA (Magnesium-Rougier)

▶ *When Should I Use This Drug?*

Acute constipation

- magnesium hydroxide is useful short term when a rapid response is required
- is equally effective and has similar adverse effects, when compared with stimulant laxatives
- choice between this agent and stimulant laxatives should be based on availability, cost, and the patient's preference
- if constipation is associated with hard, dry stools or conditions in which straining should be avoided (e.g., anorectal disorders, hernias, recovery from myocardial infarction, and cerebrovascular accident), lactulose should be chosen instead of magnesium hydroxide, as these patients likely require long-term therapy (longer than 1 week) and magnesium should be used for only occasional or short-term use

Chronic constipation

- magnesium hydroxide is for only occasional use when bulk-forming laxatives or lactulose is ineffective alone

Fecal impaction

- after the impaction is cleared, give oral magnesium citrate or sulfate to empty the colon completely
- magnesium citrate is preferable to magnesium sulfate because it is probably better tolerated by the patient (magnesium sulfate has an intensely bitter taste) and is less likely to produce fluid and electrolyte imbalance

Bowel preparation

- magnesium sulfate or citrate can be used when balanced electrolyte solutions or sodium phosphate enemas are poorly tolerated or unavailable
- there is less potential for fluid and electrolyte imbalance with balanced electrolyte solutions

Use with anthelminthics to facilitate removal of parasites

- effective at producing a liquid stool, allowing examination of the parasites without rupture of trophozoites
- magnesium is the drug of choice in this situation

Prevention of magnesium depletion

- in any patient with risk factors for inadequate intake or excessive losses in whom dietary manipulation is inadequate to counteract the negative balance
- risk factors include alcoholism; renal, gastrointestinal, and endocrine disorders; cirrhosis; and sepsis
- approximately 12 mmol of magnesium is ingested per day in patients with a normal diet

Treatment of magnesium deficiency

- when the patient has been in a negative magnesium balance and symptoms of magnesium deficiency are present
- patients with a deficit of magnesium may have normal serum magnesium concentrations, and therefore, the decision to treat should be based on the chronicity of the risk factors for a negative magnesium balance and the presence of symptoms consistent with a body magnesium deficit
- normal serum magnesium concentrations are 0.7–1.05 mmol/L

Premature labor

- used if there is a contraindication to ritodrine
- used to control preterm labor that is unresponsive to ritodrine or to decrease ritodrine requirements

Dyspepsia associated with or without duodenal or gastric ulcers and gastroesophageal reflux

- used in conjunction with aluminum hydroxide

see Antacids

Other uses

- preeclampsia

▶ When Should I Not Use This Drug?

Constipation responsive to general measures

- use increased fiber and fluid intake, exercise, and administration of bulk-forming laxatives
- regular use has the potential for fluid and electrolyte imbalance with losses via watery stools and can produce fecal urgency and incontinence

Treatment of overdose or toxic exposure

- sorbitol is preferred for this indication because it works faster, and magnesium toxicity is possible, particularly with repeated doses and compromised kidney function

▶ What Contraindications Are There to the Use of This Drug?

Intolerance of or allergic reactions to magnesium products

Symptoms of acute abdomen

- undiagnosed abdominal pain, nausea, and vomiting

Renal insufficiency

- 15–30% of magnesium ion can be absorbed, resulting in magnesium toxicity
- use lactulose, senna, or bisacodyl if renal function is impaired

Pregnancy (for use as a laxative)

- may promote sodium retention
- reduces iron absorption (Drug Ther Bull 1988;26:53–56)
- use a bulk-forming laxative instead

▶ What Drug Interactions Are Clinically Important?

Drugs that may increase the effect or toxicity of magnesium

NIFEDIPINE

- may increase the neuromuscular toxicities of magnesium
- if renal function is compromised use lactulose, senna, or bisacodyl instead of magnesium

SPIRONOLACTONE, TRIAMTERENE, AMILORIDE, ANGIOTENSIN CONVERTING ENZYME INHIBITORS

- these drugs prevent the excretion of magnesium, which can result in the accumulation of excessive potassium
- most patients do not have magnesium excretion blocked sufficiently with these drugs to warrant discontinuation of therapy

Drugs that may decrease the effect of magnesium

THIAZIDE DIURETICS, FUROSEMIDE, CARBONIC ANHYDRASE INHIBITORS, ETHACRYNIC ACID, PREDNISONE, AMPHOTERICIN B

- these drugs may cause magnesium depletion along with potassium depletion
- routine serum magnesium levels are not recommended, as they are not a good indication of total body magnesium concentrations

Drugs that may have their effect or toxicity increased by magnesium

CENTRAL NERVOUS SYSTEM DEPRESSANTS, NEUROMUSCULAR BLOCKING AGENTS

- dosage must be adjusted when administered with magnesium to avoid additive central nervous system depression or muscle weakness

Drugs that may have their effect decreased by magnesium

TETRACYCLINE

- products containing calcium, aluminum, magnesium, or iron form chelates with tetracycline; therefore, take 1 hour before or 2 hours after these drugs

▶ What Route and Dosage Should I Use?

How to administer

- $MgSO_4$ 1 g = 4 mmol of elemental magnesium = 8 mEq elemental magnesium
- magnesium glucoheptonate 75 mg = 6 mEq of elemental magnesium = 3 mmol of elemental magnesium

Orally

- take with a full glass of fluid

Parenterally

- dilute in 100 mL of IV fluid (normal saline or 5% dextrose in water [D5W]) and administer over a minimum of 4 hours
- rapid administration of magnesium results in increased urinary losses, and prolonged administration results in greater retention
- duration of infusion must be balanced with the patient's convenience

Acute constipation, chronic constipation, fecal impaction

- minimum effective dosage is 80 mEq of magnesium PO daily
- increase the dosage as needed after 24 hours by 40 mEq to a maximum of 240 mEq PO daily
- 100 mL of magnesium citrate contains approximately 80 mEq of magnesium ion
- 10 g of magnesium sulfate contains approximately 80 mEq of magnesium ion (dilute in 250 mL of water)
- 1 g of magnesium hydroxide contains approximately 35 mEq of magnesium ion (30 mL of milk of magnesia contains approximately 80 mEq of magnesium ion)

Bowel preparation, use with anthelminthics to facilitate removal of parasites

- magnesium citrate 300 mL (15 g/254 mEq of magnesium) or 1 bottle PO
- give 250–300 mL of fluid per hour for 4–6 hours before a dose and 3 hours after a dose
- magnesium sulfate 30 g (240 mEq of magnesium) or 60 mL of a 50% solution dissolved in 250 mL of water or juice

Prevention of magnesium depletion

- for patients with risk factors for a negative magnesium balance, an intake of 30 mEq/d should be started

Treatment of magnesium deficiency

Mild deficiency (asymptomatic)

- use oral administration if possible, as intramuscular administration is painful
- 6 mEq PO TID as the glucoheptonate salt (0.4 mEq/mL) can be used; however, diarrhea will limit the amount of magnesium that can be administered by mouth
- choice of magnesium salt is based on palatability and cost but the glucoheptonate is better absorbed
- if oral administration is not possible, administer 40 mEq IV daily of magnesium sulfate in D5W or normal saline over a period of 4 hours

Severe depletion (symptomatic)

- 40 mEq IV Q12H administered as 2 intermittent infusions spaced evenly during the day or as a continuous IV infusion

Premature labor

- add 40 g of magnesium sulfate to 1000 mL of D5W or half-normal saline
- give a 100 mL (4 g) loading dose IV over 20 minutes
- then infuse at a rate of 2 g/h and increase the dosage every 30 minutes by 0.5 mg/h until contractions are inhibited or 4 g/h is reached

Dosage adjustments for renal or hepatic dysfunction

- renally eliminated
- adjust the dosage on the basis of serum magnesium concentrations in patients with poor renal function

▶ *What Should I Monitor with Regard to Efficacy and Toxicity?*

Efficacy

Acute constipation, chronic constipation, fecal impaction

- magnesium hydroxide used as a laxative produces 1 bowel movement or more within 6–12 hours

Frequency of bowel movements

- for chronic constipation, compare with what is usual for each individual
- this can normally vary from 3 times a day to once a week
- assess the patient daily

Consistency of stool

- goal is soft, well-formed stools that are relatively bulky

Bowel preparation, use with anthelminthics to facilitate removal of parasites

- magnesium citrate or magnesium sulfate used as a cathartic produces watery stools within 1–3 hours

Prevention of magnesium depletion

- absence of signs and symptoms of magnesium deficiency

Treatment of magnesium deficiency

Signs and symptoms of deficiency

- the patient's symptoms of deficiency (ECG, muscle weakness, etc.) should resolve
- serum magnesium concentration is not a reliable guide to the adequacy of magnesium replacement and should not be used

Premature labor

- monitor uterine contractions continuously while intravenous dosage increases are being made and at least every hour when a stable infusion dosage has been attained
- attempt to reduce contractions to 4 per hour or fewer

Toxicity

Gastrointestinal symptoms

- cramping and diarrhea
- avoid prolonged use and question the patient regarding the frequency and consistency of stools
- when used as a laxative, magnesium can cause electrolyte and fluid disturbances (especially in the elderly) if excessive diarrhea occurs
- if diarrhea occurs, stop the magnesium and replace fluid and electrolytes as needed

Hypermagnesemia

- can occur if renal deficiency is present or when oral preparations are retained in the gut to increase overall absorption (e.g., megacolon)
- if these conditions are present or suspected, discontinue the drug administration, insert rectal tube (for retention), monitor the patient closely for magnesium toxicity, and measure serum magnesium concentrations
- signs of excessive magnesium levels include central nervous system depression, flushing, hypotension, hyporeflexia, and hypoperfusion
- muscle weakness, electrocardiographic changes, sedation, and confusion are seen with serum concentrations greater than 2 mmol/L (4 mEq/L)

▶ *How Long Do I Treat Patients with This Drug?*

Acute constipation, chronic constipation, fecal impaction

- magnesium hydroxide should not be used for longer than 1 week, its administration should be stopped as soon as constipation is controlled, and the patient should be switched to another agent if required

Prevention of magnesium depletion

- until risk factors have resolved or dietary magnesium intake has increased to offset the negative magnesium balance

Treatment of magnesium deficiency

- determination of the complete replenishment of a magnesium deficit is difficult because serum magnesium concentrations do not accurately reflect body stores
- therapy should continue until symptoms of magnesium deficiency disappear
- total dose of 100 mmol (200 mEq) given over 5 days is usually adequate to replenish magnesium stores

Premature labor

- if membranes are ruptured, do not use drug therapy for longer than 48 hours to avoid chorioamnionitis
- if membranes are intact and gestation is less than 32 weeks, continue intensive therapy for 12 hours after contractions stop, or 24 hours after the last dose of corticosteroid has been given
- if labor begins again, restart treatment or increase the infusion rate

▶ *How Do I Decrease or Stop the Administration of This Drug?*

- may be stopped abruptly
- for long-term use, substitute bulk-forming laxatives and general measures to manage constipation (increased dietary fiber and fluid intake, exercise, and so on)

▶ *What Should I Tell My Patients About This Drug?*

- oral administration can cause cramping, bloating, and diarrhea, and if this occurs, reduce the daily dosage by 50%
- cathartic doses may act within 15–30 minutes to produce watery, explosive bowel movements; therefore, stay close to a bathroom
- take with a full glass of fluid (water or juice) to prevent dehydration and to maximize laxative effect
- these drugs are not intended for regular use as laxatives
- intravenous administration may result in flushing and a sensation of warmth

▶ *Therapeutic Tips*

- give laxatives or cathartics early in the day in accordance with the desired time for onset of action
- mask the bitter taste of magnesium sulfate by adding to fruit juices and/or by chilling

Useful References

Tedesco FJ. Laxative use in constipation. Am J Gastroenterol 1985;80: 303–309
Dickerson RN. Treating hypomagnesemia. Hosp Pharm 1985;20:761–763
Gums JG. Clinical significance of magnesium: A review. DICP 1987;21: 240–246

MAPROTILINE

Lyle K. Laird and Julia Vertrees

USA (Ludiomil, others)
CANADA (Ludiomil)

▶ *When Should I Use This Drug?*

Consider an alternative agent

- maprotiline is no more effective than other antidepressants
- it has a number of toxicities (cardiovascular effects and seizures) and is more toxic than other antidepressants in overdose
- maprotiline is expensive and offers no advantages over the other antidepressants

MECLIZINE

Lynne Nakashima

USA (Antivert, Antrizine, Ru-Vert-M, Bonine)
CANADA (Bonamine; compound: Antivert)

▶ *When Should I Use This Drug?*

Motion sickness

- for mild to moderate road, air, or sea travel, especially if sedation is desired

- if sedation is not desired, use scopolamine
- almost as convenient as scopolamine, as it can be given once daily and is less expensive than scopolamine

Pregnancy

- if dietary modifications and pyridoxine therapy are unsuccessful, meclizine may be tried (Drugs 1992;43:443–463)

▶ *When Should I Not Use This Drug?*

Chemotherapy-induced nausea and vomiting

- meclizine is not usually used in chemotherapy-induced nausea and vomiting because it is generally considered no more effective than placebo (Drugs 1992;43:295–315)

▶ *What Contraindications Are There to the Use of This Drug?*

see Dimenhydrinate

▶ *What Drug Interactions Are Clinically Important?*

see Dimehydrinate

▶ *What Route and Dosage Should I Use?*

How to administer

- orally—take with food or milk or on an empty stomach; may be chewed
- parenterally—not available

Motion sickness

- 50 mg PO daily starting at least 1–2 hours before the trip
- some clinicians suggest starting this agent the day before leaving because it may have a long onset of action

Pregnancy

- 50 mg PO daily

Dosage adjustments for renal or hepatic dysfunction

- no dosage adjustments are currently recommended; the exact route of elimination has not yet been determined

▶ *What Should I Monitor with Regard to Efficacy and Toxicity?*

see Dimenhydrinate

▶ *How Long Do I Treat Patients with This Drug?*

see Dimenhydrinate

Pregnancy

- continue for 24–48 hours and assess efficacy

▶ *How Do I Decrease or Stop the Administration of This Drug?*

- may be stopped abruptly

▶ *What Should I Tell My Patients About This Drug?*

see Dimenhydrinate

Useful References

Mitchelson F. Pharmacological agents affecting emesis. A review (part 1). Drugs 1992;43:295–315
Wood CD. Antimotion sickness and antiemetic drugs. Drugs 1979;17: 471–479

MECLOFENAMATE

Kelly Jones

USA (Meclomen, various generic)
CANADA (not available)

▶ *When Should I Use This Drug?*

Consider an alternative agent

- there is no reason to use this agent for the treatment of rheumatoid arthritis because meclofenamate is toxic and not well toler-

ated when compared with other nonsteroidal antiinflammatory drugs (J Am Board Fam Pract 1989;2:257–271)

MEFENAMIC ACID

Kelly Jones

USA (Ponstel)
CANADA (Ponstan)

▶ *When Should I Use This Drug?*

Consider an alternative agent

- there is no reason to use this agent for the treatment of rheumatoid arthritis because mefenamic acid is toxic and not well tolerated as compared with other nonsteroidal antiinflammatory drugs (J Am Board Fam Pract 1989;2:257–271)
- mefenamic acid is not indicated for the treatment of rheumatoid arthritis
- mefenamic acid should not be used long term owing to side effects (diarrhea [dose related], rash, and renal toxicity are similar to those due to fenoprofen)

MEPERIDINE

Terry Baumann

USA (Demerol, various)
CANADA (Demerol, various)

▶ *When Should I Use This Drug?*

Acute pain (severe), postoperative pain

- use if there is true allergy to morphine, but it offers no advantages over morphine and has potential additional side effects in some patients (e.g., seizures in patients with renal failure)

▶ *When Should I Not Use This Drug?*

Mild to moderate pain

- unless drugs such as acetaminophen, acetaminophen-codeine, and nonsteroidal antiinflammatory drugs have been used on a regularly scheduled basis (not PRN) and are shown to be ineffective

Chronic cancer pain, chronic noncancer pain

- with moderate to severe cancer pain, use morphine, hydromorphone, methadone, or fentanyl
- metabolite of meperidine, normeperidine, accumulates with repetitive dosing and can cause central nervous system (CNS) excitation
- use methadone or fentanyl if there is a true allergy to morphine

Post–myocardial ischemia pain

- intravenous meperidine may increase the ventricular response rate, mean aortic pressure, and vascular resistance

Oral use

- is relatively ineffective orally at the dosages commonly used (50 mg PO Q4H)

▶ *What Contraindications Are There to the Use of This Drug?*

Intolerance of or allergic reaction to meperidine

- true allergies to meperidine are rare
- check that the patient has actual allergic symptoms, and if there is a true allergy, consider morphine or hydromorphone

Severe respiratory depression

- not an absolute contraindication, just start with dosages 25% of the normal initial dose and titrate up to effect while assessing the respiratory rate and oxymetry before each dose

Renal failure

- metabolite of meperidine can quickly accumulate and cause seizures

▶ *What Drug Interactions Are Clinically Important?*

see Morphine

Monoamine oxidase inhibitors

- combination of meperidine and monoamine oxidase inhibitors has caused coma, severe respiratory depression, and extreme CNS stimulation
- do not use this combination or if patient has received monoamine oxidase inhibitors during the previous 14 days

▶ *What Route and Dosage Should I Use?*

How to administer

- orally—may be administered with food or milk or on an empty stomach
- parenterally—may be administered intramuscularly, intravenously (dilute IV meperidine in 10 mL of normal saline and give over at least 1 minute), and subcutaneously

Acute pain

- 100 mg IM Q4H (not PRN), or 50 mg IM Q4H (not PRN) for elderly patients because of concerns about sedation and respiratory depression
- some patients may require Q3H dosing
- question patients frequently about the degree of pain they are having (ideally, within at most 1–2 hours after the first dose if the drug was administered via the IM route)
- if pain is unrelieved by this time and there are no signs of sedation or respiratory depression, give another dose 50% higher than the first dose
- continue this approach until pain is 75% relieved and then maintain at this dosage for 12 hours before further adjustments are made
- normal dosage increments are 100 and 150 mg
- if an immediate response (within 1–5 minutes) for severe pain is needed, use intravenously as recommended for postoperative pain

Postoperative pain

In the postanesthetic care unit

- 25 mg IV repeated every 5 minutes PRN
- adjust the dosage on the basis of the response to each dose and titrate to pain control and the desired level of sedation or respiratory rate

On the ward

Intermittent therapy

- as above for acute pain
- question the patient frequently and increase the dosage as above for acute pain on the basis of pain relief and the level of sedation

Patient-controlled analgesia

- 10 mg/bolus with a lockout time of 6 minutes
- evidence suggests that using a bolus with a baseline infusion may increase the chance of seizures
- question the patient frequently about the degree of pain
- if pain is not controlled with bolus doses, increase the bolus dose by 25–50%
- if pain relief from the bolus is adequate but the duration of pain relief is too short, decrease the lockout period

Dosage adjustments for renal or hepatic dysfunction

- hepatically metabolized to an active metabolite
- dosage adjustment is usually not required if the dose is titrated properly
- one of meperidine's metabolites (normeperidine) has been associated with seizures in patients with renal failure

Normal Dosing Interval	$C_{cr} > 60$ mL/min or 1 mL/s	C_{cr} 30–60 mL/min or 0.5–1 mL/s	$C_{cr} < 30$ mL/min or 0.5 mL/s
Q4H	adjust dosage on basis of response	do not use	do not use

▶ *What Should I Monitor with Regard to Efficacy and Toxicity?*

see Morphine

Central nervous system stimulation

- seizures, agitation, irritability, nervousness, tremors, twitches, and myoclonus are associated with the accumulation of normeperidine
- this occurs more frequently in patients with renal failure but can also occur in patients with normal renal function when using high doses for 24–48 hours

▶ *How Long Do I Treat Patients with This Drug?*

see Morphine

▶ *How Do I Decrease or Stop the Administration of This Drug?*

see Morphine

▶ *What Should I Tell My Patients About This Drug?*

see Morphine

▶ *Therapeutic Tips*

- do not use for chronic cancer pain
- in patients who will be taking regularly dosed narcotics for longer than 3–4 days, always consider prescribing narcotics in conjunction with a laxative and counsel the patient on the appropriate use of fluids and fiber intake

Useful References

see Morphine

MESALAMINE (5-AMINOSALICYLIC ACID)
Scott Whittaker

Mesalamine Suppositories

USA (Rowasa)
CANADA (Salofalk)

Mesalamine Enemas

USA (Rowasa)
CANADA (Salofalk)

Mesalamine completely enveloped by a resin (Eudragit S), which releases mesalamine in the colon

USA or CANADA (Asacol)

Mesalamine coated with a semi-permeable ethylcellulose membrane, which releases mesalamine throughout the small bowel

USA or CANADA (Pentasa)

Mesalamine completely enveloped by a resin (Eudragit L), which delivers some mesalamine to the colon and some to the small bowel

USA (Rowasa)
CANADA (Mesasal, Salofalk)

Olsalazine Sodium

USA or CANADA (Dipentum)

▶ *When Should I Use This Drug?*

Ulcerative proctitis

MESALAMINE SUPPOSITORIES

- use as initial therapy, as mesalamine (5-aminosalicylic acid [5-ASA]) suppositories are effective and are better accepted by patients than are enemas

Ulcerative colitis

MESALAMINE ENEMAS

- trial of topical 5-ASA enemas should be given to patients with mild to moderate disease limited to the rectosigmoid, as topical therapy has less frequent and severe adverse effects than does oral therapy and topical therapy provides quick relief of symptoms

- topical 5-ASA enemas should also be used in patients in combination with oral 5-ASA when minor but annoying distal symptoms persist after instituting oral therapy for 3–4 weeks

ASACOL (USA or CANADA)

- 5-ASA completely enveloped by a resin (Eudragit S), which delivers 5-ASA to the colon
- use instead of sulfasalazine in patients who are allergic to sulfa or intolerant of sulfasalazine
- nonsulfa 5-ASA products can be increased up to 4–6 g of 5-ASA per day, which is usually higher than dosages achieved with sulfasalazine
- chosen over Mesasal or Salofalk or Rowasa, as Asacol allows better delivery to the distal colon
- Pentasa releases 5-ASA throughout the small bowel but has been effective in ulcerative colitis

MESASAL, SALOFALK (CANADA), ROWASA (USA)

- 5-ASA completely enveloped by a resin (Eudragit L), which delivers some 5-ASA to the colon and some to the small bowel
- use only if above 5-ASA products are not tolerated or are ineffective
- because some 5-ASA is released in the small bowel, less 5-ASA reaches the colon and more 5-ASA is excreted in the urine, which theoretically might increase the risk of the rare renal toxicity that has been described with the use of 5-ASA preparations (Gut 1990;31:1271–1276)

DIPENTUM (USA OR CANADA)

- two 5-ASA (olsalazine) molecules bound together
- use only when other 5-ASA products are not tolerated because this product causes the highest incidence of diarrhea (Gastroenterology 1986;90:1024–1030)
- patient is usually given a trial of corticosteroids before switching to this agent

Crohn's disease
Colitis
MESALAMINE SUPPOSITORIES OR ENEMAS

- topical 5-ASA has a limited role in Crohn's disease because the majority of patients do not have left-sided colitis as their major problem
- in patients in whom the left side of the colon is the predominant site, topical therapy can be considered similar to that for ulcerative colitis (see above)

Ileitis and ileocolitis
PENTASA (USA OR CANADA)

- 5-ASA coated with a semipermeable ethylcellulose membrane, which releases 5-ASA throughout the small bowel
- preferred product for widespread disease, as 5-ASA is released throughout the small bowel
- sulfasalazine, Dipentum, and Asacol release 5-ASA in only small amounts in the small bowel and hence are not recommended when ileal disease is prominent

MESASAL, SALOFALK (CANADA), ROWASA (USA)

- use instead of Pentasa if colonic involvement is known to be more significant (based on X-ray or colonoscopy)
- decision between these agents should be based on cost

▶ When Should I Not Use This Drug?
Use in ulcerative proctitis or colitis in combination with corticosteroids

- there is no therapeutic benefit to adding 5-ASA to systemic corticosteroids in patients with a severe flare of ulcerative proctitis/colitis

▶ What Contraindications Are There to the Use of This Drug?

- intolerance of or allergy to 5-ASA or to ASA

▶ What Drug Interactions Are Clinically Important?
Drugs that may increase the effect or toxicity of mesalamine

- none

Drugs that may decrease the effect of mesalamine
LACTULOSE

- decreases the pH of colonic contents and may interfere with the dissolution of oral Asacol, Claversal, Salofalk, Mesasal, and Rowasa
- use an alternative laxative, such as magnesium hydroxide and stimulant laxatives

Drugs that may have their effect or toxicity increased by mesalamine

- none

Drugs that may have their effect decreased by mesalamine

- none

▶ What Route and Dosage Should I Use?
How to administer

- orally—must be swallowed whole and taken with food or on an empty stomach
- topically—can be given as suppository or enema, depending on the patient's preference
- parenterally—5-ASA works via topical therapy, and delivery of the drug to the colon is necessary for efficacy, and it cannot be used parenterally

Ulcerative proctitis or colitis
MESALAMINE SUPPOSITORIES

- 500 mg rectally daily at bedtime
- 500 mg rectally BID (in the morning and at bedtime) should be used if a single daily dose is ineffective after 1 week

MESALAMINE ENEMAS

- use a 4 g enema daily at bedtime and retain for as long as possible (minimum 1 hour)
- 4 g BID (in the morning and at bedtime) should be used if a single dose is ineffective after 1 week

ASACOL

- 1200 mg PO QID for flare-ups
- 400 mg PO TID for maintenance in ulcerative colitis

MESASAL, SALOFALK, ROWASA

- 1000 mg PO QID for flare-ups
- 500 mg PO TID for maintenance in ulcerative colitis

DIPENTUM

- for flare-ups, start with 1000 mg PO BID for 4 days, then increase to 1000 mg PO TID to decrease the chance of diarrhea with this product
- 500 mg PO BID for maintenance in ulcerative colitis

Crohn's disease
ORAL USE

- as above for ulcerative colitis, except that maintenance therapy is not used, because the efficacy of maintenance therapy is not established
- treat for 10–14 days after the relief of symptoms (usual course of therapy is 6–8 weeks)

PENTASA

- 1000 mg PO QID for flare-ups

Dosage adjustments for renal or hepatic dysfunction

- renally eliminated, unknown dosage modifications

▶ *What Should I Monitor with Regard to Efficacy and Toxicity?*

Efficacy

see Sulfasalazine

Toxicity

see Sulfasalazine

Nausea and headaches

- are occasionally seen; treat with nonnarcotic analgesics

▶ *How Long Do I Treat Patients with This Drug?*

see Sulfasalazine

▶ *How Do I Decrease or Stop the Administration of This Drug?*

see Sulfasalazine

▶ *What Should I Tell My Patients About This Drug?*

see Sulfasalazine

- some patients may see what appears to be unaltered capsules in the stool; in most circumstances, these are thought to be "ghosts" (empty Eudragit resin coatings, with the 5-ASA already gone)

▶ *Therapeutic Tips*

Topical use

- if a suppository or enema is not kept in place, efficacy is compromised; therefore, there is no role for suppositories during episodes of diarrhea or extreme tenesmus

Oral use

- start at a high dosage initially in acute ulcerative colitis to get maximum chance of remission

METAPROTERENOL

See Orciprenaline

METFORMIN

Christy Silvius Scott

USA (not available)
CANADA (Glucophage)

▶ *When Should I Use This Drug?*

Non–insulin-dependent diabetes

- obese patients with fasting blood glucose levels less than 230 mg/dL (13 mmol/L) (Can Med Assoc J 1992;147:697–712)
- if patients are very obese, metformin as sole therapy should be used initially as it can decrease insulin resistance in these patients, which is often the reason for their glucose intolerance (Diabetes Care 1992;15:755–772)
- metformin may be associated with weight loss or minimal weight gain and beneficial effects on lipid levels and therefore should be used as initial therapy in very obese patients and those with severe hyperlipidemias (Diabetes Care 1993;16:621–629, Diabetes Metab Rev 1979;5:233–245, Diabetes 1985;34:793–798, Diabetic Med 1990;7:510–514)
- has no potential for causing hypoglycemia (Metab Clin North Am 1989; 18:163–183)
- metformin is useful in combination with sulfonylureas if the patient has failed to respond to therapy with maximum dosages of either medication (Diabetes Care 1992;1993:621–629)
- may be used in elderly patients (older than 65 years) who do not have renal, hepatic, or cardiopulmonary insufficiency or alcoholism (Diabetic Med 1990; 7:510–514)

▶ *When Should I Not Use This Drug?*

Insulin-dependent diabetes

- patients require insulin and do not respond to oral glucose-lowering agents

Non–insulin-dependent diabetes

- in patients who are or could be adequately controlled with diet and exercise alone (N Engl J Med 1989;321:1231–1245)
- for patients who are under severe stress (trauma, surgery, or major infection), causing extreme hyperglycemia; insulin is required during these periods of metabolic decompensation
- in patients who have a fasting plasma glucose level greater than230 mg/dL (13 mmol/L) because sulfonylureas are usually thought to be more effective in this situation (Can Med Assoc J 1992;147:697–712)

▶ *What Contraindications Are There to the Use of This Drug?*

Intolerance of or allergic reaction to metformin

Moderate or severe renal dysfunction (creatinine clearance < 50 mL/ min), hepatic or cardiopulmonary insufficiency, alcoholism, severe metabolically stressful periods

- these patients are at increased risk for lactic acidosis (Diabetes Care 1987;10:118–122, Horm Metab Res 1985;17[suppl 15]: 111–115)

Pregnancy

- insulin is required to produce good control of diabetes during pregnancy if diet and exercise alone are not successful (Clin Obstet Gynecol 1981;8:353–382, The Management of Diabetes Mellitus 1990:29)
- effects on the fetus are unknown (Drug Information Reference, 3rd ed 1993:906–907)

Breast-feeding

- there is no information concerning the effects on the infant

▶ *What Drug Interactions Are Clinically Important?*

Drugs that may increase the effect or toxicity of metformin

INSULIN

- insulin also decreases blood glucose levels
- insulin therapy should be initiated in non–insulin dependent diabetes after discontinuation of the metformin-sulfonylurea combination

SULFONYLUREAS

- all sulfonylureas also decrease blood glucose levels
- sulfonylurea may be added, starting with the lowest recommended dosage if the patient has reached maximum tolerated dosages of metformin without adequate blood glucose control (Can Med Assoc J 1992;147:697–712)
- metformin may be added to a patient's therapy if maximum dosages of sulfonylurea therapy have not provided adequate blood glucose level control (Can Med Assoc J 1992;147:697–712)

ETHANOL

- inhibits gluconeogenesis by the liver, causing hypoglycemia when gluconeogenesis is required to maintain normal glucose blood levels (e.g., fasting or decreasing food intake)
- do not use metformin in alcoholic patients because they are at increased risk for lactic acidosis
- patients should limit their consumption of alcohol to an occasional 1 drink per day with food while receiving this medication

Drugs that may decrease the effect of metformin

BETA-BLOCKING AGENTS

- may block insulin secretion (owing to the inhibition of beta$_2$-receptors), occasionally causing hyperglycemia
- data suggest that beta-blockers prevent the onset of microalbuminuria in non–insulin-dependent patients and do not worsen glycemic control (Hypertension 1993;21:786–794), and these agents need not be avoided in patients with non–insulin-dependent diabetes

THIAZIDE DIURETICS

- thiazide diuretics can increase blood glucose concentrations in diabetics (and patients prone to diabetes), antagonizing the effect of oral hypoglycemics

- thiazide diuretics cause impairment of glucose tolerance, decrease insulin sensitivity, increase hemoglobin A_{1c} levels, and worsen glucose control but this effect is small and uncommon with low dosages (Ann Intern Med 1992;118:273–278)
- hyperglycemia may occur several days to months after the addition of the thiazide
- patients should monitor blood glucose levels at least weekly for 3 months after a thiazide diuretic has been added
- if administration of a thiazide diuretic is discontinued while the patient is receiving an oral hypoglycemic, blood glucose levels and symptoms of hypoglycemia should be monitored
- when used in low dosages in patients with insulin-dependent diabetes, there is little if any effect on glucose control

Drugs that may have their effect or toxicity increased by metformin

- none

Drugs that may have their effect decreased by metformin

- none

▶ What Route and Dosage Should I Use?

How to administer

- orally—take with meals (500 and 850 mg tablets); tablets are large—ensure that the patient can swallow large tablets
- parenterally—not available

Non–insulin-dependent diabetes

- 500 mg PO BID
- administer with meals to prevent or decrease gastrointestinal upset
- increase the dosage weekly by 500 mg increments until glycemic control is achieved or a maximum dosage of 3000 mg PO daily is reached (Diabetes Care 1992;15:755–772)
- most patients, however, are not able to tolerate 3000 mg/d because of gastrointestinal upset (Diabetes Care 1992;15:755–772)

Dosage adjustments for renal or hepatic dysfunction

- complete renal elimination

Normal Dosing Interval	$C_{cr} > 60$ mL/min or 1 mL/s	C_{cr} 30–60 mL/min or 0.5–1 mL/s	$C_{cr} < 30$ mL/min or 0.5 mL/s
Q12H	no adjustment needed	avoid because of risk of lactic acidosis	avoid because of risk of lactic acidosis
Q8H	no adjustment needed	avoid because of risk of lactic acidosis	avoid because of risk of lactic acidosis

▶ What Should I Monitor with Regard to Efficacy and Toxicity?

Efficacy

- primary failure is estimated to be approximately 10% in correctly selected patients (Diabetes Metab Rev 1979;5:233–245, Diabetes Care 1992;15:755–772)
see Tolbutamide

Toxicity

Gastrointestinal effects

- patients may experience diarrhea, abdominal pain, nausea, anorexia, or a metallic taste
- diarrhea is the most common side effect, occurring in approximately 20% of patients (Diabetes Care 1983;6:472–474)
- ask the patient specifically about these problems
- ensure that the patient is taking the medication with meals
- if increasing the medication dosage every week, reduce the increases to every 2–3 weeks
- these effects usually diminish with ongoing therapy (Diabetes Care 1992; 15:755–772)
- if the patient cannot tolerate these effects, discontinue the drug administration; however, fewer than 5% of patients are discontinued from therapy because of these effects (Diabetes Care 1992;15:755–772)

Lactic acidosis

- metformin, as opposed to phenformin, causes only small increases in peripheral blood lactate levels (Diabetes Care 1992; 15:755–772, Diabetes Care 1987; 10:62–67)
- reported incidence is 0–0.084 cases/1000 patient-years, of which almost all have occurred in patients in whom therapy was contraindicated (Diabetes Care 1992;15:755–772)
- strict adherence to avoiding the use of metformin in patients at risk resulted in no cases of lactic acidosis (Can Med Assoc J 1983;128:24–26)
- avoid use in patients who are at risk
- monitor renal and cardiac function with routine diabetic checkups
- if creatinine clearance decreases to 60 mL/min or 1 mL/sec or less, discontinue use
- if the patient has signs of congestive heart failure, discontinue use
- if the patient experiences hepatic dysfunction or hypoxic episodes (acutely or chronically), discontinue use

▶ How Long Do I Treat Patients with This Drug?

see Tolbutamide

▶ How Do I Decrease or Stop the Administration of This Drug?

- may be stopped abruptly, if necessary
- if satisfactory blood glucose control is maintained for 6 months, decrease the dosage by 500 mg every 2 weeks

▶ What Should I Tell My Patients About This Drug?

- take with meals, never on an empty stomach, to avoid gastrointestinal distress
- digestive tract symptoms such as loss of appetite, nausea, vomiting, stomach upset, and pain may occur early in treatment; however, do not stop taking the medication without notifying your physician
- these adverse effects often diminish or subside with time during continued therapy
- metformin may help with weight reduction; however, compliance with diet and exercise remain essential for the control of diabetes
- if a dose is missed, take it as soon as possible, but if it is remembered close to the next dose time (within 4 hours if dosed Q8H; within 6 hours if dosed Q12H), omit the missed dose
- be familiar with the signs and symptoms of hypoglycemia if you are also receiving a sulfonylurea

▶ Therapeutic Tips

- start with a low dose (e.g., 500 mg Q12H) to try to avoid or diminish gastrointestinal upset
- doses up to 3000 mg may be used, but are not usually tolerated
- remember that metformin is a useful medication, does not cause hypoglycemia, and may promote weight loss
- avoid its use in patients with decreased renal, hepatic, or cardiac function and monitor these functions during regular diabetic checkups; if a decrease in function occurs, consider discontinuation of medication administration to avoid the risk of lactic acidosis

Useful References

Bailey CJ. Biguanides and NIDDM. Diabetes Care 1992;15:755–772
Expert Committee of the Canadian Diabetes Advisory Board. Clinical practice guidelines for treatment of diabetes mellitus. Can Med Assoc J 1992;147:697–712
Vigneri R, Goldfine ID. Role of metformin in treatment of diabetes mellitus. Diabetes Care 1987;10:118–122
Pregnancy. In: Banting and Best Diabetes Centre. The Management of Diabetes Mellitus. Toronto: University of Toronto, 1990:29
Metformin. In: Leathem AM, Cadario FJ, eds. Drug Information Reference, 3rd ed. Vancouver: The B.C. Drug and Poison Information Centre, 1993:906–907

METHADONE

Terry Baumann

USA (Dolophine)
CANADA (Dolophine)

▶ When Should I Use This Drug?

Acute or chronic pain

- should be used only in patients allergic to all other opioids (excluding propoxyphene), as it offers no advantages over morphine
- it has an analgesic duration of action that is longer than that of non–sustained-release morphine, which makes it difficult to titrate, especially for acute pain
- when used for an extended period (longer than 7 days), the sedation half-life may outlast the analgesic half-life

Opioid addiction

- effective for suppressing withdrawal symptoms in a patient discontinuing an opioid regimen
- used for both detoxification and maintenance

▶ When Should I Not Use This Drug?

Mild to moderate pain

- unless drugs such as acetaminophen, acetaminophen-codeine, or nonsteroidal antiinflammatory drugs have been used on a regularly scheduled basis (not PRN) and are shown to be ineffective

▶ What Contraindications Are There to the Use of This Drug?

Intolerance of or allergic reaction to methadone

- true allergies to methadone are rare
- check that the patient has actual allergic symptoms, and if there is a true allergy, consider morphine, hydromorphone, or fentanyl

Severe respiratory depression

- not an absolute contraindication; just start with dosages 25% of the normal initial dose and titrate up to an effect while assessing respiratory rate and oxymetry before each dose

▶ What Drug Interactions Are Clinically Important?

see Morphine

▶ What Route and Dosage Should I Use?

How to administer

- orally—may be administered with food or milk or on an empty stomach
- parenterally—may be administered intramuscularly and subcutaneously

Acute pain

- 10 mg PO Q8H (not PRN), or 5 mg PO Q8H (not PRN) for elderly patients because of concerns about sedation and respiratory depression
- consider giving oral methadone if the patient is able to tolerate oral medications, as it is less expensive and has high patient and nurse acceptability, but be aware that the oral route has a slightly slower onset (30–60 minutes) than the intramuscular (15–30 minutes)
- 2.5 mg IM or SC Q8H (not PRN), or 2.5 mg IM Q8H (not PRN) for elderly patients because of concerns about sedation and respiratory depression
- question patients frequently about the degree of pain they are having (ideally, within at most 1–2 hours after the first dose if the drug was administered via the PO or the IM route)
- if pain is unrelieved by this time and there are no signs of sedation or respiratory depression, give another dose 50% higher than the first dose
- if pain continues to be unrelieved, consider switching to a faster acting agent (i.e., morphine) with a shorter duration of action
- normal dosage increments are 2.5, 5, and 10 mg
- after pain has been controlled, always include PRN doses at 50% of the maintenance dosage for breakthrough pain
- if used for longer than 4 days, increase the dosing interval to Q6H

Chronic cancer pain, chronic noncancer pain

In a patient who has received only weak opioids in the past

- 10 mg PO Q8H (not PRN), or 5 mg PO Q8H for elderly patients because of concerns about sedation and respiratory depression

- almost always give by mouth unless the patient has uncontrollable nausea or vomiting
- oral route is inexpensive and has high patient and nurse acceptability

In a patient being switched from another opioid

- determine the average daily requirements for the previous opioids and determine the 24 hour methadone equivalent
- 24 hour requirements for methadone should be divided by 3 and given every 8 hours
- if the previous opioid has not been effective, the total daily dose of methadone should be increased by 25%
- if pain is not relieved or pain returns before 8 hours, treat with a shorter-acting narcotic (morphine or hydromorphone)
- if during a 24 hour period, the patient requires more than 4 PRN doses between doses of methadone, increase the methadone dosage by 25%
- attempt to get pain at least 90% controlled

Opioid addiction

- for detoxification, 20 mg PO daily to suppress withdrawal symptoms; another 20 mg may be given the same day if symptoms reappear
- highly motivated patients may be maintained on 20–30 mg PO given once daily, but heavy opiate users may need up to 100 mg/d

Dosage adjustments for renal or hepatic dysfunction

- hepatically metabolized
- dosage adjustments are usually not needed if the dose is titrated properly

Normal Dosing Interval	$C_{cr} > 60$ mL/min or 1 mL/s	C_{cr} 30–60 mL/min or 0.5–1 mL/s	$C_{cr} < 30$ mL/min or 0.5 mL/s
Q8–12H	adjust dosage on basis of response	adjust dosage on basis of response	adjust dosage on basis of response

▶ What Should I Monitor with Regard to Efficacy and Toxicity

see Morphine

▶ How Long Do I Treat Patients with This Drug?

see Morphine

Opioid addiction

- detoxification (30–180 days)
- maintenance may last for years

▶ How Do I Decrease or Stop the Administration of This Drug?

see Morphine

▶ What Should I Tell My Patients About This Drug?

see Morphine

▶ Therapeutic Tips

see Morphine

- always order a shorter- and faster-acting analgesic for breakthrough pain when using methadone for cancer pain

Useful References

see Morphine

METHOTREXATE

Kelly Jones

USA (Rheumatrex Dose Pack, Methotrexate)
CANADA (A, generic)

▶ When Should I Use This Drug?

Severe rheumatoid arthritis

- although more experience has been obtained with intramuscular gold, methotrexate (MTX) should be chosen, as it has a longer duration of effectiveness and is likely better tolerated than gold
- has a faster onset than other disease-modifying agents, with disease suppression being seen in 2–6 weeks rather than up to 12 weeks with other agents
- there is mounting evidence that, with appropriate monitoring of dosage and response, methotrexate is well tolerated (Am J Med 1983;75[6A]:69–73, Arthritis Rheum 1988;31:167–175)

▶ When Should I Not Use This Drug?

Mild to moderate nonprogressive disease

- other agents are available that are effective and less toxic

Severe rheumatoid arthritis in unmotivated, unreliable patients

- patients must be motivated to treat their disease, should be knowledgeable enough to understand all guidelines on how to use this drug, and should realize that regular visits to the physician and monitoring are required

▶ What Contraindications Are There to the Use of This Drug?

Intolerance of or allergic reaction to methotrexate

Pregnancy and/or breast-feeding

- methotrexate has been both abortifacient and teratogenic

Conception

- pregnancy must be avoided during methotrexate therapy and after therapy for 3 months in the male and 1 month in the female patient

Hepatic disease

- patients with the following risk factors for hepatic toxicity from methotrexate should avoid the drug: history of alcohol use—past or present intake of 1–2 drinks per day, abnormal liver function test results (liver enzyme levels 2 times normal values), history of active or recent hepatitis, cirrhosis, history of intravenous drug abuse, family history of genetic hepatic disease, diabetes (insulin enhances the cytotoxic effects of methotrexate), obesity, and history of significant exposure to known hepatotoxic drugs

Severe anemia, leukopenia, or thrombocytopenia

- methotrexate worsens these conditions

Active infectious disease (e.g., tuberculosis and pyelonephritis)

- methotrexate has immunosuppressive properties

▶ What Drug Interactions Are Clinically Important?

Drugs that may increase the effect or toxicity of methotrexate

NONSTEROIDAL ANTIINFLAMMATORY DRUGS

- nonsteroidal antiinflammatory drugs (NSAIDs) decrease the clearance of methotrexate and increase the risk of toxicity
- no problem if using for rheumatoid arthritis, but the combination must not be used when high dosages (for chemotherapy) of methotrexate are being used
- it is important when patients begin methotrexate therapy that their NSAID therapy not be stopped and started (i.e., be consistent) owing to the potential for this drug interaction

RETINOIDS, KETOCONAZOLE, METHYLDOPA

- increased risk of hepatotoxicity; therefore, do not prescribe together
- if these agents are absolutely needed and no alternatives can be used, stop methotrexate administration for the duration of the therapy

SULFASALAZINE

- metabolism is inhibited by sulfonamides, and there may be enhanced toxicity of methotrexate on the bone marrow

- initiate methotrexate therapy at lowest dosage or reduce the dosage transiently to assess the effect of adding sulfasalazine to established methotrexate therapy

Drugs that may decrease the effect of methotrexate

- none

Drugs that may have their effect or toxicity increased by methotrexate

- none

Drugs that may have their effect or toxicity decreased by methotrexate

- none

▶ What Route and Dosage Should I Use?

How to administer

- orally—give with food
- parenterally—intramuscularly

Severe rheumatoid arthritis

- 7.5 mg PO weekly, with the entire dose administered as a single dose
- increase the dosage every 6 weeks (by 2.5 mg) on the basis of response up to a maximum of 20 mg/wk
- 7.5 mg IM weekly should be used only if patients cannot tolerate oral therapy or if compliance becomes an issue

Dosage adjustments for renal or hepatic dysfunction

- renally eliminated

Normal Dosing Interval	C_{cr} > 60 mL/min or 1 mL/s	C_{cr} 30–60 mL/min or 0.5–1 mL/s	C_{cr} < 30 mL/min or 0.5 mL/s
every week	no adjustment needed	decrease dosage by 50%	avoid

▶ What Should I Monitor with Regard to Efficacy and Toxicity?

Efficacy

Rheumatoid arthritis

Joint tenderness count, sedimentation rate measurements, grip strength, duration of morning stiffness, time to onset of fatigue, and the patient's report on specific functions

- patient should be assessed monthly for the first 2 months, and after symptoms are under control, the patient can be assessed every 3 months for 6 months and then every 6 months
- these variables should be used to guide drug administration initiation and discontinuation
- one study found that clinical and laboratory measures of physical well-being appeared unrelated to psychological and social measures of well-being (J Rheumatol 1991;18:650–653)
- it is important to include the patient's self-assessment of the drug's effect on their function and well-being

Toxicity

Stomatitis, malaise, headaches, nausea, and anorexia (these occur 75% of the time)

- can be decreased by giving the dose all at once and not splitting the dose over 24 hours
- if the patient continues to have problems with these side effects, it is imperative to assess the dosage (check prescription bottle for dose and directions), how the patient is taking the dose (make sure that they are *not* taking the dose every day!), and whether drug interactions are involved

Hepatotoxicity

- associated with long-term use, high dosages, and total cumulative dose of 1.5 g
- damage ranges from fibrosis (8%) to necrosis and cirrhosis
- do baseline liver enzyme and serum albumin determinations
- discontinue methotrexate therapy if liver enzyme levels increase to greater than 3 times baseline values
- decreases in serum albumin levels may precede acute hepatotoxicity

- in patients with risk factors for hepatic disease, a liver biopsy should be performed after a total cumulative dose of 1.5 g (a weekly dose of 7.5 mg takes 50 months or 4.2 years before a biopsy is required)
- biopsy should be repeated after each successive 1.5 g cumulative dose
- if the biopsy finding is grade 1 (normal; fatty infiltrate, mild; nuclear variability, mild; portal inflammation, mild) or grade 2 (fatty infiltrate, moderate to severe; nuclear variability, moderate to severe; portal tract expansion, portal tract inflammation, and necrosis, moderate to severe), continue treatment and repeat the biopsy after a 1 g cumulative dose
- if the biopsy finding is grade 3A (fibrosis, mild), continue treatment but repeat the biopsy in 6 months
- if the biopsy finding is grade 3B (fibrosis, moderate to severe) or grade 4 (cirrhosis; regenerating nodules, as well as bridging of portal tracts, must be demonstrated), stop the methotrexate administration

Nephrotoxicity

- methotrexate is not nephrotoxic; however, in patients with the possibility of renal dysfunction's developing, serum creatinine levels should be measured monthly and the dosage adjusted appropriately

Pulmonary toxicity

- most serious toxic effect with low-dose methotrexate therapy, with symptoms consisting of a persistent nonproductive dry cough, with or without dyspnea
- associated more with the divided weekly dose regimen (over 24 hours) instead of the full weekly dose regimen
- methotrexate administration should be stopped immediately and treatment with supportive care and corticosteroids should be instituted in any patient who gets a persistent or otherwise unexplained nonproductive dry cough
- do yearly chest radiograph (no data on its value, but it is strongly recommended) (Ann Intern Med 1987;107:358–366)

Bone marrow toxicity

- associated with high doses, underlying renal disease, infection, folate deficiency, and concurrent use of trimethoprim (another antifolate compound)
- get baseline complete blood count and platelet counts and repeat after 14 days of treatment, then every 4 weeks after the dosage is stable
- discontinue methotrexate administration if the neutrophil count decreases to less than 2000/mm^3 or the platelet count decreases to less than 150,000/mm^3

▶ How Long Do I Treat Patients with This Drug?

Severe rheumatoid arthritis

- there are no specific guidelines on the duration of therapy
- whether methotrexate is disease modifying is uncertain, and complete remission according to the American Rheumatism Association criteria is rarely achieved, taking up to 2 years of therapy (Arthritis Rheum 1981;24:1308–1315)
- some patients continue to improve after discontinuation of therapy with methotrexate, but most have a clinical flare 3–4 weeks later (Ann Intern Med 1987;107:358–366)
- patients with a declining therapeutic response over time have improved when the dosage was increased or when the route was switched from oral to intramuscular (J Rheumatol 1985;12[suppl 12]:35–39)
- switch to intramuscular therapy after the dosage has reached 20 mg and is still not effective

▶ How Do I Decrease or Stop the Administration of This Drug?

- may be stopped abruptly if needed

▶ What Should I Tell My Patients About This Drug?

- avoid alcohol, including beer and wine, to reduce potential hepatic toxicity

- there is the potential for hepatic toxicity, and the risk is greater if there is a history of alcoholism, insulin-dependent diabetes, and underlying hepatic disease
- during childbearing years, practice appropriate birth control
- drug interactions, especially with salicylates and other NSAIDs, are possible and do not start any new drugs without first consulting a pharmacist or a physician
- use acetaminophen instead of aspirin or other NSAIDs when you have a headache or any other minor pain
- never start or stop or change the dosage of NSAIDs without first consulting your physician
- seek medical care if you think you have an infection (immunosuppression), cough or shortness of breath (lung toxicity), or any unusual bleeding (liver or bone marrow suppression)
- once a week dosing regimen is important and daily dosing of this drug can be fatal
- read and take home the patient package insert inside of Rheumatrex (methotrexate) Dose Pack
- it is important to keep all appointments
- compliance is essential
- discuss any minor side effects such as loss of appetite, nausea (rarely vomiting), diarrhea, and mouth sores during your regular appointments

▶ Therapeutic Tips

- dose the drug on a weekly basis
- be aware of the possible drug interaction with NSAIDs
- be aware of the risk factors associated with major toxicities
- make sure that the patient is reliable and compliant

Useful References

Harris, ED. Rheumatoid arthritis: Pathophysiology and implications for therapy. N Engl J Med 1990;322:1277–1289

Kremer JM, Lee JK. The safety and efficacy of the use of methotrexate in long term therapy for rheumatoid arthritis. Arthritis Rheum 1986;29:822–831

Nesher G, Moore TL, Zuckner J. Rheumatoid arthritis in the elderly. J Am Geriatr Soc 1991;39:284–294

Tugwell P, Bennett K, Gent M. Methotrexate in rheumatoid arthritis: Indications, contraindications, efficacy, and safety. Ann Intern Med 1987; 107:358–366

Roenigk HH, Auerbach R, Maibach HI, Weinstein GD. Methotrexate in psoriasis: Revised guidelines. J Am Acad Dermatol 1988;19:145–156

Weinblatt ME, Coblyn JS, Fox DA, et al. Efficacy of low-dose methotrexate in rheumatoid arthritis. N Engl J Med 1985;312:818–822

Wilke WS, Mackenzie AH. Methotrexate therapy in rheumatoid arthritis. Drugs 1986;32:103–113

METHYLPREDNISOLONE

Karen Shalansky and Cindy Reesor Nimmo

USA (A-Methapred, Medrol, Solu-Medrol)
CANADA (Medrol, Solu-Medrol)

▶ When Should I Use This Drug?

Acute asthma or bronchitis, rheumatoid arthritis, migraine, acquired immunodeficiency syndrome with *Pneumocystis carinii* pneumonia, ulcerative colitis, skin disorders, organ transplant, collagen disease

- hydrocortisone is the parenteral corticosteroid of choice in patients unable to take oral prednisone who require short-term therapy (shorter than 3 days)
- if high-dose parenteral steroids are required for longer than 3 days, use methylprednisolone instead of hydrocortisone because methylprednisolone has less mineralocorticoid activity
- methylprednisolone is more expensive than hydrocortisone

▶ When Should I Not Use This Drug?

Oral corticosteroids can be used

- oral corticosteroids are as effective as parenteral steroids for the treatment of acute asthma
- see below under How to administer

Prevention of adrenal insufficiency

- need agent with significant mineralocorticoid and glucocorticoid effects
- use hydrocortisone

▶ What Contraindications Are There to the Use of This Drug?

see Prednisone

▶ What Drug Interactions Are Clinically Important?

see Prednisone

▶ What Route and Dosage Should I Use?

How to adminster

Orally

- there is likely no clinical difference between oral methylprednisolone and prednisone; clinicians should use prednisone as it is less expensive

Parenterally

- dilute 40 mg in 1 mL of bacteriostatic water or normal saline and dilute in a further 25–100 mL of 5% dextrose in water or normal saline and infuse over 15–30 minutes
- can be given by IV push (40 mg over 1–2 minutes)

Acute asthma, bronchitis, rheumatoid arthritis

- 40 mg IV Q6H for 24–48 hours, then taper (25% of dose every 1–2 days as tolerated) or convert to an oral prednisone regimen if oral therapy is tolerated
- to convert from parenteral methylprednisone to oral prednisone a conversion of 4 mg of methylprednisolone to 5 mg of prednisone can be used; however, most clinicians would just switch to 40–60 mg of prednisone daily
- controversy exists as to whether higher dosages (e.g., 125 mg Q6H) should be used in acute asthma attacks; several studies have shown no significant differences between high and conventional dosing (Chest 1982;82:438–440, Pediatrics 1978;61:829–831, Chest 1986;89:823–835); a faster (within 24 hours) but similar response has been found in 1 study with high-dose (125 mg Q6H) compared with medium-dose (40 mg Q6H) methylprednisone; both were significantly superior to low-dose (20 mg Q6H) methylprednisolone (Arch Intern Med 1983;143:1324–1327)

Migraine

- 40 mg IV Q8H for 24–48 hours or until the patient can take oral prednisone

AIDS with *Pneumocystis carinii* pneumonia

- 40 mg IV Q8H for 24–48 hours or until the patient can take oral prednisone

Ulcerative colitis

- 40 mg IV Q8H for 24–48 hours or until the patient can take oral prednisone

Dosage adjustments for renal or hepatic dysfunction

- hepatically metabolized
- no adjustments required; just titrate the dose to effect and toxicity

▶ What Should I Monitor with Regard to Efficacy and Toxcity?

see Prednisone

▶ How Long Do I Treat Patients with This Drug?

see Prednisone

▶ How Do I Decrease or Stop the Administration of This Drug?

see Prednisone

▶ What Should I Tell My Patients About This Drug?

see Prednisone

Useful References

Kelly HW, Murphy S. Corticosteroids for acute, severe asthma. DICP 1991;25:72–79

Siegel SC. Overview of corticosteroid therapy. J Allergy Clin Immunol 1985;76:312–320

METHYSERGIDE

Jerry Taylor

USA (Sansert)
CANADA (Sansert)

▶ When Should I Use This Drug?

Migraine prophylaxis

- used as a prophylactic agent in the management of severe recurrent headache when all other therapies have failed, because it is more toxic than other agents (fibrotic problems)
- use of this drug necessitates that the patient be under constant supervision to recognize the earliest signs and symptoms of toxicity and to prevent irreversible effects

▶ When Should I Not Use This Drug?

Migraine treatment

- is ineffective in the treatment of acute attacks of migraine

▶ What Contraindications Are There to the Use of This Drug?

Intolerance of or allergic reaction to methysergide

Peripheral vascular disease

- these patients are particularly susceptible to the vasoconstrictive complications

Severe hypertension, coronary disease, hepatic and renal failure, and pregnancy

- because of the vasoconstrictor effects seen with this drug

▶ What Drug Interactions Are Clinically Important?

Drugs that may increase the effect or toxicity of methysergide

ERGOTAMINE

- risk of arterial occlusion exists when given with high parenteral dosages of ergotamine; therefore, avoid this combination

BETA-BLOCKERS

- gangrene has been reported in a patient taking propranolol; this combination should be avoided

Drugs that may decrease the effect of methysergide

- none

Drugs that may have their effect increased by methysergide

- none

Drugs that may have their effect decreased by methysergide

- none

▶ What Route and Dosage Should I Use?

How to administer

- orally—take with food or milk
- parenterally—not available

Migraine prophylaxis

- 2 mg PO daily with a meal
- titrate at weekly intervals by 2 mg daily if necessary to a maximum of 2 mg PO QID
- if efficacy has not been demonstrated after a 3 week trial, administration of alternative agents should be initiated

Dosage adjustments for renal or hepatic dysfunction

- no dosage adjustments, as contraindicated in patients with renal or hepatic dysfunction

▶ What Should I Monitor with Regard to Efficacy and Toxicity?

Efficacy

Frequency and severity of headache

- patient with frequent migraine may need evaluation at 2–4 week intervals during the initial dose titration; then the time between visits may be extended in patients showing a response to treatment

Toxicity

Abdominal discomfort and muscle cramps

- occur in 40% of patients and commonly occur at the intiation of therapy, but symptoms are usually transient and subside within a few days or weeks

Fibrotic syndromes (retroperitoneal fibrosis, endocardial fibrosis, pleuropulmonary fibrosis)

- have been reported in 1% of patients treated continuously
- persistent reports or evidence of peripheral vasoconstriction necessitate discontinuation of drug therapy in approximately 10% of patients
- uninterrupted use of methysergide can cause fibrotic changes, but these effects rarely occur until after 7 months of continuous use
- retroperitoneal fibrosis is usually reversible if it is recognized early and therapy is discontinued; however, other fibrotic changes are less readily reversed

▶ *How Long Do I Treat Patients with This Drug?*

Migraine prophylaxis

- should not be used for longer than 6 months at a time and drug-free periods ("drug holidays") are necessary to prevent fibrotic complications

▶ *How Do I Decrease or Stop the Administration of This Drug?*

- taper slowly, reducing the dosage by 1 tablet weekly to avoid rebound headaches, and then stop for 1 month before reinstituting use if headaches recur

▶ *What Should I Tell My Patients About This Drug?*

- if you are receiving methysergide, the dosage of ergotamine required to control acute attacks of migraine may need to be reduced
- if you experience fibrotic changes or arterial spasm with manifestations such as paresthesia of the extremities or anginal pain, discontinue methysergide administration and call your physician
- report any flank pain, dysuria, and angina to help in the early detection of early fibrotic changes

▶ *Therapeutic Tips*

- discuss with the patient the therapeutic goals, the potential risks of therapy, and the requirement of interrupted therapy at intervals
- recommend an annual intravenous pyelogram in the early detection of urethral obstruction and prevention of renal damage

METOCLOPRAMIDE

Lynne Nakashima

USA (Clopra, Maxolon, Reclomide, Reglan)
CANADA (Emex, Maxeran, Reglan)

▶ *When Should I Use This Drug?*

Nausea and vomiting associated with gastric stasis

- metoclopramide increases lower esophageal sphincter tone and improves gastric emptying
- metoclopramide and domperidone have similar activity and are likely equally effective
- metoclopramide causes more frequent sedation and anticholinergic and extrapyramidal adverse effects than does domperidone
- metoclopramide is available as a parenteral agent and should be used if a parenteral promotility agent is needed
- if the oral route can be used, choose domperidone instead of metoclopramide, as it produces fewer adverse effects; the cost difference may be significant and affect this decision

Nausea and vomiting associated with migraine

- if the patient is experiencing nausea or vomiting with the headache, use metoclopramide

- metoclopramide enhances subsequent analgesic absorption, as well as providing an antimigraine effect

Chemotherapy-induced nausea and vomiting

- useful, in combination with other agents, when a patient is receiving drugs with high emetogenic potential
- low doses (10–30 mg) do not offer any advantage over other dopamine receptor antagonists (domperidone) in chemotherapy-induced nausea and vomiting, but high doses (1–2 mg/kg) are effective when used for highly emetogenic agents (Drugs 1992; 43:295–315)
- metoclopramide, in conjunction with diphenhydramine, dexamethasone, and lorazepam is a useful combination when ondansetron cannot be used
- for drugs with moderate or low emetogenic potential (Pharmacotherapy 1990;10:129–145), metoclopramide is useful if prochlorperazine cannot be used or is ineffective
- metoclopramide is likely as effective as prochlorperazine but causes akathisia, restlessness, and/or dystonic reactions in 3–5% of patients
- is more expensive than prochlorperazine

General nausea and vomiting, postoperative nausea and vomiting

- useful if agents such as prochlorperazine, perphenazine, and thiethylperazine cannot be used or are ineffective

▶ *When Should I Not Use This Drug?*

Nausea and vomiting caused by motion sickness and vestibular conditions

- does not appear useful (Drugs 1992;43:295–315)

Reflux esophagitis

- although combinations of metoclopramide and an H_2 antagonist have been used effectively in severe reflux disease, omeprazole is now considered the drug of choice, as it is effective, can be taken once daily, and is less expensive than the combination
- if a promotility agent is needed, use domperidone
- although metoclopramide is the least expensive of the promotility agents, it is associated with a large number of central nervous system (CNS) adverse effects such as sedation and has the potential to cause movement disorders

▶ *What Contraindications Are There to the Use of This Drug?*

Intolerance of or allergic reaction to metoclopramide
Parkinsonism

- may exacerbate parkinsonian symptoms

Gastrointestinal hemorrhage, mechanical obstruction, perforation

- stimulation of gastrointestinal motility may exacerbate symptoms or worsen the disease state

Tardive dyskinesia

- in patients with a history of dystonic reactions to metoclopramide or in high-risk patients (elderly or female patients) who may experience tardive dyskinesia with long-term use, metoclopramide should not be used

Pheochromocytoma

- may precipitate a hypertensive crisis

▶ *What Drug Interactions Are Clinically Important?*

Drugs that may increase the effect or toxicity of metoclopramide
CENTRAL NERVOUS SYSTEM DEPRESSANTS

- additive, sedative effects are expected when other CNS depressants (e.g., narcotic analgesics, hypnotics, and alcohol) are used
- avoid combination if possible or minimize the effects by starting with low dosages

Drugs that may decrease the effect of metoclopramide

- none

Drugs that may have their effect or toxicity increased by metoclopramide

MONOAMINE OXIDASE INHIBITORS

- may preciptiate a hypertensive crisis
- avoid concurrent use

Drugs that may have their effect decreased by metoclopramide

- none

▶ *What Route and Dosage Should I Use?*

How to administer

Orally

- take with food or milk or on an empty stomach

Parenterally

- dilute in 50 mL of normal saline or 5% dextrose in water and administer over 15 minutes
- may be administered undiluted at a rate of 5 mg/min

Nausea and vomiting associated with gastric stasis, migraine, postoperative nausea and vomiting

- 10 mg IV or IM every 3 hours when needed
- 10 mg PO every 3 hours may be used if the patient can tolerate sips of fluid

Chemotherapy-induced nausea and vomiting

Highly emetogenic drugs

- 1 mg/kg IV 30 minutes prior to chemotherapy, then 1 mg/kg IV Q3H for 3 doses
- replace parenteral metoclopramide (if patient can tolerate oral therapy) with 10 mg PO Q6H starting 6 hours after the last 1 mg/kg dose
- if emesis is uncontrolled and adverse effects are not present, increase the dosage by 20 mg increments to a maximum of 3 mg/kg until the optimum effect is obtained (Am J Hosp Pharm 1988;45:1322–1328)
- high-dose oral metoclopramide (1 mg/kg) for chemotherapy-induced nausea and vomiting has been studied (J Clin Oncol 1986;4:98–103) and no difference in efficacy was noted, but oral administration was associated with an increased incidence of diarrhea
- metoclopramide has been studied as a continuous infusion for chemotherapy-induced nausea and vomiting (Clin Pharm 1989;8:187–199) and may be useful to achieve rapid attainment and maintenance of therapeutic serum concentrations; prevention of drug accumulation, leading to decreased incidence of adverse effects; and decreased preparation and administration time and cost
- efficacy is comparable or slightly better than that with intermittent infusions and potential benefits include decreased preparation and administration costs
- if a continuous infusion is to be used, start with a loading dose of 3 mg/kg IV given over 1 hour prechemotherapy and follow with 0.5 mg/kg/h as an infusion (Clin Pharm 1986;5:150–152)

Moderate to low emetogenic drugs

- 20 mg PO 30 minutes prior to chemotherapy (give IV at same dose if the patient is already vomiting)
- follow with 20 mg PO Q6H for 24 hours and then 20 mg PO PRN for 3–4 days

Dosage adjustments for renal or hepatic dysfunction

- renally eliminated

Normal Dosing Interval	$C_{cr} > 60$ mL/min or 1 mL/s	C_{cr} 30–60 mL/min or 0.5–1 mL/s	$C_{cr} < 30$ mL/min or 0.5 mL/s
Q6H	no adjustment needed	Q8H	Q12H

- no dosage adjustment required for hepatic dysfunction

▶ *What Should I Monitor with Regard to Efficacy and Toxicity?*

Efficacy

Nausea and vomiting

Frequency of assesment depends on the severity and frequency of nausea and vomiting

Number and severity of vomiting episodes

- determine time of day, force, description of vomitus, and associated symptoms

Fluid balance (needed only if vomiting occurs for a prolonged period)

- assess jugular venous pressure and orthostatic changes in blood pressure and heart rate; any decrease in upright diastolic pressure plus a rise in heart rate of 20 bpm or greater is abnormal
- oliguria
- weight
- rising values of hematocrit and creatinine, urea, sodium, and bicarbonate levels plus decreasing potassium and chloride levels are an indication of dehydration

Toxicity

Extrapyramidal side effects

- dystonic reactions, tetany, restlessness, facial spasms, involuntary movement, torticollis, and muscular twitching occur in about 3% of patients (Pharmacotherapy 1990;10:129–145)
- patients younger than age 30 years have a higher incidence of acute extrapyramidal effects (Br Med J 1985;291:930–932)
- can usually be prevented with diphenhydramine, and diphenhydramine should be given prophylactically with metoclopramide in all patients receiving high doses (>1 mg/kg)
- give 50 mg IV (usually mixed with metoclopramide) 30 minutes prior to chemotherapy and with each dose of 1 mg/kg metoclopramide
- after the 1 mg/kg dose of metoclopramide has been given, replace the parenteral diphenhydramine with 25 mg PO Q6H
- if severe reactions occur, discontinue the metoclopramide administration

Diarrhea

- may occur in up to 45% of patients treated with high-dose (>1 mg/kg) metoclopramide (Pharmacotherapy 1990;10:129–145)
- combination regimens, including dexamethasone, generally result in a decreased incidence of diarrhea (range of 5–18%) (Med Clin North Am 1987;71:289–301, Cancer 1985;55:527–534)
- if diarrhea is moderate to severe, reduce the dosage by 50% and if diarrhea continues, stop the drug administration

Sedation

- may occur in up to 80% of patients and is usually mild
- should decrease after 1–2 days; avoid the use of other sedating medications if possible (Pharmacotherapy 1990;10:129–145)

▶ *How Long Do I Treat Patients with This Drug?*

Nausea and vomiting associated with gastric stasis

- try for a few days, and if no effect is seen, try a different agent

Nausea and vomiting associated with migraine

- 2–3 days

Postoperative nausea and vomiting

- if regular prophylactic therapy is required, treat for 24 hours
- use PRN antiemetics for 2–3 days after surgery

Chemotherapy-induced nausea and vomiting

- treat patients for 24 hours after chemotherapy, then on a PRN basis
- for cisplatin-induced nausea and vomiting, delayed symptoms may occur up to 1 week after the last dose of chemotherapy and treatment should last for up to 1 week postchemotherapy
- if there is previous experience, base the duration of use on how the patient responded the first time (e.g., if the drug was used

for 24 hours and the patient went home and experienced severe nausea and vomiting, give as a regular dose for a longer period of time)

▶ How Do I Decrease or Stop the Administration of This Drug?

- may be stopped abruptly

▶ What Should I Tell My Patients About This Drug?

- metoclopramide can be taken with food or on an empty stomach
- it takes ½–1 hour to become fully effective
- side effects include restlessness and muscle spasms, which may be controlled by diphenhydramine 25 mg Q6H; however, if severe facial or neck muscle spasms occur (uncommon), stop taking metoclopramide and go to the nearest emergency department
- drowsiness can occur but it should decrease after 1–2 days
- drowsiness may be increased if you are taking another agent that causes drowsiness (e.g., narcotic pain killers, alcohol, and some cough remedies)

▶ Therapeutic Tips

- because high dose-metoclopramide for chemotherapy-induced nausea and vomiting is usually given intravenously, inpatient administration is often necessary

Useful References

Agostinucci WA, Gannon RH, Schauer PK, et al., Continuous infusion of metoclopramide for prevention of chemotherapy-induced emesis. Clin Pharm 1986;5:150–153

Gralla RJ. Metoclopramide. A review of antiemetic trials. Drugs 1983;25 (suppl 1):63–73

Gralla RJ, Itri LM, Pisko SE, et al., Antiemetic efficacy of high-dose metoclopramide: Randomized trials with placebo and prochlorperazine in patients with chemotherapy-induced nausea and vomiting. N Engl J Med 1981;305:905–909

Merrifield KR, Chaffee BJ. Recent advances in the management of nausea and vomiting caused by antineoplastic agents. Clin Pharm 1989;8:187–199

Tortorice PV, O'Connell MB. Management of chemotherapy-induced nausea and vomiting. Pharmacotherapy 1990;10:129–145

METOLAZONE

Ian Petterson

USA (Diulo, Mykrox, Zaroxolyn)
CANADA (Zaroxolyn)

▶ When Should I Use This Drug?

Congestive heart failure or edema of other causes

- useful as an adjunct to furosemide in cases of furosemide resistance (Curr Ther Res 1977;22:686–691)
- should only be used if furosemide or hydrochlorothiazide is ineffective or not tolerated
- used if more diuresis is required than that obtained with high-dose furosemide (160 mg IV)
- effective in patients with poor renal function (creatinine clearance < 30 mL/min), whereas hydrochlorothiazide is not effective in patients with creatinine clearance less than 30 mL/min
- when metolazone, even in low doses (1.25 mg), is combined with furosemide, a dramatic diuresis may occur
- be aware that hypokalemia, hypomagnesemia, hypotension, and prerenal failure can occur with rapid diuresis

▶ When Should I Not Use This Drug?

Chronic (noncrisis) hypertension

- no advantages over hydrochlorothiazide with regard to the treatment of hypertension, unless the patient has poor renal function (creatinine clearance < 30 mL/min), as it is more expensive than hydrochlorothiazide and no more effective

Acute (crisis) hypertension

- thiazides have not been evaluated in this condition; however, they may be useful if volume overload is a contributing factor, particularly in patients with impaired renal function

Edema due to nephrotic syndrome

- this is frequently thiazide resistant; therefore, furosemide should be used as first-line therapy

▶ What Contraindications Are There to the Use of This Drug?

see Hydrochlorothiazide

▶ What Drug Interactions Are Clinically Important?

see Hydrochlorothiazide

▶ What Route and Dosage Should I Use?

How to administer

- orally—may be given with food or on an empty stomach
- parenterally—available only in an oral dosage form

Congestive heart failure or edema of other causes

- 2.5 mg PO daily as sole diuretic
- 1.25 mg PO daily if added to furosemide for diuretic synergy because of concerns about overdiuresis, electrolyte depletion, and prerenal insufficiency
- double the dosage every 3–4 days, on the basis of response, up to a maximum of 20 mg PO daily
- always administer metolazone 60 minutes prior to IV furosemide doses for maximum effects

▶ What Should I Monitor with Regard to Efficacy and Toxicity?

Efficacy

see Hydrochlorothiazide

▶ How Long Do I Treat Patients with This Drug?

Congestive heart failure or edema of other causes

- after the desired response is seen, therapy need continue only if the patient becomes refractory to furosemide again
- maintenance therapy can be given 2–3 times weekly to maintin furosemide's effectiveness

▶ How Do I Decrease or Stop the Administration of This Drug?

Congestive heart failure or edema of other causes

- tapering of the drug administration is wise because rebound salt and water retention over 1–2 weeks occurs unpredictably and can be prevented by slow withdrawal over 2–4 weeks

▶ What Should I Tell My Patients About This Drug?

see Hydrochlorothiazide

▶ Therapeutic Tips

- useful agent for congestive heart failure or edema in patients who have poor renal function
- useful in patients with poor renal function who have become refractory to furosemide

Useful Reference

Ellison DH. The physiologic basis of diuretic synergism: Its role in treating diuretic resistance. Ann Intern Med 1991;114:886–894

METOPROLOL

Robert Rangno and James McCormack

USA (Lopressor)
CANADA (Lopressor, Lopressor SR, Betaloc, Betaloc Durules, Apo-Metoprolol, Novometoprol)

▶ When Should I Use This Drug?

Myocardial infarction

- all patients (unless there are contraindications to beta-blockers) should be treated empirically with beta-blockers after a myocardial infarction (Am J Cardiol 1990;66:3C–8C) because there are

convincing data that reinfarction, sudden cardiac death, and overall mortality are reduced after myocardial infarction (MI) in patients given beta-blockers
- metoprolol has the advantage of being available as a parenteral agent, along with propranolol and atenolol (USA only)
- decision among parenteral propranolol, parenteral metoprolol, and parenteral atentolol (USA only) should be based on cost
- although parenteral therapy is usually recommended, oral administration can also be used; however, absorption of the oral agent takes about 30 minutes (some clinicians recommend the intravenous route for the first dose possibly to reduce the size of the infarction)
- some clinicians suggest that only beta-blockers with proven long-term benefits on mortality after infarction (timolol, propranolol, metoprolol, or acebutolol) should be used for post MI prophylaxis (Circulation 1991;84(suppl VI):VI-101–VI-107)

Atrial fibrillation or flutter

see Nadolol

Ventricular arrhythmias

see Nadolol

▶ When Should I Not Use This Drug?

When other beta-blockers can be used

- while metoprolol, a relatively selective beta₁-blocker, is effective in many disease states, other beta-blockers should usually be chosen over metoprolol
- metoprolol is more lipid soluble than atenolol (selective beta-blocker) or nadolol (nonselective beta-blocker)
- lipid-soluble agents (propranolol and metoprolol) have been shown to cause insomnia whereas atenolol (lipid-insoluble) does not (Circulation 1987;75:104–112)
- metoprolol has a short half-life and must be dosed at least twice daily, and while a sustained release product is available, it is usually more expensive than generic nadolol or atenolol, which can be dosed once daily

▶ What Contraindications Are There to the Use of This Drug?

see Nadolol

▶ What Drug Interactions Are Clinically Important?

see Propranolol

▶ What Route and Dosage Should I Use?

How to administer

- orally—see discussion above under When Should I Not Use This Drug?
- parenterally—metoprolol can be given by IV push

Myocardial infarction

- 5 mg IV every 2 minutes until heart rate is <60 beats/min or systolic blood pressure is <100 mm Hg or a maximum of 3 doses
- patients who tolerate the IV doses should receive 50 mg PO BID starting 2 hours after the last IV dose, increasing up to 100 mg PO BID after 3–4 days Q12H (other less lipid soluble and less frequently dosed beta-blockers should likely be chosen instead of metoprolol for long-term use)
- in patients who do not tolerate the full IV dose, begin with 25 mg orally, 15 minutes after the last IV dose, or as soon as clinical conditions allow
- metoprolol administration should be discontinued in the presence of intolerance of the drug, significant hypotension, or heart failure
- patients who experience a delay in the use of parenteral metoprolol, who do not tolerate the full early doses, or who have contraindications to early treatment with metoprolol should be started on 100 mg PO BID as soon as their clinical condition permits (Drugs 1986;31:376–429) while blood pressure and heart rate are monitored

Atrial fibrillation or flutter

- 5 mg IV every 5 minutes until the heart rate is less than 100 bpm, symptoms are alleviated, or 15 mg is reached
- do not push IV dose until a response is seen, as beta-blockers do not always work and can precipitate asystole
- if the patient is not symptomatic and rapid rate control is desired, start with 25 mg PO daily and increase every 2–3 days by 25 mg PO daily until the heart rate is controlled or a maximum dose of 200 mg/d is reached

Ventricular arrhythmias

- 50 mg PO BID (25 mg PO BID in patients with low blood pressure or heart rate < 60 bpm, or patients receiving concomitant therapy with agents that depress the function of the sinoatrial or atrioventricular nodes) and increase the dosage every 2–3 days until the patient has beta-blockade (resting heart rate and heart rate during exercise is suppressed) or a dosage of 100 mg PO BID is reached

Dosage adjustments for renal or hepatic dysfunction

- hepatically metabolized
- in general, even in patients with hepatic dysfunction, start with a low dose and titrate up to an effect

Normal Dosing Interval	C_{cr} > 60 mL/min or 1 mL/s	C_{cr} 30–60 mL/min or 0.5–1 mL/s	C_{cr} < 30 mL/min or 0.5 mL/s
Q12H	no adjustment needed	no adjustment needed	no adjustment needed

▶ What Should I Monitor with Regard to Efficacy and Toxicity?

see Nadolol

▶ How Do I Decrease or Stop the Administration of This Drug?

see Nadolol

▶ What Should I Tell My Patients About This Drug?

see Nadolol

▶ Therapeutic Tips

- beta₁ selectivity is lost above doses of 100 mg PO daily

Useful References

Benfield P, Clissold SP, Brogden RN: Metoprolol. An update review of its pharmacodynamic and pharmacokinetic properties and therapeutic efficacy, in hypertension, ischemic heart disease and related cardiovascular disorders. Drugs 1986;31:375–429

Charlap S, Lichstein E, Frishman WH. Beta-adrenergic blocking drugs in the treatment of congestive heart failure. Med Clin North Am 1989;73:373–385

Ponten J, Haggendal J, Milocco I, Waldenstrom A. Long-term metoprolol therapy and neurolepanesthesia in coronary artery surgery; withdrawal versus maintenance of beta₁-adrenoceptor blockade. Anesth Analg 1983;62:380–390

Heikkila H, Jalonen J, Laaksonen V, et al. Metoprolol medication and coronary artery bypass grafting operation. Acta Anesthesiol Scand 1984;28:677–682

METRONIDAZOLE

David Guay

USA (Flagyl, Metric, Metryl, Protostat, MetroGel)
CANADA (Flagyl, Neo-Metric, Apo-Metronidazole, Novonidazol)

▶ When Should I Use This Drug?

check antibiotic susceptibility chart (Table 4–1 in Chapter 4)

Vaginitis

- if Gram stain of a vaginal swab shows gram-positive and/or gram-negative coccobacilli, metronidazole is the drug of choice
- metronidazole covers *Gardnerella vaginalis, Mycoplasma hominis,* and other typical organisms and is less expensive than clindamycin

- if wet mount (saline) shows the presence of motile trichomonads, metronidazole is considered the drug of choice for *Trichomonas* infection

Intraabdominal infections

- for secondary peritonitis, abdominal trauma, and gangrenous or perforated appendix, metronidazole plus gentamicin is the treatment of choice (in patients with good renal function), as this combination provides excellent coverage against anaerobes and gram-negative organisms and is usually less expensive than cefoxitin or clindamycin-gentamicin

Acute or chronic osteomyelitis, cellulitis

- in combination with cloxacillin or nafcillin when both gram-positive and anaerobic organisms are suspected
- cloxacillin plus metronidazole provides a similar spectrum of activity to clindamycin and should be used if this combination is less expensive

Anaerobic sepsis

- drug of choice unless anaerobes are resistant

Anaerobic central nervous system infections

- drug of choice for organisms resistant to penicillin (*Bacteroides fragilis*), as the excellent central nervous system penetration provides a distinct advantage over clindamycin and antianaerobic beta-lactams (cefoxitin, ceftizoxime, cefotetan, and piperacillin)
- gram-positive anaerobes (*Peptococcus* and *Peptostreptococcus*) are less susceptible to metronidazole

Pseudomembranous colitis due to *Clostridium difficile*

- recommended initial treatment of choice for pseudomembranous colitis, as it is much less expensive and as effective as vancomycin (Lancet 1983;2:1043–1046)
- most effective when administered orally

Crohn's disease

- widely used in the perianal disease that may accompany Crohn's disease, although the reports of its efficacy are anecdotal
- as effective as sulfasalazine in 1 study (Gastroenterology 1982: 83:550), but it is generally used only when the other short-term agents such as mesalamine and steroids have failed because efficacy has not been definitively demonstrated and long-term toxicities (neuropathies) are common

Infective endocarditis

- if anaerobes such as *B. fragilis* are suspected or found on culture
- anaerobes are rare in endocarditis

Surgical prophylaxis

- for second-trimester instillation abortion in patients allergic to penicillins

Gastrointestinal parasitic infestations

- drug of choice for giardiasis, amebiasis, and dracunculiasis

▶ When Should I Not Use This Drug?

- infections with anaerobic cocci demonstrated to be resistant to the drug (use clindamycin)

▶ What Contraindications Are There to the Use of This Drug?

Intolerance of or allergic reaction to metronidazole

- disulfiram-like reaction may produce an "alcohol flush" in a patient who refuses to discontinue concurrent alcohol use

▶ What Drug Interactions Are Clinically Important?

Drugs that may increase the effect or toxicity of metronidazole

ALCOHOL

- metronidazole and alcohol used together may cause a disulfiram-like reaction, consisting of symptoms such as flushing, palpitation, nausea, vomiting, and tachycardia

- although this interaction does not occur frequently, patients should be told to avoid all alcohol until at least 1 day after stopping metronidazole administration
- this interaction has also been reported with the topical use of metronidazole

Drugs that may decrease the effect of metronidazole

- none

Drugs that may have their effect or toxicity increased by metronidazole

WARFARIN

- interferes with warfarin metabolism and can increase INR
- use alternative agents if possible
- if not, monitor INR every 2 days until the full extent of interaction is seen and adjust the dosage as for a warfarin dosage change
- monitor INR every 2 days when metronidazole administration is discontinued and adjust as needed

PHENYTOIN

- inhibits the metabolism of phenytoin and may produce increases in serum phenytoin concentrations
- monitor serum phenytoin measurements weekly until a new steady state is established or symptoms of toxicity occur and adjust the dosage accordingly
- when metronidazole administration is stopped, return to the previous phenytoin dosage

Drugs that may have their effect decreased by metronidazole

- none

▶ What Route and Dosage Should I Use?

How to administer

- orally—can be given with food in an attempt to minimize gastrointestinal effects
- parenterally—premixed solution contains 500 mg in 100 mL; infuse over a minimum of 20 minutes

Vaginitis

- 500 mg PO BID for bacterial vaginosis
- 2 g PO as a single dose for trichomoniasis

Intraabdominal infections, acute or chronic osteomyelitis, cellulitis, anaerobic sepsis, anaerobic central nervous system infections, infective endocarditis

- 500 mg IV Q8H
- 500 mg PO Q8H when the patient is able to tolerate oral medications

Pseudomembranous colitis due to *Clostridium difficile*

- 250 mg PO QID

Crohn's disease

- 250 mg PO TID
- 500 mg PO TID for severe or perianal disease

Surgical prophylaxis

- 500 mg IV as a single dose

Gastrointestinal parasitic infestations

Giardiasis

- 250 mg PO Q8H

Amebiasis

- 750 mg PO Q8H

Dracunculiasis

- 250 mg PO Q8H

Dosage adjustments for renal or hepatic dysfunction

- hepatically metabolized
- no dosage adjustments needed
- metabolites may accumulate in patients with renal failure, and these may be responsible for seizures and peripheral neuropathy

- use for the shortest period possible in patients with renal dysfunction

▶ What Should I Monitor with Regard to Efficacy and Toxicity?

Efficacy

- for antibiotic administration monitoring guidelines, see specific section on drug therapy

Crohn's disease

- relief of gastrointestinal symptoms, decrease in pain and discharge, and healing of fistulas and ulcers

Toxicity

Neurological effects—seizures and peripheral neuropathy

- neuropathy characterized by numbness and paresthesias can occur with long-term use
- try not to use for longer than 3 months, as many patients experience subclinical peripheral neuropathy
- if possible, stop the drug administration if it occurs
- some patients may wish to continue use of this drug for Crohn's disease, despite this adverse effect

Gastrointestinal symptoms (nausea or vomiting, metallic taste)

- question the patient about the appearance of these symptoms daily while the patient is in the hospital

Vaginal overgrowth with *Candida*

- question the patient about the appearance of symptoms of vaginitis (itching, discharge) daily while the patient is in the hospital
- if this occurs, stop the drug administration and treat with an anticandidal agent

▶ How Long Do I Treat Patients with This Drug?

Vaginitis

- 7 days for bacterial vaginosis
- single dose for trichomoniasis

Intraabdominal infections

- treatment should continue for a minimum of 10 days; however, extend if the patient has not been asymptomatic for longer than 72 hours

Cellulitis, anaerobic sepsis

- usual duration is 10 days or 4–5 days after the patient has become afebrile and has clinically improved
- if using parenteral therapy, consider switching to oral therapy after the patient has become afebrile and has clinically improved for 1–2 days

Acute or chronic osteomyelitis

- treat patients with at least 4 weeks of parenteral antibiotics after debridement surgery (the duration of therapy is based on the patient's clinical response)
- if an amputation is done proximal to the site of the infection, only prophylactic antibiotics are required (Hosp Formul 1993;28: 63–85)
- if the bone is removed and there is still evidence of soft tissue infection, the patient should receive a 2 week course of antibiotics
- treat patients with a prosthetic device for 4–6 weeks with parenteral antibiotics followed by 3–6 months of oral antibiotics
- treat patients with peripheral vascular disease with at least 4 weeks of parenteral antibiotics and follow with oral antibiotics until there is no evidence of inflammation (on the basis of clinical or radiological evidence) (Am J Med 1987;83:653–660)
- duration of parenteral antibiotic therapy prior to switching to oral therapy depends on the patient's clinical response

Anaerobic central nervous system infections

- 6–8 weeks for brain abscess

Pseudomembranous colitis due to *Clostridium difficile*

- treat for 10 days, with a minimum of 72 hours without diarrhea

Crohn's disease

- 8 weeks; in perianal disease, much longer therapy may be needed, as drainage may increase and many of the perianal symptoms quickly return when metronidazole administration is stopped

Infective endocarditis

- 6 weeks for anaerobes such as *B. fragilis*

Surgical prophylaxis

- single dose

Gastrointestinal parasitic infestations

Giardiasis

- 5 days

Amebiasis, dracunculiasis

- 10 days

▶ How Do I Decrease or Stop the Administration of This Drug?

- may be stopped abruptly

▶ What Should I Tell My Patients About This Drug?

- let your physician or pharmacist know if you have had any sort of reaction to this type of drug in the past (use trade names as cues)
- contact your physician if symptoms do not improve during next few days or weeks
- if you have shakiness, numbness, or tingling sensations in the arms or legs, contact your physician immediately
- do not drink alcoholic beverages during administration of this drug and for the day afterward
- take the medication until it is completely finished

▶ Therapeutic Tips

- use Q8H dosing regimens, not Q6H (some clinicians suggest that this agent can be dosed Q12H)
- for Crohn's disease, be prepared for early reports of side effects, but be aware that these may not persist

Useful References

Scully BE. Metronidazole. Med Clin North Am 1988;72:613–621
Hamill HA. Metronidazole, clindamycin, and quinolones. Obstet Gynecol Clin North Am 1989;16:317–328

MEXILETINE

James Tisdale

USA (Mexitil)
CANADA (Mexitil)

▶ When Should I Use This Drug?

Mexiletine should not be used without consulting a cardiologist or a cardiac electrophysiologist

Ventricular tachycardia

- prevention of recurrent symptomatic or sustained ventricular tachycardia (VT) in patients in whom therapy with quinidine, procainamide, or disopyramide alone is determined to be ineffective and in whom mexiletine is shown to suppress or to favorably modify inducible VT during electrophysiological (EP) testing or Holter monitoring
- in combination with quinidine, procainamide, or disopyramide for the prevention of symptomatic or sustained VT in patients in whom therapy with 1 of those agents alone has been ineffective, and in whom the combination has been shown to suppress or to favorably modify inducible VT during EP testing or Holter monitoring

▶ When Should I Not Use This Drug?

Asymptomatic ventricular arrhythmias

- no evidence that treatment is beneficial

Supraventricular arrhythmias

- mexiletine is not effective for the treatment of supraventricular arrhythmias

▶ *What Contraindications Are There to the Use of This Drug?*

Intolerance of or allergic reaction to mexiletine

- mexiletine is contraindicated in patients who have previously experienced hypersensitivity reactions to mexiletine or to ether-type local anesthetics

Atrioventricular nodal block

- mexiletine is contraindicated in patients with second- or third-degree atrioventricular block unless a functioning ventricular pacemaker is present

▶ *What Drug Interactions Are Clinically Important?*

Drugs that may increase the effect or toxicity of mexiletine

- none

Drugs that may decrease the effect or toxicity of mexiletine

PHENYTOIN

- phenytoin induces the hepatic metabolism of mexiletine
- patients receiving mexiletine in whom phenytoin therapy is initiated should be monitored for recurrence of arrhythmias and a serum mexiletine concentration should be obtained within 3 days of starting phenytoin

RIFAMPIN

- rifampin induces the hepatic metabolism of mexiletine
- patients receiving mexiletine in whom rifampin therapy is initiated should be monitored for recurrence of arrhythmias and a serum mexiletine concentration should be obtained within 3 days of starting rifampin

Drugs that may have their effect or toxicity increased by mexiletine

THEOPHYLLINE

- mexiletine therapy has been reported to result in elevations in plasma theophylline concentrations of approximately 100%
- in patients receiving theophylline in whom mexiletine therapy is initiated, the theophylline dosage should be decreased 50%, and a plasma theophylline concentration should be determined 3 days after the initiation of mexiletine therapy

Drugs that may have their effect or toxicity decreased by mexiletine

- none

▶ *What Route and Dosage Should I Use?*

How to administer

- orally—administer with food to minimize gastrointestinal upset
- parenterally—unavailable

Ventricular tachycardia

- start with 200 mg PO Q8H
- increase the dosage by 50 mg PO Q8H every 4 days to the maximum recommended dosage of 400 mg Q8H if arrhythmia is not controlled

Dosage adjustments for renal or hepatic dysfunction

- hepatically metabolized
- in patients with severe hepatic dysfunction, the initial dosage should be 200 mg Q12H and dosage increases may be performed as above, but doses should be administered Q12H rather than Q8H
- dosage reduction in patients with renal dysfunction is not necessary

▶ *What Should I Monitor with Regard to Efficacy and Toxicity?*

Efficacy

Ventricular tachycardia

see Quinidine

Serum concentrations

- therapeutic range of mexiletine is usually quoted as 0.75–2 μg/mL
- range of serum mexiletine concentrations required for efficacy varies widely among patients, and therefore, the therapeutic range is of relatively little use in monitoring the efficacy of mexiletine
- if therapeutic monitoring is performed use the method of monitoring target serum mexiletine concentrations (see Quinidine) (Clin Pharmacokinet 1991;20:151–166)

Toxicity

Adverse effects necessitating discontinuation of therapy occur in approximately 7–35% of patients

Nausea, vomiting, abdominal pain, and neurological adverse effects such as tremor, dizziness, fatigue, diplopia, and seizures

- mexiletine therapy should be discontinued in patients who experience seizures, new cardiac arrhythmias, or worsening of clinical arrhythmias
- mexiletine dosage should be decreased in patients who experience adverse gastrointestinal or neurological effects
- mexiletine dosage should be decreased by 50 mg Q8H unless the patient is receiving 400 mg Q8H, in which case, the dosage should be decreased by 100 mg Q8H

▶ *How Long Do I Treat Patients with This Drug?*

Ventricular tachycardia

- patients may require therapy indefinitely if contributing factors cannot be reversed

▶ *How Do I Decrease or Stop the Administration of This Drug?*

- mexiletine dosage should not be decreased or therapy discontinued without consulting a cardiologist or a cardiac electrophysiologist
- if mexiletine dosage is decreased, the patient should be monitored for recurrence of arrhythmias

▶ *What Should I Tell My Patients About This Drug?*

- mexiletine should be taken with food to minimize the likelihood of adverse gastrointestinal reactions
- if you have nausea, vomiting, abdominal pain, tremor, blurred vision, or severe fatigue, notify your physician
- if you have palpitations, shortness of breath, chest pain, or dizziness, contact your physician
- do not discontinue mexiletine therapy without consulting your physician

▶ *Therapeutic Tips*

- range of serum mexiletine concentrations required for efficacy varies widely among patients, and therefore, the therapeutic range is of relatively little use in monitoring the efficacy of mexiletine

Useful References

Monk JP, Brogden RN. Mexiletine. A review of its pharmacodynamic and pharmacokinetic properties, and therapeutic use in the treatment of arrhythmias. Drugs 1990;40:374–411

Impact Research Group. International mexiletine and placebo antiarrhythmic coronary trial: I. Report on arrhythmia and other findings. J Am Coll Cardiol 1984;4:1148–1163

Waspe LE, Waxman HL, Buxton AE, Josephson ME. Mexiletine for control of drug-resistant ventricular tachycardia: Clinical and electrophysiologic results in 44 patients. Am J Cardiol 1983;51:1175–1181

Greenspan AM, Spielman SR, Webb CR, et al. Efficacy of combination therapy with mexiletine and a type IA agent for inducible ventricular tachycardia secondary to coronary artery disease. Am J Cardiol 1985;56:277–284

MICONAZOLE

Peter Jewesson

USA (Monistat, Micatin)

CANADA (Micatin, Monistat)

▶ *When Should I Use This Drug?*

Systemic treatment of *Pseudoallescheria boydii* infections

- parenteral formulation considered to be drug of choice but comparative trials lacking
- systemic miconazole is poorly tolerated and associated with a high relapse rate; thus should be reserved for conditions not responsive to other antifungal drugs

Vaginal candidiasis

- topical miconazole/clotrimazole/terconazole are all effective and can be given as a short 3 day course of therapy
- choice between these agents should be on the basis of cost

▶ *When Should I Not Use This Drug?*

- treatment of infections involving pathogens known to be resistant to miconazole

▶ *What Contraindications Are There to the Use of This Drug?*

Intolerance or allergic reaction to miconazole or other azole agents

Pregnancy or lactation

- miconazole is teratogenic in rat model; effects on breast-feeding infant are unknown

▶ *What Drug Interactions Are Clinically Important?*

Drugs that may increase the effect or toxicity of miconazole

- none

Drugs that may decrease the effect of miconazole

RIFAMPIN AND ISONIAZID

- rifampin and isoniazid decrease serum concentrations of other azoles by stimulating hepatic metabolism
- effect may exist with miconazole when given systemically
- if existing parenteral dose ineffective, consider increasing dose to a maximum of 1200 mg IV Q8H

Drugs that may have their effect or toxicity increased by miconazole

WARFARIN

- systemic azoles interfere with warfarin metabolism and can increase PT
- use alternative agents if possible
- if not, monitor PT every 2 days until full extent of interaction is seen and adjust dose as you would with a warfarin dose change
- monitor PT every 2 days when interacting drug is discontinued and adjust as normal

CYCLOSPORINE

- although no reports of systemic miconazole inhibiting the metabolism of this agent, other azoles inhibit hepatic metabolism of cyclosporine
- expect as early as 2 days after the start of these drugs
- use alternative if possible
- monitor cyclosporine levels every other day until full extent of interaction is seen and adjust dose accordingly

PHENYTOIN

- although no reports of systemic miconazole inhibiting the metabolism of this agent, other azoles inhibit hepatic metabolism of phenytoin and may produce increases in serum phenytoin concentrations
- monitor serum phenytoin measurements weekly until a new steady-state is established or if symptoms of toxicity occur, and adjust dose accordingly
- if the azole is stopped, return to previous acceptable dose

TOLBUTAMIDE

- although there are no reports of systemic miconazole inhibiting the metabolism of this agent, other azoles inhibit hepatic metabolism of cyclosporine
- if miconazole is added to tolbutamide therapy, monitor blood glucose daily for first 3–4 days and adjust dose of tolbutamide accordingly

Drugs that may have their effect decreased by miconazole

- none

▶ *What Route and Dosage Should I Use?*

How to administer

- parenterally—dilute injectable solution in 100 mL to 250 mL of normal saline or D_5W and administer at a rate of 2 mL/min

Systemic treatment of *Pseudoallescheria boydii* infections

- 200 mg Q8H IV starting dose and increase to maximum of 25–30 mg/kg/day IV (high as 4 g daily) as tolerated by patient and according to clinical response

Vaginal candidiasis

- 200 mg vaginal suppository nightly for 3 nights

Dosage adjustment for renal or hepatic dysfunction

- eliminated by hepatic pathway
- no adjustment for renal insufficiency or dialysis

▶ *What Should I Monitor with Regard to Efficacy and Toxicity?*

Efficacy

- resolution of clinical signs and symptoms (e.g., reduced fever, inflammation, pain, erythema, associated discharge)
- negative follow-up cultures (where possible) provide additonal evidence of therapy success or failure

Toxicity

- primarily associated with systemic preparation

Cardiopulmonary toxicity

- severe anaphylactoid reactions reported after initial doses
- administer first dose with physician and anaphylaxis kit present (treat with pressor agents and antihistamines)

Thrombophlebitis

- likely associated with polyethoxylated castor oil vehicle
- administer by central vein where possible

Thrombocytosis

- elevated platelet count may occur
- monitor blood count as baseline and a minimum of once weekly during therapy
- discontinue drug if abnormality persists

Anemia

- normochromic or normocytic anemia reported
- monitor blood count at baseline and a minimum of once weekly during therapy
- discontinue drug if abnormality persists

Hyperlipidemia

- likely associated with polyethoxylated castor oil vehicle

Hyponatremia

- possibly associated with SIADH in patients with CNS infection
- monitor serum sodium concentrations a minimum of once every 72 hours while on therapy

Mild localized reactions

- stinging, erythema, urticaria, edema, desquamation, pruritus, and vesication when applied to skin

▶ *How Long Do I Treat Patients with This Drug?*

Systemic treatment of *Pseudoallescheria boydii* infections

- until clinically improved and repeat cultures, if any, are negative
- optimal duration of therapy unknown

Vaginal candidiasis

- 3 days

▶ *How Do I Decrease or Stop the Administration of This Drug?*

- may stop drug abruptly

▶ *What Should I Tell My Patients About This Drug?*

- this agent is an antifungal agent and successful therapy is contingent upon completion of the full treatment course
- some minor side effects (i.e., gastrointestinal or reversible liver changes) can be expected but these are usually self-limiting and therapy should not be stopped; contact pharmacist or physician if any symptoms arise

Useful Reference

Bennett JE. Antifungal agents. In: Mandell GL, Douglas RG, Jr, Bennett JE, eds. Principles and Practice of Infectious Diseases, 3rd ed. New York: Churchill Livingstone, 1990:361–370

MINERAL OIL

Leslie Mathews

USA (Fleet Mineral Oil Enema)
CANADA (Fleet Mineral Oil Enema)

▶ *When Should I Use This Drug?*

Fecal impaction

- mineral oil enemas are useful for impaction when sodium phosphate enemas are contraindicated, not effective, or not recommended (e.g., sensitivity to fluid and electrolyte changes, renal disease, hypocalcemia, abnormal colonic mucosa, and congestive heart failure)
- effective at softening stool when used in conjunction with sodium phosphate or tap water enemas, and manual disimpaction

▶ *When Should I Not Use This Drug?*

Chronic constipation

- avoid regular use because of impairment of normal rectal reflexes
- oil droplets can cause anal pruritus, resulting in scratching

Oral use

- associated with lipoid pneumonia and malabsorption of fat-soluble vitamins

▶ *What Contraindications Are There to the Use of This Drug?*

Intolerance of or allergic reaction to mineral oil
Symptoms of acute abdomen

- undiagnosed abdominal pain, nausea, and vomiting

▶ *What Drug Interactions Are Clinically Important?*

- none with rectal administration

▶ *What Route and Dosage Should I Use?*

How to administer

Orally

- do not use

Parenterally

- do not use

Rectally

- to administer, the patient should lie on the left side or in the knee-chest position and gently insert the prelubricated nozzle into the rectum toward the navel and squeeze the bottle slowly
- patient should remain reclining until abdominal cramping is felt, at which time rectal contents can be expelled

Fecal impaction

- 120–135 mL enema given as a single dose

Dosage adjustments for renal and hepatic dysfunction

- negligible amounts absorbed; adjustments not required

▶ *What Should I Monitor with Regard to Efficacy and Toxicity?*

Efficacy

Fecal impaction

- softens stool and elicits bowel movement within 30–60 minutes

Toxicity

Pruritus ani, hemorrhoids, cryptitis from oil leakage

- avoid large doses, divide doses, and use a stable emulsion
- monitor for perianal disease

▶ *How Long Do I Treat Patients with This Drug?*

Fecal impaction

- usually given as a single dose

▶ *How Do I Decrease or Stop the Administration of This Drug?*

- may be stopped abruptly

▶ *What Should I Tell My Patients About This Drug?*

- may leak through the anal sphincter and soil clothes; therefore, use a perineal pad when necessary
- do not use on a regular basis

Useful Reference

Tedesco FJ. Laxative use in constipation. Am J Gastroenterol 1985;80: 303–309

MINOCYCLINE

Alfred Gin and George Zhanel

USA (Minocin)
CANADA (Minocin)

▶ *When Should I Use This Drug?*

Consider an alternative agent

- minocycline offers no advantage over tetracycline or doxycycline for the treatment of any infectious disease
- minocycline also causes vestibular toxicity (dizziness, ataxia, and nausea or vomiting), which occurs commonly at the start of therapy
- minocycline has been used to eradicate the meningococcal carrier state; however, ciprofloxacin may be used for this indication

MISOPROSTOL

James McCormack and Glen Brown

USA (Cytotec)
CANADA (Cytotec)

▶ *When Should I Use This Drug?*

Prevention of nonsteroidal antiinflammatory drug–induced ulcers

- consider prophylactic therapy in patients on taking nonsteroidal antiinflammatory drugs (NSAIDs) who are older than 60 years of age, have a past history of peptic ulcer, are also receiving corticosteroids or anticoagulants, or would be poor surgical risks if ulcer complications occur (Mayo Clin Proc 1992;67:354–364)
- not required for all patients receiving NSAIDs
- misoprostol has been shown to be effective in preventing endoscopically proven NSAID ulceration (Lancet 1988;2:1277–1280), and other agents have generally been no better than placebo in preventing endoscopically proven gastric ulcers (Mayo Clin Proc 1992;67:354–364)
- at present, there is no published evidence that misoprostol prevents ulcer complications and death (Am J Gastroenterol 1991; 86:264–266)
- for all patients receiving NSAIDs ensure they are on the lowest effective dose and/or that acetaminophen in appropriate doses (up to 1 g PO QID) is ineffective

▶ *When Should I Not Use This Drug?*

Duodenal or gastric ulcers

- misoprostol is no more effective than H_2 antagonists, but is more expensive than cimetidine, is dosed 4 times per day compared with once to twice a day with other agents, and produces a higher incidence of side effects

Combination with other antiulcer medications

- no studies support combination therapy of regularly dosed upper gastrointestinal tract drugs for the treatment of peptic ulcer disease, and combinations increase cost and the chance of adverse effects (Lancet 1988;1:1383–1385, N Engl J Med 1991;325:1017–1025, Am J Gastroenterol 1993;88:675–679)

All patients taking NSAIDs

- unnecessary for primary prophylaxis in all patients as it is expensive and causes a high incidence of diarrhea (JAMA 1990;264:41–47, Br J Rheumatol 1990;29:133–136)

▶ *What Contraindications Are There to the Use of This Drug?*

Intolerance of or allergic reaction to misoprostol

Pregnancy

- 11% of women had partial or complete expulsion of uterine contents and 45% had increases in frequency and intensity of uterine contractions and bleeding when misoprostol was administered in the first trimester (Dig Dis Sci 1986;[suppl 2]:475–545)

▶ *What Drug Interactions Are Clinically Important?*

- none

▶ *What Route and Dosage Should I Use?*

How to administer

- orally—take with food or milk

Prevention of NSAID-induced ulcers

- 200 µg PO QID, and if not tolerated (diarrhea), decrease the dosage to 100 µg PO QID
- many clinicians start with 100 µg PO QID
- 200 µg QID is likely more effective at reducing the incidence of endoscopically proven ulcers than 100 µg QID

Dosage adjustments for renal or hepatic dysfunction

- hepatically metabolized
- no dosage adjustment recommendations available for hepatic dysfunction

▶ *What Should I Monitor with Regard to Efficacy and Toxicity?*

Efficacy

Prevention of NSAID-induced ulcers

- signs and symptoms of peptic ulcer disease

Toxicity

Gastrointestinal effects

Nausea and vomiting, abdominal pain

- usually minor and self-limited

Diarrhea

- is the most common adverse effect, occurring in 10% of patients, and is severe enough in 1% of patients to warrant discontinuation of therapy
- if diarrhea occurs, reduce the dosage by 50%

▶ *How Long Do I Treat Patients with This Drug?*

Prevention of NSAID-induced ulcers

- therapy should be continued for as long as the NSAID is prescribed (Br J Rheumatol 1990;29:133–136)

▶ *How Do I Decrease or Stop the Administration of This Drug?*

- may be stopped abruptly

▶ *What Should I Tell My Patients About This Drug?*

- this drug may cause diarrhea, and if it is not too severe, continue with therapy as tolerance may develop; however, if it is severe or tolerance does not develop, see your physician
- this drug should be continued while you are receiving NSAIDs, but if administration of NSAIDs is stopped, this drug should be stopped

▶ *Therapeutic Tips*

- if the patient is receiving concomitant NSAIDs, ensure that the patient is taking the lowest dosage possible of NSAIDs
- many patients, especially the elderly, require lower dosages of NSAIDs because of decreased clearance

MORICIZINE

James Tisdale

USA (Ethmozine)
CANADA (not available)

▶ *When Should I Use This Drug?*

Moricizine should not be used without consulting a cardiologist or a cardiac electrophysiologist

Ventricular tachycardia

- moricizine should be used for the suppression of recurrent, symptomatic or life-threatening ventricular tachycardia in patients in whom the following conditions apply: no history of myocardial infarction (MI) or ischemic heart disease; failure to respond to therapy with class IA (quinidine or procainamide), class IB (mexiletine or tocainide) and/or the combination of class IA and IB antiarrhythmic agents during serial drug testing in the electrophysiology laboratory or during Holter monitoring; physician and/or patient wishes to delay amiodarone or nonpharmacological therapy; and moricizine has been shown to suppress or to favorably modify inducible ventricular tachycardia during electrophysiological testing or during Holter monitoring
- use before propafenone for ventricular tachycardia, because moricizine does not have dose-dependent pharmacokinetics

▶ *When Should I Not Use This Drug?*

Asymptomatic ventricular arrhythmias

- treatment of asymptomatic ventricular arrhythmias has not been shown to be of benefit (N Engl J Med 1989;321:406–412)

Supraventricular arrhythmias

- not enough data to support its use for this indication

▶ *What Contraindications Are There to the Use of This Drug?*

Intolerance of or allergic reaction to moricizine

Atrioventricular block

- moricizine impairs conduction of electrical impulses through the atrioventricular (AV) node and, therefore, should not be used in patients with second- or third-degree AV block in the absence of a functioning ventricular pacemaker
- drug may be used in patients with first-degree AV block, but the electrocardiogram should be evaluated within 2 days for progression of AV block

Bundle branch blocks

- moricizine slows impulse conduction through the His-Purkinje system and, therefore, should not be used in patients with bifascicular or trifascicular bundle branch blocks unless a functioning ventricular pacemaker is present

History of myocardial infarction

- moricizine has been shown to adversely influence mortality if administered within 2 weeks of an acute MI (N Engl J Med 1992;327:227–233)

▶ *What Drug Interactions Are Clinically Important?*

Drugs that may increase the effect or toxicity of moricizine

CIMETIDINE

- cimetidine therapy may result in impaired clearance of moricizine of about 50%
- it is best to use an H_2 antagonist (ranitidine, famotidine, nizatidine) that has little if any effect on hepatic metabolism
- if cimetidine is being used as only a single 400 mg nighttime dose, the effect is minimal

Drugs that may decrease the effect or toxicity of moricizine

- none

Drugs that may have their effect or toxicity increased by moricizine

- none

Drugs that may have their effect or toxicity decreased by moricizine

THEOPHYLLINE

- moricizine is an inducer of hepatic oxidative metabolizing enzymes and has been shown to increase the clearance of theophylline by approximately 46–68%
- in patients receiving theophylline in whom moricizine therapy is initiated, the patient should be instructed to report worsening of respiratory symptoms, and the theophylline dosage should be increased if necessary

▶ *What Route and Dosage Should I Use?*

How to administer

- orally—administer with or without food
- parenterally—unavailable

Ventricular tachycardia

- 200 mg PO Q8H
- dosage may be increased if necessary in 72 hours to 250 mg Q8H if arrhythmia is not controlled
- dosage may be further increased if necessary to the maximum recommended dosage of 300 mg Q8H if arrhythmia is not controlled

Dosage adjustments for renal or hepatic dysfunction

- hepatically metabolized
- dosage does not need to be reduced in patients with renal dysfunction
- in patients with hepatic dysfunction titrate the dose on the basis of effect and toxicity

▶ *What Should I Monitor with Regard to Efficacy and Toxicity?*

Efficacy

Ventricular tachycardia

see Quinidine

Serum concentrations

- serum moricizine concentrations do not correlate well with efficacy and are neither necessary nor available

Toxicity

- adverse effects necessitating discontinuation of therapy occur in approximately 9% of patients

Dizziness, nausea, headache, and fatigue

- moricizine dosage should be reduced by 50 mg Q8H if patients experience dizziness or nausea
- moricizine therapy should be discontinued if patients have signs or symptoms of congestive heart failure, new cardiac arrhythmias or worsening of the clinical arrhythmia, second- or third-degree heart block, or bifascicular or trifascicular block

Congestive heart failure

- signs and symptoms should be evaluated at the first visit after the initiation of therapy

- although moricizine is considered relatively safe in patients with left ventricular dysfunction, a review reported exacerbation of congestive heart failure in 13% of treated patients with a history of left ventricular dysfunction

Electrocardiogram

- should be evaluated after 1 week of therapy to assess for prolonged PR interval (>0.2 second), prolonged duration of QRS complex (>25% increase compared with baseline values), or initiation of new arrhythmia or worsening of clinical arrhythmia
- if prolongation of the QRS interval of greater than 25% compared with baseline values occurs, the moricizine dosage should be reduced by 50 mg Q8H if patients have dizziness or nausea

▶ *How Long Do I Treat Patients With This Drug?*

Ventricular tachycardia

- moricizine therapy for recurrent, symptomatic or life-threatening ventricular tachycardia may be required indefinitely

▶ *How Do I Decrease or Stop the Administration of This Drug?*

- moricizine therapy should not be discontinued or dosage reduction performed without consulting a cardiologist or a cardiac electrophysiologist

▶ *What Should I Tell My Patients About This Drug?*

- do not discontinue this medication or change your dosage without consulting your physician
- notify your physician if you experience dizziness, nausea, fainting, palpitations, or shortness of breath while taking this medication
- because this drug may cause dizziness, do not drive or operate heavy machinery until it is determined how you will react to this medication

▶ *Therapeutic Tips*

- moricizine is capable of inducing its own hepatic metabolism, and moricizine clearance has been reported to increase by approximately 50% during the first 2 weeks of therapy
- during this period, patients should be monitored for arrhythmia recurrence and associated symptoms, and the dosage should be increased if necessary

Useful References

Kennedy HL. Noncardiac adverse effects and organ toxicity of moricizine during short- and long-term studies. Am J Cardiol 1990;65:47D–50D

Fitton A, Buckley MM-T. Moricizine. A review of its pharmacological properties, and therapeutic efficacy in cardiac arrhythmias. Drugs 1990;40:138–167

Mann HJ. Moricizine: A new class I antiarrhythmic. Clin Pharm 1990;9:842–852

MORPHINE

Terry Baumann

USA (Duramorph, MS Contin, RMS, Roxanol)
CANADA (Epimorph, Morphitec, M.O.S., MS Contin, Statex, M.O.S.-SR)

▶ *When Should I Use This Drug?*

Acute pain

- morphine is the drug of choice for severe symptoms because it is as effective and safe as other opioids when dosed appropriately
- is available in a large number of dosage forms

Chronic cancer pain

- drug of choice in all terminally ill patients when regular dosing at maximum doses with agents such as acetaminophen, acetaminophen-codeine, and nonsteroidal antiinflammatory drugs (NSAIDs) has not been effective (ensure that these drugs have been used at appropriate regular intervals)

Chronic noncancer pain

- when pain has not been responsive to other treatment modalities and agents such as acetaminophen, acetaminophen-codeine, and NSAIDs

Postoperative pain

- is the drug of choice for the treatment of postoperative pain because it is as effective as other opioids with a similar adverse effect profile, and comes in a large number of dosage forms

Post–myocardial ischemia pain

- provides analgesic effect plus reduces myocardial oxygen demand by reducing ventricular preload but blocks the patient's perception of pain, which is an important indication of ischemia

► When Should I Not Use This Drug?

Mild to moderate pain (acute or chronic)

- unless drugs such as acetaminophen, acetaminophen-codeine, and NSAIDs have been used on a regularly scheduled basis (not PRN) and are shown to be ineffective

► What Contraindications Are There to the Use of This Drug?

Intolerance of or allergic reaction to morphine

- true allergies to morphine are rare
- check that the patient has actual allergic symptoms, and if there is a true allergy, consider meperidine, methadone, or fentanyl

Respiratory depression

- not an absolute contraindication; just start with dosages 25% of the normal initial dose and titrate up to effect while assessing respiratory rate and oximetry before each dose

► What Drug Interactions Are Clinically Important?

Drugs that may increase the effect or toxicity of morphine

CENTRAL NERVOUS SYSTEM DEPRESSANTS (i.e., ALCOHOL, BENZODIAZEPINES, AND ANTIDEPRESSANTS)

- if used concomitantly, titrate the morphine dose as below but be aware of the increased potential for excessive sedation and decreased respiratory rate

Drugs that may decrease the effect of morphine

OPIOID AGONIST OR ANTAGONISTS (PENTAZOCINE, NALBUPHINE, BUPRENORPHINE, BUTORPHANOL)

- difficult to titrate the morphine dose if patients are already receiving these agents, and concomitant administration may precipitate withdrawal symptoms; therefore, never use these agents with morphine

NALOXONE

- used to reverse opioid overdose but also reverse analgesic effect

Drugs that may have their effect or toxicity increased by morphine

CENTRAL NERVOUS SYSTEM DEPRESSANTS (i.e., ALCOHOL, BENZODIAZEPINES, AND ANTIDEPRESSANTS)

- if used concomitantly, titrate the morphine dose as below but be aware of the increased potential for excessive sedation and decreased respiratory rate

Drugs that may have their effect decreased by morphine

- none

► What Route and Dosage Should I Use?

How to administer

- orally—may be administered with food or milk or on an empty stomach
- parenterally—may be administered intramuscularly, intravenously (dilute IV morphine in 10 mL of normal saline and give over at least 1 minute), subcutaneously (undiluted), epidurally (preservative-free morphine given over 1 minute by push or with an infusion device for continual infusion)

Acute pain

- 20 mg PO Q4H (not PRN), or 10 mg PO Q4H (not PRN) for elderly patients because of concerns about sedation and respiratory depression
- consider giving oral morphine if the patient is able to tolerate oral medications because it is less expensive than parenteral administration and has high patient and nurse acceptability, but the oral route has a slightly slower onset (30–60 minutes) than the intramuscular (15–30 minutes) or intravenous route (1–5 minutes)
- 10 mg IM or SC Q4H (not PRN), or 5 mg IM or SC Q4H (not PRN) for elderly patients because of concerns about sedation and respiratory depression
- question patients frequently about the degree of pain they are having (ideally, within at most 1–2 hours after the first dose if the drug was administered via the oral or intramuscular route)
- if pain is unrelieved by this time and there are no signs of sedation or respiratory depression, give another dose 50% higher than the first dose
- continue this approach until pain is 75% relieved and then maintain at this dosage for 12 hours before further adjustments are made
- normal dosage increments are 5 and 10 mg
- if an immediate response (within 1–5 minutes) for severe pain is needed, use intravenously as recommended for postoperative pain

Chronic cancer pain, chronic noncancer pain

In a patient who has received only weak opioids in the past

- 10 mg PO Q4H (not PRN), or 5 mg PO Q4H for elderly patients because of concerns about sedation and respiratory depression
- almost always give by mouth unless the patient has uncontrollable nausea or vomiting
- oral route is inexpensive and has high patient and nurse acceptability

In a patient being switched from another opioid

- determine the average daily requirements for the previously administered opioids and determine the 24 hour morphine equivalent (the accompanying table is just a guide; after switching drugs, always adjust the dosage up or down on the basis of the patient's response)

*Opioid equivalents**

Opioid	Equipotent Parenteral Doses (mg)	Equipotent Oral Doses (mg)	Duration (h)
morphine	10	20–30	4–5
meperidine	75	150	3–5
hydromorphone	1.3	4	4–5
buprenorphine	0.3	N/A	4–8
codeine	130	100	4–6
methadone	10	10–20	4–8
nalbuphine	10	N/A	3–6
propoxyphene	N/A	130	4–6
oxycodone	N/A	15	4–5
fentanyl	0.1	N/A	1–2

* See section on pain in Chapter 6 or specific drug monographs for starting doses.
N/A = not available.

- 24 hour requirements for morphine should be divided by 6 and given every 4 hours
- if the previous opioid dosage has not been effective, the total daily dose of morphine should be increased by 25–50%
- adjust the dosage as above for acute pain
- attempt to get pain at least 90% controlled
- after pain has been controlled, always order PRN doses at 25–50% of the maintenance dosage, in addition to the maintenance dosage, for breakthrough pain

Sustained-release morphine

- when good pain control is achieved with the regular-release morphine, switch to a sustained-release morphine preparation

- dosage is determined by the daily morphine requirements
- give the same total daily dose but as a sustained-release form every 12 hours
- if pain appears to return in the last 4 hours of the 12 hour dosing interval, change the interval to Q8H at the same daily dosage
- always use sustained-release morphine with an order for rapid-release oral morphine (approximately ⅙ of the sustained-release dosage) for breakthrough pain

Continuous infusion (intravenous or subcutaneous)

- initial infusion rate should be based on previous 24 hour opioid requirements
- 2–5 mg bolus may be administered hourly on a PRN basis, with a subsequent 10–20% increase in the hourly rate
- additional 5–10 mg bolus doses may be given on a PRN basis without a subsequent increase in the hourly rate when patients are subjected to or perform exceptionally painful activities

Postoperative pain

In the postanesthetic care unit

- 2.5 mg IV repeated every 5 minutes PRN
- adjust the dosage on the basis of response to each dose and titrate to pain control and the desired level of sedation or respiratory rate

On the ward

Intermittent therapy

- as above for acute pain
- use the parenteral route initially, but switch to the oral route as soon as the patient is able to take agents orally (usually 24–36 hours postoperatively)
- question the patient frequently and increase the dosage on the basis of pain relief and level of sedation (as above for acute pain)

Patient-controlled analgesia

- 1 mg/bolus with lockout time of 6 minutes
- some clinicians believe that 1–2 mg/h as an infusion with patient-controlled analgesia enables patients to sleep through the night; however, evidence suggests that using a bolus with a baseline infusion may increase the amount of narcotic used and the side effects, without improving efficacy (Anaesth Intensive Care 1991;19:555–560, Anesthesiology 1992;76:362–367)
- question the patient every 1–2 hours about the degree of pain
- if pain is not controlled with bolus doses, increase the bolus dose by 25–50%
- if pain relief from a bolus is adequate but the duration of pain relief is too short, decrease the lockout period

Epidural or intrathecal use

- can be used as an alternative to parenteral routes but these routes should be used only by anesthetists skilled in this technique
- 8 mg epidural as a single dose (0.2 mg intrathecal as a single dose) with breakthrough pain treated as above with oral or parenteral opioids
- epidural morphine can also be given as a continuous infusion

Post–myocardial ischemia pain

- 2 mg IV every 5 minutes PRN for relief of chest pain
- adjust the dosage on the basis of response to each dose and titrate to achieve pain control and an adequate level of sedation and respiratory rate
- IM injections should be avoided because they can raise creatine kinase values further, and serious IM bleeding can occur in anticoagulated patients

Dosage adjustments for renal or hepatic dysfunction

- hepatically metabolized
- dosage adjustment is usually not required if the dose is titrated properly
- one of morphine's metabolites (morphine-6-glucuronide) has been associated with respiratory depression in patients with renal failure

Normal Dosing Interval	$C_{cr} > 60$ mL/min or 1 mL/s	C_{cr} 30–60 mL/min or 0.5–1 mL/s	$C_{cr} < 30$ mL/min or 0.5 mL/s
Q4H	no adjustment needed	adjust dose on basis of response	adjust dose on basis of response

▶ *What Should I Monitor with Regard to Efficacy and Toxicity?*

Efficacy

Acute pain, chronic cancer pain, chronic noncancer pain, postoperative pain, post–myocardial ischemia pain

Subjective pain evaluation

- key to achieving effective pain control is to question patients frequently about the degree of pain they are having
- frequency of pain evaluation should be based on the knowledge of how quickly the drug should work
- 10 cm visual analog score can be used to observe trends in pain control over time and can be useful
- decision to give PRN doses or to increase the dosage should be made on the basis of the patient's assessment of the severity of pain and the duration of effect
- remember that pain is whatever the patient says it is
- when a patient's self-assessment is not possible, monitor physical signs (i.e., agitation, heart rate)

Toxicity

Respiratory depression

- significant respiratory depression is rarely seen when the dose of opioids is titrated appropriately
- assess respiratory rate before each dose during the titration period
- if respiratory rate is less than 10 breaths per minute, withhold the dose and decrease subsequent doses by 25–50%
- if respiratory depression becomes clinically important, stop the administration and give naloxone 0.1 mg IV every 2–3 minutes PRN; however, be aware that naloxone can also reverse the analgesic effect

Sedation

- assess the level of sedation before every dose during the titration period
- if the patient is overly sedated yet has good pain control, withhold the dose (or the infusion or bolus dose for patient-controlled analgesia) for 1–2 hours and decrease subsequent doses by 25%
- some sedation may be required early in therapy to gain control over severe chronic pain but patients' tolerance of the sedation develops during a few days to a week

Dizziness, euphoria, and dysphoria

- common adverse effects in first few days
- if effects persist after 2–3 days, gradually (over 1–2 days), decrease the dosage

Constipation

- most troublesome adverse effect, especially if opioids are to be used regularly for longer than 2–3 days
- for anticipated long-term therapy with narcotics, initiate prophylaxis with a fiber and bulk-forming laxative (i.e., psyllium hydrophilic mucilloid 1 teaspoon in 240 mL of fluid BID)
- if bulk-forming laxatives are contraindicated or ineffective after a 2–3 day trial, initiate stimulant laxative therapy (bisacodyl 10 mg PO daily) and titrate the dose according to response

Nausea or vomiting

- patients should not get prophylactic antinauseants, as these agents can increase the risk of sedation and confusion
- if the patient experiences nausea or vomiting, and morphine administration cannot be stopped nor the dosage reduced, try an agent such as prochlorperazine or droperidol

Postural hypotension

- warn patients about this and tell them to sit up slowly
- maintain hydration

Urinary retention

- ask patients about this postoperatively (rarely a problem in chronic or cancer pain management)
- if this occurs, the patient may need to be catheterized

Biliary tract spasm

- if this causes the patient significant discomfort, switch to another opioid
- individual patients may not experience the same intolerance when switched to an alternative agent

Psychological dependence

- not a problem in patients with chronic pain due to a terminal illness when they are treated appropriately on a regularly scheduled basis (Sci Am 1990;262:27–33)
- should not be a problem in other patients with chronic pain who are not at risk for substance abuse

Physical dependence

- not a problem with short-term use (shorter than 2 weeks); however, when opioids are used for long periods, abruptly stopping administration may precipitate withdrawal symptoms such as restlessness, rhinorrhea, sweating, muscle cramps, insomnia, nausea, diarrhea, mydriasis, and reports of pain

▶ *How Long Do I Treat Patients with This Drug?*

Acute pain, postoperative pain, post–myocardial ischemia pain

- use on a regular basis (orally or parenterally) for the expected duration of the pain (e.g., 2–3 days for postoperative pain) and then switch to acetaminophen with codeine on a regular or PRN basis and let the patient determine the need
- if the patient requests regular doses of acetaminophen with codeine, write an order for regular Q4H acetaminophen with codeine

Chronic cancer pain, chronic noncancer pain

- therapy may be needed for months to years

▶ *How Do I Decrease or Stop the Administration of This Drug?*

After long-term use (e.g., longer than 2–3 weeks) if the drug administration needs to be stopped

- reduce the total daily dosage by 25% every 3–4 days, and this should decrease withdrawal symptoms due to any physical dependence that may have developed
- if the patient exhibits signs and symptoms of withdrawal, decrease the titration rate
- morphine withdrawal is not life threatening; however, patients may exhibit signs such as restlessness, rhinorrhea, sweating, muscle cramps, insomnia, nausea, diarrhea, mydriasis, and reports of pain

▶ *What Should I Tell My Patients About This Drug?*

- using morphine with alcohol or other central nervous system depressants may cause excessive drowsiness
- initially, morphine makes some patients drowsy, so do not drive or operate heavy machinery until you know how you will react to morphine
- short-term use of opioids does not lead to dependence
- some tolerance and dependence may develop with long-term use, but you will not become addicted to opioids
- initially, get up slowly because morphine may make you feel dizzy
- if you are taking morphine regularly, increase the amount of fiber and fluid in your diet, and consider taking a laxative regularly
- initially, morphine may cause some nausea and vomiting, contact your physician if this is a problem
- patients usually begin to tolerate the drowsiness and the nausea after a few days of morphine therapy
- if you are receiving morphine for chronic pain, your family should also be told of the adverse effects and what to expect
- if you are receiving morphine for chronic pain, you and/or family members must be given counseling on the concepts of dosing adjustments

▶ *Therapeutic Tips*

- always prescribe morphine doses at regularly scheduled intervals (e.g., Q4H, never PRN)
- do not use sustained-release preparations for initial titration, as they are much more difficult to titrate than the oral solution; however, after the patient is stabilized on an appropriate dosage of oral liquid morphine, a switch to a sustained-release preparation may make the use of morphine easier for the patient
- always use sustained-release morphine with rapid-release morphine for breakthrough pain
- always give intravenous or subcutaneous morphine for severe unrelieved pain in patients with cancer and change to oral morphine after pain is controlled
- in patients who will be taking regularly dosed narcotics for longer than 3–4 days, always consider prescribing narcotics in conjunction with a laxative and counsel the patient on the appropriate use of fluids and fiber
- oral route is preferred because of better patient acceptance and decreased cost
- NSAIDs may be useful in conjunction with morphine, especially when pain is due to bone metastases
- there is no theoretical upper limit to the dosage of oral morphine (dosages as high as 100 mg Q1H have been used)

Useful References

Tuttle CB. Drug management of pain in cancer patients. Can Med Assoc J 1985;132:121–134

Twycross R, Lack S. Oral morphine in advanced cancer. Beaconsfield, Bucks, England: Beaconsfield Publishers, 1988

Baumann TJ. Pain management. In: DiPiro JT, Talbert RL, Hayes PE, et al (eds.) Pharmacotherapy: A Pathophysiologic Approach, 2nd ed. Norwalk, CT: Appleton and Lange, 1993:924–941

Melzack R. The tragedy of needless pain. Sci Am 1990;262:27–33

Recommendations of the American Pain Society on the principles of analgesic use in the treatment of acute pain and chronic cancer pain. Clin Pharm 1990;9:601–611

Stimmel B. Pain, Analgesia, and Addiction: The Pharmacology of Pain. New York: Raven, 1983

AHFS Drug Information 94. Bethesda, MD: American Society of Hospital Pharmacists, 1994.

Clinical Practice Guideline, Acute Pain Management: Operative or Medical Procedures and Trauma. Washington, DC: US Department of Health and Human Services, Public Health Service, Agency for Health Care Policy and Research; 1992.

Clinical Practice Guideline, Management of cancer pain, Washington, D.C.: US Department of Health and Human Services, Agency for Health Care Policy and Research; 1994

MULTIVITAMIN PREPARATIONS (MULTIPLE BRANDS, COMBINATIONS)
Angela Kim-Sing and Eric Yoshida

▶ *When Should I Use This Drug?*

Populations at risk

- individuals who are unable to consume a well-balanced diet as outlined in the National Food Guide (Canada's Food Guide or The Basic Four), either as a consequence of necessary dietary restriction, intestinal disease, chronic noncompliance with good eating habits should receive multivitamin preparations
- before initiating any vitamin or mineral supplementation, a thorough evaluation of the diet and diagnosis of specific micronutrients that are deficient should be undertaken
- supplementation with specific deficient nutrients should occur, rather than provision of all vitamins and minerals
- if the diet is assessed to be inadequate, supplementation before clinical presentation of deficiency is appropriate

▶ *When Should I Not Use This Drug?*

Individuals with a well-balanced diet

- adequate vitamins should first be sought in a well-balanced diet; additional vitamins in healthy individuals should not be necessary

▶ *What Contraindications Are There to the Use of This Drug?*

- intolerance or allergic reactions to vitamin preparations

▶ *What Drug Interactions Are Clinically Important?*

- none

▶ *What Route and Dosage Should I Use?*

How to administer

- orally—take with or without food or liquids
- parenterally—dilute in any IV fluid and administer over 1 hour

Populations at risk

- there are numerous multivitamin preparations commercially available over the counter and by prescription
- useful formulas should contain only vitamins and minerals for which there is an established RDA (e.g., Centrum Forte)

▶ *What Should I Monitor with Regard to Efficacy and Toxicity?*

Efficacy

- difficult to assess since used predominantly when clinical signs of deficiency are not present

Toxicity

- multivitamin/mineral products containing RDA quantities should not produce any toxicities

▶ *How Long Do I Treat Patients with This Drug?*

- therapy should continue until necessary dietary changes implemented

▶ *How Do I Decrease or Stop the Administration of This Drug?*

- may be stopped abruptly

▶ *What Should I Tell My Patients About This Drug?*

- synthetically produced vitamin compounds are absorbed and utilized to the same extent as vitamins derived from natural sources and are usually less expensive
- multivitamin and mineral supplementation does not replace good nutritional practices and does not negate totally the detrimental effects of poor eating habits

Useful References

Ivey M, Elmer G. Nutritional supplement, mineral, and vitamin products. In: Handbook of Non-Prescription Drugs, 9th ed. Washington, DC: American Pharmacy Association; 1990;447

McEvoy GK. American Hospital Formulary Service Drug Information 91. Bethesda, MD: American Society of Hospital Pharmacists, 1991

National Research Council. Recommended Dietary Allowances, 10th ed. Washington, D.C.: National Academy Press, 1989

Ovesen L. Vitamin therapy in the absence of obvious deficiency—what is the evidence? Drugs 1984;27:148–170

NABILONE

Lynne Nakashima

USA (Cesamet)
CANADA (Cesamet)

▶ *When Should I Use This Drug?*

Chemotherapy-induced nausea and vomiting

- generally used only if other treatments such as metoclopramide and ondansetron have failed
- its use has decreased since ondansetron became available because the central nervous system (CNS) effects (confusion, euphoria) of nabilone are disturbing to some patients
- nabilone has similar efficacy to dronabinol in the prevention of chemotherapy-induced nausea and vomiting (Am J Med Sci 1987;293:34–44) and is more reliably and completely absorbed from the gastrointestinal tract (Drugs 1983;25[suppl 1]:52–62)
- nabilone may be associated with fewer CNS euphoric effects than is dronabinol (Drugs 1983;25[suppl 1]:52–62; Pharmacotherapy 1990;10:129–145)

- decision between dronabinol and nabilone should be based on cost
- generally not useful after vomiting has begun

Intractable nausea and vomiting in acquired immunodeficiency syndrome

- may be useful for intractable nausea and vomiting in AIDS (Br J Clin Pharmacol 1989;28:494–495)
- useful if other agents (prochlorperazine, domperidone) are not effective (Br J Clin Pharmacol 1989;28:494–495)

▶ *When Should I Not Use This Drug?*

Other causes of nausea and vomiting

- efficacy in other forms of nausea and vomiting has not been investigated

▶ *What Contraindications Are There to the Use of This Drug?*

Intolerance of or allergic reactions to nabilone or marijuana or sesame oil

Patients with a history of psychotic disorders

- symptoms in patients with schizophrenia or bipolar disorders may be worsened

▶ *What Drug Interactions Are Clinically Important?*

Drugs that may increase the effect or toxicity of nabilone

CENTRAL NERVOUS SYSTEM DEPRESSANTS

- additive, sedative effects are expected when other CNS depressants (e.g., narcotic analgesics, hypnotics, and alcohol) are used
- avoid combination if possible or minimize by starting with low doses of CNS depressants if added to nabilone

Drugs that may decrease the effect of nabilone

- none

Drugs that may have their effect or toxicity increased by nabilone

ANTICHOLINERGICS, ANTIHISTAMINES

- additive tachycardia and hypotension may occur
- avoid combination if possible, and if these agents must be used together, use the lowest effective dosages of both agents

SYMPATHOMIMETICS

- hypertension may occur
- avoid the combination

Drugs that may have their effect decreased by nabilone

THEOPHYLLINE

- theophylline metabolism may be increased
- no empirical dosage changes are required
- if only using the combination for 24–48 hours, do not worry about the interaction
- if using the combination for longer than 24–48 hours, be aware that a reduction in the effect of theophylline may result from the interaction

▶ *What Route and Dosage Should I Use?*

How to administer

- orally—can be taken with food or milk or on an empty stomach
- parenterally—not available

Chemotherapy-induced nausea and vomiting

- give 1 mg PO 30 minutes prior to chemotherapy, followed by 1 mg PO BID for 24 hours, and then reassess the patient
- dosages can be increased to 2 mg PO BID

Dosage adjustments for renal or hepatic dysfunction

- hepatically metabolized to active metabolites
- avoid in patients with severe hepatic dysfunction

▶ What Should I Monitor with Regard to Efficacy and Toxicity?

Efficacy

Frequency of assesment depends on the severity and frequency of nausea and vomiting

Number and severity of vomiting episodes

- determine time of day, force, description of vomitus, and associated symptoms

Fluid balance (needed only if vomiting occurs for a prolonged period)

- assess jugular venous pressure and orthostatic changes in blood pressure and heart rate; any decrease in upright diastolic pressure plus a rise in heart rate of 20 bpm or greater is abnormal
- oliguria
- weight
- rising values of hematocrit and creatinine, urea, sodium, and bicarbonate levels plus decreasing potassium and chloride levels are an indication of dehydration

Toxicity

Central nervous system effects

- dizziness and ataxia occurs in about 12–65% of patients (Drugs 1985;30:127–144)
- "high" or euphoria occurs in about 27% of patients, is not always undesirable, and may be correlated with antiemetic efficacy (Pharmacotherapy 1990;10:129–145)
- dysphoria may also occur
- maximum effects occur 2 hours after a dose and abate by 24 hours
- if intolerable, discontinue nabilone administration or lower the dosage if otherwise effective

Drowsiness

- is mild to moderate and usually decreases with continued therapy (Drugs 1985;30:127–144)
- reported range is 4–89% (Drugs 1983;25[suppl 1]:52–62)
- if severe, discontinue or lower the dosage of nabilone

Orthostatic hypotension

- occurs in approximately 10% of patients
- monitor supine and upright blood pressure with the first dose and discontinue nabilone administration if severe and symptomatic

Tachycardia

- results from an anticholinergic effect and occurs in approximately 7% of patients
- tachycardia does not produce symptomatic palpitations and returns to normal on discontinuation of drug administration

Anticholinergic effects

- dry mouth, blurred vision, dizziness (Drugs 1985;30:127–144)
- if dry mouth occurs, try increasing the fluid intake or using sugarless candy or gum to keep the patient's mouth moist
- if blurred vision occurs, try using comfort drops and avoid the use of contact lenses
- if constipation occurs, increase fluid and fiber intake
- urinary retention
- if these effects are severe and intolerable, nabilone administration may need to be discontinued

▶ How Long Do I Treat Patients with This Drug?

Chemotherapy-induced nausea and vomiting

- usually, a single dose 15–30 minutes prior to chemotherapy is sufficient
- for highly emetogenic chemotherapy agents, nabilone 1 mg PO BID should be continued for 4 doses
- few data are available concerning long-term use (longer than 1 year) of cannabinoids; however, in animals treated for longer than 5 years, CNS changes are noted (Am J Dis Child 1984; 138:1109–1112)

▶ How Do I Decrease or Stop the Administration of This Drug?

- when used for short-term, intermittent therapy such as that associated with chemotherapy-induced nausea and vomiting, nabilone administration may be stopped abruptly
- abuse potential exists with any of the cannabinoids, and if this occurs, the drug administration needs to be tapered over 1–2 weeks on the basis of the patient's tolerance

▶ What Should I Tell My Patients About This Drug?

- nabilone takes 1–2 hours to become fully effective
- it can be taken with or without food
- side effects include drowsiness, which may be accentuated by other sedating medications (e.g., narcotic analgesics and alcohol)
- wait 24 hours after the last dose before attempting activities that necessitate mental alertness (e.g., driving)
- dizziness may occur; stand or rise slowly; use guardrails on staircases
- dry mouth may occur, and if it does, try increasing fluid intake or using sugarless gum or candy to keep your mouth moist
- may cause changes in mood and other adverse behavioral effects; this is a side effect of the drug and stops if the drug administration is discontinued

▶ Therapeutic Tips

- generally, younger patients tolerate and respond better to this agent than older patients

Useful References

Tortorice PV, O'Connell MB. Management of chemotherapy-induced nausea and vomiting. Pharmacotherapy 1990;10(2):129–145
Vincent BJ, Tehen P, Cohen-Solal M, Kourilsky P. Review of cannabinoids and their anti-emetic effectiveness. Drugs 1983;25(suppl 1):52–62
Ward A, Holmes B. Nabilone, a preliminary review. Drugs 1985;30:127–144

NABUMETONE

Kelly Jones

USA (Relafen)
CANADA (not available)

▶ When Should I Use This Drug?

Rheumatoid arthritis

- nabumetone can be used as an alternative for patients who fail to respond to enteric-coated aspirin or ibuprofen; however, it is more expensive
- useful in patients who have a history of noncompliance (because of once-daily dosing); however, once-daily dosing may not be preferred in patients with arthritis pain, as these patients may want to dose more than once per day (DICP 1989;23:76–85)
- most regular-release NSAIDs, including aspirin, can be taken on an every 12 hour basis when being used to treat arthritic conditions, and therefore, once-daily NSAIDs provide the advantage of only once- versus twice-daily dosing
- decision among piroxicam, tenoxicam, nabumetone, and oxaprozin (once a day NSAIDs) should be based on cost
- sustained-release NSAIDs can be used once daily, preferably in the evening to attempt reduction in morning stiffness and should be chosen if they are less expensive than piroxicam, tenoxicam, nabumetone, or oxaprozin

Osteoarthritis

- if acetaminophen, enteric-coated aspirin, or ibuprofen are not effective
- decision between this drug and other NSAIDs should be based on cost

▶ When Should I Not Use This Drug?

Acute pain, general aches and pain, dysmenorrhea

- not useful for the short-term management of general aches and pains because it is difficult to titrate owing to its long half-life and its expense

Control of acute pain associated with arthritis

- this drug should never be used initially to gain control of arthritis pain, as the long half-life does not allow dosing flexibility
- this drug should be reserved as maintenance therapy for patients with controlled disease

Combination with other nonsteroidal antiinflammatory drugs

- combinations of NSAIDs provide no increase in effectiveness compared with maximum dosages of single agents and significantly increase the risk of adverse effects

▶ *What Contraindications Are There to the Use of This Drug?*

see Ibuprofen

▶ *What Drug Interactions Are Clinically Important?*

see Ibuprofen

▶ *What Route and Dosage Should I Use?*

How to administer

- orally—take with food or milk
- parenterally—not available

Rheumatoid arthritis

- 1000 mg PO daily HS to a maximum dosage of 2000 mg PO daily
- dosages of 2000 mg daily should be divided into 2 doses

Osteoarthritis

- 1000 mg PO daily

Dosage adjustments for renal or hepatic dysfunction

- hepatically metabolized; therefore, no adjustments are needed for renal disease
- reduce the dosage by 25% in patients with a history of hepatic disease

▶ *What Should I Monitor with Regard to Efficacy and Toxicity?*

see Ibuprofen

▶ *How Do I Decrease or Stop the Administration of This Drug?*

- may be stopped abruptly if needed

▶ *What Should I Tell My Patients About This Drug?*

see Ibuprofen

▶ *Therapeutic Tips*

see Ibuprofen

Useful References

see Ibuprofen

NADOLOL

Robert Rangno and James McCormack

USA (Corgard)
CANADA (Corgard, Apo-Nadol, Syn-Nadolol)
Nadolol is a nonselective lipid-insoluble beta-blocker that can be dosed once daily • If nadolol is less expensive than atenolol, it should be considered the beta-blocker of choice for most conditions • Atenolol is similar to nadolol, except that atenolol is beta$_1$-selective and should be chosen if beta$_2$-blockade is not desired (e.g., cold extremities) or if it is less expensive than nadolol • Some clinicians suggest that only beta-blockers with proven long-term benefits on mortality after infarction (e.g., timolol, propranolol, metoprolol, or acebutolol) should be used for post-MI prophylaxis (Circulation 1991;84[suppl VI]:VI-101–VI-107)

▶ *When Should I Use This Drug?*

Acute (crisis) hypertension

- oral beta-blockers, nifedipine, and captopril have all been shown to be effective (Lancet 1985;2:34–35, Br J Clin Pharmacol 1986;

21:377–383) in the treatment of acute (crisis) hypertension and should not be considered suboptimum to parenteral therapy
- choice among these agents should be based on cost and which drug would ultimately be useful for long term control; however, many patients with more severe hypertension will require more than one drug for adequate long-term control

Chronic (noncrisis) hypertension

- beta-blockers are drugs of first choice for hypertension, especially if the patient has concomitant beta-blocker–responsive disease (e.g., ischemic heart disease, previous myocardial infarction [MI], benign familial tremor, aneurysm, atrioventricular arrhythmia, and migraine)
- there is no evidence that beta-blockers such as atenolol and nadolol result in a lower quality of life than do other agents such as the angiotensin converting enzyme inhibitors and calcium channel blockers (Circulation 1991;84[supplVI]:VI-108–VI-118)
- beta-blockers, along with angiotensin converting enzyme inhibitors and calcium channel blockers, reduce microalbuminuria in diabetic patients with essential hypertension (Hypertension 1993;21:810–815)
- nadolol can be given once daily, and the generic form (if available) is usually less expensive than calcium channel blockers and angiotensin converting enzyme inhibitors but more expensive than diuretics
- beta$_2$ blockade by nadolol may offer a distinct advantage by blockade of epinephrine (beta$_2$)–induced arrhythmia, hypokalemia, and tremor

Chronic stable angina

- beta-blockers should be the first choice therapy, in conjunction with PRN nitroglycerin, because they are inexpensive, are effective, can be given once per day, and decrease the chance of an arrhythmia, reinfarction, and sudden death after an MI
- beta-blockers are as effective as calcium channel blockers even in patients with mixed angina (angina with exercise and at rest) in which coronary vasospasm may play a role in the cause of the pain (Br Heart J 1987;57:505–511)
- calcium channel blockers are expensive and must usually be given more than once daily
- in Printzmetal's angina, an uncommon condition, calcium channel blockers may be effective when beta-blockers fail

Unstable angina

- patients with symptomatic, unstable angina who do not respond to nitrates should receive intravenous atenolol (or intravenous metoprolol in Canada, as parenteral atenolol is not available) (Clin Cardiol 1990;13:679) unless their heart rate is less than 60 bpm, their systolic blood pressure is less than 100 mmHg, or there are contraindications to the use of beta-blockers
- although parenteral therapy is usually recommended, oral administration of beta-blockers can also be used, with the realization that absorption of the agent takes about 30 minutes (some clinicians recommend the intravenous route for the first dose possibly to reduce the size of a potential or occurring infarction)
- after the initial parenteral dose, oral therapy with a beta-blocker (nadolol or atenolol) should be started

Myocardial infarction

- patients should be treated empirically with beta-blockers after an MI (Am J Cardiol 1990;66:3C–8C) because there are convincing data that reinfarction, sudden cardiac death, and overall mortality are reduced
- both selective and nonselective agents have reduced morbidity and mortality, although the absolute reduction in mortality is greater when nonselective agents are used (Lancet 1986;2:57–66, N Engl J Med 1981;304:801–807, Prog Cardiovasc Dis 1985;27:335–371)
- most beta-blockers with intrinsic sympathomimetic activity, except acebutolol (Am J Cardiol 1990;66:24C–31C), have not reduced morbidity or mortality after an MI (Am J Cardiol 1990;66:9C–20C, Prog Cardiovasc Dis 1985;27:335–371)
- nadolol and atenolol have the advantage over some of the other agents in that they can be dosed once daily and have low lipid solubility

- only timolol, propranolol, metoprolol, and acebutolol have had significant long-term effects on mortality and some clinicians suggest that only beta-blockers with proven long-term postinfarction effects should be used for post-MI prophylaxis (Circulation 1991;84[suppl VI]:VI-101–VI-107)
- beta$_2$-blockade by nadolol may offer an advantage over selective beta-blockers by blockade of epinephrine (beta$_2$)–mediated arrhythmia and hypokalemia

Atrial flutter or fibrillation, atrioventricular nodal reentrant tachycardia

- useful if the rate is not controlled with digoxin and/or is excessively rapid during exercise
- less expensive than verapamil and can be used once daily

Ventricular arrhythmias

- for long-term therapy of symptomatic benign ventricular arrhythmias (nonsustained, hemodynamically stable, not associated with structural heart disease), beta-blockers are preferable to other antiarrhythmic agents because of the benign nature of these arrhythmias and because of the relatively low incidence of adverse effects of beta-blockers compared with those of other antiarrhythmic drugs (Drugs 1974;7:118–129)
- for symptomatic premature ventricular depolarizations or nonsustained ventricular tachycardia after acute MI, beta-blockers are preferable to other antiarrhythmic agents because they suppress arrhythmias and reduce mortality in patients who have survived acute MI (JAMA 1982;247:1707–1724, N Engl J Med 1983;308:614–618)
- all beta-blockers are likely effective

Migraine prophylaxis

- effective in reducing the frequency, duration, and severity of migraines in a majority of patients and should be considered first-line chronic preventative therapy for patients who have 2 migraine attacks or more a month
- propranolol, atenolol, metoprolol, and nadolol are all effective for migraine prophylaxis and are less expensive than calcium channel blockers
- timolol and acebutolol are somewhat effective, and pindolol and oxprenolol are ineffective
- especially useful if the patient has concomitant hypertension, angina, tremor, or arrhythmia

Esophageal varices rebleeding and portal hypertension

- nadolol and propranolol decrease portal venous pressure, the incidence of esophageal rebleed, the need for transfusion, and deaths (N Engl J Med 1991;324:1532–1538)

Thyrotoxicosis

- propranolol, nadolol, and atenolol are effective and should be chosen instead of agents with intrinsic sympathomimetic activity (ISA), as it is important to control the tachycardia associated with this condition

Alcohol withdrawal syndrome

- benzodiazapines are preferable; however, beta-blockers may stop worrisome atrioventricular tachyarrhythmias

Situational anxiety such as performance anxiety in musicians, benign familial tremor

- nonselective beta-blockers are drugs of choice

Other uses

- anxiety disorders, acute panic disorder
- familial prolonged QT interval syndromes, idiopathic hypertrophic cardiomyopathy, symptomatic mitral valve prolapse, dilated cardiomyopathy

▶ *When Should I Not Use This Drug?*

Pheochromocytoma prior to alpha-blockade

- prior alpha-receptor blockade is required because nadolol blocks the vasodilator effect of peripheral beta$_2$-receptor stimulation, leaving alpha$_1$-receptor–mediated vasoconstriction unopposed

Clonidine withdrawal

- concurrent use during clonidine withdrawal can cause unacceptable increases in blood pressure (Med Clin North Am 1988;72:37–81)

▶ *What Contraindications Are There to the Use of This Drug?*

Intolerance of or allergic reaction to nadolol

Asthma or chronic bronchitis with bronchospasm

- using nadolol or any beta-blockers in such patients is potentially dangerous and alternative therapy should be chosen
- alternative therapy should also be used in patients undergoing allergy-desensitizing injections because possible bronchospasm can be made worse
- selectivity for the beta$_1$-adrenergic receptors is dose related and not absolute; consequently, a beta$_1$ selective antagonist such as atenolol should still be avoided in patients with bronchospastic disease (Drugs 1979;17:425–460)
- if there is a strong indication for a beta-blocker, such as with uncontrolled angina in a patient insufficiently responsive to maximum dosages of calcium channel blockers and nitrates, low-dose atenolol (12.5 mg PO daily), a beta$_1$-selective antagonist, may be justified in patients with asthma or chronic bronchitis; however, patients must be told to continue regular use of inhaled beta$_2$-agonists
- beta-blockers are not contraindicated in patients with chronic bronchitis with no associated bronchospasm; however, selective agents (atenolol) should be chosen and started in low doses and patients should be evaluated for worsening of their pulmonary disease

Insulin-dependent diabetes with hypoglycemic reactions

- nonselective beta-blockers should be avoided in patients who frequently have, or are at risk for, hypoglycemic reactions
- nonselective beta-blockers may mask some hypoglycemic symptoms such as palpations and tremor and may prolong hypoglycemia
- beta-blockers often increase sweating and do not alter irritability, confusion, or hunger in patients undergoing hypoglycemic reactions

Raynaud's syndrome

- nonselective beta-blockers should be avoided; however, in the presence of a strong indication, low doses of a beta$_1$-selective antagonist such as atenolol may be tried

Intermittent claudication

- beta-blockers can be used safely in the presence of intermittent claudication, provided that there is no evidence of resting leg ischemia, in which case beta-blockers, or any drug that lowers perfusion, may aggravate claudication symptoms (Arch Intern Med 1991;151:1705–1707)

Congestive heart failure

- beta-blockers have traditionally not been used in patients with congestive heart failure but old and newer data (Am J Med 1992;92:527–538) show that, when introduced slowly they often improve, not worsen, congestive heart failure symptoms, whereas some calcium channel blockers, specifically diltiazem or verapamil, may worsen congestive heart failure (Circulation 1990;82:2254–2257)

Bradycardia, atrioventricular conduction defects

- bradycardia without electrocardiographic (ECG) evidence of conduction block is not a contraindication
- beta-blocker dosage should be decreased in patients with first-degree block, and beta-blocker use should be avoided in patients with second-degree or complete block

▶ *What Drug Interactions Are Clinically Important?*

Drugs that may increase the effect or toxicity of nadolol
VERAPAMIL, DILTIAZEM, NIFEDIPINE

- beta-blockers in combination with calcium channel blockers can exacerbate cardiac conduction delay abnormalities, claudication, and heart failure

- verapamil especially should be avoided if there is ECG evidence of conduction delay or block

PHENOTHIAZINES

- additive hypotensive effects occur with high doses of phenothiazines
- monitor blood pressure and reduce the dosage of beta-blockers or phenothiazine if necessary

LEVODOPA

- beta-blockers blunt symptoms due to the positive inotropic and chronotropic effect of levodopa and may be a useful adjunct in parkinsonism

PRAZOSIN, TERAZOSIN, DOXAZOSIN

- concurrent treatment with beta-blockade increases the incidence of postural hypotension by blocking the increase in heart rate response that offsets the postural hypotension with alpha$_1$-antagonists
- start with much lower doses of alpha-antagonist given at bedtime for 1–2 weeks before increasing the dosage or switching to a morning dose

Drugs that may decrease the effect of nadolol

CLONIDINE

- severe or malignant hypertension can result if the administration of both agents is discontinued abruptly
- discontinue the use of beta-blockers at least 2 weeks before gradual clonidine withdrawal
- when switching a patient from clonidine, it must be gradually withdrawn more than 1 week before nadolol administration is started to prevent the potential threat of rebound hypertension (N Engl J Med 1981;305:678–682)

NONSTEROIDAL ANTIINFLAMMATORY DRUGS

- NSAIDs reduce the antihypertensive effect of beta-blockers and most antihypertensives by inhibiting endogenous prostaglandin synthesis
- NSAIDs such as aspirin, naproxen, and sulindac have little negative antihypertensive effect (Ann Intern Med 1994;121:289–300)

PHENYLPROPANOLAMINES (MANY ORAL COLD PREPARATIONS)

- concurrent use can result in hypertensive crisis and should be avoided
- for nasal congestion, use topical decongestants

MONOAMINE OXIDASE INHIBITORS

- contraindicated, as the combination can cause hypertensive crisis

TRICYCLIC ANTIDEPRESSANTS

- anticholinergic effects may reverse some of the bradycardiac effects of the beta-blocker, but patients are still beta-blocked
- patients should be watched for evidence of ineffective blockade such as increase in heart rate and tachycardia

Drugs that may have their effect or toxicity increased by nadolol

LIDOCAINE

- concomitant administration of propranolol or metoprolol with lidocaine may result in elevations in plasma lidocaine concentrations by reducing the clearance of lidocaine, probably as a result of decreasing cardiac output and hepatic blood flow and inhibiting hepatic enzyme levels
- if therapy with one of these drugs is initiated in a patient receiving lidocaine, the rate of lidocaine infusion should be decreased by $^1/_3$, and the patient should be monitored for arrhythmia recurrence and signs or symptoms of lidocaine toxicity
- although not studied, it should be assumed that other beta-blockers also interact with lidocaine

Drugs that may be have their effect decreased by nadolol

- none

▶ What Route and Dosage Should I Use?

How to administer

- orally—can be taken with food or milk or on an empty stomach
- parenterally—not available

Acute (crisis) hypertension

- 80 mg PO daily given immediately

Chronic (noncrisis) hypertension

- 20 mg PO daily
- increase the dosage every 4 weeks by 20 mg PO daily until an effect is seen
- dosage increase up to 80 mg PO daily may be necessary in some patients, but no benefit is likely to result from further increases
- some patients will receive an important antihypertensive effect with as little as 10 mg PO daily

Chronic stable angina, unstable angina, myocardial infarction

- 40 mg PO daily is given for the initial treatment of angina
- increases of 40 mg daily can be made every 3 days until symptoms are controlled or a maximum dosage of 240 mg PO daily is reached
- can also be titrated until exercise-induced heart rate is decreased by 15%

Atrial flutter or fibrillation, atrioventricular nodal reentrant tachycardia

- if the patient is not symptomatic (does not need parenteral therapy), start with 20 mg PO daily and increase every 2–3 days by 20 mg PO daily until the heart rate is controlled or a maximum dosage of 160 mg/d is reached

Ventricular arrhythmias

- 80 mg PO daily (40 mg PO daily in patients with low blood pressure, heart rate < 60 bpm, or concomitant therapy with agents that depress function of the sinoatrial or atrioventricular nodes) and increase every 2–3 days until the patient is beta-blocked (resting heart rate and heart rate during exercise is suppressed) or a dosage of 160 mg PO daily is reached

Migraine prophylaxis

- 20 mg PO daily
- increase the daily dosage by 20 mg PO at weekly intervals until therapeutic or toxic effects appear

Esophageal varices rebleeding and portal hypertension

- start with 20 mg PO daily and increase every 2–3 days by 20 mg PO daily until the resting heart rate is reduced by 20–25% or a maximum dosage of 160 mg/d is reached

Thyrotoxicosis, alcohol withdrawal syndrome

- give 20 mg PO and repeat at 2 hour intervals until blood pressure and heart rate are controlled

Situational anxiety such as performance anxiety in musicians

- 20 mg PO at least 1 hour before a performance

Benign familial tremor

- 20 mg PO daily
- increase the daily dosage by 20 mg PO at weekly intervals until therapeutic or toxic effects appear

Dosage adjustments for renal or hepatic dysfunction

- renally eliminated
- in general, even in patients with normal renal function, start with a low dose and titrate up to an effect

Normal Dosing Interval	C$_{cr}$ > 60 mL/min or 1 mL/s	C$_{cr}$ 30–60 mL/min or 0.5–1 mL/s	C$_{cr}$ < 30 mL/min or 0.5 mL/s
Q24H	no adjustment needed	decrease dosage by 50%	decrease dosage by 75%

▶ *What Should I Monitor with Regard to Efficacy and Toxicity?*

Efficacy

Acute (crisis) hypertension

Blood pressure

- preferably obtain intraarterial blood pressure; however, if this is not available, perform indirect (cuff) measurements every 5 minutes until the desired blood pressure is reached and then every hour, ensuring that the diastolic pressure does not go below 100 mmHg during the first 1–2 days owing to concerns about hypoperfusion
- ideal rate of blood pressure reduction in this condition is unknown; however, the goal should be to lower pressures to the desired range within 30 minutes to 2 hours

Electrocardiographic measurements

- continuous ECG monitoring is recommended until a stable blood pressure reduction has been achieved and sustained
- this is done to look for evidence of coronary ischemia, and if this occurs, treat as for angina (also consider that blood pressure may have been lowered too far)

Chronic (noncrisis) hypertension

Blood pressure

- patients with diastolic blood pressures greater than 115 mmHg or with symptoms should be evaluated again within 48 hours to ensure that at least a 5–10 mmHg drop in blood pressure has occurred
- for patients with diastolic blood pressures less than 115 mmHg, follow-up blood pressure measurements should be done within a couple of weeks
- at each visit do 2 blood pressure measurements, supine or sitting, after the patient has been resting without conversation for 5–10 minutes
- continue to do this every 4 weeks to assess the effect of each new dosage until control is achieved
- for most patients with mild hypertension once blood pressure is controlled, blood pressure measurement 2–4 times per year will be sufficient

Evidence of end-organ damage

- if blood pressure is well-controlled and no other disease states exist (e.g., diabetes), measure baseline serum creatinine, blood glucose, and serum cholesterol levels and perform urinalysis and repeat every 5 years
- repeat every year if other disease states are present

Chronic stable angina

- decreased severity, frequency, and duration of chest pain
- reduction in the use of nitroglycerin tablets
- resolution of ST segment depression should occur or the amount of total daily ischemia should be decreased on Holter monitoring
- patient should be evaluated every time the dosage of an agent needs to be increased
- patients should be reevaluated with treadmill exercise tests when symptoms change or at least every 3 years

Unstable angina

- decreased severity, frequency, and duration of chest pain
- frequency of assessment depends on the frequency of chest pain
- serial creatine kinase and ECG in the first 24 hours are used to rule out an MI
- frequency of original symptoms (e.g., shortness of breath)
- ST-T wave abnormalities should resolve and not recur

Acute myocardial infarction

- relief of chest pain and decreased frequency of chest pain
- frequency of assessment depends on the frequency of chest pain and complications of MI (cardiogenic shock, arrhythmias, and septal rupture)

Atrial flutter or fibrillation, atrioventricular nodal reentrant tachycardia, ventricular arrhythmias

- resting apical ventricular rate of 60–80 bpm is a reasonable target, although 90–100 bpm may be acceptable if the patient is asymptomatic at this heart rate
- presence or absence of symptoms related to arrhythmia (palpitations, shortness of breath, dizziness, and angina)

Migraine prophylaxis

- decrease in frequency, severity, and duration of headache

Esophageal varices rebleeding and portal hypertension

- resting heart rate and incidence of rebleeding

Thyrotoxicosis

- control of blood pressure, heart rate, and symptoms

Alcohol withdrawal syndrome

- control of blood pressure, heart rate, and symptoms

Situational anxiety such as performance anxiety in musicians, benign familial tremor

- control of symptoms

Toxicity

Heart failure or bradycardia

- obtain from history and physical examination
- uncommon if not used in patients with cardiovascular contraindications

Asthma

- can occur, and if it does, switch to a more selective agent such as atenolol or preferably use an agent from a different class

Central nervous system effects

- mental depression, sexual dysfunction, lethargy or fatigue, and nightmares can occur
- there appears to be no difference in neuropsychological side effects (perceptual motor ability, memory, or abstraction and learning) between lipid-soluble and lipid-insoluble beta-blockers (Arch Intern Med 1989;149:514–525); however, lipid-soluble agents (propranolol and metoprolol) have been shown to cause insomnia, whereas atenolol (lipid insoluble) does not (Circulation 1987;75:104–112)
- if central nervous system effects occur, reduce the dosage by 50%, or preferably use an alternative drug from another class

Hyperlipidemias

- effect of beta-blockers on low density lipoprotein and high density lipoprotein cholesterol is small, transient, and dose related and has not been shown to be of clinical significance
- main effect is to increase triglyceride levels with unknown consequences (does not occur for drugs with intrinsic sympathomimetic activity)
- there is evidence that beta-blockers reverse atherosclerosis, despite these mild effects on lipids (Am J Cardiol 1987;59:48F–52F)
- beta-blockers may not be desirable in patients with severe familial hyperlipidemias requiring lipid-lowering drug therapy; however, there is no evidence to suggest that beta-blockers enhance atherogenesis

Cold extremities

- may occur, especially when nonselective agents are used
- if these occur, switch to a more selective agent such as atenolol; if there is still a problem, switch to an agent from a different class

▶ *How Long Do I Treat Patients with This Drug?*

Acute (crisis) hypertension

- drug therapy should continue as suggested for chronic (noncrisis) hypertension

Chronic (noncrisis) hypertension

Stepped-down therapy, in general, should be considered in patients whose blood pressures during the previous few visits have been well-controlled

- approximately 50% of patients with well-controlled blood pressures successfully undergo either a reduction in dosage or number of drugs and remain so for a time, but unfortunately, this period varies from patient to patient and consistent reevaluation is necessary

- this may be explained by reversal of cardiac and vascular changes that may occur after prolonged treatment with drug therapy and may be a means of "setting back the clock" of primary hypertension evolution or may reflect an incorrect initial diagnosis
- patients most likely to have a successful reduction or discontinuation of therapy may be predicted by a low pretreatment blood pressure (mild hypertension with diastolic pressure <100 mmHg), no evidence of target organ damage, requirement of only monotherapy for blood pressure control, weight loss, salt restriction, increased exercise, and a decrease in alcohol intake
- drug administration discontinuation in patients with severe to malignant hypertension or target organ damage (e.g., MI, congestive heart failure, stroke, and renal failure) is not advised
- reassessment allows reevaluation of the efficacy of nondrug measures in the treatment of hypertension, such as reduction of weight or salt and alcohol intake
- reassessment allows hypertension to be treated with the least number of drugs in the lowest dosage (this reduces the incidence of adverse effects, reduces the frequency of drug administration, and is more cost effective)

Chronic stable angina

- maintenance drug therapy should likely be continued indefinitely; however, changes in lifestyle and the natural history of the disease will suggest reevaluation for the lowest effective dosage, replacement with a better or less expensive agent, or even drug discontinuation

Atrial flutter or fibrillation, ventricular arrhythmias

- patients with acute atrial fibrillation or flutter for which an underlying cause can be identified require rate control therapy until the underlying cause can be corrected
- patients with chronic or paroxysmal atrial fibrillation or flutter require rate control therapy indefinitely

Myocardial infarction

- prophylactic therapy should be lifelong, if tolerated, particularly in high-risk patients (Circulation 1991;84[suppl VI]:VI-101–VI-107)
- beta-blocker therapy has been shown to reduce mortality for at least 6 years after MI; therefore, beta-blockers treatment is continued as long as the patient tolerates the therapy

Migraine prophylaxis

- in the patient achieving a headache-free state, therapy should be reduced or withdrawn after 6 months to assess continued requirements
- if the patient has a return of headaches, indefinite prophylactic therapy should be considered

Esophageal varices rebleeding and portal hypertension

- treatment should be lifelong if tolerated

Thyrotoxicosis

- until effective medical or surgical therapy has been achieved

Alcohol withdrawal syndrome

- continue therapy for 2–3 days, then stop drug administration

Situational anxiety such as performance anxiety in musicians, benign familial tremor

- use as needed

▶ How Do I Decrease or Stop the Administration of This Drug?

- dosage should be reduced gradually to avoid the so-called beta-antagonist withdrawal syndrome
- dosage should be reduced by 50%, with reassessment of disease state at 2 weeks
- if the disease state is unchanged, reduce the dosage by another 50% (i.e., to 25% of the initial dose) and recheck the disease state in another 2 weeks

- if the disease state is still well controlled, stop the medication administration and recheck the disease state in 2 weeks
- so-called rebound hypertension does not occur if the dosage is gradually tapered with dosage reductions of no more than 50% at 2–4 week intervals
- sudden preoperative withdrawal can precipitate an MI (Anesth Analg 1983;62:380–390), and continued treatment is beneficial during the perioperative period (Acta Anaesthesiol Scand 1984;28:677–682)

▶ What Should I Tell My Patients About This Drug?

- should not be discontinued abruptly
- notify your physician if there is difficulty in breathing
- take at the same time each day
- may produce lassitude
- do not use if you have a history of asthma or wheezing

▶ Therapeutic Tips

- for many diseases, patients rarely require more than 20 mg/d
- patients requiring higher doses can be identified by having inadequately blocked exercise-induced tachycardia (inadequate beta-blockade); however, confirm the patient's compliance before increasing the dosage of the drug
- beta$_2$-blockade from nadolol may be particularly useful in angina, arrhythmia, migraine, and tremor

Useful References

Hell RC, Brogden RN, Pakes GE, et al. Nadolol: A review of its pharmacological properties and therapeutic efficacy in hypertension and angina pectoris. Drugs 1980;20:1–23
Frishman WH. Nadolol: A new adrenoceptor antagonist. N Engl J Med 1980;305:678–682

NAFCILLIN

John Rotschafer, Kyle Vance-Bryan, Rick Zabinski

USA (Nafcil, Nallpen, Unipen)
CANADA (not available)

▶ When Should I Use This Drug?

check antibiotic susceptibility chart (Table 4–1 in Chapter 4)
see Cloxacillin

- except oral nafcillin is not available

▶ When Should I Not Use This Drug?

see Cloxacillin

▶ What Contraindications Are There to the Use of This Drug?

see Penicillin

▶ What Drug Interactions Are Clinically Important?

see Penicillin

▶ What Route and Dosage Should I Use?

How to administer

- orally—not available
- parenterally—administer intravenously in 100 mL of IV fluid (normal saline or 5% dextrose in water) and infuse over 30 minutes

Cellulitis, pneumonia

- 1 g IV Q6H for mild to moderate infections
- 2 g IV Q6H for severe infections

Endocarditis meningitis, acute or chronic osteomyelitis

- 2 g IV Q4H

Dosage adjustments for renal or hepatic dysfunction

- eliminated mainly via the bile, and dosage adjustments are not required

▶ *What Should I Monitor with Regard to Efficacy and Toxicity?*

Efficacy

- for antibiotic administration monitoring guidelines, see specific section on drug therapy

Toxicity

see Penicillin

▶ *How Long Do I Treat Patients with This Drug?*

see Cloxacillin

▶ *How Do I Decrease or Stop the Administration of This Drug?*

- may be stopped abruptly

▶ *What Should I Tell My Patients About This Drug?*

see Penicillin

▶ *Therapeutic Tips*

see Cloxacillin

Useful Reference

Wright AJ, Wilkowske CJ. The penicillins. Mayo Clin Proc 1987;62:806–820

NALBUPHINE

Terry Baumann

USA (Nubain, various)
CANADA (Nubain, various)

▶ *When Should I Use This Drug?*

Acute pain

- use only when the patient has a true allergy to meperidine and does not tolerate morphine
- although it has been reported that nalbuphine causes less severe respiratory depression than does morphine because it is a partial agonist, if morphine (as with any opioid) is properly titrated there is likely little if any clinical difference between these drugs with regard to respiratory depression
- has a shorter duration of action than does buprenorphine and is less expensive

Postoperative pain

- drug of choice only if there is true allergy to meperidine or the patient does not tolerate morphine
- offers no advantages over morphine and is more expensive

▶ *When Should I Not Use This Drug?*

see Buprenorphine

▶ *What Contraindications Are There to the Use of This Drug?*

see Buprenorphine

▶ *What Drug Interactions Are Clinically Important?*

see Morphine

▶ *What Route and Dosage Should I Use?*

How to administer

- orally—not available
- parenterally—may be administered intramuscularly, intravenously (dilute IV nalbuphine in 10 mL of normal saline and give over at least 1 minute), or subcutaneously

Acute pain

- 10 mg IM or IV Q4H (not PRN), or 5 mg IM or IV Q4H (not PRN) for elderly patients because of concerns about sedation and respiratory depression
- question patients frequently about the degree of pain they are having (ideally within at most 1–2 hours after the first dose if the drug was administered via the IM route)

- if pain is unrelieved by this time and there are no signs of sedation or respiratory depression, give another dose 50% higher than the first dose
- continue this approach until pain is 75% relieved, and then maintain at this dosage for 12 hours before further adjustments are made
- normal dosage increments are 10, 15, and 20 mg
- if an immediate response (within 1–5 minutes) for severe pain is needed, use intravenously as recommended under postoperative pain

Postoperative pain

In the postanesthetic care unit

- 5 mg IV repeated in 30–60 minutes
- adjust the dosage on the basis of the patient's response to each dose and titrate to pain control and the desired level of sedation or respiratory rate

On the ward

Intermittent therapy

- as above for acute pain
- question the patient frequently and increase the dosage as above for acute pain on the basis of pain relief and the desired level of sedation

Patient-controlled analgesia

- 1 mg/bolus with lockout time of 6 minutes
- some clinicians believe that 1–2 mg/h as an infusion with patient-controlled analgesia enables patients to sleep through the night; however, evidence suggests that using a bolus with a baseline infusion may increase the amount of narcotic used and side effects, without improving efficacy (Anaesth Intensive Care 1991;19:555–560, Anesthesiology 1992;76:362–367)
- question patients frequently about the degree of pain they are having
- if pain is not controlled with bolus doses, increase the bolus dose by 25–50%
- if pain relief from a bolus is adequate but the duration of pain relief is too short, decrease the lockout period

Dosage adjustments for renal or hepatic dysfunction

- hepatically metabolized
- dosage adjustment is usually not required if the dose is titrated properly

▶ *What Should I Monitor with Regard to Efficacy and Toxicity?*

see Morphine

▶ *How Long Do I Treat Patients with This Drug?*

see Morphine

▶ *How Do I Decrease or Stop the Administration of This Drug?*

see Morphine

▶ *What Should I Tell My Patients About This Drug?*

see Morphine

▶ *Therapeutic Tips*

see Buprenorphine

Useful References

see Morphine

NALIDIXIC ACID

Peter Jewesson

USA (NegGram)
CANADA (NegGram)

▶ *When Should I Use This Drug?*

Consider an alternative agent

- considering the availability of other better tolerated and more effective agents, this drug is not recommended

NALOXONE
Terry Baumann

USA (Narcan, various)
CANADA (Narcan, various)

▶ *When Should I Use This Drug?*

Reversal of opioid effects

- drug of choice for intentional or unintentional opioid overdose
- naloxone is a pure opiate antagonist that reverses opioid-induced analgesia, respiratory depression, sedation, and hypotension
- it can also reverse pruritus caused by epidural or intrathecal administration of opioids
- it has no analgesic action and can precipitate withdrawal symptoms in opioid-dependent patients and does not reverse the tendency of opioids to cause constipation

▶ *When Should I Not Use This Drug?*

If it cannot be judiciously titrated

- naloxone must be titrated properly to avoid withdrawal and/or loss of pain control

▶ *What Contraindications Are There to the Use of This Drug?*

Intolerance of or allergic reaction to naloxone

- true allergies to naloxone or to morphine or its congeners (i.e., codeine, hydromorphone, oxymorphone, levorphanol, hydrocodone, oxycodone, buprenorphine, butorphanol, nalbuphine) are rare

▶ *What Drug Interactions Are Clinically Important?*

- none

▶ *What Route and Dosage Should I Use?*

How to administer

Orally

- not available

Parenterally

- can be given by the IM, IV, or SC routes
- for IV push, dilute 0.4 mg of naloxone in saline for a final volume of 10 mL or 0.04 mg/mL
- for IV infusion, dilute 2 mg of naloxone in 500 mL of normal saline or 5% dextrose solutions for a concentration of 0.004 mg/mL

Reversal of opioid effects

- 0.1 mg IV every 2–3 minutes until the desired effect is achieved (adequate analgesia without the undesired side effects)
- additional doses may be necessary depending on the amount of opioid, the time that has elapsed since the opioid was administered, and the length of action of the opioid involved
- for IV infusion, start at 0.0037 mg/kg/h, and titrate to effect (adequate analgesia without the undesired side effects)
- for opioid overdose, give 0.4 mg IV every 2–3 minutes; if there is no response after 10 mg, the respiratory depression may be caused by something other than an opioid
- after the effect is achieved, additional doses may be necessary, depending on the amount of opioid, the time that has elapsed since the opioid was administered, and the length of action of the opioid involved

▶ *What Should I Monitor with Regard to Efficacy and Toxicity?*

Efficacy

Reversal of opioid effects

- adequate analgesia without the undesired side effects
- key to achieving effective titration is to question patients frequently about the degree of pain and side effects they are having

Toxicity

- reversal of opioid effects too quickly may produce nausea, vomiting, sweating, tachycardia, and *pain*

▶ *How Long Do I Treat Patients with This Drug?*

- use as long as the undesirable effects continue

▶ *How Do I Decrease or Stop the Administration of This Drug?*

- may be stopped abruptly; however, additional doses may be necessary, depending on the amount of opioid, the time that has elapsed since the opioid was administered, and the length of action of the opioid involved

▶ *What Should I Tell My Patients About This Drug?*

- naloxone may cause withdrawal symptoms (restlessness, rhinorrhea, perspiration, muscle cramps, insomnia, and nausea) if patient is opioid dependent

▶ *Therapeutic Tips*

- carefully titrate because analgesia can easily be reversed

Useful References

see Morphine

NAPROXEN
Kelly Jones

USA (Naprosyn; sodium salt: Anaprox, Anaprox DS, Aleve)
CANADA (Naprosyn, Novonaprox, Naxen, Apo-naproxen; sodium salt: Anaprox, Anaprox DS)

▶ *When Should I Use This Drug?*

Acute pain, general aches and pain, bone pain, dysmenorrhea, cancer pain

- useful for the short-term management of general aches and pains
- only advantage over non–enteric-coated aspirin is that it causes less frequent gastrointestinal intolerance
- decision between this drug and other nonsteroidal antiinflammatory drugs (NSAIDs) should be based on cost
- sodium salt of naproxen (Anaprox) is recommended for use in dysmenorrhea because it is supposedly absorbed slightly faster; however, it is unknown whether this is a clinically important difference and the decision between these agents should be based on cost

Rheumatoid arthritis

- naproxen can be used as an alternative for patients who fail to respond to enteric-coated aspirin or ibuprofen; however, it offers no advantages over enteric-coated aspirin or ibuprofen and it is usually more expensive
- naproxen is an alternative to ibuprofen in patients taking oral anticoagulants (DICP 1989;23:76–85)

Osteoarthritis

- if acetaminophen, enteric-coated aspirin or ibuprofen are not effective
- decision between this drug and other NSAIDs should be based on cost

Migraine treatment, migraine prophylaxis

- decision between this drug and other NSAIDs should be based on cost

▶ *When Should I Not Use This Drug?*

see Ibuprofen

▶ *What Contraindications Are There to the Use of This Drug?*

see Ibuprofen

▶ *What Drug Interactions Are Clinically Important?*

see Ibuprofen

▶ *What Route and Dosage Should I Use?*

How to administer

- orally—take with food or milk
- parenterally—not available

Acute pain, general aches and pain, bone pain, dysmenorrhea
- 250–500 mg PO Q8–12H PRN
- 275–550 mg PO Q8–12H PRN (naproxen sodium)

Cancer pain
- 250 mg PO Q12H up to a maximum dosage of 1500 mg PO daily

Rheumatoid arthritis
- 500 mg PO Q12H up to a maximum dosage of 1500 mg PO daily
- 550 mg PO Q12H up to a maximum dosage of 1650 mg PO daily (naproxen sodium)

Osteoarthritis
- 250 mg PO Q12H
- 275 mg PO Q12H (naproxen sodium)

Migraine treatment
- 500 mg PO Q8H PRN up to a maximum of 500 mg PO Q8H daily

Migraine prophylaxis
- 375 mg PO Q12H

Dosage adjustments for renal or hepatic dysfunction
- hepatically metabolized; therefore, no adjustments are needed for renal disease
- reduce dosage by 25% in patients with a history of hepatic disease

▶ *What Should I Monitor with Regard to Efficacy and Toxicity?*

see Ibuprofen

▶ *How Long Do I Treat Patients with This Drug?*

see Ibuprofen

▶ *How Do I Decrease or Stop the Administration of This Drug?*

- may be stopped abruptly if needed

▶ *What Should I Tell My Patients About This Drug?*

see Ibuprofen

▶ *Therapeutic Tips*

see Ibuprofen

Useful References

see Ibuprofen

NETILMICIN
David Guay
USA (Netromycin)
CANADA (Netromycin)

▶ *When Should I Use This Drug?*
Consider an alternative agent
- netilmicin offers no advantages over gentamicin or tobramycin and is usually more expensive than gentamicin

NIACIN
Stephen Shalansky and Robert Dombrowski
USA (Nicobid, Nicolar, Niac, Slo-Niacin, Nico-400)
CANADA (various generic)

▶ *When Should I Use This Drug?*
Hypercholesterolemia
- should be considered first-line therapy for patients in whom cost is a limiting factor as niacin is less expensive than HMG-CoA reductase inhibitors and bile acid sequestrants
- while niacin does lead to a reduction in cholesterol, there is more evidence for a positive effect on cardiovascular disease, especially in primary prevention, with the HMG-CoA reductase inhibitors and bile acid sequestrants
- also chosen in patients when HMG-CoA reductase inhibitors or bile acid sequestrants are ineffective or not well tolerated
- side effects such as flushing, gastrointestinal discomfort, hyperglycemia, liver toxicity, and hyperuricemia may limit its use

Hypertriglyceridemia
- consider drug therapy only in patients with symptomatic (pancreatitis, xanthomas) hypertriglyceridemia, as there is no evidence yet to support or screen patients with asymptomatic elevated triglyceride levels (Br Med J 1992;304:394–396)
- not as effective at lowering triglycerides as fibric acid derivatives but is much less expensive and should be considered if fibric acid derivatives are not effective or tolerated

Mixed hyperlipidemias
- niacin is recommended (if it is tolerated) because it has proven efficacy in the reduction of cardiovascular disease, lowers triglyceride levels, raises high-density lipoprotein and lowers low-density lipoprotein (LDL) levels, and is less expensive than the HMG-CoA reductase inhibitors

▶ *When Should I Not Use This Drug?*
- Niacin can be used for hypercholesterolemia, hypertriglyceridemia, and mixed hyperlipidemias

▶ *What Contraindications Are There to the Use of This Drug?*
Intolerance of or allergic reaction to niacin
Arterial hemorrhaging, severe hypotension
- niacin is a vasodilator

Active hepatic disease
- niacin is metabolized hepatically

Active peptic ulcer disease
- niacin is a gastric irritant

▶ *What Drug Interactions Are Clinically Important?*
Drugs that may increase the effect or toxicity of niacin
LOVASTATIN
- niacin may increase the risk of myopathy when used in combination with lovastatin
- incidence of myopathy is increased to about 2% (Am J Cardiol 1988;62:28–34)
- niacin can be used in combination with lovastatin but niacin should be discontinued immediately if myopathy occurs (Am J Cardiol 1988;62:28–34)

ALCOHOL AND WARM DRINKS
- avoid taking niacin with alcohol or warm drinks, which may enhance flushing or pruritus

Drugs that may decrease the effect of niacin
- none

Drugs that may have their effect or toxicity increased by niacin
- none

Drugs that may have their effect decreased by niacin
- none

▶ *What Route and Dosage Should I Use?*
How to administer
- orally—give with food, avoiding hot beverages and alcohol
- parenterally—not available

Hypercholesterolemia, hypertriglyceridemia, mixed hyperlipidemias
- 100 mg PO TID with meals and increase the dosage every 2–3 days by 100 mg per dose over 2 weeks until a dosage of 500 mg PO TID is reached

- usually, at least 500 mg PO TID must be given to see an effect on lipid levels
- increase the dosage of niacin to 4 g/d if there is an inadequate response in 4 weeks
- remeasure serum lipid levels at 3 months
- if the desired total cholesterol level is achieved and niacin is well tolerated, continue the drug regimen and monitor lipid levels at 4 month intervals and then yearly
- maintenance dosages of 2–6 g/d are typical, although dosages up to 9 g/d may be necessary and can be used if tolerated
- seldom are dosages greater than 1 g PO TID used because of intolerability
- do not use sustained-release preparations, as there is an increased risk of hepatotoxicity with these agents (Am J Med 1992;92:77–81)
- if after 3 months of optimum therapy there is at least a 15% decrease in LDL or total cholesterol level, but the target level is not reached, continue niacin administration and add a second drug
- if after 3 months of optimum therapy, there is less than a 15% decrease in LDL or total cholesterol level, consider switching to or adding another agent
- if the patient is not tolerating niacin, change to another drug

▶ *What Should I Monitor with Regard to Efficacy and Toxicity?*

Efficacy

Hypercholesterolemia, hypertriglyceridemia, mixed hyperlipidemias

Total cholesterol and fractionated lipid profile

- in patients with no coronary heart disease or atherosclerotic disease and with less than 2 CHD risk factors lower total cholesterol below 240 mg/dl (6.2 mmol/L) and LDL cholesterol below 160 mg/dl (4.1 mmol/L)
- in patients with no coronary heart disease or atherosclerotic disease and with 2 or more CHD risk factors lower total cholesterol below 200 mg/dL (5.2 mmol/L) and LDL cholesterol below 130 mg/dL (3.4 mmol/L)
- for patients with coronary heart disease or atherosclerotic disease lower LDL cholesterol to below 100 mg/dL (2.6 mmol/L)
- complete lipid profiles should be measured at 1 and 3 months
- if goals are achieved, check annually

Evidence of coronary heart disease

- myocardial infarction, angina, and coronary bypass grafting

Risk factors

- reduce risk factors such as obesity and smoking
- control risk factors such as diabetes mellitus and hypertension

Toxicity

- side effects from niacin in 1119 patients were flushing (92%), pruritus (49%), rash (27%), stomach pain (14%), nausea (8%), and gout (6%) (JAMA 1975;231:360–381)

Rash and pruritus

- are transient and do not necessitate discontinuation of therapy

Flushing

- appears to be prostacycline-mediated and may be reduced by taking 325 mg of aspirin 30 minutes prior to taking niacin
- clonidine has also been shown to inhibit niacin-induced vasodilation (Lancet 1974;2:58)

Gastrointestinal symptoms

- gastrointestinal side effects include nausea, vomiting, diarrhea, heartburn, and anorexia
- adverse effects occur more commonly with sustained-release formulations than with standard products. (DICP Ann Pharmacother 1991;25:253–254)
- can aggravate peptic ulcer disease
- do not use in patients with active peptic ulcer disease

Hepatotoxicity

- severe hepatotoxicity is rare (Pharmacotherapy 1988;8:287–294)

- adverse effects on the liver are usually dose related
- sustained-release products should be avoided because they cause a higher incidence of hepatotoxicity

Atrial arrhythmias

- have rarely been reported
- monitor clinical signs and history

Increased blood glucose, uric acid, and liver enzymes (alanine aminotransferase, aspartate aminotransferase) levels

- baseline levels should be obtained
- monitor at 4–6 weeks after the start of therapy, at 6 months of therapy, and annually thereafter

▶ *How Long Do I Treat Patients with This Drug?*

Hypercholesterolemia, hypertriglyceridemia, mixed hyperlipidemias

- therapy is long term and may continue for life
- if the patient has achieved and maintained target lipid levels for 2 years, niacin administration should be discontinued and a retrial on dietary therapy alone should be tried
- recheck lipid levels at 4–6 weeks and at 3 months after drug administration has been discontinued, and restart drug therapy if target levels are not maintained

▶ *How Do I Decrease or Stop the Administration of This Drug?*

- may be stopped abruptly

▶ *What Should I Tell My Patients About This Drug?*

- common adverse reactions include gastrointestinal upset, flushing, and pruritus
- do not be alarmed by these adverse effects, which can disappear 2–6 weeks after initiating long-term high-dose therapy
- take with meals to minimize side effects
- avoid taking niacin with hot beverages or alcohol
- 325 mg of aspirin 30 minutes prior to the administration of niacin may reduce flushing
- if several doses are missed, tolerance to the flushing has to be reestablished

▶ *Therapeutic Tips*

- niacin lowers total cholesterol, LDL cholesterol, and triglycerides levels; it has also been shown to decrease mortality from CHD and reverse coronary atherosclerosis (J Am Coll Cardiol 1986;8:1245–1255, JAMA 1987;257:3233–3240)
- patients must be educated about adverse reactions, which are common and disappear as therapy with niacin continues
- patients who do not report flushing are likely not taking niacin (check to make sure that the patient has not switched to niacinamide)
- niacin is typically better tolerated in patients with a darker complexion (dark hair and eyes, and so on)
- works best on a TID basis

Useful References

Expert Panel on Detection, Evaluation, and Treatment of High Blood Cholesterol in Adults. Summary of the second report of the National Cholesterol Education Program (NCEP) expert panel on detection, evaluation, and treatment of high blood cholesterol in adults. JAMA 1993;269:3015–3023

Figge HL, Figge J, Souney PF, et al. Nicotinic acid: A review of its clinical use in the treatment of lipid disorders. Pharmacotherapy 1988;8(5):287–294

Knapp TRF, Middleton RK. Adverse effects of sustained-release niacin. DICP Ann Pharmacother 1991;25:253–254

Illingworth DR. Lipid-lowering drugs: An overview of indications and optimum therapeutic use. Drugs 1987;33:259–279

NIFEDIPINE

Stephen F. Hamilton, Stan Horton, and Udho Thadani

USA (Procardia, Procardia XL, Adalat)
CANADA (Adalat, Adalat P.A. Adalat XL, Apo-Nifed, Novonifedin, Nu-Nifed)

▶ When Should I Use This Drug?

Chronic stable angina

- calcium channel blockers are useful for patients who have no concomitant disease states and who do not tolerate or do not have complete control with nitrates and beta-blockers
- beta-blockers should be chosen instead of calcium channel blockers for new-onset angina or chronic stable angina because there is more cumulative information on the overall value of beta-blockers in these patients and beta-blockers are usually less expensive than calcium antagonists
- calcium antagonists can be used as monotherapy when contraindications to the use of beta-blockers and nitrates are present and can be added when optimum 2-drug therapy (nitrates and beta-blockers) is not adequate for symptom control (Am Heart J 1989;118:1093–1097)
- triple-drug therapy (maximum therapy) has not been shown to have advantages over optimized therapy with nitrates and beta-blockers and should be reserved for patients who are symptomatic with double (nitrates and beta-blockers)–drug therapy (J Am Coll Cardiol 1984;3:1051–1057)
- calcium channel blockers should be chosen for patients with concomitant hypertension who are unable to take beta-blockers
- calcium channel blockers should be chosen for patients with concomitant diabetes or chronic obstructive pulmonary disease asthma who cannot tolerate nitrates or in whom nitrates are ineffective
- all calcium channel blockers are equally effective; however, diltiazem is usually the best tolerated calcium channel blocker and should be chosen instead of other agents unless there are significant price differences
- calcium channel blocking agents are considered the drugs of choice for the management of Prinzmetal's variant angina

Acute (crisis) hypertension

- oral beta-blockers, nifedipine and captopril have all been shown to be effective (Lancet 1985;2:34–35, Br J Clin Pharmacol 1986;21:377–383) in the treatment of acute (crisis) hypertension and should not be considered suboptimal therapy
- these agents are also useful for the initial treatment of diastolic pressure that repeatedly exceeds 115 mmHg in patients with no target organ damage
- choice among these agents should be based on which drug would ultimately be useful for long-term control and the realization that many patients require more than 1 drug for adequate long-term control

Chronic (noncrisis) hypertension

- use only in patients who do not tolerate, do not respond to, or have contraindications to thiazide diuretics and beta-blockers because thiazide diuretics and beta-blockers have proven long-term benefit and are generally less expensive than calcium channel blockers
- calcium channel blockers are useful for hypertension in patients with ischemic heart disease if beta-blockers are not effective or tolerated and in patients with asthma, diabetes, or moderate to severe hyperlipidemias, as calcium channel blockers have no effect on these disease states
- all calcium channel blockers are equally effective; however, diltiazem is usually the best tolerated calcium channel blocker and should be chosen instead of other agents unless there are significant price differences between ditiazem and nifedipine

Raynaud's syndrome

Short-term treatment or prophylaxis, long-term

- nifedipine is the drug of choice, as it has proven efficacy and is the most studied calcium channel blocker
- diltiazem and nicardipine have been effective but have not been as extensively studied (Hypertension 1991;17:593–602)

▶ When Should I Not Use This Drug?

Migraine prophylaxis

- nifedipine can cause headaches and studies have not confirmed its effectiveness (Neurology 1989;39:284–286)

Post–myocardial infarction

- the addition of a calcium antagonist is indicated only if optimal (beta-blocker and nitrate) therapy does not control anginal symptoms
- empirical use of calcium antagonists after myocardial infarction has not shown a decrease in mortality

Atrial fibrillation or flutter, atrioventricular nodal reentrant tachycardia

- nifedipine has little if any atrioventricular nodal blocking activity and is not effective for the treatment of arrhythmias

▶ What Contraindications Are There to the Use of This Drug?

see Diltiazem

▶ What Drug Interactions Are Clinically Important?

Drugs that may increase the effect or toxicity of nifedipine

BETA-ADRENERGIC BLOCKING AGENTS

- when used concomitantly with nifedipine, these drugs increase the incidence of congestive heart failure, arrhythmia, and severe hypotension
- these agents should be used together only when anginal symptoms fail to be controlled by other drug therapy or either agent alone

Drugs that may decrease the effect of nifedipine

CALCIUM

- calcium therapy may result in antagonism of the beneficial effects and unwanted effects of calcium channel blocking agents, and therefore, concomitant use is not recommended
- calcium replacement to maintain eucalcemia is not a problem

CAFFEINE, EPINEPHRINE, ISOPROTERENOL, THEOPHYLLINE

- drugs that increase cyclic adenosine monophosphate inhibit the calcium channel blocking activity and patients should be observed for an alteration in response
- if episodic hypertension is suspected because of these agents, an ambulatory blood pressure monitor may be useful

Drugs that may have their effect or toxicity increased by nifedipine

DIGOXIN

- reports are conflicting but in general, most studies show no significant interaction
- be aware of the potential interaction, but only measure digoxin serum concentrations if toxicity is suspected

Drugs that may have their effect decreased by nifedipine

- none

▶ What Route and Dosage Should I Use?

How to administer

- orally—can be taken with food or milk or on an empty stomach (sustained-release tablets should be swallowed whole)
- parenterally—not available

Chronic stable angina

- 30 mg of nifedipine (Procardia XL, Adalat XL) PO daily, increasing the dosage weekly by 30 mg daily until symptoms are controlled or a maximum dosage of 90 mg PO daily is reached
- 10 mg of nifedipine (Adalat PA—Canada only) PO BID, increasing the dosage weekly by 20 mg daily until symptoms are controlled or a maximum dosage of 80 mg PO daily is reached
- sustained-release preparations are recommended, as they are more convenient and usually not much different in price from the regular-release products (unless generic regular-release is available)
- regular-release form is started at 10 mg PO TID and increased weekly by 10 mg PO TID until a maximum dosage of 90 mg/d is reached

Acute (crisis) hypertension

- 10 mg PO (5 mg in patients such as the elderly) in whom cerebral hypoperfusion is a potential hazard and repeat every 6 hours as needed
- do not use the sublingual route, as nifedipine is not absorbed by the oral mucosa; however, biting the capsule and swallowing the contents increases the rate of absorption by about 5–10 minutes (Am J Med 1986;81[suppl 6A]:2–5)

Chronic (noncrisis) hypertension

- 30 mg of nifedipine (Procardia XL, Adalat XL) PO daily, increasing the dosage every 4 weeks by 30 mg/d until an effect is seen or a maximum dosage of 90 mg daily is reached
- 10 mg of nifedipine (Adalat PA—Canada only) PO BID, increasing the dosage every 4 weeks by 20 mg/d until an effect is seen or a maximum dosage of 80 mg daily is reached
- sustained-release preparations are recommended, as they are more convenient and usually not much different in price from the regular-release products (unless generic regular-release drug is available)
- regular-release form is started at 10 mg PO TID, increasing the dosage every 4 weeks by 10 mg PO TID until an effect is seen or a maximum dosage of 90 mg daily is reached

Raynaud's syndrome

- for short-term treatment, 10 mg PO just prior to cold exposure or at the onset of an attack
- do not use the sublingual route, as nifedipine is not absorbed by the oral mucosa; however, biting the capsule and swallowing the contents increases the rate of absorption
- 10 mg PO Q8H for long-term prevention
- nifedipine (Adalat PA—Canada only) 10 mg PO Q12H or nifedipine (Procardia XL, Adalat XL) 30 mg PO daily may decrease the incidence of adverse effects associated with nifedipine use but may be more expensive

Dosage adjustments for renal or hepatic dysfunction

- hepatically metabolized
- specific nifedipine dosage recommendations for patients with impaired renal or hepatic function are not available
- start with a low dose and titrate to effect

▶ What Should I Monitor with Regard to Efficacy and Toxicity?

Efficacy

see Diltiazem

Acute (crisis) hypertension

Blood pressure

- preferably, obtain intraarterial blood pressure; however, if this is not available, then perform indirect (cuff) measurements every 5 minutes until the desired blood pressure is reached and then every hour, ensuring that the diastolic pressure does not go below 100 mmHg during the first 1–2 days owing to concerns about hypoperfusion
- ideal rate of blood pressure reduction in this condition is unknown; however, the goal should be to lower pressures to the desired range within 30 minutes to 2 hours

Electrocardiographic measurements

- continuous electrocardiographic monitoring is recommended until a stable blood pressure reduction has been achieved and sustained
- this is done to look for evidence of coronary ischemia, and if this occurs, treat as for angina (also consider that blood pressure may have been lowered too far)

Toxicity

see Diltiazem

▶ How Long Do I Treat Patients with This Drug?

see Diltiazem

Acute (crisis) hypertension

- drug administration discontinuation in patients with severe to malignant hypertension or target organ damage (e.g., myocardial

infarction, congestive heart failure, stroke, and renal failure) is not advised; however, continuous reassessment allows the hypertension to be treated with the least number of drugs in the lowest dosage, which reduces the incidence of adverse effects, reduces the frequency of drug administration, and is more cost effective

▶ How Do I Decrease or Stop the Administration of This Drug?

see Diltiazem

▶ What Should I Tell My Patients About This Drug?

- excessive caffeine consumption (>5 cups of coffee per day) should be avoided, as this may inhibit the action of calcium channel blocking agents
- the most common adverse effect of nifedipine is peripheral edema
- Procardia XL's nonabsorbable shell (tablet) is excreted intact in the stool

▶ Therapeutic Tips

- patients are usually more compliant with extended-release products, which are usually less expensive when the daily cost of therapy is considered
- do not use the sublingual route, as nifedipine is not absorbed by the oral mucosa; however, biting the capsule and swallowing the contents increases the rate of absorption by about 5–10 minutes (Am J Med 1986;81[suppl 6A]:2–5)
- "rescue" administration of calcium is not effective in reversing the depressant actions of nifedipine on the sinus and atrioventricular node; however, pretreatment with calcium can decrease the hypotensive effects

Useful References

Follath F. The role of calcium antagonists in the treatment of myocardial ischemia. Am Heart J 1989;118:1093–1097.

Tolins M, Weir EK, Chesler E, Pierpont GL. "Maximal" drug therapy is not necessarily optimal in chronic angina pectoris. J Am Coll Cardiol 1984;3:1051–1057

NITROFURANTOIN

George Zhanel

USA (Furadantin, Macrodantin, Furalan, Furan, Furanite, Nitrofan)

CANADA (Furadantin, Macrodantin, Apo-Nitrofurantoin, Novofuran, Nephronex)

▶ When Should I Use This Drug?

Urinary tract infection prophylaxis

- useful agent for prophylactic and suppressive therapy in patients who cannot use trimethoprim-sulfamethoxazole because of the development of resistance or sulfa allergy
- in pregnant (except at term) patients who cannot use amoxicillin

Acute urinary tract infections

- use only if organisms are resistant to or patients are allergic to trimethoprim-sulfamethoxazole or amoxicillin; nitrofurantoin must be given QID and has a greater incidence of gastrointestinal side effects than either trimethoprim-sulfamethoxazole or amoxicillin

▶ When Should I Not Use This Drug?

Non–urinary tract infections

- low serum concentrations and the absence of the therapeutically active moeity in most tissues after administration preclude use for infections other than the urinary tract (Am J Hosp Pharm 1979;36:342–351)

Pyelonephritis

- as this disease may be accompanied by bacteremia

Men with urinary tract infection

- urinary tract infections in men usually involve the prostate and do not readily respond to nitrofurantoin therapy (Ann Intern Med 1989;110:138–150)

▶ *What Contraindications Are There to the Use of This Drug?*

Intolerance of or allergic reaction to nitrofurantoin

Renal dysfunction

- combination of decreased efficacy and increased toxicity (particularly peripheral neuropathy) occurs in patients with creatinine clearance less than 40 mL/min (DICP 1985;19:540–547)

Hemolytic anemia

- more likely in patients with known glucose-6-phosphate dehydrogenase deficiency or in pregnancy at term or in infants younger than 1 month of age

▶ *What Drug Interactions Are Clinically Important?*

- none

▶ *What Route and Dosage Should I Use?*

How to administer

Orally

- should be taken with food or milk to minimize gastric upset
- use of the macrocrystalline formulation may minimize gastric upset

Parenterally

- not available

Recurrent urinary tract infection (prophylaxis)

- 50 mg PO HS

Urinary tract infection

- 100 mg PO QID

Dosage adjustments for renal or hepatic dysfunction

- renally eliminated
- does not require adjustment; however, should not be used if creatinine clearance is less than 40 mL/min because it is ineffective at this level of renal function

▶ *What Should I Monitor with Regard to Efficacy and Toxicity?*

Efficacy

- for antibiotic administration monitoring guidelines, see specific section on drug therapy

Toxicity

Allergic reactions (anaphylaxis, rash, drug fever)

- anaphylaxis is rare
- rash is uncommon and subsides when treatment is stopped
- drug fever occurs in approximately 4% of patients
- question the patient about the appearance of these symptoms daily while in the hospital or tell the patient to telephone the physician if these symptoms occur

Gastrointestinal symptoms (nausea or vomiting, anorexia)

- are frequent and dose related and may necessitate discontinuation of therapy
- decreased by administration with food or milk
- decreased with macrocrystalline formulation
- question the patient about the appearance of these symptoms daily while the patient is in the hospital

Pneumonitis (acute, subacute, chronic)

- all forms are thought to be allergic
- acute form is characterized by dyspnea at rest, nonproductive cough, fever, and rash and occurs within hours to weeks of ingestion
- subacute form occurs after 1 month of use and is characterized by progressive cough, dyspnea, orthopnea, and fever
- chronic form occurs after 6 months of use and is characterized by dyspnea on exertion, mild cough, and progressive X-ray changes
- if patients have the above signs or symptoms and they are thought to be drug related, discontinue therapy

Peripheral neuropathy

- occurs initially as paresthesias and dysesthesias, occurs more often in lower limbs than in upper limbs
- onset is days to years after the initiation of therapy
- renal dysfunction increases risk
- treatment is to discontinue medication, and complete recovery usually occurs within weeks

▶ *How Long Do I Treat Patients with This Drug?*

Urinary tract infection prophylaxis or suppression

- 50 mg HS (treatment reassessed at 6 month intervals)
- if 50 mg ineffective, can increase dose to 100 mg
- assessment of continued therapy depends on the presence of bacteriuria and the development of symptomatic infection during prophylaxis

Lower urinary tract infection

- 3 days

▶ *How Do I Decrease or Stop the Administration of This Drug?*

- may be stopped abruptly

▶ *What Should I Tell My Patients About This Drug?*

- contact your physician if symptoms do not improve during the next few days
- if you have rash, hives, fever, or difficulty with breathing, contact your physician immediately
- take this medication with food or milk
- take this medication until it is completely finished
- this medication may discolor your urine brown

▶ *Therapeutic Tips*

- ensure that renal function is normal
- in patients who fail to respond to prophylactic therapy, assess whether urine is alkalinized as this may decrease efficacy
- use amoxicillin or trimethoprim-sulfamethoxazole instead of nitrofurantoin if possible

Useful References

Gleckman R, Alvarez S, Joubert DW. Drug therapy reviews: Nitrofurantoin. Am J Hosp Pharm 1979;36:342–351
D'Arcy PF. Nitrofurantoin. DICP 1985;19:540–547
Holmberg L, Boman G, Böttinger LE, et al. Adverse reactions to nitrofurantoin. Am J Med 1980;69:733–738

NITROGLYCERIN

Stephen F. Hamilton, Stan Horton, and Udho Thadani

Nitroglycerin

USA (Nitrogard, Nitro-Bid, Nitrocap, Nitrocine Timecaps, Nitroglyn, Nitrong, Tridil, Nitrostat, Transderm-Nitro, Nitro-Dur, Nitrolingual Spray)
CANADA (Nitrogard, Nitro-Bid, Nitroglyn, Nitrol, Nitrong, Tridil, Nitrostat, Transderm-Nitro, Nitro-Dur, Nitrolingual Spray)

Isosorbide Dinitrate

USA (Isordil, Sorbitrate)
CANADA (Isordil, Sorbitrate, APO-ISDN, Cedocard-SR, Coronex)

Isosorbide Mononitrate

USA (ISMO)
CANADA (IMDUR-SR)

▶ *When Should I Use This Drug?*

Suspected angina

SUBLINGUAL NITROGLYCERIN

- any patient with suspected anginal symptoms should have sublingual nitroglycerin available and be instructed in its use for acute symptomatic relief of angina

- sublingual and lingual nitroglycerin are used because of their rapid onset of action
- relatively easy for patient to carry
- efficacy is well established
- sublingual is inexpensive but loses potency when exposed to light and air
- nitroglycerin tablets and nitroglycerin spray are equally effective
- nitroglycerin spray is more expensive per dose than the tablets; however, if nitroglycerin spray is used only infrequently, it may be more cost effective than infrequent use of tablets if the tablets routinely become outdated (nitroglycerin tablets outdate after 6 months, whereas the spray is good for 3 years)
- sublingual nitroglycerin is also useful for prevention before planned exercise that may bring on symptoms
- sublingual isosorbide dinitrate is not recommended, as it necessitates metabolism and its onset of action is slower than nitroglycerin

Chronic stable angina

ISOSORBIDE MONONITRATE, ISOSORBIDE DINITRATE, NITROGLYCERIN

- oral nitrates have a long history of efficacy and safety, low cost, and lack of serious side effects and should be used in patients in whom beta-blockers are ineffective or not tolerated (Postgrad Med 1992;91:307–318)
- development of tolerance during long-term therapy is, however, a major limitation
- beta-blockers should be the first choice, in conjunction with PRN nitroglycerin, because they are inexpensive, are effective, can be given once per day, and decrease the chance of an arrhythmia and sudden cardiac death after myocardial infarction
- nitrates are initial drugs of choice for chronic stable angina in patients with chronic obstructive pulmonary disease or asthma, congestive heart failure, and diabetes, as nitrates do not worsen these disease states
- in congestive heart failure, nitrates may be used even when mitral regurgitation is present
- oral isosorbide dinitrate, isosorbide mononitrate, and transdermal preparations reduce the frequency of angina and increase exercise tolerance
- isosorbide mononitrate has dependable bioavailability because it does not require conversion from dinitrate to mononitrate and has proven efficacy in dosages that tend to circumvent tolerance
- isosorbide dinitrate has been widely studied, but there are inadequate data proving that tolerance is circumvented after the second and third dose of the day during 3 times daily therapy (Am J Cardiol 1992;70:43B–53B)
- halitosis (bad breath), flushing, and rash have not been reported with the isosorbide mononitrate, but have been with isosorbide dinitrate
- nitroglycerin tablets and capsules are popular products; however, the evidence of their efficacy and dosing regimens are extrapolated from studies with poor controls or presumed from knowledge of other nitrate products (their use is not recommended)

TRANSDERMAL NITROGLYCERIN

- nitroglycerin patches are more expensive than generic oral isosorbide dinitrate and should be used only if the patient cannot tolerate oral medications or does not like taking pills
- nitroglycerin ointment is inconvenient and messy to use, and its only advantage is that the effect can be stopped relatively quickly by wiping it off

Unstable angina, acute myocardial infarction

SUBLINGUAL NITROGLYCERIN

- sublingual nitroglycerin can be safely given if systolic blood pressure is at least 90 mmHg and doses can be repeated every 5 minutes
- multiple doses may be required and can be given as long as systolic blood pressure is at or above 90 mmHg

INTRAVENOUS NITROGLYCERIN

- all patients who remain symptomatic after sublingual nitroglycerin or have recurrent pain should receive intravenous nitroglyc-

erin for 48 hours (Clin Cardiol 1990;13:679–686) and the dose should be titrated to appropriate reductions in blood pressure
- with titration upward, it is thought that intravenous dosing overcomes the problem of nitrate tolerance

ISOSORBIDE MONONITRATE, ISOSORBIDE DINITRATE, TRANSDERMAL NITROGLYCERIN

- switch to a nonparenteral form of nitrate preparation after the patient is stabilized (usually after 48 hours of intravenous therapy or freedom from pain for 24 hours)
- decision between oral route and transdermal route should be based on the patient's preference and cost
- transdermal patch may be more convenient initially for the nursing staff (once-daily application)

Congestive heart failure

Acute pulmonary edema

- sublingual nitroglycerin may be useful in reducing preload in patients slow to respond to diuretic therapy
- nitroglycerin ointment or a patch can be used if there is a delay in getting parenteral nitroglycerin
- there is a danger of decreasing preload, which leads to decreased cardiac output and forward failure

Mild to moderate chronic congestive heart failure

- nitrates in conjunction with hydralazine may prolong survival but should be used only in patients intolerant of angiotensin converting enzyme inhibitors (N Engl J Med 1986;314: 1547–1552)

Perioperative hypertension associated with cardiovascular procedures

- produces controlled hypotension during surgical procedures

▶ *When Should I Not Use This Drug?*

Migraine

- vasodilators such as nitrates may worsen a migraine headache and should be avoided

Acute myocardial infarction (long-acting forms of nitrates)

- long-acting dosage forms should not be used in patients with acute myocardial infarction because the effects are difficult to terminate rapidly if excessive hypotension or bradycardia occurs

Right ventricle inferior infarcts

- have a high incidence of nodal bradycardia and hypotension (similar to the Bezold-Jarisch reflex) that may be accentuated by nitrates

Functional or organic gastrointestinal hypermotility or malabsorption syndrome

- extended-release preparations should not be used in patients with these conditions because these agents may not be absorbed completely
- topical nitroglycerin preparations should not be applied in the area of the chest where defibrillation paddles are to be placed because of their high resistance and low electrical conductivity

▶ *What Contraindications Are There to the Use of This Drug?*

Intolerance of or allergic reaction to nitrates

Severe anemia

- potential for reducing hemoglobin level and impairing oxygen delivery

Heart trauma

- pericardial trauma or constrictive pericarditis can worsen with a decrease in preload

Cerebral hemorrhage

- may increase intracranial pressure similar to the increase seen in intraocular pressure

Postural hypotension, systolic pressure of less than 90 mmHg, hypovolemia

- nitrates decrease blood pressure and increase the chance of postural hypotension and/or severe hypotension

Angle closure or open angle glaucoma

- intraocular pressure is at most increased only briefly and drainage of aqueous humor from the eye is not impeded so nitrates can be used
- ophthalmological consultation should be obtained and pressures measured if long-term use is required

Head injury

- to avoid increases in intracranial pressure

▶ *What Drug Interactions Are Clinically Important?*

Drugs that may increase the effect or toxicity of nitroglycerin

ALCOHOL

- may cause hypotension so patients should avoid alcohol at the time of the peak effects from nitrate doses

Drugs that may decrease the effect of nitroglycerin

- none

Drugs that may have their effect or toxicity increased by nitroglycerin

- none

Drugs that may have their effect decreased by nitroglycerin

HEPARIN

- intravenous nitroglycerin may antagonize the anticoagulant effect of heparin when these drugs are administered concomitantly
- partial thromboplastin time (PTT) should be monitored within 6 hours of the addition of intravenous nitroglycerin to ensure adequate anticoagulation
- if intravenous nitroglycerin therapy is discontinued in patients receiving heparin, reductions in heparin dosage may be necessary; therefore, PTT should be checked at 6 hours after stopping intravenous nitroglycerin administration

▶ *What Route and Dosage Should I Use?*

How to administer

Orally

- bioavailability is not significantly affected by food, but the rate of absorption is slowed

Sublingually

- placed under the tongue at the onset of symptoms

Lingual spray

- dose should be sprayed onto the tongue, and the mouth should be closed immediately after each dose

Parenterally

- 25–50 mg should be prepared in 250 mL glass containers of either 5% dextrose or normal saline injection
- because standard polyvinyl chloride administration sets adsorb 40–80% of the nitroglycerin in solution, special nitroglycerin IV administration sets should be used (unfiltered)

Topically

- apply to the upper body, as this provides better absorption
- rotate sites to avoid skin irritation

Suspected angina

SUBLINGUAL NITROGLYCERIN

- 0.4 mg (0.3 mg in Canada owing to different available dosage forms) placed under the tongue at the onset of symptoms or for prophylaxis before planned exercise as prevention
- patients should discontinue the activity that produced the symptoms and be seated until symptoms resolve
- this dose should be repeated at 5 minute intervals, and if the symptoms are not relieved within 3 doses (15 minutes), the patient should seek emergency medical assistance

LINGUAL NITROGLYCERIN SPRAY

- one spray on the tongue at the onset of symptoms or for prophylaxis before planned exercise as prevention

- patients should discontinue the activity that produced the symptoms and be seated until symptoms resolve
- this dose should be repeated at 5 minute intervals, and if the symptoms are not relieved within 3 doses (15 minutes), the patient should seek emergency medical assistance
- spray should not be inhaled

Chronic stable angina

ISOSORBIDE MONONITRATE (QUICK RELEASE PRODUCT)

- 20 mg PO at 8 AM and 3 PM is effective and avoids tolerance for the regular release tablets (Ann Intern Med 1994;120:353–359)
- increase dose to 40 mg PO with the same dosage schedule after 1 week of therapy if symptoms are not controlled

ISOSORBIDE DINITRATE (QUICK RELEASE PRODUCT)

- 30 mg PO at 7 AM and 12 noon avoids tolerance for the subsequent 7 AM dose, but the 12 noon dose may not be as effective

TRANSDERMAL NITROGLYCERIN

- 0.4 mg/h for 12–14 h/d applied to provide coverage during the time of maximum symptoms
- dose titration is essential, and the dose can be increased every 2–3 days until symptoms are controlled or a maximum of 0.8 mg/h for 12–14 h/d has been given
- large doses cover a large surface area and are unacceptable to many patients (J Am Coll Cardiol 1989;13:786–795)

Unstable angina, acute myocardial infarction

SUBLINGUAL NITROGLYCERIN

- as above
- can be safely given if systolic blood pressure is at least 90 mmHg, and can be repeated every 5 minutes
- several doses may be required and can be given as long as systolic blood pressure is at or above 90 mmHg

INTRAVENOUS NITROGLYCERIN

- start with a constant infusion of 10 μg/min
- infusion rate can be increased by 10 μg/min (by 25 μg/min when the dosage has reached 50 μg/min) every 5–10 minutes until the signs and symptoms of ischemia are absent or mean arterial blood pressure is decreased by 10% in previously normotensive patients (30% in previously hypertensive patients), keeping systolic blood pressure at or above 90 mmHg
- if the increase in heart rate is more than the decrease in systolic blood pressure, there may be a detrimental effect on the double product (heart rate times systolic blood pressure, which is a bedside estimate of myocardial oxygen demand and should decrease with effective therapy) and the dosage should be decreased
- there is no absolute maximum dosage, and dosages of 200 μg/min or higher may be required provided hypotension is avoided
- if invasive monitoring is available and pulmonary capillary wedge pressure (PCWP) is elevated, a decrease in PCWP of 10–30% is a reasonable goal

Congestive heart failure

Acute pulmonary edema

SUBLINGUAL NITROGLYCERIN

- 0.4 mg (0.3 mg in Canada owing to different available dosage forms) placed under the tongue or 1 spray on the tongue every 3 minutes until symptoms improve or systolic blood pressure is less than 90 mmHg

Mild to moderate chronic congestive heart failure

- see above under chronic stable angina
- the only dose studied in regard to morbidity and mortality associated with congestive heart failure is isosorbide dinitrate 60 mg PO QID

Perioperative hypertension associated with cardiovascular procedures

INTRAVENOUS NITROGLYCERIN

- start with 50 μg/min and increase every 5 minutes by 25–50 μg/min until the desired blood pressure is reached

Dosage adjustments for renal or hepatic dysfunction

- hepatically metabolized
- no specific dosage adjustments are necessary in patients with renal impairment or hepatic insufficiency

▶ *What Should I Monitor with Regard to Efficacy and Toxicity?*

Efficacy

Suspected angina

- relief of chest pain should be evaluated for the efficacy of sublingual nitroglycerin at 5 minute intervals, and if the symptoms are not relieved within 3 doses (15 minutes), the patient should seek emergency medical assistance

Chronic stable angina

- relief of chest pain and decreased frequency of chest pain
- patient should be evaluated every time the dosage of an agent needs to be increased
- patients should be reevaluated with treadmill exercise tests when symptoms change or at least every 3 years

Unstable angina

- relief of chest pain and decreased frequency of chest pain
- frequency of assessment depends on frequency of chest pain
- serial creatine kinase determination and electrocardiographic evaluation in the first 24 hours are used to rule out a myocardial infarction
- frequency of original symptoms (e.g., shortness of breath)
- ST-T wave abnormalities should resolve and not recur

Acute myocardial infarction

- relief of chest pain and decreased frequency of chest pain
- frequency of assessment depends on the frequency of chest pain and complications of myocardial infarction (cardiogenic shock, arrhythmias, and septal rupture)
- ST-T wave abnormalities should resolve and not recur

Congestive heart failure

- look for relief of dyspnea, orthopnea, paroxysmal nocturnal dyspnea, and ankle edema
- jugular venous pressure, rales, edema, liver size, weight, chest X-ray, and urea, creatinine, and serum sodium levels

Perioperative hypertension associated with cardiovascular procedures

- measure blood pressure every 5 minutes and increase the dosage every 5 minutes by 25–50 μg/min until the desired blood pressure is reached

Toxicity

Blood pressure

- systolic blood pressure less than 90 mmHg associated with evidence of inadequate cerebral (increasing confusion, agitation), renal (decreasing urine output), or peripheral (cold extremities) perfusion
- blood pressure should be monitored every 5 minutes during therapy for acute conditions and every 20–30 minutes thereafter
- if low systolic pressure and symptoms occur, reduce the dosage to the previous level, and elevate the foot of the bed
- if severe, withhold the dose and give 100 mL aliquots of normal saline until blood pressure is stabilized

Heart rate

- increase in heart rate greater than 10 bpm
- if the increase in heart rate is more than the decrease in systolic blood pressure, there may be a detrimental effect on myocardial oxygen demand and the dosage should be decreased

Headache

- headache is most frequent early in therapy and usually diminishes rapidly and may disappear within several days to weeks if treatment is continued
- patients should be warned about this adverse effect and told it subsides in 2–3 days
- nitrate headaches may be treated with acetaminophen 650 mg PO or acetaminophen with codeine
- patient should sit and apply an ice pack to the head at the first sign of headache to reduce the headache pain

Allergic reactions, palpitations, rash, blurred vision, gastrointestinal effects

- if rash occurs, the nitrate administration should be discontinued
- cross-sensitivity among the drugs may occur
- discontinue if blurred vision or dry mouth occurs
- gastrointestinal upset may be controlled by temporarily reducing the dosage

▶ *How Long Do I Treat Patients with This Drug?*

Suspected angina

- initial treatment with sublingual nitroglycerin should continue as long as patients are suspected or known to have angina
- patients should be evaluated within 4 weeks with some provocative test such as a symptom-limited exercise treadmill test or an exercise test with thallium

Chronic stable angina

- maintenance drug therapy should likely be continued indefinitely; however, changes in lifestyle and the natural history of the disease should suggest continual reevaluation for the lowest effective dosage, replacement with a better or less expensive agent, or even drug administration discontinuation

Unstable angina

- maintenance drug therapy should likely be continued indefinitely

Acute myocardial infarction

- intravenous nitrates are replaced with oral nitrates after the patient is stabilized for 48 hours, and these are continued indefinitely, as for patients with chronic stable angina

Congestive heart failure

- after an acute event, administration of nitrates should be discontinued and the patient should be assessed for the need for long-term vasodilator therapy

Perioperative hypertension associated with cardiovascular procedures

- continue therapy until the hypertension is controlled or therapy has been given for 24 hours

▶ *How Do I Decrease or Stop the Administration of This Drug?*

- there have been reports of anginal attacks that are more easily provoked and of rebound hemodynamic effects that occur soon after nitrate withdrawal in angina patients
- when discontinuing IV nitroglycerin therapy, the dose should be titrated downward while another nitroglycerin dosage form (oral or topical) is being titrated upward (e.g., apply a nitrate patch, and 15 minutes later, start decreasing nitroglycerin infusion by 10 μg/min every 5 minutes until the infusion is stopped or symptoms recur); if symptoms recur, add a further patch and continue to decrease the infusion
- when discontinuation of oral nitroglycerin therapy is planned, supplementary doses of sublingual nitroglycerin should be made available during dosage reduction

▶ *What Should I Tell My Patients About This Drug?*

- headache is most frequent early in therapy, generally diminishes rapidly, and usually disappears within several days if treatment is continued
- nitrate headaches may be treated with acetaminophen 650 mg PO
- alcohol may enhance the blood pressure–lowering effects, causing dizziness and loss of consciousness

- transient flushing of head and neck may occur
- consult your physician or go to a hospital emergency room immediately if chest pain is not relieved after 3 sublingual nitroglycerin doses approximately every 5 minutes, because the inability of these drugs to relieve chest pain may indicate acute myocardial infarction
- extended-release isosorbide dinitrate products should not be chewed
- sublingual nitroglycerin should be kept in its original bottle
- new prescription of sublingual nitroglycerin should be obtained 6 months after opening the bottle because the potency of nitroglycerin is lost when it is exposed to light and air

▶ Therapeutic Tips

- if syncope occurs, the patient should be placed in the recumbent position and measures should be initiated to facilitate venous return (e.g., head low [Trendelenburg's] position, deep breathing) and increase recovery rate
- tolerance of nitrates appears to be associated with high and/or sustained plasma drug concentrations and frequent administrations; however, nitrate tolerance does not develop to the same degree in all patients
- some evidence suggests that the development of tolerance can be prevented or minimized by use of the lowest effective dosage of nitrate and an intermittent dosing schedule with a nitrate-free interval of 10–12 hours
- if patients experience an increase in frequency and severity of angina during the nitrate-free interval, the use of concomitant antianginal therapy with another class of drugs (calcium channel blocking agents, beta-adrenergic blocking agents) designed to provide maximum coverage during the nitrate-free interval should be considered
- if nitrate tolerance is suspected in patients with unstable angina, the dosage of nitrates should be increased or patients should be started on a regimen of intravenous nitroglycerin
- bradycardia and hypotension can occur with sublingual or intravenous nitrate administration (Circulation 1976;54:624–628, Arch Intern Med 1981;141:984, Cardiology 1981;67:180–189) and are probably more frequent in inferior infarcts associated with right ventricular infarction
- cases of heart block have also been reported (Am J Med 1976;60:922–927), and this reaction is similar to the Bezold-Jarisch reflex, and IV atropine 0.5–1 mg is needed and should be used to increase blood pressure and heart rate simultaneously
- oral and topical nitrates should not be used together in the same patients (maximize the dose by 1 of the 2 routes)

Useful References

Parker JO, Farrell B, Lahey KA, Moe G. Effect of intervals between doses on the development of tolerance to isosorbide dinitrate. N Engl J Med 1987;316:1440–1444

Morse JR, Mesto RW. Double-blind crossover comparison of the antianginal effects of nifedipine and isosorbide dinitrate in patients with exertional angina receiving propranolol. J Am Coll Cardiol 1985;6:1395–1401

Thadani U. Nitrate tolerance, how to prevent it or minimize its effects. Postgrad Med 1992;91:307–318

Thadani U, IS-5MN Study Group. Isosorbide-5-mononitrate (IS-5MN) in angina pectoris: Efficacy of AM and PM doses, lack of tolerance and zero hour effects during eccentric BID therapy (abstract). Circulation 1991;84[suppl II]:II730

Bassan MM. The daylong pattern of the antianginal effect of long-term three times daily administered isosorbide dinitrate. J Am Coll Cardiol 1990;16:936–940

NIZATIDINE

James McCormack and Glen Brown

USA (Axid)
CANADA (Axid)

▶ When Should I Use This Drug?

All H₂ antagonists have equivalent efficacy and toxicity (N Engl J Med 1990;323:1749–1755) • The decision among these agents should be based on cost

see Ranitidine

▶ When Should I Not Use This Drug?

Stress ulcer prophylaxis

- not available as a parenteral form

see Ranitidine

▶ What Contraindications Are There to the Use of This Drug?

- intolerance of or allergic reaction to nizatidine

▶ What Drug Interactions Are Clinically Important?

see Ranitidine

▶ What Route and Dosage Should I Use?

How to administer

- orally—may be given with food or on an empty stomach
- parenterally—not available

Dyspepsia or duodenal or gastric ulcers

- 300 mg PO at bedtime or with the evening meal
- 150 mg PO BID if the patient has frequent daytime ulcer pain

Prevention of peptic ulcer disease recurrence

- 150 mg PO at bedtime

Gastroesophageal reflux

- 150 mg PO BID
- 150 mg PO at bedtime if the patient has only nighttime symptoms

Dosage adjustments for renal or hepatic dysfunction

- renally eliminated

Normal Dosing Interval	$C_{cr} > 60$ mL/min or 1 mL/s	C_{cr} 30–60 mL/min or 0.5–1 mL/s	$C_{cr} < 30$ mL/min or 0.5 mL/s
Q12H	no adjustment needed	Q24H	Q24H and decrease dosage by 50%
Q24H	no adjustment needed	decrease dosage by 50%	decrease dosage by 75%

▶ What Should I Monitor with Regard to Efficacy and Toxicity?

see Cimetidine

▶ How Long Do I Treat Patients with This Drug?

see Cimetidine

▶ How Do I Decrease or Stop the Administration of This Drug?

- may be stopped abruptly
- if the patient requires prophylactic therapy, decrease the dosage from 300 mg PO HS to 150 mg PO HS

▶ What Should I Tell My Patients About This Drug?

see Ranitidine

▶ Therapeutic Tips

see Ranitidine

NORFLOXACIN

Peter Jewesson

USA (Noroxin)
CANADA (Noroxin)

▶ When Should I Use This Drug?

check antibiotic susceptibility chart (Table 4–1 in Chapter 4)

Lower urinary tract infections

- norfloxacin should be reserved for the treatment of urinary tract infections when patients are known or suspected to be intolerant of trimethoprim-sulfamethoxazole and amoxicillin, or when pathogens associated with the infections are known or suspected to be resistant to trimethoprim-sulfamethoxazole and amoxicillin, because norfloxacin is more expensive than these agents and no more effective if the organisms are sensitive

- ciprofloxacin 250 mg PO Q12H should be used instead of norfloxacin 400 mg PO Q12H if it is less expensive, except if the patient is taking theophylline (drug interaction with ciprofloxacin)

Enteric infections

- norfloxacin is at least as active as previously used agents, is usually better tolerated, but is more expensive
- drug of choice for severe shigellosis, traveler's diarrhea, and salmonellosis if less expensive than ciprofloxacin
- use trimethoprim-sulfamethoxazole for mild infections, as it is effective and less expensive

▶ When Should I Not Use This Drug?

Systemic infections

- norfloxacin should not be used for systemic infections
- only ciprofloxacin and other newer fluoroquinolones, which achieve adequate systemic concentrations, should be used for systemic infections

▶ What Contraindications Are There to the Use of This Drug?

see Ciprofloxacin

▶ What Drug Interactions Are Clinically Important?

Drugs that may increase the effect or toxicity of norfloxacin

- none

Drugs that may decrease the effect of norfloxacin

ANTACIDS, FERROUS SULFATE

- magnesium—or aluminum—containing antacids or ferrous sulfate reduce the absorption of fluoroquinolones
- avoid concomitant use or space doses by 3 hours or longer

SUCRALFATE

- sucralfate contains aluminum salts and has been demonstrated to reduce the bioavailability of fluoroquinolones
- avoid concomitant use or space doses by 3 hours or longer

Drugs that may have their effect or toxicity increased by norfloxacin

- none

Drugs that may have their effect decreased by norfloxacin

- none

▶ What Route and Dosage Should I Use?

How to administer

- orally—on an empty stomach, or with food if gastrointestinal intolerance occurs

Lower urinary tract infections

- 400 mg PO Q12H

Enteric infections

- 400 mg PO Q12H

Dosage adjustments for renal or hepatic dysfunction

- renally eliminated

Normal Dosing Interval	$C_{cr} > 60$ mL/min or 1 mL/s	C_{cr} 30–60 mL/min or 0.5–1 mL/s	$C_{cr} < 30$ mL/min or 0.5 mL/s
Q12H	no adjustment needed	no adjustment needed	Q24H

▶ What Should I Monitor with Regard to Efficacy and Toxicity?

see Ciprofloxacin

▶ How Long Do I Treat Patients with This Drug?

see Ciprofloxacin

▶ How Do I Decrease or Stop the Administration of This Drug?

- may be stopped abruptly

▶ What Should I Tell My Patients About This Drug?

see Ciprofloxacin

▶ Therapeutic Tips

- always consider efficacy, toxicity, and cost when determining the role of norfloxacin relative to other available agents
- reserve use for difficult to treat infections involving susceptible pathogens, as overuse likely results in the development of resistance over time

Useful Reference

Paton JH, Reeves DS. The fluoroquinolone antibiotics. Drugs 1988;36; 193–228

NORTRIPTYLINE

Lyle K. Laird and Julia Vertrees

USA (Aventyl, Pamelor)
CANADA (Aventyl)

▶ When Should I Use This Drug?

Major depression, dysthymia, generalized anxiety disorder

- nortriptyline is as effective as other antidepressants, and although imipramine is usually chosen for these disorders, nortriptyline is the tricyclic antidepressant that causes the least orthostatic hypotension and should be chosen for patients with concerns about falling (e.g., the elderly) and patients with orthostatic hypotension
- nortriptyline has a recognized and well-documented reduced risk of causing orthostatic hypotension (Pharmacol Clin 1970;2:68–71)
- nortriptyline is not as well studied as other antidepressants for panic disorders and chronic pain syndromes

▶ When Should I Not Use This Drug?

see Imipramine

▶ What Contraindications Are There to the Use of This Drug?

see Imipramine

Pregnancy

- adequate human studies have not been performed

▶ What Drug Interactions Are Clinically Important?

see Imipramine

▶ What Route and Dosage Should I Use?

How to administer

- orally—can be given with food or on an empty stomach
- parenterally—not available

Major depression, dysthymia, generalized anxiety disorders

- 25 mg PO daily at bedtime
- increase after 3 days to 50 mg PO daily at bedtime
- increase to 75 mg PO daily at bedtime after 1 week and leave at this dosage for 10–14 days
- if target symptoms are not improving after 3 weeks of therapy, continue to increase the daily dosage by 25 mg at weekly intervals until a response is seen or a maximum dosage of 150 mg PO daily has been reached
- in geriatric patients and patients with a seizure history, start with 12.5 mg PO at bedtime, and in general, dosages should be approximately 50% of those used in younger patients
- nortriptyline has a long duration of action; hence, long-acting or sustained-release products are unnecessary and once-daily dosing is appropriate in adults

- after the patient has experienced a therapeutic response, the dosage should be maintained at that level for 6–9 months because relapses may occur if dosage reduction is attempted

Dosage adjustments for renal or hepatic dysfunction

- hepatically metabolized
- start with low doses as for a geriatric patient
- decreased renal function does not necessitate dosage adjustments

▶ *What Should I Monitor with Regard to Efficacy and Toxicity?*

see Imipramine

Efficacy
Plasma concentration monitoring

see Imipramine

- nortriptyline is perhaps the only antidepressant with a reasonably accepted therapeutic range; at steady state conditions, a 12 hour postdose plasma concentration of 50–150 ng/mL is likely to correlate with clinical efficacy (Clin Pharmacokinet 1987;13: 381–392)

▶ *How Long Do I Treat Patients with This Drug?*

see Imipramine

▶ *What Should I Tell My Patients About This Drug?*

see Imipramine

▶ *Therapeutic Tips*

see Imipramine

Useful References

Bryant SG, Brown CS. Major depressive disorders. In: Young LY, Koda-Kimble MA, eds. Applied Therapeutics: The Clinical Use of Drugs, 4th ed. Vancouver, WA: Applied Therapeutics, 1988:1231–1253

Wells BG, Hayes PE. Depressive illness. In: DiPiro JT, Talbert RL, Hayes PE, et al, eds. Pharmacotherapy: A Pathophysiologic Approach. New York: Elsevier, 1989:748–764

NYSTATIN

Peter Jewesson

USA (Candex, Moronal)
CANADA (Mycostatin, Nadostine, Nilstat, Nyaderm, Flagystatin (with metronidazole))

▶ *When Should I Use This Drug?*

Oropharyngeal candidiasis

- topical agents should initially be used because they are associated with less toxicity and there is less potential for drug interactions
- unfortunately, compliance with these regimens may be poor, and this often mandates a change to systemic antifungal therapy such as ketoconazole, fluconazole, or itraconazole (see below under esophageal candidiasis)
- nystatin and cotrimazole are likely equally effective
- clotrimazole is preferred over nystatin as the initial treatment of oropharyngeal candidiasis as it is usually better tolerated; however, clotrimazole is usually more expensive than nystatin
- patients with severe disease may need to be treated with ketoconazole/fluconazole/amphotericin B

▶ *When Should I Not Use This Drug?*

Esophageal candidiasis

- topical agents are usually not effective for esophageal candidiasis and oral agents such as ketoconazole or fluconazole should be used

Vaginal candidiasis

- topical miconazole/clotrimazole/terconazole are considered

more effective than nystatin (Obstet Gynecol 1976;48:491) and can be given as a short 3 day course of therapy

Bowel sterilization (selective decontamination) for immunocompromised patients

- nystatin prophylaxis has not been proven to improve outcomes and may lead to selection of resistant organisms

▶ *What Contraindications Are There to the Use of This Drug?*

- intolerance or allergic reaction to nystatin

▶ *What Drug Interactions Are Clinically Important?*

- none

▶ *What Route and Dosage Should I Use?*

Oropharyngeal candidiasis

- 1 vaginal tablet (100,000 units) dissolved slowly in the mouth TID (up to 5 times/d depending on response)
- the suspension is generally less effective due to decreased contact time but can be used at 500,000 units swish and swallow QID
- choice of the above is dependent on patient preference and compliance

Dosage adjustment for renal/liver dysfunction

- no systemic absorption, therefore no dosage adjustment needed for renal or hepatic dysfunction

▶ *What Should I Monitor with Regard to Efficacy and Toxicity?*

Efficacy
Oropharyngeal candidiasis

- reduction in pain, disappearance of lesions
- assess symptoms daily if in hospital or at least weekly as an outpatient

Toxicity

- possible local irritation but no significant toxicity as there is no systemic absorption

▶ *How Long Do I Treat Patients with This Drug?*

Oropharyngeal candidiasis

- 1 week and at least 2 days after the symptoms have resolved
- patient should begin to respond within a few days
- continuous therapy may be required in patients with frequent relapses

▶ *How Do I Decrease or Stop the Administration of This Drug?*

- may be stopped abruptly

▶ *What Should I Tell My Patients About This Drug?*

- this agent is an antifungal agent and successful therapy is contingent upon good compliance and completion of the full treatment course
- some minor side effects (i.e., local irritation) may occur—contact pharmacist or physician if any unusual symptoms arise

▶ *Therapeutic Tips*

- increased contact with oral mucosa will increase effectiveness
- compliance with high dose prophylactic oral regimens is typically poor and not associated with increased efficacy

Useful References

Bennett JE. Antifungal agents. In: Mandell GL, Douglas RG Jr, Bennett JE, eds. Principles and Practice of Infectious Diseases, 3rd ed. New York: Churchill Livingstone, 1990;361–370

Degregorio MW, et al. Candida infections in patients with acute leukemia. Ineffectiveness of nystatin prophylaxis and relationship between oropharyngeal and systemic candidiasis. Cancer 1982;50:2870

OMEPRAZOLE

James McCormack and Glen Brown

USA (Prilosec)
CANADA (Losec)

▶ *When Should I Use This Drug?*

Gastric or duodenal ulcers

- high costs and unknown long-term effects of omeprazole relegate it to a second-line regimen at present because most patients respond to other less expensive agents
- use in patients who have not responded to a 12 week course of H_2 antagonists

Gastroesophageal reflux

- for mild to moderate disease after therapy with nondrug measures and H_2 antagonists has failed
- 90–100% of patients who fail to respond to therapy with H_2 antagonists heal with omeprazole
- drug of choice for severe disease, as it is more effective than H_2 antagonists and motility agents in the treatment of severe or erosive esophagitis

Zollinger-Ellison syndrome

- omeprazole is the proven drug of choice (N Engl J Med 1990;323:1749–1755)
- need large doses of H_2 antagonists at frequent intervals, which can be inconvenient, is costly, and potentially causes a higher incidence of adverse effects

▶ *When Should I Not Use This Drug?*

Initial treatment of duodenal or gastric ulcers

- although ulcers heal slightly faster with omeprazole than H_2 antagonists, there are no obvious advantages of omeprazole for the initial treatment of peptic ulcer disease, as H_2 antagonists are effective and less expensive (N Engl J Med 1991;324:965–975)

Combination with other antiulcer medications

- no studies to support combination therapy of regularly dosed upper gastrointestinal drugs for the treatment of peptic ulcer disease, and it increases cost and the chance of adverse effects (Lancet 1988;1:1383–1385, N Engl J Med 1991;325:1017–1025, Am J Gastroenterol 1993;88:675–679)

▶ *What Contraindications Are There to the Use of This Drug?*

- intolerance of or allergic reaction to omeprazole

▶ *What Drug Interactions Are Clinically Important?*

Drugs that may increase the effect or toxicity of omeprazole

- none

Drugs that may decrease the effect of omeprazole

- none

Drugs that may have their effect or toxicity increased by omeprazole

BENZODIAZEPINES

- omeprazole may inhibit the metabolism of benzodiazepines
- if benzodiazepines are used regularly, monitor the patient for increased sedation and decrease the dosage if needed

WARFARIN

- interferes with warfarin metabolism and can increase INR
- use alternative agents if possible and if not possible, monitor INR every 2 days until the full extent of the interaction is seen and adjust the dosage as for a warfarin dosage change
- monitor INR every 2 days when administration of the interacting drug is discontinued and adjust as for a warfarin dosage change

PHENYTOIN

- inhibits metabolism of phenytoin and may produce increases in serum phenytoin concentrations

- monitor serum phenytoin concentrations weekly until a new steady state is established or symptoms of toxicity occur, and adjust the phenytoin dosage accordingly
- if administration of the inhibitor is stopped, return to previous dosage

Drugs that may have their effect decreased by omeprazole

KETOCONAZOLE

- decreased gastric acidity reduces ketoconazole absorption
- use an alternative antifungal (fluconazole)

IRON

- adjust the dosage on the basis of the clinical and laboratory response to iron

▶ *What Route and Dosage Should I Use?*

How to administer

- orally—can be given with food or on an empty stomach

Gastric or duodenal ulcers

- 20 mg PO daily (Digestion 1990;47[suppl 1]:64–68, N Engl J Med 1991;324:965–975)

Gastroesophageal reflux

- start with 20 mg PO daily for mild to moderate disease
- start with 40 mg PO daily for severe disease

Zollinger-Ellison syndrome

- 40 mg PO daily up to 120 mg PO Q8H

Dosage adjustments for renal or hepatic dysfunction

- hepatically metabolized
- no dosage adjustment recommendations are available for hepatic dysfunction; however, start with 20 mg PO daily and titrate to response

▶ *What Should I Monitor with Regard to Efficacy and Toxicity?*

Efficacy

Duodenal or gastric ulcer

- relief of symptoms such as epigastric pain or discomfort, belching, burning, bloating, fullness, and nausea and vomiting

Gastroesophageal reflux

- decrease in reflux episodes

Toxicity

Adverse effects are infrequent

Gastric carcinoid tumors

- with long-term use, hypergastrinemia may occur in a small number of patients treated with omeprazole, and it also has the potential to cause gastric tumors (in animal studies); however, no long-term studies have established the risk/benefit ratio
- no special monitoring is recommended at present

▶ *How Long Do I Treat Patients with This Drug?*

Gastric or duodenal ulcers

- 4 weeks (Digestion 1990;47[suppl 1]:64–68, N Engl J Med 1991;324:965–975)
- if the ulcer has not healed at 4 weeks, continue therapy and evaluate again at 8 weeks
- if the ulcer has not healed at 8 weeks, increase the dosage to 40 mg and treat for a further 4 weeks

Gastroesophageal reflux

- give omeprazole for 4 weeks, and if there is no response, continue for another 4 weeks
- if there is still no response, increase the dosage by 20 mg PO daily
- after symptoms are controlled, cut back the dosage by 50% every few weeks to identify the lowest effective dosage (some patients will be controlled with as little as 20 mg PO Q 2–3 days)

- most patients with gastroesophageal reflux experience relapse; therefore, after healing has occurred, omeprazole may have to be continued indefinitely

Zollinger-Ellison syndrome

- drug therapy is lifelong

▶ *How Do I Decrease or Stop the Administration of This Drug?*

- may be stopped abruptly

▶ *What Should I Tell My Patients About This Drug?*

- it may take several days for this drug to relieve stomach pain
- if no relief of symptoms is seen in 7 days, contact your physician
- if symptoms are not completely resolved after 4 weeks, contact your physician
- this drug may interact with many medications; therefore, check with your physician or pharmacist before using other medications
- take the drug for the full 4 weeks even if symptoms disappear after 1–2 weeks

▶ *Therapeutic Tips*

- do not use omeprazole for the initial treatment of peptic ulcer disease, as it is more expensive than alternative therapies

Useful Reference

Maton PN. Omeprazole. N Engl J Med 1991;324:965–975

ONDANSETRON

Lynne Nakashima

USA (Zofran)
CANADA (Zofran)

▶ *When Should I Use This Drug?*

Chemotherapy-induced nausea and vomiting

- drug of choice when a patient is receiving drugs with high emetogenic potential
- although ondansetron is expensive, it is the most effective agent available for preventing nausea and vomiting in patients receiving highly emetogenic therapy and other therapy is often not effective
- expense of ondansetron must be compared with the cost of preparing the parenteral 3- or 4-agent regimens and the cost of "rescue" medications (Eur J Cancer 1993;29A[3]:303–306)
- ondansetron is well tolerated by most patients
- ondansetron, in combination with dexamethasone, is more effective than ondansetron alone (J Clin Oncol 1991;9:675–678)
- ondansetron can be used for patients who experience intolerable extrapyramidal side effects or sedation with phenothiazine antiemetic agents, as it does not cause extrapyramidal side effects or sedation (Hosp Pharm 1991;26:252–253)

▶ *When Should I Not Use This Drug?*

Nausea and vomiting due to other causes

- ondansetron is expensive, and its use for other indications should be limited pending further experience

▶ *What Contraindications Are There to the Use of This Drug?*

- intolerance of or allergic reaction to ondansetron

▶ *What Drug Interactions Are Clinically Important?*

- no clinically significant drug interactions have been reported
- ondansetron is metabolized by the cytochrome P-450 system; therefore, inhibitors or inducers of this enzyme system may affect the clearance of ondansetron (Eur J Clin Oncol 1989; 25[suppl 1]:575–577)

▶ *What Route and Dosage Should I Use?*

How to administer

- orally—take with food or milk or on an empty stomach

- parenterally—give in 50 mL of 5% dextrose in water or normal saline and infuse in over 15 minutes

Chemotherapy-induced nausea and vomiting

- 8 mg PO 30 minutes prior to chemotherapy (give intravenously at same dosage if the patient is already vomiting)
- use oral dosing before chemotherapy, unless the patient has preexisting nausea and vomiting because the oral dose is half the cost of intravenous therapy and equally effective
- follow the prechemotherapy dose with 8 mg PO Q8H starting 4 hours after chemotherapy and continue for 2 days

Dosage adjustments for renal or hepatic dysfunction

- hepatically metabolized
- no dosage adjustments are currently recommended

▶ *What Should I Monitor with Regard to Efficacy and Toxicity?*

Efficacy

Frequency of assessment depends on the severity and frequency of nausea and vomiting

Number and severity of vomiting episodes

- determine time of day, force, description of vomitus, and associated symptoms

Fluid balance (only needed if vomiting occurs for a prolonged period)

- assess jugular venous pressure and orthostatic changes in blood pressure and heart rate; any decrease in upright diastolic pressure plus a rise in heart rate of 20 bpm or greater is abnormal
- oliguria
- weight
- rising values of hematocrit and creatinine, urea, sodium, and bicarbonate levels plus decreasing potassium and chloride levels are an indication of dehydration

Toxicity

Headache

- of mild to moderate severity in approximately 15–20% of patients (Ann Intern Med 1990;113:834–840)
- discontinue therapy if acetaminophen 650 mg PO is ineffective in controlling symptoms

Constipation

- of mild to moderate severity in approximately 10% of patients (Ann Intern Med 1990;113:834–840)
- if constipation occurs, increase the fluid intake and try a laxative

Lightheadedness, dizziness, faintness

- may occur; therefore, tell the patient to rise slowly and to use guardrails on stairways

Liver function tests

- total bilirubin values may increase above the normal range; this is usually asymptomatic and rapidly returns to normal levels after discontinuation of therapy (J Clin Oncol 1990;8:731–735)
- liver enzyme values may increase above the normal range in approximately 30% of patients (J Clin Oncol 1990;8:731–735)
- none of these elevated liver function test results were associated with clinical symptoms and none necessitated discontinuation of therapy (J Clin Oncol 1990;8:731–735)
- no need for routine monitoring; however, if monitoring liver function tests for chemotherapy, consider ondansetron as a possible cause if values rise above normal levels

▶ *How Long Do I Treat Patients with This Drug?*

Chemotherapy-induced nausea and vomiting

- ondansetron is usually continued for 48 hours after chemotherapy
- breakthrough nausea and vomiting should be treated with a rescue antiemetic such as prochlorperazine 10 mg PO or PR Q6H PRN

▶ *How Do I Decrease or Stop the Administration of This Drug?*

- may be stopped abruptly

▶ *What Should I Tell My Patients About This Drug?*

- headache may occur, and if this occurs, try acetaminophen 650 mg every 4 hours as needed
- if lightheadedness, dizziness, or faintness occurs, try rising slowly and use guardrails on stairways
- these effects are temporary and stop after you finish taking the drug
- constipation may also occur, and increasing fluid intake may help alleviate the problem

▶ *Therapeutic Tips*

- oral ondansetron should be used in place of IV ondansetron whenever possible, as it is less expensive

Useful References

Burnette PK, Perking J. Parenteral ondansetron for the treatment of chemotherapy-and-radiation induced nausea and vomiting. Pharmacotherapy 1992;12:120–131

Cubeddu LX, Hoffman IS, Fuenmayor NT, et al. Efficacy of ondansetron and the role of serotonin in cisplatin-induced nausea and vomiting. N Engl J Med 1990;322:810–816

Einhorn LH, Nagy C, Werner K, Finn AL. Ondansetron: A new antiemetic for patients receiving cisplatin chemotherapy. J Clin Oncol 1990; 8:731–735

Merrifield KR, Chaffee BJ. Recent advances in management of nausea and vomiting caused by antineoplastic agents. Clin Pharm 1989;8:187–199

Mike RJ, Heel RC. Ondansetron. Therapeutic use as an antiemetic. Drugs 1991;41:574–595

Chaffee BJ, Tankanow RM. Ondansetron—The first of a new class of antiemetics. Clin Pharm 1991;10:430–436

Perez EA, Gandara DR. Advances in the control of chemotherapy-induced emesis. Ann Oncol 1992;3(suppl 3):S47–S50

ORCIPRENALINE, METAPROTERENOL

Karen Shalansky and Cindy Reesor Nimmo

USA (Alupent, Dey-Lute Metaproterenol Sulfate, Metaprel)
CANADA (Alupent)

▶ *When Should I Use This Drug?*

Consider an alternative agent

- orciprenaline (Canada) or metaproterenol (USA) is less beta$_2$ selective than salbutamol or terbutaline, resulting in a higher incidence of cardiac stimulation (Med Lett 1991;33:9–12)

Useful References

Kelly HW. New beta$_2$-adrenergic agonist aerosols. Clin Pharm 1985; 4:393–403

McFadden ER. Clinical use of beta-adrenergic agonists. J Allergy Clin Immunol 1985;76:352–356

ORPHENADRINE

Ruby Grymonpre

USA (Disipal, Marflex, Norflex [extended release], Orflagen [extended release])
CANADA (Disipal, Norflex)

▶ *When Should I Use This Drug?*

Consider an alternative agent

- antihistamine orphenadrine is probably effective for parkinsonism through its anticholinergic and sedative properties
- orphenadrine is not a recommended antiparkinsonian agent, as there has been greater clinical experience with the other anticholinergic agents and there appears to be no real advantage to using orphenadrine instead of other anticholinergics

OXACILLIN

John Rotschafer, Kyle Vance-Bryan, and Rick Zabinski

USA (Bactocill, Prostaphlin)
CANADA (not available)

▶ *When Should I Use This Drug?*

Consider an alternative agent

- identical indications to those of cloxacillin and offers no advantages over cloxacillin
- likely causes more hepatotoxicity than do other penicillinase-resistant penicillins

OXAPROZIN

Kelly Jones

USA (Daypro)
CANADA (not available)

▶ *When Should I Use This Drug?*

Rheumatoid arthritis

- oxaprozin can be used as an alternative for patients who fail to respond to enteric-coated aspirin or ibuprofen; however, it is more expensive
- useful in patients who have a history of noncompliance (because it has once-daily dosing); however, once-daily dosing may not be preferred in patients with arthritis pain, as these patients may want to dose more than once per day (DICP 1989;23:76–85)
- most regular-release nonsteroidal antiinflammatory drugs (NSAIDs), including aspirin, can be taken on an every 12 hour basis when being used to treat arthritic conditions, and therefore once-daily NSAIDs provide only the advantage of once versus twice daily dosing
- decision among piroxicam, tenoxicam, nabumetone, and oxaprozin (once a day NSAIDs) should be based on cost
- sustained-release NSAIDs can be used once daily, preferably in the evening to attempt reduction in morning stiffness, and should be chosen if they are less expensive than piroxicam, tenoxicam, nabumetone, or oxaprozin

Osteoarthritis

- if acetaminophen, enteric-coated aspirin or ibuprofen are not effective
- decision between this drug and other NSAIDs should be based on cost

▶ *When Should I Not Use This Drug?*

Acute pain, general aches and pain, dysmenorrhea

- not useful for the acute management of general aches and pains because it is difficult to titrate owing to its long half-life and because it is expensive

Control of acute pain associated with arthritis

- this drug should never be use initially to gain control of arthritis pain, as the long half-life does not allow dosing flexibility
- this drug should be reserved as maintenance therapy for those with controlled disease

Combination with other NSAIDs

- combinations of NSAIDs provide no increase in effectiveness compared with maximum dosages of single agents and significantly increases the risk of adverse effects

▶ *What Contraindications Are There to the Use of This Drug?*

see Ibuprofen

▶ *What Drug Interactions Are Clinically Important?*

see Ibuprofen

▶ *What Route and Dosage Should I Use?*

How to administer

- orally—take with food or milk
- parenterally—not available

Rheumatoid arthritis

- 1200 mg PO daily HS to a maximum dosage of 1800 mg PO daily as a divided dose (BID)

Osteoarthritis

- 600 mg PO daily HS to a maximum of 1800 mg PO daily as a divided dose (BID)

Dosage adjustments for renal or hepatic dysfunction

- hepatically metabolized; therefore, no adjustments are needed for renal disease
- reduce dosage by 25% in patients with a history of hepatic disease

▶ *What Should I Monitor with Regard to Efficacy and Toxicity?*

see Ibuprofen

▶ *How Do I Decrease or Stop the Administration of This Drug?*

- may be stopped abruptly if needed

▶ *What Should I Tell My Patients About This Drug?*

see Ibuprofen

▶ *Therapeutic Tips*

see Ibuprofen

Useful References

see Ibuprofen

OXAZEPAM

Steven Stanislav, Patricia Marken, and Jonathan Fleming

USA (Serax)
CANADA (Serax, Apo-Oxazepam, Oxazepam, Novoxapam, PMS Oxazepam, Zapex)

▶ *When Should I Use This Drug?*

Generalized anxiety disorder

- benzodiazepines have been considered first-line therapy owing to extensive research and over 30 years' clinical experience
- predictors of response to benzodiazepines are acute symptoms, a precipitating stressful event, high level of psychic and somatic anxiety, absence of or low level of depression, no previous drug treatment, good response to previous therapy, and expectation of recovery or desire for medication
- benzodiazepines have an effect immediately to within several days, whereas buspirone's effect is delayed for 2–4 weeks
- all benzodiazepines are equally effective; therefore, the choice is based on the patient's previous response and the cost
- agents with an intermediate duration of action (lorazepam or oxazepam) are preferred because they allow easier dose titration by both the patient and the physician
- onset of action for lorazepam is a little faster (15–45 minutes versus 45–90 minutes) than that of oxazepam (likely because it is absorbed faster) but this difference is probably not important when these agents are dosed long term

Transient situational insomnia, short-term insomnia (up to 3 weeks' duration)

- all of the marketed benzodiazepines have sedative properties and can be used as hypnotics
- they differ in their pharmacokinetics, side effect profile, capacity to cause discontinuation syndromes (e.g., rebound insomnia), and cost
- lorazepam, oxazepam, and temazepam are equally effective, although there are fewer data on the use of lorazepam and oxazepam as hypnotics
- oxazepam is absorbed slightly slower than lorazepam and must be given 60–90 minutes before retiring, whereas lorazepam can be given 30–40 minutes before retiring
- decision should also include cost (lorazepam and oxazepam are available as generics and are usually less expensive)

Acute psychosis

- short-term therapy with benzodiazepines can be used to control initial agitation and decrease the need for initial high doses of antipsychotics

- lorazepam is usually chosen for this condition because it is available in a parenteral formulation

▶ *When Should I Not Use This Drug?*

Transient and short-term insomnia when it is important to avoid daytime sedation or effects on psychomotor performance, such as for the management of jet lag

- oxazepam has a moderately long half-life; therefore, use triazolam, which has fewer hangover effects

▶ *What Contraindications Are There to the Use of This Drug?*

see Lorazepam

▶ *What Drug Interactions Are Clinically Important?*

see Lorazepam

▶ *What Route and Dosage Should I Use?*

How to administer

- orally—can be taken with food or milk or on an empty stomach
- parenterally—not available

Generalized anxiety disorder

- start with 15 mg PO BID
- if no excessive sedation occurs, increase the dosage by 15 mg increments every 3–4 days up to 30 mg PO TID (this dosage controls these disorders in most people) or until symptoms are well under control

Transient situational insomnia, short-term insomnia (up to three weeks' duration)

- give 15 mg PO to be taken 60 minutes before retiring and increase to 30 mg only if the lower dosage is ineffective

Acute psychosis

- 60 mg PO Q1H until settled

Dosage adjustments for renal or hepatic dysfunction

- hepatically metabolized
- no dosage adjustments for organ dysfunction are recommended; however, always start with lowest dose and titrate to response

▶ *What Should I Monitor with Regard to Efficacy and Toxicity?*

see Lorazepam

▶ *How Long Do I Treat Patients with This Drug?*

see Lorazepam

▶ *How Do I Decrease or Stop the Administration of This Drug?*

see Lorazepam

▶ *What Should I Tell My Patients About This Drug?*

see Lorazepam

▶ *Therapeutic Tips*

see Lorazepam

- to treat initial insomnia, give 60 minutes before the anticipated retiring time

Useful Reference

Gillin JC, Byerley WF. The diagnosis and management of insomnia, N Engl J Med 1990;322:239–248

OXTRIPHYLLINE

Karen Shalansky and Cindy Reesor Nimmo

USA (Choledyl, Choledyl SA)
CANADA (Choledyl, Choledyl SA)

▶ *When Should I Use This Drug?*

Consider an alternative agent

- oxtriphylline contains 65% theophylline and offers no advantage over other theophylline preparations and should be used only if it is less expensive

OXYCODONE

Terry Baumann

USA (Roxicodone; combination: Percodan, Percocet, Tylox, various)
CANADA (Roxicodone; combination: Percodan, Percocet, Tylox, various)

▶ *When Should I Use This Drug?*

Acute pain, cancer pain, chronic noncancer pain

- for moderate symptoms if treatment with nonopioid agents (acetaminophen or nonsteroidal antiinflammatory drugs [NSAIDs]) is not effective after titrating rapidly to maximum doses
- in general, codeine should be chosen instead of oxycodone, as oxycodone provides no clinical advantages over codeine
- oxycodone can be used instead of codeine, as it may have placebo value in patients who are convinced that a codeine product does not work
- oxycodone provides no advantages over morphine

▶ *When Should I Not Use This Drug?*

Severe pain

- use morphine or hydromorphone
- not available as an injection

▶ *What Contraindications Are There to the Use of This Drug?*

see Morphine

▶ *What Drug Interactions Are Clinically Important?*

see Morphine

▶ *What Route and Dosage Should I Use?*

How to administer

- orally—may be administered with food or milk or on an empty stomach
- parenterally—not available

Acute pain, cancer pain, chronic noncancer pain

- 5 mg PO Q4H in combination with at least 325 mg of acetaminophen, 300 mg of aspirin, or another NSAID
- use 2.5 mg of oxycodone in the elderly
- do not use the acetaminophen or aspirin combination for more than 5 days in a round-the-clock fashion because of the possible acetaminophen or aspirin toxicity

Dosage adjustments for renal or hepatic dysfunction

- hepatically metabolized
- dosage adjustment is usually not required if the dose is titrated properly

▶ *What Should I Monitor with Regard to Efficacy and Toxicity?*

see Morphine

▶ *How Long Do I Treat Patients with This Drug?*

see Morphine

- do not use the acetaminophen or aspirin combination for more than 5 days in a round-the-clock fashion because of the possible acetaminophen or aspirin toxicity
- may be used indefinitely on a PRN basis as long as maximum daily aspirin or acetaminophen dosages are not exceeded

▶ *How Do I Decrease or Stop the Administration of This Drug?*

see Morphine

▶ *What Should I Tell My Patients About This Drug?*

see Morphine

▶ *Therapeutic Tips*

see Morphine

- be aware that when oxycodone is used in combination products with acetaminophen or aspirin in a round-the-clock fashion, possible acetaminophen or aspirin toxicity may occur owing to the possible ingestion of large amounts of acetaminophen and/or aspirin

Useful References

see Morphine

OXYTOCIN

Glenda Meneilly

USA (Pitocin, Syntocinon)
CANADA (Pitocin, Syntocinon)

▶ *When Should I Use This Drug?*

Induction of labor

- for augmentation of labor when nondrug measures, such as amniotomy (artificial rupture of membranes) and nipple stimulation, are unsuccessful when there is documentation of progressive dilation to at least 3 cm and effacement
- oxytocin should be used as inital treatment (instead of prostaglandin gel) if Bishop's score is greater than 5 (favorable cervix) or patients are gravida 3 or greater
- when prolongation of pregnancy is dangerous to fetus
- induction should be considered at 37–38 weeks' gestation in patients with mild chronic hypertension or pregnancy-induced hypertension
- induction is undertaken immediately if severe pregnancy-induced hypertension (eclampsia) or uncontrolled chronic hypertension (mean arterial pressure > 126 mmHg) is present
- induction should be considered in pregnant diabetics who have poorly controlled blood glucose despite maximal therapy, progression of nephropathy or retinopathy, or patients who have previously delivered a macrosomic (large) fetus
- prolonged pregnancy or dysfunctional labor

Induction of labor for abortion

- for second trimester pregnancies that do not abort with prostaglandins

Control or prevention of postpartum bleeding

- for all patients, who are bleeding heavily or the uterus is not contracting
- ergonovine maleate or methylergonovine maleate produces stronger and more sustained uterine contractions and is usually preferred for this indication

Evaluation of fetal well-being

- oxytocin challenge test (contraction stimulation test)
- used when the results of a nonstress test are nonreactive or suspicious

Promotion of milk let-down

- administered as nasal solution
- may enhance the onset of lactation in women who deliver prematurely
- oxytocin nasal spray is expensive and frequently ineffective

▶ *When Should I Not Use This Drug?*

Bishop's score of 4 or less

- induction usually fails in these patients, as the uterus is not responsive to oxytocin
- these patients should first be treated with prostaglandin E₂ gel

▶ *What Contraindications Are There to the Use of This Drug?*

- intolerance of or allergic reaction to oxytocin
- induction should *not* be undertaken in the presence of fetal distress, placenta previa, cephalopelvic disproportion, or any condi-

tion in which there is a predisposition to uterine rupture, such as overdistention of the uterus due to multiple gestation or polyhydramnios or a previous history of traumatic delivery
- if labor is indicated, oxytocin is *not* contraindicated

▶ What Drug Interactions Are Clinically Important?

- none

▶ What Route and Dosage Should I Use?

How to administer

- orally—not available
- parenterally—administer by intravenous infusion using a constant rate infusion pump to ensure accurate drug administration and piggyback oxytocin into the main intravenous catheter near the intravenous insertion site, as this prevents large amounts of oxytocin from being infused after the infusion has been stopped
- add oxytocin to nonhydrating fluids such as lactated Ringer's solution or normal saline
- oxytocin infusion rates vary with both the indication for use and the type of patient
- to deliver 1 mU/min, add 10 units of oxytocin to 1 L of IV fluid (solution will contain 1 mU in each 0.1 mL)
- if the pump delivers 10 drops/mL, set at 1 drop/min for oxytocin 1 mU/min
- nasally—hold squeeze bottle in upright position: with the patient in a sitting position, spray once into each nostril
- can be given IM if IV route not possible

Induction of labor

Preterm patient

- start with infusion rate of 1 mU/min and increase by 2 mU/min every 30 minutes; infusion rates of 20–40 mU/min may be required
- although older oxytocin dosing regimens increased the dosage exponentially (2, 4, 8, 16, and so on) every 15–20 minutes, evidence has shown that arithmetic (2, 4, 6, 8, 10, and so on) increases at intervals of 30–60 minutes result in equally effective induction of labor with less uterine hyperstimulation (Obstet Gynecol 1990;75:757–761)

Term patient, patient with favorable cervix or preexisting uterine activity

- start with infusion rate of 0.5 mU/min and increase by 1 mU/min every 30 minutes, with an infusion rate of 2–8 mU/min usually being sufficient to achieve cervical dilation of 1 cm/h, and a dosage of more than 20 mU/min at term is rarely needed (Obstet Gynecol Surv 1988;43:730–743)

Induction of labor for abortion

- start with an infusion of 20 mU/min and increase by 10 mU/min every 15 minutes to a maximum of 100 mU/min

Control or prevention of postpartum bleeding

- add 20 units (40 units if bleeding heavily) to 1000 mL of normal saline and administer at 125 mL/h after delivery of the placenta
- if the IV route is not possible, give 10 units IM
- if blood loss is greater than 500 mL, administer 0.2 mg of methylergonovine maleate IM simultaneously

Evaluation of fetal well-being

- infuse 0.5 mU/min initially
- increase by 1 mU/min every 15 minutes until 3 contractions occur within 10 minutes, each 40–60 seconds long

Promotion of milk let-down

- oxytocin nasal spray (40 units/mL) has been used for postpartum breast engorgement
- 1 spray instilled into 1 or both nostrils 2–3 minutes before nursing or pumping breasts

Dosage adjustments for renal or hepatic dysfunction

- metabolized in the liver and kidney, and metabolites are eliminated renally

- no dosage adjustments are required, because the dose is titrated to an effect

▶ What Should I Monitor with Regard to Efficacy and Toxicity?

Efficacy

Induction of labor

Cervical dilation rate

- desired cervical dilation rate of 1 cm/h can be used as a guide for increasing oxytocin infusion rates

Uterine activity

- monitor with every oxytocin dosage change or at least every 30 minutes
- at an effective dosage, uterine contractions occur every 3–4 minutes, with a duration of about 60 seconds
- if hyperstimulation occurs (6 contractions or more in 10 minutes for a total of 20 minutes), discontinue the oxytocin infusion, turn the patient to the left lateral position, and administer oxygen
- wait at least 15 minutes before restarting, and restart the infusion at $^1/_2$ the previous rate and evaluate the patient at least every 30 minutes

Induction of labor for abortion

- patient should have regular contraction of uterus and successful evacuation of uterus

Control and prevention of postpartum bleeding

- contraction of uterus and decreased bleeding
- effect should be seen within 10 minutes

Evaluation of fetal well-being

- production of 3 contractions within 10 minutes
- persistent late decelerations in fetal heart rate with most contractions, decreased variability, and no accelerations indicate poor fetal and uteroplacental reserve
- no late decelerations in fetal heart rate, good baseline variability, and acceleration with fetal movement indicate good fetal and uteroplacental reserve

Promotion of milk let-down

- increased milk production beginning within 1–2 minutes and lasting 20 minutes

Toxicity

Many of the adverse effects are dose related, so carefully controlled infusion rates are crucial (Br J Obstet Gynaecol 1985;92:1120–1126)

Fetal distress

- recurrent late-onset decelerations, recurrent severe variable decelerations, or fetal tachycardia seen on fetal heart rate tracing
- monitor the patient with an electronic fetal monitor
- fetal distress is due to decreased blood flow in a hyperstimulated uterus
- stop the infusion, administer oxygen to the patient, and place the patient in left lateral position
- restart the infusion at $^1/_2$ the previous rate when fetal well-being is ensured
- avoid prolonged infusion rates if other potential signs of fetal compromise, such as meconium staining of amniotic fluid or vaginal bleeding, are present

Hypotension (maternal)

- monitor maternal blood pressure and vital signs every 30 minutes and after increases in the infusion rate
- after prolonged infusion, a mild rise in blood pressure and heart rate may occur
- if hypotension occurs, stop the oxytocin infusion and slowly infuse isotonic saline

Uterine hyperstimulation

- monitor maternal contractions continuously during infusion
- if contractions last longer than 90 seconds, or their frequency is greater than every 2–3 minutes, discontinue the infusion, administer oxygen, and place the patient in the left lateral position

- wait 15 minutes before restarting the infusion at $\frac{1}{2}$ the previous rate
- establish fetal well-being (fetal heart rate tracing) before restarting the infusion)

Water intoxication

- manifested by nausea, vomiting, oliguria, and potentially seizures, this is due to the antidiuretic effect of oxytocin
- water intoxication is most commonly seen after administration of large doses (40–50 mU/min) in electrolyte-free solutions (5% dextrose in water) over several hours
- if high doses are required, increase the concentration, not the flow rate, and administer the drug in normal saline or 5% dextrose in lactated Ringer's solution

▶ How Long Do I Treat Patients with This Drug?

Induction of labor

- during induction or augmentation after adequate labor has been established, the infusion rate should be decreased to the lowest effective rate or discontinued
- if no active labor occurs after 12 hours of oxytocin infusion, stop the infusion and allow the patient to rest overnight
- this may be repeated for up to 3 days
- restart the infusion protocol from the beginning the next morning
- do not continue oxytocin infusions in preeclamptic patients for more than 6–8 hours
- patients with dysfunctional labor should be reassessed after 2 hours
- patients with adequate uterine activity who have no progress in cervical dilation after 3–4 hours of infusion should be reassessed

Induction of labor for abortion

- until delivery is achieved

Control or prevention of postpartum bleeding

- for prevention, a single dose is adequate
- for control of bleeding, oxytocin administration should be continued for 15 minutes and then the patient should be evaluated for surgical management

Evaluation of fetal well-being

- until 3 contractions (each 40–60 seconds long) occur within 10 minutes

Promotion of milk let-down

- until breast-feeding is established

▶ How Do I Decrease or Stop the Administration of This Drug?

- may be stopped abruptly
- discontinuation of the infusion results in a gradual decline in uterine activity over 20 minutes, commencing 10–15 minutes after the infusion is stopped

▶ What Should I Tell My Patients About This Drug?

- this drug is used to stimulate contractions of your uterus
- notify a nurse or a physician if you have nausea or vomiting or feel lightheaded

▶ Therapeutic Tips

- when oxytocin infusion rates are increased too rapidly or at less than 30 minute intervals, there is a 2-fold increase in the frequency of discontinuing or decreasing the oxytocin infusion because of hyperstimulation or fetal distress (Am J Obstet Gynecol 1982;144:899–905)
- most of the adverse effects are dose related; therefore, use the minimum effective dose
- supine position increases the risk of fetal hypoxemia and may slow cervical dilation–repositioning the patient to the left lateral position alone may be effective in reversing fetal distress or hyperstimulation
- if induction is not successful on the first day, allowing patients to rest overnight, and restarting the infusion the next morning may improve uterine sensitivity

Useful Reference

Brindley BA, Sokol RJ. Induction and augmentation of labor: Basis and methods for current practice. Obstet Gynecol Surv 1988;43:730–743

PARALDEHYDE

Jonathan Fleming

USA (not available)
CANADA (Paraldehyde)

▶ When Should I Use This Drug?

Consider an alternative agent

- there are more effective and safer hypnotics available
- decomposes on storage, especially when opened; necessitates the use of glass syringes; and has significant adverse effects (foul taste and gastric irritation when given orally; tissue necrosis, nerve damage, and sterile abscesses when injected)
- pulmonary complications (7% of an oral dose is exhaled through the lungs) in patients with and without pulmonary disease are not uncommon (JAMA 1943;121:187–190, Chest 1982;82:371–372)

PENBUTOLOL

Robert Rangno and James McCormack

USA (Levatol)
CANADA (not available)

▶ When Should I Use This Drug?

Consider an alternative agent

- nonselective beta-blocker with mild partial agonist activity
- as effective as other beta-blockers
- as with other beta-blockers with partial agonist activity, this agent may cause less bradycardia; however, the clinical benefit (if any) over other available agents is unknown (Med Lett 1989;31:70–71)

PENICILLAMINE

Kelly Jones

USA (Cuprimine, Depen)
CANADA (Cuprimine, Depen)

▶ When Should I Use This Drug?

Severe rheumatoid arthritis

- after failure with azathioprine therapy
- azathioprine should be chosen before penicillamine because it works more quickly than penicillamine (8–10 weeks versus 6 months) and penicillamine has a number of toxicities that may not be reversible on discontinuation of the drug administration

▶ When Should I Not Use This Drug?

Mild to moderate nonprogressive disease

- other agents are available that are effective and less toxic

Severe rheumatoid arthritis in unmotivated, unreliable patients

- patients must be motivated about treating their disease and should be knowledgeable enough to understand all guidelines on how to use this drug and realize that regular visits and monitoring are required

▶ What Contraindications Are There to the Use of This Drug?

Intolerance of or allergic reaction to penicillamine

- drug is not contraindicated if patients are allergic to penicillins

Pregnancy and lactation

- relationship to fetal anomalies has been observed and several authors suggest avoiding use during lactation (Scand J Rheumatol 1985;14:1–7)

▶ What Drug Interactions Are Clinically Important?

Drugs that may increase the effect or toxicity of penicillamine

- none

Drugs that may decrease the effect of penicillamine

IRON SALTS, ANTACIDS

- reduce bioavailability from 35% to 66%
- avoid concomitant use of agents or take penicillamine 1 hour before or 2 hours after these drugs

Drugs that may have their effect or toxicity increased by penicillamine

- none

Drugs that may have their effect or toxicity decreased by penicillamine

DIGOXIN

- reduction of digoxin levels that necessitate an increase in the digoxin dosage
- monitor for a decrease in the effect of digoxin and increase the dosage if needed

▶ *What Route and Dosage Should I Use?*

How to administer

- orally—take 1 hour before or 2 hours after meals
- parenterally—not available

Severe rheumatoid arthritis

- 250 mg PO daily for 2 months and increase to 500 mg PO daily for 2 months, then increase to 750 mg/d
- available as capsules and tablets, and the choice is based on the patient's preference
- at dosages greater than 500 mg daily, split the dose (500 mg every morning, 250 mg every evening)
- dosages greater than 1 g daily do not markedly increase efficacy (Med Clin North Am 1986;70:285–304)

Dosage adjustments for renal or hepatic dysfunction

- renally eliminated

Normal Dosing Interval	$C_{cr} > 60$ mL/min or 1 mL/s	C_{cr} 30–60 mL/min or 0.5–1 mL/s	$C_{cr} < 30$ mL/min or 0.5 mL/s
Q24H	no adjustment needed	avoid	avoid

▶ *What Should I Monitor with Regard to Efficacy and Toxicity?*

Efficacy

Severe rheumatoid arthritis

Joint tenderness count, sedimentation rate measurements, grip strength, duration of morning stiffness, time to onset of fatigue, and patient's report on specific functions

- patient should be assessed monthly for the first 2 months, and after symptom control, the patient can be assessed every 3 months for 6 months and then every 6 months
- these measures should be used to guide drug administration initiation and discontinuation
- one study found that clinical and laboratory measures of physical well-being appeared to be unrelated to psychological and social measures of well-being (J Rheumatol 1991;18:650–653)
- it is important to include the patient's self-assessment of the drug's effect on their function and well-being

Toxicity

Gastrointestinal effects

- occur early in therapy and are related to increasing the dose too quickly

Cutaneous effects

- early eruptions are characterized by a morbilliform rash, and if this occurs, stop the drug administration, restart at a lower dosage and increase the dosage slowly
- late eruptions are scaly, pruritic, or bullous eruptions
- bullous eruptions are the most severe form and can begin after 6–9 months of treatment; if they occur, the drug administration should be stopped and not restarted

Hypogeusia

- occurs early in therapy and usually clears after 3 months of therapy

Hematological toxicity

- thrombocytopenia (4%), leukopenia (2%), and anemia
- these reactions occur commonly in the first year of therapy
- decrease in hemoglobin level may precede a drop in platelet and/or leukocyte counts (Clin Pharm 1987;6:475–491)
- do baseline complete blood count and platelet count and recheck weekly for 8 weeks, then every 2 weeks for 6 months, and then monthly thereafter
- discontinue the drug administration if the platelet count is less than $100,000/mm^3$, white blood cell count is less than $4000/mm^3$, or the monocyte count rises to greater than $500/mm^3$

Renal toxicity

- hematuria and proteinuria (6–32%)
- may be related to the duration of therapy and the rate of increase in dosage (Semin Arthritis Rheum 1986;15:261–281)
- can be mild (<1 g/d of protein) or progress to a nephrotic syndrome (>2 g/d of protein)
- do baseline urinalysis and recheck weekly for 8 weeks, then every 2 weeks for 6 months, and then monthly thereafter
- if the protein spillage is less than 1 g, continue therapy if the patient is benefiting
- discontinue the drug administration immediately if patients are spilling more than 1 g/d and do not restart the therapy

Polymyositis, myasthenia gravis, Goodpasture's syndrome, Sjögren's syndrome, drug-induced systemic lupus erythematosus

- these diseases usually subside when the drug is withdrawn, but this is not always the case

▶ *How Long Do I Treat Patients with This Drug?*

Severe rheumatoid arthritis

- response necessitates 4–6 months of total treatment
- continue therapy as long as the drug is tolerated and effective (Med Clin North Am 1986;70:285–304)
- up to 50% stop therapy with penicillamine after 1 year owing to the drug's toxicity
- try to keep the dosage as low as possible to minimize side effects; however, dosages lower than 500 mg daily are less efficacious (Clin Pharm 1987;6:475–491)

▶ *How Do I Decrease or Stop the Administration of This Drug?*

- may be stopped abruptly

▶ *What Should I Tell My Patients About This Drug?*

- take on an empty stomach (1 hour before or 2 hours after a meal)
- watch for any unusual bleeding or bruising or skin eruptions; if they occur, contact your physician
- taste disturbances are transient and disappear in 3 months
- always make sure to keep appointments for close monitoring to reduce potential toxic effects

▶ *Therapeutic Tips*

- take 1 hour before or 2 hours after meals
- capsules (Cuprimine) and tablets (Depen) are available; let the patient decide on the dosage form
- prescribe only a 2 week supply with no refill so that the patient comes back for monitoring and follow-up
- penicillin allergy does not preclude the use of penicillamine
- prior development of proteinuria from gold may be a risk factor for using penicillamine

Useful Reference

Pugh MC, Pugh CB. Current concepts in clinical therapeutics: Disease-modifying drugs for rheumatoid arthritis. Clin Pharm 1987;6:475–491

PENICILLIN

John Rotschafer, Kyle Vance-Bryan, and Rick Zabinski

Penicillin G Potassium (Benzyl Penicillin Potassium)

Penicillin G Sodium (Benzyl Penicillin Sodium, Crystalline Penicillin)

USA (Hyasorb, M-Cillin B, Paclin G, Pentids, Pfizerpen, SK-Penicillin G)
CANADA (Crystapen, Megacillin, Novopen G)

Penicillin V (Phenoxymethyl Penicillin)

USA (Beepen-VK, Betapen-VK, Dowpen VK, Ledercillin VK, Paclin VK, Penapar VK, Pen-Vee K, Pfizerpen VK, Robicillin VK, Ro-Cillin VK, Suspen, VK-Penicillin VK, Uticillin VK, V-Cillin-K, Veetids)
CANADA (Apo-Pen-VK, Ledercillin VK, Nadopen-V, Novopen-VK, Pen-Vee, PVF K, V-Cillin K, VC-K 500)

Penicillin G Procaine (Aqueous Procaine Penicillin G [APPG], Benzylpenicillin Procaine, Procaine Benzylpenicillin, Procaine Penicillin G)

USA (Crysticillin A.S., Duracillin AS, Pfizepen-AS, Wycillin)
CANADA (Ayercillin, Wycillin)

Penicillin G Benzathine (Benzathine Benzylpenicillin, Benzathine Penicillin G, Benzylpenicillin Benzathine, Dibenzylethylenediamine Benzylpenicillin)

USA (Bicillin L-A, Permapen)
CANADA (Bicillin, Megacillin Suspension)

▶ When Should I Use This Drug?

check antibiotic susceptibility chart (Table 4–1 in Chapter 4)

Meningitis

- penicillin is the drug of choice if gram stain of the cerebrospinal fluid shows gram-positive diplococci (*Streptococcus pneumoniae*) or gram-negative diplococci (*Neisseria meningitidis*) because penicillin is effective against these organisms, is well tolerated, and is inexpensive

Endocarditis

- as sole therapy for penicillin-sensitive streptococci (minimum inhibitory concentration [MIC] < 0.1 mg/L) if the patient is 65 years or older, has renal or auditory impairment, and has no prosthetic valve (JAMA 1989;261:1471–1477)

Use in conjunction with gentamicin for:

- penicillin-sensitive streptococci (MIC < 0.1 mg/L) if the patient is younger than 65 years and has no renal or auditory impairment
- intermediately sensitive streptococci (MIC 0.1–1.0 mg/L)
- penicillin-sensitive enterococci
- penicillin-sensitive diphtheroids (JK diptheroids, a frequent cause of endocarditis, are often penicillin resistant and necessitate vancomycin)
- culture-negative cases
- native valve endocarditis, if the patient is acutely ill with cardiovascular or neurological complications
- as empirical therapy, in conjunction with gentamicin for native valve endocarditis; however, if the patient is 65 years or older or has auditory or renal dysfunction, just use penicillin

Pneumonia

- penicillin is the drug of choice for pneumonia if Gram stain of the sputum shows gram-positive diplococci (*S. pneumoniae*) because penicillin is effective against *S. pneumoniae,* is well tolerated, and is inexpensive
- drug of choice for aspiration pneumonia (community acquired), as it provides good coverage against gram-positive organisms (other than staphylococci) and anaerobes typically found in the lung
- penicillin is also less expensive and better tolerated than clindamycin

Cellulitis

- drug of choice if only streptococcal organisms are suspected or proven because penicillin has good activity against group A beta-hemolytic streptococcus
- penicillin is effective, is well tolerated, and is less expensive than cloxacillin or clindamycin and is usually better tolerated than erythromycin

Erysipelas

- penicillin has activity against the organism that causes erysipelas (group A streptococci)

Genital ulcers (syphilis)

- penicillin is the drug of choice for syphilis (if there is clinical suspicion and lesions are suggestive of syphilis [usually painless with raised border and indurated base] or dark-field microscopy shows corkscrew spirochetes)
- penicillin is less expensive than ceftriaxone or doxycycline

Prophylaxis of pneumococcal infections

- in children with anatomical or functional asplenia and in individuals with hypogammaglobulinemia or in adults who have undergone splenectomy owing to trauma

Prophylaxis of recurrent rheumatic fever

- drug of choice

Streptococcal throat infection

- drug of choice as it decreases the risk of complications due to streptococcal throat infection

Anthrax (*Bacillus anthracis* infection)

- penicillin is the drug of choice

Systemic infections caused by *Streptococcus pneumoniae, S. viridans, S. pyogenes, S. bovis,* penicillin-sensitive *Staphylococcus aureus, Neisseria meningitidis, Pasteurella multocida, Clostridium perfringens,* other *Clostridium, Fusobacterium,* or anaerobic streptococci

- penicillin is the drug of choice (regardless of the site) if infection is caused by one of these organisms because it is inexpensive and is well tolerated

▶ When Should I Not Use This Drug?

Staphylococcal infections

- use cloxacillin or nafcillin or cefazolin because most staphylococcal organisms produce beta-lactamases and are not sensitive

Gram-negative infections

- infections caused by *Klebsiella pneumoniae, S. aureus, Pseudomonas* spp., *Acinetobacter* spp., *Enterobacter* spp., *Serratia marcescens, Citrobacter* spp., and *Bacteroides fragilis* cannot be treated with penicillin because it has little if any useful activity against these organisms

Enterococcal infections

- although penicillin has good activity against enterococcal organisms, ampicillin is usually more active and is not much more expensive than penicillin

Oral use (except for prophylaxis of pneumococcal infections, prophylaxis of recurrent rheumatic fever, and mild infections)

- oral penicillin G is not recommended because penicillin G undergoes some degradation by gastric acid and blood levels are lower than those obtained with penicillin V
- penicillin V is not a substitute for parenterally administered penicillin G when such therapy is needed, and amoxicillin should be used for mild infections due to penicillin-susceptible organisms of the throat or respiratory tract, as amoxicillin is better absorbed from the gastrointestinal tract and provides higher, more sustained serum concentrations than does penicillin V
- amoxicillin also has the advantage of TID rather than QID dosing and can be taken with food or on an empty stomach, which improves compliance

Lyme disease (early stage)

- use oral doxycycline for individuals 9 years of age or older and oral amoxicillin for individuals younger than 9 years of age

Prophylaxis of bacterial endocarditis prior to dental procedure

- use amoxicillin because it is better absorbed from the gastrointestinal tract and provides higher, more sustained serum concentrations than does penicillin V

▶ *What Contraindications Are There to the Use of This Drug?*

Intolerance of or allergic reaction to penicillins

- if the patient states an allergy to penicillins or cephalosporins, check that the patient has actual allergic symptoms
- in patients reporting a true allergy-like reaction to penicillins, penicillins and cephalosporins should not be used
- although experience to date may indicate that many patients who say they are allergic to penicillin do not have problems when they receive a cephalosporin, this is usually because the patient was not truly allergic to penicillins (Rev Infect Dis 1983;5: S368–S379)

▶ *What Drug Interactions Are Clinically Important?*

Drugs that may increase the effect or toxicity of penicillin

PROBENECID

- may potentiate seizures when used with high dosages of aqueous penicillin G intravenously
- produces higher and prolonged serum concentrations of penicillins when administered before or simultaneously with these agents

AMINOGLYCOSIDES

- synergistic bactericidal effects have been reported for combinations of a penicillin and an aminoglycoside; however, penicillins are physically and/or chemically incompatible with aminoglycosides
- if concomitant therapy is indicated, in vitro mixing of penicillins and aminoglycosides should be avoided
- body fluids likely to contain both antibiotics should be processed as soon as possible (if processing is delayed, keep samples frozen to minimize inactivation)

Drugs that may decrease the effect of penicillin

OTHER BETA-LACTAM ANTIBIOTICS

- reports from in vitro studies indicate that the antibacterial activity of penicillins may be additive, synergistic, or antagonistic when penicillins are combined with other beta-lactams
- if therapeutic failure occurs in any patient receiving 2 beta-lactams, antagonism, via in vitro sensitivity tests, should be ruled out as a possible cause of failure
- in patients with life-threatening infections in which combination beta-lactam therapy is being considered, consider performing in vitro tests to rule out antagonism

Drugs that may have their effect or toxicity increased by penicillin

- none

Drugs that may have their effect decreased by penicillin

ORAL CONTRACEPTIVES

- unwanted pregnancies have been seen in patients receiving penicillins and oral contraceptives; therefore, additional means of birth control should be recommended during that menstrual cycle

▶ *What Route and Dosage Should I Use?*

How to administer

Orally

- take on an empty stomach because acid degrades oral penicillin G and decreases the absorption of penicillin V

Parenterally

- aqueous penicillin G (sodium or potassium salt) administered intravenously in any convenient amount of normal saline or 5% dextrose in water and given over 30–60 minutes
- more rapid infusions may cause high central nervous system levels and toxicity in elderly and renally compromised patients
- sodium penicillin G contains approximately 2 mEq of sodium per 1 million units
- potassium penicillin G contains 1.7 mEq of potassium per 1 million units
- procaine penicillin must be given intramuscularly (pseudoanaphylaxis is seen when it is given intravenously)
- benzathine penicillin must be given intramuscularly
- aspirate the injection site to avoid injection into blood vessel
- give intramuscular injections into the gluteus maximus or into the midlateral thigh

400,000 units = 250 mg

Meningitis

- 4 million units IV Q4H

Endocarditis

- 4 million units IV Q4H
- 5 million units IV Q4H for intermediately sensitive streptococci (MIC 0.1–1.0 mg/L)

Pneumonia

- 600,000 units IV Q6H for pneumococcal pneumonia (500 mg PO QID if treated orally)
- 1 million units IV Q6H for moderate illness
- 2 million units IV Q4H for aspiration pneumonia

Cellulitis, erysipelas

- 250–300 mg (depending on available dosage form) of penicillin V PO Q6H for mild infections
- 2 million units IV Q6H for severe infections

Genital ulcers (syphilis)

- 2.4 million units IM of benzathine penicillin as a single dose for syphilis of less than 1 year's duration
- 2.4 million units IM of benzathine penicillin weekly for 3 weeks for syphilis of greater than 1 year's duration
- 2 million units IV Q4H for 10 days for neurosyphilis followed by penicillin G benzathine 2.4 million units IM once weekly for 3 weeks

Prophylaxis of pneumococcal infections

- 1.2 million units of benzathine penicillin every 4 weeks

Strep throat

- 250–300 mg (depending on available dosage form) of penicillin V PO Q12H for 10 days

Prophylaxis of recurrent rheumatic fever

- 1.2 million units of penicillin G benzathine every 4 weeks

Anthrax (*bacillus anthracis* infection)

- 2 million units IV Q4H for 4 days, then oral penicillin V 250–300 mg (depending on available dosage form) PO Q6H for a total of 10 days

Dosage adjustments for renal or hepatic dysfunction

- renally eliminated

Normal Dosing Interval	C_{cr} > 60 mL/min or 1 mL/s	C_{cr} 30–60 mL/min or 0.5–1 mL/s	C_{cr} < 30 mL/min or 0.5 mL/s
Q4H	no adjustment needed	Q6H	Q8H
Q6H	no adjustment needed	Q8H	Q12H
Q12H	no adjustment needed	Q24H	Q24H and decrease dosage by 50%
Q24H	no adjustment needed	Q24H and decrease dosage by 50%	Q24H and decrease dosage by 75%

▶ *What Should I Monitor with Regard to Efficacy and Toxicity?*

Efficacy

- for antibiotic administration monitoring guidelines, see specific section on drug therapy

Toxicity

Allergic reactions (rash, angioedema, anaphylaxis, and so on)

- morbilliform rash (5–10%); fatal anaphylactic reaction (1/50,000)
- rashes occur more commonly in patients taking ampicillin
- question the patient about the appearance of these symptoms daily while the patient is in the hospital
- if patients are not hospitalized, tell them that if they experience rash, itching, hives, wheezing, or difficulty in breathing, they should contact their physician immediately
- to avoid the risk of progression of the cutaneous symptoms, penicillin therapy should be discontinued if any allergic rash occurs
- for specific treatment, see discussion of drug-induced skin rash or anaphylaxis in Chapter 11

Gastrointestinal symptoms—diarrhea or pseudomembranous colitis

- question the patient about the appearance of these symptoms on a daily basis while the patient is in the hospital
- if patients are not hospitalized, tell them that penicillins can cause diarrhea, and if the diarrhea is severe, they should contact their physician
- for specific treatment, see discussion of drug-induced diarrhea in Chapter 11

Seizures

- seen in patients receiving high doses of parenteral ampicillin in conjunction with decreased renal function; therefore, ensure that the dosage is adjusted for the patient's renal function
- also may occur when high dosages of aqueous penicillin G are given intravenously with probenecid; be aware of this interaction

Interstitial nephritis

- characterized by hematuria and oliguria
- can occur but is rare, and drug administration must be discontinued

Jarisch-Herxheimer reaction

- frequently occurs when penicillin G is used to treat syphilis (50% of those treated for primary syphilis, 75% of those treated for secondary syphilis, and 30% of those treated for neurosyphilis) and may also occur when penicillin is used to treat other spirochetal infections (e.g., Lyme disease)
- reaction occurs 2–12 hours after the initiation of therapy and consists of headache, fever, chills, sweating, sore throat, myalgia, arthralgia, malaise, increased heart rate, and increased blood pressure
- reaction generally subsides within 12–24 hours and is presumably caused by the release of pyrogens from killed organisms

Nervous system effects

- inadvertent injection of penicillin G preparations into or near nerves can result in neurological damage; deep intragluteal injections should be avoided to avoid sciatic nerve irritation and dysfunction
- inadvertent IV administration of procaine penicillin may cause an immediate toxic reaction consisting of bizarre behavior, visual disturbances, unusual tastes, anxiety, confusion, agitation, depression, weakness, dizziness, palpitation, seizures, hallucinations, combativeness, and fear of impending death as a result of the free procaine found in the preparation

▶ *How Long Do I Treat Patients with This Drug?*

Meningitis

- 7 days for patients who respond quickly if meningitis is caused by *S. pneumoniae;* however, treat for 10 days if the patient responds slowly

Endocarditis

- 4 weeks for penicillin-sensitive streptococci (MIC < 0.1 mg/L) if the patient is 65 years or older or has renal or auditory impairment and no prosthetic valve
- 2 weeks (gentamicin for 2 weeks) for penicillin-sensitive streptococci (MIC < 0.1 mg/L) if the patient is younger than 65 years and has no renal or auditory impairment
- 4 weeks (6 weeks if there is a prosthetic valve, symptoms longer than 3 months, or negative culture) plus gentamicin for 2 weeks for penicillin-sensitive streptococci (MIC < 0.1 mg/L)
- 4 weeks for both drugs for intermediately sensitive streptococci (MIC 0.1–1.0 mg/L), enterococci, and penicillin-sensitive diphtheroids

Pneumonia

- usual duration of therapy is 10 days or 4–5 days after the patient has become afebrile and has clinically improved
- consider switching to oral amoxicillin (500 mg PO Q8H) after the patient has become afebrile and has clinically improved for 1–2 days

Cellulitis, erysipelas

- treat for a total of 10 days
- depending on clinical improvement, initial parenteral therapy may be switched to oral therapy for the remainder of the 10 days

Genital ulcers (syphilis)

- single dose for syphyllis of less than 1 year's duration
- penicillin G benzathine IM weekly for 3 weeks for syphilis of greater than 1 year's duration, unless there is neurological involvement
- penicillin IV Q4H for 10–14 days followed by penicillin G benzathine 2.4 million units IM once weekly for 3 weeks for the treatment of neurosyphilis

Prophylaxis of pneumococcal infections

- indefinitely for hypogammaglobulinemia or splenectomy

Streptococcal throat infection

- 10 days of therapy is required to reduce chance of complications due to streptococcal throat infection

Prophylaxis of recurrent rheumatic fever

- should be continued for at least 5 years after the last rheumatic attack and until the patients have reached their early twenties; however, treatment may need to be continued indefinitely (Principles and Practice of Infectious Diseases, 3rd ed., 1990:1534)

Anthrax (*Bacillus anthracis* infection)

- 3–4 days IV, then oral for a total of 10 days

▶ *How Do I Decrease or Stop the Administration of This Drug?*

- may be stopped abruptly

▶ *What Should I Tell My Patients About This Drug?*

- have you ever had an allergic reaction to a penicillin? if so, describe the reaction and how long ago it happened
- if you have rash, itching, hives, wheezing, or difficulty with breathing, contact your physician immediately
- penicillins can cause diarrhea, and if the diarrhea is severe, contact your physician
- if you use oral contraceptives, they may not work as well when you take a penicillin; therefore, use additional means of birth control during the entire month that you are taking penicillins

▶ *Therapeutic Tips*

- penicillins can cause falsely elevated urine glucose levels; patients should recheck their results with a qualitative test (e.g., glucose oxidase)
- false-positive or falsely elevated results in turbidimetric measurements of urinary and serum proteins that use sulfosalicylic acid or trichloroacetic acid may occur; simply be aware that this interaction may occur

- false-positive Coombs' reactions have occurred with large intravenous doses of penicillins; simply be aware that this interaction may occur
- do not administer intramuscularly, as intramuscular aqueous penicillin G is painful
- use procaine penicillin only if oral therapy with amoxicillin is not an option
- avoid accidental intravenous administration of intramuscular penicillin G procaine by aspirating at the injection site; if blood is aspirated, pull the needle out, apply local pressure, and try another injection site
- in general, the amount of sodium in the penicillin G sodium is unimportant unless the patient is receiving greater than 12 million units/d and has a condition necessitating sodium restriction such as congestive heart failure

Useful References

Wright AJ, Wilkowske CJ. The penicillins. Mayo Clin Proc 1987;62:806–820
Neu HC. Penicillins. In: Mandell, Douglas, Bennett. Principles and Practice of Infectious Diseases, 3rd ed. New York: Wiley, 1990:230–246
Bisno AL, Dismukes WE, Durack DT, et al. Antimicrobial treatment of infective endocarditis due to viridans streptococci, enterococci, and staphylococci. JAMA 1989;261:1471–1477

PENTAMIDINE

Ann Beardsell

USA (Pentam, Pentacarinat, Nebupent)
CANADA (Pentacarinat, Pentam, Pneumopent)

▶ *When Should I Use This Drug?*

Pneumocystis carinii pneumonia

Treatment

- should be used instead of trimethoprim-sulfamethoxazole in patients known to react to sulfa drugs who require intravenous therapy (e.g., for severe *P. carinii* pneumonia [PCP]) or who cannot take oral medications
- trimethoprim in combination with either sulfamethoxazole or dapsone is preferred to pentamidine because of the cost of pentamidine

Prophylaxis

- used for prophylaxis against PCP via the aerosol form as well as intravenously
- reasonable option for patients intolerant of sulfa drugs or those who have evidence of bone marrow dysfunction
- aerosol form is most commonly used, although the intravenous form is used in some patients resistant to aerosol pentamidine and/or intolerant of other regimens (use intravenously only as a last choice when nothing else is effective)

▶ *When Should I Not Use This Drug?*

Aerosolized route to treat *Pneumocystis carinii* pneumonia

- aerosolized administration has not been effective for the treatment of active disease (Ann Intern Med 1990;113:195–202, 203–209)

▶ *What Contraindications Are There to the Use of This Drug?*

- intolerance of or allergic reaction to pentamidine

▶ *What Drug Interactions Are Clinically Important?*

Drugs that may increase the effect or toxicity of pentamidine

NEPHROTOXIC AGENTS (AMINOGLYCOSIDES, AMPHOTERICIN B, CISPLATIN, VANCOMYCIN, AND SO ON)

- concomitant use of parenteral pentamidine increases the potential nephrotoxicity of both medications
- if used concurrently, monitor serum creatinine and urea levels every 2–3 days and ensure adequate hydration
- if serum creatinine and BUN begin to rise, discontinue the other nephrotoxic medication until pentamidine treatment is completed, adjust the pentamidine dosage or dosing interval, or switch pentamidine to intravenous or oral trimethoprim-sulfamethoxazole if the patient is not allergic to sulfa drugs (for allergy and a mild case of PCP, switch to oral dapsone-trimethoprim combination)

ZIDOVUDINE

- may potentiate the bone marrow suppressant actions of both drugs, resulting in neutropenia and anemia
- monitor complete blood cell count (CBC) and differential count every 2–3 days and reduce the dosage of zidovudine by 100–300 mg daily if the white blood cell count (WBC) and/or granulocyte count decreases significantly
- if the WBC is less than 1.5/mm^3, the granulocyte count is less than 0.8/mm^3, or the hemoglobin B level is less than 8 g/dL, withhold zidovudine administration until PCP is resolved and laboratory values return to preinfection levels

Drugs that may decrease the effect of pentamidine

- none

Drugs that may have their effect increased by pentamidine

- none

Drugs that may have their effect decreased by pentamidine

- none

▶ *What Route and Dosage Should I Use?*

How to administer

- orally—not available
- inhaled—use via nebulizer
- parenterally—diluted in 50–500 mL of 5% dextrose in water (at least 250 mL if tolerable); the intravenous route is most commonly used, although pentamidine can be administered by intramuscular injection, but this route is painful and can cause sterile abscesses
- to minimize hypotension and renal dysfunction, each dose should be administered over a minimum of 60 minutes but preferably 2–3 hours

Pneumocystis carinii pneumonia

Treatment

- 4 mg/kg IV daily

Prophylaxis

Aerosol route

- can be used for primary and secondary prophylaxis
- dosage depends on the type of nebulizer used
- 60 mg every 2–3 days for 5 doses followed by 60 mg every 2 weeks via ultrasonic nebulizer (FisoNeb) or 300 mg per month via continuous, flow-driven nebulizer (Respirgard II), whichever is available
- routine premedication with salbutamol is recommended to decrease the risk of bronchospasm

Intravenous route

- 4 mg/kg every 4 weeks

Dosage adjustments for renal/hepatic dysfunction

- method of elimination not really known

Normal Dosing Interval	C$_{cr}$ > 60 mL/min or 1 mL/s	C$_{cr}$ 30–60 mL/min or 0.5–1 mL/s	C$_{cr}$ < 30 mL/min or 0.5 mL/s
Q24H	no adjustment needed	no adjustment needed	**Severe infections:** 4 mg/kg daily for 7–10 days, then reduce to alternate-day therapy for remainder of 14 doses **Less severe infection:** 4 mg/kg IV on alternate days for 14 doses

► *What Should I Monitor with Regard to Efficacy and Toxicity?*

Efficacy

Pneumocystis carinii pneumonia

Treatment

- for treatment of acute infection, efficacy is determined by improvement of clinical symptoms such as clearing of chest X-ray, improved oxygenation, and resolution of fever and cough
- if no improvement is seen within 5 days of initiating therapy, addition of corticosteroids must be considered (if the patient is not already receiving them) and, if there is still no improvement, switch to trimethoprim-sulfamethoxazole

Prophylaxis

- no development of primary PCP; marked reduction in secondary or recurrent episodes
- before starting PCP prophylaxis, a chest X-ray should be obtained to ensure that there is no active pulmonary disease
- pulmonary function test consisting of simple spirometry is also advisable to rule out asthma in patients who will be treated with aerosolized pentamidine
- no specific ongoing monitoring is required over that necessary for the follow-up of patients taking antiretroviral therapy
- PCP can occur despite adequate prophylaxis, and its presentation may be atypical

Toxicity

Most adverse effects are associated with the intravenous use of pentamidine • Because there are few alternatives to pentamidine, especially in sulfa-allergic patients, most adverse effects are treated symptomatically to maintain the patient on therapy unless the toxicity is life-threatening • Aerosolized pentamidine has few or no systemic effects, but the most common local effect is irritation of the airway and coughing

Renal effects

- incidence of nephrotoxicity with pentamidine is significant (25%) and appears to be more common in patients with acquired immunodeficiency syndrome (AIDS) and/or those who are dehydrated
- is gradual in onset, with a mild to moderate increase in serum creatinine and/or blood urea nitrogen (BUN) level, usually early in the second week of therapy, and resolves after treatment is completed or discontinued
- acute renal failure or severe renal insufficiency necessitating discontinuation of therapy is uncommon but has occurred
- monitor serum creatinine and BUN levels prior to starting treatment and every 2–3 days during treatment
- if creatinine clearance decreases to below 35 mL/min, dosage adjustment may be required as outlined above
- ensure that the patient is well hydrated

Hypoglycemia or hyperglycemia

- effects on blood glucose levels, while the mechanism is unclear, are thought to result from a direct toxic effect on the beta cells of the pancreas
- hypoglycemia, which can be severe, may occur after the first few doses but more frequently develops after the first week of treatment or even several days after treatment has been completed
- hyperglycemia and possibly insulin-dependent diabetes mellitus may also occur, not necessarily preceded by hypoglycemia, and may develop several months after treatment
- most common with intravenous use of pentamidine but has been reported with aerosol use
- monitor serum glucose levels prior to treatment and every 2–3 days during treatment
- if serum glucose levels become a problem and a change of therapy to another drug regimen is not possible, hypoglycemia should be treated by increased glucose intake in IV fluids, and hyperglycemia may necessitate oral hypoglycemic agents or insulin

Hematological effects

- leukopenia and thrombocytopenia may occur
- monitor CBC and platelet counts every 3 days during therapy

- if the leukocyte and/or platelet counts are less than 1000/mm^3 and less than 20,000/mm^3, respectively, alternative therapy should be considered

Gastrointestinal effects

- nausea, vomiting, diarrhea, abdominal pain, decreased appetite, and an unpleasant metallic taste are all common with short-term treatment and, to a lesser extent, with monthly prophylaxis and aerosolized treatment
- treat symptomatically

Hepatic effects

- elevated liver function test results may occur with intravenous pentamidine treatment but usually resolve after the infection has been treated

Cardiovascular effects

- moderate to severe hypotension can develop suddenly after 1 dose or more slowly during the 2 week treatment period
- administer each dose with large fluid volumes (if tolerable) over several hours with the patient lying down at the beginning of the infusion
- monitor blood pressure before and after the infusion
- ventricular tachycardia, electrocardiographic abnormalities, and facial flushing have also been reported

Nervous system

- confusion and hallucinations have been reported with pentamidine, but the effects of the infection and suboptimum oxygenation may play a role in these reactions
- dizziness (unrelated to hypotension) with both intravenous and aerosolized use

Respiratory effects

- cough and/or bronchospasm is common with aerosolized use, although bronchospasm has been reported with parenteral use and may be severe enough to necessitate discontinuation of therapy
- pretreatment with a bronchodilator, such as salbutamol inhaler, helps to reduce bronchospasm and cough and enables patients to continue with therapy
- because of the release of the drug into the air by the nebulizers, there is concern about occupational exposure, although never clearly defined, in clinics where patients go to use the equipment; hence, caution is advised for workers continually exposed, especially those who are pregnant, and special vents and/or compartments have been designed
- incidence of pneumothorax appears to be higher in patients receiving aerosolized pentamidine, and therefore, any complaints of chest pain should be followed up by an assessment for possible pneumothorax

► *How Long Do I Treat Patients with This Drug?*

Pneumocystis carinii pneumonia

Treatment

- for 14–21 days (14 days is usually adequate)
- if the patient responds slowly, give for 21 days
- if the patient is clinically improving and is afebrile after 5–7 days of therapy, intravenous pentamidine may be switched to a combination of oral dapsone (100 mg PO daily) and trimethoprim (200–300 mg PO QID) for the remainder of the 14 days, which allows the patient to be treated at home

Prophylaxis

- for primary and secondary prophylaxis, treatment is indefinite as long as it is tolerated

► *How Do I Decrease or Stop the Administration of This Drug?*

- may be stopped abruptly

► *What Should I Tell My Patients About This Drug?*

Intravenous route

- as this drug may cause you to feel dizzy and lightheaded, sit up slowly and dangle your legs over the side of the bed for a few

minutes before attempting to stand, and if these symptoms become severe, tell your physician immediately
- pentamidine may also cause you to have a metallic taste in your mouth, which may last for up to 1 month after therapy but eventually disappears
- after you finish the treatment, if you notice that you are excessively thirsty or are urinating more than usual, let your physician know immediately

Aerosol route
- little, if any, of this drug is absorbed into the body
- you may find that the aerosolized drug irritates your throat and lungs and causes you to cough
- if you have problems breathing in the mist, talk to your physician, as he or she can prescribe another medication to help to open up the lung passages
- aerosolized pentamidine may leave a metallic or bad taste in your mouth after use; sucking a hard candy or lozenge afterward helps to alleviate this

▶ *Therapeutic Tips*

Intravenous route
- ensure that the patient is kept quite hydrated to minimize renal problems
- use larger volumes for dilution, and administer the dose over several hours to reduce hypotension
- monitor all laboratory work carefully and regularly
- after the patient is stable and feeling better, further treatment in a medical daycare setting or conversion to oral therapy and discharge to the home can be contemplated
- early concomitant use of corticosteroids in moderate to severe infections may speed the recovery period
- monitor blood glucose levels and blood pressure even after the treatment is completed

Aerosol route
- have trained personnel instruct the patient on the use and care of the machine and the mixing of medication

PENTAZOCINE
Terry Baumann

USA (Talwin)
CANADA (Talwin)

▶ *When Should I Use This Drug?*

Consider an alternative agent
- psychomimetic adverse effects (dysphoria, hallucinations, sense of unreality, depersonalization, and nervousness) have made the use of pentazocine obsolete (J Pain Symptom Manage 1987; 2:35–44)

PENTOBARBITAL
Jonathan Fleming

USA (Nembutal)
Canada (Nembutal, Novo-pentobarb)

▶ *When Should I Use This Drug?*

Consider an alternative agent
- barbiturates are contraindicated in the management of insomnia (Report of the Expert Advisory Committee on the Short and Intermediate Acting Barbiturates, 1985)
- their effects on sleep architecture (reduction in rapid eye movement sleep and delta sleep), safety (risk of dependence and abuse, lethality in overdosage), lack of efficacy (tolerance to hypnotic effects develops within 2 weeks), and significant withdrawal reactions (rebound insomnia) make them unsuitable for use

Useful References

Lapierre YD (chairman). Report of the Expert Advisory Committee on the Short and Intermediate Acting Barbiturates. Ottawa, Ontario: Health Protection Branch, Information Letter 679, April 1985

PENTOXIFYLLINE
Richard Ogilvie

USA (Trental)
CANADA (Trental)

▶ *When Should I Use This Drug?*

Intermittent claudication related to chronic occlusive arterial disease of the limbs
- generally useful only if the disease is of moderate severity (Am J Surg 1990;160:266–270)

Trophic leg ulcers due to chronic peripheral vascular disease
- in conjunction with other therapy (Drugs 1987;34:50–97)

▶ *When Should I Not Use This Drug?*

Very mild or very severe cases of intermittent claudication
- patients are unlikely to benefit (Am J Surg 1990;160:266–270)
- severe claudication (resting pain, leg ulcers) should prompt investigation for possible angioplastic or surgical intervention rather than drug therapy

Cerebrovascular disorders and vasoocclusive crises of sickle cell disease
- unproven benefit

▶ *What Contraindications Are There to the Use of This Drug?*

Intolerance of or allergic reaction to pentoxifylline or other xanthines

Acute myocardial infarction or acute hemorrhage
- worsening of coronary artery disease is possible

Acute hemorrhage
- may worsen bleeding

Severe hepatic disease
- metabolized by the liver

▶ *What Drug Interactions Are Clinically Important?*

Drugs that may increase the effect or toxicity of pentoxifylline

THEOPHYLLINE, SYMPATHOMIMETICS
- concurrent use may lead to increased central nervous system stimulation
- avoid the combination if possible; however, if the combination must be used, alert the patient to possible adverse effects and decrease the dosage of theophylline by 25% if they occur

CIMETIDINE
- inhibits pentoxifylline metabolism
- switch to ranitidine or other H₂ antagonist if the combination must be used, as these agents have less of an effect on metabolism

Drugs that may decrease the effect of pentoxifylline
- none

Drugs that may have their effect or toxicity increased by pentoxifylline

ANTIHYPERTENSIVES
- antihypertensive effect may be enhanced; therefore, monitor blood pressure every 2–3 days until the full extent of interaction is seen and adjust the dosage of antihypertensive medication accordingly

WARFARIN
- may prolong INR, and pentoxifylline also inhibits platelet aggregation
- use alternative agents if possible
- if not, monitor INR every 2 days until the full extent of interaction is seen and adjust the dosage as for a warfarin dosage change
- monitor INR every 2 days when administration of the pentoxifylline is discontinued and adjust warfarin dose as usual

HYPOGLYCEMIC AGENTS

- hypoglycemic effect may be enhanced; therefore, monitor blood glucose levels every 2–3 days (if not already doing this) until the full extent of the interaction is seen, and adjust the dosage of the hypoglycemic agent accordingly

Drugs that may have their effect decreased by pentoxifylline

ADENOSINE

- methylxanthine compounds inhibit the effect of adenosine, perhaps by competitively blocking adenosine-sensitive receptors
- patients receiving pentoxifylline may require unusually high doses of adenosine or may not respond at all
- use an initial dose of 12 mg rather than 6 mg

▶ What Route and Dosage Should I Use?

How to administer

- orally—take with meals to reduce gastrointestinal side effects

Intermittent claudication related to chronic occlusive arterial disease of the limbs, trophic leg ulcers due to chronic peripheral vascular disease

- 400 mg PO TID as a controlled-release formulation

Dosage adjustments for renal or hepatic dysfunction

- hepatically metabolized
- no dosage adjustments needed for renal dysfunction
- avoid in severe hepatic dysfunction

▶ What Should I Monitor with Regard to Efficacy and Toxicity?

Efficacy

Intermittent claudication related to chronic occlusive arterial disease of the limbs, trophic leg ulcers due to chronic peripheral vascular disease

- improvement may be seen after 2–4 weeks; assess efficacy at 4 week intervals
- subjective improvement in pain-free walking distance
- objective improvement in pain-free treadmill walking distance (2 mph [3.2 kph] at 12.5% or 7.1 degree inclination)
- an improvement by 80–100 m for everyday walking should be expected (Circulation 1989;80:1549–1556)

Toxicity

Gastrointestinal symptoms

- 5% of patients discontinue therapy because of nausea, vomiting, dyspepsia, belching, bloating, and flatulence

Central nervous system effects

- dizziness, nervousness, and agitation
- decrease the dosage to 400 mg PO BID

Cardiovascular effects

- flushing, palpitations
- decrease the dosage to 400 mg PO BID

▶ How Long Do I Treat Patients with This Drug?

Intermittent claudication related to chronic occlusive arterial disease of the limbs, trophic leg ulcers due to chronic peripheral vascular disease

- if an improvement of at least 25–50% is not seen after 8 weeks of therapy, stop the drug administration
- if improvement is noted at 8 weeks, continue therapy for 6 months followed by a 2 month drug-free period for reassessment of need for continued therapy
- reassessment is needed, as the patient may improve with drug therapy, which increases the ability to exercise and may decrease the need for the drug regimen

▶ How Do I Decrease or Stop the Administration of This Drug?

- may be stopped abruptly

▶ What Should I Tell My Patients About This Drug?

- this drug is adjunctive therapy to regular dynamic leg exercise and discontinuation of inhalation of cigarette smoke, both active (personal smoking) and passive (secondhand smoke)
- it should be taken with meals to reduce adverse gastrointestinal effects

▶ Therapeutic Tips

- trial off drug after 6 months is recommended because of the cost
- reassessment is important because statistically demonstrable improvement may not always be clinically important and is unpredictable, and also, the patient may improve with drug therapy, which increases the ability to exercise and may decrease the need for the drug (Ann Intern Med 1990;113:135–146)

Useful References

Ward A, Clissold SP. Pentoxifylline. Drugs 1987;34:50–97

Radack K, Wyderski RJ. Conservative management of intermittent claudication. Ann Intern Med 1990;113:135–146

Lindgärde F, Jelnes R, Björkman H, et al. Conservative drug treatment in patients with moderately severe chronic occlusive peripheral arterial disease. Circulation 1989;80:1549–1556

AbuRahma AF, Woodruff BA. Effects and limitations of pentoxifylline therapy in various stages of peripheral vascular disease of the lower extremity. Am J Surg 1990;160:266–270

PERPHENAZINE

Lynne Nakashima

USA (Trilafon, generics)

Canada (Apo-Perphenazine, Trilafon, PMS Perphenazine)

▶ When Should I Use This Drug?

Consider an alternative agent

- although this drug is effective, it provides no advantage over other available agents
- usually expensive and should likely be used only if the patient has responded to it in the past

PHENELZINE

Lyle K. Laird and Julia Vertrees

USA (Nardil)

Canada (Nardil)

▶ When Should I Use This Drug?

Major Depression, atypical depression, dysthymia

- phenelzine is most often used as a second-line agent in patients who have failed to respond to other antidepressants or who cannot tolerate their side effects
- useful in patients with atypical depression characterized by anxiety, feeling of tension, tremor, cardiovascular or gastrointestinal symptoms, phobias and panic attacks, or reverse vegetative symptoms, such as increased sleep, increased appetite, increased weight, increased libido, and reversed diurnal variation (feeling best in the morning)

Panic disorders

- useful in patients resistant to benzodiazepines or tricyclic antidepressants

Migraine prophylaxis

- use only in patients who fail to benefit from less toxic prophylactic agents such as beta-blockers and tricyclic antidepressants

▶ When Should I Not Use This Drug?

Patients taking long-term medications that could potentially interact

- phenelzine interacts with a number of drugs, and other agents should be tried instead

Bipolar disorder, depression

- patients who have this illness (also known as manic depression) may be at risk of exacerbating the manic phase of the illness if given antidepressants (Arch Gen Psychiatry 1979;36:555–559)

Depression after a bereavement

- in cases of depressed mood that do not meet the definition of clinical depression (e.g., an otherwise depressed feeling that follows a normal periodic fluctuation in mood or a depression due to bereavement and less than 2 weeks in duration)

▶ *What Contraindications Are There to the Use of This Drug?*

Intolerance of or allergic reaction to phenelzine

The following are absolute contraindications to the use of phenelzine:

Active alcoholism

- all alcoholic beverages should be avoided, as this helps to minimize the chances of hypertensive crisis (Lancet 1988;1:879)

Pheochromocytoma

- pressor substances from these tumors can change blood pressure when monoamine oxidase (MAO) inhibitors are used

Severe hepatic dysfunction

- phenelzine may precipitate hepatic precoma in cirrhotic patients who are sensitive to the effects of phenelzine

Severe renal dysfunction

- renal elimination may be decreased, leading to cumulative effects

The following are relative contraindications (i.e., other antidepressants are ineffective or not tolerated, phenelzine may be used, but monitoring for potential adverse effects must be done):

Hypertension

- concurrent use of MAO inhibitors in patients already taking antihypertensive medication is not recommended owing to the potential for excessive hypotension
- hypertensive crises due to the ingestion of tyramine-containing foods may be more severe in a patient with preexisting hypertension
- evaluate blood pressure twice weekly initially in patients with hypertension until the effect of this agent on blood pressure has been seen

Congestive heart failure

- phenelzine can cause both hypertension and hypotension, which could potentially worsen congestive heart failure (see above)

Sympathectomy

- patients who have undergone sympathectomy may be more sensitive to the hypotensive effects of MAO inhibitors (see above)

Cardiovascular and/or cerebrovascular disease

- ischemia may be worsened by MAO inhibitor–induced hypotension (see above)

Schizophrenia

- phenelzine may cause excessive stimulation in schizophrenics

Severe or frequent headaches

- headache is 1 of the first signs of a hypertensive reaction to an MAO inhibitor, which could be masked by severe or frequent headaches, although this agent can be effective in the prophylaxis of migraines

Seizure disorder history

- seizure pattern may be altered by an effect on seizure threshold

Pregnancy

- human studies have not been done

▶ *What Drug Interactions Are Clinically Important?*

Drugs that may increase the effect or toxicity of phenelzine

TRICYCLIC ANTIDEPRESSANTS

- results in gastrointestinal complaints, symptoms of central nervous system (CNS) excitability; hyperthermia; cardiovascular events, including dysrhythmia; seizures; and coma

- most likely to occur if the tricyclic antidepressant is added to an MAO inhibitor regimen
- combination may be used, after monotherapy has been tried, if both tricyclic antidepressant and the MAO inhibitor are started together or if MAO inhibitor is added to the tricyclic antidepressant regimen
- if the patient is receiving an MAO inhibitor, and a tricyclic antidepressant is to be added, the patient should be MAO inhibitor free for at least 2 weeks prior to starting the new combination regimen (J Clin Psychopharmacol 1981;1:264–282)

AMPHETAMINE, DEXTROAMPHETAMINE, METHAMPHETAMINE

- several case reports describe rapid onset of headache and severe hypertension (hypotension, hyperpyrexia, and seizures in 1 case) when patients taking MAO inhibitors have been given amphetamines; additionally, there are reports of fatal cerebral hemorrhage
- concurrent use of these medications should be avoided; the risk of this reaction may persist for several weeks after stopping MAO inhibitor administration

SYMPATHOMIMETICS (PHENYLEPHRINE, DOPAMINE, PHENYLPROPANOLAMINE, PSEUDOEPHEDRINE)

- direct or mixed-acting sympathomimetics may result in severe headache, hypertension, and hyperpyrexia and possibly hypertensive crisis when administered concurrently with MAO inhibitors; minimum, if any, interaction has been noted with MAO inhibitors and direct-acting sympathomimetics
- concurrent use of these medications should be avoided

LEVODOPA

- hypertensive reactions have appeared within 1 hour after administration of levodopa to patients taking MAO inhibitors; the effect appears to be dose related; also reported are flushing, lightheadedness, and palpitations, with the theoretical possibility of cardiac arrhythmias
- concurrent use should be avoided

MEPERIDINE

- adverse effects (agitation, seizures, diaphoresis, fever, coma, and respiratory depression) have been reported with the combination of medications; the reaction is unpredictable and additionally may occur 2–3 weeks after discontinuation of MAO inhibitor administration
- deaths have been reported in patients reacting to this combination
- avoid meperidine in patients with a history of taking MAO inhibitors
- other opioid analgesics can be used if required, but use lower initial dosages and more gradual titration while monitoring the patient for this reaction

FLUOXETINE

- concurrent administration of fluoxetine and an MAO inhibitor or administration of an MAO inhibitor shortly after discontinuing fluoxetine therapy may lead to a serotonin syndrome, including CNS irritability, increased muscle tone, shivering, myoclonus, and altered consciousness
- manufacturer recommends a 5 week interval between discontinuing fluoxetine therapy and beginning an MAO inhibitor regimen

ANESTHETICS

- concomitant use can result in hypotension
- discontinue use 2 weeks prior to surgery
- if this is not possible, avoid the use of pressor agents owing to the risk of hypertensive reactions
- most anesthetists are not concerned as long as they know the patient has been taking an MAO inhibitor so that they can titrate blood pressure as needed

Drugs that may decrease the effect of phenelzine

- none

Drugs that may have their effect or toxicity increased by phenelzine

INSULIN

- hypoglycemic response to insulin may be potentiated and delay recovery from hypoglycemia
- increased blood glucose monitoring is warranted during concurrent administration, with adjustment of the insulin dosage as required

SULFONYLUREAS

- MAO inhibitors may enhance the hypoglycemic action of sulfonylureas
- increased blood glucose monitoring is warranted during concurrent administration, with adjustment of the sulfonylurea dosage as required to achieve euglycemia until the sulfonylurea dosage is reestablished

Drugs that may have their effect decreased by phenelzine

- none

▶ *What Route and Dosage Should I Use?*

How to Administer

- orally—on an empty stomach or with food or milk
- parenterally—not available

Major depression, atypical depression, dysthmia

- 30 mg PO daily (15 mg PO BID) and increase by 15 mg/d at 5–7 day intervals until 60 mg PO daily is reached (a starting dosage of up to 1 mg/kg/d has been advocated by some clinicians (Arch Gen Psychiatry 1973;29:407–413)
- maintain this dosage for 2 weeks, and if no response occurs, increase the daily dosage by 15 mg at weekly intervals to a maximum of 90 mg PO daily (or 1 mg/kg/d, whichever is less)
- give the full daily dose by noon if possible; but give the last dose before supper, at the latest, to avoid insomnia
- therapeutic trial is usually considered to be at least 45 mg/d for 4 weeks

Panic disorders

- lower dosages are usually required
- 15 mg PO daily

Migraine prophylaxis

- 15 mg PO BID and increase as needed to 15 mg PO TID after 2–4 weeks

Dosage adjustments for renal or hepatic dysfunction

- hepatically metabolized
- no dosage adjustment guidelines are available
- in patients with renal or hepatic dysfunction, start with the lowest available dosage and titrate the dose on the basis of efficacy and toxicity

▶ *What Should I Monitor with Regard to Efficacy and Toxicity?*

Efficacy

Major depression, atypical depression, dysthmia

Sleep disturbance

- is the first symptom to improve (after 10–14 days) and should be assessed weekly

Nervousness, somatic complaints, appetite, feelings of helplessness and hopelessness, depressed mood

- tend to improve more slowly over 2–3 weeks
- close friends or relatives notice signs of improvement before the patient is aware of changes
- adequate clinical response should not be expected for at least 4 weeks
- after they are stable, patients should be clinically assessed for target symptoms at least monthly (or weekly if clinical decompensation is suspected)

Plasma concentrations

- plasma levels are not useful for routinely monitoring the efficacy or toxicity of MAO inhibitor therapy

Panic disorders

Target symptoms

- monitor changes in shortness of breath, choking or smothering sensations, dizziness, palpitations or chest pain, trembling, nausea, depersonalization, tingling, and fear of impending doom
- should see initial response within several days
- after they are stable, patients should be clinically assessed for target symptoms at least monthly (or weekly if clinical decompensation is suspected)

Migraine prophylaxis

Frequency and severity of headache

- patient with frequent migraine may need evaluation at 2–4 week intervals during initial dosage titration; then the interval between follow-up visits may be extended in patients showing a response to treatment

Toxicity

Orthostatic hypotension

- orthostatic hypotension is the most common cardiovascular effect and is found even with therapeutic dosages
- treatment of orthostatic hypotension includes having the patient rise slowly from supine or sitting positions and wear support stockings and ensuring that adequate fluid intake is being maintained
- reduce the dosage if orthostatic hypotension persists

Hypertension

- hypertensive crisis may produce the following symptoms: severe headache, palpitations, neck stiffness, nausea, vomiting, dilated pupils, sweating, and chest pain
- if these symptoms occur, immediate therapy with antihypertensive agents should be instituted

Syndrome of inappropriate secretion of antidiuretic hormone

- transient edema may occur; however, if it persists, check electrolyte levels for the possibility of SIADH

Mild headache without increased blood pressure

- can be treated with acetaminophen or aspirin
- measure blood pressure, especially if headache is persistent or intolerable

Decreased sexual ability

- decrease the dosage or discontinue medication administration if it persists

Decreased and increased appetite (due to carbohydrate craving)

- alert the patient to this potential side effect

Central nervous system stimulation (muscle twitching during sleep, restlessness, agitation, trouble with sleeping)

- decrease the dosage and ensure that the drug is given in the morning

Anticholinergic effects

Dry Mouth

- increase fluid intake and/or use sugarless chewing gum or hard candies

Constipation

- increase fluid and fiber in diet, and if needed, use a laxative

Blurred vision

- reduce the dosage; if there is no resolution of symptoms, switch to a drug with less severe anticholinergic properties

Urinary hesitancy

- reduce the dosage, and if it persists, stop the drug administration

► *How Long Do I Treat Patients with This Drug?*

Major depression, atypical depression, dysthymia

- antidepressant therapy is generally continued for 6 months after the patient is symptom free, or for 6 months after the usual natural duration of an individual's depressive episodes if known
- selected patients may need continuous antidepressant therapy if depression recurs consistently on stopping antidepressant therapy

Panic disorders

- as is the case for generalized anxiety disorder, studies suggest that panic disorders are a chronic illness with waxing and waning symptoms
- no long-term follow-up studies longer than 6 months exist, and the efficacy of drug therapy after 6 months is unknown, but patients receiving long-term therapy do experience relapse when drug administration is discontinued
- some clinicians recommend at least a 6 month symptom-free period prior to attempting discontinuation (J Clin Psychiatry 1990;51:11–15)
- concurrent behavioral or desensitization therapy after drug administration discontinuation may decrease the risk of relapse

Migraine prophylaxis

- in the patient achieving a headache-free state, therapy should be reduced or withdrawn after 6 months to assess continued requirements
- if patient has a return of headaches, indefinite prophylactic therapy should be considered

► *How Do I Decrease or Stop the Administration of This Drug?*

- MAO inhibitors need to be tapered over 2–3 weeks at the end of therapy to decrease the risk of rebound depression and to avoid a possible withdrawal syndrome consisting of agitation, confusion, irritability, drowsiness, tachycardia, hallucination, headache, nausea, severe nightmares, difficulty in talking, sweating, and shivering
- effects of MAO inhibitors may persist for up to 2 weeks after stopping administration of the medication; therefore, dietary and other medication restrictions should continue for 2 weeks

► *What Should I Tell My Patients About This Drug?*

- this drug has significant interactions with foods and the recommended diet needs to be followed (Can J Psychiatry 1984; 29:707–711, Psychiatr Clin North Am 1984;7:549–546, J Am Diet Assoc 1986;86:1059–1064)
- small amounts of normally harmless pressor amines in foods can lead to a hypertensive crisis (often termed the cheese reaction) because MAO inhibitors also inhibit gut MAO, which normally breaks down these amines (principally tyramine) before they can reach the systemic circulation
- 6 mg of tyramine may produce a mild crisis; 10–25 mg may produce severe headaches and possibly intracranial hemorrhage
- although any food rich in aromatic amino acids can become high in tyramine if aging, contamination, prolonged storage, or spoilage occurs, only 4 foods clearly warrant absolute prohibition: aged cheese (Cheddar, bleu, Swiss), pickled fish (herring), concentrated yeast extracts (brewer's yeast), and broad bean pods (Italian broad beans or fava beans)
- insufficient evidence exists to prohibit alcohol completely, as tyramine content varies from beverage to beverage (even among Chianti wines), but the use of alocoholic beverages is still not recommended
- keep tyramine intake below 5 mg, begin diet therapy and diet counseling before drug therapy, monitor the patient's compliance, recommend preparation and consumption of only fresh foods, and continue the diet for 4 weeks after drug therapy to allow full recovery of gut MAO
- this drug can cause some anticholinergic effects
- headache may be the first indication of a hypertensive reaction to tyramine
- this drug interacts with several other medications, especially over the counter cough and cold medications and appetite suppressants; therefore, check with your physician or pharmacist before using other medications

► *Therapeutic Tips*

- avoid in patients who are unlikely to adhere to dietary restrictions
- patients not responsive to 1 MAO inhibitor may be responsive to another
- MAO inhibitors' psychomotor effects can lead to insomnia and other sleep disturbances and therefore they are usually not given at night (give the daily dose before noon)

PHENOBARBITAL

William Parker and Jonathan Fleming

USA (Luminal, Phenobarbital [various], Solfoton)
CANADA (Phenobarbital [various])

► *When Should I Use This Drug?*

Generalized seizures (no primary focus)

Tonic-clonic seizures

- use only if valproic acid, phenytoin, or carbamazepine is not effective
- phenobarbital is effective but has a greater potential for causing sedation or behavioral disturbances than do the other drugs

Partial seizures (with or without secondarily generalized tonic-clonic seizures)

- use only if valproic acid, phenytoin, or carbamazepine is not effective
- phenobarbital is effective but has a greater potential for causing sedation or behavioral disturbances than do the other drugs

Status epilepticus

- use only if the patient is still having seizures 1 hour after the intravenous benzodiazepine and phenytoin load
- usefulness is limited by slow onset of action

► *When Should I Not Use This Drug?*

Use in conjunction with primidone

- phenobarbital should not be used concurrently with primidone (5–25% of primidone is metabolized to phenobarbital); the phenobarbital/primidone ratio is highly variable and phenobarbital may lead to excessive sedation when combined with primidone during long-term therapy

Absence seizures

- may worsen absence seizures

Insomnia

- phenobarbital is contraindicated in the management of insomnia because of safety factors (tolerance, lethality in overdosage, risk of abuse, and drug-drug interactions [N Engl J Med 1990;322: 239–241])
- barbiturate effects on sleep architecture (reduction in rapid eye movement sleep and delta sleep), safety (risk of dependence and abuse, lethality in overdosage), lack of efficacy (tolerance of hypnotic effects develops within 2 weeks), and significant withdrawal reactions (rebound insomnia) make them unsuitable for use

► *What Contraindications Are There to the Use of This Drug?*

Intolerance of or allergic reaction to phenobarbital

Porphyria

- avoid use because phenobarbital induces hepatic cytochrome P-450 and increases hepatic heme turnover, which can exacerbate symptoms of acute intermittent porphyria and porphyria variegata

Severe respiratory disease

- phenobarbital may cause worsening of dyspnea or airway obstruction

▶ *What Drug Interactions Are Clinically Important?*

Drugs that may increase the effect of phenobarbital

VALPROIC ACID, PHENYTOIN, CIMETIDINE, AND CHLORAMPHENICOL

- may inhibit phenobarbital metabolism, necessitating a decrease in phenobarbital dosage
- their concurrent use need not be avoided; however, patients should be monitored to ensure effective anticonvulsant control and to avoid possible phenobarbital toxicity

CENTRAL NERVOUS SYSTEM DEPRESSANTS (ALCOHOL, BENZODIAZEPINES, ANTIDEPRESSANTS, ANTIPSYCHOTICS, AND SO ON)

- if used concomitantly, there is increased potential for excessive sedation
- give daily phenobarbital dose at bedtime and/or reduce the drug dosages

Drugs that may decrease the effect of phenobarbital

DIURETICS

- alkalinization of the urine and use of diuretics may decrease serum phenobarbital levels and result in decreased efficacy
- if seizure frequency increases, monitor serum phenobarbital concentrations and adjust the dosage as required

Drugs that may have their effect increased by phenobarbital

PHENYTOIN

- may inhibit metabolism
- if signs and symptoms of toxicity occur, monitor serum concentrations and adjust the dosage of phenytoin on the basis of serum concentrations

Drugs that may have their effect decreased by phenobarbital

THEOPHYLLINE, WARFARIN, RIFAMPIN, QUINIDINE, OTHER ANTIEPILEPTICS, ANTIARRYTHMICS, METHADONE, MEPERIDINE, ORAL CONTRACEPTIVES

- phenobarbital is a potent enzyme inducer and increases the elimination of many drugs metabolized by the liver
- be aware of the potential for decreased effects of these agents
- for patients taking oral contraceptives, use an alternative form of birth control

▶ *What Route and Dosage Should I Use?*

How to administer

Orally

- give on an empty stomach

Parenterally

- give intravenously at a rate not to exceed 60 mg/min
- barbiturate solutions are extremely alkaline; therefore, avoid perivascular extravasation or intraarterial injection
- intramuscular injection should not exceed a volume of 5 mL at any one site owing to possible tissue damage

Generalized seizures (no primary focus), partial seizures (with or without secondarily generalized tonic-clonic seizures)

- 30 mg PO TID, increasing by 60 mg/d every 5 days until seizure control is achieved or side effects become intolerable or a maximum dosage of 250 mg PO daily is reached
- maintenance dosage can be consolidated into a single nightly dose because of the drug's long half-life
- takes 2–3 weeks to reach steady state concentration

Status epilepticus

- give 250 mg IV at a maximum rate of 60 mg/min and repeat in 30 minutes if seizures are not controlled, to a maximum dosage of 20 mg/kg
- maximum drug effect may not be seen for up to 30 minutes, so give the drug time to work before reinjecting, to avoid overdose

Dosage adjustments for renal or hepatic dysfunction

- hepatically metabolized (~65%)
- no first-pass metabolism; metabolites are inactive; downward dosage adjustment may be necessary if significant hepatic impairment develops
- about 30% is excreted unchanged in the urine; dosage reduction may be necessary if renal function decreases
- if the dose is titrated upward on the basis of efficacy and adverse effects, no specific dosage adjustments are needed

▶ *What Should I Monitor with Regard to Efficacy and Toxicity?*

Efficacy

Generalized seizures (no primary focus), partial seizures (with or without secondarily generalized tonic-clonic seizures)

Seizure frequency

- reduction in frequency and severity of seizures

Serum concentrations

- accepted therapeutic range is 15–40 μg/mL (65–170 μmol/L); occasionally, patients respond to lower or higher concentrations
- steady state concentration is reached in 14–21 days after the maintenance dosage is attained
- except when desired after a loading dose, do not obtain phenobarbital concentrations for 3–4 weeks after starting therapy unless side effects occur
- because of low protein binding (~50%), free drug concentrations are not useful
- because of the long half-life, there are minimal peak to trough fluctuations with once-daily dosing
- trough serum concentrations are preferred unless the patient reports side effects a few hours after the dose

Toxicity

Serious adverse effects to phenobarbital are rare, but mild adverse effects occur frequently

Behavioral disturbances (hyperexcitability, confusion, depression) and cognitive impairment (impaired short-term memory, decreased memory concentration)

- occur frequently, particularly in children and the elderly
- these reactions may not respond to dosage reduction and may necessitate switching to another anticonvulsant

Sedation and central nervous system side effects

- are frequent, are dose related, and tend to decrease or disappear with continued use
- minimize by starting with low dosages, gradually increasing the dosage, giving a single dosage at bedtime, and avoiding concomitant administration of central nervous system (CNS) depressants

Respiratory depression

- IV administration may produce severe respiratory depression, and provisions for respiratory support should be made

Dysarthria, ataxia, nystagmus

- with serum levels greater than 40 μg/mL (170 μmol/L)

Stupor, coma

- with serum levels greater than 70 μg/mL (300 μmol/L)

Physical and psychological dependence

- may also occur, especially in alcoholic patients and those known to be dependent on other drugs; use of a nonbarbiturate, nonbenzodiazepine anticonvulsant is recommended

▶ *How Long Do I Treat Patients with This Drug?*

Generalized seizures (no primary focus), partial seizures (with or without secondarily generalized tonic-clonic seizures)

- 4 year seizure-free period is recommended before attempting to withdraw phenytoin administration
- factors promoting complete withdrawal include a seizure-free period of 2–4 years, complete seizure control within 1 year of

onset, an onset of seizures between 2 and 35 years of age, and a normal electroencephalogram
- patients should not drive during withdrawal and for 3–4 months after, and this may make it difficult for some patients to try withdrawal
- prior to withdrawal, patients should be advised that about ⅓ experience relapse, and if this occurs, the patient and the physician will know that the drug is still necessary
- factors associated with a poor prognosis in stopping the drug administration despite a seizure-free period include a history of a high frequency of seizures, repeated episodes of status epilepticus, multiple seizure types, and the development of abnormal mental functioning

Status epilepticus
- after seizures are controlled, therapy should be initiated with a first-line agent

▶ *How Do I Decrease or Stop the Administration of This Drug?*
- phenobarbital can usually be safely withdrawn from patients with intractable epilepsy who are maintained on appropriate nonbarbiturate anticonvulsants
- sudden withdrawal is to be avoided, especially during long-term, high-dose therapy
- withdrawal is best done over several months
- decrease the dosage by 30 mg daily each month until withdrawal is complete
- seizure relapse is most common during withdrawal or the first 3 months after withdrawal
- if seizures recur, reinstitute treatment with the same drugs used previously
- simultaneous substitution of another anticonvulsant may be necessary during phenobarbital withdrawal; the dosage of the new agent should be gradually increased as phenobarbital is gradually withdrawn, to maintain adequate seizure control
- if multiple-anticonvulsant therapy is used, the drugs should be withdrawn 1 at a time

▶ *What Should I Tell My Patients About This Drug?*
- using phenobarbital with alcohol or other CNS depressants may cause excessive drowsiness and ataxia
- initially, phenobarbital may make some patients drowsy and unsteady on their feet, so take in small, frequent doses or take the largest dose at bedtime; do not undertake activities requiring mental alertness or physical coordination until you know how you will react to phenobarbital
- these effects should lessen with time
- behavioral disturbances and cognitive impairment may develop while using phenobarbital; notify your physician, who may decrease the dosage or change to another anticonvulsant
- abrupt discontinuation of therapy may result in the precipitation of seizures, so do not stop taking phenobarbital or reduce the dosage without prior advice from your physician
- you should avoid situations that could be dangerous or life-threatening if further seizures occur

▶ *Therapeutic Tips*
- patients adapt to CNS sedation due to phenobarbital; however, patients who have the drug therapy withdrawn or changed to another antiepileptic after long-term use often notice an improvement in sensorium
- do not give the drug more frequently than once per day after the dose has been titrated
- give dose at bedtime
- serum concentrations can help clinicians to decide when phenobarbital is causing some low-level CNS depression

Useful References

Pugh CB, Garnett WR. Current issues in the treatment of epilepsy. Clin Pharm 1991;10:335–358
Parker WA. Epilepsy. In: Herfindal ET, Gourley DR, Hart LL, eds. Clinical Pharmacy and Therapeutics, 4th ed. Baltimore: Williams & Wilkins, 1988:570–592

Levy RH, Wilensky AJ, Friel PN. Other antiepileptic drugs. In: Evans WE, Schentag JJ, Jusko WJ, eds. Applied Pharmacokinetics. Principles of Therapeutic Drug Monitoring, 2nd ed. Spokane WA: Applied Therapeutics, 1986:540–569

PHENOLPHTHALEIN
Leslie Mathews

USA (Ex-Lax, Phenolax, Evac-Q-Tabs, Evac-U-Gen, Prulet; combination: Correctol, Feen-A-Mint, Agoral, Alophen)
CANADA (Ex-Lax, Neo-Prunex, Evac-Q-Kwik, Alophen; combination: Doxidan, Calcium Docuphen, Mucinum, Agarol, Alophen)

▶ *When Should I Use This Drug?*
Consider an alternative agent
- action of a single dose may last 3–4 days because up to 15% of the dose is enterohepatically recirculated (Am J Gastroenterol 1985;80:303–309)
- often abused because it empties the colon thoroughly after use, disrupting normal stooling patterns, and this results in progressively higher dosages being taken to maintain a daily bowel movement
- excessive cramping and fluid loss can occur with normal doses
- dehydration and electrolyte imbalance occur often with overuse; osteomalacia (due to impaired absorption of vitamin D and calcium), protein-losing gastroenteropathy, hyperaldosteronism, and hypokalemia can occur with long-term use (Hosp Pharm 1988;23:565–573)
- fixed drug eruptions and other dermatological reactions can occur in the hypersensitive patient (Drug Evaluations, 6th ed 1986:983)
- fatal anaphylactic reactions (rare) can occur
- can cause morphological changes in the epithelium of the gut and, with long-term use, produce a "cathartic colon" (Postgrad Med 1988;83:339–349)

Useful References

Tedesco FJ. Laxative use in constipation. Am J Gastroenterol 1985;80: 303–309
Rousseau P. Treatment of constipation in the elderly. Postgrad Med 1988; 83:339–349
Tolstoi LG. Nutritional problems related to stimulant laxative abuse. Hosp Pharm 1988;23:565–573

PHENYLBUTAZONE
Kelly Jones

USA (various generic, Azolid, Butazolidin)
CANADA (various generic)

▶ *When Should I Use This Drug?*
Consider an alternative agent
- there is no reason to use this agent in the treatment of rheumatoid arthritis today
- there are better tolerated nonsteroidal antiinflammatory drugs (NSAIDs) with less severe side effects
- phenylbutazone carries a warning in the package insert stating that phenylbutazone or oxyphenbutazone should be used only when other NSAIDs have failed to be effective, owing to the increased risk of agranulocytosis and aplastic anemia

PHENYLPROPANOLAMINE
Penny Miller

USA (Prolamine, Dexatrim; combination: Triaminic, Genex, Rhinocaps)
CANADA (combination products only: Contac.C, Ornade, Sine-Off N.D., Corsym)

▶ *When Should I Use This Drug?*
Nasal congestion
- nasal congestion resulting from eustachian tube dysfunction during air travel, deep sea diving, the common cold, allergic rhinitis, sinusitis, and rebound congestion due to overuse of topical decongestants

- phenylpropanolamine is effective and safe when given in recommended dosages (Health Protection Branch. Third Report of the Expert Advisory Committee on Nonprescription Cough and Cold Remedies. Health and Welfare Canada, 1989), but is available in Canada only in combination products, and abuse has been reported
- use in place of pseudoephedrine only if combination products are required for multiple symptoms and if these combination products are less expensive
- acute psychotic reactions and excessive central nervous system stimulation have occurred in patients taking high doses of phenylpropanolamine combined with antihistamines or diphenylpyraline (Am Fam Physician 1989;39:201–206, Br J Psychiatry 1989;151:548–550)
- when used as an oral decongestant, rebound congestion and tachyphylaxis may occur within a few days, and this is not seen with pseudophedrine (American Hospital Formulary Service, Drug Information, ASHP, Bethesda, MD, 1993:752)

▶ *When Should I Not Use This Drug?*

Serous otitis media (otitis media with effusion) to improve eustachian tube function

- lack of efficacy has been demonstrated (Pediatrics 1978;61: 679–684, N Engl J Med 1983;308:297–301)

Central nervous system stimulation

- risk of hypertension and palpitations is too great when high doses are used for central nervous system stimulation

Appetite suppression

- lack of efficacy as a weight reducing agent

▶ *What Contraindications Are There to the Use of This Drug?*

see Pseudoephedrine

▶ *What Drug Interactions Are Clinically Important?*

see Pseudoephedrine

▶ *What Route and Dosage Should I Use?*

How to administer

- orally—can be given with food or on an empty stomach

Nasal congestion

- 25 mg PO Q4H PRN to a maximum of 150 mg PO daily

Dosage adjustments for renal or hepatic dysfunction

- no adjustment needed

▶ *What Should I Monitor with Regard to Efficacy and Toxicity?*

see Pseudoephedrine

▶ *How Long Do I Treat Patients with This Drug?*

see Pseudoephedrine

▶ *How Do I Decrease or Stop the Administration of This Drug?*

see Pseudoephedrine

▶ *What Should I Tell My Patients About This Drug?*

see Pseudoephedrine

▶ *Therapeutic Tips*

see Pseudoephedrine

Useful References

USPDI 1993, U.S. Pharmacopeial Convention, Rockville, MD, 1993
American Hospital Formulary Service, Drug Information, ASHP, Bethesda, MD, 1993:1675
Health Protection Branch. Third Report of the Expert Advisory Committee on Nonprescription Cough and Cold Remedies. Health and Welfare Canada, 1989

PHENYTOIN

William Parker

USA (Phenytoin [various], Dilantin, Diphenylan)
CANADA (Dilantin)

▶ *When Should I Use This Drug?*

Generalized seizures (no primary focus)

Tonic-clonic seizures

- phenytoin should be used if valproic acid or carbamazepine is not effective or tolerated
- valproic acid is effective and is better tolerated than phenytoin or carbamezepine
- phenytoin and carbamazepine cause a greater incidence of central nervous system (CNS) adverse effects
- if the electroencephalogram shows partial seizures, which secondarily generalize, either phenytoin or carbamezepine is the drug of choice
- many clinicians prefer carbamazepine to phenytoin as initial therapy owing to fewer adverse effects, easier dose titration, and fewer cosmetic side effects than with phenytoin
- carbamazepine is more expensive than phenytoin and must be dosed twice a day, compared with once-daily dosing for phenytoin
- phenytoin is the drug of choice if an agent must be given parenterally (other agents are not available as parenteral agents)

Partial seizures (with or without secondarily generalized tonic-clonic seizures)

- phenytoin and carbamazepine are equally effective, and the decision between these agents is as above for generalized seizures

Status epilepticus

- phenytoin administration should be started as soon as possible after the initial dose of the benzodiazepine
- may not be needed after the history has been determined, but it is best to give the patient a phenytoin load initially and then decide in 12–24 hours whether the patient requires maintenance phenytoin therapy

Arrhythmia due to digoxin toxicity

- drug of first choice for the treatment of arrhythmias due to digitalis intoxication

Ventricular tachycardia and paroxysmal atrial tachycardia

- in patients failing to respond to conventional antiarrhythmics or to cardioversion

Trigeminal neuralgia

- may be useful in patients who fail to respond to or cannot tolerate carbamazepine
- patients who fail to respond to carbamazepine likely do not respond to phenytoin, but it can be given prior to trying surgery

▶ *When Should I Not Use This Drug?*

Absence seizures

- phenytoin is ineffective and may increase the frequency of seizures

Young women and children

- should be avoided if possible owing to the possibility of cosmetic problems (hirsutism, gingival hyperplasia, and coarsening of facial features) and the possibility of reducing cognitive performance

Alcohol withdrawal seizures

- phenytoin is not effective in the prevention of alcohol withdrawal seizures (Ann Emerg Med 1991;20:520–522, Am J Med 1989; 87:645–648)
- diazepam is the drug of choice

▶ *What Contraindications Are There to the Use of This Drug?*

Intolerance of or allergic reaction to phenytoin

Sinus bradycardia, sinoatrial block, second- or third-degree atrioventricular block, or Stokes-Adams syndrome

- intravenous use of the drug should be avoided because the propylene glycol (40%) in the diluent can cause cardiovascular toxicity and exacerbate the underlying condition

Porphyria

- avoid use because phenytoin induces hepatic cytochrome P-450 and increases hepatic heme turnover, which can exacerbate symptoms of acute intermittent porphyria and porphyria variegata

▶ *What Drug Interactions Are Clinically Important?*

Drugs that may increase the effect or toxicity of phenytoin

CIMETIDINE

- inhibits metabolism of phenytoin and may increase serum phenytoin concentrations by 50% or more
- use ranitidine or famotidine in place of cimetidine, which may avoid an increase in phenytoin levels

DISULFIRAM, CHLORAMPHENICOL, ISONIAZID, AND OTHER INHIBITORS OF CYTOCHROME P-450

- inhibit metabolism of phenytoin and may produce increases in serum phenytoin concentrations
- monitor serum phenytoin measurements weekly until a new steady state concentration is established or symptoms of toxicity occur, and adjust the dosage accordingly
- if administration of the inhibitor is stopped, return to the previous dosage of phenytoin

Drugs that may decrease the effect of phenytoin

THEOPHYLLINE

- may decrease the absorption and steady state serum phenytoin concentration
- dosage adjustment and increased monitoring are not required if an antiepileptic drug is being added
- if theophylline is added, monitor serum phenytoin concentrations weekly until a steady state concentration is established, and adjust the phenytoin dosage accordingly

FOLIC ACID

- administration of 5 mg/d or more of folic acid to patients previously stabilized on phenytoin may result in increased seizure frequency and lowered serum phenytoin concentrations, whereas long-term administration of phenytoin may cause low serum folate concentrations and symptoms of folic acid deficiency in some patients
- patients receiving phenytoin should be observed for symptoms of folic acid deficiency, and if necessary, folic acid 1 mg/d may be added as supplemental therapy with monitoring for decreased phenytoin concentrations

RIFAMPIN, PHENOBARBITAL, CARBAMAZEPINE, AND OTHER INDUCERS OF HEPATIC CYTOCHROME P-450 ENZYMES

- may decrease steady state serum phenytoin concentrations
- dosage adjustment and increased monitoring are not required if an antiepileptic drug is being added
- if interacting drugs are added, monitor serum phenytoin concentrations weekly until a steady state concentration is established, and adjust the dosage accordingly

ENTERAL FEEDING

- high-protein diet supplements administered by an enteral tube can impair the absorption of phenytoin from the suspension
- phenytoin may also adsorb to the polyvinyl chloride in nasogastric tubes
- effect may be reduced by stopping enteral feeding before the phenytoin dose and/or diluting the suspension with sterile water or normal saline and then irrigating the tubing after the dose with at least 30 mL of diluent before resuming the feeding
- serum phenytoin concentrations should be monitored weekly while the patient is receiving supplementation until a steady state concentration has been established

Drugs that may have their effect or toxicity increased by phenytoin

- none

Drugs that may have their effect decreased by phenytoin

THEOPHYLLINE

- theophylline clearance may be increased by 75% after 10 days of concurrent phenytoin administration
- interaction may result in loss of asthma control
- use an alternative agent for chronic asthma, if possible, in patients with seizures necessitating phenytoin therapy
- if phenytoin must be added, measure the theophylline concentrations every 5 days and adjust the theophylline dosage accordingly

CYCLOSPORINE

- phenytoin can reduce cyclosporine serum concentrations, possibly by increasing its hepatic metabolism, and can cause organ rejection
- avoid the combination if possible; otherwise monitor serum cyclosporine levels every 3–5 days and adjust the dosage accordingly, until a new steady state concentration has been established

ORAL CONTRACEPTIVES

- phenytoin can increase the hepatic metabolism of the estrogenic component of oral contraceptives, leading to spotting and possibly loss of efficacy
- increasing the dosage of the estrogen may reduce bleeding, but efficacy may still be affected, and an alternative method of contraception should be used while the patient is receiving phenytoin

▶ *What Route and Dosage Should I Use?*

How to administer

- orally—take with food or milk
- parenterally—give a direct intravenous injection (50 mg/min) or dilute with normal saline to a concentration of 25 mg/mL and infuse through an intravenous volume control set with inline filter (maximum of 50 mg/min)
- never give intramuscularly, as it is absorbed slowly and incompletely via this route and is painful

Generalized seizures (no primary focus), partial seizures (with or without secondarily generalized tonic-clonic seizures), status epilepticus, trigeminal neuralgia

Tablets and suspension contain phenytoin acid, whereas the capsules (sustained release) and parenteral forms contain phenytoin sodium, which is 92% phenytoin

Oral use with no loading dose

- 300 mg PO HS daily
- adjust on the basis of response and serum concentration (see below)
- 400 mg PO HS daily if the patient weighs greater than 70 kg
- to reduce initial gastrointestinal or CNS side effects, start the dosage slowly (100 mg PO HS daily for 3 days), and increase to 200 mg PO HS daily for 3 days and then to 300 mg PO HS daily (400 mg if the patient weighs >70 kg)
- once-daily dosing is appropriate if capsules (sustained release) are used
- if tablets or suspension is used, the daily dose must be split and given BID
- in patients who clear the drug rapidly, have side effects, or tend to forget some doses, phenytoin should be given in 2 divided doses

Oral loading dose

- oral loading dose should be used in patients when rapid (within 8–12 hours) attainment of effective serum concentrations is needed (for a patient who has had several recent seizures)
- without a loading dose, steady state serum concentrations may not be achieved for a couple of weeks
- 15 mg/kg (usually 1 g given PO as 400 mg, 300 mg, and 300 mg administered at 3 hour intervals)
- initiate the maintenance dosage the following day

Intravenous use (if the oral route is not available or if status epilepticus is present)

- 15 mg/kg IV given no faster than 50 mg/min (see below)
- start the maintenance dosage the following day

- if only the parenteral route is available, give 100 mg IV TID or 200 mg IV Q12H as the maintenance dosage

Arrhythmia due to digoxin toxicity, ventricular tachycardia, paroxysmal atrial tachycardia

- 100 mg direct IV injection (50 mg/min) every 5 minutes until arrhythmia is controlled, undesirable effects appear, or a maximum dose of 1 g is reached
- follow-up oral dose is 300 mg PO daily

Dosage adjustments for renal or hepatic dysfunction

- hepatically metabolized; however, hypoalbuminemia and uremia (creatinine clearance < 30 mL/min) significantly increase the fraction of unbound drug

Normal Dosing Interval	C_{cr} > 60 mL/min or 1 mL/s	C_{cr} 30–60 mL/min or 0.5–1 mL/s	C_{cr} < 30 mL/min or 0.5 mL/s
Q24H if sustained-release capsules used Q8–12H if given parenterally	no adjustment needed	no adjustment needed	target concentrations should be reduced to 5–10 mg/L and are equivalent to the usual therapeutic phenytoin concentrations of 10–20 mg/L

▶ **What Should I Monitor with Regard to Efficacy and Toxicity?**

Efficacy

Generalized seizures (no primary focus), partial seizures (with or without secondarily generalized tonic-clonic seizures), status epilepticus

Reduction in seizure frequency

- monitor for a reduction in seizure frequency (a seizure diary can be used)

Serum concentrations

- serum phenytoin concentration in target range (see below)

Pharmacokinetic monitoring

- serum concentration monitoring is important because phenytoin displays dose-dependent, saturable metabolism, which occurs within the therapeutic range, and small increases in dosage can result in large disproportionate increases in steady state serum concentrations
- prior to ordering any serum concentration determinations, ensure that the patient is receiving an appropriate dose for age, weight, renal or hepatic function, and disease state
- usual target range for serum phenytoin concentrations is 10–20 mg/L (40–80 μmol/L); however, some patients achieve complete seizure control at serum concentrations below 10 mg/L (40 μmol/L)
- in patients with low serum albumin levels, the fraction of unbound phenytoin is increased
- in general, if a patient's serum albumin level is approximately 35 g/dL, the free amount of phenytoin is about 25% greater than that seen in a patient with a normal serum albumin levels
- if the serum albumin level is 30, 25, or 20 g/dL, the free fraction of phenytoin is approximately 50%, 75%, and 100% greater, respectively
- trough concentrations (just before a maintenance dose) are preferred, and if serum concentrations are not measured at a trough, this must be taken into account

Admission concentrations

- determine a concentration in all patients who have signs and symptoms of toxicity or seizures and/or in those in whom poor compliance is suspected
- concentrations (unless ordered immediately) may not be reported until the following day, but the admission concentration is useful

retrospectively as a guide to determining whether drug was responsible for adverse effects and/or the drug was at a therapeutic concentration at the time of hospital admission

Concentrations without a loading dose

- if a loading dose has not been used, serum concentrations should be monitored no more frequently than once weekly until steady state concentration has been achieved
- when phenytoin administration is started or the daily dosage is changed, most patients take 10 days or more to reach a steady state concentration

Concentrations with an oral or intravenous loading dose

- measure the serum concentration the morning after the load, as this concentration is used to determine the adequacy of the load but, more importantly, is the starting point for the assessment of the appropriateness of the maintenance dosage
- level 2–3 days after the start of a maintenance dosage provides information about the adequacy of the maintenance dosage
- if the level at 2–3 days is greater than the level measured the morning after the load, one does not know how high the concentration will be at steady state but can tell how fast the concentration could possibly rise, and therefore, one knows when to measure the next level
- assuming that the maintenance dose does not change, the rate of rise in the serum concentration is always decreasing (e.g., if the serum concentration has gone up 3 mg/L in the 3 days since the load, the concentration cannot increase by more than 3 mg/L during the next 3 days)
- conversely, if the concentration has decreased by 3 mg/L since the load (while the patient is receiving a maintenance dosage), the concentration will not fall by more than 3 mg/L during the next 3 days

Dosage adjustment guidelines

- using serum levels as a guide, increase in 50–100 mg/d increments every week until desired concentrations are achieved

Arrhythmia due to digoxin toxicity, ventricular tachycardia and paroxysmal atrial tachycardia

- monitor for resolution of the arrhythmia or the appearance of undesirable side effects or until a total of 1 g is given

Trigeminal neuralgia

Pain relief

- usually, a response is seen within 48 hours; the drug should not be used preventively during periods of remission
- therapeutic serum concentration for trigeminal neuralgia has not been defined

Toxicity

Nausea, vomiting, epigastric pain, and anorexia

- up to 50% of patients experience gastrointestinal intolerance, especially with once-daily dosing
- start doses gradually
- if these symptoms occur, give smaller doses in a divided regimen and give with food

Drowsiness, fatigue, incoordination and similar central nervous system depressant effects

- commonly seen, especially in the first few days but frequently decrease or disappear during continued therapy
- minimize by avoiding concomitant administration of CNS depressants and by starting with low doses, gradually increasing the dosage and giving the daily dose at bedtime

Nystagmus, slurred speech, ataxia, blurred vision, and dizziness

- appear frequently with serum levels between 20 and 40 μg/mL (80 and 160 μmol/L), with confusional states, mood changes, and possible exacerbation of seizures at concentrations greater than 40 μg/mL (160 μmol/L)

Gingival hyperplasia

- may occur in up to 50% of patients with long-term use; therefore, recommend good oral hygiene, gum massage, and regular dental visits to help to minimize this problem

Vitamin D deficiency, osteomalacia, folic acid deficiency, hypertrichosis, carbohydrate intolerance, coarsening of facial features

- except for hypertrichosis and coarsening of facial features, which may be irreversible, the other effects generally respond well to conventional interventions (vitamin D, calcium, and folic acid replacement; dietary management; and/or insulin therapy)

Stevens-Johnson syndrome, exfoliative dermatitis, erythema multiforme

- phenytoin is associated with rare but serious hypersensitivity or idiosyncratic reactions resulting in skin reactions
- most hypersensitivity reactions occur within the first 2 months of therapy
- discontinue phenytoin administration if these reactions are present

Hepatitis, bone marrow suppression, and various lymphadenopathies

- routine laboratory monitoring is not indicated, and patients should be monitored on clinical grounds such as unexplained bruising, infection, fever, nausea, vomiting, scleral icterus, and so on

Burning, pain at the intravenous access site, bradycardia, dizziness, and hypotension

- may be seen with IV phenytoin therapy; slowing the rate of infusion may minimize these complications
- IV administration at greater than 50 mg/min may result in cardiovascular collapse and/or CNS depression

▶ *How Long Do I Treat Patients with This Drug?*

Status epilepticus, generalized tonic-clonic and simple complex seizures, partial complex seizures, myoclonic, akinetic, tonic seizures

- 4 year seizure-free period is recommended before attempting to withdraw phenytoin therapy
- factors promoting complete withdrawal include a seizure-free period of 2–4 years, complete seizure control within 1 year of onset of therapy, an onset of seizures between 2 and 35 years of age, and a normal electroencephalogram
- patients should not drive during withdrawal and for 3–4 months after, and this may make it difficult for some patients to try withdrawal
- prior to withdrawal, patients should be advised that about one third experience relapse, and if this occurs, the patient and the physician will know that the drug is still necessary
- factors associated with a poor prognosis in stopping drug therapy despite a seizure-free period include a history of a high frequency of seizures, repeated episodes of status epilepticus, multiple seizure types, and the development of abnormal mental functioning
- neurosurgical use of phenytoin may be discontinued after surgery, although some patients need to continue the phenytoin regimen or be switched to another anticonvulsant for clinical control

Arrhythmia due to digoxin toxicity

- after 2–3 days, the digoxin serum concentration drops to a safe level in most individuals and the phenytoin administration can then be stopped

Ventricular tachycardia and paroxysmal atrial tachycardia

- after the arrhythmia is under control, the patient should be switched to conventional antiarrhythmics for maintenance therapy

Trigeminal neuralgia

- if there is no improvement in the frequency or severity of attacks within several days, stop phenytoin therapy, as it is likely not effective

▶ *How Do I Decrease or Stop the Administration of This Drug?*

- sudden withdrawal is to be avoided, especially after long-term, high-dose therapy
- withdrawal is best done over several months
- decrease the dosage by 100 mg daily each month until withdrawal is complete

- seizure relapse is most common during withdrawal or the first 3 months after withdrawal
- if seizures recur, reinstitute treatment with the same drugs used previously
- if multiple-anticonvulsant therapy is being used, drugs should be withdrawn 1 at a time

▶ *What Should I Tell My Patients About This Drug?*

- using phenytoin with alcohol or other CNS depressants may cause excessive drowsiness and ataxia
- initially, phenytoin may make some patients drowsy and unsteady on their feet, so take in small doses and do not undertake activities requiring mental alertness or physical coordination until you know how you react to phenytoin; this effect should lessen with time
- using phenytoin may cause nausea or loss of appetite early in therapy, so start with a small dose and take with food if necessary
- good oral hygiene, gum massage, and regular dental visits may help to prevent gum tenderness, bleeding, or enlargement
- shake phenytoin suspensions vigorously before administration, to resuspend adequately
- unexplained weakness, fatigue, repeated vomiting, yellowing of the eyes, easy bruisability, fever, and loss of seizure control may be early signs of drug-induced toxicity and should be reported immediately
- you may be overly sensitive to the combination of this drug with alcohol or other CNS depressants and you should not drive or operate heavy machinery until you know how you react to these agents
- abrupt stoppage of therapy may result in the precipitation of seizures, so do not stop taking phenytoin or reduce the dosage without prior advice from your physician
- avoid situations that could be dangerous or life-threatening if further seizures should occur

▶ *Therapeutic Tips*

- monitoring of the patient and serum drug level is recommended when changing the phenytoin dosage form or brand
- absorption of a suspension is impaired in patients receiving concurrent enteral tube feedings
- similarly, drug is lost when given via a nasogastric tube because of adherence to the polyvinyl chloride tubing
- minimize drug loss by stopping the feeding before and after the dose, diluting the suspension with sterile water or normal saline, and irrigating the tube with at least 30 mL of diluent after administration
- oral suspensions must be shaken vigorously to resuspend adequately
- a great degree of pharmacokinetic variability exists among patients, and all dosing must be based on serum concentrations
- consolidated doses, which improve patient compliance, should be attempted after the patient has been stabilized on a multiple-dose regimen for at least 1 month
- the higher the dose, the greater the likelihood that multiple dosing is needed
- only the extended-release capsules should be used in once-daily dosing
- phenytoin is highly protein bound and may be displaced by other highly protein bound drugs, but no dosage adjustment is necessary, and problems occur when clinicians react to a lower total phenytoin concentration without considering the free fraction (an initial increase in free phenytoin is followed by an increase in clearance, a fall in total phenytoin concentrations, and the reestablishment of normal free phenytoin concentrations)

Useful References

Pugh CB, Garnett WR. Current issues in the treatment of epilepsy. Clin Pharm 1991;10:335–358

Parker WA. Epilepsy. In: Herfindal ET, Gourley DR, Hart LL, eds. Clinical Pharmacy and Therapeutics, 4th ed. Baltimore: Williams & Wilkins, 1988:570–592

Winter ME, Tozer TN. Phenytoin. In: Evans WE, Schentag JJ, Jusko WJ, eds. Applied Pharmacokinetics. Principles of Therapeutic Drug Monitoring, 2nd ed. Spokane WA: Applied Therapeutics, 1986:493–539

PHOSPHORUS

Angela Kim-Sing and Eric Yoshida

USA (Neutra Phos, Neutra Phos K, K-Phos Neutral tabs, Uro-KP-Neutral tabs, Fleet Phospho-Soda, Potassium phosphate, Sodium phosphate)
CANADA (Phosphate-Sandoz, Potassium phosphate)

▶ *When Should I Use This Drug?*

Treatment of phosphorus deficiency

- treat underlying cause of phosphate deficiency (alcoholism, ingestion of phosphate binding antacids, diabetic ketoacidosis, malabsorption)
- serum phosphate concentrations are not a reliable indicator of body stores
- phosphorus depletion can affect respiratory, cardiovascular, neuromuscular, and hematological systems
- symptoms include malaise, muscular weakness, paresthesias, confusion, obtundation, anorexia, bone pain, and stiffness, and progress in severe depletion to include irritability, ataxia, tremors, platelet and leukocyte dysfunction, seizures, coma, cardiomyopathy, EEG changes, and respiratory failure
- individuals with moderate (0.3–0.7 mmol/L) or severe hypophosphatemia (<0.3 mmol/L) should receive supplementation, especially if symptomatic or if asymptomatic with phosphate < 0.3 mmol/L

▶ *When Should I Not Use This Drug?*

Hyperphosphatemia

- if serum phosphate concentrations are normal or elevated, additional phosphate supplementation is not indicated as it can increase the risk of extra-skeletal (soft tissue) calcification with calcium

Moderate hypophosphatemia (serum phosphate concentration 0.7 to 1.0 mmol/L)

- if no underlying risk factors for phosphate depletion (e.g., alcoholic), hypophosphatemia is often transient and will resolve with resumption of dietary intake

Renal impairment

- serum phosphate may accumulate depending on the severity of renal failure; therefore, supplementation should be guided by serum phosphate monitoring

Hyperkalemia

- potassium phosphate is the most widely available salt for parenteral administration and consideration of the potassium content (4.4 mEq K^+ for every 3 mmol of phosphorus) is required if phosphate is administered parenterally

▶ *What Contraindications Are There to the Use of This Drug?*

- intolerance or allergic reaction to phosphorus

▶ *What Drug Interactions Are Clinically Important?*

Drugs that may increase the effect or toxicity of phosphorus

- none

Drugs that may decrease the effect or phosphorus

ALUMINUM, MAGNESIUM, OR COMBINATION-CONTAINING ANTACIDS AND SUCRALFATE

- bind to phosphate in the gastrointestinal tract and prevent absorption of phosphate
- space administration of drugs apart by 2 hours

CATECHOLAMINES, SALBUTAMOL (ALBUTEROL), TERBUTALINE

- can increase distribution of phosphate into tissue or bone
- unlikely to induce clinically relevant hypophosphatemia in patients with normal phosphate stores

ACETAZOLAMIDE, FUROSEMIDE, THEOPHYLLINE, GLUCOCORTICOIDS, DOPAMINE, ESTROGEN

- can increase renal elimination of phosphate
- unlikely to induce clinically relevant hypophosphatemia in patients with normal phosphate stores

Drugs that may have their effect or toxicity increased by phosphorus

- none

Drugs that may have their effect decreased by phosphorus

- none

▶ *What Route and Dosage Should I Use?*

How to administer

- orally—capsules must be dissolved in water; dilute liquid preparation in 120 ml of water or 500 ml of tube feeding to prevent diarrhea
- parenterally—dilute in IV fluid (100 ml for every 4 mmol of potassium phosphate) of NS or D_5W and infuse over a minimum of 4 hours

Treatment of phosphorus deficiency

- oral replacement is the preferred route
- phosphorus should be ordered in mmol as it is a polyvalent anion; ordering phosphate in mEq can lead to dosing errors
- give approximately 16 mmol (depends on product) of phosphate PO TID of the least expensive and most palatable phosphate product
  Neutra Phos capsules (8 mmol phosphorus and 7 mEq of potassium and 7 mEq of sodium per capsule
  Neutra Phos K capsules (8 mmol phosphorus and 14 mEq of potassium per capsule)
  K-Phos Neutral tablets (8 mmol phosphorus and 13 mEq of sodium per tablet)
  Uro-KP-Neutral tablets (8 mmol phosphorus and 1 mEq of potassium and 10 mEq of sodium per tablet)
  Fleet Phospho-Soda (4.1 mmol phosphorus and 4.8 mEq of sodium/mL)
- if patient symptomatic, vomiting, unable to tolerate the oral route or if serum phosphate concentration is < 0.3 mmol/L, patient should be supplemented intravenously
- 0.08 mmol/kg of phosphate IV infused over 4–6 hours if uncomplicated and of recent onset
- 0.16 mmol/kg of phosphate IV infused over 4–6 hours if prolonged and multifactorial
- increase dose by 25% if symptomatic
- decrease dose by 25% if patient hypercalcemic to avoid calcium-phosphate precipitation into tissues
- subsequent phosphate administration should be determined by patient's response to the initial dose
- alternatively, could repeat dosing every 12 hours until serum phosphate concentration normalized
- choice of either sodium or potassium salt depends on need for these agents: potassium phosphate (3 mmol phosphate and 4.4 mEq of potassium/ml; sodium phosphate (3 mmol phosphate and 4.0 mEq of sodium/ml)

Dosage adjustments for renal/hepatic dysfunction

- renally eliminated
- in patients with renal dysfunction, give 50% of the recommended dose above and base additional doses on serum phosphate measurement

▶ *What Should I Monitor with Regard to Efficacy and Toxicity?*

Efficacy

Serum phosphate concentration

- serum phosphate concentrations should be assessed at 6 hours following IV infusions and phosphate administration repeated until the concentration has normalized
- for moderate hypophosphatemia treated with oral supplements, the serum concentration should be evaluated in 1 week to ensure concentration is rising, and if it is rising regular measurement is not required

- if patient severely malnourished, aggressive carbohydrate supplementation can precipitously decrease serum phosphate concentration, which can be fatal (refeeding syndrome); therefore, parenteral nutrition solutions with adequate phosphate should be started slowly and increased gradually in these patients

Signs and symptoms of deficiency

- any signs or symptoms of phosphate deficiency (described above) should resolve as phosphate concentration increases and phosphate deficit is replaced

Toxicity

Hypocalcemia and hyperkalemia

- serum potassium, phosphate, and calcium should be monitored daily following each intravenous phosphate dose
- excessive phosphate concentration or infusion rate may produce hypocalcemia, possibly resulting in tetany, neuromuscular abnormalities, paresthesias, arrhythmias, heart block, weakness, and/or confusion
- potassium phosphate is the most widely available salt for parenteral administration and consideration should be given to the potassium content (4.4 mEq K^+ for every 3 mmol of phosphorus)

Diarrhea

- oral supplements may cause diarrhea, and reducing the dosage transiently may help resolve the problem
- if patient unable to tolerate phosphate supplementation, excellent sources of dietary phosphate include dairy products, chicken, fish, and red meat

▶ *How Long Do I Treat Patients with This Drug?*

Treatment of phosphorous deficiency

- length of treatment depends on severity and etiology of hypophosphatemia
- usually treat until serum concentrations are stable within normal range

▶ *How Do I Decrease or Stop the Administration of This Drug?*

- may be stopped abruptly

▶ *What Should I Tell My Patients About This Drug?*

- oral phosphate supplements may cause diarrhea, and reducing the dosage transiently may help resolve this problem

▶ *Therapeutic Tips*

- diarrhea may limit oral phosphate dose
- if patient unable to tolerate phosphate supplementation, excellent sources of dietary phosphate include dairy products, chicken, fish, and red meat.

Useful References

Brown GR, Greenwood JK. Drug and nutrition-induced hypophosphatemia: Mechanisms and relevance in the critically ill. Ann Pharmacother 1994;28:626–632

Dickerson RN. Treating hypophosphatemia. Hosp Pharm 1985;20:920–925

Lloyd CW, Johnson CE. Management of hypophosphatemia. Clin Pharm 1988;7:123–128

Solomon SM, Kirby DF. The refeeding syndrome: A review. J Parenteral Enteral Nutr 1990;14:90–97

Lentz RD, Brown DM, Kjellstrand CM. Treatment of severe hypophosphatemia. Ann Intern Med 1978;89:941–944

Vannatta JB, Whang R, Papper S. Efficacy of intravenous phosphorus therapy in the severely hypophosphatemic patient. Arch Intern Med 1981;141:885–887

PIMOZIDE

Juan Avila and Patricia Marken

USA (Orap)
CANADA (Orap)

▶ *When Should I Use This Drug?*

Tourette's syndrome

- this drug is effective but is likely the second choice after haloperidol (greater cardiovascular effects than haloperidol and there have been reports of sudden death associated with the use of pimozide)

▶ *When Should I Not Use This Drug?*

Acute psychosis therapy, maintenance psychosis therapy, manic phase of bipolar illness

- although this drug is effective, it provides no advantages over other available agents

see Chlorpromazine

▶ *What Contraindications Are There to the Use of This Drug?*

see Chlorpromazine

▶ *What Drug Interactions Are Clinically Important?*

see Thiothixene

▶ *What Route and Dosage Should I Use?*

How to administer

- orally—take with food or milk or on an empty stomach
- parenterally—not available

Tourette's syndrome

- give 1 mg PO daily and increase every 4–7 days up to a maximum dosage of 20 mg PO daily

Dosage adjustments for renal or hepatic dysfunction

- hepatically metabolized
- no specific dosage adjustments are needed; just start with a low dose and titrate to effect

▶ *What Should I Monitor with Regard to Efficacy and Toxicity?*

Efficacy

Tourette's syndrome

- reduction of relief of symptoms

Toxicity

see Chlorpromazine

▶ *How Long Do I Treat Patients with This Drug?*

Tourette's syndrome

- lifelong therapy may be needed

▶ *How Do I Decrease or Stop the Administration of This Drug?*

see Chlorpromazine

▶ *What Should I Tell My Patients About This Drug?*

see Chlopromazine

▶ *Therapeutic Tips*

see Chlorpromazine

Useful References

Kane JM. The current status of neuroleptic therapy. J Clin Psychiatry 1989;50:322–328

Hemstrom CA, Evans RL, Lobeck FG. Haloperidol decanoate: A depot antipsychotic. DICP 1988;22:290–295

Coryell W, Kelly M, Perry PJ, Miller DD. Haloperidol plasma levels and acute clinical change in schizophrenia. J Clin Psychopharmacol 1990;10:397–402

Alexander B. Antipsychotics: How strict the formulary? DICP 1988;22:324–326

PINDOLOL

Robert Rangno and James McCormack

USA (Visken)
CANADA (Visken, Apo-Pindol, Novo-Pindol, Syn-Pindolol, Nu-Pindol

▶ When Should I Use This Drug?

Consider an alternative agent

- pindolol is a nonselective agent with high lipid solubility that needs to be dosed more frequently than once daily
- offers no advantages over atenolol and nadolol
- pindolol has more intrinsic sympathomimetic activity than does acebutolol
- partial agonist activity can cause tremor, palpitations, and failure of control of nocturnal angina
- pindolol's high lipid solubility may increase the risk of central nervous system and sleep disturbances
- its use in patients after a myocardial infarction increases the risk of sudden death and reinfarction (Am J Cardiol 1990;66:3C–8C)
- pindolol is reported to be more ''lipid friendly'' than some other beta-blockers but the lipid changes of all beta-blockers are usually slight, are short lived, and have no proven consequences

PIPERACILLIN

John Rotschafer, Kyle Vance-Bryan, and Rick Zabinski

USA (Pipracil)
CANADA (Pipracil)

▶ When Should I Use This Drug?

check antibiotic susceptibility chart (Table 4–1 in Chapter 4)

Presumed or proven infections caused by *Pseudomonas aeruginosa* or other susceptible gram-negative bacilli

- should be chosen instead of ceftazidime and imipenem only if it is less expensive
- piperacillin has the disadvantage of usually being dosed Q4H, whereas other antipseudomonal agents can be dosed less frequently

Treatment of mixed aerobic-anaerobic bacterial infections

- equally effective as second-generation cephalosporins (cefoxitin, cefotetan, and ceftizoxime)
- piperacillin, however, covers *P. aeruginosa* and enterococci, which are not covered by cefoxitin, cefotetan, or ceftizoxime
- decision between piperacillin and the cephalosporins above should be based on cost and the differences in coverage
- piperacillin has the disadvantage of usually being dosed Q4H (Q6H for less serious infections), whereas other agents can be dosed less frequently

Febrile neutropenic patients

- piperacillin in conjunction with tobramycin is useful empirical antimicrobial therapy for febrile neutropenic patients if *P. aeruginosa* is suspected

▶ When Should I Not Use This Drug?

Staphyloccocal infections

- use cloxacillin, nafcillin, or cefazolin because most staphylococcal organisms produce beta-lactamases and are not sensitive to piperacillin

Infections caused by single organisms

- in general, piperacillin should be reserved for infections presumed or proved to be caused by mixed organisms

▶ What Contraindications Are There to the Use of This Drug?

see Penicillin

▶ What Drug Interactions Are Clinically Important?

see Penicillin

▶ What Route and Dosage Should I Use?

How to administer

- orally—not available
- parenterally—administer intravenously in 100 mL of IV fluid (normal saline or 5% dextrose in water) and infuse over 30 minutes

Systemic infections

Severe infections, central nervous system infections such as meningitis, endocarditis

- 3 g IV Q4H

Moderate infections such as mixed aerobic-anaerobic infections

- 2 g IV Q4H

Mild infections such as soft tissue infections

- 1 g IV Q6H

Dosage adjustments for renal or hepatic dysfunction

- renally eliminated

Normal Dosing Interval	C_{cr} > 60 mL/min or 1 mL/s	C_{cr} 30–60 mL/min or 0.5–1 mL/s	C_{cr} < 30 mL/min or 0.5 mL/s
Q4H	no adjustment needed	Q6H	Q8H
Q6H	no adjustment needed	Q8H	Q12H

▶ What Should I Monitor with Regard to Efficacy and Toxicity?

Efficacy

- for antibiotic administration monitoring guidelines, see specific section on drug therapy

Toxicity

see Penicillin

Interstitial nephritis

- characterized by hematuria and oliguria
- can occur but is rare and the drug administration must be discontinued if it occurs

Hypokalemia, hepatotoxicity, decreased platelet aggregation

- these occur rarely, and monitoring is not required but the clinician should be aware that they can occur

▶ How Long Do I Treat Patients with This Drug?

Pneumonias

- usual duration of therapy is 10 days or 4–5 days after the patient has become afebrile and has clinically improved

Meningitis

- 21 days (stop aminoglycoside treatment after 10 days because of increased risk of toxicity) if meningitis is caused by gram-negative organisms

Intraabdominal infections

- treatment should continue for 10 days; however, extend treatment if the patient has not been asymptomatic for 72 hours

Febrile neutropenic patients

- if the patient is afebrile for 72 hours, no causative agent is found, and the total granulocyte count is greater than 500/μL, discontinue antibiotic therapy after 7 days of treatment (J Infect Dis 1990;161:381–396)
- if the patient remains neutropenic, continue antibiotic therapy until the patient is afebrile for 5 days
- if the patient is clinically unwell, continue antibiotic therapy until the granulocyte count is less than 500/μL (J Infect Dis 1990;161:381–396)

▶ How Do I Decrease or Stop the Administration of This Drug?

- may be stopped abruptly

▶ *What Should I Tell My Patients About This Drug?*

see Penicillin

▶ *Therapeutic Tips*

- can use as a single agent for mild infections; however, use as combination therapy with aminoglycosides for more serious gram-negative infections
- during therapy, be aware of the risk of the development of resistant organisms, especially if treatment is for pseudomonal infection
- do not use in combination with imipenem, as this combination provides no clinical advantages
- for serious infections, use maximum dosages of the drug
- do not use, especially as a single agent, for enterococcal infections

see Penicillin

Useful References

Wright AJ, Wilkowske CJ. The penicillins. Mayo Clin Proc 1987;62:806–820

Barriere SL, Conte JE Jr. Manual of Antibiotics and Infectious Diseases, 7th ed. Philadelphia: Lea & Febiger, 1992

PIRENZEPINE

James McCormack and Glen Brown

USA (not available)
CANADA (Gastrozepin)

▶ *When Should I Use This Drug?*

Consider an alternative agent

- although pirenzepine has fewer adverse effects than do other anticholinergics, it is no more effective and has more adverse effects than do other drugs used to treat peptic ulcer disease

PIROXICAM

Kelly Jones

USA (Feldene)
CANADA (Feldene, Apo-Piroxicam, Novopirocam)

▶ *When Should I Use This Drug?*

Rheumatoid arthritis

- piroxicam can be used as an alternative for patients who fail to respond to enteric-coated aspirin or ibuprofen; however, it is more expensive
- piroxicam is a preferred agent for patients at risk for hepatotoxicity, as piroxicam is the least toxic to the liver (J Am Board Fam Pract 1989;2:257–271)
- useful in patients who have a history of noncompliance (because it has once-daily dosing); however, once-daily dosing may not be preferred in patients with arthritis pain, as these patients may want to dose more than once per day (DICP 1989;23:76–85)
- most regular-release nonsteroidal antiinflammatory drugs (NSAIDs), including aspirin, can be taken on an every 12 hour basis when being used to treat arthritic conditions, and therefore once-daily NSAIDs provide the advantage of only once- versus twice-daily dosing
- decision among piroxicam, tenoxicam, nabumetone, and oxaprozin (once a day NSAIDs) should be based on cost
- sustained-release NSAIDs can be used once daily, preferably in the evening to attempt reduction in morning stiffness, and should be chosen if they are less expensive than piroxicam, tenoxicam, nabumetone, or oxaprozin
- piroxicam is considered harsh on the stomach and should not be used in patients believed to be at high risk for gastrointestinal toxicity (J Am Board Fam Pract 1989;2:257–271)

Osteoarthritis

- if acetaminophen enteric-coated aspirin or ibuprofen are not effective
- decision between this drug and other NSAIDs should be based on cost

▶ *When Should I Not Use This Drug?*

Acute pain, general aches and pains, dysmenorrhea

- not useful for the acute management of general aches and pains because it is difficult to titrate because of its long half-life and its expense

Control of acute pain associated with arthritis

- this drug should never be used initially to gain control of arthritis pain, as the long half-life does not allow dosing flexibility
- this drug should be reserved for use as maintenance therapy for patients with controlled disease

Combination with other NSAIDs

- combinations of NSAIDs provide no increase in effectiveness compared with maximum dosages of single agents and significantly increase the risk of adverse effects

▶ *What Contraindications Are There to the Use of This Drug?*

see Ibuprofen

▶ *What Drug Interactions Are Clinically Important?*

see Ibuprofen

▶ *What Route and Dosage Should I Use?*

How to administer

- orally—take with food or milk
- parenterally—not available

Rheumatoid arthritis

- 10 mg PO at HS to a maximum dosage of 20 mg PO at HS

Osteoarthritis

- 10 mg PO at HS

Dosage adjustments for renal or hepatic dysfunction

- hepatically metabolized; therefore, no adjustments are needed for renal disease
- reduce the dosage by 25% in patients with a history of hepatic disease

▶ *What Should I Monitor with Regard to Efficacy and Toxicity?*

see Ibuprofen

▶ *How Do I Decrease or Stop the Administration of This Drug?*

- may be stopped abruptly if needed

▶ *What Should I Tell My Patients About This Drug?*

see Ibuprofen

▶ *Therapeutic Tips*

see Ibuprofen

▶ *Useful References*

see Ibuprofen

POLYETHYLENE GLYCOL–ELECTROLYTE SOLUTION

Leslie Mathews

USA (GoLYTELY, Colyte)
CANADA (GoLYTELY, Klean-Prep)

▶ *When Should I Use This Drug?*

Fecal impaction

- used to clean the bowel after impaction has been cleared with enemas and/or manual disimpaction (Gastroenterol Clin North Am 1990; 19:405–418, Age Ageing 1986;15:182–184)

Acute constipation

- use only when osmotic or stimulant laxatives are ineffective or contraindicated
- relatively safe for elderly patients, poorly hydrated patients, or those at risk for circulatory overload (Clin Pharm 1985;4: 414–424)

Chronic constipation

- smaller dosages are being investigated for this indication (Am J Gastroenterol 1990;85:261–265)
- further study regarding possible toxicity with absorption of polyethylene glycol is needed
- consider use only when all other treatment fails

Bowel preparation

- drug of choice for bowel preparation for colonoscopy, barium enema examination, and elective colorectal surgery because as effective or better than standard hydration, cathartic, enema regimens and causes the best and most complete evacuation of the gastrointestinal tract (Gastroenterology 1983;84:1512–1516)
- patients prefer polyethylene glycol–electrolyte solution (PEG-ES) to enema or cathartic preparation because it is more convenient (5 hours versus 3 days), is more rapidly active, and causes less discomfort (Clin Pharm 1985;4:414–424)

▶ When Should I Not Use This Drug?

On same day as barium enema examination

- can interfere with coating of barium on the wall of the colon
- instead, use the night before a barium enema study or use in conjunction with bisacodyl (Clin Pharm 1985;4:414–424)

▶ What Contraindications Are There to the Use of This Drug?

Intolerance of or allergic reaction to polyethylene glycol–electrolyte solution

Intestinal obstruction, perforation

- increased activity of the gut caused by this agent could worsen these conditions

Gastric retention

- increased risk of aspiration, given the large volumes that are used

Toxic megacolon, toxic colitis

- greater fluid absorption is likely with abnormal bowel mucosa (Clin Pharm 1985;4:414–424) and the effects of possible absorption of polyethylene glycol are unknown

Aspiration risk

- impaired gag reflex, decreased level of consciousness

▶ What Drug Interactions Are Clinically Important?

- none, although PEG-ES may affect the absorption of sustained-release products by decreasing gut transit time, but this is likely not clinically important unless it is used regularly for chronic constipation

▶ What Route and Dosage Should I Use?

How to administer

- orally—give on an empty stomach
- parenterally—do not use

Fecal impaction, acute constipation

- guidelines unclear to date
- suggest 2 L given orally or via nasogastric tube
- give another 2 L the following day if the first 2 L is not effective (Age Ageing 1986;15:182–184)

Chronic constipation

- start with 240 mL/d and increase as needed to 480 mL/d

Bowel preparation

- 4 L (1 gallon) given orally over 3 hours (240 mL every 10–15 minutes), given 4–5 hours before colonoscopy

- give the night before surgery or barium enema study
- can be given by nasogastric tube (20–30 mL/min)
- patient should fast for 3–4 hours prior to administration
- patient should not ingest any solids after administration or before examination

Dosage adjustments for renal or hepatic dysfunction

- negligible amounts are absorbed from the gastrointestinal tract (Gastroenterology 1986;90:1914–1918)
- initial data suggest that this agent is safe for patients with chronic renal failure (Clin Pharm 1985;4:414–424)

▶ What Should I Monitor with Regard to Efficacy and Toxicity?

Efficacy

Fecal impaction, acute constipation, chronic constipation, bowel preparation

- produces liquid stool within 30–60 minutes

Toxicity

Gastrointestinal symptoms

- nausea occurs in 20% of patients and is transient
- abdominal bloating occurs in 10% of patients
- chilling the solution improves the salty taste
- measure the patient's temperature after ingestion of 2 L or more of the chilled solution, especially in the elderly, owing to the risk of hypothermia (Med Lett 1985;27:39–40)
- monitor patients with nasogastric administration for regurgitation and aspiration (observe the patient during the first few minutes of administration, and if regurgitation or aspiration occurs or is suspected, discontinue the drip infusion and check the position of the tube)

Esophageal tear due to severe vomiting

- has not occurred with PEG-ES but has with other whole bowel irrigation solutions
- decrease the rate of administration with persistent nausea
- use antiemetics; discontinue administration with persistent vomiting

Colonic explosion due to hydrogen and methane gas formation

- has not occurred with PEG-ES but has with whole bowel irrigation solutions containing mannitol (Gastroenterology 1979;77:1307–1310); therefore, do not add sweetening agents to the preparation

▶ How Long Do I Treat Patients with This Drug?

Fecal impaction, acute constipation

- 1–2 days

Chronic constipation

- guidelines are unclear, but it should be safe for long-term use because it does not significantly affect water and electrolyte balance (Am J Gastroenterol 1990;85:261–265)

Bowel preparation

- continue until rectal return is clear (usually requires 4 L over 3 hours)

▶ How Do I Decrease or Stop the Administration of This Drug?

- may be stopped abruptly

▶ What Should I Tell My Patients About This Drug?

- it produces diarrhea (large amounts) starting 30–60 minutes after the first dose
- you may also experience cramping, abdominal bloating, and gas
- nausea and occasional vomiting can occur, and if so, drink the solution more slowly (240 mL over 20–25 minutes)
- refrigerate the solution to improve the taste and prevent nausea
- contact your physician if vomiting or abdominal pain is persistent

- do not add anything (including sweeteners) to the solution
- fast for 3–4 hours prior to administration
- do not ingest any solids after administration of the solution or before the examination

▶ Therapeutic Tips

- chill the solution to improve its unpleasant, salty taste
- be wary of hypothermia when large volumes are given
- sweeteners or other additives may alter the osmolality of the solution or introduce substances capable of fermentation by gut bacteria, producing potentially explosive gases

Useful References

Michael KA, DiPiro JT, Bowden TA, Tedesco FJ. Whole-bowel irrigation for mechanical colon cleansing. Clin Pharm 1985;4:414–424

Andorsky RI, Goldner F. Colonic lavage solution (polyethylene glycol electrolyte lavage solution) as a treatment for chronic constipation: A double-blind, placebo-controlled study. Am J Gastroenterol 1990;85:261–265

Puxty JAH, Fox RA. GoLYTELY: A new approach to faecal impaction in old age. Age Ageing 1986;15:182–184

POTASSIUM

Eric Yoshida and Angela Kim-Sing

USA (K-Lyte, Micro-K, K-Lor, generics)
CANADA (Slow-K, K-Dur, generics)

▶ When Should I Use This Drug?

Prevention of potassium depletion

- depletion is usually a consequence of increased urinary losses (e.g., diuretics, amphotericin B, corticosteroid therapy), fecal losses (e.g., diarrhea), and poor oral intake (e.g., postsurgery, anorexia nervosa)
- monitor serum potassium concentration in patients with these risk factors and supplement their diet if serum potassium is less than 3.5 mEq/L
- cellular potassium shifts (e.g., metabolic alkalosis, beta-adrenergic effects) may be clinically significant in patients with depleted total body stores

Treatment of potassium deficiency

- when serum potassium concentration is less than 3.5 mEq/L or less than 4.0 mEq/L if at risk for cardiac arrhythmia (e.g., post MI, concurrent antiarrhythmic therapy, including digoxin)

▶ When Should I Not Use This Drug?

At a dose of less than 20 mEq/d

- doses less than 20 mEq/d are not sufficient to maintain or increase serum potassium concentrations

▶ What Contraindications Are There to the Use of This Drug?

Intolerance or allergic reaction to potassium

Severe renal insufficiency/end stage renal disease

- potassium supplements should not be used at all if the patient is normokalemic
- if the patient is hypokalemic, administer a single dose with follow-up potassium serum concentration within 12 hours; subsequent doses should be guided by serum potassium and creatinine concentrations

▶ What Drug Interactions Are Clinically Important?

Drugs that may increase the effect or toxicity of potassium

SPIRONOLACTONE, TRIAMTERENE, AMILORIDE, TRIMETHOPRIM

- these agents directly inhibit renal excretion of potassium
- monitor potassium serum concentration within 1 week after interacting drugs are initiated; discontinue/avoid potassium supplements and/or discourage excessive dietary potassium intake
- unless patient remains hypokalemic on these potassium sparing agents, this combination should be avoided

ANGIOTENSIN-CONVERTING ENZYME INHIBITORS (CAPTOPRIL, ENALAPRIL, LISINOPRIL, QUINAPRIL, RAMIPRIL)

- angiotensin-converting enzyme inhibitors interfere with aldosterone-induced potassium excretion and can lead to hyperkalemia
- this will be enhanced by combining potassium supplements and angiotensin-converting enzyme inhibitors, especially in the context of renal insufficiency
- unless patient remains hypokalemic when angiotensin-converting enzyme inhibitors are used, this combination should be avoided
- if this combination is used, check serum potassium concentrations when the angiotensin-converting enzyme is started and weekly until the extent of potassium retention is seen

CYCLOSPORINE, FK506

- these immunosuppressants have considerable nephrotoxicity and decrease potassium excretion via decreased glomerular filtration rate
- monitor potassium serum concentrations 3 times a week for the first 2 weeks after starting potassium and only use potassium if patient is hypokalemic
- discontinue/avoid potassium supplements and/or discourage excessive dietary potassium intake where warranted

Drugs that may decrease the effect of potassium

RESIN-BINDING AGENTS

- resin binding agents (e.g., cholestyramine, sodium polystyrene, calcium resonium) prevent potassium absorption
- sodium polystyrene (Kayexalate)/Calcium resonium are used in the treatment of hyperkalemia
- space oral potassium supplements by 2 hours with cholestyramine administration

THIAZIDE DIURETICS (e.g., HYDROCHLOROTHIAZIDE, CHLORTHALIDONE, METOLAZONE) AND LOOP DIURETICS (e.g., FUROSEMIDE, ETHACRYNIC ACID)

- the effect with thiazide diuretics is dose dependent but incidence and magnitude are very low on 12.5–25 mg PO daily of hydrochlorothiazide or equivalent
- effect is quite variable but ranges between a drop of 0.1–0.6 mEq/L within the first week and is maximal by the end of 1 month
- furosemide causes less hypokalemia than thiazides (i.e., 40 mg PO daily of furosemide versus 50 mg PO daily of hydrochlorothiazide) (Arch Intern Med 1983;143:1694–1699) because of furosemide's relatively short duration of action (4–6 hours) compared to that seen with hydrochlorothiazide (18–24 hours)
- in patients receiving any diuretics, monitor the potassium levels at 2 weeks and at the end of 1 month
- once stable, repeat measurement only if dose/disease state changes occur
- if serum potassium decreases to less than 3.5 mEq/L (or < 4.0 mEq/L while on digoxin) supplement by increasing dietary potassium and restricting sodium intake

AMPHOTERICIN B

- results from renal tubular defect
- supplement therapy for all patients with minimum of 40 mmol potassium chloride (not in same IV bag) daily and adjust according to serum potassium concentration
- monitor serum potassium concentrations twice weekly

CORTICOSTEROIDS

- increased potassium excretion secondary to mineralocorticoid effect
- monitor serum potassium concentration when corticosteroid therapy initiated and monitor potassium levels at 2 weeks and at the end of 1 month
- once stable, repeat measurement only if dose/disease state changes occur

- if serum potassium decreases to less than 3.5 mEq/L (or < 4.0 mEq/L while on digoxin) supplement by increasing dietary potassium and restricting sodium intake

Drugs that may have their effect or toxicity increased by potassium

- none

Drugs that may have their effect decreased by potassium

- none

▶ What Route and Dosage Should I Use?

How to administer

- orally—take with 250 mL of water or juice
- parenterally

  usually ordered as potassium chloride (KCl), in multiples of 10 or 20 mEq to a maximum of 60 mEq, to each liter of maintenance IV fluids (normal saline, Ringer's lactate, 5% dextrose etc.) and administered at rate desired depending on IV fluid needs (e.g., KCL 40 mEq per liter of normal saline at 100 ml/h)

  KCl boluses may be administered in a critical care setting with cardiac monitoring in doses of 10 mEq/h

Prevention of potassium depletion

- in a patient with normal renal function, approximately 20 mEq/d is required; however, this must be individualized for each patient depending on dietary potassium intake and degree of potassium losses with diuretics, diarrhea, etc.
- a variety of oral dosage forms and products are commercially available (extended release tablet, solution, or effervescent tablet) and selection should be based on safety, palatability, potassium content, and cost
- slow release potassium chloride products preferred over other dosage forms to reduce the incidence of gastrointestinal irritation
- enteric-coated preparations should be avoided because of small bowel toxicity reported with their use
- wax-matrix or microencapsulated polymers minimize gastric irritation but have also been associated with gastric irritation and bleeding
- most liquid potassium formulations have an unpleasant taste and aftertaste and may produce nausea, heartburn, and diarrhea, which may affect compliance

Treatment of potassium deficiency

Mild to moderate deficiency (potassium greater than 3.0 mEq/L and asymptomatic)

- a 1 mEq reduction in serum potassium concentration generally implies a body deficit of 100–200 mEq potassium)
- 20 mEq PO TID as initial treatment
- 60 mEq as an IV infusion over 24 hours with maintenance intravenous fluids
- the oral route is safest and most economical
- potassium chloride should be used if hypokalemia is diuretic-induced since an associated chloride deficit is usually present
- other potassium salts (acetate, bicarbonate, citrate, and/or gluconate) are appropriate for treatment of conditions where bicarbonate loss is associated with potassium loss (diarrhea, renal potassium wasting in renal tubular acidosis)

Severe depletion (serum potassium concentration < 3.0 mEq/L); may be symptomatic (e.g., weakness) and at increased risk for cardiac arrhythmias

- give 20–40 mEq PO as a liquid preparation immediately and repeat in 2–4 hours with further doses guided by serial serum potassium concentrations
- if the parenteral route is required add 60 mEq KCl to a liter of IV fluid and infuse at a maximum rate of 20 mEq/h
- KCL boluses in doses of 10 mEq/100 mL IV over 1 hour may be given in a critical care setting with continuous ECG monitoring

Dosage adjustments for renal or hepatic dysfunction

- in patients with estimated creatinine clearance <30 mL/min, recheck serum potassium concentration after each 20–30 mEq IV potassium supplement to ensure hyperkalemia is avoided

- subsequent doses should be guided by serum potassium concentration and dietary intake

▶ What Should I Monitor with Regard to Efficacy and Toxicity?

Efficacy

Prevention and treatment of potassium deficiency

Serum potassium

- for patients with severe deficiency or on high dose intravenous diuretics, potassium may need to be monitored daily until stable
- in patients receiving any oral diuretics, monitor the potassium levels at 2 weeks and at the end of 1 month
- once stable, repeat measurement only if dose/disease state changes occur

Signs and symptoms

- signs and symptoms of hypokalemia (ECG changes, muscle weakness) should resolve when potassium is > 3.0 mEq/L

Toxicity

Hyperkalemia

- can easily occur if potassium supplements are given indiscriminately without serum potassium monitoring, especially in the setting of renal impairment (including prerenal failure secondary to hypovolemia) or in combination with potassium-sparing agents or ACE inhibitors.
- significant hyperkalemia is present with a serum potassium > 6.0 mEq/L
- with a serum potassium >6.5 mEq/L, intravenous fluids, loop diuretics such as furosemide, sodium bicarbonate, and IV insulin with glucose (e.g., 10 U of regular insulin added to 250 ml of 10% dextrose, given as a bolus) are recommended
- with ECG changes associated with hyperkalemia or serum potassium of 7.0 mEq/L or greater, 10 ml of 10% calcium gluconate, which has cardioprotective effects, is recommended in addition to the above therapy
- an ECG recording should always be obtained with a potassium > 6.5 mEq/L; ECG changes including peaked T waves, ST segment depression, and widened QRS complex are the most significant indications of hyperkalemia
- a sine wave ECG pattern is an ominous sign of hyperkalemic cardiotoxicity and requires immediate treatment

Gastrointestinal irritation

- symptoms of gastric irritation (dyspepsia, abdominal pains) may occur with oral potassium products; "pill" esophagitis and esophageal ulcers were originally described with enteric preparations but have also been reported with wax-matrix extended release preparations
- likewise, small intestinal ulcers, described with enteric preparations, have been described with the wax-matrix, extended release tablets
- some liquid potassium solutions contain sorbitol as a sweetener and may result in an osmotic diarrhea

▶ How Long Do I Treat Patients with This Drug?

Prevention of potassium depletion

- until risk factors for potassium deficiency have been resolved or dietary intake has been increased to compensate for negative balance

Treatment of potassium deficiency

- until body deficit replenished (e.g., serum potassium concentrations normalized and symptoms resolved)

▶ How Do I Decrease or Stop the Administration of This Drug?

- may be stopped abruptly

▶ What Should I Tell My Patients About This Drug?

- must be taken with food or a full glass of water
- oral tablets should be swallowed whole, not chewed or crushed

- patients may notice portions of the wax-matrix tablet in their stool
- liquid solutions, powders, and effervescent tablets must be diluted or dissolved in water or juice to minimize the gastrointestinal irritation

▶ Therapeutic Tips

- doses of less than 20 mEq/d, with normal renal function, in patients with poor oral intake may not be sufficient to prevent deficiency
- with refractory hypokalemia, consider coexistent hypomagnesemia or other medical causes (e.g., hyperaldosteronism in a hypertensive patient)
- salt substitutes (potassium chloride approximately 50–60 mEq/teaspoonful) may be economical alternatives for some patients; however, specific amount should be specified for daily use
- avoid solid oral dosage forms due to increased risk of ulceration; patients at increased risk include those with gastroparesis, esophageal strictures, achalasia, and intestinal hypomotility

Useful References

Greenberg S, Reiser IW, Porush JG. Trimethoprim-sulfamethoxazole induces reversible hyperkalemia. Ann Intern Med 1993;119:291–295

Krishna GG. Hypokalemic states: Current clinical issues. Semin Nephrol 1990;10:515–524

Leier CV, Deicas L, Metra M. Clinical relevance and management of major electrolyte abnormalities in congestive heart failure: Hyponatremia, hypokalemia and hypomagnesemia. Am Heart J 1994;128:564–574

Modest GA, Price B, Mascoli N. Hyperkalemia in elderly patients receiving standard doses of trimethoprim-sulfamethoxazole. Ann Intern Med 1994;20:437

Stanaszek WF, Romankiewicz JA. Current approaches to management of potassium deficiency. Drug Intell Clin Pharm 1985;19:176–184

PRAVASTATIN

Stephen Shalansky and Robert Dombrowski

USA (Pravachol)
CANADA (Pravachol)

▶ When Should I Use This Drug?

see Lovastatin

▶ When Should I Not Use This Drug?

see Lovastatin

▶ What Contraindications Are There to the Use of This Drug?

see Lovastatin

▶ What Drug Interactions Are Clinically Important?

No significant drug interactions have been reported (Clin Pharm 1992;11:677–689) • A higher incidence of myopathy has not been seen when used in combination with cyclosporine, gemfibrozil, or niacin

▶ What Route and Dosage Should I Use?

How to administer

- orally—can be given with food or on an empty stomach, as bioavailability is not increased by food
- parenterally—not available

Hypercholesterolemia, mixed hyperlipidemias

- start with 10 mg PO daily given before bed
- double the dosage if an adequate response has not been seen within 4 weeks
- dosage range is 20–80 mg daily
- dosages greater than 20 mg/d are more effective when given twice daily (JAMA 1986;256:2829–2834)
- pravastatin may be given once daily to enhance compliance
- if after 3 months of optimum therapy, there is at least a 15% decrease in LDL or total cholesterol levels, but the target level is not reached, continue pravastatin administration and add a second drug

- if after 3 months of optimum therapy, there is less than a 15% decrease in LDL or total cholesterol levels, consider switching to or adding another agent
- if the patient is not tolerating pravastatin, change to another drug

Dosage adjustments for renal or hepatic dysfunction

- hepatically metabolized
- do not use in severe hepatic dysfunction
- no dosage adjustments for renal dysfunction

▶ What Should I Monitor with Regard to Efficacy and Toxicity?

Efficacy

see Lovastatin

Toxicity

see Lovastatin

- causes less insomnia than does lovastatin (Clin Pharmacol Ther 1991;50:730–737)

▶ How Long Do I Treat Patients with This Drug?

see Lovastatin

▶ How Do I Decrease or Stop the Administration of This Drug?

- may be stopped abruptly

▶ What Should I Tell My Patients About This Drug?

see Lovastatin

▶ Therapeutic Tips

- pravastatin has a steep dose-response curve, and many patients show a significant LDL level lowering with 10 mg PO daily
- drug is more effective if given twice daily compared with once daily in the evening, but patients may be more compliant on once-daily dosing
- doses given once daily are more effective if given in the evening versus the morning (Clin Pharmacol Ther 1986;40:338–343)

Useful References

McKenney JM. Lovastatin: A new cholesterol lowering agent. Clin Pharm 1988;7:21–36

Jungnickel PW, Cantral KA, Maloley PA. Pravastatin: A new drug for the treatment of hypercholesterolemia. Clin Pharm 1992;11:677–689

PREDNISONE

Karen Shalansky, Cindy Reesor Nimmo, and Scott Whittaker

USA (Cortan, Deltasone, Medicorten, Orasone, Panasol-S, Prenicen, Sterapred Unipak)
CANADA (Deltasone, Winpred, Apo-Prednisone)

▶ When Should I Use This Drug?

Acute asthma, bronchitis

- add to therapy in patients demonstrating an incomplete response or inability to maintain complete response after 30 minutes of aggressive bronchodilator therapy (DICP 1991;25:72–79)
- oral corticosteroids are as effective as parenteral corticosteroids in the treatment of asthma in the emergency department and are less expensive (JAMA 1988;260:527–529, Lancet 1986;1:181–184)
- short 3 day bursts of prednisone therapy should be considered early in the course of upper respiratory tract infections if the patient has a history of severe exacerbations during viral illnesses (DICP 1991;25:72–79), as the cost and risk are negligible and this regimen may decrease long-term consequences

Chronic asthma, emphysema, bronchitis

- use only if symptoms remain uncontrolled with maximally tolerated doses of inhaled beta2-agonists, inhaled ipratropium bromide, high-dose inhaled corticosteroids, and theophylline

- should be used only after inhalers have failed because of the long-term adverse effects associated with oral corticosteroids
- prednisone is the preferred oral corticosteroid owing to intermediate half-life (12–30 hours), allowing once-daily dosing

Prevention of adrenal insufficiency

- during periods of increased stress (e.g., infection, surgery, and pregnancy) in patients maintained on greater than 5 mg/d for longer than 2 months, or within 1 year of systemic steroid therapy withdrawal

Rheumatoid arthritis

- because disease-modifying antirheumatic drugs are classically slow in onset, corticosteroids should be used when the administration of disease-modifying drugs is initiated and then tapered and discontinued when disease activity is controlled
- systemic corticosteroids are also useful short term when patients have disease flares
- should also be used when patients' symptoms are severe and disrupting their quality of life
- prednisone is useful in patients when systemic manifestations of rheumatoid arthritis such as vasculitis, pericarditis, and scleritis become clinically important

Migraine

- to bring prolonged migraine attacks under control and to lessen the need for narcotics
- when a migraine continues for longer than 36 to 48 hours (status migraine), a short course of steroids may be useful

Acquired immunodeficiency syndrome with *Pneumocystis carinii* pneumonia

- should be added to the initial treatment in patients with moderate to severe respiratory depression defined by an arterial oxygen partial pressure less than 75 mmHg while the patient is breathing room air

Ulcerative colitis

- if the disease is active (>6 bloody bowel movements per day) with systemic signs and symptoms (fever, weight loss)
- oral prednisone is effective but because of long-term adverse effects, it should be used (other than for acute episodes) only in patients with mild disease who fail to respond to other therapy

Crohn's disease

- severe Crohn's disease, regardless of the site of disease, should be treated with corticosteroids
- mild and moderate Crohn's disease is also often treated with prednisone when the disease involves the small intestine, and until other medications are shown to be effective in small intestinal disease, steroids are the drug of first choice

Gout

- initial drug of choice for an acute attack of gout in patients with a history of aspirin allergy and renal failure as these patients are at risk for nonsteroidal antiinflammatory drug (NSAID)–induced nephrotoxicity (Semin Arthritis Rheum 1990;19:329–336)

Other uses

- skin disorders
- organ transplant
- collagen disease

▶ *When Should I Not Use This Drug?*

Long-term for mild to moderate asthma, chronic obstructive pulmonary disease, or rheumatoid arthritis

- long-term use should be avoided in these patients if possible, owing to the severe adverse effect profile

Patients with severe asthma who are not receiving maximum doses of inhaled corticosteroids

- patients who require oral corticosteroids must be given inhaled corticosteroids, which should decrease the total amount of systemic corticosteroids required

▶ *What Contraindications Are There to the Use of This Drug?*

Intolerance of or allergic reaction to prednisone

Viral, fungal, or active or quiescent tuberculosis infections

- corticosteroids depress the body's immune system and its ability to fight infections and should not be used unless absolutely required

Vaccinations

- poor response due to lack of antibody production and possible neurological complications
- avoid live viral vaccines (e.g., varicella vaccine)

Osteoporosis, psychoses, diabetes mellitus, or glaucoma

- corticosteroids may potentiate these conditions; therefore, use in the lowest possible dosages

▶ *What Drug Interactions Are Clinically Important?*

Drugs that may increase the effect or toxicity of prednisone

ORAL CONTRACEPTIVES

- estrogens may inhibit the metabolism of prednisone, resulting in higher serum levels of prednisone
- monitor patients for an increase in the toxic effects of prednisone

AMPHOTERICIN B

- amphotericin B may potentiate potassium loss; monitor serum potassium levels twice weekly for patients receiving this combination

Drugs that may decrease the effect of prednisone

PHENYTOIN, BARBITURATES, RIFAMPIN

- enhance microsomal enzymes, which metabolize prednisone
- may reduce corticosteroid effect, necessitating higher dosages of prednisone
- titrate the dose to response as indicated below

Drugs that may have their effect or toxicity increased by prednisone

- none

Drugs that may have their effect decreased by prednisone

SALICYLATES

- corticosteroids enhance renal excretion of aspirin (acetylsalicylic acid)
- salicylate levels may decrease by 30% after 4 weeks of concomitant therapy
- monitor serum salicylate level after 1 month if a prolonged course of prednisone is anticipated and adjust the salicylate dosage accordingly

▶ *What Route and Dosage Should I Use?*

How to administer

- orally—take with food or milk
- parenterally—not available

Acute asthma, bronchitis

- 40 mg PO daily (Br Med J 1986;292:1045–1047)
- some clinicians suggest higher dosages (60 mg PO Q8H) for the first 1–2 days (Am Rev Respir Dis 1993;147:1306–1310)
- continue prednisone therapy for 1 week (3–4 days if the patient improves rapidly) and then taper the dosage over 1 week by reducing the dosage daily by 5 mg as tolerated

Chronic asthma

- patients should be maintained on high-dose inhaled corticosteroids to minimize the dose of systemic prednisone
- give 40 mg PO daily for 5 days then decrease by 5 mg every 2 days
- taper the dosage to the minimum required to maintain control of symptoms
- try to maintain a dosage of less than 10 mg/d to reduce long-term side effects

- give as a single morning dose to lessen hypothalamic-pituitary-adrenal (HPA) axis suppression (J Allergy Clin Immunol 1985; 76:312–320)
- after the patient is stabilized, attempt alternate-day dosing to minimize toxicity and HPA axis suppression
- note that alternate-day dosing may not be as effective in controlling asthma (N Engl J Med 1989;321:1517–1527)

Converting to alternate-day therapy

- if the patient is receiving divided daily doses, convert to a single daily morning dose
- increase the daily dosage by a particular increment (usually 5 mg/d) on 1 day, and decrease the daily dosage by the same increment on the next day until 0 mg/d is reached on the alternate day

Example: the patient is taking 15 mg of prednisone every morning

day 1	20 mg	day 5	30 mg
day 2	10 mg	day 6	0 mg
day 3	25 mg	day 7	30 mg
day 4	5 mg	day 8	0 mg

- after alternate-day dosing has been achieved, attempts should be undertaken to decrease the dosage to the minimum level that is consistent with disease control

Converting to inhaled corticosteroids

In patients not previously maintained on corticosteroid inhaler therapy

- initiate high-dose inhaled corticosteroid therapy and taper prednisone administration as tolerated over a minimum of 2 weeks, as maximum effect from inhaled steroids does not occur until 1–4 weeks
- high-dose inhaled coriticosteroids are preferable to oral prednisone and must be used together to minimize the dose of oral prednisone (J Allergy Clin Immunol 1990;85:1098–1111)

Prevention of adrenal insufficiency in patients currently or previously receiving corticosteroids

- 100 mg/d in 4 divided doses for 72 hours after major surgery and for 24 hours after minor surgery; resume at a dosage 10–15% above that taken just before the emergency (J Allergy Clin Immunol 1985; 76:312–320)

Rheumatoid arthritis

- 5 mg PO daily
- increase the dosage to 7.5 mg PO daily if 5 mg is not effective
- higher dosages are usually avoided owing to concerns about toxicity (N Engl J Med 1990;322:1277–1289)

Migraine

- 40 mg PO daily 4 days, then taper by 5 mg daily every 2 days

AIDS with *Pneumocystis carinii* pneumonia

- 40 mg PO BID for 1 week, followed by 40 mg PO daily for 1 week, and followed by 20 mg PO daily for 1 week

Ulcerative colitis, Crohn's disease

- 40 mg PO daily for 1–2 weeks, depending on the patient's response
- decrease the dosage to 30 mg PO daily for 1 week and then reduce the daily dosage by 5 mg every week

Gout

- 40 mg PO daily for 3–4 days and then taper by 5 mg/d

Dosage adjustments for renal or hepatic dysfunction

- hepatically metabolized
- no adjustments are required; just titrate the dose to effect and toxicity

▶ *What Should I Monitor with Regard to Efficacy and Toxicity?*

Efficacy

Acute asthma

For severe acute asthma, assess the patient after each dose of inhaled bronchodilator until improvement is seen

Heart rate, degree of respiratory distress, and presence of cyanosis
Pulmonary function tests

Peak expiratory flow rate

- should be measured before treatment if possible
- measured after treatment to assess the effect of treatment
- patients with an acute attack should be given a peak flow gauge and should record peak expiratory flow rate (PEFR) at least twice daily

Arterial blood gases

- if the patient has a PEFR less than 40% of predicted values or is not responding to treatment
- repeat within 24 hours if the blood carbon dioxide level is elevated or the patient is fatiguing

Chronic asthma

Frequency of as-needed beta$_2$-agonist use
Pulmonary function tests

- can be used to assess the effectiveness of long-term therapy; however, some patients taking bronchodilators (salbutamol, ipratropium bromide, theophylline) do not have a demonstrable effect on pulmonary function test results but become clinically improved (increased walking distance, decreased use of PRN medications, and so on)
- patients taking either oral or inhaled corticosteroids should have administration of medications continued only if a positive measurable response is seen after the institution of these agents

Peak expiratory flow rate

- peak flowmeter should be used by patients who experience severe attacks with little warning and patients who have symptoms of breathlessness or chest tightness repeatedly or require regular Q6H to Q8H beta$_2$-agonist therapy (J Allergy Clin Immunol 1990;85:1098–1111)
- establish best PEFR early in therapy
- usually measured on walking and before bed, and before and after beta$_2$-agonist administration (minimum of twice daily [e.g., AM and PM]) and is the best of 3 measurements on each occasion
- daily variation should be less than 20% and ideally less than 10%
- patients should be instructed to double the dosage of inhaled corticosteroids if PEFR is less than 75% of the best value, start a short course of oral steroids if PEFR is less than 50% of the best result, and call their physician if PEFR is less than 25% of the best value (Postgrad Med J 1991;67:1–3)

Rheumatoid arthritis

Joint tenderness count, sedimentation rate measurements, grip strength, duration of morning stiffness, time to onset of fatigue, and patient's report on specific symptoms

- patient's symptoms and x-rays should be assessed monthly for the first 2 months, and after the disease is under control, the patient can be assessed every 3 months for 6 months and then every 6 months
- these variables should be used to guide drug administration
- one study found that clinical and laboratory measures of physical well-being appeared to be unrelated to psychological and social measures of well-being (J Rheumatol 1991;18:650–653)
- it is important to include the patient's self-assessment of the drug's effect on the patient's ability to function and well-being

Migraine

- relief of pain should be seen in 8–12 hours

AIDS with *Pneumocystis carinii* pneumonia

- improvement in blood gas values

Ulcerative colitis

Signs and symptoms

- diarrhea, urgency, tenesmus, blood per rectum, abdominal pain, fever, and weight status should improve
- symptoms begin to improve with steroid (topical or oral) therapy within a week, but improvement with mesalamine (5-aminosalicylic acid [5-ASA]) therapy may take a few days longer

Crohn's disease

Signs and symptoms

- diarrhea, abdominal pain, fever, abdominal distention and tenderness, size of mass (if present), and appetite
- these symptoms may persist for 2–3 weeks before improvement is seen, and complete relief of symptoms may not occur

Gout

- reduction in pain and swelling typically occurs within 12–48 hours for agents used for acute treatment; however, if the attack is already established (e.g., 48 hours), response to treatment is slower

Toxicity

Short term (early onset)

Fluid and electrolyte disturbances

- sodium and fluid retention, hypokalemia, hypocalcemia may occur; may aggravate preexisting heart failure or hypertension; monitor electrolyte levels and blood pressure twice weekly during hospitalization and every 6 months during long-term therapy

Hyperglycemia

- may exacerbate diabetes or unmask latent diabetes
- monitor blood glucose levels twice weekly while the patient is hospitalized and then every 6 months
- patient should be made aware of the potential signs of diabetes (increased thirst, hunger, and urination)

Increased susceptibility to infection

- use the lowest dosage possible and administer the best available treatment for infection

Acute psychosis

- increased risk in patients with preexisting psychological disorder receiving dosages greater than 40 mg/d

Gastric upset (abdominal pain, gastritis)

- take with food or milk

Peptic ulcer disease

- corticosteroid-treated patients have a 1.8% incidence of peptic ulcers compared with 0.8% incidence in control subjects (N Engl J Med 1983;309:21–24); gastrointestinal prophylaxis has not been shown to be effective
- do not use prophylaxis unless the patient is receiving steroids with NSAIDs (Br Med J 1992;304:654–655)

Long term (late onset)

Cushing's syndrome

- buffalo hump, moon facies, striae, acne, hirsutism, obesity
- use the lowest dosage possible

Hypothalamic-pituitary-adrenal axis suppression

- with longer than 3 weeks of continuous therapy (Chest 1992; 101:418S–421S), steroid dosages should be tapered downward

Osteoporosis, osteonecrosis

- maintain adequate calcium in the diet (1 g of elemental calcium per day); this condition may also occur with multiple bursts of systemic corticosteroids (DICP 1991;25:72–79)

Subcapsular cataracts

- greater incidence if the patient maintained on greater than 15 mg PO daily of prednisone equivalents for longer than 1 year
- annual ophthalmological examination is recommended

Muscle wasting, cramping

- associated with high-dose corticosteroids

▶ *How Long Do I Treat Patients with This Drug?*

Acute asthma, bronchitis

- continue prednisone administration until significant improvement is seen (usually 3–4 days) and then taper the dosage over 1 week

Chronic asthma, emphysema, bronchitis

- always consider alternative therapy
- attempt to taper the dosage to the minimum effective level every 3 months in well-controlled patients

Prevention of adrenal insufficiency

- 72 hours after major surgery and 24 hours after minor surgery

Rheumatoid arthritis

- always consider alternative therapy
- attempt to taper the dosage to the minimum effective level every 3 months in well-controlled patients
- taper off prednisone when other therapy such as the disease-modifying agents can be used to get the disease under control

Migraine

- use daily for 4 days, then taper by 5 mg daily every 2 days

AIDS with *Pneumocystis carinii* pneumonia

- 2 weeks

Ulcerative colitis

- for lesser forms of colitis, prednisone may be used in dosages of 20 mg or higher for 6 months, and if there is no effect and if 5-ASA preparations have not worked, a 5 day course of intravenous hydrocortisone in the hospital should be considered

Crohn's disease

- prednisone for acute disease is used for about 2 weeks and then tapered over about 6 weeks

Gout

- give full dose for 3–4 days and then taper by 5 mg daily over the next 8 days

▶ *How Do I Decrease or Stop the Administration of This Drug?*

Dosage tapering is always required

- key is to go slow and watch for exacerbation of disease and symptoms of withdrawal (anorexia, nausea or vomiting, lethargy, headache, dizziness, arthralgia, eosinophilia, hypotension, hyperthermia, hypoglycemia, hyponatremia, and hyperkalemia)

Short-term therapy (less than 1 month)

- taper by 5 mg increments every 1–2 days (as tolerated) until therapy discontinued or the lowest effective dosage reached
- in patients that worsen as the dose is decreased below 10 mg/day, taper dose in 2.5 mg increments every 2 days

Long-term therapy

- taper by 5 mg/wk until 10 mg/d is reached
- subsequent dosages should be decreased by 2.5 mg/wk until therapy is discontinued or the lowest effective dosage is reached
- any reduction in dosage may result in exacerbation of disease (West J Med 1980;133:383–391)
- if withdrawal symptoms occur, increase the dosage again and taper more gradually (1 mg/wk)

▶ *What Should I Tell My Patients About This Drug?*

- do not stop taking this drug abruptly
- always make sure that you have an adequate supply on hand
- take single daily doses with your morning meal and take multiple daily doses with food or milk to avoid stomach upset
- if you forget a dose, take it as soon as you remember on the *same* day; otherwise go back to your normal daily dosage
- for alternate-day dosing, take the dose as soon as you remember on the *same* day, then resume your normal dosage schedule; if you do not remember until the next day, take the dose that morning, skip the next day's dose, and then resume your normal dosage schedule
- inform all health care professionals (e.g., dentist) that you are taking prednisone

- call your physician if you have bone or joint pain, black tarry stools, visual disturbances, or any other unusual symptoms that do not go away

▶ *Therapeutic Tips*

- for chronic asthma, never use oral corticosteroids without inhaled corticosteroids
- there is no therapeutic gain to adding 5-ASA compounds to prednisone during short-term therapy of ulcerative colitis
- it is always best to taper the administration of corticosteroids, even if they are used for only a short period, to decrease the risk of exacerbation of the disease state

Useful References

Kelly HW, Murphy S. Corticosteroids for acute, severe asthma. DICP 1991; 25:72–79
Siegel SC. Overview of corticosteroid therapy. J Allergy Clin Immunol 1985; 76:312–320
Garber EK, Fan PT, Bluestone R. Realistic guidelines of corticosteroid therapy in rheumatic disease. Semin Arthritis Rheum 1981;11:231–255

PRIMIDONE

William Parker

USA (Mysoline)
CANADA (Apo-Primidone, Mysoline, PMS Primidone)

▶ *When Should I Use This Drug?*

Generalized seizures (no primary focus)

Tonic-clonic seizures

- use only if valproic acid, phenytoin, carbamazepine, and phenobarbital are ineffective

Partial seizures (with or without secondarily generalized tonic-clonic seizures)

- use only if valproic acid, phenytoin, carbamazepine, and phenobarbital are ineffective
- primidone is used mainly as an adjunct to other anticonvulsants, offering little clinical benefit over more conventional agents

▶ *When Should I Not Use This Drug?*

see Phenobarbital

▶ *What Contraindications Are There to the Use of This Drug?*

see Phenobarbital

▶ *What Drug Interactions Are Clinically Important?*

see Phenobarbital

▶ *What Route and Dosage Should I Use?*

How to administer

- orally—on an empty stomach
- parenterally—not available

Generalized seizures (no primary focus), partial seizures (with or without secondarily generalized tonic-clonic seizures)

- initial adult dosage is 125 mg nightly for 3 days, increasing by 125 mg/d increments every 3 days until seizure control is achieved or side effects become intolerable; the usual maintenance dosage is 250 mg PO TID
- because of the short half-lives of primidone and its active metabolite phenylethylmalonamide (PEMA), primidone should be given in divided doses

Dosage adjustments for renal or hepatic dysfunction

- hepatically metabolized with variable amounts going to active metabolites phenobarbital (5–25%) and PEMA (30–70%), depending on the duration of therapy and concomitant anticonvulsant therapy; downward dosage adjustment may have to be made if significant hepatic impairment is present
- up to 50% of primidone and 80% of PEMA are excreted unchanged in the urine; dosage reduction may be necessary if the serum creatinine level rises more than 50% over baseline values

- if the dose is titrated upward on the basis of efficacy and adverse effects, no specific dosage adjustments are needed

▶ *What Should I Monitor with Regard to Efficacy and Toxicity?*

Efficacy

Generalized seizures (no primary focus), partial seizures (with or without secondarily generalized tonic-clonic seizures)

Seizure frequency

- reduction in frequency and severity of seizures

Serum concentrations

- accepted therapeutic range is 15–40 μg/mL (65–170 μmol/L) of phenobarbital and 6–12 μg/mL (27–55 μmol/L) of primidone (PEMA concentrations are not routinely monitored); occasionally, patients respond to lower or higher concentrations
- primidone steady state is reached 4–7 days after the maintenance dosage is attained; phenobarbital steady state concentration is not reached for 14–21 days because of its much longer half-life (3–5 days versus 10–12 hours)
- because of low protein binding (~25% primidone, ~50% phenobarbital), free drug concentrations are not necessary
- trough levels are preferred unless patients report side effects (then measure the concentration at the time of the adverse effect)

Toxicity

see Phenobarbital

▶ *How Long Do I Treat Patients with This Drug?*

see Phenobarbital

▶ *How Do I Decrease or Stop the Administration of This Drug?*

- primidone therapy can usually be safely withdrawn from patients with intractable epilepsy who are maintained on appropriate nonbarbiturate anticonvulsants
- sudden withdrawal is to be avoided, especially during long-term, high-dose therapy
- withdrawal is best done over several months
- decrease the dosage by 250 mg daily each month until withdrawal is complete
- seizure relapse is most common during withdrawal or the first 3 months after withdrawal
- if seizures recur, reinstitute treatment with the same drugs used previously
- simultaneous substitution of another anticonvulsant may be necessary during phenobarbital therapy withdrawal; administration of the new agent should be gradually increased as primidone is gradually withdrawn to maintain adequate seizure control
- if multiple-anticonvulsant therapy is present, drugs should be withdrawn 1 at a time

▶ *What Should I Tell My Patients About This Drug?*

see Phenobarbital

▶ *Therapeutic Tips*

- it is rare that a patient taking primidone needs supplemental doses of phenobarbital, a practice that should be avoided because it often leads to increased adverse central nervous system effects

Useful References

Pugh CB, Garnett WR. Current issues in the treatment of epilepsy. Clin Pharm 1991;10:335–358
Parker WA. Epilepsy. In: Herfindal ET, Gourley DR, Hart LL, eds. Clinical Pharmacy and Therapeutics, 4th ed. Baltimore: Williams & Wilkins, 1988:570–592

PROBENECID

C. Wayne Weart

USA (Benemid, Probalan, generics)
CANADA (Benemid, Benuryl)

▶ *When Should I Use This Drug?*

Prophylaxis of acute gouty arthritis

- patients who excrete less than 600 mg/24 h of uric acid, have good renal function (glomerular filtration rate > 50 mL/min) and no history of nephrolithiasis, and are deemed candidates for uric acid–lowering therapy can be treated with either probenecid or allopurinol
- probenecid and allopurinol are the preferred agents and are considered equally effective in these patients, and the choice largely depends on the patient's preference (cost and frequency of administration factors) and adverse effects

Adjuvant therapy with antibiotics

- to elevate and prolong plasma concentrations of selected antibiotics when they are given either orally or parenterally
- used for penicillin, ampicillin, amoxicillin, and some cephalosporins (Clin Pharmacokinet 1993;24:289–300, J Antimicrob Chemother 1993; 31:1009–1011)

▶ *When Should I Not Use This Drug?*

Acute gout attack

- has no analgesic or antiinflammatory activity and may exacerbate and prolong the acute attack

Prophylactic therapy in patients with renal insufficiency

- in patients with renal insufficiency (i.e., creatinine clearance < 50 mL/min) or a history of renal stones (uric acid– or calcium-containing stones), probenecid increases urinary concentrations of uric acid and may cause stone formation

Probenecid should not be used with antibiotics in patients with renal impairment

- these patients tend to have elevated concentrations of antimicrobials without probenecid

▶ *What Contraindications Are There to the Use of This Drug?*

Intolerance of or allergic reaction to probenecid

History of uric acid kidney stones

- probenecid may increase the risk of urate or calcium renal stones if the baseline 24 hour urine uric acid measurement is elevated

▶ *What Drug Interactions Are Clinically Important?*

Drugs that may increase the effect or toxicity of probenecid

- none

Drugs that may decrease the effect of probenecid

SALICYLATES

- high doses of salicylates (serum levels > 50 μg/mL) may inhibit the uricosuric effect of probenecid
- avoid taking aspirin or other salicylates

Drugs that may have their effect or toxicity increased by probenecid

ACYCLOVIR, ALLOPURINOL, BARBITURATES, BENZODIAZEPINES, CLOFIBRATE, DAPSONE, DYPHYLLINE, METHOTREXATE, NONSTEROIDAL ANTIINFLAMMATORY DRUGS, PENICILLAMINE, SULFONYLUREAS, ZIDOVUDINE, RIFAMPIN, PENICILLINS, NALIDIXIC ACID, CEPHALOSPORINS

- inhibits renal tubular secretion of these drugs
- do not use together unless increased concentrations are desired

Drugs that may have their effect decreased by probenecid

- none

▶ *What Route and Dosage Should I Use?*

How to administer

- orally—with food or milk to reduce stomach upset
- parenterally—not available

Prophylaxis of acute gouty arthritis

- give 250 mg PO BID and increase the dosage weekly by 250 mg daily until the serum uric acid concentration is less than 6 mg/dL or the total daily dose reaches 3 g
- slow dose titration is recommended to prevent or minimize the risk of mobilization gout and to avoid sudden excretion of large amounts of uric acid through the kidney

Penicillin or cephalosporin therapy

- 500 mg PO QID

Dosage adjustments for renal or hepatic dysfunction

- renally eliminated

Normal Dosing Interval	$C_{cr} > 60$ mL/min or 1 mL/s	C_{cr} 30–60 mL/min or 0.5–1 mL/s	$C_{cr} < 30$ mL/min or 0.5 mL/s
Q12H	no adjustment needed	avoid, as it may not be effective	avoid
Q6H	no adjustment	avoid	avoid

▶ *What Should I Monitor with Regard to Efficacy and Toxicity?*

Efficacy

Prophylaxis of acute gouty arthritis

Serum uric acid level

- measure at baseline and repeat weekly until appropriate dosage has been determined to reduce the serum uric acid level below 6 mg/dL
- after uric acid stabilizes on a given dose of probenecid measure every 6–12 months

24 hour urine uric acid determination

- before starting therapy to determine whether probenecid therapy is needed

Number of attacks

- number of acute gouty attacks should decrease

Toxicity

Renal function

- serum creatinine levels at baseline and then yearly

Uric acid stones

- liberal fluid intake is recommended to minimize the risk of uric acid stone formation until serum uric acid levels are maintained in the normal range and tophaceous deposits disappear

Headache, anorexia, nausea and vomiting

- decrease the dosage if these occur
- if they continue, stop the drug administration and switch to an alternative agent

Fever, dermatitis, anaphylaxis, pruritus, anemia, hemolytic anemia

- discontinue the drug administration if these occur

Nephrotic syndrome, hepatic necrosis, uric acid stones, or renal colic

- if hematuria or costovertebral angle tenderness occurs, suspect renal stones

▶ *How Long Do I Treat Patients with This Drug?*

Prophylaxis of acute gouty arthritis

- uric acid–lowering therapy is usually continued indefinitely, but consideration should be given to reduced dosage of probenecid in older patients, patients with reduced renal function, or obese patients who have successfully attained ideal body weight
- generally not able to withdraw uric acid–lowering therapy but may be able to reduce the dosage as long as the serum uric acid level is maintained below 6 mg/dL

Penicillin or cephalosporin therapy

- for the duration of antimicrobial therapy

▶ *How Do I Decrease or Stop the Administration of This Drug?*

- may be stopped abruptly
- reduce the daily dosage by 500 mg increments every 4 months when titrating the dose downward

▶ *What Should I Tell My Patients About This Drug?*

- drink at least 6–8 full (8 ounce) glasses of water each day to reduce the risk of kidney stones
- may take each dose with food to reduce gastrointestinal upset
- avoid taking large doses of aspirin, which may antagonize the effects of probenecid (if an analgesic or antipyretic is needed, use acetaminophen)

▶ *Therapeutic Tips*

- start with low dosages and gradually increase the dosage until serum uric acid levels are maintained at less than 6 mg/dL
- low-dose colchicine should be given concurrently for the first 3 months to reduce the risk of mobilization gout
- fixed combination products of probenecid and colchicine do not allow individual titration of the agents, so do not use them

Useful References

Simkin PA. Management of gout. Ann Intern Med 1979;90:812–816
Wallace SL, Singer JZ. Treatment. In: Primer on Rheumatic Diseases. 9th ed. Atlanta: Arthritis Foundation, 1988:202–206
Wallace SL, Singer JZ. Therapy in gout. Rheum Dis Clin North Am 1988; 14:441–457
Wisner DE, Simkin PA. Management of gout and hyperuricemia. Prim Care, 1984;11:283–294

PROBUCOL

Stephen Shalansky and Robert Dombrowski

USA (Lorelco)
CANADA (Lorelco)

▶ *When Should I Use This Drug?*

Hypercholesterolemia

- used by lipid specialists to accelerate regression of xanthomas in patients with familial hypercholesterolemia

▶ *When Should I Not Use This Drug?*

First-line agent for hypercholesterolemia

- do not use as a first-line agent, as there are no studies evaluating its effect on cardiovascular morbidity or mortality
- probucol decreases high density lipoprotein (HDL) cholesterol by 15–25% (Ann Intern Med 1982;96:475–482)
- HDL is inversely related to the incidence of coronary heart disease (CHD) (Am J Med 1977;62:707–714)
- there are no long-term studies assessing probucol's effect on CHD risk

Hypertriglyceridemia

- probucol has little effect on triglycerides

▶ *What Contraindications Are There to the Use of This Drug?*

- intolerance of or allergic reaction to probucol

▶ *What Drug Interactions Are Clinically Important?*

- none

▶ *What Route and Dosage Should I Use?*

How to administer

- orally—give with meals to enhance bioavailability
- parenterally—not available

Hypercholesterolemia

- 500 mg PO BID

- if after 3 months of therapy the drug is tolerated and there has been at least a 15% decrease in lipid levels but not to the desired level, continue the drug administration and add second-line agent
- if adding another drug, monitor as if initiating therapy
- if the drug is not tolerated or there is less than a 15% decrease in the total cholesterol level, stop probucol therapy and start a different drug

Dosage adjustments for renal or hepatic dysfunction

- metabolic fate unknown
- no dosage adjustment necessary in renal failure
- no information in hepatic failure

▶ *What Should I Monitor with Regard to Efficacy and Toxicity?*

Efficacy

Hypercholesterolemia

Total cholesterol and fractionated lipid profile

- in patients with no coronary heart disease or atherosclerotic disease and with less than 2 CHD risk factors, lower total cholesterol below 240 mg/dL (6.2 mmol/L) and LDL cholesterol below 160 mg/dL (4.1 mmol/L)
- in patients with no coronary heart disease or atherosclerotic disease and with 2 or more CHD risk factors, lower total cholesterol below 200 mg/dL (5.2 mmol/L) and LDL cholesterol below 130 mg/dL (3.4 mmol/L)
- for patients with coronary heart disease or atherosclerotic disease, lower LDL cholesterol to below 100 mg/dL (2.6 mmol/L)
- complete lipid profiles should be measured at 1 and 3 months
- if goals are acheived, then check annually

Evidence of coronary heart disease

- myocardial infarction, angina, and coronary bypass grafting

Risk factors

- reduce risk factors such as obesity and smoking
- control risk factors such as diabetes and hypertension

Xanthomas

- look for regression of xanthomas

Toxicity

Gastrointestinal symptoms

- include diarrhea, flatulence, abdominal pain, and nausea and vomiting
- diarrhea is the most commonly reported side effect (10–26%)
- tolerance of these side effects may develop

Cardiovascular effects

- a number of studies have reported a prolonged QT interval in patients given probucol, but this has not been associated with an increased incidence of arrhythmias or sudden death (Drugs 1989;37:761–800)
- electrocardiogram should be performed within the first month of therapy and yearly thereafter

▶ *How Long Do I Treat Patients with This Drug?*

Hypercholesterolemia

- therapy is long term and may continue for life
- if xanthomas have resolved and the patient has achieved and maintained target lipid levels for 2 years, administration pf this drug should be discontinued and a trial of dietary therapy alone should be attempted
- recheck lipid levels at 4–6 weeks and at 3 months after the drug administration has been discontinued, and restart drug therapy if target levels are not maintained

▶ *How Do I Decrease or Stop the Administration of This Drug?*

- may be stopped abruptly

▶ *What Should I Tell My Patients About This Drug?*

- take this medication with meals

- patients may experience some gastrointestinal side effects (nausea, constipation, diarrhea, and abdominal pain), and in most patients, tolerance of these side effects develops within the first few months

Useful References

Expert Panel on Detection, Evaluation, and Treatment of High Blood Cholesterol in Adults. Summary of the second report of the National Cholesterol Education Program (NCEP) expert panel on detection, evaluation, and treatment of high blood cholesterol in adults. JAMA 1993;269: 3015–3023

Knodel LC, Talbert RL. Adverse effects of hypolipidemic drugs. Med Toxicol 1987;2:10–32

Illingworth DR. Lipid-lowering drugs: An overview of indications and optimum therapeutic use. Drugs 1987;33:259–279

Buckley MM-T, Goa KL, Price AH, et al. Probucol: A reappraisal of its pharmacological properties and therapeutic use in hypercholesterolemia. Drugs 1989;37:761–800

Zimetbaum P, Eder H, Frishman W. Probucol: Pharmacology and clinical application. J Clin Pharmacol 1990;30:3–9

Howard PA. Probucol in hypercholesterolemia. DICP 1989;23:880–881

PROCAINAMIDE

James Tisdale

USA (procainamide hydrochloride, Promine, Pronestyl, Pronestyl-SR, Procan SR, Rhythmin)
CANADA (Procan SR, Pronestyl, Pronestyl-SR)

▶ When Should I Use This Drug?

Atrial fibrillation or flutter

- procainamide may be administered intravenously for conversion of atrial fibrillation to sinus rhythm in patients in whom rapid cardioversion is desired, but in whom electrical cardioversion is not desired (Br Heart J 1980;44:589–595) because quinidine should not be given intravenously, as it is not well tolerated (causes hypotension)
- procainamide therapy should not be administered until control of ventricular response has been achieved with agents that inhibit the conduction of impulses through the atrioventricular (AV) node
- oral procainamide therapy may be used for pharmacological conversion of atrial fibrillation to sinus rhythm in patients with a past history of myocardial infarction (MI) or moderate left ventricular dysfunction in whom quinidine therapy is not successful or well tolerated or is contraindicated
- procainamide may be used for the prevention of episodes of paroxysmal atrial fibrillation or flutter in patients with a past history of MI or moderate left ventricular dysfunction in whom quinidine therapy is not successful or well tolerated or is contraindicated
- intravenous procainamide should be used for control of ventricular rate and conversion to sinus rhythm in patients with atrial fibrillation or flutter who are known to have a ventricular preexcitation syndrome such as Wolff-Parkinson-White syndrome because procainamide also blocks conduction in the accessory pathway and, unlike digoxin or verapamil, does not increase ventricular rate in this situation (Cardiol Clin 1990;8:503–521)

Atrioventricular nodal reentrant tachycardia

- procainamide therapy should be used for the long-term prevention of recurrent episodes of paroxysmal supraventricular tachycardia (PSVT) due to AV nodal reentry in patients with a history of MI or left ventricular dysfunction in whom empirical therapy with digoxin, alone or in combination with propranolol, or quinidine therapy has been unsuccessful, poorly tolerated, or contraindicated

Wolff-Parkinson-White syndrome

- procainamide should be used for the prevention of atrial fibrillation or flutter and/or PSVT due to AV reentry in patients with Wolff-Parkinson-White syndrome in whom flecainide, disopyramide, and quinidine have been proved ineffective and in whom procainamide has been shown to be effective during electrophysiolgical (EP) testing

Ventricular premature depolarizations

- procainamide may be used for the empirical management of symptomatic, benign ventricular premature depolarizations in patients in whom therapy with beta-adrenergic receptor blocking agents or quinidine has been unsuccessful or poorly tolerated; however, in this situation, consultation of a cardiac electrophysiologist for assessment and selection of therapy is appropriate

Ventricular tachycardia

- procainamide should be administered intravenously for the short-term management of symptomatic nonsustained or sustained ventricular tachycardia in patients in whom lidocaine therapy has been unsuccessful or is poorly tolerated (Circulation 1963;28:486–491)
- intravenous procainamide should be administered immediately after the induction of a symptomatic or sustained ventricular tachycardia during a baseline EP study, and the EP study should be repeated immediately after the administration of procainamide (Circulation 1983;67:30–37)
- oral procainamide therapy should be administered for the long-term prevention of ventricular tachycardia in patients in whom intravenous procainamide therapy suppressed inducible ventricular tachycardia during EP testing and in whom quinidine therapy is contraindicated or poorly tolerated (Circulation 1983;67: 30–37, Circulation 1973;47:1204–1210)
- oral procainamide should be administered for the long-term prevention of ventricular tachycardia in patients in whom the drug suppressed ventricular tachycardia during Holter monitoring if an EP study is not performed

▶ When Should I Not Use This Drug?

Atrial fibrillation or flutter

- procainamide should not be administered to patients who have atrial fibrillation or flutter of longer than 1 year in duration, as successful conversion to sinus rhythm is highly unlikely (Ann Intern Med 1966;65:216–224)
- procainamide should not be administered to patients with an enlarged left atrium (>45 mm as determined by echocardiography), as successful conversion to sinus rhythm is highly unlikely (Circulation 1976;53:273–279)

Asymptomatic ventricular arrhythmias

- no evidence that treatment is beneficial

Ventricular tachycardia

- oral procainamide therapy should not be administered during serial drug testing in the EP laboratory in patients in whom intravenous procainamide therapy failed to suppress inducible ventricular tachycardia (J Am Coll Cardiol 1984;4:1247–1254, Am J Cardiol 1985;56:883–886)

▶ What Contraindications Are There to the Use of This Drug?

Intolerance of or allergic reaction to procainamide

- procainamide should not be administered to patients who have previously demonstrated hypersensitivity to the drug or to procaine or chemically related local anesthetic agents (Clin Ther 1985;7:618–640)

Atrioventricular nodal block

- procainamide is contraindicated in patients with second- or third-degree AV block in whom a functioning ventricular pacemaker is not present (Clin Ther 1985;7:618–640)

Myasthenia gravis

- procainamide may interfere with neuromuscular conduction and has been reported to exacerbate symptoms of myasthenia gravis (Mt Sinai J Med 1976;43:10–14)

Long QT syndrome

- procainamide therapy may result in prolongation of QT intervals on surface electrocardiogram (ECG) and should be avoided in patients with congenital long QT syndrome

Previous procainamide-induced systemic lupus erythematosus–like syndrome

- procainamide is contraindicated in patients who have previously experienced systemic lupus erythematosus–like syndrome associated with procainamide therapy

Previous torsades de pointes associated with class IA antiarrhythmic agents

- procainamide should not be used in patients who have previously experienced torsades de pointes in association with class IA antiarrhythmic drug use

▶ *What Drug Interactions Are Clinically Important?*

Drugs that may increase the effect or toxicity of procainamide

CIMETIDINE

- cimetidine reduces the renal tubular secretion of procainamide and its active metabolite, *N*-acetylprocainamide (NAPA) by approximately 40 and 25%, respectively, resulting in increased serum procainamide and NAPA concentrations (Eur J Clin Pharmacol 1983;25:339–345)
- ranitidine reduces the renal tubular secretion of procainamide and NAPA, resulting in increased serum procainamide and NAPA concentrations (Br J Clin Pharmacol 1984;18:175–181); however, the magnitude of this interaction appears to be smaller than that demonstrated in association with cimetidine

TRIMETHOPRIM

- trimethoprim reduces the renal tubular secretion of procainamide and NAPA by approximately 47% and 13%, respectively, resulting in increased serum procainamide and NAPA concentrations (Clin Pharmacol Ther 1988;44:467–477)

AMIODARONE

- amiodarone reduces the renal clearance of procainamide and NAPA (Clin Pharmacol Ther 1987;41:603–610) and increases serum procainamide and NAPA concentrations by approximately 57% and 32%, respectively (Am J Cardiol 1984;53: 1264–1267)
- if amiodarone therapy is initiated in patients receiving procainamide, the procainamide dosage should be reduced by ⅓ and the patient should be closely monitored for signs and symptoms of procainamide toxicity
- if a target serum concentration has been determined in the past, measure a serum concentration within 2–3 days and ensure that the drug concentration remains above this target level (see Quinidine)

Drugs that may decrease the effect or toxicity of procainamide

- none

Drugs that may have their effect increased by procainamide

CLASS IA OR III ANTIARRHYTHMICS, PHENOTHIAZINES, ANTIPSYCHOTICS, ERYTHROMYCIN

- avoid combination if possible
- if not, monitor QT interval and if it increases > 25%, stop the interacting drug

Drugs that may have their effect decreased by procainamide

- none

▶ *What Route and Dosage Should I Use?*

How to administer

Orally

- can administer with or without food

Parenterally

- by direct bolus (<20 mg/min) or continuous infusion in normal saline or dextrose solutions
- although the American Heart Association recommends an infusion rate of 20 mg/min to avoid procainamide-induced hypotension, in situations in which more rapid procainamide administra-

tion may be desired (in the EP laboratory, for example), procainamide has been safely infused at a rate of 50 mg/min (J Am Coll Cardiol 1991;17:1581–1586)

Atrial fibrillation or flutter, atrioventricular nodal reentrant tachycardia, Wolff-Parkinson-White syndrome, ventricular premature depolarizations, ventricular tachycardia

Intravenous administration

- 17 mg/kg IV (12 mg/kg in patients with renal failure) administered at a rate of 20 mg/min (Eur J Clin Pharmacol 1978;13:303–308)
- maintenance infusion of 2.8 mg/kg/h (1.9 mg/kg/h in patients with moderate CHF; 1 mg/kg/h in patients with renal failure) should follow the loading dose

Oral administration

- after a patient has been stabilized on intravenous procainamide (conversion to sinus rhythm), the total daily dosage of oral procainamide should approximate the total daily intravenous dosage, divided Q4H if a conventional-release preparation is used or Q6H if a sustained-release preparation is used (most clinicians use the sustained-release preparation)
- when oral procainamide therapy is desired in a patient not receiving intravenous procainamide therapy, an initial daily dosage of 50 mg/kg PO divided Q4H (conventional-release preparations) or Q6H (sustained-release preparations) is recommended (most clinicians use the sustained-release preparation, as there is likely no clinical difference and it allows a more convenient dosing schedule) (JAMA 1971;215:1454–1460)

Dosage adjustments for renal or hepatic dysfunction

- 40–60% renally eliminated with an active metabolite (NAPA), which is 85% renally eliminated

Normal Dosing Interval	C_{cr} > 60 mL/min or 1 mL/s	C_{cr} 30–60 mL/min or 0.5–1 mL/s	C_{cr} < 30 mL/min or 0.5 mL/s
Q4H (conventional release)	no adjustment needed	Q6H	Q8H
Q6H (sustained release)	no adjustment needed	Q8H	Q12H

▶ *What Should I Monitor with Regard to Efficacy and Toxicity?*

Efficacy

Serum concentrations

- therapeutic range of procainamide is usually quoted as 4–10 μg/mL
- although NAPA concentrations are routinely monitored, a therapeutic range has not been established
- range of serum procainamide concentrations required for efficacy varies widely among patients, and therefore, the therapeutic range is of relatively little use in monitoring the efficacy of procainamide
- if therapeutic monitoring is performed, use the method of monitoring target serum procainamide and NAPA concentrations (see Quinidine) (Clin Pharmacokinet 1991;20:151–166)

Toxicity

Adverse effects necessitating discontinuation of therapy occur in approximately 41–61% of patients

Cardiovascular effects

- monitor for AV block or bradycardia with a repeated electrocardiogram after the initiation of therapy
- evaluate prolonged PR interval (>0.2 second), prolonged duration of QRS complex and QT intervals (>25% compared to with baseline levels), and initiation of new arrhythmia or worsening of clinical arrhythmia

Hypotension

- can occur with a rapid intravenous infusion; infuse at a rate no greater than 20 mg/min

Hematological effects

- neutropenia has been reported in approximately 0.5% of patients (Circulation 1984;70[suppl II]:446)
- monitor complete blood counts weekly during the first 3 months of therapy, and every 3–6 months thereafter

Systemic lupus erythematosus–like symptoms

- monitor for signs and symptoms of systemic lupus erythematosus–like syndrome (arthralgias, fever, rash, pleuritis, and pericarditis), which may occur in 20–50% of patients receiving long-term oral procainamide therapy
- if these symptoms occur, obtain an antinuclear antibody test, and if the result is positive, procainamide administration should be discontinued

▶ *How Long Do I Treat Patients with This Drug?*

see Quinidine

▶ *How Do I Decrease or Stop the Administration of This Drug?*

- procainamide administration may be stopped abruptly
- dosage reduction should not be done without consulting a cardiologist or a clinical electrophysiologist
- decrease the dosage if clinical presentation of toxicities occurs or if QRS or QT interval increases by greater than 25% of baseline value

▶ *What Should I Tell My Patients About This Drug?*

- if you experience nausea, vomiting, anorexia, fever, sore throat, joint pain, rash, palpitations, shortness of breath, chest pain, or dizziness, contact your physician
- do not discontinue procainamide therapy without consulting your physician

Useful References

Anderson JL. Conventional and sustained-release procainamide: Update on pharmacology and clinical uses. Clin Ther 1985;7:618–640

Lima JJ, Conti DR, Goldfarb AL, et al. Pharmacokinetic approach to intravenous procainamide therapy. Eur J Clin Pharmacol 1978;13:303–308

Waxman HL, Buxton AE, Sadowski LM, Josephson ME. The response to procainamide during electrophysiologic study for sustained ventricular tachyarrhythmias predicts the response to other medications. Circulation 1983;67:30–37

Fenster PE, Comes KA, Marsh R, et al. Conversion of atrial fibrillation to sinus rhythm by acute intravenous procainamide infusion. Am Heart J 1983;106:501–504

Woosley RL, Drayer DE, Reidenberg MM, et al. Effect of acetylator phenotype on the rate at which procainamide induces antinuclear antibodies and the lupus syndrome. N Engl J Med 1978;298:1157–1159

PROCATEROL

Karen Shalansky and Cindy Reesor Nimmo

USA (not available)
CANADA (Pro-Air)

▶ *When Should I Use This Drug?*

Consider an alternative agent

- is a long-acting beta$_2$-agonist, which provides no apparent clinical advantage over other available agents, unless it is being used on a regular basis (beta-agonists should primarily be used for symptomatic relief)
- this agent could be considered in a patient who continues to have nighttime symptoms despite optimal use of inhaled corticosteroids and a dose of salbutamol/albuterol at bedtime

PROCHLORPERAZINE

Lynne Nakashima

USA (Compazine)
CANADA (Stemetil)

▶ *When Should I Use This Drug?*

Chemotherapy-induced nausea and vomiting

- for drugs with moderate or low emetogenic potential

- when given intravenously, prochlorperazine is a reasonably effective agent, which is likely as effective as metoclopramide and probably causes less frequent extrapyramidal effects
- is less expensive than metoclopramide
- efficacy as a single agent for chemotherapy-induced nausea and vomiting ranges from 10–15% (Am J Med Sci 1987;293:34–44)

General nausea and vomiting, postoperative nausea and vomiting

- prochlorperazine shows some efficacy in the prevention of nausea and vomiting due to a variety of causes such as anesthetics, opioids, radiation, cancer, and drug toxicity (Drugs 1983;25 [suppl 1]:35–51)
- prochlorperazine, perphenazine, and thiethylperazine are likely equally effective and the decision among them should be based on cost and availability
- these agents likely cause less sedation than does dimenhydrinate
- prochlorperazine is extremely useful because it is available in different dosage forms (oral, intravenous, intramuscular, and rectal); if 1 route of administration is unacceptable, there are options for other routes

▶ *When Should I Not Use This Drug?*

Motion sickness

- prochlorperazine and related compounds are not effective in preventing motion sickness (Drugs 1992;43:295–315)

▶ *What Contraindications Are There to the Use of This Drug?*

Intolerance of or allergic reaction to phenothiazines

Central nervous system depression or comatose states

- may exacerbate central nervous system (CNS) depression and delay recovery

Blood dyscrasias

- may increase the risk of agranulocytosis; however, this agent is still used in patients with chemotherapy- or radiation-induced emesis

Pheochromocytoma

- may precipitate a hypertensive crisis

Suspected or established subcortical brain damage

- may precipitate a hyperthermic reaction

Seizures

- may lower the seizure threshold and precipitate seizures

Angle closure glaucoma

- may cause an increase in intraocular pressure, leading to an acute attack of glaucoma

Bladder neck or urethral obstruction

- may precipitate or aggravate urinary retention

Pyloroduodenal obstruction

- may decrease motility and tone, leading to obstruction and gastric retention

▶ *What Drug Interactions Are Clinically Important?*

Drugs that may increase the effect or toxicity of prochlorperazine

CENTRAL NERVOUS SYSTEM DEPRESSANTS

- additive, sedative effects are expected when other CNS depressants (e.g., narcotic analgesics, hypnotics, and alcohol) are used
- avoid the combination if possible or minimize these effects by starting with low dosages

Drugs that may decrease the effect of prochlorperazine

- none

Drugs that may have their effect or toxicity increased by prochlorperazine

- none

Drugs that may have their effect decreased by prochlorperazine

- none

▶ *What Route and Dosage Should I Use?*

How to administer

Orally

- take with food or milk or on an empty stomach

Parenterally

- may be administered via an intravenous or intramuscular route
- for intravenous use, dilute to 1 mg/mL and administer at a rate not exceeding 1 mg/min

Chemotherapy-induced nausea and vomiting

- 10 mg PO 30 minutes prior to chemotherapy (give intravenously at the same dosage if the patient is already vomiting)
- follow with 10 mg PO Q6H for 24 hours and then 10 mg PO PRN for 3–4 days

General nausea and vomiting, postoperative nausea and vomiting

- 10 mg IV or IM every 3 hours when needed
- 10 mg PO every 3 hours may be used if the patient can tolerate sips of fluid
- can also be used rectally 25 mg Q6H (only 10 mg suppository is available in Canada)

Dosage adjustments for renal or hepatic dysfunction

- hepatically metabolized
- no dosage adjustment required; titrate the dose to effect

▶ *What Should I Monitor with Regard to Efficacy and Toxicity?*

Efficacy

Nausea and vomiting

Frequency of assessment depends on the severity and frequency of nausea and vomiting

Number and severity of vomiting episodes

- determine time of day, force, description of vomitus, and associated symptoms

Fluid balance (needed only if vomiting occurs for a prolonged period)

- assess jugular venous pressure and orthostatic changes in blood pressure and heart rate; any decrease in upright diastolic pressure plus a rise in heart rate of 20 bpm or greater is abnormal
- oliguria
- weight changes
- rising values of hematocrit and creatinine, urea, sodium, and bicarbonate levels plus decreasing potassium and chloride levels are an indication of dehydration

Toxicity

Extrapyramidal reactions

- dystonic reactions, tetanus, restlessness, facial spasms, involuntary movement, torticollis, and muscular twitching (Drugs 1983;25[suppl 1]:35–51)
- routine prophylaxis with diphenhydramine is not usually recommended; however, diphenhydramine 25 mg PO every 4 hours can be used to control symptoms if they occur
- if severe facial or neck muscle spasms occur, diphenhydramine 25 mg IV should be given

Sedation

- is usually mild and decreases after 1–2 days of use
- avoid other sedating medications if possible

Hypotension

- most often associated with intravenous administration and suggests hypovolemia (Clin Pharm 1989;8:187–199)
- use slow rate of infusion
- may administer while the patient is recumbent

- tell patients to avoid rising quickly
- ensure that the patient is well hydrated

Anticholinergic effects

- dry mouth, blurred vision, dizziness (Drugs 1983;25[suppl 1]:35–51)
- if dry mouth occurs, try increasing fluid intake or using sugarless candy or gum to keep the patient's mouth moist
- if blurred vision occurs, try using comfort drops and avoid the use of contact lenses
- if constipation occurs, increase fluid and fiber intake
- urinary retention
- if these effects are severe and intolerable, prochlorperazine therapy may need to be discontinued

Hypersensitivity

- cholestatic jaundice is the most common serious hypersensitivity reaction (Drugs 1983;25[suppl 1]:35–51)
- incidence of about 1.4% (Drugs 1983;25[suppl 1]:35–51)
- monitor alkaline phosphatase and total and conjugated bilirubin levels at baseline and then monthly if using long-term high-dose therapy
- discontinue prochloperazine therapy if this occurs

Hematological effects

- pancytopenia, leukopenia, agranulocytosis, thrombocytopenic purpura, and eosinophilia can occur (Drugs 1983;25[suppl 1]: 35–51)
- monitor complete blood count at baseline and then monthly if using long-term (longer than 1 month) high-dose therapy
- discontinue prochlorperazine administration if this occurs

▶ *How Long Do I Treat Patients with This Drug?*

Chemotherapy-induced nausea and vomiting

- prochlorperazine is usually continued PRN for 5 days after the last dose of chemotherapy

Postoperative nausea and vomiting

- treatment may be required for 24 hours after surgery; then PRN antiemetic use may be useful

General nausea and vomiting

- therapy should be continued on a PRN basis until vomiting is controlled and the underlying pathophysiological change is treated

▶ *How Do I Decrease or Stop the Administration of This Drug?*

- may be stopped abruptly

▶ *What Should I Tell My Patients About This Drug?*

- prochlorperazine can be taken with or without food
- it takes 1/2–1 hour to become fully effective
- if both tablets and suppositories are prescribed, use suppositories if you are vomiting
- restlessness or muscle spasms may occur and can be controlled with diphenhydramine
- if severe facial or neck muscle spasms occur, stop taking prochlorperazine and go to a hospital emergency department
- drowsiness may also occur; avoid activities requiring you to be mentally alert (this may be increased if you are taking other medications that cause drowsiness)
- dry mouth may also occur; therefore, use sugarless candy or gum and try to increase fluid intake

▶ *Therapeutic Tips*

- antiemetic effect of prochlorperazine may be dose related (Am J Med Sci 1987;293:34–44)
- high-dose prochlorperazine appears to be equivalent to high-dose metoclopramide (Eur J Cancer 1992;28A[11]:1798–1802); however, clinical experience with high-dose prochlorperazine is limited, and as a result, prochlorperazine is usually used for mildly to moderately emetogenic antineoplastic regimens

Useful References

Craig JB, Powell BL. Review: The management of nausea and vomiting in clinical oncology. Am J Med Sci 1987;293:34–44

Gralla RJ, Tyson LB, Kris MG, Clark RA. The management of chemotherapy-induced nausea and vomiting. Med Clin North Am 1987;71:289–301

Merrifield KR, Chaffee BJ. Recent advances in the management of nausea and vomiting caused by antineoplastic agents. Clin Pharm 1989;8:187–199

Wampler G. The pharmacology and clinical effectiveness of phenothiazines and related drugs for managing chemotherapy-induced emesis. Drugs 1983;25(suppl 1):35–51

PROCYCLIDINE

Ruby Grymonpre

USA (Kemadrin)
CANADA (Kemadrin, Procyclid)

▶ When Should I Use This Drug?

Parkinson's disease

- anticholinergics have been used as first-line therapy for patients with mild Parkinson's disease (tremor as the predominant symptom) and good cognitive function; however, anticholinergics are now most often used as adjuncts to levodopa therapy when tremor is a problem
- there is no difference among benztropine, trihexyphenidyl, procyclidine, and biperiden with respect to efficacy; however, benztropine may have a greater sedative effect than some of the other anticholinergic agents (Clin Pharmacokinet 1987;13:141–178)
- trihexyphenidyl is more stimulating than the other agents
- benztropine is the only agent that can be given once daily, whereas trihexyphenidyl, with the exception of the sustained-release product, and procyclidine may need to be given more frequently
- decision among these agents should be based on cost, compliance issues, and the patient's response

▶ When Should I Not Use This Drug?

see Benztropine

▶ What Contraindications Are There to the Use of This Drug?

see Benztropine

▶ What Drug Interactions Are Clinically Important?

see Benztropine

▶ What Route and Dosage Should I Use?

How to administer

- orally—can be taken with food or milk or on an empty stomach but best to take in a similar fashion each time
- parenterally—available

Parkinson's disease

- 2.5 mg PO TID
- increase the dosage at weekly intervals by 2.5 mg to a usual dosage of 5 mg 3 times a day
- if necessary, a maximum daily dosage of 45–60 mg in 3 equally divided doses may be employed

Dosage adjustments for renal or hepatic dysfunction

- hepatic metabolism
- no dosage adjustment is required; just start with a low dose and titrate up to effect or toxicity

▶ What Should I Monitor with Regard to Efficacy and Toxicity?

see Benztropine

▶ How Long Do I Treat Patients with This Drug?

see Benztropine

▶ How Do I Decrease or Stop the Administration of This Drug?

see Benztropine

▶ What Should I Tell My Patients About This Drug?

see Benztropine

▶ Therapeutic Tips

see Benztropine

PROGESTINS (Progesterone, Norgestrel, Norethindrone, Norethindrone Acetate, Ethynodiol Diacetate, Levonorgestrel, Norgestimate, Medroxyprogesterone, Desogestrel)

Deborah Stier Carson

USA (Provera, Cycrin, Amen, Ovrette, Norlutin, Norlutate, Aygestin)
CANADA (Provera, Norlutate, PMS-progesterone)

▶ When Should I Use This Drug?

Prevention of osteoporosis or bone loss, treatment of osteoporosis (low bone mass and fractures)

- estrogen replacement plus cyclic medroxyprogesterone should be recommended, particularly in women with an intact uterus, to prevent endometrial cancer from unopposed estrogen stimulation
- in women unwilling to accept the resumption of menstruation, continuous estrogen and progestin therapy can be prescribed; however, there are few data on continuous use regarding risk of endometrial cancer and effects on levels of lipids and lipoproteins (Am J Med 1990;162:1534–1542, Obstet Gynecol 1990;75[suppl 4]:59S–76S)
- although it is not recommended, unopposed estrogen therapy provides a positive reduction in cardiovascular disease that outweighs the increased risk of endometrial cancer from unopposed estrogen therapy (N Engl J Med 1991;325:800–802)
- in women without an intact uterus, medroxyprogesterone should be used only in patients with low bone density (some progestins may promote new bone formation)

Hormonal contraception

see discussion of birth control in Chapter 7

Dysmenorrhea

- oral contraceptives are the drugs of choice for the initial treatment of dysmenorrhea, especially in women who desire contraception as well

see discussion of birth control in Chapter 7

Other uses

- dysfunctional uterine bleeding, endometriosis, benign breast disease, and functional ovarian cysts

▶ When Should I Not Use This Drug?

Pregnancy test

- progestin withdrawal should not be used as a pregnancy test because of concerns about teratogenicity

Women without a uterus

- progestins are generally not needed in women who do not have a uterus
- can be used if patient has low bone density, as some progestins promote new bone formation

▶ What Contraindications Are There to the Use of This Drug?

Intolerance of or allergic reaction to progestins

Absolute contraindications

- known or suspected pregnancy
- known or suspected cancer of the breast, except in appropriately selected patients being treated for metastatic disease
- undiagnosed abnormal genital bleeding
- active thrombophlebitis or thromboembolic disorder or a history thereof

- cerebrovascular accident or a history thereof
- benign or malignant hepatic tumor or a history thereof
- impaired hepatic function at present time

Strong relative contraindications (can be used if there are no useful alternatives)

- renal dysfunction, as progestins may aggravate fluid retention
- diabetes, as progestins may alter glucose metabolism
- history of ectopic pregnancy
- mental depression
- hyperlipidemia
- previous cholestasis during pregnancy

▶ *What Drug Interactions Are Clinically Important?*

Drugs that may increase the effect or toxicity of progestins

- none

Drugs that may decrease the effect of progestins

- none

Drugs that may have their effect or toxicity increased by progestins

- none

Drugs that may have their effect decreased by progestins

BROMOCRIPTINE

- progestins may cause amenorrhea and/or galactorrhea, thereby interfering with the effects of bromocriptine

▶ *What Route and Dosage Should I Use?*

How to adminster

- orally—take with food or milk
- parenterally—not available

Prevention of osteoporosis or bone loss, treatment of osteoporosis (low bone mass and fractures)

- 10 mg PO daily for 12 consecutive days each month (usually days 1–12) in women who have an intact uterus
- 10 mg dose likely has a greater effect on the endometrium; however, if it is not tolerated, 5 mg PO daily may be used
- 2.5 mg PO daily in combination with estrogen can be used to reduce cyclic withdrawal bleeding
- continuous administration of progestins reduces cyclic withdrawal bleeding; however, many women still experience irregular spotting and bleeding for up to 12 months
- indicators such as lipid profiles, blood glucose levels and blood pressure suggest that a continuous regimen is as safe as cyclic regimens for the prevention of osteoporosis and cardiovascular disease but no long-term data are available
- levonorgestrel and norgestrel tend to be androgenic, and their use is not recommended for postmenopausal therapy

Hormonal contraception, dysmenorrhea

see discussion of birth control in Chapter 7

Dosage adjustments for renal or hepatic dysfunction

- hepatically metabolized
- no dosage adjustments for renal dysfunction
- avoid in patients with active hepatic disease

▶ *What Should I Monitor with Regard to Efficacy and Toxicity?*

see Estrogens

▶ *How Long Do I Treat Patients with This Drug?*

see Estrogens

▶ *How Do I Decrease or Stop the Administration of This Drug?*

- administration of progestins does not need to be tapered if the decision is made to discontinue their use
- depending on the status of the endometrium, uterine bleeding may be experienced at irregular times after progestin therapy is stopped

▶ *What Should I Tell My Patients About This Drug?*

see Estrogens

▶ *Therapeutic Tips*

- progestins, especially synthetic compounds, have the ability to negate or minimize the beneficial effects of estrogens on serum lipids
- natural progesterone and medroxyprogesterone (2.5–5 mg PO daily) have little effect on serum lipid levels
- continuous progestin administration reduces cyclic withdrawal bleeding; however, many women still experience irregular spotting and bleeding for up to 12 months
- indicators such as lipid profiles, blood glucose levels, and blood pressure suggest that a continuous regimen is as safe as cyclic regimens for the prevention of osteoporosis and cardiovascular disease but no long-term data are available

PROMETHAZINE

Lynne Nakashima

USA (Phencen-50, Phenergan, Prometh-50, Phenameth, Prothazine, V-Gan 25)

CANADA (Histantil, Phenergan)

▶ *When Should I Use This Drug?*

Motion sickness

- for mild to moderate road, air, or sea travel, especially if sedation is desired (Drugs 1979;17:471–479)
- decision between dimenhydrinate and promethazine should be based on cost
- if sedation is not desired, use scopolamine

Postoperative nausea and vomiting

- should be chosen for patients undergoing ear surgery owing to its anticholinergic and antihistaminic activity (Can Anaesth Soc J 1984;31:407–415)

▶ *When Should I Not Use This Drug?*

Chemotherapy-induced nausea and vomiting

- promethazine is not usually used in chemotherapy-induced nausea and vomiting because it is generally considered no more effective than placebo (Drugs 1992;43:295–315)

Common cold

- should not be used for cold symptoms, as it offers no advantages over antihistamines and has marked anticholinergic and sedative effects and a potential to cause dystonic reactions

▶ *What Contraindications Are There to the Use of This Drug?*

see Prochlorperazine

▶ *What Drug Interactions Are Clinically Important?*

see Prochlorperazine

▶ *What Route and Dosage Should I Use?*

How to administer

Orally

- take with food to prevent gastrointestinal discomfort

Parenterally

- may be administered via an intramuscular or intravenous route
- for intravenous use, dilute to 25 mg/mL and administer at a rate not exceeding 25 mg/min

Motion sickness

- 25 mg PO BID starting 1–2 hours before the trip
- continue therapy for the duration of the trip

Postoperative nausea and vomiting

- 25 mg IV or IM every 3 hours when needed

- 25 mg PO every 3 hours may be used if the patient can tolerate sips of fluid

Dosage adjustments for renal or hepatic dysfunction

- hepatically metabolized
- no dosage adjustment required; titrate the dose to effect

▶ What Should I Monitor with Regard to Efficacy and Toxicity?

see Prochlorperazine

▶ How Long Do I Treat Patients with This Drug?

see Prochlorperazine

▶ How Do I Decrease or Stop the Administration of This Drug?

- may be stopped abruptly

▶ What Should I Tell My Patients About This Drug?

- promethazine may be taken with food to reduce stomach irritation

see Prochlorperazine

Useful Reference

Wood CD. Antimotion sickness and antiemetic drugs. Drugs 1979;17: 471–479

PROPAFENONE

James Tisdale

USA (Rythmol)
CANADA (Rythmol)

▶ When Should I Use This Drug?

Propafenone should not be used without consulting a cardiologist or a cardiac electrophysiologist

Ventricular tachycardia

- propafenone should be used for the suppression of recurrent, symptomatic or life-threatening ventricular tachycardia in patients in whom the following conditions apply: there is failure to respond to therapy with class IA (quinidine or procainamide), class IB (mexiletine or tocainide), and/or the combination of class IA and IB antiarrhythmic agents during serial drug testing in the electrophysiology (EP) laboratory; the physician and/or the patient wishes to delay amiodarone or nonpharmacological therapy; flecainide is contraindicated; moricizine is contraindicated or not well tolerated; and propafenone has suppressed or favorably modified inducible ventricular tachycardia during EP testing or during Holter monitoring

Atrial fibrillation or flutter

- propafenone should be used for the prevention of episodes of atrial fibrillation or flutter only in patients in whom therapy with quinidine, procainamide, disopyramide, flecainide, and sotalol has been unsuccessful, poorly tolerated, or contraindicated and who wish to delay amiodarone therapy

Atrioventricular nodal reentrant tachycardia

- propafenone should be used for the prevention of episodes of paroxysmal supraventricular tachycardia only in patients in whom therapy with digoxin, beta-adrenergic receptor blocking agents (beta-blockers), verapamil, quinidine, procainamide, disopyramide, and flecainide has been unsuccessful, poorly tolerated, or contraindicated and who wish to delay amiodarone therapy

▶ When Should I Not Use This Drug?

Asymptomatic ventricular arrhythmias

- treatment of asymptomatic ventricular arrhythmias has not been shown to be of benefit (N Engl J Med 1989;321:406–412)

▶ What Contraindications Are There to the Use of This Drug?

Intolerance of or allergic reaction to propafenone

Acute congestive heart failure

- propafenone has negative inotropic activity and may depress the function of the left ventricle, and therefore the drug should not be used in patients with acute exacerbations of congestive heart failure

Sinus bradycardia

- propafenone has beta-receptor blocking activity and should therefore be avoided in patients with sinus bradycardia

Sick sinus syndrome

- owing to propafenone's beta-blocking activity, the drug should not be used in patients with sick sinus syndrome unless a functioning pacemaker is present

Atrioventricular block

- propafenone impairs conduction of electrical impulses through the atrioventricular (AV) node and therefore should not be used in patients with second- or third-degree AV block unless a functioning ventricular pacemaker is present
- propafenone may be used in patients with first-degree AV block, but the electrocardiogram should be monitored closely for progression of AV block

Bundle branch blocks

- propafenone slows impulse conduction through the His-Purkinje system and therefore should not be used in patients with bifascicular or trifascicular blocks unless a functioning ventricular pacemaker is present

Asthma

- in view of the beta-blocking activity of propafenone, the drug should not be used in patients with asthma or other conditions in which bronchospasm is present

▶ What Drug Interactions Are Clinically Important?

Drugs that may increase the effect or toxicity of propafenone

- none

Drugs that may decrease the effect of propafenone

- none

Drugs that may have their effect or toxicity increased by propafenone

DIGOXIN

- propafenone may increase digoxin concentrations by up to 88%
- when propafenone therapy is added in patients receiving digoxin, decrease the digoxin dosage by 50% when starting propafenone therapy and make further dosage changes on the basis of clinical response
- if digoxin toxicity is suspected, measure a digoxin serum concentration

WARFARIN

- propafenone increases warfarin concentrations by 40%
- if propafenone is added, monitor INR every 2 days until the full extent of interaction is seen and adjust the dosage as for a warfarin dosage change (Clin Pharmacokinet 1991;21:1–10)

METOPROLOL

- propafenone increases metoprolol concentrations 2–5 times, prolongs its duration, and may have additive beta-blocking effects
- metoprolol dosages should be decreased by 50%, and monitor for PR prolongation and heart rate

Drugs that may have their effect decreased by propafenone

- none

▶ What Route and Dosage Should I Use?

How to administer

- orally—food may enhance absorption; therefore, administration should be consistent with or without food
- parenterally—not available

Ventricular tachycardia, atrial fibrillation or flutter, atrioventricular nodal reentrant tachycardia

- 150 mg PO Q8H; the dosage may be increased to the maximum recommended dosage of 300 mg Q8H after an additional 4 days if arrhythmia is not controlled

Dosage adjustments for renal or hepatic dysfunction

- hepatically metabolized
- in patients with severe hepatic disease, initial and maintenance propafenone dosages should be reduced by 50%
- dosage reduction in patients with renal dysfunction is not necessary

▶ What Should I Monitor with Regard to Efficacy and Toxicity?

Efficacy

Ventricular tachycardia, atrial fibrillation or flutter, atrioventricular nodal reentrant tachycardia

see Quinidine

- serum propafenone concentrations do not correlate well with efficacy and are neither necessary nor available

Toxicity

Adverse effects necessitating discontinuation of therapy occur in approximately 3–7% of patients

Taste disturbances (15–20%), dizziness or lightheadedness (12%), constipation, nausea, and vomiting

- if these occur, dosage reduction is warranted, except for taste disturbances, which often resolve over time without dosage adjustment

Congestive heart failure

- patient should be assessed during the first week of therapy and every 3–6 months afterward for evidence of congestive heart failure (shortness of breath, crackles, orthopnea, and paroxysmal nocturnal dyspnea)

Electrocardiogram

- evaluation at 1 week should assess prolonged PR interval (>0.2 second), prolonged duration of QRS complex (>25% increase compared with baseline values), and initiation of new arrhythmias or worsening of clinical arrhythmia

▶ How Long Do I Treat Patients with This Drug?

Ventricular tachycardia, atrial fibrillation or flutter, atrioventricular nodal reentrant tachycardia

- treatment with propafenone may be required indefinitely

▶ How Do I Decrease or Stop the Administration of This Drug?

- propafenone therapy should not be discontinued or dosage reduction performed without consulting a cardiologist or a cardiac electrophysiologist
- daily dosage of propafenone should be decreased if patient experiences dizziness, lightheadedness, constipation, nausea, vomiting, and/or prolongation of the QRS complex of greater than 25% compared with baseline values
- if the dosage is reduced, patient should be instructed to report changes in symptoms or pulse rate
- propafenone therapy should be discontinued abruptly if patient has congestive heart failure, symptomatic bradycardia, symptomatic first-degree AV block, second- or third-degree AV block, bifascicular or trifascicular block, new cardiac arrhythmias, or worsening of clinical arrhythmia

▶ What Should I Tell My Patients About This Drug?

- do not discontinue this medication or change your dosage without consulting your physician
- notify your physician if you experience dizziness, lightheadedness, disturbances in taste, nausea, vomiting, constipation, fainting, palpitations, or shortness of breath while taking this medication
- because this drug may cause dizziness, do not drive or operate heavy machinery until it is determined how you react to this medication

▶ Therapeutic Tips

- hepatic metabolism of propafenone is dose or concentration dependent (saturable), and therefore plasma concentrations may increase disproportionately after dosage increases
- patients should be monitored for the occurrence of adverse effects for several days after an increase in propafenone dosage

Useful References

Chow MSS, Lebsack C, Hilleman D. Propafenone: A new antiarrhythmic agent. Clin Pharm 1988;7:869–877

Parker RB, McCollam PL, Bauman JL. Propafenone: A novel type Ic antiarrhythmic agent. DICP 1989;23:196–203

Funck-Bretano C, Kroemer HK, Lee JT, Roden DM. Propafenone. N Engl J Med 1990;322:518–525

PROPOXYPHENE

Terry Baumann

USA (Darvon, Dolene, various combinations: Darvocet-N 100, Wygesic, various)
CANADA (Darvon, Dolene, Novopropoxyn, various)

▶ When Should I Use This Drug?

Acute pain

- for moderate acute pain not relieved by a nonopiate analgesic (acetaminophen or nonsteroidal antiinflammatory drugs [NSAIDs]) given regularly and/or the patient has a true allergy to morphine or codeine
- not as effective as morphine
- propoxyphene should not be used alone because it produces a far better effect when used with acetaminophen or NSAIDs

▶ When Should I Not Use This Drug?

Severe pain, cancer pain, chronic noncancer pain

- is ineffective for the treatment of severe or chronic pain

Single therapy

- propoxyphene produces only a weak analgesic effect when used alone

▶ What Contraindications Are There to the Use of This Drug?

Intolerance of or allergic reaction to propoxyphene

- true allergies to propoxyphene are rare
- check that the patient has actual allergic symptoms, and if there is a true allergy, consider morphine or codeine with acetaminophen

Severe respiratory depression

- not an absolute contraindication; just start with dosages 25% of the normal initial dosage and titrate up to effect while assessing respiratory rate and oxymetry before each dose

▶ What Drug Interactions Are Clinically Important?

see Morphine

Drugs that may have their effect or toxicity increased by propoxyphene

CARBAMAZEPINE, WARFARIN, TRICYCLIC ANTIDEPRESSANTS

- propoxyphene may raise serum levels of these compounds
- choose an alternative pain medication

▶ What Route and Dosage Should I Use?

How to administer

- orally—may be administered with food or milk or on an empty stomach
- parenterally—not available

Acute pain

- 100 mg of the napsylate salt or 65 mg of the hydrochloride salt PO Q4H in combination with at least 325 mg of acetaminophen, 300 mg of aspirin, or an NSAID
- when using acetaminophen or aspirin combination for more than 5 days in a round-the-clock fashion, be aware of possible acetaminophen or aspirin toxicity

Dosage adjustments for renal or hepatic dysfunction

- hepatically metabolized

Normal Dosing Interval	C$_{cr}$ > 60 mL/min or 1 mL/s	C$_{cr}$ 30–60 mL/min or 0.5–1 mL/s	C$_{cr}$ < 30 mL/min or 0.5 mL/s
Q4–6H	no adjustment needed	adjust dosage on basis of response	adjust dosage on basis of response

▶ What Should I Monitor with Regard to Efficacy and Toxicity?

see Morphine

▶ How Long Do I Treat Patients with This Drug?

see Morphine

▶ How Do I Decrease or Stop the Administration of This Drug?

see Morphine

▶ What Should I Tell My Patients About This Drug?

see Morphine

▶ Therapeutic Tips

- most effective when used with peripheral-acting nonopiate analgesics (acetaminophen or NSAIDs)
- questionable efficacy when used alone or in dosages less than those mentioned above
- be aware that when propoxyphene is used in combination products with acetaminophen or aspirin in a round-the-clock fashion, possible acetaminophen or aspirin toxicity may occur owing to the possible ingestion of large amounts of acetaminophen or aspirin
- in patients who will be taking regularly dosed narcotics for longer than 3–4 days, always consider prescribing narcotics in conjunction with a laxative and counsel the patient on the appropriate use of fluids and fiber

Useful References

see Morphine

PROPRANOLOL

Robert Rangno and James McCormack

USA (Inderal, Inderal LA, generics)
CANADA (Inderal, Inderal LA, Apo-Propranolol, Novopranol)

▶ When Should I Use This Drug?

Myocardial infarction

- all patients should be treated empirically with beta-blockers after a myocardial infarction (unless there are contraindications to the use of beta-blockers) (Am J Cardiol 1990;66:3C–8C), because there are convincing data that reinfarction, sudden cardiac death, and overall mortality are reduced after myocardial infarction
- propranolol has the advantage of being available as a parenteral agent, along with metoprolol and atenolol (USA only)

- decision among parenteral propranolol, parenteral metoprolol, and parenteral atenolol should be based on cost
- although parenteral therapy is usually recommended, oral administration can also be used, with the realization that absorption of the agent takes about 30 minutes (some clinicians recommend the intravenous route for the first dose possibly to reduce the size of the infarction)
- some clinicians suggest that only beta-blockers with proven long-term benefits on mortality after infarction (timolol, propranolol, metoprolol, or acebutolol) should be used for post-MI prophylaxis (Circulation 1991;84[suppl VI]:VI-101–VI-107)

Atrial fibrillation or flutter

see Nadolol

▶ When Should I Not Use This Drug?

When other beta-blockers can be used

- while propranolol, a nonselective beta-blocker, is effective in many disease states, other beta-blockers should usually be chosen over propranolol
- propranolol is more lipid soluble than atenolol (selective beta-blocker) or nadolol (nonselective beta-blocker)
- lipid-soluble agents (propranolol and metoprolol) have been shown to cause insomnia whereas atenolol (lipid insoluble) does not (Circulation 1987;75:104–112)
- propranolol in most cases causes more decrease in quality of life measurements than the other beta-blockers (Circulation 1991;84[suppl VI]:VI-108–VI-118)
- propranolol has a short half-life and must be dosed at least twice daily, and while a sustained-release product is available, it is usually more expensive than generic nadolol or atenolol
- oral propranolol has a high variability in systemic bioavailability (Circulation 1991;84[suppl VI]:VI-108–VI-118)
- oral propranolol has totally unpredictable fifty-fold variability of oral systemic bioavailability secondary to large first-pass liver metabolism (Clin Pharmacol Ther 1985;38:509–518), such that a significant proportion of patients will not realize adequate beta-blockade and conversely others could have adverse effects from excessive blockade (this phenomenon is even further accentuated with the sustained-release preparations)
- there is a much greater chance of clinically important drug interactions with propranolol versus non-hepatically metabolized beta-blockers such as atenolol and nadolol

▶ What Contraindications Are There to the Use of This Drug?

see Nadolol

▶ What Drug Interactions Are Clinically Important?

see Nadolol, in addition to the following

Drugs that may increase the effect or toxicity of propranolol

CIMETIDINE

- cimetidine can decrease the metabolism of propranolol to a varying degree owing to the effect cimetidine has on hepatic metabolism
- it is best to use an H$_2$ antagonist (ranitidine, famotidine, nizatidine) that has little if any effect on hepatic metabolism or use a beta-blocker that is not hepatically metabolized (e.g., nadolol, atenolol)

Drugs that may decrease the effect of propranolol

RIFAMPIN

- decreases plasma concentrations of propranolol
- evaluate the patient within 2–3 days of starting rifampin administration, and increase the dosage of propranolol if a clinical change in response to propranolol is seen

▶ What Route and Dosage Should I Use?

How to administer

- orally—see discussion above under When Should I Not Use This Drug?

- parenterally—propranolol can be given by IV push at a rate no greater than 1 mg/min

Myocardial infarction

- 1 mg IV over 2 minutes, and follow with another 1 mg IV 2–3 minutes later unless heart rate is < 60 beats/min or systolic blood pressure is less than 100 mmHg
- patients who tolerate the IV doses should receive 40 mg PO Q8H starting 2 hours after the last IV dose, increasing the dose up to 60 mg PO TID after 3–4 days (other less lipid-soluble, less frequently dosed beta-blockers should likely be chosen instead of propranolol for long-term use)

Atrial fibrillation or flutter

- 1 mg IV every 2 minutes until heart rate is less than 130 bpm (100 bpm if angina or congestive heart failure is present) or 0.1 mg/kg (7–10 mg) is reached

Dosage adjustment for renal or hepatic dysfunction

- hepatically metabolized
- in general, even in patients with hepatic dysfunction, start with a low dose and titrate up to an effect

Normal Dosing Interval	C_{cr} > 60 mL/min or 1 mL/s	C_{cr} 30–60 mL/min or 0.5–1 mL/s	C_{cr} < 30 mL/min or 0.5 mL/s
Q12H	no adjustment needed	no adjustment needed	no adjustment needed

▶ What Should I Monitor with Regard to Efficacy and Toxicity

Efficacy

Myocardial infarction

- decreased severity, frequency, and duration of chest pain
- frequency of assessment depends on the frequency of chest pain and complications of myocardial infarction (cardiogenic shock, arrhythmias, and septal rupture)

Toxicity

see Nadolol

▶ How Do I Decrease or Stop the Administration of This Drug?

see Nadolol

▶ What Do I Tell My Patients About This Drug?

- should not be discontinued abruptly
- notify your physician if there is difficulty in breathing
- may produce lassitude and sleep disturbances

▶ Therapeutic Tips

- interpatient variability in plasma concentrations of drug after oral administration of propranolol is wide, and therefore, patience is required in adjusting the dosage until adequate therapeutic response is obtained

Useful References

Tyrer P. Current status of beta-blocking drugs in the treatment of anxiety disorders. Drugs 1988;36:773–783

Feely J, Peden N. Use of beta-adrenoceptor blocking drugs in hyperthyroidism. Drugs 1984;27:425–446

Lewis JA, Davis JM, Allsopp D, Cameron HA. Beta-blockers in portal hypertension: An overview. Drugs 1989;37(suppl 2):62–69

Frishman WH. Beta-adrenergic blockers. Med Clin North Am 1988;71:37–81

Wood AJJ, Vestal RE, Spannuth CL, et al. Propranolol disposition in renal failure. Br J Clin Pharmacol 1980;10:561–566

Stone WJ, Walle T. Massive propranolol metabolite retention during maintenance hemodialysis. Clin Pharmacol Ther 1980;28:449–455

PROTRIPTYLINE

Lyle K. Laird and Julia Vertrees

USA (Vivactil)
CANADA (Triptil)

▶ When Should I Use This Drug?

Consider an alternative agent

- protriptyline is as effective as other antidepressants for depression; however, it likely offers no advantages over any of the other agents
- protriptyline is the most stimulating tricyclic antidepressant, but with the advent of fluoxetine, protriptyline is likely only an alternative in patients who do not respond to other agents

Useful References

Bryant SG, Brown CS. Major depressive disorders. In: Young LY, Koda-Kimble MA, eds. Applied Therapeutics: The Clinical Use of Drugs, 4th ed. Vancouver, WA: Applied Therapeutics, 1988:1231–1253

Wells BG, Hayes PE. Depressive illness. In: DiPiro JT, Talbert RL, Hayes PE, et al, eds. Pharmacotherapy: A Pathophysiologic Approach. New York: Elsevier, 1989:748–764

PSEUDOEPHEDRINE

Penny Miller

USA (Sudafed, Cenafed, Sufedrin)
CANADA (Sudafed, Eltor)

▶ When Should I Use This Drug?

Nasal congestion

- nasal congestion resulting from eustachian tube dysfunction during air travel, deep sea diving, the common cold, allergic rhinitis, sinusitis, and rebound congestion resulting from overuse of topical decongestants
- has proven efficacy, a low vasopressor effect, and low abuse potential; is available as single-entity oral preparations; and is inexpensive

▶ When Should I Not Use This Drug?

Serous otitis media (otitis media with effusion) to improve eustachian tube function

- lack of efficacy has been demonstrated (Pediatrics 1978;61: 679–684, N Engl J Med 1983;308:297–301)

Central nervous system stimulation

- at dosages required for central nervous system stimulation, the risk of hypertension and palpitations is too high

Appetite suppression

- lack of efficacy as a weight reduction aid (Self Medication. Reference for Health Professionals 1992, Canadian Pharmaceutical Association, Ottawa, 1992)

Sole therapy in allergic reactions of the nasal cavities

- decongestants provide symptomatic relief of congestion only and do not affect the cause of the allergic reaction
- antihistamines should be the mainstay of therapy because they block histamine release
- decongestants should be considered only as adjunctive temporary treatment because of their sympathetic side effects and the potential for rebound congestion with topical decongestants

▶ What Contraindications Are There to the Use of This Drug?

Intolerance of or allergic reaction to pseudoephedrine

Ischemic heart disease

- stimulation of beta-receptors in the heart can cause tachycardia and worsen angina; therefore, use topical decongestants

Hypertension

- systolic and diastolic blood pressure may be increased, although pseudoephedrine is the decongestant least likely to cause this effect
- use topical decongestants rather than oral agents

Hyperthyroidism

- increased blood pressure and tachycardia may be enhanced; therefore, use topical decongestants

Patients receiving monoamine oxidase inhibitors

- hypertensive crisis may result, and therefore, avoid all sympathomimetics

Diabetes mellitus

- increased blood glucose levels may occur owing to beta$_2$-adrenergic stimulation; therefore, use topical decongestants

Prostatic hypertrophy

- urinary retention may occur; therefore, use topical decongestants

Pregnancy

- animal studies have revealed teratogenic effects

Breast-feeding

- infants have increased sensitivity to sympathomimetic agents; therefore, use topical decongestant only after saline drops have failed

Glaucoma (closed angle)

- may precipitate an attack

▶ *What Drug Interactions Are Clinically Important?*

Drugs that may increase the effect or toxicity of pseudoephedrine

MONOAMINE OXIDASE INHIBITORS

- severe hypertension and possible crisis can occur, resulting from increased storage and release of norepinephrine; therefore, avoid concurrent use

CARBONIC ANHYDRASE INHIBITORS OR ANTACIDS

- increased pseudoephedrine toxicity results in decreased renal excretion owing to alkaline urine; therefore, avoid concurrent use

Drugs that may decrease the effect of pseudoephedrine

- none

Drugs that may have their effect or toxicity increased by pseudoephedrine

DIGOXIN

- increased tendency for cardiac arrhythmia; therefore, avoid concurrent use

Drugs that may have their effect decreased by pseudoephedrine

BETA-BLOCKERS

- increased pressor effects of pseudoephedrine; therefore, avoid concurrent use

▶ *What Route and Dosage Should I Use?*

How to administer

- orally—can be given with food or on an empty stomach

Nasal congestion

- 60 mg PO Q6H PRN to a maximum of 240 mg PO daily
- higher dosages result in nervousness, dizziness, or sleeplessness
- single-entity products are preferred; however, if 2 symptoms or more are bothersome and treatment is desired, a combination of the above with an appropriate antihistamine or analgesic is considered acceptable (Health Protection Branch. First Report of the Expert Advisory Committee on Nonprescription Cough and Cold Remedies. Health and Welfare Canada, 1988:23–24)

Dosage adjustments for renal or hepatic dysfunction

- no adjustment needed

▶ *What Should I Monitor with Regard to Efficacy and Toxicity?*

Efficacy

Nasal congestion

- reduced nasal congestion occurs within 30 minutes and persists for 4–6 hours

- decreased ear pain associated with eustachian tube dysfunction during air travel and deep sea diving

Toxicity

- adverse effects are infrequent if dosages do not exceed maximum recommended daily dosages

Central nervous system effects

- include nausea, vomiting, sweating, vertigo, tremor, nervousness, apprehension, and insomnia
- depending on the severity of symptoms, dosages of pseudoephedrine should be decreased or its use discontinued if these symptoms occur

Cardiovascular effects

- increased systolic and diastolic blood pressure and increased cardiac output
- may increase blood pressure in normal individuals (Am Fam Physician 1985;31:183–187)
- patients with hypertension should use topical decongestants

▶ *How Long Do I Treat Patients with This Drug?*

Nasal congestion

- for the common cold, treat as long as the cold persists, about 7 days on a PRN basis
- for allergic rhinitis, occasional use for up to 7 days when stuffiness is not controlled with antihistamines alone
- for sinusitis, treat when symptoms are most evident, for up to 7 days
- for rebound congestion from topical decongestants, treat on a regular basis for 1–2 weeks

▶ *How Do I Decrease or Stop the Administration of This Drug?*

- may be stopped abruptly
- tolerance and physical dependence are not a reported clinical problem

▶ *What Should I Tell My Patients About This Drug?*

- do not take more than the recommended dosage
- do not take this medication if you are now taking or have taken monoamine oxidase inhibitors in the past 2 weeks or if you are taking antihypertensive medication
- if nervousness, insomnia, headaches, or fast pounding heartbeat occurs, discontinue therapy
- discontinue therapy if urination is difficult or painful (important for men older than 50 years old with benign prostatic hypertrophy)

▶ *Therapeutic Tips*

- ensure that maximum daily dosages are not exceeded
- unlike antihistamines, decongestants do not dry up nasal secretions
- in patients taking pseudoephedrine, routine physical examinations may show increased blood pressure and heart rate, so ensure that blood pressure is taken after the patient has been off the drug for at least a few days
- unlike topical decongestants, pseudoephedrine produces little if any rebound congestion (AHFS Drug Information 1992:705)
- sustained-release products may not always release drugs consistently, and although, theoretically, they should produce more constant serum drug concentrations with less dramatic swings (thereby diminishing the likelihood of adverse reactions), they should be tried only if the patient has adverse effects with the less expensive nonsustained preparations

Useful References

USPDI 1993, US Pharmacopeial Convention, Rockville, MD, 1993

American Hospital Formulary Service, Drug Information ASHP, Bethesda, MD, 1993

Health Protection Branch. First Report of the Expert Advisory Committee on Nonprescription Cough and Cold Remedies—Antihistamines, Nasal Decongestants and Anticholinergics; Health and Welfare Canada, August, 1988

PYRAZINAMIDE

Ann Beardsell

USA (Pyrazinamide)
CANADA (Tebrazid, PMS Pyrazinamide)

▶ *When Should I Use This Drug?*

Tuberculosis

- used as first-line agent in the treatment of *Mycobacterium* tuberculosis
- must be used in conjunction with other antituberculosis agents to prevent the development of resistance and to promote a shorter infective period

▶ *When Should I Not Use This Drug?*

Single agent in the treatment of tuberculosis

- must be used in conjunction with other agents to prevent resistance

▶ *What Contraindications Are There to the Use of This Drug?*

Intolerance of or allergic reaction to pyrazinamide

Hepatic disease

- pyrazinamide may potentiate hepatic disease

▶ *What Drug Interactions Are Clinically Important?*

Drugs that may increase the effect or toxicity of pyrazinamide

PROBENECID

- blocks the excretion of pyrazinamide, which may result in higher incidence of toxicity to pyrazinamide
- use probenecid only if unavoidable
- if the combination is used, monitor for signs and symptoms of toxicity and discontinue pyrazinamide or probenecid if toxicities occur

Drugs that may decrease the effect of pyrazinamide

- none

Drugs that may have their effect or toxicity increased by pyrazinamide

- none

Drugs that may have their effect decreased by pyrazinamide

ALLOPURINOL, COLCHICINE, PROBENECID, SULFINPYRAZONE

- pyrazinamide may precipitate gout by increasing serum uric acid levels, thereby reducing the efficacy of concurrent medications used for gout
- monitor serum uric acid levels monthly initially, and adjust the dosages of antigout medications if uric acid concentrations increase or symptoms of gout are present

▶ *What Route and Dosage Should I Use?*

How to administer

- orally—take with food or milk or on empty stomach
- parenterally—not available

Tuberculosis

- numerous regimens exist, involving different combinations and dosages of drugs
- 15–35 mg/kg PO daily in 3 divided doses to a maximum of 3 g daily (dosage depends on the regimen being followed)

Dosage adjustments for renal or hepatic dysfunction

- hepatically metabolized (no adjustments needed for renal dysfunction)

▶ *What Should I Monitor with Regard to Efficacy and Toxicity?*

Efficacy

Tuberculosis

- disease improvement or resolution of symptoms such as fevers, sweats, and weight loss

Toxicity

Hepatic effects

- hepatotoxicity (jaundice, hepatitis, hepatomegaly, and splenomegaly) is common with pyrazinamide, and liver function test results (aspartate aminotransferase, alanine aminotransferase, and bilirubin levels) must be followed monthly and drug therapy discontinued if values are above normal levels and are continuing to rise after 2 consecutive tests

Hyperuricemia

- pyrazinamide inhibits the renal excretion of urates, which may result in nongouty polyarthralgia or acute gout; therefore, monitor serum uric acid levels monthly
- hyperuricemia may be controlled by the use of uricosuric agents; however, pyrazinamide therapy should be discontinued if acute gouty arthritis occurs or if hyperuricemia is severe (serum uric acid concentrations ≥ 12–13 mg/dL or 700 μmol/L)

Gastrointestinal effects

- nausea, vomiting, and anorexia may occur but usually resolve with ongoing therapy
- treat symptomatically

Other effects

- malaise, arthralgia, fever, and photosensitivity may occur but are less common
- treat symptomatically

▶ *How Long Do I Treat Patients with This Drug?*

Tuberculosis

- 6 to 9 months, depending on the regimen

▶ *How Do I Decrease or Stop the Administration of This Drug?*

- may be stopped abruptly

▶ *What Should I Tell My Patients About This Drug?*

- it is important to take this medication on a regular basis and not to miss doses
- do not stop taking this medication, even if you feel better, until told to do so by your physician
- if you miss a dose, take it as soon as you remember unless it is time for your next dose, in which case you should just skip the forgotten dose and not double up doses
- notify your physician if your symptoms do not improve after several weeks on the medication
- contact your physician immediately if you notice a yellowing of your skin or eyes or if you have any pain and swelling of your joints, especially the big toe
- do not take this medication by itself, as it should always be used in combination with other antituberculous medications
- if you are diabetic, it is important to note that this medication may cause false results with the urine ketone tests
- check with your physician before altering diet and/or medications for diabetes
- this medication may cause you to be more sensitive to sunlight, and therefore, at first, avoid too much sun and use sunscreen until you see how you react

▶ *Therapeutic Tips*

- if gastrointestinal upset occurs in patients taking numerous antimycobacterial agents, stop the administration of all drugs, and restart with just 1 or 2 drugs and slowly add back the rest
- if gastrointestinal upset reappears, stop therapy with the last drug added

QUINAPRIL

Jack Onrot and James McCormack

USA (Accupril)
CANADA (Accupril)

▶ *When Should I Use This Drug?*

see Enalapril

▶ *When Should I Not Use This Drug?*

see Enalapril

▶ *What Contraindications Are There to the Use of This Drug?*

see Captopril

▶ *What Drug Interactions Are Clinically Important?*

see Captopril

▶ *What Route and Dosage Should I Use?*

How to administer

- orally—can be administered with or without food
- parenterally—not available

Congestive heart failure

- 2.5 mg PO daily
- rapidity of dosage escalation depends on the severity of symptoms
- dosage may be increased daily if necessary
- no value in exceeding a total daily dosage of 40 mg

Chronic (noncrisis) hypertension

- 2.5 mg PO daily
- increase the dosage by 2.5 mg PO daily every 4 weeks until adequate blood pressure is achieved or a maximum daily dosage of 20 mg is reached
- limited value in exceeding a total daily dosage of 20 mg (dosages as high as 40 mg PO daily have been used)
- for some patients, the antihypertensive effect may be diminished before 24 hours and twice-daily dosing may be required (Inpharma 1993;881:5)

Dosage adjustments for renal or hepatic dysfunction

- renally eliminated
- titrate the dose to clinical response and not concurrent renal or hepatic function

▶ *What Should I Monitor with Regard to Efficacy and Toxicity?*

see Captopril

▶ *How Long Do I Treat Patients with This Drug?*

see Captopril

▶ *How Do I Decrease or Stop the Administration of This Drug?*

see Captopril

▶ *What Should I Tell My Patients About This Drug?*

see Captopril

▶ *Therapeutic Tips*

see Captopril

QUINIDINE

James Tisdale

USA (Quinidine Sulfate, Cin-Quin, Quinora, Quinidex Extentabs, Quinidine Gluconate, Quinaglute Dura-Tabs, Quinatime, Quin-Release, Duraquin, Cardioquin)
CANADA (Quinidine Sulfate, Apo-Quinidine, Novo-Quinidin, Quinidex, Biquin, Quinidine Gluconate, Quinaglute, Quinate, Cardioquin)

▶ *When Should I Use This Drug?*

Atrial fibrillation or flutter

Conversion to sinus rhythm

- drug of choice for pharmacological conversion of relatively new-onset (less than 1 year) atrial fibrillation or flutter in patients in whom direct current cardioversion is considered undesirable

- quinidine should be considered the drug of choice because it is the agent for which the most efficacy data exist (N Engl J Med 1992;326:1264–1271)
- quinidine should not be administered until control of ventricular response has been achieved with an agent that inhibits conduction of impulses through the atrioventricular (AV) node

Maintenance of sinus rhythm

- drug of choice for the maintenance of sinus rhythm after cardioversion in patients with paroxysmal atrial fibrillation or flutter
- quinidine therapy may be preferable to therapy with procainamide, as more data supporting the efficacy of quinidine exist (Am Heart J 1986;111:1150–1161)
- meta-analysis has suggested that quinidine therapy may be associated with a significantly higher incidence of mortality than is placebo (Circulation 1990;82:1106–1116), and the use of quinidine in atrial fibrillation or flutter is being reevaluated
- until these findings are confirmed in a prospective study, and until the effects of other antiarrhythmic drugs on mortality are determined in this population, quinidine should remain a first-line agent for the prevention of recurrent atrial fibrillation or flutter

Atrioventricular nodal reentrant tachycardia

- quinidine may be used for long-term prevention of episodes of paroxysmal supraventricular tachycardia (PSVT) due to AV nodal reentry in patients with structural heart disease in whom empirical therapy with digoxin or beta-blockers has failed, is contraindicated, or is not tolerated

Wolff-Parkinson-White syndrome

- quinidine should be used for the prevention of atrial fibrillation or flutter and/or PSVT in patients with Wolff-Parkinson-White syndrome in whom quinidine has been proven effective during electrophysiological (EP) testing (Circulation 1977;55:15–22)

Ventricular premature depolarizations

- quinidine may be used for the empirical management of symptomatic, benign ventricular premature depolarizations (VPDs) in patients in whom VPDs or symptoms have not been suppressed with beta-adrenergic receptor blocking agents
- in this situation, however, consultation of an electrophysiologist for assessment and selection of therapy should be done to assess the risk of sudden cardiac death and determine the need for EP testing

Ventricular tachycardia

- quinidine should be used during serial drug testing in the EP laboratory in patients with inducible ventricular tachycardia that is suppressed after intravenous procainamide administration (Am J Cardiol 1985;56:883–886)
- if ventricular tachycardia continues to be suppressed during EP testing while the patient is receiving quinidine, the patient should be discharged from the hospital on quinidine therapy (N Engl J Med 1980;303:1073–1077)
- if ventricular tachycardia is suppressed on Holter monitoring in patients who do not undergo EP testing, the patient should be maintained on quinidine therapy

▶ *When Should I Not Use This Drug?*

Atrial fibrillation or flutter (of longer than 1 year's duration or in patients with an enlarged left atrium)

- quinidine should not be administered to patients who have atrial fibrillation or flutter of longer than 1 year in duration, as successful conversion to sinus rhythm is highly unlikely (Ann Intern Med 1966;65:216–224)
- quinidine should not be administered to patients with an enlarged left atrium (>45 mm as determined by echocardiography), as successful conversion to sinus rhythm is highly unlikely (Circulation 1976;53:273–279)

Asymptomatic ventricular arrhythmias

- no evidence that treatment is beneficial

Ventricular tachycardia if procainamide therapy has failed

- quinidine should not be administered during serial drug testing in the EP laboratory in patients in whom intravenous procainamide therapy failed to suppress inducible ventricular tachycardia (J Am Coll Cardiol 1987;9:882–889) because it is unlikely to be beneficial

▶ *What Contraindications Are There to the Use of This Drug?*

Intolerance of or allergic reaction to quinidine or cinchona derivatives

Atrioventricular nodal block

- quinidine is contraindicated in patients with incomplete or complete AV block in whom a functioning pacemaker is not present

Myasthenia gravis

- quinidine may interfere with neuromuscular conduction, and has been reported to exacerbate symptoms of myasthenia gravis (Mt Sinai J Med 1976;43:10–14)

Long QT syndrome

- quinidine therapy may result in prolongation of QT intervals on surface electrocardiogram and should be avoided in patients with congenital long QT syndrome (Am Heart J 1986;111:1088–1093)

Previous torsades de pointes associated with class IA antiarrhythmic agents

- quinidine should not be used in patients who have previously experienced torsades de pointes in association with a class IA antiarrhythmic drug

▶ *What Drug Interactions Are Clinically Important?*

Drugs that may increase the effect or toxicity of quinidine

AMIODARONE

- amiodarone increases serum quinidine concentrations
- if amiodarone therapy is initiated in patients taking quinidine therapy, the quinidine dosage should be reduced by 25–50%
- if a target serum concentration has not been determined, monitor the patient over the next few days for either adverse effects or arrhythmia recurrence
- if a target serum concentration has been determined in the past, measure a serum concentration within 2–3 days and ensure that the drug concentration remains above this target level

ACETAZOLAMIDE OR ANTACID

- agents that alkalinize the urine may result in increases in the proportion of un-ionized quinidine, resulting in increased renal tubular reabsorption of the drug (Ann Intern Med 1969;71:927–933)

CIMETIDINE

- cimetidine therapy inhibits the hepatic metabolism of quinidine, resulting in increased serum quinidine concentrations (Am J Cardiol 1983;52:172–175)
- switch to ranitidine or other H_2 antagonist if a combination must be used, as these agents have less of an effect on metabolism

Drugs that may decrease the effect of quinidine

PHENOBARBITAL, PHENYTOIN, RIFAMPIN

- may induce the hepatic metabolism of quinidine, resulting in decreased serum quinidine concentrations (N Engl J Med 1976;294:699–702, N Engl J Med 1981;304:1466–1469)
- after the initiation of phenobarbital, phenytoin, or rifampin therapy, the patient should be monitored for arrhythmia recurrence
- if a target serum concentration has been determined in the past, measure a serum concentration within 2–3 days and ensure that the drug concentration remains above this target level

Drugs that may have their effect or toxicity increased by quinidine

DIGOXIN

- quinidine therapy has been reported to result in 2- to 3-fold elevations in serum digoxin concentrations, which may occur as early as several hours after the initiation of quinidine therapy (N Engl J Med 1979;301:400–404, Int J Cardiol 1981;1:109–116)

- when quinidine therapy is added in patients receiving digoxin, decrease the digoxin dosage by 50% when starting quinidine therapy and make further dosage changes on the basis of clinical response
- if digoxin toxicity is suspected, measure a serum concentration

WARFARIN

- quinidine may potentiate the hypoprothrombinemic effects of warfarin (Ann Intern Med 1968;68:511–517)
- monitor INR every 2 days until the full extent of interaction is seen and adjust the dosage as for a warfarin dosage change

Drugs that may have their effect decreased by quinidine

- none

▶ *What Route and Dosage Should I Use?*

How to administer

- orally—may be taken with or without food
- parenterally—avoid because of hypotensive effects
- efficacy and toxicity of quinidine are related primarily to the amount of quinidine base administered
- different salts of quinidine contain different amounts of quinidine base
- the relative amounts of quinidine base in different quinidine salts is as follows:

quinidine gluconate 324 mg = 200.9 mg of quinidine base (62%)

quinidine sulfate 200 mg = 166 mg of quinidine base (83%)

quinidine polygalacturonate 275 mg = 165 mg of quinidine base (60%)

quinidine bisulfate 250 mg = 166 mg of quinidine base (66%)

- selection of a quinidine salt should be based on the dosing schedule and cost
- bisulfate products (not available in the USA) allow twice-daily administration (versus Q6H for the sulfate)
- quinidine gluconate (TID administration) may be the most cost effective quinidine salt in the USA

Atrial fibrillation or flutter, atrioventricular nodal reentrant tachycardia, Wolff-Parkinson-White syndrome

- 200 mg of quinidine sulfate PO Q2H until conversion is achieved or a maximum dosage of 1200 mg PO in 12 hours is reached (Am J Cardiol 1986;58:496–498)
- follow the loading dose with a longer-acting agent such as 324 mg PO TID of quinidine gluconate or 500 mg PO BID of quinidine bisulfate (not available in the USA)
- although an intravenous form of quinidine is available, intravenous administration of quinidine is not recommended, because severe hypotension may result

Ventricular premature depolarizations, ventricular tachycardia

- give 324 mg PO TID of quinidine gluconate and increase to 486 mg PO TID in 48 hours if it is well tolerated and arrhythmia is not suppressed (can be increased to 648 mg PO TID in another 48 hours if needed)
- give 500 mg PO BID of quinidine bisulfate, and increase to 750 mg PO BID in 48 hours if it is well tolerated and arrhythmia is not suppressed (can be increased to 1000 mg PO BID in another 48 hours if needed)

Dosage adjustments for renal or hepatic dysfunction

- hepatically metabolized (50–90%)
- dosage reduction is not required in patients with renal dysfunction
- no recommendations for hepatic dysfunction (titrate the dose on the basis of effectiveness and toxicity)

▶ *What Should I Monitor with Regard to Efficacy and Toxicity?*

Efficacy

Atrial fibrillation or flutter, atrioventricular nodal reentrant tachycardia, Wolff-Parkinson-White syndrome, ventricular premature depolarizations, ventricular tachycardia

Electrocardiography or Holter monitoring

- presence or absence of arrhythmia and reduced frequency of arrhythmia episodes

- should promote cardioversion within 12–24 hours; if not, continue quinidine administration until electrical cardioversion can be performed or switch to another drug

Vital signs

- symptoms associated with arrhythmia (palpitations, shortness of breath, chest pain, or syncope)

Serum quinidine concentration

- for each patient, there may exist a specific threshold concentration above which a desired effect is seen
- some clinicians recommend measuring the drug concentration associated with therapeutic success to serve as a target for long-term therapy (Clin Pharmacokinet 1991;20:151–166)
- these clinicians suggest that subsequent failure of therapy could be evaluated on the basis of maintenance of drug concentrations above this established benchmark
- however, this assumes that the threshold for efficacy does not change with time
- serum quinidine concentration can be determined when efficacy is determined (a target concentration)
- if the patient experiences a recurrence of the arrhythmia being treated, a serum quinidine concentration should be determined, and if it is below the previously determined target level, the dose should be increased to elevate the serum quinidine concentration to the previously determined target level
- if the patient experiences no arrhythmia recurrences, a serum quinidine concentration should be determined every 6 months, and if it is below the previously determined target level, the dose should be increased to elevate the serum quinidine concentration to the previously determined target level (Clin Pharmacokinet 1991;20:151–166)

Toxicity

Adverse effects necessitating discontinuation of therapy occur in approximately 5–36% of patients

Nausea, vomiting, diarrhea, cinchonism (tinnitus, blurred vision, confusion, and delirium)

- dose-related and commonly seen early in therapy
- quinidine dosage should be reduced in patients who experience adverse gastrointestinal effects or signs or symptoms of cinchonism
- if the dosage is reduced, recurrence of arrhythmias must be closely monitored

Rash, fever

- question the patient after 1 week
- if a rash occurs, drug administration discontinuation is usually needed

Anaphylaxis

- extremely uncommon with quinidine, and if it occurs, the drug should never be used again in that patient

Hemolytic anemia, thrombocytopenia

- question the patient regarding any bruising at the first visit; measure red blood cell and platelet values prior to and 1 month after the initiation of therapy

Hepatitis

- question and examine the patient at each visit for signs of jaundice or hepatic tenderness
- obtain liver enzyme concentrations every 6 months, and if the increase is greater than 2–3 times over baseline values, it may be best to stop quinidine administration and try a different agent

Electrocardiogram

- monitor for prolonged PR interval (>0.2 second), prolonged duration of the QT interval (>25% compared with baseline values), and initiation of new arrhythmia or worsening of clinical arrhythmia at 1 week after the initiation of quinidine therapy and every 3–6 months thereafter
- quinidine dosage should be reduced in patients with prolongation of the QT interval greater than 25% compared with baseline values

▶ *How Long Do I Treat Patients with This Drug?*

Atrial fibrillation or flutter, atrioventricular nodal reentrant tachycardia, ventricular premature depolarizations, ventricular tachycardia

- patients treated for the prevention of episodes of atrial fibrillation or flutter, PSVT, or ventricular tachyarrhythmias may require therapy indefinitely if contributing factors cannot be reversed

Wolff-Parkinson-White syndrome

- patients with Wolff-Parkinson-White syndrome require therapy until arrhythmia cure can be achieved using catheter ablation techniques
- if arrhythmia cure cannot be achieved, therapy may be required indefinitely

▶ *How Do I Decrease or Stop the Administration of This Drug?*

- may be stopped abruptly
- do not decrease the dosage or discontinue therapy without consulting a cardiologist or a cardiac electrophysiologist

▶ *What Should I Tell My Patients About This Drug?*

- if you experience nausea, vomiting, diarrhea, ringing of the ears or any other hearing disturbances, blurred vision, confusion, rash, bruising, or fever, notify your physician
- if you have palpitations, shortness of breath, chest pain, or dizziness, contact your physician
- do not discontinue quinidine therapy without consulting your physician

▶ *Therapeutic Tips*

- quinidine can have idiosyncratic proarrhythmic effects unrelated to the dosage or the duration of therapy
- lightheadedness or dizziness in the first few days of therapy may be the result of tachyarrhythmias induced by quinidine

Useful References

Cohen IS, Jick H, Cohen SI. Adverse reactions to quinidine in hospitalized patients: Findings based on data from the Boston Collaborative Drug Surveillance Program. Prog Cardiovasc Dis 1977;20:151–163

Greenblatt DJ, Pfeifer HJ, Ochs HR, et al. Pharmacokinetics of quinidine in humans after intravenous, intramuscular and oral administration. J Pharmacol Exp Ther 1977;202:365–378

Boissel JP, Wolf E, Gillet J, et al. Controlled trial of a long-acting quinidine for maintenance of sinus rhythm after conversion of sustained atrial fibrillation. Eur Heart J 1981;2:49–55

DiMarco JP, Garan H, Ruskin JN. Quinidine for ventricular arrhythmias: Value of electrophysiologic testing. Am J Cardiol 1983;51:90–95

Coplen SE, Antman EM, Berlin JA, et al. Efficacy and safety of quinidine therapy for maintenance of sinus rhythm after cardioversion. A meta-analysis of randomized control trials. Circulation 1990;82:1106–1116

RAMIPRIL

Jack Onrot and James McCormack

USA (Altace)
CANADA (Altace)

▶ *When Should I Use This Drug?*

see Enalapril

▶ *When Should I Not Use This Drug?*

see Enalapril

▶ *What Contraindications Are There to the Use of This Drug?*

see Captopril

▶ *What Drug Interactions Are Clinically Important?*

see Captopril

▶ *What Route and Dosage Should I Use?*

How to administer

- orally—can be administered with or without food
- parenterally—not available

Congestive heart failure

- 1.25 mg PO daily
- rapidity of dosage escalation depends on the severity of symptoms
- in general, increase doses weekly, however, dosages may be increased daily if necessary
- no value in exceeding a total daily dosage of 20 mg

Chronic (noncrisis) hypertension

- 1.25 mg PO daily
- increase dosage by 1.25 mg PO daily every 4 weeks until adequate blood pressure is achieved or a daily dosage of 10 mg is reached
- limited value in exceeding a total daily dosage of 10 mg (dosages as high as 20 mg PO daily have been used)
- for some patients, the antihypertensive effect may be diminished before 24 hours and twice-daily dosing may be required (Inpharma 1993;881:5)

Dosage adjustments for renal or hepatic dysfunction

- renal and biliary elimination
- titrate the dosage to clinical response and not concurrent renal or hepatic function

▶ **What Should I Monitor with Regard to Efficacy and Toxicity?**

see Captopril

▶ **How Long Do I Treat Patients with This Drug?**

see Captopril

▶ **How Do I Decrease or Stop the Administration of This Drug?**

see Captopril

▶ **What Should I Tell My Patients About This Drug?**

see Captopril

▶ **Therapeutic Tips**

see Captopril

RANITIDINE

James McCormack and Glen Brown

USA (Zantac)
CANADA (Zantac, Apo-Ranitidine, Novo-Ranidine)

▶ **When Should I Use This Drug?**

Dyspepsia, duodenal or gastric ulcers, prevention of peptic ulcer disease recurrence, gastroesophageal reflux

- use cimetidine unless the patient is taking drugs that specifically interact with cimetidine
- ranitidine appears to have less potential to affect hepatic metabolism; however, be aware that hepatic metabolism interactions have been reported with all H_2 antagonists (Arch Intern Med 1991;151:810–815)
- if the patient is taking drugs that have the potential to interact with cimetidine, choose ranitidine, famotidine, or nizatidine, whichever is the least expensive

Stress ulcer prophylaxis

- for patients with extensive burns, central nervous system injury, prolonged hypotension, sepsis, uncorrectable coagulopathy, acute respiratory failure (undergoing ventilation) or hepatic failure (Am J Gastroenterol 1990;85:95–96) who cannot receive sucralfate by gastric administration
- use the least expensive parenteral H_2 antagonist

▶ **When Should I Not Use This Drug?**

Prior to anesthesia for prophylaxis of aspiration pneumonitis

- cimetidine, which is less expensive than ranitidine, can be used for this indication, even in patients taking interacting drugs because cimetidine will be used for only 1 dose
  see Cimetidine

▶ **What Contraindications Are There to the Use of This Drug?**

- intolerance of or allergic reaction to ranitidine

▶ **What Drug Interactions Are Clinically Important?**

Drugs that may increase the effect or toxicity of ranitidine

- none

Drugs that may decrease the effect of ranitidine

ANTACIDS

- antacids decrease absorption of H_2 antagonists; therefore do not take antacids within 1 hour of taking an H_2 antagonist

Drugs that may have their effect or toxicity increased by ranitidine

- none

Drugs that may have their effect decreased by ranitidine

KETOCONAZOLE, IRON

- decreased gastric acidity reduces ketoconazole and iron absorption (Clin Pharm 1988;7:228–233)
- administer ketoconazole or iron at least 2 hours prior to H_2 antagonists, and be aware that absorption of ketoconazole or iron may still be decreased to some extent

▶ **What Route and Dosage Should I Use?**

How to administer

Orally

- may be given with food or on an empty stomach

Parenterally

- dilute to 20 mL and inject over not less than 5 minutes
- dilute to 100 mL and infuse over 15–20 minutes

Dyspepsia or duodenal or gastric ulcers

- 300 mg PO at bedtime or with the evening meal is as effective as 150 mg PO BID and is more convenient for the patient (Curr Ther Res 1986;40:893–897)
- 150 mg PO BID if the patient has frequent daytime ulcer pain

Prevention of peptic ulcer disease recurrence

- 150 mg PO at bedtime

Gastroesophageal reflux

- 150 mg PO BID
- 150 mg PO at bedtime if the patient has only nighttime symptoms

Stress ulcer prophylaxis

- give 50 mg IV Q8H or 0.125 mg/kg/h IV as continuous infusion and titrate to maintain gastric pH of greater than 4 at all times
- infusion is not clinically superior (although it does produce better pH control) to intermittent therapy and should be used only if it is more practical or economical than intermittent injections
- analysis of aspirates of gastric fluid should be done Q4H and the dosage increased in 25 mg increments to maintain gastric pH of greater than 4 at all times

Dosage adjustments for renal or hepatic dysfunction

- renally eliminated

Normal Dosing Interval	$C_{cr} > 60$ mL/min or 1 mL/s	C_{cr} 30–60 mL/min or 0.5–1 mL/s	$C_{cr} < 30$ mL/min or 0.5 mL/s
Q8H	no adjustment needed	Q12H	Q24H
Q12H	no adjustment needed	Q24H	Q24H and decrease dosage by 50%
Q24H or by infusion	no adjustment needed	decrease dosage by 50%	decrease dosage by 75%

▶ *What Should I Monitor with Regard to Efficacy and Toxicity?*

see Cimetidine

▶ *How Long Do I Treat Patients with This Drug?*

see Cimetidine

▶ *How do I Decrease or Stop the Administration of This Drug?*

- may be stopped abruptly

▶ *What Should I Tell My Patients About This Drug?*

- it may take several days for this drug to relieve stomach pain
- if no relief of symptoms is seen in 7 days, contact your physician
- if symptoms are not completely resolved after 6 weeks, contact your physician
- for peptic ulcer disease, take the drug for the full 6 weeks, even if symptoms disappear after 1–2 weeks
- contact your physician if you have any excessive dizziness or confusion

▶ *Therapeutic Tips*

- ensure that the drug dosage has been adjusted for renal function
- anyone who has been taking any full-dose H₂ antagonist regimen for longer than 8 weeks must be evaluated to determine need for continued therapy
- at least 50% of patients being given H₂ antagonists for longer than 8 weeks are receiving them for inappropriate indications (J Am Geriatr Soc 1987;35:1023–1027, DICP 1987;21:452–458)
- use only 150 mg PO at bedtime for prevention of ulcer recurrence

RIFAMPIN (RIFAMPICIN)

Ann Beardsell

USA (Rifadin, Rimactane)
CANADA (Rifadin, Rimactane, Rofact)

▶ *When Should I Use This Drug?*

Mycobacterium avium infection

- used in conjuction with other antimycobacterial agents owing to the rapid development of resistance when only 1 drug is used alone
- *Mycobacterium avium–intracellulare* is less sensitive and responsive to these agents and response may be slow

Tuberculosis

- is a major agent in the treatment of pulmonary and extrapulmonary tuberculosis and is always used in inital treatment unless the organism is resistant or rifampin is contraindicated
- used in combination with other antituberculosis drugs, depending on the type and sensitivity of the organism and the protocol being used to prevent resistance to any 1 of the drugs

Meningococcus carriers

- used as prophylaxis against meningococcal meningitis by eradicating nasopharyngeal *Neisseria meningitidis* in asymptomatic carriers

Haemophilus influenzae carriers

- used as prophylaxis against *H. influenzae* type B infection by eradicating oronasopharyngeal *H. influenzae* type B in carriers and contacts of patients with *H. influenzae*

Leprosy

- used in combination with other antiinfectives (dapsone, clofazimine, and possibly ethionamide)

▶ *When Should I Not Use This Drug?*

Single agent in the treatment of tuberculosis

- as a single agent, because resistance rapidly develops when it is used alone

▶ *What Contraindications Are There to the Use of This Drug?*

- intolerance of or allergic reaction to rifampin

▶ *What Drug Interactions Are Clinically Important?*

Drugs that may increase the effect or toxicity of rifampin

- none

Drugs that may decrease the effect of rifampin

- none

Drugs that may have their effect or toxicity increased by rifampin

- none

Drugs that may have their effect decreased by rifampin

CHLORAMPHENICOL, CLOFIBRATE, CORTICOSTEROIDS, CYCLOSPORINE, DAPSONE, DIAZEPAM, DIGOXIN, ESTROGENS, KETOCONAZOLE, ORAL CONTRACEPTIVES, ORAL ANTICOAGULANTS, PHENYTOIN, THEOPHYLLINE, VERAPAMIL

- rifampin is one of the most powerful inducers of microsomal hepatic enzymes and can increase the metabolism of a number of drugs, and the efficacy of all these drugs may be compromised, resulting in loss of control of the disease state being treated

ORAL CONTRACEPTIVES

- patients requiring rifampin and taking oral contraceptives should be advised to use other forms of birth control

VERAPAMIL

- may substantially reduce the oral bioavailability of verapamil by increasing first-pass metabolism via the induction of hepatic microsomal enzymes
- be aware of this effect and monitor within a few days for reduced clinical efficacy or for toxicity whenever concomitant administration of these agents is initiated or discontinued, respectively (adjust the dosage of verapamil on the basis of changes in effect or toxicity)
- patients may require a switch to a different agent

WARFARIN

- interferes with warfarin metabolism and can decrease INR
- use alternative agents if possible
- if not, monitor INR every 2 days until the full extent of interaction is seen, and adjust the dosage as for a warfarin dosage change
- monitor INR every 2 days when administration of the rifampin is discontinued and adjust as for a dosage change of warfarin

KETOCONAZOLE

- concomitant use of rifampin and ketoconazole may result in therapeutic levels of rifampin but subtherapeutic levels of ketoconazole, regardless of the spacing of drug administration times
- if the existing dosage is ineffective, consider increasing the dosage
- if this does not work, fluconazole may be tried, but rifampin may also decrease serum concentrations of fluconazole

▶ *What Route and Dosage Should I Use?*

How to administer

- orally—should be administered on an empty stomach 1 hour before or 2 hours after meals
- parenterally—parenteral form available through the emergency drug release program of Health Protection Branch (Canada)

Mycobacterium avium infection

- 600 mg PO daily

Tuberculosis

- 10 mg/kg (up to 600 mg) PO daily

Meningococcal prophylaxis

- 600 mg PO daily for 4 days

Haemophilus influenzae **prophylaxis**

- 20 mg/kg PO daily (up to 600 mg) for 4 days

Leprosy

- 600 mg PO daily for 6 months

Dosage adjustments for renal or hepatic dysfunction

- hepatically metabolized
- no dosage adjustments are required

▶ *What Should I Monitor with Regard to Efficacy and Toxicity?*

Efficacy

***Mycobacterium avium* infection**

Signs and symptoms

- fevers, chills, night sweats, malaise, fatigue, weight loss, abdominal pain, and diarrhea
- there are few or no physical signs to follow, other than body weight or possibly the presence of a lesion in patients with localized disease (e.g., regional lymphadenopathy)
- patients should also be advised to report new or worsening diarrhea while taking such regimens, because *Clostridium difficile* colitis is a possible complication
- patients should be assessed every 1–2 weeks during the first 1–2 months of treatment

Complete blood count

- monthly or more frequently if there is severe disease, to detect progressive anemia and cytopenias due to bone marrow involvement, which may persist despite treatment

Blood cultures

- to document reduction or clearance of mycobacteremia, particularly in patients who have persistent symptoms

Tuberculosis

- disease improvement or resolution of symptoms such as fevers, sweats, and weight loss

Leprosy

- tissue stain smears, which should become negative with time
- skin lesions may take 8–12 weeks to show improvement, depending on the severity of disease

Toxicity

Discoloration of body tissues

- may color body fluids such as saliva, sputum, tears, sweat, urine, and feces reddish orange, which is of no concern except that soft contact lenses may be permanently stained

Gastrointestinal effects

- these are the most common type of adverse effects and include nausea, vomiting, diarrhea, heartburn, epigastric distress, anorexia, abdominal cramps and pain, and gas
- treat symptomatically, but if gastrointestinal upset continues, rifampin may be given with food
- if gastrointestinal effects are severe, discontinue rifampin administration (in general, severe gastrointestinal upset is rare but more commonly seen in patients with human immunodeficiency virus infection who have *M. avium* infection)

Hepatic

- rifampin can cause transient elevations in liver function test results early in treatment, but they usually return to normal values
- monitor aspartate aminotransferase, alanine aminotransferase, bilirubin, and alkaline phosphatase levels monthly, especially in patients with preexisting hepatic dysfunction, concomitant administration of hepatotoxic medications, and history of concurrent alcohol intake
- in rare cases in which jaundice and hepatitis occur, discontinue rifampin therapy

Dermatological effects

- are usually mild in nature, occur early in treatment, and include flushing, rash, and itching of the face and neck
- treat symptomatically

Hypersensitivity

- some patients experience an influenza-like syndrome consisting of fever, chills, headache, dizziness, and bone pain
- reaction is most commonly seen with intermittent therapy (given twice weekly or stopped and then restarted), occurs after several months, and is more prevalent in women
- syndrome can be controlled by reducing the dosage or changing to a daily regimen
- if shortness of breath, hemolytic anemia, or renal failure occur, discontinue the drug administration permanently

Neurological effects

- headache, confusion, ataxia, fatigue, drowsiness, numbness, muscle weakness, and joint pain have been seen, especially early in therapy
- manage symptomatically

▶ *How Long Do I Treat Patients with This Drug?*

***Mycobacterium avium* infection**

- indefinitely as tolerated

Tuberculosis

- 6 or 9 months, depending on the regimen

Meningococcal prophylaxis

- 4 days

***Haemophilus influenzae* prophylaxis**

- 4 days

Leprosy

- 6 months

▶ *How Do I Decrease or Stop the Administration of This Drug?*

- may be stopped abruptly

▶ *What Should I Tell My Patients About This Drug?*

- rifampin is generally well tolerated
- take this medication on an empty stomach, 1 hour before or 2 hours after meals; if you experience stomach upset, you may try taking it with food
- if nausea, vomiting, and diarrhea occur, they are usually transient and should resolve in 2–4 weeks; however, if the symptoms persist, contact your physician
- rifampin causes body fluids, such as sweat, urine, saliva, sputum, tears, and feces, to turn red orange, and soft contact lenses should not be worn, as they will be stained permanently

▶ *Therapeutic Tips*

- patients having difficulty in swallowing the capsules can mix powder in a small amount of applesauce or jam
- commonly, the cause of gastrointestinal upset in combination therapies

RITODRINE

Glenda Meneilly

USA (Yutopar)
CANADA (Yutopar)

▶ *When Should I Use This Drug?*

Premature labor

- if the onset of labor is between 24 and 32 weeks' gestation with documented uterine contractions occurring every 7–10 minutes for 30–60 minutes, each lasting 30 seconds; with ruptured membranes or intact membranes, if there are documented cervical

changes or cervical effacement of 80% or dilation of more than 2 cm
- if the patient has not responded to bed rest, oral hydration, or mild sedation
- drug of choice if the patient does not have cardiac disease (arrythmias or congestive heart failure), suspected infection, or hyperthyroidism
- the greatest worldwide experience in tocolysis is with ritodrine, and ritodrine is the only drug approved by the US Food and Drug Administration for the treatment of preterm labor
- because perinatal morbidity and mortality are not altered, the indication for tocolysis is to delay delivery long enough to administer glucocorticoids to the mother to hasten fetal pulmonary maturation

▶ When Should I Not Use This Drug?

Any time immediate delivery is indicated

- major maternal illness that cannot be controlled, eclampsia or severe preeclampsia, abruptio placenta, severe fetal anomaly (incompatible with life), and fetal demise
- if ritodrine is used in the presence of ruptured membranes, there should be no evidence of chorioamnionitis

▶ What Contraindications Are There to the Use of This Drug?

Intolerance of or allergic reaction to ritodrine

Maternal history of cardiac disease, especially arrhythmias or congestive heart failure

- beta-agonists cause fluid overload through an antidiuretic effect at high doses
- beta-agonists may also cause cardiac arrhythmias

Maternal hyperthyroidism

- owing to enhanced cardiovascular beta-adrenergic response

▶ What Drug Interactions Are Clinically Important?

Drugs that may increase the effect or toxicity of ritodrine

CORTICOSTEROIDS

- corticosteroids may potentiate the risk of pulmonary edema
- while no extra monitoring is required, the clinician should be aware of the increased risk with this combination

MAGNESIUM

- magnesium may potentiate the cardiovascular effects of ritodrine
- while no extra monitoring is required, the clinician should be aware of the increased risk with this combination

Drugs that may decrease the effect of ritodrine

BETA BLOCKERS

- beta-adrenergic blocking agents antagonize the effects of ritodrine
- if they must be used together, give a beta$_1$-selective blocker such as atenolol

Drugs that may have their effect or toxicity increased by ritodrine

- none

Drugs that may have their effect decreased by ritodrine

- none

▶ What Route and Dosage Should I Use?

How to administer

Orally

- take with food or milk to reduce stomach irritation

Parenterally

- administer by intravenous infusion in 5% dextrose in water, using an infusion control device
- can be given intramuscularly if there is not intravenous access

Premature labor

- dilute 150 mg in 500 mL of 5% dextrose in water and start the infusion at 20 mL/h (100 μg/min)

- increase by 50 μg/min (10 mL/h) every 15 minutes until uterine contractions stop, to a maximum of 350 μg/min (70 mL/h)
- maintain the infusion rate for 1 hour, then decrease the infusion by 50 μg/min every 30 minutes to achieve the lowest infusion rate that sustains inhibition (Am J Obstet Gynecol 1990;162:429–437)

Dosage adjustments for renal or hepatic dysfunction

- hepatically metabolized
- in patients with hepatic disease, start with 50 μg/min and increase by 25 μg/min every 15 minutes

▶ What Should I Monitor with Regard to Efficacy and Toxicity?

Efficacy

Premature labor

Uterine activity

- monitor uterine contractions continually while intravenous dosage increases are being made, and at least every hour when a stable infusion dosage has been attained
- attempt to reduce contractions to 4 per hour or less

Cervical dilation and effacement

- monitor cervical dilation and effacement 1–2 hours after the initiation of therapy and then no more frequently than every 12 hours
- attempt to maintain less than 4 cm dilation and 80% effacement

Toxicity

Cardiovascular effects

- do a baseline electrocardiogram (ECG) prior to therapy to rule out maternal cardiac disease
- measure the maternal and fetal heart rate every 15 minutes
- decrease the infusion rate by 25% if the maternal heart rate is greater than 130 bpm or the fetal heart rate is greater than 160 bpm)
- increased maternal systolic blood pressure and decreased diastolic blood pressure (monitor blood pressure and decrease the infusion rate if the blood pressure is less than 90/50)
- if chest pain occurs, reduce the dosage, and do an ECG and chest X-ray

Pulmonary effects

- shortness of breath or pulmonary edema due to activation of renin-angiotensin system (incidence, 3–9%) (N Engl J Med 1992; 327:349–351)
- limit total fluid intake to 80 mL/h; do not infuse ritodrine in saline solutions
- monitor fluid status in patients concurrently receiving corticosteroids
- incidence of pulmonary edema is higher if maternal infection is present (Am J Obstet Gynecol 1988;159:723–728)

Metabolic effects

- maternal hyperglycemia and hypokalemia can occur
- measure blood glucose and electrolyte levels every 12 hours (every 6 hours in diabetics) during intravenous therapy and treat with insulin or/and potassium replacement

Other effects

- palpitations, tremor, nausea, vomiting, headaches, nervousness, and anxiety
- decrease the infusion rate if symptoms are intolerable

▶ How Long Do I Treat Patients with This Drug?

Premature labor

- ritodrine intravenous infusion should continue until 12 hours after uterine activity has ceased, or 24 hours after the last dose of corticosteroids

▶ How Do I Decrease or Stop the Administration of This Drug?

- may be stopped abruptly
- when contractions have ceased for 12 hours, decrease the infusion rate by 50 μg/min every 30 minutes until the drug is discontinued

- if contractions recur, increase infusion rate to previous effective dose

▶ What Should I Tell My Patients About This Drug?

- you may experience some palpitations, nausea, headache, or flushing while you are taking this medication
- notify your physician of any dizziness, palpitations, chest pain or tightness, or difficulty in breathing
- notify your physician immediately if contractions begin or your water breaks
- do not take any over the counter cold products without consulting your pharmacist or physician

▶ Therapeutic Tips

- tachycardia, hypotension, and nausea may respond to a decrease in infusion rate
- to minimize the incidence of circulatory overload or pulmonary edema, avoid the use of saline solutions
- keep intravenous fluids to a minimum and use the lowest effective infusion rate

Useful References

Caritis SN, Darby MJ, Chan L. Pharmacologic treatment of preterm labor. Clin Obstet Gynecol 1988;31:429–437

Higby K, Xenakis EM-J, Paverstein CJ. Do tocolytic agents stop preterm labor? A critical and comprehensive review of efficacy and safety. Am J Obstet Gynecol 1993;168:1247–1259

Canadian Preterm Labor Investigators Groups. Treatment of preterm labor with the beta-adrenergic agonist ritodrine. N Engl J Med 1992;327:308–312

SALBUTAMOL, ALBUTEROL (IN USA)

Karen Shalansky and Cindy Reesor Nimmo

USA (Proventil, Ventolin)
CANADA (Novosalmol, Ventodisks, Ventolin)

▶ When Should I Use This Drug?

Acute asthma or acute exacerbation of chronic obstructive pulmonary disease, chronic asthma, or chronic obstructive pulmonary disease

- first-line treatment for intermittent, short-term, or long-term relief of reversible obstructive diseases
- it is beta$_2$-selective, works quickly (within minutes), is safe for short-term use, and is inexpensive
- terbutaline may be used if it is less expensive than salbutamol
- fenoterol is not recommended, as it has been associated with a substantially higher incidence of side effects (Clin Pharm 1985;4:393–403, Chest 1978;73:348–351, Am Rev Respir Dis 1989;139:176–180) and a possible increase in asthmatic deaths (Lancet 1989;1:917–922, N Engl J Med 1992;326:501–506)

Exercise-induced asthma

- effective, well tolerated, and less expensive than cromolyn
- salbutamol is also useful if the patient experiences breakthrough wheezing

▶ When Should I Not Use This Drug?

Allergic rhinitis, cough, or cold symptoms

- unless there is evidence of bronchoconstrictive disease (e.g., wheezing)

Oral therapy

- oral salbutamol should not be used in adults, as it offers no benefit over inhaled salbutamol and causes more side effects

▶ What Contraindications Are There to the Use of This Drug?

Intolerance of or allergy to salbutamol
Preexisting tachyarrhythmias or ischemic heart disease

- salbutamol may exacerbate preexisting cardiac tachyarrhythmias or provoke myocardial ischemia by increasing inotropy and chronotropy
- this is not an absolute contraindication if the patient absolutely requires salbutamol

- for the first few doses, monitor for increases in heart rate and the development of chest pain, and if they occur, stop the drug administration and try other alternatives

▶ What Drug Interactions Are Clinically Important?

Drugs that may increase the effect or toxicity of salbutamol

- none

Drugs that may decrease the effect of salbutamol

BETA-BLOCKERS

- beta-blockers (even beta$_1$-selective and partial agonist agents) are a definite contraindication in patients with asthma, as they can cause bronchoconstriction, antagonism of the effect of salbutamol, and worsening of asthma

Drugs that may have their effect or toxicity increased by salbutamol

- none

Drugs that may have their effect decreased by salbutamol

- none

▶ What Route and Dosage Should I Use?

How to administer

Orally

- do not use

Inhaled

- dilute each nebulized dose to 4 mL with normal saline (water, half-normal saline, or hypertonic saline may be used), place in the nebulizer, and use an airflow rate of 6–8 L/min
- for metered-dose inhalers (MDIs), see patient instructions below

Parenterally

- dilute 5 mg or 10 mg in 250 mL of IV fluid to make a 20 μg/mL or 40 μg/mL dilution, respectively

Acute asthma or acute exacerbation of chronic obstructive pulmonary disease

- aggressive therapy is indicated in an acute attack
- in acute exacerbations of airflow obstruction, there is decreased penetration, deposition, and duration of action of aerosols in the peripheral airways, necessitating higher dosages for emergency treatment (N Engl J Med 1986;315:870–874)

Metered-dose inhaler

- MDIs have been shown to be as effective as nebulizers with salbutamol for the treatment of acute asthma (Chest 1987;91:804–807) and are currently the preferred mode of inhalation owing to the reduced cost and improved efficiency and speed of drug delivery (Chest 1989;95:888–894)
- patients who are unable to coordinate the inhalation of an MDI may benefit from the use of an extension device
- 4 puffs over 2 minutes, then 1 puff every minute until side effects such as tremor occur or until breathlessness and flow rates improve
- repeat 4 puffs every 20–30 minutes for 3 doses then every 1–2 hours until the patient is stable; maintain with 2 puffs every 4–6 hours
- beta$_2$-agonists administered by an MDI or by a nebulizer are equally effective (Chest 1987;91:804–807)
- MDI should be used with an extension device or facemask for acute asthma
- nebulizer should be used in patients who are distressed or require oxygen to be given at the same time as the salbutamol
- each puff of salbutamol releases 100 μg of active drug

Nebulizer

- nebulizer should be used for patients who are distressed or require oxygen to be given at the same time as the salbutamol
- 5 mg repeated every 20 minutes for 3 doses, then every 1–2 hours until the patient is stable
- use 2.5 mg if patients experience side effects such as tremor and tachycardia

- maintain with 2.5 mg every 4–6 hours
- each dose is delivered over 10–15 minutes

Intravenous use

- use in patients who do not respond to inhalation therapy (Thorax 1977;32:555–558)
- initiate at 5 μg/min, and increase by 5–10 μg/min at 15–30 minute intervals to 30–40 μg/min as tolerated (heart rate < 120 bpm)

Chronic asthma or chronic obstructive pulmonary disease

Metered-dose inhaler

- administer 1–2 puffs every 4–6 hours as needed
- if patients require more than 2 inhalations daily on a regular basis, it is now recommended to initiate low-dose inhaled steroid and maintain salbutamol on a PRN basis; continual use of a beta-agonist may lead to deterioration of asthma control (Lancet 1990;336:1391–1395)
- may require extension device in patients with difficulty in coordination

Rotahaler or Diskhaler

- may be preferred to an MDI if patients have difficulty in coordination
- 100 μg by MDI is equivalent to 200 μg by powder delivery system
- administer 1–2 inhalations (200–400 μg) every 4–6 hours as needed

Nebulizer

- 1.25–2.5 mg every 4–6 hours as required
- drug may be diluted immediately prior to use or may be prepared in bulk if normal saline with a preservative (e.g., benzalkonium chloride 0.01%) is used
- bulk solution is stable for 6 months but should be discarded 1 month after opening the bottle

Exercise-induced asthma

- inhale 1–2 puffs about 10 minutes prior to exercise

▶ What Should I Monitor with Regard to Efficacy and Toxicity?

Efficacy

Acute asthma or acute exacerbation of chronic obstructive pulmonary disease

For severe acute asthma, assess the patient after each dose of inhaled bronchodilator and until improvement is seen

Heart rate, degree of respiratory distress, and presence of cyanosis
Peak expiratory flow rate

- should be measured before treatment if possible
- measure after treatment to assess the effect of treatment
- patients with an acute attack should be given a peak flow gauge and should record peak expiratory flow rate (PEFR) at least twice daily

Forced expiratory volume in 1 second

- assess once to determine the reversibility of bronchoconstriction
- reversibility is indicated by an increase of 15–20% in forced expiratory volume in 1 second (FEV_1) after bronchodilator use

Arterial blood gases

- if the patient has a PEFR less than 40% of predicted value or is not responding to treatment
- repeat within 24 hours if blood carbon dioxide level is elevated or the patient is fatiguing

Chronic asthma or chronic obstructive pulmonary disease

Frequency of as needed beta$_2$-agonist use
Pulmonary function tests

- can be used to assess effectiveness of long-term therapy; however, some patients taking salbutamol do not have a demonstrable effect on pulmonary function tests but become clinically improved (increased walking distance, decreased use of PRN medications)

Peak expiratory flow rate

- peak flowmeter should be used by patients who experience severe attacks with little warning and patients who have symptoms of breathlessness or chest tightness repeatedly or require regular Q6H to Q8H beta$_2$-agonist therapy (J Allergy Clin Immunol 1990;85:1098–1111)
- establish best PEFR early in therapy
- usually measured on waking and before bed and before and after beta$_2$-agonist dose (minimum of twice daily [e.g., morning and evening]) and is the best of 3 measurements on each occasion
- daily variation should be less than 20% and ideally less than 10%

Toxicity

Side effects are generally dose related and occur more frequently with systemic formulations but can still be seen with repeated doses of inhaled salbutamol

Tachycardia (common), palpitations (uncommon), arrhythmias (rare)

- measure heart rate and blood pressure prior to each dose if being given more frequently than every 4 hours
- continuous ECG monitoring should be done during intravenous therapy
- due to beta$_2$ effects
- reduce the dosage to minimally effective levels if these effects occur

Tremor (up to 20% of patients)

- due to beta$_2$ effects
- may improve with continued use; if not, reduce the dosage to minimally effective levels

Hypokalemia, gluconeogenesis (more prominent with parenteral use)

- due to beta$_2$ effects (hypokalemia may be caused by an insulin-enhanced uptake of potassium [N Engl J Med 1989;321:1517–1527])
- hospitalized patients should have potassium levels determined at least twice weekly if receiving parenteral therapy

Headache (up to 7% of patients)

- may be relieved by acetaminophen

Dry mouth

- if this develops after inhaler use, rinse the mouth with warm water

Tolerance (clinical importance is controversial)

- may develop with prolonged use owing to a decrease in beta$_2$-receptor responsiveness
- may be reversed by steroids, which potentiate beta$_2$-agonist responsiveness and upgrade beta$_2$-receptors (Applied Therapeutics: The Clinical Use of Drugs, 5th ed 1992:15-1–15-24, J Allergy Clin Immunol 1985;76:312–320)

▶ How Long Do I Treat Patients with This Drug?

Acute asthma or acute exacerbation of chronic obstructive pulmonary disease

- continue frequent dosing of bronchodilators until pulmonary function returns to normal or the best result achievable is obtained on pulmonary function tests
- after full control has been achieved (absence of night and morning symptoms, normalization of or maximization of pulmonary function, or peak flow readings), the dosage should be reduced to the minimum necessary (PRN) to maintain control of the disease

Chronic asthma or chronic obstructive pulmonary disease

- after control of the disease or best pulmonary function test result is achieved and the lowest level of effective treatment is established, the patient should be reassessed every 1–6 months, depending on the severity of the disease
- administer indefinitely as long as the patient continues to obtain benefit from the drug with minimum toxicity

▶ How Do I Decrease or Stop the Administration of This Drug?

- may be discontinued abruptly; however, tapering is rational and may prevent psychological rebound
- recurrence of symptoms is not rebound, rather verification of usefulness

▶ What Should I Tell My Patients About This Drug?

- if your symptoms persist even after your usual doses, notify your physician
- you may experience tremor, but this often improves as you continue to take the medication
- if you have a headache, it can be relieved by 1 or 2 doses of acetaminophen
- if the headaches occur frequently or are severe, contact your physician
- dry mouth may be relieved by rinsing with warm water after you use the inhaler
- contact your physician if you experience a fast heart rate (palpitations)
- MDI and rotahaler should be rinsed with warm water at least every 2 weeks

Metered-dose inhaler

1. place the canister firmly into the outer shell
2. shake well; remove the cap
3. exhale to a normal relaxed expiration
4. place the tip of the mouthpiece—either 2 fingerbreadths in front of the widely opened mouth or between the teeth and lips
5. breathe in slowly, and at the same time press the canister to release 1 puff of the drug
6. continue to inhale as deeply as possible—hold the breath for as long as is comfortable (5–10 seconds)
7. breathe out to a normal relaxed resting position
8. if a second inhalation is prescribed, repeat the same procedure with the second puff, 30 seconds after the first

Diskhaler

1. remove the outer blue cover
2. grasp the white cartridge and gently pull—squeeze the ribbed sides to remove the cartridge unit
3. place the disk on the cartridge wheel with the numbers face up; slide the cartridge back into the body
4. gently push in and pull out the loaded cartridge—the disk rotates—continue this step until the number 8 appears in the indicator window
5. lift the rear edge of the diskhaler lid to a 90 degree angle—this pierces both the top and the bottom of the blister
6. exhale to a normal relaxed expiration
7. keeping the disk level, place the mouthpiece between the teeth and lips
8. breathe in quickly—hold breath for as long as possible (5–10 seconds)
9. if a second inhalation is prescribed, repeat steps 4–8 (the next blister to appear should be number 7) 30 seconds after the last inhalation
10. each disk has 8 blisters of drug—to replace a disk, follow steps 1–3, removing the old disk

Rotahaler

1. hold the rotahaler by the mouthpiece and twist the barrel until it stops
2. press a rotacap into the raised square hole with the clear end pointed down
3. keep the barrel level with the white dot marked on the side and twist the barrel in the opposite direction to pierce the capsule
4. exhale to a normal expiration
5. place the mouthpiece between the teeth and lips and tilt the head back
6. breathe in quickly—hold the breath for as long as possible (5–10 seconds)
7. if a second inhalation is prescribed, repeat the procedure after 30 seconds

Extension device (e.g., aerochamber) (for use with metered-dose inhalers)

1. remove the mouthpiece covers from the inhaler and the extension device
2. shake the inhaler well and insert into the large rubber ring on the extension device
3. exhale to a normal relaxed expiration, then place the mouthpiece of the extension device between the teeth and lips—do not cover the small holes on either side of the mouthpiece
4. activate the MDI into the extension device
5. breathe in slowly and deeply—hold your breath for 5–10 seconds—breathe out slowly to normal relaxed resting position
6. if you are unable to take a deep breath, breathe in and out normally for 3 or 4 breaths
7. if a second inhalation is prescribed, the same procedure is repeated with the second puff, at least 30 seconds after the first

▶ Therapeutic Tips

- if salbutamol is not effective, ensure that the proper technique has been followed
- 2 most important variables for proper use of an MDI are speed of inhalation (slow, deep inhalation) and duration of breath-holding (at least 5–10 seconds)
- use an MDI with or without an extension device whenever possible because other delivery systems are more expensive
- need exponential increases in puffs to produce further improvement in bronchodilation (e.g., 2 to 4 puffs, 4 to 8 puffs) (Clin Pharm 1985;4:393–403)
- use as necessary for acute symptoms, but not regularly in the absence of symptoms, as continuous bronchodilator therapy leads to a greater decline in FEV_1 than does intermittent use (Br Med J 1991;303:1426–1431)
- oral salbutamol should not be used in adults, as it offers no benefit over inhaled salbutamol and causes more side effects

Useful References

Kelly HW. New β2-adrenergic agonist aerosols. Clin Pharm 1985;4:393–403
McFadden ER. Clinical use of beta-adrenergic agonists. J Allergy Clin Immunol 1985;76:352–356
Young LY, Kimble MA, eds. Applied Therapeutics: The Clinical Use of Drugs. 4th ed. Vancouver, WA: Applied Therapeutics, 1988:372

SALMETEROL

Karen Shalansky and Cindy Reesor Nimmo

USA (Serevent)
CANADA (Serevent)

▶ When Should I Use This Drug?

Consider an alternative agent

- is a long-acting beta₂-agonist that provides no apparent clinical advantage over other available agents, unless it is being used on a regular basis (beta-agonists should primarily be used for symptomatic relief)
- this agent could be considered in a patient who continues to have nighttime symptoms despite optimal use of inhaled corticosteroids and a dose of salbutamol/albuterol at bedtime

SALSALATE

Kelly Jones

USA (Disalcid, various generics, Salflex, Salsitab, Mono-Gesic, Arthra-G)
CANADA (not available)

▶ When Should I Use This Drug?

Acute pain, general aches and pain, bone pain

- useful for the short-term management of general aches and pains
- only advantage over non–enteric-coated aspirin is that it causes less gastrointestinal intolerance
- decision between this drug and other nonsteroidal antiinflammatory drugs (NSAIDs) should be based on cost

Rheumatoid arthritis

- not considered first line, as this agent is less effective than the NSAIDs
- should be used as an alternative for patients with rheumatoid arthritis who cannot tolerate the adverse effects on the gastrointestinal system and kidneys from nonaspirin NSAIDs, as nonacetylated salicylates (salsalate, diflunisal, choline salicylate–magnesium salicylate) are less likely to affect the gastrointestinal tract than is aspirin (Gastroenterology 1990;99:1616–1621)
- can be used as an alternative when platelet function is important, as nonacetylated salicylates have no appreciable effect on platelets (J Am Board Fam Pract 1989;2:257–271)
- decision among nonacetylated salicylates should be based on cost

Osteoarthritis

- if acetaminophen and ibuprofen are not effective
- decision between this drug and other NSAIDs should be based on cost

▶ *When Should I Not Use This Drug?*

see Ibuprofen

▶ *What Contraindications Are There to the Use of This Drug?*

see Aspirin

▶ *What Drug Interactions Are Clinically Important?*

see Ibuprofen

▶ *What Route and Dosage Should I Use?*

In acute cases, higher dosages of nonacetylated salicylates should be used to bring the disease under control

How to administer

- orally—take with food or milk
- parenterally—not available

Acute pain, general aches and pain, bone pain

- 500 mg PO Q8–12H PRN

Rheumatoid arthritis

- 500 mg PO BID and increase to a maximum of 3000 mg PO daily

Osteoarthritis

- 500 mg PO BID

Dosage adjustments for renal or hepatic dysfunction

- hepatically metabolized; therefore, no adjustments are needed for renal disease
- reduce the dosage by 25% in patients with a history of hepatic disease

▶ *What Should I Monitor with Regard to Efficacy and Toxicity?*

see Aspirin

▶ *How Long Do I Treat Patients with This Drug?*

see Aspirin

▶ *How Do I Decrease or Stop the Administration of This Drug?*

- may be stopped abruptly if needed

▶ *What Should I Tell My Patients About This Drug?*

see Aspirin

▶ *Therapeutic Tips*

see Aspirin

Useful References

see Aspirin

SCOPOLAMINE

Lynne Nakashima

USA (Transdermscop)
CANADA (Transderm-V)

▶ *When Should I Use This Drug?*

Motion sickness

- is useful for nausea and vomiting related to motion sickness and is an equally effective alternative to dimenhydrate or meclizine (Drugs 1979;17:471–479, Clin Pharmacol Ther 1981;29:414–419)
- for travel on rough seas and for extended journeys (Pharmacotherapy 1982;2:29–31)
- more convenient than dimenhydrate, as it can be applied every 3 days
- causes less sedation than does dimenhydrate but causes a high incidence of anticholinergic effects, and confusion and psychosis in the elderly has been reported
- for mild to moderate road, air, or sea travel, especially if sedation is desired, use dimenhydrate
- also effective after nausea has started (Drugs 1992;43:443–463)

▶ *When Should I Not Use This Drug?*

Chemotherapy-induced nausea and vomiting

- not effective as a single agent for the prophylaxis of chemotherapy-induced nausea and vomiting (Drugs 1987;34:136–149, Cancer Treat Rep 1982;66:1975–1976)
- no more effective than placebo (Drugs 1992;43:295–315)

▶ *What Contraindications Are There to the Use of This Drug?*

Intolerance of or allergic reaction to scopolamine

Confusion and psychosis

- confusion and psychosis in the elderly have been reported; therefore, scopolamine should not be used in patients with these symptoms

Glaucoma, gastroparesis, urinary bladder neck obstruction, constipation, tachyarrythmias

- anticholinergic effects of this drug may worsen these conditions

▶ *What Drug Interactions Are Clinically Important?*

Drugs that may increase the effect or toxicity of scopolamine

ANTICHOLINERGIC AGENTS (ANTIDEPRESSANTS, ANTIPSYCHOTICS)

- additive effects with other anticholinergics
- avoid combination if possible; if not, use the lowest effective dosage of each agent

Drugs that may decrease the effect of scopolamine

- none

Drugs that may have their effect or toxicity increased by scopolamine

- none

Drugs that may have their effect decreased by scopolamine

- none

▶ *What Route and Dosage Should I Use?*

How to administer

- orally—not available
- parenterally—not available
- topically—apply transdermal patch to hairless, intact skin (usually behind the ear)

Motion sickness

- apply a 1.5 mg patch at least 4 hours before anticipated exposure to motion
- change every 72 hours as needed

Dosage adjustments for renal or hepatic dysfunction

- no dosage adjustments are currently recommended
- metabolism and excretion are not fully determined

▶ *What Should I Monitor with Regard to Efficacy and Toxicity?*

Efficacy

Motion sickness

Number and severity of vomiting episodes

- determine time of day, force, description of vomitus, and associated symptoms

Toxicity

Anticholinergic effects

- dry mouth, confusion, drowsiness, urinary retention, constipation, blurred vision (Pharmacotherapy 1982;2:29–31)
- if dry mouth occurs, try increasing the fluid intake or using sugarless candy or gum
- if blurred vision occurs, try using comfort drops and avoid the use of contact lenses
- if excessive drowsiness, confusion, symptoms of psychosis, or blurred vision occurs, remove the patch and wash the site

▶ *How Long Do I Treat Patients with This Drug?*

Motion sickness

- treatment should continue for the duration of susceptibility to motion sickness

▶ *How Do I Decrease or Stop the Administration of This Drug?*

- may be stopped abruptly

▶ *What Should I Tell My Patients About This Drug?*

- patch should be applied 4 hours before anticipated need
- wash and dry the hands and the hairless intact area of skin where the patch will be applied (usually behind the ear) before the application, expose the adhesive surface, avoid touching this surface, place on the skin, and wash the hands
- patch should remain in place for a maximum of 72 hours; the patch may be removed prior to 72 hours if it is no longer required
- if the patch becomes dislodged, remove the patch and avoid touching the adhesive surface and wash the application site thoroughly with soap and water
- if a second patch is needed, reapply the patch to a different site
- if you experience a dry mouth, try increasing fluid intake or using sugarless candy or gum to keep the mouth moist

▶ *Therapeutic Tips*

- it is useful to test the tolerance of this medication at a convenient time before the voyage if possible

Useful References

Cronin CM, Sallan SE, Wolfe L. Transdermal scopolamine in motion sickness. Pharmacotherapy 1982;2:29–31
Wood CD. Antimotion sickness and antiemetic drugs. Drugs 1979; 17:471–479

SECOBARBITAL

Jonathan Fleming

USA (Seconal Sodium, generics)
CANADA (Seconal Sodium)

▶ *When Should I Use This Drug?*

Consider an alternative agent

- barbiturates are contraindicated in the management of insomnia (Report of the Expert Advisory Committee on the Short and Intermediate Acting Barbiturates, 1985)
- their effects on sleep architecture (reduction in rapid eye movement sleep and delta sleep), safety (risk of dependence and abuse, lethality in overdosage), lack of efficacy (tolerance of hypnotic effects develops within 2 weeks), and significant withdrawal reactions (rebound insomnia) make them unsuitable for use

Useful Reference

Lapierre YD (chairman). Report of the Expert Advisory Committee on the Short and Intermediate Acting Barbiturates. Ottawa, Ontario: Information Letter 679, Health Protection Branch, April 1985

SELEGILINE

Ruby Grymonpre

USA (Eldepryl)
CANADA (Eldepryl)

▶ *When Should I Use This Drug?*

Parkinson's disease

- although there is a suggestion that selegiline halts the progression of the disease, there is no firm evidence to substantiate these claims (Drugs 1990;39:646–651)
- despite the lack of definitive evidence that selegiline delays the progression of Parkinson's disease, it has now become common to use it early in the course of treatment, either before or at the same time that levodopa administration is started
- selegiline can also be added to levodopa therapy as adjunct therapy when the patient's condition deteriorates with dosages of levodopa (with a decarboxylase inhibitor) of greater than 700 mg PO daily

▶ *When Should I Not Use This Drug?*

Initial single therapy

- owing to the relatively high costs associated with selegiline, and the lack of definitive evidence that it delays the progression of Parkinson's disease, this agent is not recommended as an initial single drug for the treatment of Parkinson's disease but is commonly used as such
- patients unresponsive to levodopa therapy should be reevaluated for whether Parkinson's disease is the correct diagnosis before trying alternative dopaminergic agents

▶ *What Contraindications Are There to the Use of This Drug?*

- intolerance of or allergic reaction to selegiline

▶ *What Drug Interactions Are Clinically Important?*

Drugs that may increase the effect or toxicity of selegiline

AMPHETAMINES AND SYMPATHOMIMETIC AMINES

- should be avoided because selegiline is metabolized to amphetamine and there are additive stimulant effects

MEPERIDINE

- combined use of selegiline with opiates, particularly meperidine, should be avoided because fatal reactions have been reported with the combination of meperidine and other irreversible monoamine oxidase (MOA) inhibitors

Drugs that may decrease the effect of selegiline

- none

Drugs that may have their effect or toxicity increased by selegiline

LEVODOPA

- adjust the levodopa dose downward if insomnia or hallucinations or other central nervous system effects become a problem

Drugs that may have their effect decreased by selegiline

- none

▶ *What Route and Dosage Should I Use?*

How to administer

- orally—take with food or milk
- parenterally—not available

Parkinson's disease

- 5 mg PO BID, with breakfast and lunch (to minimize nausea and insomnia)
- it is questionable whether higher dosages are of any benefit, and controlled studies have not been conducted on dosages greater than 10 mg PO daily (Am Fam Physician 1990;41:589–591)
- at a dosage higher than 20–25 mg, selegiline begins to lose its MAO B selectivity and, as is the case for the nonselective MAO inhibitors, may produce potentially fatal hypertensive crises if it is taken with food high in tyramine or sympathomimetic medications
- after several days of treatment with selegiline, attempt to reduce the levodopa or carbidopa dosage by 10–30%
- reduction in the levodopa dosage is usually not practical unless selegiline is added late in therapy

Dosage adjustments for renal or hepatic dysfunction

- hepatically metabolized
- dosage adjustment is not required

▶ What Should I Monitor with Regard to Efficacy and Toxicity?

Efficacy

Parkinson's disease

Signs and symptoms

- assess symptoms weekly during the titration period
- after the patient has been stabilized, assess the patient every 3 months

Toxicity

At recommended dosage, selegiline has few side effects and side effects are generally due to the potentiation of levodopa effects

see Levodopa

Insomnia

- avoid bedtime administration of selegiline

▶ How Long Do I Treat Patients with This Drug?

Parkinson's disease

- although selegiline's efficacy deteriorates over time (6–12 months in most patients and by 24 months), long-term therapy is recommended
- when there appears to be no further benefit, selegiline administration can be stopped

▶ How Do I Decrease or Stop the Administration of This Drug?

- selegiline administration should not be discontinued abruptly unless severe adverse reactions occur
- decrease the selegiline dosage at weekly intervals by 2.5 mg until 5 mg PO daily is reached, then stop the drug therapy

▶ What Should I Tell My Patients About This Drug?

- taking this drug with food reduces any nausea or vomiting you may be experiencing
- it is best to take the last dose of this drug before 4 PM to avoid sleep disturbances
- contact your physician if symptoms do not improve within the next 1–2 days

▶ Therapeutic Tips

- some clinical trials suggest that initial monotherapy with selegiline may extend the time before levodopa therapy is needed; however, other studies suggest that selegiline monotherapy is ineffective and concomitant levodopa therapy is necessary
- whether selegiline slows the progression of Parkinson's disease also needs further study
- it is expensive but causes few side effects, so many clinicians are using it early in the disease
- it can provide symptomatic benefit but is relatively ineffective late in the course of the disease

Useful References

Golbe LI, Langston JW, Shoulson I. Selegiline and Parkinson's disease: Protective and symptomatic considerations. Drugs 1990;39:646–651
Calesnick B. Selegiline for Parkinson's disease. Am Fam Physician 1990;41:589–591

SENNA

Leslie Mathews

USA (Senokot, Fletcher's Castoria, Senolax, Gentlax, Nytilax; combination: Senokot-S, Prompt)
CANADA (Senokot, Glysennid, Sennoside A and B, Mucinum-Herbal, X-Prep; combination: Mucinum, Senokot/S, Prodiem)

▶ When Should I Use This Drug?

Acute constipation

- when bulk-forming laxatives or osmotic laxatives are ineffective or contraindicated
- to provide a more rapid effect than with a bulk-forming laxative
- all stimulant laxatives are equally effective and are less expensive than agents such as lactulose
- although some authors advocate the use of senna instead of any of the other stimulants, claiming that it is the mildest and that standardized senna is the most physiological of all the nonfiber laxatives, (Pharmacology 1988;36[suppl 1]:230–236), no good studies confirm or deny these claims
- should be used only short term, as other agents are safer and more effective for long-term treatment
- decision about which stimulant laxative (bisacodyl, senna, cascara) to use should be based on availability and cost

Chronic constipation

- occasional use in patients with an absent or poor defecation reflex or severely delayed gut transit or in patients with severe debilitation or terminal illness (if long-term use is required, use lactulose)
- useful for bedridden, anorexic patients who are unable to tolerate fluids (and therefore bulk-forming laxatives cannot be used)
- patients with neurogenic constipation (e.g., due to spinal cord injury or multiple sclerosis) often require stimulation of the gut, frequently in conjunction with stool softeners and regular stimulation of the rectal mucosa with suppositories and/or enemas to prevent fecal impaction

▶ When Should I Not Use This Drug?

see Bisacodyl

▶ What Contraindications Are There to the Use of This Drug?

- intolerance of or allergic reaction to senna

see Bisacodyl

▶ What Drug Interactions Are Clinically Important?

▶ What Route and Dosage Should I Use?

How to administer

- orally—take with a full glass of water
- rectally—remove the wrapper, moisten the suppository with lukewarm water, and insert the tapered end high and against the wall of the rectum

Acute constipation, chronic constipation

- senna preparations containing senna leaf are not recommended, as they are less stable and reliable than crystalline senna glycosides or standardized concentrations of senna pod (Self Medication: A Reference for the Health Professional, 3rd ed 1988: 327–336)
- 15 mg PO daily
- increase the dosage as needed after 24 hours by 7.5 mg to a maximum of 60 mg PO daily
- use the lowest recommended dosage on the label, for example, syrup, 10 mL; granules or sennosides, 15 mg PO daily (eg., Senokot granules, 1 teaspoon (3 g daily) equivalent to 15 mg of active senna glycosides or Nytilax [calcium salts of sennosides A and B], 2 tablets HS)
- 30 mg daily as a suppository

▶ What Should I Monitor with Regard to Efficacy and Toxicity?

see Bisacodyl (except that bisacodyl is much more notorious for causing anorectal symptoms and this effect is rarely mentioned in reports about senna suppositories)

▶ How Long Do I Treat Patients with This Drug?

see Bisacodyl

▶ *How Do I Decrease or Stop the Administration of This Drug?*

see Bisacodyl

▶ *What Should I Tell My Patients About This Drug?*

- discontinue its use with diarrhea or relief of constipation
- decrease the dosage by 50% with persistent abdominal cramps
- notify your physician if constipation persists after 1 week of use
- prolonged use can cause serious side effects and can lead to laxative dependency and loss of normal bowel function
- complete bowel emptying can occur
- you may not have another bowel movement for 2–3 days after use
- take at bedtime to produce effects by morning
- suppositories or enemas may cause burning; therefore, stop their use with anal swelling or pain
- insert the suppository against the wall of the rectum rather than into stool, and defecation will occur within an hour
- urine may appear yellowish brown or red with this drug
- take each dose with a full glass of water

▶ *Therapeutic Tips*

- give dose at bedtime, especially with the elderly, to avoid nocturnal fecal incontinence
- low doses are usually effective
- senna pod preparations cause less cramping than do senna leaf preparations
- suppositories should be given at room temperature

Useful References

Tedesco FJ. Laxative use in constipation. Am J Gastroenterol 1985; 80:303–309

Rousseau P. Treatment of constipation in the elderly. Postgrad Med 1988;83:339–349

Godding EW. Laxatives and the special role of senna. Pharmacology 1988;36(suppl 1):230–236

Clarke C, ed. Self Medication: A Reference for the Health Professional, 3rd ed. Canadian Pharmaceutical Association, Ottawa, 1988:330

SIMVASTATIN

Stephen Shalansky and Robert Dombrowski

USA (Zocor)
CANADA (Zocor)

▶ *When Should I Use This Drug?*

Hypercholesterolemia

see Lovastatin

▶ *When Should I Not Use This Drug?*

see Lovastatin

▶ *What Contraindications Are There to the Use of This Drug?*

see Lovastatin

▶ *What Drug Interactions Are Clinically Important?*

see Lovastatin

▶ *What Route and Dosage Should I Use?*

How to administer

- orally—can be given with food or on an empty stomach; however, the drug is better absorbed with food
- parenterally—not available

Hypercholesterolemia

- start with 10 mg PO daily given with the evening meal
- increase the dosage to 20 mg PO daily if there is inadequate response after 4 weeks
- dosage range is 10–80 mg daily
- dosages greater than 10 mg/d are more effective when divided and given twice daily (JAMA 1986;256:2829–2834)

- simvastatin may be given once daily to enhance compliance
- if after 3 months of optimum therapy, there is at least a 15% decrease in LDL or total cholesterol levels, but the target level is not reached, continue simvastatin therapy and add a second drug
- if after 3 months of optimum therapy, there is less than a 15% decrease in LDL or total cholesterol levels, consider switching to or adding another agent
- if the patient is not tolerating simvastatin, change to another drug

Dosage adjustments for renal or hepatic dysfunction

- hepatically metabolized
- do not use in severe hepatic dysfunction
- no dosage adjustments for renal dysfunction

▶ *What Should I Monitor with Regard to Efficacy and Toxicity?*

see Lovastatin

▶ *How Long Do I Treat Patients with This Drug?*

see Lovastatin

▶ *How Do I Decrease or Stop the Administration of This Drug?*

- may be stopped abruptly

▶ *What Should I Tell My Patients About This Drug?*

see Lovastatin

▶ *Therapeutic Tips*

- drug is more effective if given twice daily compared with once daily in the evening, but patients may be more compliant with once-daily dosing
- doses given once daily are more effective if given in the evening instead of the morning (Clin Pharmacol Ther 1986;40:338–343)

Useful Reference

Mauro VF, MacDonald JL. Simvastatin: A review of its pharmacology and clinical use. DICP Ann Pharmacother 1991;25:257–264

SODIUM PHOSPHATE

Leslie Mathews

USA (Fleet Enema, Fleet Phospho-soda, K-Phos)
CANADA (Fleet Enema, pHos-pHaid, Phosphate-Sandoz; combination: GentL-Tip)

▶ *When Should I Use This Drug?*

Fecal impaction

- drug of choice for severe impaction after or instead of manual disimpaction
- is convenient, is easier to administer than many enemas because it is premixed and the nozzle is prelubricated, uses a low volume, and uses less nursing time than other enemas
- as effective as tap water or saline enemas (Handbook of Nonprescription Drugs, 8th ed 1986:73–90)

Acute constipation

- last resort when oral laxatives and glycerin or stimulant suppositories are ineffective

Chronic constipation

- for occasional use when oral laxatives and glycerin suppositories are ineffective, especially in the elderly who are unable to pass soft putty-like stool
- for patients at risk for toxic megacolon (e.g., with significant autonomic dysfunction from cerebrovascular accident or Parkinson's disease)
- to help retrain a cathartic-dependent colon if distention of the rectum may help promote defecatory reflex (Postgrad Med 1988;83:339–349)

Bowel preparation

- before surgery or diagnostic examinations when the patient cannot take an oral agent
- use polyethylene glycol–electrolyte solution (PEG-ES [GoLYTELY]) or osmotic laxatives and suppositories instead because sodium phosphate (Fleet) enemas may cause mucosal damage (friability, sloughing of the rectal epithelium, redness) and impede interpretation of barium enema or sigmoidoscopy results (Applied Therapeutics: The Clinical Use of Drugs, 4th ed 1988:101–122)
- patients prefer PEG-ES preparation enema to cathartic preparation because it is more convenient (5 hours versus 3 days), is more rapidly active, and causes less discomfort (Clin Pharm 1985;4:414–424)
- some patients are unable to retain enemas, resulting in lower-quality study films and inadequate bowel preparation
- significant toxicity can occur with use (fluid and electrolyte imbalance and rectal or colonic injury)

▶ *When Should I Not Use This Drug?*

Long-term use

- may contribute to poor rectal tone, increased risk of fecal incontinence, dependence, and phosphate poisoning

Lavage solution for the treatment of iron overdose

- too toxic and likely of no benefit

▶ *What Contraindications Are There to the Use of This Drug?*

Intolerance of or allergic reaction to sodium phosphate

Symptoms of acute abdomen

- undiagnosed abdominal pain, nausea, and vomiting

Congestive heart failure, marked dehydration or preexisting electrolyte disturbances, edema, cirrhosis

- fatal case of hyperphosphatemic, hypocalcemic coma in a 91-year-old patient occurred after he received 1 sodium phosphate enema (Isr J Med Sci 1989;25:237–238)
- 2 sodium phosphate enemas given to an adult with polycystic kidney disease resulted in hypocalcemic tetany (Lancet 1985; 2:1433)

Patients sensitive to fluid and electrolyte changes (e.g., patients who are elderly, have a colostomy, cardiac disease, hypertension, sodium restriction, or convulsive disorders; or patients using diuretics or other drugs that may affect serum electrolyte levels)

- single doses are likely safe; however, repeated doses are not recommended in these patients

Renal disease, hypocalcemia, or abnormal colonic mucosa

- accumulation of phosphate is possible (South Med J 1985;78: 1241–1242, Lancet 1985;2:1433)

▶ *What Drug Interactions Are Clinically Important?*

- none

▶ *What Route and Dosage Should I Use?*

How to administer

Orally

- do not use

Parenterally

- do not use

Rectally

- to administer, the patient lies on the left side or in the knee-chest position and gently inserts the prelubricated nozzle into the rectum toward the navel and squeezes the bottle slowly
- patient should remain reclining until abdominal cramping is felt, at which time rectal contents can be expelled

Fecal impaction

- one 120 mL enema per rectum daily (some formulations are 118 mL)

- repeat once if ineffective (e.g., not retained until abdominal cramping felt or little or no stool evacuated)

Acute constipation, chronic constipation

- one 120 mL enema per rectum as needed

Bowel preparation

- one 120 mL enema per rectum given at least 2 hours before the procedure

Dosage adjustments for renal or hepatic dysfunction

- dosage adjustments (e.g., small volume) likely make it ineffective

Normal Dosing Interval	C$_{cr}$ > 60 mL/min or 1 mL/s	C$_{cr}$ 30–60 mL/min or 0.5–1 mL/s	C$_{cr}$ < 30 mL/min or 0.5 mL/s
single dose	no adjustment needed	no adjustment needed	avoid

▶ *What Should I Monitor with Regard to Efficacy and Toxicity?*

Efficacy

Fecal impaction, acute constipation, chronic constipation, bowel preparation

- watery evacuation within 5–30 minutes, depending on the retention time
- may be ineffective if not administered correctly and/or not retained long enough
- if ineffective, do a digital examination to assess the need for manual disimpaction or a repeated enema

Toxicity

Fluid and electrolyte imbalance

- particularly dehydration, hypernatremia, hyperphosphatemia, and hypocalcemia with long-term use
- to prevent, give the dose with extra fluids, avoid repeated doses, and ensure that the enema is fully expelled
- hyperphosphatemia or hypocalcemia can occur with repetitive enemas that are retained, even in patients with normal renal function; therefore, avoid repeating enemas, particularly in patients with abnormal colonic mucosa (e.g., diverticulitis)
- ask the nursing staff to report retained enemas and insert a rectal tube if retained longer than 1 hour
- monitor fluid and electrolyte levels if the patient is at risk or becomes symptomatic or the enema is retained
- monitor for symptoms of dehydration such as dry skin and mucous membranes, poor skin turgor, oliguria, cracked lips, confusion, and hypotension
- monitor for symptoms of hypernatremia such as nausea, vomiting, diarrhea, thirst, weakness, restlessness, dizziness, headache, convulsions, hypotension, and tachycardia

Rectal trauma, colonic perforation (rare)

- ensure that the nozzle is well lubricated, insert gently, and avoid force

Poor rectal tone, fecal incontinence

- avoid long-term use of enemas

▶ *How Long Do I Treat Patients with This Drug?*

Fecal impaction, acute constipation, chronic constipation, bowel preparation

- usually given as a single dose
- for treating intractable constipation and bowel retraining, an enema may be needed daily or every 3–4 days

▶ *How Do I Decrease or Stop the Administration of This Drug?*

- may be stopped abruptly

▶ *What Should I Tell My Patients About This Drug?*

- do not use if you are experiencing abdominal pain, nausea, and vomiting

- frequent, prolonged use may lead to dehydration, electrolyte disturbances, and dependence
- to administer the enema, lie on your left side or in a knee-chest position, gently insert the prelubricated nozzle into the rectum toward the navel, and squeeze the bottle
- remain reclining for a few minutes until abdominal cramping is felt, at which time rectal contents can be expelled
- drink extra fluids after the enema to prevent dehydration

▶ Therapeutic Tips

- to administer the enema, the patient should lie on the left side with the knees bent or assume a knee-chest position
- sitting position is incorrect, as this allows for clearing of the rectum only
- flow of enema solution should be slow to avoid excessive cramping and premature discharge

Useful References

Elliot DL, Watts WJ, Girard DE. Constipation—Mechanisms and management of a common clinical problem. Postgrad Med 1983;74:143–149

Rousseau P. No soapsuds enemas! Postgrad Med 1988;83:352–353

Rohack JJ, Bhasker RM, Subramanyam K. Hyperphosphatemia and hypocalcemic coma associated with phosphate enema. South Med J 1985;78:1241–1242

Handbook of Nonprescription Drugs, 8th ed. American Pharmaceutical Association, 1986:85

Young LY, Koda-Kimble MA, eds. Applied Therapeutics: The Clinical Use of Drugs, 4th ed. Applied Therapeutics, Vancouver, WA, 1988:101–122

SOTALOL

James Tisdale

USA (Betapace)
CANADA (Sotacor)

Sotalol is a beta-blocker that prolongs the QT interval on electrocardiogram in contrast to other nonselective beta-antagonists; thus, it has both class II and class III antiarrhythmic activity

▶ When Should I Use This Drug?

Atrial fibrillation or flutter

- sotalol should be used for the maintenance of sinus rhythm in patients with paroxysmal atrial fibrillation in whom quinidine, procainamide, and flecainide have been ineffective, are poorly tolerated, or are contraindicated

Atrioventricular nodal reentrant tachycardia

- sotalol should be used for the long-term prevention of episodes of atrioventricular (AV) nodal reentrant tachycardia in patients in whom therapy with digoxin, other beta-blocking agents without class III activity, verapamil, quinidine, procainamide, disopyramide, or flecainide has been ineffective, is poorly tolerated, or is contraindicated

Ventricular arrhythmias

- sotalol should be used for the suppression of premature symptomatic ventricular contractions in patients who fail to respond to therapy with other beta-blockers, class IA or class IB antiarrhythmic agents
- sotalol should be used for the suppression of symptomatic or life-threatening ventricular tachyarrhythmias in patients in who fail to respond to therapy with quinidine or procainamide (class IA), mexiletine or tocainide (class IB), and/or the combination of these agents during serial drug testing in the electrophysiology laboratory

Chronic (noncrisis) hypertension

- has efficacy in mild to moderate hypertension and may have advantage in treating hypertension complicated by atrial fibrillation or flutter or in maintaining stability after conversion to sinus rhythm and in the presence of the Wolff-Parkinson-White syndrome (Drugs 1987;34:311–349)
- sotalol should be used only for the treatment of hypertension in patients who have a clear second indication (resistant arrhythmias) because torsades de pointes has been reported to occur in 3–5% of patients receiving this agent (Med Lett 1993;34:27–28)

▶ When Should I Not Use This Drug?

see Nadolol

Asymptomatic ventricular arrhythmias

- treatment of asymptomatic ventricular arrhythmias has not been of benefit and may be harmful with some drugs (N Engl J Med 1989;321:406–412)

▶ What Contraindications Are There to the Use of This Drug?

see Nadolol

Sick sinus syndrome, sinus bradycardia, or atrioventricular nodal block in the absence of a functioning pacemaker

- because sotalol is a beta-blocker, it may decrease sinus node activity and conduction through the AV node

Long QT syndrome or history of torsades de pointes in association with antiarrhythmic drugs

- because sotalol may prolong QT intervals on surface electrocardiogram (ECG), the drug is contraindicated in patients with long QT syndrome or history of torsades de pointes

▶ What Drug Interactions Are Clinically Important?

see Nadolol

Drugs that may increase the effect or toxicity of sotalol

- effects of sotalol and other agents that prolong QT intervals on surface ECG (quinidine, procainamide, disopyramide, and amiodarone) may be additive

▶ What Route and Dosage Should I Use?

How to administer

- orally—can be taken with food or milk or on an empty stomach (food slightly decreases the bioavailability of sotalol but not to a clinically important degree [Am J Cardiol 1990;65:12A–21A])
- parenterally—not available

Atrial flutter or fibrillation, atrioventricular nodal reentrant tachycardia, ventricular arrhythmias, chronic (noncrisis) hypertension

- start with 80 mg PO BID
- dosage may be increased to 160 mg PO BID in 3 days if needed to control arrhythmia
- dosage may be increased to the maximum recommended level of 240 mg PO BID if necessary (risk of torsades de pointes is substantially higher at this dosage)
- dosages for hypertension can be given once daily

Dosage adjustment for renal or hepatic dysfunction

- renally eliminated
- in general, even in patients with renal dysfunction, start with a low dose and titrate up to an effect

Normal Dosing Interval	$C_{cr} > 60$ mL/min or 1 mL/s	C_{cr} 30–60 mL/min or 0.5–1 mL/s	$C_{cr} < 30$ mL/min or 0.5 mL/s
Q12H	no adjustment needed	Q24H	Q36–48H

▶ What Should I Monitor with Regard to Efficacy and Toxicity?

Efficacy

see Nadolol

Atrioventricular nodal reentrant tachycardia

- frequency or duration of episodes (may be evaluated by ambulatory ECG or by the patients' reports of the frequency of symptoms)
- patients should be assessed every few weeks during the first few months of therapy and every few months thereafter

Ventricular arrhythmias

- intermittent ECG or Holter monitoring for the presence or absence of arrhythmia; reduced frequency of arrhythmia episodes

- symptoms associated with arrhythmia (palpitations, shortness of breath, chest pain, and syncope) should resolve with successful suppression of arrhythmia

Toxicity

see Nadolol

Electrocardiogram

- evaluate ECG within 1 week of inititiation of therapy for prolongation of PR interval (>0.2 second), signs of second- or third-degree AV block, prolongation of QT interval (>25% compared with baseline values), new cardiac arrhythmias (such as torsades de pointes), or worsening of the patient's clinical arrhythmia
- sotalol dosage should be reduced by 80 mg PO BID in patients with prolongation of the QT interval to greater than 25% compared with baseline values
- sotalol therapy should be discontinued abruptly in patients who experience new cardiac arrhythmias (such as torsades de pointes) or worsening of the clinical arrhythmia
- torsades de pointes has been reported to occur in 3–5% of patients receiving this agent (Med Lett 1993;34:27–28)

▶ How Long Do I Treat Patients with This Drug?

see Nadolol

Atrioventricular nodal reentrant tachycardia

- unless a nonpharmacological arrhythmia cure (such as radiofrequency ablation or surgery) is attempted and achieved, therapy is required indefinitely

Ventricular arrhythmias

Acute episodes

- treatment should continue until the underlying cause of the arrhythmia can be corrected
- if no correctable cause exists, therapy should continue until the patient can be evaluated for oral therapy
- if the patient is to undergo electrophysiological testing, the administration of antiarrhythmic drugs should be discontinued at least 5 half-lives prior to the baseline study (i.e., 10 days), if the patient can tolerate the discontinuation of therapy

Long-term oral therapy

- therapy may be required indefinitely if contributing factors cannot be reversed

▶ How Do I Stop or Decrease the Administration of This Drug?

see Nadolol

- sotalol therapy should not be discontinued or dosage reduction performed without consulting a cardiologist or a cardiac electrophysiologist
- sotalol therapy should be discontinued abruptly in patients who experience new cardiac arrhythmias (such as torsades de pointes) or worsening of the clinical arrhythmia

▶ What Should I Tell My Patients About This Drug?

see Nadolol

▶ Therapeutic Tips

- sotalol can cause AV block and polymorphic ventricular tachycardia (torsades de pointes) in overdose, especially in the presence of impaired renal function

Useful References

Singh BN, Deedwania P, Nademanee K, et al. Sotalol. A review of its pharmacodynamic and pharmacokinetic properties, and therapeutic use. Drugs 1987;34:311–349

Carmeliet E. Electrophysiologic and voltage clamp analysis of effects of sotalol on isolated cardiac muscle and Purkinje fibres. J Pharmacol Exp Ther 1985;232:817–825

Tisdale JE, Chow MSS. Sotalol: An adrenergic beta-receptor blocking agent with class III antiarrhythmic activity. Hosp Formul 1989;24:485–497

SPIRONOLACTONE

Ian Petterson

USA (Aldactone)
CANADA (Aldactone, Novospiroton)

▶ When Should I Use This Drug?

Chronic (noncrisis) hypertension

- alone produces only a modest lowering of blood pressure, although it has more of an effect than does either amiloride or triamterene
- blood pressure reduction is additive with thiazide diuretics
- use in combination with thiazide diuretics only to prevent or treat hypokalemia
- use only if there is documented hypokalemia or the patient is at high risk for adverse effects due to hypokalemia (e.g., cardiac arrhythmias, muscle weakness, and concomitant digoxin administration)
- useful in patients requiring a diuretic who have diabetes, as spironolactone does not adversely affect glucose levels

Hypokalemia

- in dosages of 25–75 mg/d, it is more effective than oral potassium supplementation (Eur J Clin Pharm 1986;30:535–540) or triamterene for the treatment of hypokalemia due to thiazide or loop diuretics (Br J Clin Pharm 1982;14:256–263)

Hypomagnesemia

- maintains magnesium as well as potassium levels (Drugs 1984; 28[suppl 1]:161–166)

Primary hyperaldosteronism

- considered drug of choice in the long-term preoperative treatment of primary hyperaldosteronism (Conn's and Cushing's syndromes)
- more effective than amiloride in the management of hypertension and electrolyte abnormalities associated with primary hyperaldosteronism (Clin Pharm Ther 1980;27:317–323)

Congestive heart failure

- used only in addition to other diuretics
- useful if hypokalemia persists despite the use of angiotensin converting enzyme inhibitors as spironolactone is more effective at maintaining potassium than potassium supplements
- spironolactone is preferable to the other potassium-sparing diuretics, as it has the most diuretic effect plus antagonizes the vascular effect of secondary aldosteronism

Ascites associated with hepatic cirrhosis

- considered the diuretic of choice because of increased production and decreased metabolism of aldosterone in patients with ascites
- effective in 75% of cases
- can be given in conjunction with a thiazide or loop diuretic if more rapid diuresis is required

Hirsutism

- in women with either idiopathic or polycystic ovary disease, spironolactone can be tried to treat hirsutism

▶ When Should I Not Use This Drug?

Concomitant use of potassium-sparing agent or potassium supplement (amiloride, triamterene, or angiotensin converting enzyme inhibitor)

- risk of hyperkalemia and inappropriate duplication of therapy
- use only if the patient is still hypokalemic despite maximum doses of other potassium-sparing agents

Renal tubular acidosis

- high risk of life-threatening hyperkalemia

▶ What Contraindications Are There to the Use of This Drug?

Intolerance of or allergic reaction to spironolactone

Acute or chronic renal failure

- risk of hyperkalemia is increased as renal function decreases

Hyperkalemia (potassium level > 5 mmol/L)

- risk of life-threatening hyperkalemia is high

▶ *What Drug Interactions Are Clinically Important?*

Drugs that may increase the effect or toxicity of spironolactone

POTASSIUM-SPARING DIURETICS OR POTASSIUM SUPPLEMENTS

- risk of hyperkalemia is increased when either agent is used concurrently with spironolactone
- do not use these agents together

ANGIOTENSIN CONVERTING ENZYME INHIBITORS

- little reason to use together because both drugs are effective potassium-sparing agents
- risk of hyperkalemia is increased when both agents are used together
- do not use together unless the patient remains hypokalemic with appropriate dosages of angiotensin converting enzyme inhibitors

Drugs that may decrease the effect of spironolactone

NONSTEROIDAL ANTIINFLAMMATORY DRUGS

- avoid combination if possible, and if not, monitor serum creatinine and potassium levels and weight at baseline and every 4 days for 2–3 weeks, then every 2 weeks for 8 weeks, then every month for 3 months, and then as needed (J Musculoskel Med 1991;8:31–46)

Drugs that may have their effect or toxicity increased by spironolactone

- none

Drugs that may have their effect decreased by spironolactone

- none

▶ *What Route and Dosage Should I Use?*

How to administer

- orally—usually given once daily and bioavailability is enhanced with food
- parenterally—not available

Chronic (noncrisis) hypertension, hypokalemia, hypomagnesemia

- always start with a low dosage (25 mg PO daily) and titrate to effect
- dosages greater than 75 mg PO daily do not produce additional antihypertensive effect and increase the chance of side effects (e.g., gynecomastia) (Am J Cardiol 1987;60:820–825)

Primary hyperaldosteronism

- start with 100 mg PO daily and may increase by 50% per week to control hypertension and hypokalemia

Congestive heart failure

- 50 mg PO daily
- double the dosage weekly, on the basis of response, up to a maximum of 400 mg PO daily

Ascites associated with hepatic cirrhosis

- start with 100 mg PO daily and may increase the dosage weekly by 50% on the basis of response

Hirsutism

- 100 mg PO daily

Dosage adjustments for renal or hepatic dysfunction

- hepatically metabolized
- dosage adjustment is not required, but the drug should be avoided if severe hepatic disease is present and when creatinine clearance is less than 20 mL/min to avoid life-threatening hyperkalemia

▶ *What Should I Monitor with Regard to Efficacy and Toxicity?*

Efficacy

Chronic (noncrisis) hypertension, hypokalemia, hypomagnesemia, congestive heart failure

- measure serum potassium level and realize that the maximum effect is seen after 7–10 days of therapy

Primary hyperaldosteronism

- measure blood pressure and potassium levels weekly until these have normalized

Ascites associated with hepatic cirrhosis

- treatment needs to proceed slowly to prevent acid-base, fluid, and electrolyte imbalances, which can precipitate hepatic encephalopathy
- 3 primary goals of therapy are weight loss of 0.3–1 kg/d, urine output of 300–1000 mL/d over daily input, and patient comfort

Hirsutism

- regression is generally evident after 2 months of treating hirsutism and maximum effect is seen after 6 months

Toxicity

Hyperkalemia

- significant if potassium level is greater than 6 mmol/L or has risen dramatically since the initiation of therapy
- occurrence of 8–10% in normal patients (especially with higher dosages) and 25% in the elderly or in patients with renal dysfunction
- stop drug therapy if the patient becomes hyperkalemic but realize that potassium levels may still rise for up to 3 days after the drug administration is stopped
- if patients exhibit electrocardiographic changes, regardless of the potassium level, the drug regimen should be stopped
- if mild hyperkalemia develops (potassium level of 5–5.9 mEq/L), decrease the dosage by 50%; if the potassium level is unchanged in 3 days, decrease the dosage further and reevaluate the use of the drug

Gynecomastia, mastalgia, and impotence

- occurs in 50% of male patients and is related to the dosage and the duration of therapy (i.e., generally seen only in patients receiving dosages exceeding 75 mg/d over several months)
- reversible on discontinuation of therapy or dosage reduction but may take several months
- mastalgia is a more common complaint and can be seen even at low dosages (25–75 mg/d)

Gastrointestinal effects

- mild nausea occurs in 20% of patients; therefore, take the drug with food

▶ *How Long Do I Treat Patients with This Drug?*

Chronic (noncrisis) hypertension, congestive heart failure

- use until the reason for persistent hypokalemia is removed

Hypokalemia, hypomagnesemia

- until precipitating factors can be reversed

Primary hyperaldosteronism

- drug therapy is lifelong unless surgical correction is possible

Ascites associated with hepatic cirrhosis

- treat until the cause of the exacerbation of ascites is gone
- treatment may be lifelong if ascites is due to alcoholic cirrhosis; however, always reevaluate for the lowest effective dosage

Hirsutism

- treatment may continue indefinitely unless the cause of hirsutism is eliminated

▶ *How Do I Decrease or Stop the Administration of This Drug?*

- may be stopped abruptly

▶ *What Should I Tell My Patients About This Drug?*

- because this drug helps to maintain your potassium balance, you should avoid taking any potassium supplements
- you may experience some nausea or stomach upset, but taking it with food should alleviate this

- if gastrointestinal discomfort persists, contact your physician, as it may indicate an electrolyte abnormality
- you may notice some dizziness or fatigue-like symptoms but they will likely go away in a few days
- (men) should report any breast tenderness or swelling
- (women) may notice some menstrual irregularities

▶ Therapeutic Tips

- before adding any potassium-sparing diuretic or potassium supplement, consider dosage reduction of the thiazide or loop diuretic
- never exceed 75 mg daily for hypertension, especially in men, because greater dosages have no greater antihypertensive effect and present a greater risk of mastalgia, gynecomastia, and impotence
- not as useful as amiloride for the initial treatment or prevention of hypokalemia caused by thiazide diuretics because it causes more side effects
- avoid in renal failure because of the risk of serious hyperkalemia
- do not start with a fixed-combination product (e.g., Aldactazide)
- titrate each drug separately and then use a combination if appropriate
- may be able to decrease the dosage of a concurrently administered diuretic
- do not use in combination with other potassium-sparing agents, potassium supplements, or angiotensin converting enzyme inhibitors unless the patient remains hypokalemic with these therapies

Useful References

Nader C, Thompson JR, Alpern RJ. Complications of diuretic use. Semin Nephrol 1988;8:365–387

Krishna GG, Shulman MD, Narins RG. Clinical use of potassium sparing diuretics. Semin Nephrol 1988;8:354–364

Skluth HA, Gums JG. Spironolactone—A re-evaluation. DICP 1990;24:52–59

Jeunemaitre X, Chatellier G, Kreft-Jais C, et al. Efficacy and tolerance of spironolactone in essential hypertension. Am J Cardiol 1987;60:820–825

STREPTOKINASE

Stephen F. Hamilton, Stan Horton, and Udho Thadani

USA (Kabikinase, Streptase)
CANADA (Kabikinase, Streptase)

▶ When Should I Use This Drug?

Acute myocardial infarction

- all appropriate patients with a suspected or proven myocardial infarction should receive thrombolytic therapy
- appropriate patients are those without contraindications to thrombolytic therapy with pain lasting 12 hours or less and ST segment elevation in 2 contiguous leads
- much research is underway and similar patients older than 75 years seem to benefit as much as or more than younger patients, but major and fatal bleeding complications are higher
- streptokinase is the drug of first choice because it has efficacy in reducing mortality that is equivalent to that of tissue plasminogen activator and it is less expensive
- streptokinase is the drug of first choice unless patients have received streptokinase or anistreplase (anisoylated plasminogen streptokinase activator complex) or have been treated for a streptococcal infection within the previous year because these patients have streptococcal antibodies that neutralize the streptokinase

Acute massive pulmonary embolism, acute deep vein thrombosis

- streptokinase should be considered in patients with massive pulmonary embolism who are hemodynamically unstable as long as they are not prone to bleeding (Chest 1992;102[suppl]::408S–425S), although there is no evidence that this changes mortality or morbidity
- diagnosis should be objectively confirmed by pulmonary angiography or pulmonary scan for pulmonary embolism or ascending venography for deep vein thrombosis
- therapy should be initiated as soon as possible after the onset of the thromboembolic episode, preferably no later than 7 days

▶ When Should I Not Use This Drug?

Patients with streptococcal infections or previous streptokinase treatment within the previous 12 months

- these patients may have elevated levels of streptokinase antibodies and have a likelihood of resistance to streptokinase therapy or increased allergic effects
- if thrombin time does not differ substantially from the normal control value (less than 1.5 times control value) after 4 hours of streptokinase therapy, the drug administration should be discontinued because excessive resistance is present

▶ What Contraindications Are There to the Use of This Drug?

Intolerance of or allergic reaction to streptokinase

Absolute contraindications

- active internal bleeding, suspected aortic dissection, diabetic hemorrhagic retinopathy, any other ophthalmic hemorrhages, history of cerebrovascular accident known to be hemorrhagic, recent head trauma, known intracranial neoplasm, pregnancy, blood pressure greater than 200/120 mmHg, history of allergic reactions to any thrombolytic agent, and trauma or surgery within less than 2 weeks

Relative contraindications (if evidence of a myocardial infarction is strong enough, thrombolytic therapy should still be used)

- history of severe hypertension, history of cerebrovascular accident, significant hepatic dysfunction, active peptic ulcer, patients taking oral anticoagulants, prolonged or traumatic cardiopulmonary resuscitation, and surgery or trauma within greater than 2 weeks to 6 months

▶ What Drug Interactions Are Clinically Important?

Drugs that may increase the effect or toxicity of streptokinase

WARFARIN, HEPARIN

- warfarin or heparin may increase the risk of hemorrhage

ASPIRIN

- low-dose aspirin therapy concomitantly with thrombolytics has been associated with greater reductions in short-term and long-term mortality and the overall risk of stroke than those produced by streptokinase therapy alone
- concurrent therapy is associated with an increased risk of major bleeding, primarily at arterial puncture sites, and a slight increase in the incidence of confirmed intracranial hemorrhage

Drugs that may decrease the effect of streptokinase

AMINOCAPROIC ACID

- inhibits the streptokinase-induced activation of plasminogen and can be used to reverse the fibrinolytic effects of streptokinase
- use only if the effects of thrombolytic agents need to be reversed, such as after a major bleed

Drugs that may have their effect or toxicity increased by streptokinase

- none

Drugs that may have their effect decreased by streptokinase

- none

▶ What Route and Dosage Should I Use?

How to administer

Parenterally

- is most stable at a pH of 6–8 and should be used immediately after reconstitution because the solution contains no preservatives
- 20 mL of diluent (normal saline injection or dextrose 5% injection) should be added slowly and the vial gently rolled and tilted while avoiding shaking because foaming may result
- further dilution with normal saline injection or dextrose 5% injection, to a final volume of 125 mL
- streptokinase solutions should be filtered with an 0.8 μm or larger filter

- if administration is delayed, reconstituted streptokinase should be refrigerated at 2–4°C and used or discarded after 24 hours

Acute myocardial infarction

- 1.5 million units IV over 1 hour via a controlled infusion device (Lancet 1987;2:871–874, Lancet 1988;2:349–360)

Deep vein thrombosis, pulmonary embolism

- start with a loading dose of 250,000 IU over a 30 minute period to neutralize antistreptococcal antibodies
- follow the loading dose with a maintenance infusion of 100,000 IU/h for 24–72 hours (Chest 1992;102[suppl]:408S–425S) and measure a thrombin time 2–4 hours after the start of treatment
- this dose should maintain the thrombin time at 1.5–5 times the normal control value in most patients
- if thrombin time is less than 1.5 times the normal control value at 4 hours, an excessive resistance to streptokinase is present and the drug administration should be discontinued

Dosage adjustments for renal or hepatic dysfunction

- no dosage adjustment is required

▶ What Should I Monitor with Regard to Efficacy and Toxicity?

Efficacy

Acute myocardial infarction

- reduction of chest pain
- reduction of ST segment elevation
- reperfusion arrhythmias
- patients receiving thrombolytic therapy for acute myocardial infaction should be continuously monitored by telemetry for possible arrhythmias during and immediately after administration of the drug, and antiarrhythmic therapy for bradycardia and/or ventricular irritability should be available during administration of the drug

Deep vein thrombosis

Limb circumference, swelling, tenderness, perfusion

- assess the patient daily

Pulmonary embolism

Apprehension, cough, pleuritic chest pain, hemoptysis

- assess the patient daily

Toxicity

Hemorrhagic tendency

- watch for bleeding and apply prophylactic pressure dressings to previous puncture sites
- chance of hemorrhage with streptokinase is greater than that with heparin (J Med Technol 1985;2[2]:89–93)
- baseline prothrombin time, partial thromboplastin time, and thrombin time to detect the presence of any preexisting hemostatic problems
- 4 hour thrombin time greater than 5 suggests fibrinogen depletion or disseminated intravascular coagulation
- thrombin time less than 1.5 suggests a resistance to streptokinase

Signs of excessive bleeding (such as gross bleeding at the puncture site or hypotension)

- if uncontrolled bleeding occurs, thrombolytic therapy should be discontinued
- blood loss should be replaced with packed red blood cells, preferentially to whole blood

Allergic reactions

- streptokinase is antigenic; thus, anaphylaxis and other allergic reactions are possible
- monitor for elevated or lowered blood pressure or asthmatic symptoms
- infusion should be stopped in the presence of anaphylaxis, hypertensive emergencies, or hypotension

Blood pressure and heart rate

- measure every 15 minutes until stable
- occasionally, bradycardia and hypotension occur during successful thromboytic therapy, and they are more frequent with an inferior infarction associated with right ventricular infarcts
- 0.5–1 mg of atropine given intravenously usually restores heart rate and blood pressure
- hypotension that is not due to bleeding or anaphylaxis is usually transient and may be related to the rate of streptokinase infusion
- infusion rate should not exceed 500 units/kg/min in normotensive patients to avoid severe hypotension, and in hemodynamically unstable patients, the infusion rate should not exceed 200–250 units/kg/min
- if hypotension develops and other causes are not apparent, stop the infusion, elevate the patient's legs and administer saline until systolic blood pressure is greater than 90 mmHg; then restart streptokinase infusion at a slower rate

▶ How Long Do I Treat Patients with This Drug?

Acute myocardial infarction

- a single dose given over 1 hour

Deep vein thrombosis, pulmonary embolism

- given over 24 hours for pulmonary embolism and 72 hours for deep vein thrombosis (Chest 1992;102[suppl]:408S–425S)
- heparin should be restarted when the streptokinase therapy is stopped and the partial thromboplastin time or thrombin time is 1.5 times control values or less

▶ How Do I Decrease or Stop the Administration of This Drug?

- may be abruptly stopped

▶ What Should I Tell My Patients About This Drug?

- complete medication history is important to evaluate the potential drug interactions that may potentiate bleeding problems
- complete medical problem history is important to evaluate potential risk and contraindications to thrombolytic therapy
- compliance with strict bed rest or other measures is important to minimize bleeding
- may cause severe hypersensitivity reactions, including anaphylaxis, especially in patients who have had prior streptokinase therapy or a recent streptococcal infection

▶ Therapeutic Tips

- use of acetaminophen rather than aspirin is recommended for febrile reactions due to streptokinase

Useful References

Gruppo Italiano. per lo.Studio della Streptochi nasi nell'Infarto Miocardico (GISSI). Long-term effects of intravenous thrombolysis in acute myocardial infarction: Final report of the GISSI Study. Lancet 1987; 2:871–874

ISIS-2 (Second Internation Study of Infarct Survival) Collaborative Group. Randomized trial of intravenous streptokinase, oral aspirn, both or neither among 17, 187 cases of suspected acute myocardial infarction: ISIS-2. Lancet 1988;2:349–360

Wilcox RG, Von Der LIppe G, Olsson CG, et al. Trial of tissue plasminogen activator for mortality reduction in acute myocardial infarction: Anglo Scandinavian Study of Early Thrombolysis (ASSET). Lancet 1988; 2:525–530

SUCRALFATE

James McCormack and Glen Brown

USA (Carafate)
CANADA (Sulcrate)

▶ When Should I Use This Drug?

Duodenal or gastric ulcers

- use if H₂ antagonists or omeprazole cannot be used because of intolerance or documented drug interactions
- sucralfate needs to be given twice daily and is more expensive than cimetidine

Prevention of peptic ulcer disease recurrence

- use sucralfate if the patient is unable to tolerate H_2 antagonists

Stress ulcer prophylaxis

- for patients with extensive burns, central nervous system injury, prolonged hypotension, sepsis, uncorrectable coagulopathy, or acute respiratory or hepatic failure (Am J Gastroenterol 1990; 85:95–96)
- when oral or nasogastric administration is possible, sucralfate is favored over parenteral H_2 antagonists because there is a lower risk of nosocomial infection and sucralfate is less expensive

▶ *When Should I Not Use This Drug?*

In combination with other antiulcer medications

- no studies support combination therapy of regularly dosed upper gastrointestinal drugs for the treatment of peptic ulcer disease, and combinations only increase the cost and the chance of adverse effects (Lancet 1988;1:1383–1385, N Engl J Med 1991; 325:1017–1025, Am J Gastroenterol 1993;88:675–679)

Prevention of nonsteroidal antiinflammatory drug–induced ulcers

- sucralfate does not appear to be any better than placebo

▶ *What Contraindications Are There to the Use of This Drug?*

- intolerance of or allergic reaction to sucralfate

▶ *What Drug Interactions Are Clinically Important?*

Drugs that may increase the effect or toxicity of sucralfate

- none

Drugs that may decrease the effect of sucralfate

ANTACIDS

- may interfere with the effect of sucralfate on the mucosa; therefore, do not take antacids within 30 minutes of taking sucralfate

Drugs that may have their effect or toxicity increased by sucralfate

- none

Drugs that may have their effect decreased by sucralfate

PHENYTOIN, TETRACYCLINE, CIPROFLOXACIN, NORFLOXACIN, FAT-SOLUBLE VITAMINS

- a number of drugs have been shown to have their absorption decreased by sucralfate
- to minimize this effect, administer these drugs at least 3 hours before or after sucralfate administration

▶ *What Route and Dosage Should I Use?*

How to administer

- orally—take with a glass of water

Duodenal or gastric ulcers

- 2 g PO BID has been shown to be as effective as 1 g PO QID (Am J Med 1987;83[suppl 3B]:86–90)

Prevention of duodenal or gastric ulcer recurrence

- 1 g PO BID

Stress ulcer prophylaxis

- 1 g PO or via nasogastric tube QID

Dosage adjustments for renal or hepatic dysfunction

- not absorbed orally; therefore, no dosage adjustments are needed
- long-term use in patients with renal failure should be avoided because of potential accumulation of aluminum

▶ *What Should I Monitor with Regard to Efficacy and Toxicity?*

Efficacy

Duodenal or gastric ulcer

- relief of symptoms such as epigastric pain or discomfort, belching, burning, bloating, fullness, and nausea and vomiting

- if there is no relief after 1 week, endoscopy or reendoscopy is recommended
- for duodenal ulcers, reendoscopy is not needed unless symptoms persist
- for gastric ulcers, reendoscopy is recommended to ensure that complete healing has occurred because loss of symptoms is well described in malignant ulcers

Stress ulcer prophylaxis

- absence of blood in gastric aspirates
- if aspirate contains blood, the need for endoscopy should be evaluated

Toxicity

Gastrointestinal effects

- constipation is the most common side effect
- if constipation occurs, increase fluid and fiber intake

▶ *How Long Do I Treat Patients with This Drug?*

Duodenal or gastric ulcers

- 6 weeks
- if there is satisfactory response, stop the drug
- if there is no response at this time, continue therapy for another 6 weeks
- if there is still no response, consider alternative therapy such as omeprazole

Prevention of peptic ulcer disease recurrence

- indefinitely; however, consideration should be given to a trial off drug in patients who have remained symptom free for longer than 2 years unless the peptic ulcer disease was associated with complications (bleeding, perforation, and so on)

Stress ulcer prophylaxis

- after a patient is no longer at risk for hypoperfusion or is receiving consistent feeding by gastric administration, stress ulcer prophylaxis is not needed
- in general, if a patient is no longer in an intensive care unit or burn ward and has sepsis or central nervous system injury, prophylaxis can be stopped

▶ *How Do I Decrease or Stop the Administration of This Drug?*

- may be stopped abruptly

▶ *What Should I Tell My Patients About This Drug?*

- this drug may cause constipation; therefore, increase fiber and fluid intake
- this drug may interact with some medications; therefore, check with your physician or pharmacist before using other medications

SULFINPYRAZONE

C. Wayne Weart

USA (Anturane, generics)
CANADA (Antazone, Anturan, Apo-Sulfinpyrazone, Novopyrazone)

▶ *When Should I Use This Drug?*

Prophylaxis of acute gouty arthritis

- probenecid is the preferred agent in patients who excrete less than 700 mg/24 h of uric acid, as it has fewer adverse gastrointestinal and hematological effects than does sulfinpyrazone
- no real advantages over other agents such as allopurinol and is generally not used

▶ *When Should I Not Use This Drug?*

Acute gout attack

- has no analgesic or antiinflammatory activity and may exacerbate and prolong the acute attack

Prophylactic therapy in patients with renal insufficiency

- in patients with renal insufficiency (i.e., creatinine clearance less than 50 mL/min) or a history of renal stones (uric acid– or calcium-containing stones), sulfinpyrazone increases urinary concentrations of uric acid and may cause stone formation

Angina, myocardial infarction, transient ischemic attacks, atherosclerosis, thromboemboli, arteriovenous dialysis shunts, and prosthetic heart valves

- inhibits platelet aggregation and prolongs platelet survival time; however, these effects are generally not impressive
- not approved indications and its use is not recommended

▶ What Contraindications Are There to the Use of This Drug?

Intolerance of or allergic reaction to sulfinpyrazone or phenylbutazone

Patients with a history of uric acid renal stones

- sulfinpyrazone may increase the risk of urate or calcium renal stones if baseline 24 hour urine uric acid level is elevated

Patients with a history of gastrointestinal ulceration

- significant risk of gastrointestinal distress and activation of peptic ulcer disease

Patients with a history of blood dyscrasias

- may worsen these conditions

▶ What Drug Interactions are Clinically Important?

Drugs that may increase the effect or toxicity of sulfinpyrazone

- none

Drugs that may decrease the effect of sulfinpyrazone

NIACIN

- may reduce the uricosuric effect of sulfinpyrazone
- avoid combination, as niacin can increase uric acid concentrations

SALICYLATES

- may reduce the uricosuric effect of sulfinpyrazone
- avoid the administration of aspirin and salicylates and consider acetaminophen

Drugs that may have their effect or toxicity increased by sulfinpyrazone

WARFARIN

- may enhance the activity of warfarin
- use alternative agents if possible because of the possible gastrointestinal toxicity and platelet inhibition effect
- if not, monitor INR every 2 days until the full extent of interaction is seen and adjust the dosage as for a warfarin dosage change
- monitor INR every 2 days when administration of the interacting drug is discontinued and adjust as needed

ORAL HYPOGLYCEMICS

- can displace the sulfonylurea from albumin and also may reduce clearance
- if these drugs are added to therapy, treat as if a dosage change of the oral hypoglycemic has been made

Drugs that may have their effect decreased by sulfinpyrazone

THEOPHYLLINE

- may enhance plasma clearance of theophylline and thus lower theophylline levels

VERAPAMIL

- sulfinpyrazone may increase the clearance of verapamil and reduce its effectiveness
- if the clinical effect of verapamil decreases, increase the dosage of verapamil
- avoid combination if possible

▶ What Route and Dosage Should I Use?

How to administer

- orally—take with food or milk
- parenterally—not available

Prophylaxis of acute gouty arthritis

- give 100 mg PO daily and gradually increase the dosage by 100 mg weekly until the serum uric acid concentration is less than 6 mg/dL or the total daily dose reaches 800 mg
- slow dosage titration is recommended to prevent or minimize the risk of mobilization gout and to avoid sudden excretion of large amounts of uric acid through the kidney
- wait 2–3 weeks after an acute gouty attack to initiate therapy to lower uric acid concentrations, as urate-lowering therapy may exacerbate the acute gouty attack

Dosage adjustments for renal or hepatic dysfunction

Normal Dosing Interval	C_{cr} > 60 mL/min or 1 mL/s	C_{cr} 30–60 mL/min or 0.5–1 mL/s	C_{cr} < 30 mL/min or 0.5 mL/s
Q12H	no adjustment needed	avoid, as it may not be effective	avoid

▶ What Should I Monitor with Regard to Efficacy and Toxicity?

Efficacy

Prophylaxis of acute gouty arthritis

Serum uric acid level

- measure at baseline and repeat weekly until an appropriate dosage has been determined to reduce serum uric acid levels to less than 6 mg/dL
- after levels are stable measure every 6–12 months

24 hour urine uric acid levels

- before starting therapy to determine whether probenecid therapy is needed

Number of attacks

- number of acute gouty attacks should decrease

Toxicity

24 hour urine uric acid levels

- sulfinpyrazone may increase the risk of urate or calcium renal stones if the baseline 24 hour urine uric acid level is elevated
- if the 24 hour urine uric acid levels with sulfinpyrazone therapy do not exceed 700 mg/d, sulfinpyrazone dosage may not be adequate or the drug is not effective
- liberal fluid intake and an alkaline urine are desired to minimize the risk of uric acid stone formation until serum uric acid levels are maintained in the normal range and tophaceous deposits disappear

Gastrointestinal distress, gastrointestinal blood loss

- significant risk of gastrointestinal distress and activation of peptic ulcer disease
- if this occurs, stop the drug administration and try an alternative agent

Blood dyscrasias

- allopurinol may cause agranulocytosis, thrombocytopenia, leukopenia, and/or aplastic anemia
- monitor complete blood count at baseline and remeasure with suspected toxicity

▶ How Long Do I Treat Patients with This Drug?

Prophylaxis of acute gouty arthritis

- uric acid–lowering therapy is usually continued indefinitely but consideration should be given to reduced dosage of sulfinpyrazone as patients age or experience reduced renal function or as obese patients successfully attain ideal body weight
- generally not able to withdraw uric acid–lowering therapy but may be able to reduce the dosage as long as the serum uric acid level is maintained below 6 mg/dL

▶ How Do I Decrease or Stop the Administration of This Drug?

- may be stopped abruptly

- reduce the daily dosage by 100 mg increments every 4 months when titrating the dose downward
- may go to as little as 200 mg/d in divided doses as long as serum uric acid levels do not go above 6 mg/dL

▶ What Should I Tell My Patients About This Drug?

- drink at least 6–8 full (8 ounce) glasses of water each day to reduce the risk of renal stones
- take each dose with food to reduce gastrointestinal upset
- avoid taking large doses of aspirin, which may antagonize the effects of sulfinpyrazone (if an analgesic or antipyretic is needed, try acetaminophen)

▶ Therapeutic Tips

- start out with low doses (e.g., 100 mg PO daily) and gradually increase the dosage until serum uric acid levels are maintained less than 6 mg/dL
- low-dose colchicine should be given concurrently for the first 3 months to reduce the risk of mobilization gout

Useful References

Simkin PA. Management of gout. Ann Intern Med 1979;90:812–816

Tate G, Schumacher HR. Clinical features. In: Primer on Rheumatic Diseases. 9th ed. Atlanta: Arthritis Foundation, 1988:198–202

Wallace SL, Singer JZ. Treatment. In: Primer on Rheumatic Diseases. 9th ed. Atlanta: Arthritis Foundation, 1988:202–206

Wallace SL, Singer JZ. Therapy in gout. Rheum Dis Clin North Am 1988;14:441–457

SULFASALAZINE (5-AMINOSALICYLIC ACID BOUND TO SULFAPYRIDINE)

Scott Whittaker and Kelly Jones

USA (Azulfidine, generics)
CANADA (Salazopyrin, S.A.S. Enteric-500, S.A.S.-500)

▶ When Should I Use This Drug?

Ulcerative colitis

- in disease limited to the rectosigmoid, if urgency and tenemus limit the retention time for enemas and thus the effectiveness of these agents, oral mesalamine (5-aminosalicylic acid [5-ASA]) should be used
- in patients with mild to moderate disease not limited to the rectosigmoid, and perhaps as high as the splenic flexure, or patients unable to retain enemas, oral 5-ASA should be used as first-line therapy
- all patients with established ulcerative colitis should receive maintenance therapy with some 5-ASA agent, unless they refuse to take this medication long term
- in patients with mild to moderate ulcerative colitis who are not allergic to sulfa, sulfasalazine is the 5-ASA drug of choice because sulfasalazine is as effective and much less expensive than the new 5-ASA medications.
- there are rare, but serious side effects with sulfasalazine, which has led some gastroenterologists to use the newer non–sulfa-containing 5-ASA preparations, but there is no evidence that these new preparations are more effective than sulfasalazine (Gut 1991;32:462–463)
- sulfasalazine requires bacterial action to split (activate); therefore, it is useful only in colonic inflammatory disease

Crohn's disease

- sulfasalazine is effective for Crohn's disease involving the colon (Gastroenterology 1979;77:847–869)
- in patients with mild to moderate Crohn's colitis without small bowel involvement who are not sulfa allergic, sulfasalazine is the drug of choice, as it is effective and less expensive than the other agents

Moderate rheumatoid arthritis

- as a second-line agent in moderate disease if symptoms persist with little sign of remission after a 1 month trial with nonsteroidal antiinflammatory drugs

- sulfasalazine is used in patients who fail to respond to 6 months of oral gold therapy (auranofin) for the treatment of mild rheumatoid arthritis
- this agent may be preferable to gold in patients with mild disease who are classically noncompliant with office visits and follow-up laboratory work
- this drug is safe, with a study reporting no fatalities in 900 patients treated for 11 years (Br Med J 1986;293:420–423), although some researchers believe that sulfasalazine has more side effects than does hydroxychloroquine (Postgrad Med 1990;87:79–92)
- sulfasalazine is easy to administer and is inexpensive

▶ When Should I Not Use This Drug?

Ulcerative proctitis or colitis in combination with corticosteroids

- there is no therapeutic benefit to adding 5-ASA to systemic corticosteroids in patients with a severe flare of ulcerative proctitis or colitis

Crohn's disease with small bowel involvement or severe disease being treated with corticosteroids

- not useful in patients with small bowel involvement because 5-ASA is not released in the small bowel
- there is no therapeutic gain to adding 5-ASA compounds to prednisone during short-term therapy, except in the first 6 weeks (Ann Intern Med 1991;114:445–450)

Severe rheumatoid arthritis

- not as effective as methotrexate and intramuscular gold

▶ What Contraindications Are There to the Use of This Drug?

Intolerance of or allergy to sulfa drugs, acetylsalicylic acid, or sulfasalazine

Men who wish to have children

- sulfasalazine may cause oligospermia and alter sperm function

▶ What Drug Interactions Are Clinically Important?

Drugs that may increase the effect or toxicity of sulfasalazine

- none

Drugs that may decrease the effect of sulfasalazine

- none

Drugs that may have their effect or toxicity increased by sulfasalazine

METHOTREXATE

- metabolism is inhibited by sulfonamides, and there may be enhanced toxicity of methotrexate on the bone marrow
- initiate methotrexate therapy at the lowest dosage or reduce the dosage transiently to assess the effect of adding sulfasalazine to established methotrexate therapy

WARFARIN

- interferes with warfarin metabolism and can increase INR
- use alternative agents if possible
- if not, monitor INR every 2 days until the full extent of interaction is seen and adjust the dosage as for a warfarin dosage change
- monitor INR every 2 days when administration of the interacting drug is discontinued and adjust as for a warfarin dosage change

ORAL HYPOGLYCEMICS

- can reduce the metabolism of oral hypoglycemics
- if sulfasalazine is added to therapy, treat as if a dosage change of the oral hypoglycemic has been made

Drugs that may have their effect decreased by sulfasalazine

FOLIC ACID

- sulfasalazine may interfere with the absorption and efficacy of folic acid, but folic acid is not routinely administered unless evidence of deficiency exists

▶ What Route and Dosage Should I Use?

How to administer

- orally—take with food
- parenterally—not available

Ulcerative colitis

- give 1 g PO BID and increase every 4 days by 1 g/d until 4 g/d is reached (in 4 divided doses) or the patient experiences intolerable side effects
- dosage greater than 4 g/d is usually not well tolerated; however, a dosage up to 6 g may be used if the patient can tolerate it
- 1 g PO BID as a maintenance dosage after remission has been induced for ulcerative colitis
- use an enteric-coated product if gastrointestinal symptoms are a problem

Crohn's disease

- as above for ulcerative colitis, except that maintenance therapy is generally not used, because the efficacy of maintenance therapy is not well established; however, new information may alter this recommendation
- treat for 10–14 days beyond relief of symptoms (usual course of therapy is 6–8 weeks)

Moderate rheumatoid arthritis

- 500 mg PO BID of the enteric-coated product for 2 weeks, then increase to 1000 mg PO BID for 2 weeks, and if necessary, increase to 1500 mg PO BID at 6 weeks
- this slow increase in dosage reduces the incidence of side effects (J Rheumatol 1988;16:5–8)

Dosage adjustments for renal or hepatic dysfunction

- renally eliminated, unknown dosage modifications

▶ What Should I Monitor with Regard to Efficacy and Toxicity?

Efficacy

Ulcerative colitis

- in general, patients should be seen within 2 weeks of starting therapy, particularly if steroids are being employed, because tapering of steroid administration should begin no later than 2 weeks after starting therapy

Signs and symptoms

- diarrhea, urgency, tenesmus, blood per rectum, abdominal pain, fever, and weight status should improve
- symptoms begin to improve with steroids (topical or oral) within a week, but may take a few days longer with 5-ASA

Laboratory variables

- indicators of inflammation (increased white blood cell count, including left shift) and of blood loss from ulceration (decreased hemoglobin) should improve in 1 week
- in severely ill hospitalized patients, these counts are done daily
- in less ill outpatients, these are repeated after a week

Crohn's disease

- treat for 1–2 weeks and reassess the patient

Signs and symptoms

- diarrhea, abdominal pain, fever, abdominal distention and tenderness, decreased size of mass (if present), and increased appetite
- these symptoms may persist for 2–3 weeks before improvement is seen and complete relief of symptoms may not occur

Laboratory variables

- indicators of inflammation (increased white blood cell count, including left shift) and of blood loss from ulceration (decreased hemoglobin) should improve in 1 week
- in severely ill hospitalized patients, these counts are done daily
- in less ill outpatients, these are repeated after a week

Rheumatoid arthritis

Joint tenderness count, sedimentation rate measurements, grip strength, duration of morning stiffness, time to onset of fatigue, and patient's report on specific symptoms

- patient's symptoms and X-rays should be assessed monthly for the first 2 months, and after the disease is under control, the patient can be assessed every 3 months for 6 months and then every 6 months
- these variables should be used to guide drug administration starting and stopping
- one study found that clinical and laboratory measures of physical well-being appeared to be unrelated to psychological and social measures of well-being (J Rheumatol 1991;18:650–653)
- it is important to include the patient's self-assessment of the drug's effect on their function and well-being

Toxicity

Nausea, epigastric distress, and headaches

- are frequent, particularly at higher dosages (4 g or higher)
- reduction of the dosage may alleviate toxicities, and a slow increase in subsequent dosages may avoid toxic symptoms
- to prevent gastrointestinal side effects, use enteric-coated product and increase the dosage slowly, and if the patient still has symptoms, decrease the dosage and give 4 times a day, and if symptoms persist, stop the drug administration for 7 days and reinstate at a lower dose

Hepatitis and pancreatitis

- rare, but ask the patient at each visit about the presence of new abdominal pains and examine for jaundice

Stevens-Johnson syndrome, hemolytic anemia and leukopenia, agranulocytosis

- occur rarely, but are severe potential side effects
- complete blood count with differential and platelet counts at baseline, then every 2 weeks for 8 weeks, then monthly for 6 months, and then every 2 months thereafter

Transverse myelitis, convulsions, peripheral neuropathy

- occur rarely, but ask the patient at each visit about signs of muscle weakness or unusual sensations in the limbs

Hypersensitivity

- can occur, but are rare
- these reactions involve urticaria and serum sickness–type reactions and the drug administration should be discontinued

Serum creatinine levels

- changes in renal function can occur but are rare
- in patients with severe renal disease, measure serum creatinine levels every 2 weeks for 6 weeks to evaluate the impact of the drug on renal function

▶ How Long Do I Treat Patients with This Drug?

Ulcerative colitis

- in cases of an acute flare-up of inflammatory bowel disease, after the maximum dosage tolerated has been reached, the drug is continued at that dosage and there is no need to taper
- for maintenance therapy of ulcerative colitis, the drug administration is continued indefinitely, as relapses occur in only 20% of the patients taking the drug versus 73% of the patients receiving no therapy (Lancet 1965;2:185–188)
- some patients who have had infrequent flares (e.g., every few years) with no maintenance therapy (patients either are undiagnosed or have refused maintenance), use drug therapy just for treatment of flares of the disease

Crohn's disease

- total of a 6–8 week course of sulfasalazine for acute disease is all that is usually necessary
- for the patient with Crohn's disease that is in remission, the drug administration may be stopped abruptly 10–14 days after the patient is symptom free

Moderate rheumatoid arthritis

- this drug should be given at least a 3 month trial at 3 g/d before resorting to other therapies; improvement should be noted by 8 weeks
- sulfasalazine can be used indefinitely as long as the patient tolerates the drug and is receiving relief of symptoms
- patients whose disease is not controlled or becomes progressive (noted radiographic changes) should have the drug stopped and another agent tried
- studies suggest long-term safety (Br Med J 1986;293:420–423)

▶ *How Do I Decrease or Stop the Administration of This Drug?*

- may be stopped abruptly

▶ *What Should I Tell My Patients About This Drug?*

Ulcerative colitis, Crohn's disease

- drug may take several days to few weeks for control of symptoms
- if there is worsening of symptoms in the first week, return for reevaluation
- you should be seen at 2 weeks for reevaluation
- if you have Crohn's disease, the drug administration should be continued for approximately 2 weeks after complete relief of symptoms
- if you are receiving maintenance therapy for ulcerative colitis, the drug should be continued, even though you feel perfectly well
- be aware of the increase in relapse rates of ulcerative colitis after discontinuation of the medication regimen

Moderate rheumatoid arthritis

- take the medication after a meal
- check stool for enteric-coated tablet (some patients lack intestinal esterases that degrade the coating)
- monitor for any unusual symptoms such as unusual bleeding, fever, and malaise
- drug may cause a yellow-orange discoloration of the urine; it can also stain contact lenses
- take with a full glass of water to prevent possible crystalluria from the sulfur component

▶ *Therapeutic Tips*

- start at a relatively low dosage of 1 g BID in the acute and build up over a period of several days, increasing the dosage roughly every 4 days by 1 g until the maximum dosage of 6 g/d is given or until the patient is intolerant, which often begins at about 4 g of drug per day
- do not increase the dosage after the dose-related side effects (nausea and headache) develop
- if the patient finds the drug in the stool after taking the enteric-coated product the non–enteric-coated product should be used
- go low and go slow with the dosing

SULINDAC
Kelly Jones

USA (Clinoril, various generics)
CANADA (Clinoril, Apo-Sulin, Novosundac)

▶ *When Should I Use This Drug?*

Acute pain, general aches and pain, bone pain, dysmenorrhea, cancer pain

- useful for the short-term management of general aches and pains
- only advantage over non–enteric-coated aspirin is that it causes less gastrointestinal intolerance
- decision between this drug and other nonsteroidal antiinflammatory drugs (NSAIDs) should be based on cost

Rheumatoid Arthritis

- sulindac can be used as an alternative for patients who fail to respond to ibuprofen; however, it is more expensive

---

- sulindac is generally believed to have the least adverse effect on the kidney; however, all NSAIDs have the potential to cause adverse renal effects (N Engl J Med 1991;324:1716–1725)
- sulindac is a prodrug and must be converted to active drug in the liver (sulindac sulfide)
- when sulindac is excreted in the kidney, it is proposed that the drug is converted back to its prodrug state and is less likely to affect renal prostaglandins (JAMA 1982;248:2864–2867); however, this mechanism has been debated over the years
- sulindac is the preferred agent in patients taking lithium if patients are unable to tolerate enteric coated aspirin
- among NSAIDs, aspirin and sulindac appear to have the least hypertensive effect (Ann Intern Med 1994;121:289–300) however, all NSAIDs likely have the potential to worsen blood pressure control and blood pressure should be measured at every follow-up visit in patients who are hypertensive or borderline hypertensive
- sulindac is considered harsh on the stomach and should not be used in patients at high risk for gastrointestinal toxicity (J Am Board Fam Pract 1989;2:257–271)

Osteoarthritis

- if acetaminophen, aspirin, or ibuprofen are not effective
- decision between this drug and other NSAIDs should be based on cost

▶ *When Should I Not Use This Drug?*

Combination with other nonsteroidal antiinflammatory drugs

- combinations of NSAIDs provide no increase in effectiveness compared with maximum doses of single agents and significantly increase the risk of adverse effects

▶ *What Contraindications Are There to the Use of This Drug?*

see Ibuprofen

▶ *What Drug Interactions Are Clinically Important?*

see Ibuprofen

▶ *What Route and Dosage Should I Use?*

How to administer

- orally—take with food or milk
- parenterally—not available

Acute pain, general aches and pain, bone pain, dysmenorrhea

- 150–200 mg PO Q12H PRN

Rheumatoid arthritis, cancer pain

- 150 mg PO Q12H up to a maximum dosage of 400 mg PO daily

Osteoarthritis

- 150 mg PO Q12H

Dosage adjustments for renal or hepatic dysfunction

- hepatically metabolized; therefore, no adjustments are needed for renal disease
- reduce dosage by 25% in patients with a history of hepatic disease

▶ *What Should I Monitor with Regard to Efficacy and Toxicity?*

see Ibuprofen

▶ *How Long Do I Treat Patients with This Drug?*

see Ibuprofen

▶ *How Do I Decrease or Stop the Administration of This Drug?*

- may be stopped abruptly if needed

▶ *What Should I Tell My Patients About This Drug?*

see Ibuprofen

▶ *Therapeutic Tips*

see Ibuprofen

Useful References

see Ibuprofen

SUMATRIPTAN

Jerry Taylor

USA (Imitrex)

CANADA (Imitrex)

▶ *When Should I Use This Drug?*

Migraine treatment

- should be used in patients who have failed to respond to simple analgesics or who have moderate to severe symptoms especially in patients with contraindications to ergot compounds
- is effective and well tolerated when given as single subcutaneous or oral dose (JAMA 1991;265:2831–2835) but does not work in all patients and it is expensive
- appears to be more effective and safer than ergotamine, but further comparative trials are needed (Eur Neurol 1991;31: 314–322)
- no comparative trials have been done between parenteral sumatriptan and other effective parenteral regimens (dihydroergotamine ± metoclopramide)
- oral sumatriptan has been shown to be more effective than the combination of aspirin and metoclopramide (Br Med J 1991; 303:1491)
- approximately 50% of patients respond within 2 hours of an oral dose (Lancet 1991;338:782–783) and 70% of patients within 1 hour of subcutaneous administration

▶ *When Should I Not Use This Drug?*

Migraine prophylaxis

- no evidence that it is effective in the prevention of migraines

▶ *What Contraindications Are There to the Use of This Drug?*

Intolerance of or allergic reaction to sumatriptan

Hypertension and angina

- mild increases in systolic and diastolic blood pressure or potential for peripheral vasoconstriction may aggravate underlying conditions

▶ *What Drug Interactions Are Clinically Important?*

- none

▶ *What Route and Dosage Should I Use?*

How to administer

- orally—take with food or milk or on an empty stomach
- parenterally—infuse over 10 minutes in normal saline
- subcutaneously—patients may be instructed to use an autoinjector device to give an injection to their thigh

Migraine treatment

- 100 mg PO as early as possible after the start of the attack
- 6 mg SC as early as possible after the start of the attack if the patient is unable to use the oral route or the oral product is not available
- if the initial dose is not effective, repeated doses are not likely to be effective (N Engl J Med 1991;325:316–321)
- if the initial dose is effective but headache returns, repeat the dose (maximum of 3 doses orally or 2 subcutaneously per 24 hours)

Dosage adjustments for renal or hepatic dysfunction

- extensively metabolized by the liver, and dosage adjustments in renal failure are not required

- reductions have been suggested in hepatic disease; however, no specific recommendations have been provided

▶ *What Should I Monitor with Regard to Efficacy and Toxicity?*

Efficacy

Migraine treatment

Relief of pain and other symptoms such as prodromal, aura, and gastrointestinal effects

- assess the patient hourly during the early stage of migraine attacks

Toxicity

Sensation of heaviness and pressure in the chest and warmth or tingling in the head or extremities

- mild symptoms are noticed in approximately 50% of patients and last approximately 10–30 minutes (N Engl J Med 1991; 325:316–321)

▶ *How Long Do I Treat Patients with This Drug?*

Migraine treatment

- give as a single dose, as administration of a second dose does not appear to improve the benefits (N Engl J Med 1991;325:316–321); however, if the initial dose is effective and the headache returns (e.g., within 24 hours), a repeated dose may be useful

▶ *How Do I Decrease or Stop the Administration of This Drug?*

- may be stopped abruptly

▶ *What Should I Tell My Patients About This Drug?*

- proper timing of dose administration is most important
- effect with the oral form is seen within 2 hours
- effect with the parenteral form is seen within 1 hour
- side effects are mild and transient and often disappear within 30 minutes of the injection
- pain at the site of the injection may occur

▶ *Therapeutic Tips*

- 2–3 trials of this drug should be given because occasionally different migraine episodes (e.g., different triggers) may respond differently to this drug
- 30–40% of patients have recurrence of symptoms 24 hours after the initial dose
- does not work for everyone and rescue medication should be given to the patient who has not had an adequate response

Useful References

Peroutka SJ. The pharmacology of current anti-migraine drugs. Headache 1990;30(suppl 1):5–11

Humphrey PPA, Feniuk W, Perren MJ. Anti-migraine drugs in development: Advances in serotonin receptor pharmacology. Headache 1990;30(suppl 1):12–16

TEMAZEPAM

Jonathan Fleming

USA (Restoril)

CANADA (Restoril)

▶ *When Should I Use This Drug?*

Transient situational insomnia, short-term insomnia

- this is an all-purpose hypnotic, which covers the whole sleep period
- all of the marketed benzodiazepines have sedative properties and can be used as hypnotics
- they differ in their pharmacokinetics, side effect profile, capacity to cause discontinuation syndromes (e.g., rebound insomnia), and cost
- lorazepam, oxazepam, and temazepam are equally effective, although there are fewer data on the use of lorazepam and oxazepam as hypnotics

- lorazepam, as with other high-potency, short-acting benzodiazepines, is associated with worse rebound effects than less potent or longer-acting compounds (not important if being used for just a few nights)
- decision should also include cost (lorazepam and oxazepam are available as generics and are usually less expensive)

Long-term treatment of insomnia

- effective in the intermittent treatment of long-term insomnia if the use of alternative, behavioral techniques for controlling insomnia is ineffective
- although studies on the efficacy of long-term use of hypnotics are scant and many sleep laboratory studies show a loss of hypnotic effect (tolerance) by the fourth week of continuous use, about 10% of patients benefit from continuous or intermittent use of hypnotics and long-term users often report high satisfaction with their sleep and few adverse effects (Age Ageing 1984;13:335–343)
- continued, intermittent medication use (provided there is demonstrable benefit) may be the most sensible approach

Periodic limb movement disorder

- clonazepam, temazepam (Sleep 1986;9:385–392), nitrazepam (Can J Neurol Sci 1986;13:52–54), levodopa (Clin Neuropharmacol 1986;9:456–463), and trazodone (Sleep Res 1988;17:39) have demonstrated efficacy in managing this disorder
- although there are more scientific data for clonazepam and temazepam, trazodone (on the basis of clinical experience) may have an advantage over these agents in that patients do not appear to become tolerant of its effects

▶ When Should I Not Use This Drug?

Transient and short-term insomnia when it is important to avoid daytime sedation or effects on psychomotor performance such as for the management of jet lag

- temazepam has a moderately long half-life; therefore, use triazolam, which has fewer hangover effects

▶ What Contraindications Are There to the Use of This Drug?

see Lorazepam

▶ What Drug Interactions Are Clinically Important?

see Lorazepam

▶ What Route and Dosage Should I Use?

How to administer

- orally—1–1½ hours before retiring

Transient situational insomnia, short-term insomnia, long-term insomnia

- 15 mg PO 1–1½ hours prior to retiring
- increase to 30 mg only if the lower dosage is clearly ineffective

Dosage adjustments for renal or hepatic dysfunction

- hepatically metabolized
- no dosage adjustments for organ dysfunction are recommended; however, always start with the lowest dose and titrate to response

▶ What Should I Monitor with Regard to Efficacy and Toxicity?

see Lorazepam

▶ How Long Do I Treat Patients with This Drug?

see Lorazepam

▶ How Do I Decrease or Stop the Administration of This Drug?

see Lorazepam

▶ What Should I Tell My Patients About This Drug?

- hard gelatin capsule affects the absorption rate; if being used for initial insomnia, it should be taken 1–1½ hours prior to the planned retiring time

- rebound insomnia may occur, and transitory sleep disturbance on withdrawal is to be expected and is not an indication to restart the medication regimen
- report any adverse effects as soon as they occur
- increasing the dosage can lead to unwanted side effects, and if the dosage is not effective, consult your physician before increasing the dosage on your own
- do not use with alcohol
- should be stopped if you are planning to become pregnant
- disturbances in memory may occur, particularly for material learned just prior to the sleep period or during the sleep period (e.g., physicians may forget orders given during the night, students may forget information learned that night)
- sedative properties are additive if it is used with over the counter antihistamines; increased sedation may occur
- note the improvements in your sleep performance and daytime functioning so that these can be evaluated at the follow-up visit

▶ Therapeutic Tips

- this is an all-purpose hypnotic, which covers the whole sleep period and is a good first-line medication
- if the drug is used for managing initial insomnia, ensure that it is given early enough because of the slow absorption rate
- is effective in the management of periodic leg movements during sleep (Sleep 1986;9:385–392), but try trazodone first because it may not lead to tolerance

Useful References

Hosie HE, Nimmo WS. Temazepam absorption in patients before surgery. Br J Anaesth 1991;66:20–24

Ngen CC, Hassan R. A double-blind placebo-controlled trial of zopiclone 7.5 mg and temazepam 20 mg in insomnia. Int Clin Psychopharmacol 1990;5:165–171

Mitler MM, Browman CP, Menn SJ, et al. Nocturnal myoclonus: Treatment efficacy of clonazepam and temazepam. Sleep 1986;9:385–392

TENOXICAM

Kelly Jones

USA (not available)
CANADA (Mobiflex)

▶ When Should I Use This Drug?

Rheumatoid arthritis

- tenoxicam can be used as an alternative for patients who fail to respond to enteric coated aspirin or ibuprofen; however, it is more expensive
- useful in patients who have a history of noncompliance (because of its once-daily dosing); however, once-daily dosing may not be preferred in patients with arthritis pain, as these patients may want to dose more than once per day (DICP 1989;23:76–85)
- most regular-release nonsteroidal antiinflammatory drugs (NSAIDs), including aspirin, can be taken on an every 12 hour basis when being used to treat arthritic conditions, and therefore, once-daily NSAIDs provide the advantage of only once- versus twice-daily dosing
- decision among piroxicam, tenoxicam, nabumetone, and oxaprozin (once a day NSAIDs) should be based on cost
- sustained-release NSAIDs can be used once daily, preferably in the evening, to attempt a reduction in morning stiffness and should be chosen if they are less expensive than piroxicam, tenoxicam, nabumetone, or oxaprozin

Osteoarthritis

- if acetaminophen, enteric coated aspirin or ibuprofen are not effective
- decision between this drug and other NSAIDs should be based on cost

▶ When Should I Not Use This Drug?

Acute pain, general aches and pain, dysmenorrhea

- not useful for the short-term management of general aches and pains because it is difficult to titrate owing to its long half-life

Control of acute pain associated with arthritis

- this drug should never be used initially to gain control of arthritis pain, as the long half-life does not allow dosing flexibility
- this drug should be reserved as maintenance therapy for those with controlled disease

Combination with other nonsteroidal antiinflammatory drugs

- combinations of NSAIDs provide no increase in effectiveness compared with maximum dosages of single agents and significantly increase the risk of adverse effects

▶ *What Contraindications Are There to the Use of This Drug?*

see Ibuprofen

▶ *What Drug Interactions Are Clinically Important?*

see Ibuprofen

▶ *What Route and Dosage Should I Use?*

How to administer

- orally—take with food or milk
- parenterally—not available

Rheumatoid arthritis

- 10 mg PO at HS to a maximum dosage of 20 mg PO at HS

Osteoarthritis

- 10 mg PO at HS

Dosage adjustments for renal or hepatic dysfunction

- hepatically metabolized; therefore, no adjustments are needed for renal disease
- reduce dosage by 25% in patients with a history of hepatic disease

▶ *What Should I Monitor with Regard to Efficacy and Toxicity?*

see Ibuprofen

▶ *How Do I Decrease or Stop the Administration of This Drug?*

- may be stopped abruptly if needed

▶ *What Should I Tell My Patients About This Drug?*

see Ibuprofen

▶ *Therapeutic Tips*

see Ibuprofen

Useful References

see Ibuprofen

TERBUTALINE

Karen Shalansky and Cindy Reesor Nimmo

USA (Brethaire, Brethine, Bricanyl)
CANADA (Bricanyl)

▶ *When Should I Use This Drug?*

Acute asthma or acute exacerbation of chronic obstructive pulmonary disease, chronic asthma or chronic obstructive pulmonary disease

- use only if less expensive than salbutamol
- first-line treatment for intermittent, short-term, or long-term relief of reversible obstructive diseases
- it is beta$_2$-selective, works quickly, is safe, and is inexpensive
- similar in efficacy and duration to salbutamol (albuterol)
- if the patient does not respond to the inhalation route or if the inhalation is not effective, subcutaneous terbutaline has been shown to be more effective than subcutaneous epinephrine (J Asthma 1989;26:287–290)

Exercise-induced asthma

- well tolerated, less expensive, and equally effective as cromolyn
- is also useful if the patient experiences breakthrough wheezing

▶ *When Should I Not Use This Drug?*

Allergic rhinitis, cough or cold symptoms

- unless there is evidence of bronchoconstrictive disease (e.g., wheezing)

Oral therapy

- oral terbutaline should not be used in adults, as it offers no benefit over inhaled beta-agonists and causes more side effects

▶ *What Contraindications Are There to the Use of This Drug?*

see Salbutamol

▶ *What Drug Interactions Are Clinically Important?*

see Salbutamol

▶ *What Route and Dosage Should I Use?*

How to administer

Orally

- do not use

Inhaled

- for metered-dose inhalers (MDIs), see patient instructions below
- for turbuhalers, see patient instructions below

Parenterally

- available for subcutaneous use only (usually given into lateral deltoid area)

Acute asthma or acute exacerbation of COPD

- aggressive therapy is indicated in an acute attack
- in acute exacerbations of airflow obstruction, there is decreased penetration, deposition, and duration of action of aerosols in the peripheral airways, necessitating higher doses for emergency treatment (N Engl J Med 1986;315:870–874)

Metered-dose inhaler

- MDIs are as effective as nebulizers for the treatment of acute asthma (Chest 1987;91:804–807) and are currently the preferred mode of inhalation owing to reduced cost and improved efficiency and speed of drug delivery (Chest 1989;95:888–894)
- patients who are unable to coordinate the inhalation of an MDI may benefit from the use of an extension device
- 4 puffs during 2 minutes, then 1 puff every minute until side effects, such as tremor, occur or until breathlessness and flow rates improve (up to 12 puffs); repeat 4 puffs every 20–30 minutes for 3 doses, then every 1–2 hours until the patient is stable; maintain with 2 puffs every 4–6 hours (Chest 1989;95:888–894, J Allergy Clin Immunol 1990;85:1098–1111)
- need exponential increases in puffs to produce further improvement in bronchodilation (e.g., 2 to 4 puffs, 4 to 8 puffs) (Clin Pharm 1985;4:393–403)
- each puff of terbutaline via an MDI releases 200 μg of active drug

Subcutaneous

- 0.25 mg subcutaneously every 15 minutes for 3 doses as needed

Chronic asthma or COPD

Metered-dose inhaler

- administer 1–2 puffs every 4–6 hours as needed
- if patients require greater than 2 inhalations daily on a regular basis, it is now recommended to initiate low-dose inhaled steroids and maintain terbutaline on a PRN basis; continuous use of a beta-agonist may lead to deterioration of asthma control (Lancet 1990;336:1391–1395)
- may require extension device in patients with difficulty in coordination

Turbuhaler

- may be preferred to an MDI if patients have difficulty in coordination

- 100 μg by MDI is equivalent to 200 μg by powder delivery system
- administer 1–2 inhalations (500–1000 μg) every 4–6 hours as needed
- each puff of terbutaline via a turbuhaler contains 500 μg

Exercise-induced asthma

- inhale 1–2 puffs about 10 minutes prior to exercise

▶ *What Should I Monitor with Regard to Efficacy and Toxicity?*

see Salbutamol

▶ *How Long Do I Treat Patients with This Drug?*

see Salbutamol

▶ *How Do I Decrease or Stop the Administration of This Drug?*

see Salbutamol

▶ *What Should I Tell My Patients About This Drug?*

see Salbutamol

Turbuhaler

1. unscrew and remove the cover
2. holding the Turbuhaler upright, turn the colored grip fully in 1 direction and then back again until it clicks
3. exhale to a normal relaxed expiration, then place the mouthpiece between the teeth and lips
4. breathe in quickly and deeply through your mouth—hold your breath for 5–10 seconds—breathe out slowly to a normal relaxed resting position
5. replace the cover and screw it shut
6. if the Turbuhaler is dropped, the dose is lost and it must be reloaded by turning the colored grip (see step 2)

▶ *Therapeutic Tips*

see Salbutamol

TERFENADINE

Penny Miller

USA (Seldane)
CANADA (Seldane)

▶ *When Should I Use This Drug?*

Seasonal allergic rhinitis, chronic (perennial) rhinitis, chronic dermatological allergies (atopic dermatitis, chronic urticaria, pruritus of unknown cause)

- all antihistamines are considered to have relatively the same efficacy in preventing or treating allergic reactions; however, there is great interpatient variation in the response to a given antihistamine
- selection of any particular antihistamine is based on the degree of sedation and anticholinergic effects, plus convenience of dosing and cost
- terfenadine is useful if the patient has sedative effects or would be sensitive to the sedative effects from less expensive antihistamines such as chlorpheniramine
- choice among astemizole, terfenadine, and loratadine should be based on cost and onset of action (astemizole has a slow onset of action)
- does not impair psychomotor activity or potentiate ethanol's central nervous system effects, such as sedation, decreased visual discrimination, and slowed reaction times
- it does not lower the seizure threshold (unlike diphenhydramine or chlorpheniramine)
- demonstrates little or no anticholinergic side effects (antihistamine effects are responsible for the relief of allergic symptoms)

Acute dermatological allergies (e.g., hives and allergic conjunctivitis caused by allergens or food)

- antihistamines relieve pruritus and prevent further extension of the lesions

- if sedation from an antihistamine is a problem, choose either loratadine or terfenadine, whichever is the least expensive
- if mild sedation would not be a problem, use chlorpheniramine as an HS dose, which is less expensive than terfenadine

▶ *When Should I Not Use This Drug?*

Common cold

- for the symptoms of sneezing and runny nose, terfenadine is not effective because it has little or no anticholinergic effects, unlike chlorpheniramine

▶ *What Contraindications Are There to the Use of This Drug?*

- intolerance of or allergic reaction to terfenadine
- severe hepatic disease
- preexisting cardiac disease or metabolic disease that may cause electrolyte disturbances as these conditions may increase the risk of cardiac toxicity with this agent

▶ *What Drug Interactions Are Clinically Important?*

Drugs that may increase the effect or toxicity of terfenadine

KETOCONAZOLE, ERYTHROMYCIN, CIPROFLOXACIN, FLUCONAZOLE, CIMETIDINE, DISULFIRAM, METRONIDAZOLE

- these drugs decrease the metabolism of terfenadine and patients taking these combinations have, in rare circumstances, experienced life-threatening cardiac events (arrhythmias)
- do not use these products in combination with terfenadine

PREDNISONE, DIURETICS, B$_2$ AGONISTS

- these agents can lower serum potassium
- hypokalemia may increase the risk of cardiac toxicity from terfenadine
- avoid the combination and choose an alternative antihistamine (e.g., chlorpheniramine or loratadine)

Drugs that may decrease the effect of terfenadine

- none

Drugs that may have their effect or toxicity increased by terfenadine

TRICYCLIC ANTIDEPRESSANTS, PHENOTHIAZINES, ANTIARRHYTHMICS

- these agents can prolong the QT interval and this may increase the risk of cardiac toxicity when combined with terfenadine
- avoid the combination and choose an alternative antihistamine (e.g., chlorpheniramine or loratadine)

Drugs that may have their effect decreased by terfenadine

- none

▶ *What Route and Dosage Should I Use?*

How to administer

- orally—take on an empty stomach or with food or milk
- parenterally—not available

Seasonal allergic rhinitis, chronic (perennial) rhinitis, chronic dermatological allergies (atopic dermatitis, chronic urticaria, pruritus of unknown cause)

- 60 mg PO daily
- increase the dosage to 120 mg PO daily if an effect is not seen in 2–3 days

Acute dermatological allergies (e.g., hives and allergic conjunctivitis caused by allergens or food)

- 60 mg PO daily on a PRN basis for symptoms

Dosage adjustments for renal or hepatic dysfunction

- hepatically metabolized
- no dosage adjustments for renal dysfunction are required; titrate dose up to an effect
- avoid use in patients with hepatic dysfunction

What Should I Monitor with Regard to Efficacy and Toxicity?

Efficacy
- see Chlorpheniramine

Toxicity

Mild fatigue, headache, dry mouth and sedation
- can occur but less often than with chlorpheniramine and likely not clinically significant

Cardiac arrhythmias
- serious cardiac arrhythmias (ventricular tachycardia, torsades de pointes, ventricular fibrillation) and QT prolongation, hypotension, palpitations, and syncope have occurred with dosages 2 or 3 times above the recommended levels and at normal dosages in patients with significant hepatic dysfunction and/or with concomitant administration of drugs that inhibit hepatic metabolism
- avoid the use of this drug in patients who have hepatic dysfunction or are taking interacting drugs, and do not exceed recommended dosages

How Long Do I Treat Patients with This Drug?

see Chlorpheniramine

How Do I Decrease or Stop the Administration of This Drug?

- may be stopped abruptly
- when being used for chronic allergic symptoms, drug administration should likely be tapered (decrease the dosage by 25% every week)

What Should I Tell My Patients About This Drug?

- episodes of syncope, dizziness, chest pain, shortness of breath, and/or palpitations should be reported to your physician
- do not exceed the recommended daily dosage of 120 mg PO

Therapeutic Tips

- useful for patients who cannot tolerate the sedative or anticholinergic effects of diphenhydramine or chlorpheniramine and in whom there is no risk of cardiac arrhythmias (Med Lett 1992; 34:9–10)

Useful References

Mann KV, Crowe JP, Tietze KJ. Drug reviews. Non-sedating histamine H1 receptor antagonists. Clin Pharm 1989;8:331–344
Sutherland D. Antihistamine agents—New options or just more drugs? On Continuing Practice 1991;18:31–36
Estelle F, Simmons R, Simons KJ. Pharmacokinetic optimization of histamine H1-receptor antagonist therapy. Clin Pharmacokinet 1991;21: 372–393

TETRACYCLINE

Alfred Gin and George Zhanel

USA (Achromycin, Delfamicin, Panmycin, Sumycin, Tetracyn, Tetralan, others)
CANADA (Achromycin, Apo-Tetra, Novo-tetra, Nu-tetra, Tetracyn)

When Should I Use This Drug?

Both tetracycline and doxycycline are equally effective • Doxycycline has the advantages of less frequent dosing (BID for doxycycline versus QID for tetracycline), can be used in patients with decreased renal function, and may be taken with food and should be recommended unless tetracycline is less expensive • Parenteral tetracycline is no longer available

check antibiotic susceptibility chart (Table 4–1 in Chapter 4)

Urethritis
- tetracycline as sole therapy can be used if urethral discharge shows increased polymorphonuclear neutrophils (PMNs) and no diplococci (no *Neisseria gonorrhoeae*), as tetracycline is effective against *Chlamydia trachomatis*
- tetracycline should be used in combination with cefixime if urethral discharge or endocervical discharge shows increased PMNs and gram-negative intracellular diplococci or if no results are available, as this combination covers both *N. gonorrhoeae* and *Chlamydia*

Cervicitis
- regardless of the results of cervical stain, tetracycline, in combination with cefixime, is the drug of choice, as this combination covers both *N. gonorrhoeae* and *Chlamydia,* which are usually present

Genital ulcers
- drug of choice in penicillin-allergic patients, if there is clinical suspicion and lesions are suggestive (usually painless) of syphilis and/or dark-field microscopy shows corkscrew spirochetes

Pelvic inflammatory disease
- use in combination with cefoxitin, cefotetan, or ceftizoxime for the treatment of inpatient pelvic inflammatory disease, as tetracycline provides good coverage against *Chlamydia*
- for outpatient treatment, tetracycline can be combined with ceftriaxone or ciprofloxacin if the patient is penicillin allergic

Acne
- oral tetracycline is effective against *Propionibacterium acnes* and should be used when topical agents are ineffective or not tolerated

Lyme disease
- drug of choice for the treatment of the early stage of disease but ceftriaxone is recommended in late disease, especially in patients with neurological disease

Rickettsial infection
- tetracycline is the drug of choice for Rocky Mountain spotted fever, Q fever, typhus fever, and tick bite fever

***Vibrio* infections**
- tetracycline is the drug of choice for *Vibrio cholerae*

Pneumonia
- useful in patients with proven atypical pneumonias (*Mycoplasma, Legionella*) who cannot tolerate erythromycin

When Should I Not Use This Drug?

Gram-negative infections
- many gram-negative organisms are resistant to the tetracyclines

What Contraindications Are There to the Use of This Drug?

Intolerance of or allergic reaction to tetracyclines

Renal failure
- tetracycline causes an increase in blood urea nitrogen level but no decrease in glomerular filtration rate
- not a true contraindication, but doxycycline should be used in patients with poor renal function

Pregnancy or lactation
- may cause permanent tooth discoloration and depression of skeletal growth in the newborn and hepatotoxicity in the mother

Children (younger than 8 years of age)
- may cause permanent tooth discoloration and depression of skeletal growth

What Drug Interactions Are Clinically Important?

Drugs that increase the effect or toxicity of tetracycline
- none

Drugs that decrease the effect of tetracycline

ANTACIDS, MILK, IRON, CALCIUM
- products containing calcium, aluminum, magnesium, or iron form chelates with tetracycline; therefore, take an hour before or 2 hours after these drugs

Drugs that have their effect or toxicity increased by tetracycline

- none

Drugs that have their effect decreased by tetracycline

- none

▶ *What Route and Dosage Should I Use?*

How to administer

- orally—take with a full glass of water 1 hour before meals or 2 hours after
- parenterally—not available

Urethritis, cervicitis, genital ulcers

- 500 mg PO Q6H

Pelvic inflammatory disease

- 500 mg PO Q6H

Acne

- 250 mg PO Q12H until a response is seen and then reduce to the lowest effective dosage

Lyme disease, rickettsial infection, *Vibrio* infections

- 500 mg PO Q6H

Pneumonia

- 500 mg PO QID if the patient is moderately ill

Dosage adjustments for renal or hepatic dysfunction

- renally eliminated
- tetracycline is renally eliminated and should not be used in patients with creatinine clearance less than 30 mL/min (use doxycycline)

Normal Dosing Interval	$C_{cr} > 60$ mL/min or 1 mL/s	C_{cr} 30–60 mL/min or 0.5–1 mL/s	$C_{cr} < 30$ mL/min or 0.5 mL/s
Q6H	no adjustment needed	Q8H	use doxycycline

▶ *What Should I Monitor With Regard to Efficacy and Toxicity?*

Efficacy

- for antibiotic administration monitoring guidelines, see specific section on drug therapy

Toxicity

Gastrointestinal symptoms (nausea and vomiting, diarrhea)

- common side effect, occurring in approximately 5% of patients
- question the patient about the appearance of these symptoms on a daily basis while the patient is in the hospital
- if these symptoms occur, try reducing the dosage or switch to doxycycline

Esophagitis

- tetracyclines can cause esophageal ulceration if these agents get lodged in the esophagus
- always take with a glass of water to ensure esophageal clearing

Allergic reactions (rashes, urticaria, fever)

- occur in a small percentage of patients
- question the patient about the appearance of these symptoms on a daily basis while the patient is in the hospital

Superinfection

- oral and anogenital candidiasis is common
- if this occurs, discontinue the drug administration if possible or treat with topical antifungals

Hepatoxicity

- rare occurrence; more common in pregnancy
- monitor aminotransferase and bilirubin levels weekly in patients with renal impairment or those who are pregnant

Nephrotoxicity

- in patients with renal failure, tetracycline may cause further increases in blood urea nitrogen; therefore, use doxycycline if needed in patients with renal failure

▶ *How Long Do I Treat Patients with This Drug?*

Urethritis, cervicitis

- 7 days

Genital ulcers

- 14 days

Pelvic inflammatory disease

- for a total of 10–14 days (PO and IV therapy)

Acne

- indefinite at a low dosage

Lyme disease

- 3 weeks, especially in patients with neurological disease

Rickettsial infection

- 2–3 weeks and potentially months in patients with Q fever

***Vibrio* infections**

- 7–10 days

Prevention of postoperative infections

- single dose

Pneumonia

- if caused by *Mycoplasma* or *Legionella,* a 14 day course of therapy should be given (Clin Chest Med 1991;12:237–242, Ann Intern Med 1987;106:341–345)
- *Legionella* infection can necessitate 3 weeks if the patient responds slowly

▶ *How Do I Decrease or Stop the Administration of This Drug?*

- may be stopped abruptly

▶ *What Should I Tell My Patients About This Drug?*

- tetracycline may cause your skin to be more sensitive to sunlight; therefore, avoid sun exposure or protect yourself with clothing or sunscreen (need a product that protects against both ultraviolet A and B rays)
- avoid taking tetracycline with milk, antacids, iron-containing vitamin products, or calcium supplements
- take tetracycline 1 hour before or 2 hours after meals
- take the medication until it is completed
- take with a full glass of water

▶ *Therapeutic Tips*

- sunscreens, if needed, must contain both a para-aminobenzoic acid ester and a benzophenone to provide adequate protection to prevent photosensitivity
- tetracycline should be taken with a full glass of water

Useful References

Francke EL, Neu HC. Chloramphenicol and tetracycline. Med Clin North Am 1987;71:1155–1166

Wilson WR, Cockerill FR III. Tetracyclines, chloramphenicol, erythromycin and clindamycin. Mayo Clin Proc 1987;62:906–915

THEOPHYLLINE

Karen Shalansky and Cindy Reesor Nimmo

USA (Accurbron, Aerolate, Aquaphyllin, Asmalix, Bronkodyl, Constant-T, Elixophyllin, Lanophyllin, Quibron-T Dividose, Respbid, Slo-bid Gyrocaps, Slo-phyllin Gyrocaps, Somophyllin-T, Sustaire, Theo-24, Theo-Dur, Theo-Dur Sprinkle, Theobid Duracaps, Theochron, Theoclear, Theolair, Theo-Sav, Theospan-SR, Theostat 80, Theovent, Uniphyl)

CANADA (Elixophyllin, Pulmophylline, Quibron-T/SR, Slo-Bid, Somophyllin-12, Theochron, Theo-Dur, Theolair, Theo-SR, Uniphyl)

▶ *When Should I Use This Drug?*

Acute asthma, acute exacerbation of chronic obstructive pulmonary disease

- use only after appropriate dosages of beta₂-agonists, ipratropium, and corticosteroids have been tried (Am Rev Respir Dis 1980; 22:365–371)
- some clinicians suggest that theophylline is of no benefit in acute asthma when appropriate dosages of beta₂-agonists, ipratropium, and corticosteroids have been tried and that theophylline only increases the risk of toxicity (Chest 1990;98:1–3); however, some trials do suggest that theophylline provides some clinical benefit (Ann Intern Med 1993;119:1155–1160)

Chronic asthma, chronic obstructive pulmonary disease

- for chronic asthma, use only after appropriate doses of beta₂-agonists, cromolyn, and inhaled corticosteroids have been tried (N Engl J Med 1989;321:1517–1527, Chest 1990;97[27 suppl]: 19S–23S)
- some patients derive subjective improvement of chronic obstructive pulmonary disease (COPD) that is not achieved with inhaled bronchodilators (Chest 1990;97:19S–23S, Chest 1985;88:112S–117S)

Nocturnal asthma

- for nocturnal asthma, the first-line prophylactic treatment is inhaled corticosteroids, and only if symptoms are still present should theophylline be added

▶ *When Should I Not Use This Drug?*

First-line therapy for obstructive pulmonary disease

- weak bronchodilator with a narrow therapeutic range, serious toxicity, and several drug interactions, as a result it has fallen from first-line therapy of obstructive pulmonary diseases (Chest 1990;98:1–2)
- ensure that other agents in full dosages have been used

Noncompliant patients

- because this drug is usually used for long-term therapy, a noncompliant patient does not usually benefit from this drug and serum level monitoring is difficult if not impossible

▶ *What Contraindications Are There to the Use of This Drug?*

Intolerance of or allergic reaction to xanthine preparations, including any salt of theophylline

Cardiac tachyarrythmias, seizure disorders

- it is best to avoid theophylline, as this drug may exacerbate these conditions
- if it is considered essential to use theophylline, monitor theophylline levels and maintain in lower end of therapeutic range and continue use only if there is demonstrable efficacy

▶ *What Drug Interactions Are Clinically Important?*

Drugs that may increase the effect or toxicity of theophylline

CIMETIDINE

- inhibits microsomal enzymes, which metabolize theophylline
- theophylline levels may increase by 20–40%; onset of interaction 24–72 hours
- if an H₂ antagonist is necessary, prescribe an alternative H₂ antagonist that does not interact (e.g., ranitidine and famotidine)

CIPROFLOXACIN, ERYTHROMYCIN

- similar interaction as cimetidine
- theophylline levels may increase up to 100% with concomitant ciprofloxacin administration, and to 20–40% with erythromycin administration, after 3–5 days of concomitant therapy

- toxicity due to increased theophylline levels can be life threatening
- use an alternative antibiotic if possible; if not, and the combination will be used for longer than 3 days, measure the theophylline level on day 3, and then twice weekly, until the extent of interaction is known
- in patients started on ciprofloxacin therapy, reduce the dosage empirically by 30–50% (depending on the ease of adjusting the dosage form)
- adjust the dosage on the basis of theophylline levels

Drugs that may decrease the effect of theophylline

PHENYTOIN

- metabolism of phenytoin or theophylline may be enhanced, resulting in decreased serum levels of either drug
- monitor serum levels of both drugs as for a dosage change (i.e., at least weekly)

RIFAMPIN

- metabolism of theophylline may be enhanced, resulting in decreased serum levels of theophylline; onset of interaction 48–72 hours
- monitor serum theophylline levels on day 3, and then twice weekly until the extent of the interaction is known
- adjust the dosage on the basis of theophylline levels

Drugs that may have their effect or toxicity increased by theophylline

- none

Drugs that may have their effect decreased by theophylline

- none

▶ *What Route and Dosage Should I Use?*

How to administer

Orally

- should be taken with food or milk to decrease gastrointestinal upset

Parenterally

- loading dose: give in 50–100 mL of 5% dextrose in water (D5W) or normal saline (NS) at a rate of 25 mg/min (20–30 minutes)
- maintenance dosage: give in 500–1000 mL of D5W, NS, or combination of fluids and administer via an infusion control device

Chronic asthma, COPD

- theophylline = aminophylline × 0.80 = oxtriphylline × 0.65
- initiate with 200 mg PO BID of a sustained-release preparation, as these are preferred owing to decreased administration times
- increase the dosage by 25% increments if tolerated, every 3 days until a therapeutic response occurs or one reaches 800 mg/d or a maximum dosage of 13 mg/kg, whichever is less
- Theo-Dur and Slo-Bid Gyrocaps show least peak-trough fluctuations when administered either to children or adults (Applied Pharmacokinetics 1986:1116–1119)
- capsules (e.g., Slo-bid Gyrocaps) may be opened and sprinkled on food or applesauce for children; Theo-Dur Sprinkles show decreased absorption when opened and are therefore not recommended for young children
- Uniphyl may be administered once daily at midevening (8 PM) on an empty stomach for nocturnal asthma; peak serum levels occur early in the morning and may provide better nocturnal bronchodilation than occurs during the daytime (Ration Drug Ther 1988;22:1–5)
- Uniphyl should be used only in patients with nocturnal asthma, as it does not provide effective serum concentrations throughout the entire day when given as a single daily dose
- sustained-release products are initially given every 12 hours to healthy nonsmoking adults, and every 8 hours to adult smokers owing to a faster clearance of the drug

Acute asthma, acute exacerbation of COPD (in patients unable to take oral medications)

- following are guidelines for IV theophylline (to convert to dosages of parenteral aminophylline, multiply parenteral theophylline dosages by 1.25)

Intravenous loading dose

- 5 mg/kg (unless the patient is morbidly obese) over 20–30 minutes; remember to round the dose to closest 50 mg
- if the patient is currently taking theophylline, give half a loading dose (2.5 mg/kg)
- each 1 mg/kg of theophylline results in a predicted increase of 2 mg/L (11 μmol/L) in serum theophylline levels

Intravenous maintenance dose

- 0.4 mg/kg/h in healthy nonsmoking adults
- 0.7 mg/kg/h for healthy smoking adults, as smoking induces hepatic enzymes and this effect is seen for 3 months to 2 years after cessation of smoking
- 0.2 mg/kg/h in patients with congestive heart failure and/or hepatic disease, as metabolism in these patients is decreased
- remember to round the dose to the nearest 5 mg/h

Switch to oral therapy

- do as soon as the patient is able to take oral medications
- take the total daily theophylline parenteral dose and divide the dose by 2 and give this every 12 hours as a sustained-release product
- stop the infusion and start the sustained-release preparation at the same time

Dosage adjustments for renal or hepatic dysfunction

- hepatically metabolized
- reduce the dosage in patients with hepatic disease (see above)

▶ *What Should I Monitor with Regard to Efficacy and Toxicity?*

Efficacy

Acute asthma, acute exacerbation of COPD

Heart rate, degree of respiratory distress, and presence of cyanosis

Peak expiratory flow rate
- should be measured before treatment if possible
- measured after treatment to assess the effect of treatment
- patients with an acute attack should be given a peak flow gauge and should record peak expiratory flow rate (PEFR) at least twice daily

Forced expiratory volume in 1 second
- assess once to determine the reversibility of bronchoconstriction
- reversibility is indicated by an increase of 15–20% in forced expiratory volume in 1 second after bronchodilator

Arterial blood gas values
- if patient has a PEFR less than 40% of predicted or is not responding to treatment
- repeat within 24 hours if blood carbon dioxide level is elevated or patient is fatiguing

Chronic asthma, COPD

Frequency of as needed beta$_2$-agonist use

Pulmonary function tests
- can be used to assess the effectiveness of long-term therapy; however, some patients taking bronchodilators (salbutamol, ipratropium, theophylline) do not have a demonstrable effect on pulmonary function test results but will become clinically improved (increased walking distance, decreased use of PRN medications)

Peak expiratory flow rate
- a peak flowmeter should be used by patients who experience severe attacks with little warning and patients who have symptoms of breathlessness or chest tightness repeatedly or who require regular Q6H to Q8H beta$_2$-agonist therapy (J Allergy Clin Immunol 1990;85:1098–1111)
- establish best PEFR early in therapy
- usually measured on waking and before bed and before and after beta$_2$-agonist administration (minimum of twice daily, i.e., morning and evening) and is the best of 3 measurements on each occasion
- daily variation should be less than 20% and ideally less than 10%

Serum theophylline levels
- usual therapeutic range is 10–20 mg/L (55–110 μmol/L); however, some patients experience a benefit at serum concentrations less than this
- best to start with low dosage and adjust the dosage on the basis of an evaluation of clinical response
- peak levels are not useful for dosage adjustment, as the time to peak levels and actual peak values may vary significantly from day to day; therefore, for routine monitoring, obtain trough levels
- useful to obtain peak levels only if signs and symptoms of toxicity are present at the time when the peak level is achieved
- conventional release tablet or liquid—peak level, 1–2 hours after a dose
- sustained-release tablet or capsule—peak level, 4–6 hours after a dose
- once-daily sustained-release capsule—peak level, 12 hours after a dose
- a trough level measured after 48–72 hours of regular dosing provides a concentration at steady state, and further dosage adjustments should be based on this concentration and an evaluation of efficacy
- after the patient is stabilized on therapy, a concentration every 6 months, with concomitant assessment of efficacy, is warranted

Toxicity

- fewer than 8% of patients appear to have an absolute intolerance of theophylline at therapeutic levels

Gastrointestinal effects

- nausea, vomiting, diarrhea, anorexia, and gastroesophageal reflux can occur
- transient intolerance of theophylline is common if large initial doses are used, instead of the slow titration method
- if toxicity is mild but persistent, measure the concentration and reduce the dosage if it is elevated
- if the concentration is not elevated and symptoms continue, decrease the dosage by 25% or consider stopping the drug administration
- gastrointestinal complications are seen at concentrations of 20–30 mg/L (110–165 mmol/L) and can occur at concentrations less than this

Central nervous system effects

- nervousness, insomnia, or headache can occur and frequently occur at concentrations greater than 20 mg/L (110 mmol/L), and if they occur, adjust the dosage as above for gastrointestinal toxicity
- if seizures occur, stop the drug administration, measure the concentration, and reduce the dosage accordingly; if concentrations are not above 20–25 mg/L (110–135 mmol/L), consider other causes and/or alternative therapy
- seizures may occur without any other signs of toxicity

Cardiac effects

- tachycardia (100–120 bpm), premature atrioventricular contractions, and atrial fibrillation
- if premature beats are present, stop the drug administration, measure the concentration, and reduce the dosage accordingly; if concentrations are not above 20–25 mg/L (110–135 mmol/L), consider other causes and/or alternative therapy

Serum theophylline levels

- usual therapeutic range is 10–20 mg/L (55–110 μmol/L); however, some patients experience toxicity within the normal therapeutic range
- draw concentration whenever toxicity is suspected and empirically reduce the dosage by 25% until results are available

▶ *How Long Do I Treat Patients with This Drug?*

Acute asthma, acute exacerbation of COPD

- after an acute asthmatic episode has subsided (pulmonary function test results return to normal or the best result and symptoms are absent), patients should continue to take theophylline for long-term therapy only after appropriate dosages of beta$_2$-agonists, cromolyn, and inhaled corticosteroids have been tried

Chronic asthma, COPD

- after control or the best result is achieved and the lowest level of effective treatment is established, the patient should be reassessed every 1–6 months, depending on severity of the symptoms
- theophylline may be continued indefinitely as long as patient continues to obtain benefit from the drug with minimum toxicity
- always consider a dose reduction and/or discontinuation to re-evaluate benefit or need

▶ How Do I Decrease or Stop the Administration of This Drug?

- may be stopped abruptly

▶ What Should I Tell My Patients About This Drug?

- you will require periodic blood tests to monitor the effectiveness of this medication
- you may take this drug with food or milk if an upset stomach occurs
- upset stomach, nervousness, or headache may occur with initial use of this drug but often disappear with continued use
- contact your physician if you experience a rapid heart rate, confusion, or continued upset stomach or if any other intolerable side effect develops

▶ Therapeutic Tips

- use only after full dosages of safer or more effective agents have been used
- do not use theophylline-containing combination products
- transient intolerance of theophylline is common if large initial doses are used; therefore, start with a low dose and increase slowly
- consider discontinuing periodically to validate usefulness
- to convert from intravenous aminophylline to oral theophylline, take the hourly infusion rate of aminophylline, multiply by 10, and give this dosage as a sustained-release theophylline preparation every 12 hours (e.g., for an aminophylline infusion of 30 mg/h, give sustained-release theophylline at 300 mg Q12H)

Useful References

Hendeles L, Weinberger M. Theophylline. "A state of the art" review. Pharmacotherapy 1983;3:2–44

Ellis E, Hendeles L. Theophylline. In: Taylor WJ, Caviness MHD, eds. A Textbook for the Clinical Application of Therapeutic Drug Monitoring. Irving, TX, Abbott Laboratories, 1986:185–201

Edwards PJ, Zarowitz BJ, Slaughter RL. Theophylline. In: Evans WE, Schentag JJ, Jusko WJ, eds. Applied Pharmacokinetics: Principles of Therapeutic Drug Monitoring, 3rd ed. Vancouver, WA: Applied Therapeutics Inc, 1992:13-1–13-38

THIETHYLPERAZINE

Lynne Nakashima

USA (Norzine, Torecan)
CANADA (Torecan)

▶ When Should I Use This Drug?

General nausea and vomiting, postoperative nausea and vomiting, chemotherapy-induced nausea and vomiting

- prochlorperazine, perphenazine, and thiethylperazine are likely equally effective and the decision among them should be based on cost and availability
- these agents likely cause less sedation than does dimenhydrinate
- thiethylperazine cannot be given intravenously

▶ When Should I Not Use This Drug?

see Prochlorperazine

▶ What Contraindications Are There to the Use of This Drug?

see Prochlorperazine

▶ What Drug Interactions Are Clinically Important?

see Prochlorperazine

▶ What Route and Dosage Should I Use?

How to administer

- orally—can be taken with or without food
- parenterally—administer as a deep IM injection; do not use intravenously or subcutaneously

General nausea and vomiting, postoperative nausea and vomiting, chemotherapy-induced nausea and vomiting

- 10 mg IM every 3 hours when needed
- 10 mg PO every 3 hours may be used if the patient can tolerate sips of fluid
- can also be used rectally 10 mg Q8H

Dosage adjustments for renal or hepatic dysfunction

- hepatically metabolized
- no dosage adjustment is required; titrate the dose to effect

▶ What Should I Monitor with Regard to Efficacy and Toxicity?

see Prochlorperazine

▶ How Long Do I Treat Patients with This Drug?

see Prochlorperazine

▶ How Do I Decrease or Stop the Administration of This Drug?

- may be stopped abruptly

▶ What Should I Tell My Patients About This Drug?

see Prochlorperazine

Useful References

Tortorice PV, O'Connell MB. Management of chemotherapy-induced nausea and vomiting. Pharmacotherapy 1990;10:129–145

Wampler G. The pharmacology and clinical effectiveness of phenothiazines and related drugs for managing chemotherapy-induced emesis. Drugs 1983;25[suppl 1]:35–51

THIORIDAZINE

Juan Avila and Patricia Marken

USA (Mellaril, generic)
CANADA (Mellaril, Apo-Thioridazine, Novoridazine)

▶ When Should I Use This Drug?

Acute psychosis therapy (if prompt control is required)

- in the acutely psychotic and agitated patient, use for rapid tranquilization with the goal of quietly calming a dangerous patient
- thioridazine is a low-potency antipsychotic with high anticholinergic activity
- thioridazine produces more sedation and orthostatic hypotension than do the medium- or high-potency antipsychotic, but produces a low incidence of extrapyramidal or dystonic reactions
- drug of choice if sedation is required if it is less expensive than chlorpromazine
- should be used only in patients who have not responded to other antipsychotics, as it is no more effective than other agents but is more expensive
- no parenteral form is available
- when a patient has a previous history of response to this agent

Maintenance psychosis therapy

- to ameliorate the symptoms of psychosis, including hallucinations, delusions, formal thought disorder, bizarre behavior, agitation, and/or hyperactivity
- should be used only in patients who have not responded to other antipsychotics, as it is no more effective than other agents but is more expensive

Manic phase of bipolar illness

- antipsychotics are often also required for adequate sedation and behavioral control and are usually preferred to benzodiazepines for acutely manic patients with concurrent psychoses; however, there is some evidence that high-dose benzodiazepines may be equally efficacious with less frequent adverse effects (J Clin Psychopharmacol 1985;5:109–113)
- decision as to when to choose this agent is as above for acute psychosis therapy

▶ *When Should I Not Use This Drug*

see Chlorpromazine

▶ *What Contraindications Are There to the Use of This Drug?*

see Chlorpromazine

▶ *What Drug Interactions Are Clinically Important?*

see Fluphenazine

▶ *What Route and Dosage Should I Use?*

How to administer

- orally—take with food or milk or on an empty stomach
- parenterally—not available

Acute psychosis therapy (if prompt control is required), manic phase of bipolar illness

- 100 mg PO every 30–60 minutes until control is achieved or the patient does not tolerate drug (usually 2–3 doses)
- start a maintenance dose after an adequate response has been seen (see below)
- titrate to sedative effect or cerebellar side effects (ataxia, slurred speech)

Maintenance psychosis therapy

- 150 mg PO BID
- 75 mg PO BID in smaller or elderly patients
- increase the dosage every 2 weeks until an appropriate response has been seen
- typical maintenance dosage is 300–400 mg PO daily given as a single dose
- maximum daily oral dose is 800 mg because of the risk of pigmentary retinopathy

Dosage adjustments for renal or hepatic dysfunction

- hepatically metabolized
- no specific dosage adjustments; just start with a low dose and titrate to effect

▶ *What Should I Monitor with Regard to Efficacy and Toxicity?*

see Chlorpromazine

▶ *How Long Do I Treat Patients with This Drug?*

see Chlorpromazine

▶ *How Do I Decrease or Stop the Administration of This Drug?*

see Chlorpromazine

▶ *What Should I Tell My Patients About This Drug?*

see Chlorpromazine

Useful References

Black JL, Richelson E, Richardson JW. Antipsychotic agents: A clinical update. Mayo Clin Proc 1985;60:777–789
Kane JM. The current status of neuroleptic therapy. J Clin Psychiatry 1989;50(9):322–328

THIOTHIXENE

Juan Avila and Patricia Marken

USA (Navane)
CANADA (Navane)

▶ *When Should I Use This Drug?*

Acute psychosis therapy (if prompt control is required)

- in the acutely psychotic and agitated patient, use for rapid tranquilization with the goal of quietly calming a dangerous patient
- thiothixene is a medium-potency antipsychotic with moderate anticholinergic activity
- thiothixene produces a moderate amount of sedation and orthostatic hypotension (less than that seen with chlorpromazine) and a medium incidence of acute extrapyramidal or dystonic reactions
- drug of choice in the young, otherwise healthy patient if it is less expensive than loxapine
- one disadvantage is that it must be given more frequently than once daily
- is available in a parenteral form
- when a patient has a previous history of response to this agent

Maintenance psychosis therapy

- to ameliorate the symptoms of psychosis, including hallucinations, delusions, formal thought disorder, bizarre behavior, agitation, and/or hyperactivity
- drug of choice in the young, otherwise healthy patient if it is less expensive than thiothixene
- one disadvantage is that it must be given more frequently than once daily

Manic phase of bipolar illness

- antipsychotics are often also required for adequate sedation and behavioral control and are usually preferred to benzodiazepines for acutely manic patients with concurrent psychoses; however, there is some evidence that high-dose benzodiazepines may be equally efficacious with less adverse effects (J Clin Psychopharmacol 1985;5:109–113)
- decision as to when to choose this agent is as above for acute psychosis therapy

▶ *When Should I Not Use This Drug?*

see Chlorpromazine

▶ *What Contraindications Are There to the Use of This Drug?*

see Chlorpromazine

▶ *What Drug Interactions Are Clinically Important?*

Drugs that may increase the effect or toxicity of thiothixene

CENTRAL NERVOUS SYSTEM DEPRESSANTS (OPIATES, BARBITURATES, GENERAL ANESTHETICS, ALCOHOL)

- excessive sedation and central nervous system (CNS) depression may occur if used concomitantly
- start with low dosages of both agents to avoid excessive sedation or CNS depression, and adjust dosages on the basis of clinical presentation

Drugs that may decrease the effect of thiothixene

- none

Drugs that may have their effect or toxicity increased by thiothixene

- none

Drugs that may have their effect decreased by thiothixene

ANTICONVULSANTS (PHENYTOIN, PHENOBARBITAL)

- thiothixene may lower the seizure threshold and dosage adjustments of anticonvulsants may be necessary when the drugs are used concomitantly, but no adjustments should be made unless seizures develop

▶ *What Route and Dosage Should I Use?*

How to administer

- orally—take with food or milk or on an empty stomach
- parenterally—IM only (not available in Canada)

Acute psychosis therapy (if prompt control is required), manic phase of bipolar illness

- 10–20 mg PO or 4–10 mg IM (if the patient will not take oral medication) every 30–60 minutes until control is achieved or the patient does not tolerate the drug (usually 2–3 doses)
- start a maintenance dosage after an adequate response has been seen (see below)

Maintenance psychosis therapy

- 5 mg PO BID
- 2 mg PO BID in smaller or elderly patients
- increase the dosage every 2 weeks until an appropriate response has been seen
- typical maintenance dosage is 30 mg PO daily given as a single daily dose
- maximum daily oral dosage is 60 mg

Dosage adjustments for renal or hepatic dysfunction

- hepatically metabolized
- no specific dosage adjustments; just start with a low dose and titrate to effect

▶ *What Should I Monitor with Regard to Efficacy and Toxicity?*

see Chlorpromazine

▶ *How Long Do I Treat Patients with This Drug?*

see Chlorpromazine

▶ *How Do I Decrease or Stop the Administration of This Drug?*

see Chlorpromazine

▶ *What Should I Tell My Patients About This Drug?*

see Chlorpromazine

▶ *Therapeutic Tips*

see Chlorpromazine

Useful References

Black JL, Richelson E, Richardson JW. Antipsychotic agents: A clinical update. Mayo Clinic Proc 1985;60:777–789

Kane JM. The current status of neuroleptic therapy. J Clin Psychiatry 1989;50(9):322–328

Alexander B. Antipsychotics: How strict the formulary? DICP 1988;22:324–326

TICARCILLIN

John Rotschafer, Kyle Vance-Bryan, and Rick Zabinski

USA (Ticar)
CANADA (Ticar)

▶ *When Should I Use This Drug?*

Consider an alternative agent

- owing to high sodium content and generally inferior in vitro susceptibility profile against many important nosocomial gram-negative organisms and enterococci compared with the case with piperacillin
- piperacillin should be used instead of ticarcillin (Infect Dis Clin North Am 1989;3:571–594, Rev Infect Dis 1984;6:13–32, Ann Intern Med 1982;97:755–760)

Useful Reference

Wright AJ, Wilkowske CJ. The penicillins. Mayo Clin Proc 1987;62:806–820

TICARCILLIN-CLAVULANATE

John Rotschafer, Kyle Vance-Bryan, and Rick Zabinski

USA (Timentin)
CANADA (Timentin)

▶ *When Should I Use This Drug?*

check antibiotic susceptibility chart (Table 4–1 in Chapter 4)

Treatment of mixed aerobic-anaerobic bacterial infections

- ticarcillin-clavulanate should be considered for empirical therapy when coverage against *S. aureus,* gram-negative bacilli, and anaerobes is desired
- ticarcillin-clavulanate can be chosen instead of combinations of antibiotics (e.g., clindamycin, gentamicin, ampicillin) if it is less expensive
- piperacillin and ticarcillin-clavulanate have similar spectrums; except that ticarcillin-clavulanate has activity against penicillinase-producing staphylococci and ampicillin-resistant *Haemophilus influenzae*
- although piperacillin can be used as a single agent for mild infections, combination therapy with aminoglycosides is recommended for more serious gram-negative infections
- in contrast, ticarcillin-clavulanate has an advantage over piperacillin in that it can be used as a single agent for moderate to severe infections (except those caused by *Pseudomonas aeruginosa*)
- decision between ticarcillin-clavulanate and other agents (e.g., imipenem and piperacillin) should be based on cost and frequency of administration
- ticarcillin-clavulanate has the disadvantage of usually being dosed Q4H (Q6H for less serious infections), whereas other similar agents can be dosed less frequently
- also considered one of the antibiotics of choice for *Stenotrophomonas multophilia*

▶ *When Should I Not Use This Drug?*

Infections caused by single organisms

- in general, ticarcillin-clavulanate should be reserved for infections presumed or proved to be caused by mixed organisms

▶ *What Contraindications Are There to the Use of This Drug?*

see Penicillin

▶ *What Drug Interactions Are Clinically Important?*

see Penicillin

▶ *What Route and Dosage Should I Use?*

How to administer

- orally—not available
- parenterally—administer intravenously in 100 mL of IV fluid (normal saline or 5% dextrose in water) and infuse over 30 minutes

Systemic infections (dose based on ticarcillin content)

Severe infections

- 3.0 g IV Q4H

Moderate infections such as mixed aerobic-anaerobic infections

- 1.5 g IV Q4H (some clinicians suggest 3 g IV Q6H)

Mild infections such as soft tissue infections

- 1.5 g IV Q6H

Dosage adjustments for renal or hepatic dysfunction

- renally eliminated

Normal Dosing Interval	C_cr > 60 mL/min or 1 mL/s	C_cr 30–60 mL/min or 0.5–1 mL/s	C_cr < 30 mL/min or 0.5 mL/s
Q4H	no adjustment needed	Q6H	Q8H
Q6H	no adjustment needed	Q8H	Q12H

▶ *What Should I Monitor with Regard to Efficacy and Toxicity?*

see Piperacillin

▶ *How Long Do I Treat Patients with This Drug?*

see Piperacillin

▶ *How Do I Decrease or Stop the Administration of This Drug?*

- may be stopped abruptly

▶ *What Should I Tell My Patients About This Drug?*

see Penicillin

▶ *Therapeutic Tips*

- owing to high sodium content (5.2 mEq of sodium per gram) of ticarcillin-clavulanate, use piperacillin instead of ticarcillin-clavulanate when sodium restriction is required (Infect Dis Clin North Am 1989;3:571–594, Rev Infect Dis 1984;6:13–32, Ann Intern Med 1982;97:755–760)
- for serious infections, use maximum dosages of the drug

see Penicillin

Useful Reference

Wright AJ, Wilkowske CJ. The penicillins. Mayo Clin Proc 1987;62:806–820

TICLOPIDINE

J. Chris Bradberry

USA (Ticlid)
CANADA (Ticlid)

▶ *When Should I Use This Drug?*

Transient ischemic attacks

- use if aspirin is contraindicated or is ineffective in reducing attacks
- although ticlopidine was slightly more effective than aspirin (13% incidence of stroke for aspirin versus 10% for ticlopidine), ticlopidine had a higher incidence of adverse effects (diarrhea, rash, and severe neutropenia) (N Engl J Med 1989;321:501–507)
- ticlopidine is far more expensive (drug cost and toxicity evaluation) and less convenient to take than aspirin

Completed stroke

- drug of choice for male patients after a completed stroke is aspirin
- in female patients, there is a suggestion that ticlopidine is slightly more effective (Neurology 1992;42:111–115)
- some clinicians suggest that ticlopidine should be used in patients with significant neurological deficit

▶ *When Should I Not Use This Drug?*

Secondary prevention of stroke in patients who cannot take anticoagulants

- evidence to support the use of ticlopidine in this area is not available

▶ *What Contraindications Are There to the Use of This Drug?*

Intolerance of or allergic reaction to ticlopidine

Neutropenia and thrombocytopenia

- ticlopidine causes neutropenia in approximately 1% of patients

Hemostatic problems or bleeding diathesis

- ticlopidine can worsen these conditions

Hepatic disease

- can cause elevated hepatic enzyme levels and may worsen hepatic disease

▶ *What Drug Interactions Are Clinically Important?*

Drugs that may increase the effect or toxicity of ticlopidine

- none

Drugs that may decrease the effect of ticlopidine

- none

Drugs that may have their effect or toxicity increased by ticlopidine

THEOPHYLLINE

- ticlopidine may decrease theophylline clearance (Clin Pharmacol Ther 1988;41:358–362)
- use alternative agents if possible; if not, and the combination will be used for longer than 3 days, measure the theophylline level every 2 days until the extent of interaction is known

DRUGS METABOLIZED BY THE LIVER

- ticlopidine may reduce the clearance of drugs metabolized by the liver, but no clear recommendations can be made at this time

ASPIRIN OR OTHER AGENTS THAT INHIBIT PLATELET ACTIVITY

- do not use in combination, as there may be a potentiation of the effect on platelet aggregation

Drugs that may have their effect decreased by ticlopidine

- none

▶ *What Route and Dosage Should I Use?*

How to administer

- orally—take with food or milk to minimize gastrointestinal discomfort
- parenterally—not available

Transient ischemic attacks, completed stroke

- 250 mg PO BID

Dosage adjustments for renal or hepatic dysfunction

- hepatically metabolized
- dosage adjustments in renal dysfunction are not needed
- no guidelines are available for dosage adjustments in patients with hepatic dysfunction

▶ *What Should I Monitor with Regard to Efficacy and Toxicity?*

Efficacy

Transient ischemic attacks

- assess the patient monthly initially and tell the patient to contact the physician if any future transient ischemic attacks occur (loss of vision in 1 eye, dizziness, weakness on one side, or numbness in the face, arm, or leg)
- if no transient ischemic attacks during the first 3 months, assess the patient every 6 months thereafter

Completed stroke

- no efficacy variables other than absence of future strokes

Toxicity

Complete blood count and liver function tests

- baseline and every 2 weeks for the first 3 months of therapy
- neutropenia (0.8%) and hepatic toxicity (4.4%) have been reported
- if these adverse effects occur, stop the drug administration
- both effects are reversible, with neutropenia resolving within 1–3 weeks of drug administration discontinuation

Gastrointestinal effects

- diarrhea occurs in 20% of patients; try a temporary reduction in dosage or administer with food

Rash

- occurs in 10–15% of patients and the drug administration should be stopped if a rash occurs
- many rashes do not recur on rechallenge

▶ *How Long Do I Treat Patients with This Drug?*

Transient ischemic attacks

- until more information is available, the drug administration should be stopped if the incidence of transient ischemic attacks or stroke accelerates or does not decrease
- if effective, continue therapy indefinitely

Completed stroke

- evidence exists for benefit for up to 2–3 years and therapy should likely be continued indefinitely

▶ *How Do I Decrease or Stop the Administration of This Drug?*

- may be stopped abruptly

▶ *What Should I Tell My Patients About This Drug?*

- because of its effect on platelets, you should report any abnormal bleeding or bruising
- if you notice an increase in infections, report this to your physician
- if you experience stomach upset or diarrhea, remember to take this drug with food and this should help
- if stomach upset or diarrhea continues or a rash develops, contact your physician

▶ *Therapeutic Tips*

- if a patient with transient ischemic attacks is aspirin intolerant, ticlopidine should be used
- if the patient fails to respond to aspirin, ticlopidine should be used
- studies show greater effectiveness in secondary stroke prevention and in treatment of women as compared with the case with aspirin; however, more confirming information is needed in this regard

Useful References

Gent M, Easton JD, Hachinski VC, et al. The Canadian-American Ticlopidine Study (CATS) in thromboemboblic stroke. Lancet 1989;2:1215–1220

Hasr WK, Easton JD, Adams HP, et al. A randomized trial comparing ticlopidine hydrochloride with aspirin for the prevention of stroke in high-risk patients. N Engl J Med 1989;321:501–507

Robert S, Miller AJ, Fagan SC. Ticlopidine: A new antiplatelet agent for cardiovascular disease. Pharmacotherapy 1991;11:317–325

TIMOLOL

Robert Rangno and James McCormack

USA (Blocadren, generics)
CANADA (Blocadren, Apo-Timol)

▶ *When Should I Use This Drug?*

Consider an alternative agent

- although this nonselective drug has more complete and predictable bioavailability than does propranolol, timolol's half-life is relatively short and therefore BID dosing, at least, is necessary
- has higher lipid solubility than does nadolol or atenolol and may produce more sleep disturbances than agents such as atenolol and nadolol
- although timolol has the most impressive data for post–myocardial infarction reduction of deaths and recurrent myocardial infarctions, other nonselective beta-blockers (e.g., nadolol) should be equally effective

TISSUE PLASMINOGEN ACTIVATOR (ALTEPLASE)

Stephen F. Hamilton, Stan Horton, and Udho Thadani

USA (Activase)
CANADA (Activase)

▶ *When Should I Use This Drug?*

Acute myocardial infarction

- all appropriate patients with a suspected or proven myocardial infarction should receive thrombolytic therapy
- appropriate patients are those without contraindications to thrombolytic therapy and with pain lasting 12 hours or less and ST segment elevation in 2 contiguous leads
- much research is underway and similar patients older than 75 years seem to benefit as much as or more than younger patients, but the risk of major and fatal bleeding complications are higher

- streptokinase is the drug of first choice because of equivalent efficacy to alteplase in reducing mortality in the majority of large scale comparative trials and it is much less expensive
- alteplase is the drug of choice if patients have received streptokinase or anistreplase (anisoylated plasminogen streptokinase activator complex) or have been treated for a streptococcal infection within the previous year because these patients have streptococcal antibodies that neutralize the streptokinase
- may be better for hypotensive patients, as streptokinase causes a higher incidence of hypotension than does alteplase, although thrombolytic agent–induced hypotension is uniformly transient and easily managed with intravenous fluids (Pharmacotherapy 1992;12:440–444)
- may be more beneficial than streptokinase in young patients with large anterior myocardial infarctions (N Engl J Med 1993;329:673–682)

▶ *When Should I Not Use This Drug?*

Streptokinase can be used

- streptokinase is much less expensive than alteplase

▶ *What Contraindications Are There to the Use of This Drug?*

Intolerance of or allergic reaction to alteplase

Absolute contraindications

- active internal bleeding, suspected aortic dissection, diabetic hemorrhagic retinopathy, any other opthalmic hemorrhages, history of cerebrovascular accident known to be hemorrhagic, recent head trauma, known intracranial neoplasm, pregnancy, blood pressure greater than 200/120 mmHg, history of allergic reactions to any thrombolytic agent, and trauma or surgery within less than 2 weeks

Relative contraindications (if evidence of a myocardial infarction is strong enough, thrombolytic therapy should still be used)

- history of severe hypertension, history of cerebrovascular accident, significant hepatic dysfunction, active peptic ulcer, patients taking oral anticoagulants, prolonged or traumatic cardiopulmonary resuscitation, surgery or trauma within greater than 2 weeks to 6 months

▶ *What Drug Interactions Are Clinically Important?*

Drugs that may increase the effect or toxicity of alteplase

ASPIRIN

- low-dose aspirin concomitantly with thrombolytic agents has been associated with greater reductions in short-term and long-term mortality and overall risk of stroke than those produced by streptokinase therapy alone
- concurrent therapy was associated with an increased risk of major bleeding, primarily at arterial puncture sites, and a slight increase in the incidence of confirmed intracranial hemorrhage

Drugs that may decrease the effect of alteplase

- none

Drugs that may have their effect or toxicity increased by alteplase

- none

Drugs that may have their effect decreased by alteplase

- none

▶ *What Route and Dosage Should I Use?*

How to administer

Parenterally

- 50 mg of drug is reconstituted with 50 mL of sterile water for injection and used as 1 mg/mL concentration or may be further diluted in normal saline injection or 5% dextrose injections to no more than 0.5 mg/mL (precipitates at lower concentrations)
- reconstituted alteplase should be used immediately or discarded after 24 hours
- do not use bacteriostatic water for injection, as this has preservatives that interact with the alteplase molecule

Acute myocardial infarction

- 15 mg IV bolus, followed by 0.75 mg/kg (not to exceed 50 mg) over 30 minutes; then 0.5 mg/kg (up to 35 mg) over the next 60 minutes (N Engl J Med 1993;329:673–682)

Dosage adjustments for renal or hepatic dysfunction

- no dosage adjustment is required

▶ *What Should I Monitor with Regard to Efficacy and Toxicity?*

see Streptokinase

▶ *How Long Do I Treat Patients with This Drug?*

Acute myocardial infarction

- single dose given over 3 hours

▶ *How Do I Decrease or Stop the Administration of This Drug?*

- may be abruptly stopped

▶ *What Should I Tell My Patients About This Drug?*

- complete medication history is important to evaluate the potential drug interactions that may potentiate bleeding problems
- complete medical problem history is important to evaluate potential risks of and contraindications to thrombolytic therapy
- compliance with strict bed rest or other measures to minimize bleeding is important

Useful References

Gruppo Italiano. per lo.Studio della Streptochi nasi nell'Infarto Miocardico (GISSI). Long-term effects of intravenous thrombolysis in acute myocardial infarction: Final report of the GISSI Study. Lancet 1987; 2:871–874

ISIS-2 (Second Internation Study of Infarct Survival) Collaborative Group. Randomized trial of intravenous streptokinase, oral aspirin, both or neither among 17,187 cases of suspected acute myocardial infarction: ISIS-2. Lancet 1988;2:349–360

Wilcox RG, Von Der Lippe G, Olsson CG, et al. Trial of tissue plasminogen activator for mortality reduction in acute myocardial infarction: Anglo-Scandinavian Study of Early Thrombolysis (ASSET). Lancet 1988; 2:525–530

TOBRAMYCIN

David Guay

USA (Nebcin, generics)
CANADA (Nebcin, generics)

▶ *When Should I Use This Drug?*

check antibiotic susceptibility chart (Table 4–1 in Chapter 4)

Upper urinary tract infection (pyelonephritis), acute or chronic bacterial prostatitis, pneumonias, intraabdominal infection, endocarditis, cellulitis, meningitis, gram-negative shock, febrile neutropenia

- tobramycin should be used in these infections only if they are suspected or documented to be caused by *Pseudomonas aeruginosa* or organisms proved to be resistant to gentamicin and sensitive to tobramycin
- although tobramycin is more expensive than gentamicin, tobramycin's minimum inhibitory concentrations, especially for *Pseudomonas,* are lower than those for gentamicin (J Infect Dis 1976;134[suppl]:S3–S19
- gentamicin resistance usually parallels tobramycin resistance but differences in susceptibility can exist
- if *Pseudomonas* is suspected, ensure that the patient is receiving tobramycin in combination with another agent that has antipseudomonal activity (a penicillin, cephalosporin, or quinolone)

▶ *When Should I Not Use This Drug?*

see Gentamicin

▶ *What Contraindications Are There to the Use of This Drug?*

see Gentamicin

▶ *What Drug Interactions Are Clinically Important?*

see Gentamicin

▶ *What Route and Dosage Should I Use?*

How to administer

- orally—not absorbed
- parenterally—dilute in 100 mL of saline or 5% dextrose in water and infuse over 30 minutes
- can be given intramuscularly if the intravenous route is not available

Dosages depend on the patient's size, the severity of the illness, and renal function • Round the dose up to nearest 20 mg dose (e.g., 60, 80, 100, 120, 140, 160 mg, and so on) to allow ease of administration

Upper urinary tract infection (pyelonephritis), acute or chronic bacterial prostatitis, pneumonias, cellulitis, acute or chronic osteomyelitis, intraabdominal infections, endocarditis

- 1.5 mg/kg IV Q8H for mild to moderate illness
- 2 mg/kg IV Q8H for severe illness

Meningitis

- 2 mg/kg IV Q8H plus 7.5 mg intrathecally or intraventricularly Q24H if the patient fails to respond to IV therapy

Gram-negative shock

- 2.5 mg/kg IV Q8H

Febrile neutropenia

- 2 mg/kg IV Q8H

Dosage adjustments for renal or hepatic dysfunction

- renally eliminated

Normal Dosing Interval	$C_{cr} > 60$ mL/min or 1 mL/s	C_{cr} 30–60 mL/min or 0.5–1 mL/s	$C_{cr} < 30$ mL/min or 0.5 mL/s
Q8H	no adjustment needed	Q12H	Q24H

▶ *What Should I Monitor with Regard to Efficacy and Toxicity?*

Efficacy

- for antibiotic administration monitoring guidelines, see specific section on drug therapy

Toxicity

see Gentamicin

▶ *How Long Do I Treat Patients with This Drug?*

see Gentamicin

▶ *How Do I Decrease or Stop the Administration of This Drug?*

- may be stopped abruptly

▶ *What Should I Tell My Patients About This Drug?*

- see Gentamicin

▶ *Therapeutic Tips*

- ensure that organism sensitivity mandates tobramycin use rather than gentamicin
- see Gentamicin

TOCAINIDE

James Tisdale

USA (Tonocard)
CANADA (Tonocard)

▶ When Should I Use This Drug?

Tocainide should not be used without consulting a cardiologist or a cardiac electrophysiologist

Ventricular tachycardia

- should be used for the prevention of recurrent ventricular tachycardia if it has been shown to suppress inducible ventricular tachycardia in the electrophysiology laboratory or on Holter monitor
- tocainide should be tried only if mexiletene is poorly tolerated and quinidine or procainamide have failed to suppress inducible ventricular tachycardia during serial drug testing in the electrophysiology laboratory or on Holter monitor
- if partial suppression of inducible ventricular tachycardia has been achieved with quinidine or procainamide, tocainide may be added to the regimen if it has been shown to suppress inducible ventricular tachycardia in the electrophysiology laboratory or on Holter monitor and if patients do not tolerate therapy with mexiletine

▶ When Should I Not Use This Drug?

Supraventricular arrhythmias

- tocainide is not effective for the management of supraventricular arrhythmias

Asymptomatic ventricular arrhythmias

- no evidence that treatment is beneficial

▶ What Contraindications Are There to the Use of This Drug?

Intolerance of or allergic reaction to tocainide

- tocainide is contraindicated in patients who have previously experienced hypersensitivity to tocainide or to amide-type local anesthetics

Atrioventricular block

- tocainide is contraindicated in patients with second- or third-degree atrioventricular block unless a functioning ventricular pacemaker is present

▶ What Drug Interactions Are Clinically Important?

Drugs that may increase the effect or toxicity of tocainide

- none

Drugs that may decrease the effect of tocainide

CIMETIDINE

- cimetidine has been reported to reduce the bioavailability of tocainide, thereby reducing plasma tocainide concentrations (J Clin Pharmacol 1988;28:640–643)
- ranitidine does not influence plasma tocainide concentrations; therefore, use ranitidine instead of cimetidine

RIFAMPIN

- rifampin has been reported to induce the hepatic metabolism of tocainide, thereby reducing plasma tocainide concentrations (Clin Pharm 1989;8:200–205)
- if rifampin therapy is initiated in patients stabilized with tocainide, the patient should be monitored for arrhythmia recurrence
- if a target serum concentration has been determined in the past, measure a serum concentration within 2–3 days and ensure that the drug concentration remains above this target

Drugs that may have their effect or toxicity increased by tocainide

- none

Drugs that may have their effect decreased by tocainide

- none

▶ What Route and Dosage Should I Use?

How to administer

- orally—can administer with or without food
- parenterally—unavailable

Ventricular tachycardia

- 400 mg PO Q8H
- increase the dosage to 600 mg PO Q8H after 3 days if the response is inadequate
- dosage may be increased to 800 mg PO Q8H after another 3 days if the response is still inadequate
- most patients do not tolerate dosages greater than 600 mg PO Q8H

Dosage adjustments for renal or hepatic dysfunction

- renally and hepatically eliminated

Normal Dosing Interval	$C_{cr} > 60$ mL/min or 1 mL/s	C_{cr} 30–60 mL/min or 0.5–1 mL/s	$C_{cr} < 30$ mL/min or 0.5 mL/s
Q8H	no adjustment needed	Q12H	Q24H

▶ What Should I Monitor with Regard to Efficacy and Toxicity?

Efficacy

Ventricular tachycardia

Serum concentrations

- therapeutic range of tocainide is usually quoted as 4–10 μg/mL
- range of serum tocainide concentrations required for efficacy varies widely among patients, and therefore, the therapeutic range is of relatively little use in monitoring the efficacy of tocainamide
- if therapeutic monitoring is performed, use the method of monitoring target serum tocainide concentrations (see Quinidine) (Clin Pharmacokinet 1991;20:151–166)

see Quinidine

Toxicity

Adverse effects necessitating discontinuation of therapy occur in approximately 10–20% of patients (Mayo Clin Proc 1987;62:1033–1050)

- assess the patient regularly for nausea, vomiting, anorexia, diarrhea, or signs of any hypersensitivity reactions such as rash, fever, arthralgia, and myalgia

Central nervous system effects

- tremor, dizziness, lightheadedness, confusion, ataxia, nystagmus, paresthesias, agitation, or seizures may occur
- reduce the dosage by 200 mg per dose (e.g., 600 mg PO Q8H to 400 mg PO Q8H) for central nervous system effects and discontinue the drug administration if seizures develop

Pulmonary fibrosis

- monitor by questioning patients about symptoms of shortness of breath at each visit
- reported in less than 1% of patients
- tocainide should be discontinued if this occurs

Hematological effects

- anemia, neutropenia, and thrombocytopenia may occur in less than 1% of patients
- patients receiving tocainide should have complete blood counts determined at weekly intervals during the first 3 months of therapy and every 6 weeks thereafter
- tocainide administration should be discontinued if hematological abnormalities occur

Cardiovascular effects

- perform continuous electrocardiograms (ECGs) until patient is stabilized, then every 3–6 months do ECGs
- if symptoms of worsening arrhythmia occur, continuous ECG monitoring is indicated

▶ How Long Do I Treat Patients with This Drug?

Ventricular tachycardia

- patients may require therapy indefinitely if contributing factors cannot be reversed

▶ How Do I Decrease or Stop the Administration of This Drug?

- tocainide therapy should not be discontinued or dosage reduction performed without consulting a cardiologist or a cardiac electrophysiologist
- tocainide therapy can be discontinued abruptly if ineffective or poorly tolerated

▶ What Should I Tell My Patients About This Drug?

- if you experience nausea, vomiting, anorexia, diarrhea, fever, sore throat, joint pain, tremor, dizziness, lightheadedness, confusion, difficulty in walking, numbness, agitation or convulsions, fever, sore joints or muscles, palpitations, shortness of breath, or chest pain, contact your physician
- do not discontinue tocainide therapy without consulting your physician

▶ Therapeutic Tips

- avoid until other antiarrhythmics have been demonstrated to be ineffective
- range of serum tocainide concentrations required for efficacy varies widely among patients, and therefore, the therapeutic range is of relatively little use in monitoring the efficacy of tocainide

Useful Reference

Roden DM, Woosley RL. Tocainide. N Engl J Med 1986;315:41–45
Lalka D, Meyer MB, Duce BR, Elvin AT. Kinetics of the oral antiarrhythmic lidocaine congener, tocainide. Clin Pharmacol Ther 1976;19:757–766
Adhar GC, Swerdlow CD, Lance BL, et al. Tocainide for drug-resistant ventricular tachyarrhythmias. J Am Coll Cardiol 1988;11:124–131

TOLAZAMIDE

Christy Silvius Scott

USA (Tolinase, Tolamide, generic)
CANADA (not available)

▶ When Should I Use This Drug?

Consider an alternative agent

- offers no advantages over other available agents and has active metabolites that are retained in renal insufficiency
- more favorable agents to use include tolbutamide, glyburide, and gliclazide

Useful Reference

Gerich JE. Oral hypoglycemic agents. N Engl J Med 1989;321:1231–1245

TOLBUTAMIDE

Christy Silvius Scott

USA (Orinase, Oramide, generic)
CANADA (Orinase, Mobenol, Apo-Tolbutamide, Novobutamide)

▶ When Should I Use This Drug?

Non–insulin-dependent diabetes

- obese (>120% of ideal body weight) and/or older patients (older than 40 years) with moderate hyperglycemia and without significant symptoms
- obese diabetics are in a state of insulin resistance; therefore, large dosages of insulin may be required and euglycemia may be difficult to achieve with insulin (N Engl J Med 1989;321:1231–1245)
- shortest duration of action (6–10 hours) and least potent agent; therefore, administered 2 or 3 times a day
- probably associated with the fewest serious adverse effects of all the sulfonylureas (Drugs 1981;22:211–245, N Engl J Med 1989;321:1231–1245)
- causes 5 times fewer hypoglycemic reactions than do glyburide and chlorpropamide (Diabetes Care 1989;12:203–208, Drugs 1981;22:211–245, N Engl J Med 1989;321:1231–1245)
- less expensive than glyburide, gliclazide, and glipizide but has the disadvantage of having to be dosed 2–3 times daily

- useful for patients who have developed severe hypoglycemia with the other agents despite dosage reductions or for patients at high risk for hypoglycemia (N Engl J Med 1989;321:1231–1245) and patients who cannot afford more expensive agents
- patient risk factors for hypoglycemia include age older than 60 years, malnourishment, alcoholism, renal or hepatic dysfunction, and adrenal insufficiency (N Engl J Med 1989;321:1231–1245)
- metabolized to inactive compounds and, therefore, may be safely used in patients with renal insufficiency and the elderly

▶ When Should I Not Use This Drug?

Insulin-dependent diabetes

- requires insulin and does not respond to oral hypoglycemics

Non–insulin-dependent diabetes

- in patients who are or could be adequately controlled with diet and exercise alone (N Engl J Med 1989;321:1231–1245)
- in patients who are under severe stress (trauma, surgery, major infection) that is causing extreme hyperglycemia; insulin is required during these periods of metabolic decompensation

▶ What Contraindications Are There to the Use of This Drug?

Intolerance of or allergic reaction to tolbutamide or other sulfonylureas and sulfa medications

- allergy to sulfonamides is not an absolute contraindication; the cross-sensitivity of sulfonamides is approximately 17% and the sulfonylureas are structurally different (Applied Therapeutics: The Clinical Use of Drugs, 5th ed. 1993:Chap. 72, pages 1–53)

Pregnancy

- insulin is required to produce good control of diabetes during pregnancy if diet and exercise alone are not successful (Clin Obstet Gynecol 1981;8:353–382); there is also risk to the fetus if sulfonylureas are used during pregnancy (Drugs in Pregnancy and Lactation, 4th ed. 1994)

Breast-feeding

- there is no information concerning the effects on the infant (Drugs in Pregnancy and Lactation, 4th ed. 1994)

▶ What Drug Interactions Are Clinically Important?

Drugs that may increase the effect or toxicity of tolbutamide

INSULIN

- insulin also decreases blood glucose levels
- insulin therapy should be initiated in non–insulin-dependent diabetes after discontinuation of the administration of oral hypoglycemics (Diabetes Care 1992;13:1240–1262)
- oral hypoglycemics should be added to the insulin regimen slowly, beginning with the lowest available dosage
- may lengthen hypoglycemic episodes in experimentally induced hypoglycemia; however, the clinical importance of this, particularly with selective beta-blockers, is not well described
- may block insulin secretion owing to inhibition of beta-receptors), occasionally causing hyperglycemia; however, this is not usually clinically relevant
- in general, cardioselective beta-blockers can be used in patients with diabetes because CNS symptoms are usually unaltered and sweating is enhanced; however, symptoms such as palpitation and tremors are decreased or diminished
- nonselective beta-blockers should be avoided in diabetic patients
- if a beta-blocker must be used, choose a cardioselective agent (atenolol, metoprolol, or acebutolol) in low dosages to maintain their cardioselectivity
- particularly when the benefits outweigh the risks (e.g., post-myocardial infarction) beta-blockers should not be avoided in diabetic patients (Diabetes Care 1983;6:285–290, Eur HJ 1989;10:423–428)

ETHANOL

- inhibits gluconeogenesis by the liver, causing hypoglycemia when gluconeogenesis is required to maintain normal glucose blood levels (e.g., fasting state or decreased food intake)
- avoid the use of glyburide (and all long-acting sulfonylureas) in alcoholic patients; tolbutamide may be a more useful medication
- patients should limit their consumption of alcohol to an occasional 1 drink per day with food while receiving this medication

PHENYLBUTAZONE, OXYPHENBUTAZONE

- increases the action of tolbutamide, acetohexamide, and chlorpropamide by interfering with elimination of the parent compound and/or its metabolites; it is assumed to occur possibly with all sulfonylureas
- patients should be told of the potential for an interaction and to be more aware of signs and symptoms of hypoglycemia when phenylbutazone is added
- dosage of oral hypoglycemics should be decreased if hypoglycemia occurs

SALICYLATES

- may enhance the glucose-lowering effects of oral hypoglycemics
- lower dosages (e.g., for headaches and myocardial infarction prophylaxis) probably have minimum effects
- high dosages (e.g., for rheumatoid arthritis) may cause hypoglycemia in combination with sulfonylureas
- patients should be told of the potential for an interaction and of the need for greater awareness of signs and symptoms of hypoglycemia when salicylates are added
- dosage of sulfonylureas should be decreased if hypoglycemia is noted

SULFONAMIDES

- hypoglycemia has been reported in patients receiving a sulfonamide (sulfisoxazole, sulfamethizole, and trimethoprim-sulfamethoxazole) and glyburide, tolbutamide, chlorpropamide, or glipizide
- patients should be told of the potential for an interaction and of the need for greater awareness of signs and symptoms of hypoglycemia when sulfonamide is added

MONOAMINE OXIDASE INHIBITORS

- may enhance the glucose-lowering effects of sulfonylureas and increase the duration of hypoglycemia
- patients should be told of the potential for an interaction and of the need for greater awareness of signs and symptoms of hypoglycemia when a sulfonamide is added
- blood glucose levels should be monitored for hyperglycemia after monoamine oxidase inhibitor therapy is discontinued

Drugs that may decrease the effect of tolbutamide

BETA-ADRENERGIC BLOCKERS

- may block insulin secretion (owing to inhibition of $beta_2$-receptors), occasionally causing hyperglycemia
- see above for other effects caused by beta-blocking agents

THIAZIDE DIURETICS

- thiazide diuretics can increase blood glucose concentrations in diabetics (and patients prone to diabetes), antagonizing the effect of oral hypoglycemics
- thiazide diuretics cause impairment of glucose tolerance, decrease insulin sensitivity, increase hemoglobin A_{1c} (HbA$_{1c}$) levels, and produce worsening of glucose level control but this effect is small and uncommon with low dosages (Ann Intern Med 1992;118:273–278)
- hyperglycemia may occur several days to months after the addition of thiazide diuretics
- patients should monitor blood glucose levels at least weekly for 3 months after a thiazide diuretic has been added
- if administration of a thiazide diuretic is discontinued while the patient is receiving an oral hypoglycemic, blood glucose levels and symptoms of hypoglycemia should be monitored
- in patients with insulin-dependent diabetes, there is little if any effect on glucose control when thiazide diuretics are used in low dosages

- data suggest that diuretics, when used long term, prevent the onset of microalbuminuria in non–insulin-dependent patients and do not worsen glycemic control (Hypertension 1993;21:786–794)

RIFAMPIN

- decreases serum concentrations of glyburide and tolbutamide, and therefore, may reduce their action
- little information is known about other sulfonylureas and rifampin interactions
- patient should monitor for hyperglycemia after rifampin has been added, and for hypoglycemia after rifampin administration has been discontinued

CORTICOSTEROIDS

- corticosteroids may cause hyperglycemia and increased doses of sulfonylureas may be necessary
- after corticosteroids are discontinued, the patient should be told to be more aware of signs and symptoms of hypoglycemia

Drugs that may have their effect or toxicity increased by tolbutamide

- none

Drugs that may have their effect decreased by tolbutamide

- none

▶ What Route and Dosage Should I Use?

How to administer

- orally—because tolbutamide is short acting, it may be best to administer the dose 30 minutes prior to meals, especially the breakfast meal (Diabetes Care 1992;15:737–754); it is best to administer the tablets round the clock (e.g., Q8H or Q12H, not BID or TID)

Non–insulin-dependent diabetes

- 250 mg PO BID
- increase the dosage weekly by 250 mg increments until glycemic control or a maximum daily dosage of 3000 mg is reached
- daily dosages greater that 1500 mg should be divided TID
- average daily dosage is 1500 mg (N Engl J Med 1989;321:1231–1245)

Dosage adjustments for renal or hepatic dysfunction

- metabolized to inactive compounds

Normal Dosing Interval	$C_{cr} > 60$ mL/min or 1 mL/s	C_{cr} 30–60 mL/min or 0.5–1 mL/s	$C_{cr} < 30$ mL/min or 0.5 mL/s
Q8H	no adjustment necessary	no adjustment necessary	Q12H
Q12H	no adjustment necessary	no adjustment necessary	Q24H

▶ What Should I Monitor with Regard to Efficacy and Toxicity?

Efficacy

Non–insulin-dependent diabetes

Blood glucose measurements preprandial

- patients with poorly controlled non–insulin-dependent diabetes should be taught self-monitoring of blood glucose levels
- although it is controversial, patients should self-monitor blood glucose levels at least before breakfast (fasting) and dinner (Can Med Assoc J 1992;147:697–712; Diabetes Care 1993;16:60–64)
- some studies suggest that self-monitoring of glucose levels in patients with non–insulin-dependent diabetes is not helpful in the overall treatment of the disease (Br Med J 1992;305:1171–1172, 1194–1196, Am J Med 1986;81:830–835, Diabetes Care 1990;13:1044–1050)
- 80–120 mg/dL (4.4–6.7 mmol/L) is considered excellent control
- 120–140 mg/dL (6.7–7.8 mmol/L) is considered acceptable control
- 140–180 mg/dL (7.8–10 mmol/L) is considered fair control
- greater than 180 mg/dL (>10 mmol/L) is considered poor control (N Engl J Med 1989;321:1231–1245)

- random plasma glucose measurement may be useful for comparison with a simultaneous capillary blood glucose measurement obtained and determined by the patient every 4–6 months to assess self-monitoring technique (Can Med Assoc J 1992;147:697–712)
- frequency and scheduling of self-tests must be individualized to the goals and the agents used for treatment, the extent of blood glucose fluctuation, and the patient's willingness to self-monitor

Urine glucose level (Diabetes Care 1993;16[suppl 2]:39)

- if the patient is not willing to self-monitor blood glucose levels, urine glucose testing should be used; however, there are many limitations to this type of testing
- normal renal threshold for glucose is 180 mg/dL (10 mmol/L)
- renal threshold may be increased in patients with diabetes of long duration
- urine concentration may affect the results
- reflects only an average level of blood glucose since the last voiding
- hypoglycemia cannot be detected
- color tests used for urine testing are not accurate

Glycosylated hemoglobin (e.g., HbA₁c) (HbA_{1c}) (N Engl J Med 1989;321:1231–1245, Can Med Assoc J 1992;147:697–712)

- glycosylated hemoglobin is expressed as a percentage of total hemoglobin level
- hemoglobin is slowly and irreversibly glycosylated throughout the life of the red blood cell; the amount that is glycosylated depends on blood glucose concentrations
- because the life of a red blood cell is approximately 120 days, measuring HbA_{1c} more frequently than 4 times per year is not beneficial
- best index of glycemic control because it reflects the mean blood glucose values during the preceding 6–10 weeks
- HbA_{1c} level should be determined in all diabetics at least every 6 months, and preferably every 3 months in patients with non–insulin-dependent diabetes with poor glycemic control
- HbA_{1c} values of 6–8% suggest good glucose control
- HbA_{1c} values of 8–11% suggest fair glucose control
- HbA_{1c} values of 11–13% suggest poor glucose control
- upper limit of normal varies from laboratory to laboratory: in general, a HbA_{1c} value within 1% of the upper limit reflects good control; within 1–3%, acceptable control; and greater than 3% above normal, poor control
- goal of therapy is to have HbA_{1c} values suggesting good control

Symptoms

- reduction in symptoms such as polyuria, polydypsia, yeast and urinary tract infections

Toxicity

Hypoglycemia

- may occur in up to 20% of patients (Diabetes Care 1989;12:203–208) and is the most common, severe adverse reaction of the sulfonylureas (N Engl J Med 1989;321:1231–1245, Diabetes Care 1992;15:737–754); permanent neurological sequela and death may occur if hypoglycemia is severe
- some studies suggest that glyburide causes the highest incidence of hypoglycemia (Diabetes Care 1989;12:203–208, Br Med J 1988;296:949–950)
- incidence of hypoglycemia with gliclazide is less than with glyburide and chlorpropamide (Diabetes Care 1989;12:203–208)
- glipizide causes approximately 50% less hypoglycemia than does glyburide (Drugs 1981;22:211–245)
- although the incidence of hypoglycemia is less with tolbutamide compared with other agents, patients still need to be aware of the potential for this adverse reaction
- ask whether the patient has experienced any symptoms of hypoglycemia: sweaty palms, generalized sweating, tremors, hunger, palpitations, anxiety, irritability, restlessness, loss of concentration, confusion, visual disorders, headache, restless sleep, and nightmares
- if these symptoms occur, the patient should be instructed to take in simple carbohydrates: ½ cup of orange juice or nondiet soda,

2 sugar cubes, 6 Life-Savers, or 2 glucose tablets followed by a longer acting carbohydrate (e.g., milk or a sandwich) to replete glycogen stores and decrease risk of a hypoglycemic reaction

- if consistent hypoglycemic episodes are not severe, reduce the dosage by 50% and monitor the patient for hypoglycemic episodes
- if the patient has a severe episode of hypoglycemia (coma, seizures), discontinue administration of the medication and monitor blood glucose levels Q6H for at least 48 hours, give 50 mL of 50% glucose IV rapidly; a 10% glucose infusion may be necessary to maintain glucose concentrations of 90–180 mg/dL (5–10 mmol/L) (Br Med J 1988;296:949–950, N Engl J Med 1989;321:1231–1245)
- investigate the reason for hypoglycemia
- if medication is still required, switch to a shorter-acting agent such as tolbutamide or reinstitute at the lowest available dosage
- educate the patient on factors contributing to hypoglycemia (fasting or decreased food intake, vomiting, excessive exercise, alcohol consumption)
- be aware of drug interactions that may increase the action of sulfonylureas

Weight gain

- weight gain is common in patients attaining glucose control (Diabetologia 1983;24:404–411)
- patients should be instructed to weigh themselves weekly, and they should be weighed at regular office visits
- if weight gain occurs, the importance of diet and exercise should be emphasized to aid in controlling the disease

Gastrointestinal effects (AHFS Drug Information 1994:2072–2075, Curr Ther Res 1959;1:69–75, Drugs 1981;22:295–320)

- gastrointestinal upset, including dyspepsia, nausea, epigastric fullness, and heartburn, occurs in approximately 1–2% of patients
- this appears to be dose related and may be minimized by decreasing the dose

Dermatological effects (AHFS Drug Information 1994;2072–2075, Curr Ther Res 1959;1:69–75, Drugs 1981;22:295–320)

- allergic skin reactions, including pruritus, erythema, uricaria, and maculopapular eruptions, occur in about 1–2% of patients
- these reactions may dissipate with ongoing therapy
- if the patient experiences a persistent allergic skin reaction, tolbutamide therapy should be discontinued
- other sulfonylureas may have cross-sensitivity but can be tried
- metformin (if available) is an alternative in allergy situations
- photosensitivity reactions may also occur; advise sunscreen use

▶ *How Long Do I Treat Patients with This Drug?*

Non–insulin-dependent diabetes

- continue therapy until adequate control is achieved or the maximum daily dosage (3000 mg) is reached (N Engl J Med 1989;321:1231–1245)
- approximately ⅓ of all patients with non–insulin-dependent diabetes receiving sulfonylureas fail to respond to therapy, most often owing to dietary noncompliance (N Engl J Med 1989;321:1231–1245)
- if only a partial response has been seen with maximum doses of the first agent, add metformin if available (Can Med Assoc J 1992;147:697–712, N Engl J Med 1989;321:1231–1245)
- if maximum dosages have been tried without adequate glucose control, a trial with glyburide, gliclazide, or glipizide is warranted (N Engl J Med 1989;321:1231–1245)
- patients who do not respond to oral agents should be treated with insulin (Diabetes Care 1990;13:1240–1262, Can Med Assoc J 1992;147:697–712)
- patients responding satisfactorily to sulfonylurea treatment should have a trial of dosage reduction after 6 months of therapy to determine whether a lower dosage is acceptable (N Engl J Med 1989;321:1231–1245)
- patients with good glycemic control on modest dosages of an oral agent may maintain satisfactory control after withdrawal of the drug administration (N Engl J Med 1989;321:1231–1245)

- patients need to have the importance of diet and exercise reemphasized so that a trail without oral therapy can occur

▶ How Do I Stop or Decrease the Administration of This Drug?

- may be stopped abruptly, if necessary
- if satisfactory glucose levels have been maintained for 6 months, decrease the dosage by 250 mg every 2 weeks

▶ What Should I Tell My Patients About This Drug?

- obese patients should reduce weight to allow oral hypoglycemic agents to be maximally effective
- weight gain may reduce the ability of oral hypoglycemics to lower blood glucose levels
- exercise helps to reduce weight and enhances the blood glucose-lowering effects of glyburide
- if a dose is missed, take it as soon as possible, but if it is remembered close to the next dose time (e.g., within 4 hours if dosed Q8H, within 6 hours if dosed Q12H, within 12 hours if dosed Q24H), omit the missed dose (i.e., do not double up on doses)
- you may be more sensitive to the sun; use sunscreen (UVA and UVB coverage)
- ensure that you and family members are familiar with the signs and symptoms of hypoglycemia; discuss at each visit
- know the common causes of low blood glucose levels, such as missed meals, poor eating habits, excessive exercise, and alcohol consumption
- for mild hypoglycemia, oral ingestion of a simple carbohydrate (orange or apple juice) is recommended
- confirmation of hypoglycemia with glood glucose level is recommended
- for severe cases with loss of consciousness, family and friends should seek emergency medical assistance before administering anything orally (the patient may choke)

▶ Therapeutic Tips

- remember that this is a potent agent; initiate therapy with low doses and keep dosage increments small
- hypoglycemic reactions may be severe and prolonged, resulting in convulsions and coma and subsequent neurological deficits and death
- to assess continuing benefit, use a withdrawal trial of glyburide in selected patients with excellent control every 6 months
- reemphasize the crucial importance of the diabetic diet and a weight loss program for obese patients, which should include exercise
- avoid concomitant use of drugs reported to affect blood glucose level control and those with potential to interact with sulfonylureas

Useful References

American Hospital Formulary Service. AHFS Drug Information 1993. Bethesda, MD: American Society of Hospital Pharmacists, 1993

Gerich JE. Oral hypoglycemic agents. N Engl J Med 1989;321:1231–1245

Groop LC. Sulfonylureas in NIDDM. Diabetes Care 1992;15:737–754

Hansten PD, Horn JR. Drug Interactions and Updates. Philadelphia: Lea & Febiger, 1993

Tatro DS, ed. Drug Interaction Facts. St Louis: Facts and Comparisons, 1995

Koda-Kimble MA. Diabetes mellitus. In: Koda-Kimble MA, Young LY, eds. Applied Therapeutics: The Clinical Use of Drugs. 5th ed. Vancouver, WA: Applied Therapeutics, 1992;Chapter 72, pages 1–53

Briggs GG, Freeman RD, Yaffe SJ, eds. Drugs in Pregnancy and Lactation, 3rd ed. Baltimore: Williams & Wilkins, 1994

TOLMETIN

Kelly Jones

USA (Tolectin)
CANADA (Tolectin)

▶ When Should I Use This Drug?

Acute pain, general aches and pain, bone pain, dysmenorrhea, cancer pain

- useful for the short-term management of general aches and pains

- only advantage over non–enteric-coated aspirin is that it causes less gastrointestinal intolerance
- decision between this drug and other nonsteroidal antiinflammatory drugs (NSAIDs) should be based on cost

Rheumatoid arthritis

- tolmetin can be used as an alternative for patients who fail to respond to enteric coated aspirin or ibuprofen; however, it is more expensive
- tolmetin is an alternative to ibuprofen in patients taking oral anticoagulants. (DICP 1989;23:76–85)
- tolmetin may be less toxic to the liver than other NSAIDs such as indomethacin or diclofenac
- second only to indomethacin with regard to gastrointestinal upset and central nervous system adverse effects

Osteoarthritis

- if acetaminophen, enteric coated aspirin or ibuprofen are not effective
- decision between this drug and other NSAIDs should be based on cost

▶ When Should I Not Use This Drug?
Combination with other NSAIDs

- combinations of NSAIDs provide no increase in effectiveness compared with maximum dosages of single agents and significantly increase the risk of adverse effects

▶ What Contraindications Are There to the Use of This Drug?

see Ibuprofen

▶ What Drug Interactions Are Clinically Important?

see Ibuprofen

▶ What Route and Dosage Should I Use?
How to administer

- orally—take with food or milk
- parenterally—not available

Acute pain, general aches and pain, bone pain, dysmenorrhea

- 200–400 mg PO Q6–8H PRN

Cancer pain

- 200 mg PO Q8H up to a maximum dosage of 2000 mg PO daily

Rheumatoid arthritis

- 400 mg PO Q8H up to a maximum dosage of 2000 mg PO daily

Osteoarthritis

- 200 mg PO Q8H

Dosage adjustments for renal or hepatic dysfunction

- hepatically metabolized; therefore, no adjustments are needed for renal disease
- reduce dosage by 25% in patients with a history of hepatic disease

▶ What Should I Monitor with Regard to Efficacy and Toxicity?

see Ibuprofen

▶ How Long Do I Treat Patients with This Drug?

see Ibuprofen

▶ How Do I Decrease or Stop the Administration of This Drug?

- may be stopped abruptly if needed

▶ *What Should I Tell My Patients About This Drug?*

see Ibuprofen

▶ *Therapeutic Tips*

see Ibuprofen

Useful References

see Ibuprofen

TRANYLCYPROMINE

Lyle K. Laird and Julia Vertrees

USA (Parnate)
CANADA (Parnate)

▶ *When Should I Use This Drug?*

Major depression, atypical depression, dysthmia

- tranylcypromine is used in patients in whom phenelzine is not effective or tolerated

▶ *When Should I Not Use This Drug?*

see Phenelzine

▶ *What Contraindications Are There to the Use of This Drug?*

see Phenelzine

▶ *What Drug Interactions Are Clinically Important?*

see Phenelzine

▶ *What Route and Dosage Should I Use?*

How to administer

- orally—can be taken on an empty stomach or with food or milk
- parenterally—not available

Major depression, atypical depression, dysthmia

- 10 mg PO BID (given in the morning and afternoon)
- maintain this dosage for 2 weeks, and if there is no response, increase the daily dosage by 10 mg at weekly intervals to a maximum of 60 mg PO daily
- give the full daily dose before noon if possible, but at the latest before supper
- dosages greater than 30 mg PO daily are often associated with increased adverse effects and rarely provide increased efficacy
- in geriatric patients, start with 5 mg PO BID and increase up to a maximum of 45 mg/d

Dosage adjustments for renal or hepatic dysfunction

- hepatically metabolized
- no dosage adjustment guidelines are available
- in patients with renal or hepatic dysfunction, start with the lowest available dosage and titrate the dose on the basis of efficacy and toxicity

▶ *What Should I Monitor with Regard to Efficacy and Toxicity?*

see Phenelzine

▶ *How Long Do I Treat Patients with This Drug?*

see Phenelzine

▶ *How Do I Decrease or Stop the Administration of This Drug?*

see Phenelzine

▶ *What Should I Tell My Patients About This Drug?*

see Phenelzine

▶ *Therapeutic Tips*

see Phenelzine

TRAZODONE

Lyle K. Laird, Julia Vertrees, and Jonathan Fleming

USA (Desyrel, Trialodine, others)
CANADA (Desyrel)

▶ *When Should I Use This Drug?*

Periodic limb movement disorder

- clonazepam, temazepam (Sleep 1986;9:385–392), nitrazepam (Can J Neurol Sci 1986;13:52–54), levodopa (Clin Neuropharmacol 1986;9:456–463), and trazodone (Sleep Res 1988;17:39) have demonstrated efficacy in managing this disorder
- although there are more scientific data for clonazepam and temazepam, trazodone may have an advantage over these agents in that, on the basis of clinical experience, patients do not appear to become tolerant of its effects

▶ *When Should I Not Use This Drug?*

Major depression

- trazodone is no more effective than other antidepressants, is associated with a high incidence of orthostasis and sedation, has a number of active metabolites, is usually dosed more frequently than once daily, and offers no advantages over the other antidepressants

see Imipramine

▶ *What Contraindications Are There to the Use of This Drug?*

Intolerance of or allergic reaction to trazodone

Pregnancy

- human studies have not been done

Cardiac disease

- trazodone may potentiate ventricular arrhythmias, premature ventricular contractions, and ventricular tachycardia

▶ *What Drug Interactions Are Clinically Important?*

ALCOHOL

- about 20% of insomniacs may take alcohol and sleeping pills concurrently to aid sleep (Confin Psychiatry 1977;15:151–172) and this can produce additive sedative effects
- concurrent use of alcohol may increase the risk of transient global amnesia (JAMA 1987;258:945–946)
- avoid combination

OTHER DRUGS

- no other clinically important drug interactions have been reported, but there are case reports of interactions with fluoxetine, phenytoin, and warfarin

▶ *What Route and Dosage Should I Use?*

How to administer

- orally—can be given with food or on an empty stomach
- parenterally—not available

Periodic limb movement disorder

- start with 50 mg PO 40 minutes before retiring and increase up to a maximum of 150 mg PO HS

Dosage adjustments for renal or hepatic dysfunction

- renally eliminated
- no dosage adjustment guidelines are available
- in patients with renal or hepatic dysfunction, start with the lowest available dosage and titrate the dose on the basis of efficacy and toxicity

▶ *What Should I Monitor with Regard to Efficacy and Toxicity?*

Efficacy

Periodic limb movement disorder

Establish baseline sleep performance

- prior to starting the drug administration, the patient should be forewarned that a course of treatment will be provided and the patient should be monitored each week, at least by telephone, to quantify side and therapeutic effects

- have the patient quantify the current sleep performance for 2 days in a diary, noting the time of retiring, the time to fall asleep after lights out, the estimated number of awakenings and the duration and time of the longest awakening, the time of awakening, and the total sleep time, as this assists in making the diagnosis and in having a baseline measure against which to assess any improvements

Initial monitoring for efficacy should be weekly at first

- ensure that the patient is following good sleep hygiene and getting up at the same time each day, avoiding naps and horizontal rests, and limiting or discontinuing caffeine, alcohol, nicotine, or recreational drug use
- quantify and note subjective improvements in daytime performance; if none are apparent, stop the hypnotic regimen and try behavioral interventions
- particularly in the elderly, ensure that there is no impairment in coordination on awakening during the night for washroom visits or on awakening in the morning

Toxicity

see Imipramine (produces less severe anticholinergic effects than does imipramine)

Priapism

- although this is rare (1/15,000–30,000), patients should be told about this adverse effect
- should this occur, stop the drug immediately

▶ How Long Do I Treat Patients with This Drug?
Periodic limb movement disorder

- chronic disorder necessitating long-term drug therapy
- there are no clinical studies on the long-term use of sleep-promoting medicines for this condition; however, clinical experience suggests that treatment be continued as long as it is effective
- if tolerance develops (this is rare), intermittent use (e.g., weekday nights, alternate days) or drug-free periods ("drug holidays"): taper over 1 week and stop for 2 weeks should be tried if necessary to prevent or delay the development of tolerance

▶ What Should I Tell My Patients About This Drug?

see Imipramine

- although priapism is rare (1/15,000–30,000), patients should be told about this adverse effect and told to seek medical attention if this occurs

▶ Therapeutic Tips

- trazodone is not related to any currently available antidepressants
- dosage is individualized by titration; serum concentrations are not useful clinically

TRIAMCINOLONE ACETONIDE

Karen Shalansky and Cindy Reesor Nimmo

USA (Azmacort)
CANADA (Azmacort)

▶ When Should I Use This Drug?
Consider an alternative agent

- triamcinolone acetonide provides no advantages over the other inhaled corticosteroids
- triamcinolone acetonide has not been well studied, and unless it is less expensive than the other agents, there is no reason to use it

TRIAMTERENE

Ian Petterson

USA (Dyrenium; combination: Dyazide, Maxizide)
CANADA (Dyrenium; combination: Dyazide, Novotriamzide, Apo-Triazide)

▶ When Should I Use This Drug?
Consider an alternative agent

- triamterene exhibits little, if any, antihypertensive or diuretic activity on its own and is therefore usually used in combination with a thiazide diuretic
- augments all of the biochemical adverse effects of the thiazide diuretics (i.e., increased urea, uric acid, and glucose levels)
- is not as effective a potassium-sparing agent as spironolactone
- triamterene, in combination products, is combined with only 25 mg of hydrochlorothiazide, and this low dose of hydrochlorothiazide may account for the low incidence of hypokalemia seen with these combinations
- interstitial nephritis has been reported with triamterene but not with amiloride or spironolactone

Useful References

Nader C, Thompson JR, Alpern RJ. Complications of diuretic use. Semin Nephrol 1988;8:365–387
Krishna GG, Shulman MD, Narins RG. Clinical use of potassium sparing diuretics. Semin Nephrol 1988;8:354–364
Ryan MP. Magnesium and potassium-sparing diuretics. Magnesium 1986;5:282–292
Dyckner T, Wester P. Potassium-sparing diuretics. Acta Med Scand 1985;707(suppl):79–83

TRIAZOLAM

Jonathan Fleming

USA (Halcion)
CANADA (Halcion, Apo-Triazolam)

▶ When Should I Use This Drug?
Transient situational insomnia, short-term insomnia

- with its short duration of action, triazolam is useful for the short-term management (2–3 days) of stress-related insomnia when it is important to avoid daytime sedation or effects on psychomotor performance such as jet lag, as it has less hangover effect than does temazepam, lorazepam, or oxazepam
- triazolam was recently removed from the market in the United Kingdom and other countries
- regulatory authorities in the USA and Canada have changed the packaging and package insert for this medication and the 0.5 mg dosage has been removed
- at dosages of 0.25 mg or less, there is likely no difference between this agent and other benzodiazepines, as the spontaneously reported adverse drug reactions have occurred with dosage of 0.5 mg or higher

▶ When Should I Not Use This Drug?
Transient and short-term insomnia complicated by terminal insomnia (last third of the night)

- in patients with maintenance insomnia characterized by last third of the night awakenings, triazolam's rapid elimination results in less of hypnotic effect in the last third of the night and has been noted to cause early morning insomnia in some patients (Science 1983;220:95–97)
- avoid in the elderly who are mostly troubled by last third of the night awakenings

Long-term insomnia

- when long courses (longer than 3 weeks of continuous use) are planned, as loss of efficacy (tolerance of the hypnotic effect) has been shown to occur as early as 2 weeks (J Clin Pharmacol 1976;16:399–406) and discontinuation syndromes with triazolam are more prominent with protracted use, especially if the dosage has been increased to more than 0.5 mg

▶ What Contraindications Are There to the Use of This Drug?
Intolerance of or allergic reaction to triazolam

- previous adverse responses to triazolam (anterograde amnesia, paradoxical excitement, and so on) or other benzodiazepines

Patients with chronic obstructive pulmonary disease and sleep-related breathing disorders (particularly obstructive sleep apnea)

- these conditions are worsened by the use of hypnotics

Pregnant or lactating female patients

- because effects are unknown

Patients with a history of abusing benzodiazepines or alcohol

- concurrent alcohol use increases amnestic effects (JAMA 1987; 258:945–946)

▶ *What Drug Interactions Are Clinically Important?*

Drugs that may increase the effect or toxicity of triazolam

ALCOHOL

- about 20% of insomniacs may take alcohol and sleeping pills concurrently to aid sleep (Confin Psychiatry 1977;15:151–172) and this can produce additive sedative effects
- concurrent use of alcohol may increase the risk of transient global amnesia (JAMA 1987;258:945–946)
- avoid combination

CENTRAL NERVOUS SYSTEM DEPRESSANTS

- additive sedative effects are expected when concomitant central nervous system depressants are used
- avoid combination if possible or minimize by starting with low, divided daily doses of CNS depressants and allow tolerance to develop before dosage increases

Drugs that may decrease the effect of triazolam

- none

Drugs that may have their effect or toxicity increased by triazolam

- none

Drugs that may have their effect decreased by triazolam

- none

▶ *What Route and Dosage Should I Use?*

How to administer

- orally—40 minutes prior to retiring

Transient situational insomnia, short-term insomnia

- 0.125 mg PO 40 minutes prior to retiring
- increase to 0.25 mg only if the lower dosage is clearly ineffective
- do not increase above 0.25 mg, as there is an increased risk of adverse side effects (memory effects) and discontinuation problems
- use only 0.125 mg in the elderly

Dosage adjustments for renal or hepatic dysfunction

- hepatically metabolized
- no dosage adjustments for organ dysfunction are recommended; however, always start with the lowest dose and titrate to response

▶ *What Should I Monitor with Regard to Efficacy and Toxicity?*

Efficacy

Transient situational insomnia, short-term insomnia

Shortening of the time taken to fall asleep and improved sleep efficiency

- quantify through the use of a sleep diary and compare with pretreatment sleep performance

Improved daytime function

- quantify by comparing changes in the symptoms (e.g., anxiety, tension, and fatigue) with treatment with baseline values

Toxicity

Changes in higher cortical functioning (amnesia, confusion, agitation, hyperexcitability)

- these are dose dependent, with substantial behavioral and cognitive side effects being reported with 4 times (1 mg) the recommended adult dosage (Clin Pharmacol Ther 1986;40:378–386)

- use only at the lowest effective dosage and for the shortest possible time period

Early morning insomnia (Science 1983;220:95–97) **and late afternoon anxiety** (Br Med J 1982:942)

- treatment with triazolam 0.5 mg has been associated with these side effects and appears to be related to triazolam's short half-life
- use an agent with a longer duration of action, such as temazepam and oxazepam

Prominent morning confusion and/or daytime sleepiness in snoring patients

- should raise suspicion that obstructive sleep apnea has been missed in diagnosis and is being aggravated by nocturnal sedation

Depression

- patients with masked clinical depression may report marked affective changes (depression) on using sedatives (anxiolytics or hypnotics)
- assess suicidal risk because, although rare, fatal overdosages of triazolam have been reported in older, debilitated patients (Br Med J 1988;297:719)

Discontinuation syndrome

- frequently, patients increase the dosage, often without consultation, and are then at risk for amnestic effects and a more severe discontinuation syndrome, including rebound insomnia and rapid eye movement sleep rebound, causing nightmares, awakenings, and withdrawal anxiety

▶ *How Long Do I Treat Patients with This Drug?*

Transient situational insomnia, short-term insomnia

- use for the shortest period possible
- triazolam is suitable for promoting sleep outside the usual nocturnal sleep period (e.g., with jet lag and shift work), as it is relatively free of hangover effects (Clin Pharmacol Ther 1986;40:314–320)
- tolerance of triazolam's hypnotic effect can occur early, so short courses are preferred
- regulatory authorities recommend limiting treatment to 14 days

▶ *How Do I Decrease or Stop the Administration of This Drug?*

see Lorazepam

▶ *What Should I Tell My Patients About This Drug?*

- rebound insomnia may occur, so transitory sleep disturbance on withdrawal of therapy is expected and is not an indication to restart the medication administration
- report any adverse effects as soon as they occur
- increasing the dosage can lead to unwanted side effects so if the dosage is not effective, consult your physician before increasing it on your own
- do not use with alcohol
- stop therapy if you are planning to become pregnant
- disturbances in memory may occur, particularly for material learned just prior to the sleep period or during the sleep period (e.g., physicians may forget orders given during the night, students may forget information learned that night)
- sedative properties are additive if used with over the counter antihistamines
- note the improvements in your sleep performance and daytime functioning so that these can be evaluated at the follow-up visit

▶ *Therapeutic Tips*

- adverse media publicity about this drug (particularly side effects of higher dosages) may necessitate patient education, but when it is used in the recommended dosage for short periods, it is a useful drug
- rebound insomnia and withdrawal anxiety can be prominent when withdrawal is abrupt after long periods of use; therefore, discuss benzodiazepine discontinuation syndromes with the patient and the strategy you plan to use for handling this

- use for only short periods (2–3 days)
- ideal for managing jet lag and sleep disruption caused by shift work (use for first 3 days of adjustment)
- some clinicians recommend that patients with chronic insomnia not use the medication each night but rather, after a good night's sleep with the drug, go 1 or 2 nights without it to decrease tolerance, habituation, and withdrawal problems

Useful References

Kales JD, Kales A. Clinical selection of benzodiazepine hypnotics. Psychiatr Med 1987;4:229–241

Bixler EO, Kales A, Manfredi RL, et al. Next-day memory impairment with triazolam use. Lancet;1991:827–831

TRIHEXYPHENIDYL

Ruby Grymonpre

USA (Artane, Artane Sequels [extended-release], Trihexane, Trihexidyl Hydrochloride, Trihexy-2, Trihexy-5)
CANADA (Artane, Artane Sequels)

▶ When Should I Use This Drug?

Parkinson's disease

- anticholinergics have been used as first-line therapy for patients with mild Parkinson's disease (tremor as the predominant symptom) and good cognitive function; however, anticholinergics are now most often used as adjuncts to levodopa therapy when tremor is a problem
- there is no difference among benztropine, trihexyphenidyl, procyclidine, and biperiden with respect to efficacy; however, benztropine may have a greater sedative effect than some of the other anticholinergic agents (Clin Pharmacokinet 1987;13:141–178)
- trihexyphenidyl is more stimulating than the other agents
- benztropine is the only agent that can be given once daily, whereas trihexyphenidyl, with the exception of the sustained-release product, and procyclidine may need to be given more frequently
- decision among these agents should be based on cost, compliance issues, and the patient's response

▶ When Should I Not Use This Drug?

see Benztropine

▶ What Contraindications Are There to the Use of This Drug?

see Benztropine

▶ What Drug Interactions Are Clinically Important?

see Benztropine

▶ What Route and Dosage Should I Use?

How to administer

- orally—with food or milk or on an empty stomach
- parenterally—not available

Parkinson's disease

- 1 mg PO on day 1
- increase the dosage by 2 mg increments weekly to a maximum dosage of 6–10 mg PO daily in 2 divided doses
- extended-release capsules (5 mg) should not be used in initial therapy or until an effective maintenance dosage has been established
- extended-release capsules can be administered as a single daily dose if this is desirable for the patient
- elixir form is available for patients who are unable to swallow capsules or tablets

Dosage adjustments for renal or hepatic dysfunction

- hepatically metabolized
- no dosage adjustment is required; just start with a low dose and titrate up to effect or toxicity

▶ What Should I Monitor with Regard to Efficacy and Toxicity?

see Benztropine

▶ How Long Do I Treat Patients with This Drug?

see Benztropine

▶ How Do I Decrease or Stop the Administration of This Drug?

see Benztropine

▶ What Should I Tell My Patients About This Drug?

see Benztropine

▶ Therapeutic Tips

see Benztropine

TRIMETHOPRIM-SULFAMETHOXAZOLE (TMP/SMX, CO-TRIMOXAZOLE)

George Zhanel and Ann Beardsell

USA (Bactrim, Bethaprim, Cotrim, Septra, Sulfatrim)
CANADA (Apo-Sulfatrim, Bactrim, Novotrimel, Protrin, Roubac, Septra)

▶ When Should I Use This Drug?

check antibiotic susceptibility chart (Table 4–1 in Chapter 4)

Upper urinary tract infection

- trimethoprim-sulfamethoxazole is equally effective to other agents if organisms are sensitive, provides convenient twice-daily dosing, and is less expensive than the newer agents
- patients who are mild to moderately ill with pyelonephritis may be treated orally if they are reliable and compliant (Am J Med 1988;85:793–798)

Lower urinary tract infection (cystitis), asymptomatic bacteriuria, catheter-related infection

- drug of choice for cystitis, asymptomatic bacteriuria, and catheter-related infection (Am J Med 1988;85:793–798, Ann Intern Med 1987;106:341–345)
- is equally effective to other agents (may be better than amoxicillin) if organisms are sensitive, provides convenient twice-daily dosing, and is less expensive than newer agents

Recurrent lower urinary tract infection

- drug of choice for prophylaxis or suppression of urinary tract infection, as it is effective and inexpensive

Acute or chronic bacterial prostatitis

- patients who are mild to moderately ill, reliable, and compliant may be treated orally (Am J Med 1988;85:793–798)
- trimethoprim-sulfamethoxazole penetrates the prostate well, provides convenient twice-daily dosing, and is less expensive than the newer agents

Otitis media

- if a patient is allergic to amoxicillin or has failed to respond to repeated courses of amoxicillin
- one advantage over amoxicillin is that it allows BID dosing versus TID dosing with amoxicillin

Pneumonia

- trimethoprim-sulfamethoxazole has good activity against pneumococcus and ampicillin-resistant *Haemophilus influenzae* and is less expensive than agents such as cefuroxime axetil and amoxicillin-clavulanate and is better tolerated than erythromycin
- trimethoprim-sulfamethoxazole has good activity against many gram-negative organisms
- trimethoprim-sulfamethoxazole is useful in mild to moderately ill patients with or without underlying disease states when a Gram stain of sputum shows gram-positive diplococci (*Streptococcus*

pneumoniae) or gram-negative coccobacilli (*H. influenzae*) and the patient is penicillin allergic
- can also be used for *Legionella* if erythromycin or tetracycline cannot be used or tolerated

Pneumocystis carinii pneumonia

- used instead of trimethoprim-dapsone if there is known dapsone intolerance, or if the initial hemoglobin level is below 110 g/L, because dapsone is known to produce methemoglobinemia and hemolytic anemia in a dose-related fashion
- if concomitant bacterial infection is present or suspected, trimethoprimsulfamethoxazole is preferred because of its inherent antimicrobial activity
- trimethoprim in combination with either sulfamethoxazole or dapsone is preferred to pentamidine because of the cost of pentamidine

Pneumocystis carinii pneumonia prophylaxis

- trimethoprim-sulfamethoxazole is the drug of choice for prophylaxis, as it is effective, more convenient, and less expensive than aerosolized pentamidine

Enteric infections

- drug of choice for mild to moderate shigellosis or traveler's diarrhea if the patient is not sulfa allergic, as it is effective and less expensive than the quinolones
- administration of antibiotics should be initiated when diarrhea develops and should not be used for prophylaxis because of the risk of adverse effects and the development of resistance

▶ *When Should I Not Use This Drug?*
Anaerobic infections

- trimethoprim-sulfamethoxazole has virtually no anaerobic activity

Pseudomonas aeruginosa infections

- although trimethoprim-sulfamethoxazole has broad gram-negative bacillary activity, it demonstrates poor activity against *P. aeruginosa*

▶ *What Contraindications Are There to the Use of This Drug?*
Intolerance of or allergic reaction to sulfonamides or trimethoprim

- do not use if the patient states a true allergy to either component

Pregnancy or lactation

- sulfonamides may cause kernicterus if used in the third trimester of pregnancy or in newborns

Severe renal insufficiency

- in patients with creatinine clearance less than 15 mL/min, use an alternative agent to prevent exacerbation of renal dysfunction (Med Clin North Am 1987;71:1177–1194)

▶ *What Drug Interactions Are Clinically Important?*

- none

▶ *What Route and Dosage Should I Use?*
How to administer

- orally—should be taken with food or milk to minimize gastric upset
- parenterally—IV—dilute each 5 mL of trimethoprim-sulfamethoxazole (80 mg/400 mg) in 125 mL of 5% dextrose in water or normal saline

Upper urinary tract infection

- 160 mg/800 mg of trimethoprim-sulfamethoxazole (1 double-strength tablet) PO BID

Lower urinary tract infection (cystitis), asymptomatic bacteriuria, catheter-related infection

- 160 mg/800 mg of trimethoprim-sulfamethoxazole PO BID

Recurrent lower urinary tract infection

- 40 mg/200 mg PO HS or after intercourse in women whose infections occur in association with sexual activity
- alternative in the compliant patient is treatment initiated by the patient at the first signs or symptoms at a dosage as above for lower urinary tract infection

Acute or chronic bacterial prostatitis

- 160 mg/800 mg of trimethoprim-sulfamethoxazole PO BID

Otitis media

- 10 mg trimethoprim/50 mg sulfamethoxazole/kg/day divided in BID PO doses

Pneumonia

- 160 mg/800 mg PO BID if the patient is moderately ill
- 160 mg/800 mg IV Q8H if the patient is severely ill

Pneumocystis carinii pneumonia

- for treatment, 20 mg/kg/d of trimethoprim IV or PO (if it can be tolerated) divided into 4 daily doses
- when using trimethoprim-sulfamethoxazole, this equals approximately 2 double-strength tablets QID
- use intravenously only if there is intolerance of oral trimethoprim-sulfamethoxazole

Pneumocystis carinii pneumonia prophylaxis

- for prophylaxis, 160 mg/800 mg of trimethoprim-sulfamethoxazole PO daily

Enteric infections

- 160 mg/800 mg of trimethoprim-sulfamethoxazole PO BID

Dosage adjustments for renal or hepatic dysfunction

- renally eliminated

Normal Dosing Interval	$C_{cr} > 60$ mL/min or 1 mL/s	C_{cr} 30–60 mL/min or 0.5–1 mL/s	$C_{cr} < 30$ mL/min or 0.5 mL/s
Q8H	no adjustment needed	Q12H	avoid
Q12H	no adjustment needed	Q24H	avoid

▶ *What Should I Monitor with Regard to Efficacy and Toxicity?*
Efficacy

- for antibiotic administration monitoring guidelines, see specific section on drug therapy

Toxicity

Allergic reactions (rash, urticaria, severe cutaneous reactions)

- minor rash occurs in approximately 3% of patients
- severe cutaneous reactions (erythema multiforme, toxic epidermal necrolysis, and exfoliative dermatitis) are rare
- question the patient about the appearance of these symptoms on a daily basis while the patient is in the hospital
- if these above reactions occur, discontinue the drug administration

Gastrointestinal symptoms (nausea or vomiting, diarrhea)

- occur in less than 5% of patients
- question the patient about the appearance of these symptoms on a daily basis while the patient is in the hospital
- if these reactions occur, reduce the dosage (if possible)

Hematological disorders (anemia, leukopenia, thrombocytopenia)

- these reactions are rare
- monitor hemoglobin level, white blood cell count, and platelet count in patients receiving this drug for longer than 14 days

Patients with human immunodeficiency virus infection or acquired immunodeficiency syndrome

- adverse effects, including allergic reactions, gastrointestinal symptoms, hematological disorders, and hepatotoxicity, occur in approximately 50% of patients (Ann Intern Med 1986;105:37–44)

▶ *How Long Do I Treat Patients with This Drug?*

Lower urinary tract infections, asymptomatic bacteriuria

- 3 days if uncomplicated

Catheter-related bacteriuria

- 5 days

Upper urinary tract infection

- 14 days total (IV and PO)

Recurrent lower urinary tract infection

- use prophylaxis for 6 months, then discontinue and reassess

Acute or chronic bacterial prostatitis

- 30 days for treatment of acute prostatitis
- for chronic disease, give for 6 weeks as initial treatment

Otitis media

- 10 days

Pneumonia

- usual duration of therapy is 10 days or 4–5 days after the patient has become afebrile and has clinically improved
- consider switching to an oral agent after the patient has become afebrile and has clinically improved for 1–2 days

***Pneumocystis carinii* pneumonia**

- for treatment, 14 days of therapy is usually adequate
- 21 days if the patient responds slowly

***Pneumocystis carinii* pneumonia prophylaxis**

- continue for life or as long as the patient tolerates drug therapy

Enteric infections

- 5 days

▶ *How Do I Decrease or Stop the Administration of This Drug?*

- may be stopped abruptly

▶ *What Should I Tell My Patients About This Drug?*

- if you have a rash, itching, hives, wheezing, or difficulty in breathing, contact your physician immediately
- if you have signs and symptoms of a viral illness (fever, cough, sore throat), contact your physician immediately
- take the medication until it is completely finished

▶ *Therapeutic Tips*

- use the oral formulation if possible because of good bioavailability
- in patients with HIV infection or AIDS, adverse effects with trimethoprim-sulfamethoxazole occur in more than 50% of patients
- do not use in patients with a creatinine clearance of less than 15 mL/min

Useful References

Safrin S, Siegel D, Black D. Pyelonephritis in adult women: Inpatient versus outpatient therapy. Am J Med 1988;85:793–798

Stamm WE, McKevitt M, Counts GW. Acute renal infection in women: Treatment with trimethoprim-sulfamethoxazole or ampicillin for 2 or 6 weeks. Ann Intern Med 1987;106:341–345

Wharton JM, Coleman DL, Wofsy CB, et al. Trimethoprim-sulfamethoxazole or pentamidine for *Pneumocystis carinii* pneumonia in acquired immunodeficiency syndrome. Ann Intern Med 198;105:37–44

Hughes WT, Armstron D, Bodey GP, et al. Guidelines for the use of antimicrobial agents in neutropenic patients with unexplained fever. J Infect Dis 1990;161:381–396

Foltzer MA, Reese RE. Trimethoprim-sulfamethoxazole and other sulfonamides. Med Clin North Am 1987;71:1177–1194

Cockerill FR, Edson RS. Trimethoprim-sulfamethoxazole. Mayo Cln Proc 1987;62:921–929

TRIMIPRAMINE

Lyle K. Laird and Julia Vertrees

USA (Surmontil, others)
CANADA (Surmontil, Apo-Trimip, Rhotrimine)

▶ *When Should I Use This Drug?*

Consider an alternative agent

- trimipramine is as effective as other antidepressants for depression; however, it offers no advantages over any of the other agents

Useful References

Bryant SG, Brown CS. Major depressive disorders. In: Young LY, Koda-Kimble MA, eds. Applied Therapeutics: The Clinical Use of Drugs, 4th ed. Vancouver, WA: Applied Therapeutics, 1988:1231–1253

Wells BG, Hayes PE. Depressive illness. In: DiPiro JT, Talbert RL, Hayes PE, et al, eds. Pharmacotherapy: A Pathophysiologic Approach. New York: Elsevier, 1989:748–764

VALPROIC ACID

William Parker, Steven Stanislav, and Patricia Marken

Valproate Sodium

USA (Depakene, Myproic Acid)
CANADA (Depakene)

Valproic Acid

USA (Depakene, Deproic)
CANADA (Depakene)

Divalproex Sodium

USA (Depakote)
CANADA (Epival)

▶ *When Should I Use This Drug?*

Generalized seizures (no primary focus)

Tonic-clonic seizures

- valproic acid is effective and is better tolerated than phenytoin or carbamazepine
- less frequent central nervous system (CNS) side effects than with phenytoin or carbamazepine
- also useful if the patient has generalized and absence seizures, as valproic acid treats both seizure types

Absence seizures

- ethosuximide is preferred by some clinicians to valproic acid because of the risk of serious hepatotoxicity and pancreatitis with valproic acid, although this is much lower in adults than in children
- can be used if a contraindication to the use of ethosuximide is present or ethosuximide is ineffective
- drug of choice if multiple seizures are present because ethosuximide is effective for only absence seizures

Myoclonic seizures (including juvenile myoclonic epilepsy)

- drug of choice, as it is the most effective agent for juvenile myoclonic epilepsy

Partial seizures (with or without secondarily generalized tonic-clonic seizures)

- valproic acid is not as effective as carbamazepine and phenytoin, but is an alternative for patients who do not respond to or cannot tolerate phenytoin or carbamazepine (N Engl J Med 1992; 327:765–771)

Status epilepticus

- may be useful for status epilepticus refractory to intravenous diazepam or lorazepam when it is administered by rectal enema

Prophylactic therapy for bipolar disorder (started in conjunction with short-term therapy)

- consider as first-line agent when contraindications to the use of lithium and carbamazepine exist or the patient cannot tolerate or is unresponsive to lithium and carbamazepine
- alternative agent if the patient does not tolerate or has no response with lithium or carbamazepine
- possible synergy with concurrent lithium therapy (J Clin Psychiatry 1988;49:13–18)
- limited data from open, uncontrolled studies suggest possible efficacy as monotherapy or as an adjunct to lithium or carbamazepine
- moderate to marked response reported in several uncontrolled studies; long-term studies are lacking
- possibly more effective in rapid cyclers (Am J Psychiatry 1990;147:431–434)
- consider as possible first-line agent in patients with concurrent seizure disorder (Am J Psychiatry 1989;146:840–847)

▶ *When Should I Not Use This Drug?*

Mild, behavioral dyscontrol or psychotic agitation

- may respond equally well to temporary therapy with other agents (e.g., antipsychotics and sedative-hypnotics)
- try lithium and/or carbamazepine first unless the patient has a history of positive response to valproate sodium; valproate sodium appears less effective for schizoaffective disorders than for bipolar disorder

▶ *What Contraindications Are There to the Use of This Drug?*

Intolerance of or allergic reaction to valproate

Severe hepatic dysfunction

- use only if therapy alternative drugs has failed in patients who may be at greater risk for hepatotoxicity (use of multiple anticonvulsants, presence of congenital metabolic disorders, age older than 10 years)
- avoid use if possible in children younger than 2 years (use as a single agent if valproic acid must be given)
- frequency of fatal hepatoxicity increases in children younger than 2 years receiving valproic acid with other anticonvulsants, especially if congenital metabolic disorders are present or severe neurological disease is present (risk may be 1/500 in such patients)

▶ *What Drug Interactions Are Clinically Important?*

Drugs that may increase the effect or toxicity of valproic acid

PHENOBARBITAL, PRIMIDONE, CARBAMAZEPINE

- coadministration with valproic acid may result in increased sedation, CNS depression, and neurological toxicity with or without increased serum levels of either drug
- start with lower valproate sodium dosage (250 mg/d) and monitor for excessive sedation and/or signs of neurological toxicity (obtain serum level of barbiturate at the first signs or symptoms of toxicity) and decrease the valproate sodium dosage

SALICYLATES

- concurrent use of salicylates may increase free valproate sodium concentrations and decrease metabolism of valproate sodium
- if concurrent therapy is indicated, start with low doses of both drugs and titrate
- intermittent use of salicylates is not likely to be a problem

Drugs that may decrease the effect of valproic acid

- none

Drugs that may have their effect or toxicity increased by valproic acid

PHENYTOIN

- may increase or decrease the steady state phenytoin concentration and increase the free fraction of phenytoin

- do not adjust the phenytoin dosage unless toxicity occurs or seizures are exacerbated and are associated with changes in serum concentration

PHENOBARBITAL

- may increase serum phenobarbital concentrations, which may cause increased sedation
- monitor serum concentrations if sedation occurs and adjust the dosage if necessary

CENTRAL NERVOUS SYSTEM DEPRESSANTS (ALCOHOL, BENZODIAZEPINES, ANTIDEPRESSANTS, ANTIPSYCHOTICS)

- if used concomitantly, there is increased potential for excessive sedation
- give the greatest dosage at bedtime and/or reduce the drug dosages if possible

WARFARIN

- valproate sodium may alter INR
- if valproate sodium is started in a patient receiving maintenance anticoagulation therapy, monitor prothrombin time every 2 days until the full extent of the interaction is seen and adjust the dosage as for a warfarin dosage change

Drugs that have their effect decreased by valproic acid

- none

▶ *What Route and Dosage Should I Use?*

How to administer

- orally—take with food or milk
- parenterally—not available

There is no difference in clinical efficacy between valproic acid and divalproex sodium • Divalproex sodium is enteric coated and may afford less gastrointestinal side effects, although it is still recommended to take it with food (some clinicians always use the enteric-coated product because of the concern for gastrointestinal upset)

Generalized seizures (no primary focus), partial seizures (with or without secondarily generalized tonic-clonic seizures)

- 15 mg/kg/d as a starting dosage
- if an immediate response is not needed, it is best to start the dosage at 500 mg PO HS and increase by 500 mg daily every 5–7 days to minimize gastrointestinal side effects
- final total daily dose depends on the frequency of seizures and the patient's ability to tolerate the drug
- patients with primary generalized seizures require 1500–2000 mg PO daily divided BID–TID depending on tolerance
- patients with juvenile myoclonic epilepsy generally require lower dosages
- patients previously receiving valproic acid can be initiated on divalproex sodium (enteric coated) at the same daily dosage
- divalproex sodium is often the agent used on a BID regimen to reduce the incidence of gastrointestinal upset

Status epilepticus

- 500 mg of valproic acid syrup diluted 1 : 1 with water as a single-dose retention enema

Prophylactic therapy for bipolar disorder

- start with 250 mg PO BID
- increase the dosage by 250 mg every week on the basis of clinical response, adverse effects, and serum concentrations (serum level for optimum response is not well established; a few studies suggest a target range of 50–100 μg/mL)

Dosage adjustments in renal or hepatic dysfunction

- hepatically metabolized
- for patients with hepatic disease, start with 250 mg/d and titrate the dose to serum level; avoid the use of valproate sodium in significant hepatic dysfunction

▶ *What Should I Monitor with Regard to Efficacy and Toxicity?*

Efficacy

Generalized seizures (no primary focus), partial seizures (with or without secondarily generalized tonic-clonic seizures)

Seizure frequency

- reduction in the frequency and severity of seizures

Prophylactic therapy for bipolar disorder

Target symptoms

- improvement in agitation; decreased sleep; rapid, pressured speech with flight of ideas for manic phase; or symptoms of depression

Symptoms of psychoses

- auditory or visual hallucinations; delusional or disorganized thinking

Serum concentrations

- serum concentration monitoring is less useful as a therapeutic tool with valproic acid than with other anticonvulsants
- they may be useful to assess compliance, possible toxicity, or unexplained increases in seizure
- accepted therapeutic range is 50–100 μg/mL (350–700 μmol/L); some patients require a minimum therapeutic level of 70 μg/mL (470 μmol/L) and peak levels greater than 100 μg/mL (700 μmol/L)
- valproate sodium serum concentration–clinical response relationships are not well established for bipolar disorder; therefore, maintain at the lowest effective dosage; several reports suggest a therapeutic range of 50–100 μg/mL
- it may take several weeks at a given serum concentration for full therapeutic benefits to develop; these effects may also persist for several days after the drug administration is stopped and serum levels have declined below detectable limits
- serum valproic acid concentrations may vary by as much as 100% over a single dosing interval; always check valproic acid levels at the same time in relationship to drug dosing
- in patients receiving valproic acid with multiple anticonvulsants, valproic acid serum concentrations may not be able to be increased to as high a level as desired because of enhanced hepatic metabolism and enzyme induction by other anticonvulsants
- hypoalbuminemia, severe hepatic or renal disease, and pregnancy may increase the unbound fraction of valproic acid
- serum concentration–dose relationship is curvilinear (concentration/dose ratio decreases with increasing dosage) owing to an increased free fraction and increased clearance
- steady state concentration is reached in 2–4 days after the maintenance dose is attained
- trough levels are preferred
- enteric coating on divalproex sodium tablets delays absorption, so trough levels may be shifted and occur 2–4 hours after the next dose

Toxicity

Hepatotoxicity

- incidence is rare in older children and adults receiving monotherapy
- most deaths have occurred in patients who were younger than 2 years of age, were mentally handicapped, or were receiving multiple anticonvulsants and early in the course of therapy
- clinical symptoms of hepatic dysfunction damage usually precede liver function test changes and transient rise in liver function test results are common in during first 6 months and typically return to baseline levels
- hyperammonemia is common (50%) but does not necessarily imply hepatic damage
- minor elevations in aminotransferase and lactate dehydrogenase levels also occur frequently (50%) and appear to be dose related and nontoxic
- baseline liver function tests should be performed

- because asymptomatic, benign elevations in hepatic enzymes are common early in therapy, and symptoms of hepatic damage (malaise, weakness, lethargy, anorexia, vomiting) usually precede laboratory changes, frequent liver function tests during early therapy are unlikely to detect serious hepatotoxicity
- monitor patients on clinical grounds for signs and symptoms of hepatotoxicity
- discontinuation of valproate sodium administration is not necessary unless clinical symptoms emerge or hepatic enzyme levels are greater than 3 times baseline values
- educate patients to identify early signs or symptoms of hepatic damage

Hematological effects

- up to 40% of patients may experience mild dose-dependent thrombocytopenia, although other hematological side effects are rare and are infrequently clinically significant
- minimize by dosage reduction and avoidance of other agents known to affect platelet counts and bleeding times
- baseline platelet count should be performed
- coagulation tests should be monitored prior to surgery

Transient alopecia and hair changes

- may be seen but usually disappear with continued drug use or dosage reduction

Central nervous system effects

- sedation and drowsiness often occur early in therapy and resolve within several weeks; monitor for persistent or increased drowsiness or signs of neurological toxicity (ataxia, tremor, nystagmus), especially with concomitant use of barbiturates and other CNS depressants
- fine tremor is sometimes experienced by patients but is usually well tolerated

Gastrointestinal side effects (nausea, vomiting, anorexia, abdominal cramps, diarrhea)

- occurs in 25% of patients, especially during the initiation of therapy
- minimize by starting therapy at 25–30% of the usual 15 mg/kg/d starting dosage, increase weekly, take with food, and/or use the enteric-coated formulation
- may cause weight gain
- valproic acid is a rare cause of pancreatitis

▶ *How Long Do I Treat Patients with This Drug?*

Generalized seizures (no primary focus), partial seizures (with or without secondarily generalized tonic-clonic seizures)

- 4 year seizure-free period is recommended before attempting to withdraw valproic acid therapy
- factors promoting complete withdrawal include a seizure-free period of 2–4 years, complete seizure control within 1 year of onset, an onset of seizures between 2 and 35 years of age, and a normal electroencephalogram
- patients should not drive during withdrawal and for 3–4 months after, and this may make it difficult for some patients to try withdrawal
- prior to withdrawal, patients should be advised that about $\frac{1}{3}$ experience relapse, and if this occurs, the patient and the physician will know that the drug is still necessary
- factors associated with a poor prognosis in stopping the drug administration, despite a seizure-free period, include a history of a high frequency of seizures, repeated episodes of status epilepticus, multiple seizure types, and the development of abnormal mental functioning

Prophylactic therapy for bipolar disorder

- adequate trial period (typically 3–4 weeks at therapeutic serum concentrations; some patients require up to 6 weeks for full response) is necessary to evaluate efficacy
- duration of therapy is not well defined
- at the minimum, treatment should continue until symptoms resolve, the patient is euthymic, and sleep normalizes (some clinicians recommend continuing therapy for several months after symptoms resolve)

- prophylactic or maintenance therapy should be continued in rapid cyclers (more than 4 episodes per year) and probably in patients with history of recurrent bipolar disorder (at least 1 episode a year) with marked severity and substantial disruption of functioning

▶ *How Do I Decrease or Stop the Administration of This Drug?*

- sudden withdrawal is to be avoided, especially after long-term, high-dose therapy
- withdrawal is best done over several months
- decrease the dosage by 500 mg daily each month until withdrawal is complete
- seizure relapse is most common during withdrawal or the first 3 months after withdrawal
- if seizures recur, reinstitute treatment with the same drugs used previously
- if multiple anticonvulsant therapy is present, drugs should be withdrawn one at a time
- for psychiatric disorders, most patients do not experience a withdrawal syndrome or rebound phenomenon on abrupt discontinuation of therapy; however, certain individuals may have increased risks of recurrence of symptoms after discontinuation (Br J Psychiatry 1986;149:498–501)
- it is best to taper the drug withdrawal; decrease the daily dosage by 250 mg every week and monitor the patient weekly for the first few weeks (monitoring for early relapse) and then monthly after that (monitoring for late relapse)

▶ *What Should I Tell My Patients About This Drug?*

- notify your physician at once if you experience extreme malaise or vomiting, yellowish pigmenting of skin or eyes, a change in the color of urine or stool, or severe gastrointestinal pain
- you may be overly sensitive to the combination of this drug with alcohol or other CNS depressants, and you should not drive or operate heavy machinery until you know how you react to these agents
- avoid the use of other CNS depressant drugs while taking valproate sodium
- you make take valproate sodium with food to minimize stomach irritation
- tablets and capsules should be swallowed whole, not chewed or crushed, to avoid local irritation of the mouth and throat
- contents of capsules containing coated particles of divalproex sodium may be sprinkled on a small amount of semisolid food immediately prior to administration; the mixture should not be chewed
- drug syrup should not be mixed with carbonated drinks because valproic acid may be liberated, causing local irritation and an unpleasant taste
- tell patients that tremor and some weight gain are frequent side effects

▶ *Therapeutic Tips*

- start therapy gradually to minimize gastrointestinal upset
- do not chew, break, or crush tablets or capsules because this may irritate your mouth or throat
- obtain trough valproate levels to ensure consistency in follow-up monitoring; product formulation and ingestion with food affect the time of peak drug level; however, trough levels remain fairly consistent
- transient liver function test result elevations are common (especially in first 6 months of therapy) and usually do not require drug administration discontinuation unless they are more than 3 times baseline values or the patient has clinical signs of hepatotoxicity (see above)
- most patients can be treated BID
- therapeutic range is not helpful as a guide to therapy

Useful References

Pugh CB, Garnett WR. Current issues in the treatment of epilepsy. Clin Pharm 1991;10:335–358
Parker WA. Epilepsy. In: Herfindal ET, Gourley DR, Hart LL, eds. Clinical Pharmacy and Therapeutics, 4th ed. Baltimore: Williams & Wilkins, 1988:570–592

Levy RH, Wilensky AJ, Friel PN. Other antiepileptic drugs. In: Evans WE, Schentag JJ, Jusko WJ, eds. Applied Pharmacokinetics: Principles of Therapeutic Drug Monitoring. Spokane WA: Applied Therapeutics, 1986;540–569
Post RM. Introduction: Emerging perspectives on valproate in affective disorders. J Clin Psychiatry 1989;50[3]:3–12
Calabrese JR, Delucchi GA. Spectrum of efficacy of valproate in 55 patients with rapid-cycling bipolar disorder. Am J Psychiatry 1990;147:431–434

VANCOMYCIN

George Zhanel

USA (Vancocin, Vancoled, Vancor)
CANADA (Vancocin)

▶ *When Should I Use This Drug?*

check antibiotic susceptibility chart (Table 4–1 in Chapter 4)

Pneumonia

- nafcillin and cloxacillin are usually the drugs of choice for sensitive gram-positive staphyloccocal organisms, as they are less expensive than vancomycin
- vancomycin should be used if Gram stain shows gram-positive cocci in clusters (*Staphylococcus aureus*) if the patient is allergic to penicillin and/or resistant organisms are suspected

Acute or chronic osteomyelitis

- as empirical therapy until sensitivities are known in patients with osteomyelitis if prosthetic joints are involved
- vancomycin has activity against the common organisms causing osteomyelitis in patients with prosthetic joints (*S. aureus* and *S. epidermidis*) (Infect Dis Clin North Am 1989;3:329–338)
- if organisms are not methicillin resistant, switch to cloxacillin or nafcillin after sensitivities are known

Meningitis

- if Gram stain shows gram-positive cocci in clusters (*S. aureus* or *S. epidermidis*), use vancomycin
- although cloxacillin or nafcillin can be effective, these agents should not be used until sensitivities have been determined
- vancomycin should be used in patients with suspected shunt infections if Gram stain is not yet available or Gram stain shows no organisms, as it covers either *S. aureus* or *S. epidermidis* until culture and sensitivity testing results are known
- use in conjunction with ceftazidime in patients who are severely ill with suspected shunt infections to cover *S. aureus*, *S. epidermidis*, and gram-negative organisms (*Pseudomonas* possible) until culture and sensitivity testing results are known

Endocarditis

Vancomycin should be used for the following:

- penicillin-resistant diphtheroids
- penicillin-sensitive streptococci (minimum inhibitory concentration [MIC] < 0.1 mg/L) and a history of an immediate-type hypersensitivity reaction to penicillin
- methicillin-resistant *S. aureus* with a native valve
- *S. aureus* and a history of an immediate-type hypersensitivity reaction to penicillin

Vancomycin should be used in conjunction with gentamicin for the following:

- methicillin-resistant *S. aureus* with a prosthetic valve
- penicillinase-producing enterococcus
- patients with a history of an immediate-type hypersensitivity to penicillin and with penicillin-sensitive streptococci (MIC < 0.1 mg/L) who are younger than 65 years and have no renal or auditory impairment
- penicillin-resistant streptococci (MIC ≥ 2.0 mg/L)
- gentamicin-sensitive diphtheroids
- culture-negative endocarditis if the patient has a history of an immediate-type hypersensitivity to penicillin

Vancomycin in conjunction with gentamicin and rifampin should be used after culture and sensitivity testing if the following are present:

- methicillin-resistant *S. aureus* or *S. epidermidis* if the patient does not respond to vancomycin and gentamicin

- for staphylococcus resistant to gentamicin, use another aminoglycoside; and for resistance to all aminoglycosides, omit aminoglycosides

Vancomycin in conjunction with gentamicin should be used empirically if the patient is acutely ill or has cardiovascular or neurological complications for the following:

- native valve endocarditis if the patient is penicillin allergic
- new valvular insufficiency or suspected IV drug abuser
- prosthetic valve endocarditis

Bacterial endocarditis prophylaxis

- for dental, oral, or respiratory tract procedures as an alternative to amoxicillin in penicillin-allergic patients unable to take oral medications (JAMA 1990;264:2919–2922)

Prevention of postoperative infections

- use in combination with gentamicin for neurosurgery
- in patients with penicillin allergy or in institutions in which there is a high incidence of infection with coagulase-negative *Staphylococcus* species or methicillin-resistant *Staphylococcus* species, use vancomycin for cardiac surgery, noncardiac surgery, peripheral vascular surgery, and orthopedic surgery

Pseudomembranous colitis

- use in patients with proven metronidazole-resistant *Clostridium difficile* or without adequate response to metronidazole
- metronidazole is as effective as vancomycin and less expensive (Lancet 1983;2:1043–1046)

▶ *When Should I Not Use This Drug?*

Methicillin-sensitive infections

- vancomycin is no more effective than cloxacillin or nafcillin or cefazolin for infections caused by methicillin-sensitive organisms

Non–beta-lactam allergic patients

- check true allergy status, and use cloxacillin or nafcillin or cefazolin if possible

Infection prevention in neutropenic patients

- not effective as an oral nonabsorbable antibiotic

Gram-negative bacillary infections

- infections caused by *Escherichia coli*, *Klebsiella pneumoniae*, *Enterobacter* sp., *Pseudomonas aeruginosa*, and *Bacteroides fragilis*, because vancomycin has no activity against these organisms

Empirical therapy for febrile neutropenic patients

- unless methicillin-resistant staphylococcus organisms have previously caused infection in a particular patient, vancomycin is likely not needed as empirical therapy

▶ *What Contraindications Are There to the Use of This Drug?*

Intolerance of or allergic reaction to vancomycin

- if the patient states hypersensitivity to vancomycin, check that this is a true hypersensitivity reaction and not a histamine-related event (e.g., red man syndrome [see below])

▶ *What Drug Interactions Are Clinically Important?*

Drugs that may increase the effect of vancomycin

AMINOGLYCOSIDES

- there is a suggestion that using these 2 agents together increases the risk of toxicity (Antimicrob Agents Chemother 1983;23:138–141)
- no dosage adjustments are necessary; however, monitoring of renal and auditory function is warranted (see below)

Drugs that may decrease the effect of vancomycin

HEPARIN

- in intravenous solutions, concurrent use of heparin (at high concentrations) with vancomycin can inactivate vancomycin; therefore, do not mix together

Drugs that may have their effect increased by vancomycin

- none

Drugs that may have their effect decreased by vancomycin

- none

▶ *What Route and Dosage Should I Use?*

How to administer

Orally

- take with food or milk or on an empty stomach

Parenterally

- dilute vancomycin in 100 mL of 5% dextrose in water or normal saline when given intravenously
- after it is diluted, administer vancomycin over at least 1 hour (to avoid red man syndrome and to decrease the incidence of thrombophlebitis)
- if dosages are greater than 1000 mg, infuse the drug over 2 hours

Pneumonia, acute or chronic osteomyelitis

- 15 mg/kg Q12H

Meningitis

- 20 mg/kg Q12H

Endocarditis

- 15 mg/kg Q12H

Bacterial endocarditis prophylaxis

- 1 g IV 1 hour prior to the procedure

Prevention of postoperative infections

- 15 mg/kg as a single dose

Pseudomembranous colitis

- 125 mg PO Q6H
- 500 mg PO Q6H is no more effective than 125 mg PO Q6H (Am J Med 1989;86:15–19)

Dosage adjustments for renal or hepatic dysfunction

- renally eliminated

Normal Dosing Interval	C_{cr} > 60 mL/min or 1 mL/s	C_{cr} 30–60 mL/min or 0.5–1 mL/s	C_{cr} < 30 mL/min or 0.5 mL/s
Q12H	no adjustment needed	Q24H	give a single dose and base further doses on serum concentration measurements

▶ *What Should I Monitor with Regard to Efficacy and Toxicity?*

Efficacy

- for antibiotic administration monitoring guidelines, see specific section on drug therapy

Toxicity

Allergic reactions

- question the patient about the appearance of these signs and symptoms on a daily basis while the patient is in the hospital
- chills occur in approximately 5% of patients
- thrombophlebitis occurs in approximately 6% of patients
- these reactions are less frequent if the drug is infused at a slow rate (over at least 1 hour) and in a large volume of fluid
- if the dose is greater than 1000 mg, infuse the drug over 2 hours
- rash occurs in approximately 4% of patients

Nephrotoxicity

- occurs in less than 5% of patients
- usually transient and reversible on adjusting or discontinuing therapy

- avoid concomitant use of nephrotoxic drugs if possible (e.g., aminoglycosides, amphotericin B, and furosemide)
- monitor serum creatinine levels 3 times weekly while the patient is taking vancomycin
- if serum creatinine level increases (i.e., by >50% of baseline values), attempt to identify and remove other causes of renal dysfunction (hypotension, shock, other nephrotoxic agents, and so on)
- if no other cause can be found, consideration should be given to discontinuing the drug administration if the infection is not life threatening; or if vancomycin is still required, adjust the dosage according to renal function using the guidelines above
- no correlation between nephrotoxicity and peak levels
- fair to poor correlation between trough levels and toxicity

Ototoxicity

- occurs in less than 2% of patients, although there is controversy about whether vancomycin as single therapy is ototoxic (Antimicrob Agents Chemother 1989;33:791–796)
- question the patient about the appearance of tinnitus, hearing loss, and balance problems on a daily basis while the patient is in the hospital
- if the patient has any of these symptoms, serious consideration must be given to discontinuing vancomycin therapy
- usually auditory instead of vestibular (Clin Pharmacokinet 1986;11:257–282)
- tinnitus and high-tone hearing loss precede deafness
- hearing often continues to deteriorate despite discontinuation of therapy

Red man syndrome (red neck syndrome)

- incidence is approximately 5–11%
- occurs as tingling and flushing of the face, neck, upper trunk, back, and arms, which may be associated with hypotension
- owing to rapid infusion over less than 1 hour and/or doses greater than 1000 mg
- can be prevented by administering antihistamines before vancomycin and/or increasing the duration of the infusion (longer than 1 hour) (Clin Pharmacokinet 1986;11:257–282)
- red man syndrome subsides quickly after the infusion is stopped

Vancomycin serum levels

- therapeutic range: peaks, 30–40 mg/L; troughs, 5–10 mg/L
- considerable controversy exists about the clinical utility of vancomycin levels (Clin Pharm 1987;6:652–654, 655–658)
- there is little, if any, evidence that maintaining vancomycin levels within a therapeutic range decreases the risk of toxicity or improves outcome compared with basing dosage adjustment on renal function
- obtain trough levels in patients receiving longer than 7 days of therapy, patients taking concomitant nephrotoxins (aminoglycosides, amphotericin B), elderly patients (older than 65 years), hypotensive patients, or those with significant renal compromise (creatinine clearance < 50 mL/min)

▶ How Long Do I Treat Patients with This Drug?

Pneumonia

- usual duration of therapy is 10 days or 4–5 days after the patient has become afebrile and has clinically improved
- consider switching to oral agents after the patient has become afebrile and has clinically improved for 1–2 days

Acute osteomyelitis

- treat patients without a prosthetic device for 4 weeks with parenteral antibiotics
- treat patients with a prosthetic device for 4–6 weeks with parenteral antibiotics, followed by 3–6 months of oral antibiotics
- treat patients with peripheral vascular disease with 4 weeks of parenteral antibiotics, followed by 6 weeks of oral antibiotics (Am J Med 1987;83:653–660)

Chronic osteomyelitis

- treat with 4–6 weeks of parenteral antibiotics, followed by 2 months of oral antibiotics

Meningitis

- 7 days for patients who respond quickly if meningitis is caused by *Streptococcus pneumoniae,* however, treat for 10 days if the patient responds slowly
- if the infection is shunt associated, treat for at least 14 days

Endocarditis

- 4 weeks for methicillin-resistant *S. aureus* with native valve and for penicillin-sensitive streptococci (MIC < 0.1 mg/L)
- some clinicians suggest that the duration of therapy for right-sided *S. aureus* endocarditis be 4 weeks and that left-sided *S. aureus* endocarditis be treated for 4–6 weeks, depending on the clinical response (Infect Dis Clin North Am 1993;7:53–68)
- 6 weeks for penicillin-resistant diphtheroids or for methicillin-resistant *S. aureus* or *S. epidermidis,* in conjunction with rifampin administration, if the patient does not respond to vancomycin and gentamicin alone
- 4 weeks for penicillinase-producing enterococcus, penicillin-sensitive streptococci (MIC < 0.1 mg/L) if the patient is younger than 65 years and has no renal or auditory impairment, intermediately sensitive streptococci (MIC 0.1–1.0 mg/L), penicillin-resistant streptococci (MIC ≥ 2.0 mg/L), enterococci, penicillin-sensitive diptheroids, or culture-negative endocarditis

Bacterial endocarditis prophylaxis

- single dose

Prevention of postoperative infections

- single dose

Pseudomembranous colitis

- usual duration is 7 days, and therapy for longer than 10 days is rarely necessary

▶ How Do I Decrease or Stop the Administration of This Drug?

- may be stopped abruptly

▶ What Should I Tell My Patients About This Drug?

- during drug infusion, let your physician know if you feel any tingling or flushing or if you feel faint
- if you have ringing in the ears or if your ability to hear decreases, contact your physician
- if you have a rash, contact your physician

▶ Therapeutic Tips

- ensure that the dosing interval is adjusted for renal function, especially in the elderly and in patients with preexisting renal dysfunction
- every 12 hour dosing is preferable to every 6–8 hour dosing because it allows less frequent dosing intervals in most patients with normal renal function
- ensure that the drug is infused over at least 1 hour

Useful References

Matzke GR, Zhanel GG, Guay DR. Clinical pharmacokinetics of vancomycin. Clin Pharmacokinet 1986;11:257–282
Cheung RP, Dipiro JT. Vancomycin: An update. Pharmacotherapy 1986;6:153–169

VERAPAMIL

Stephen F. Hamilton, Stan Horton, and Udho Thadani

USA (Calan, Isoptin, Calan SR, Isoptin SR, Verelan)
CANADA (Isoptin, Isoptin-SR, Apo-Verap, Novo-Veramil, Nu-Verap)

▶ When Should I Use This Drug?

Chronic stable angina

- if there are no concomitant disease states, calcium channel blockers are useful in patients who do not tolerate or do not have complete control with nitrates and beta-blockers
- beta-blockers should be chosen instead of calcium channel blockers for new-onset angina or chronic stable angina because there

is more cumulative information for the overall value of beta-blockers in these patients and they are less expensive than calcium antagonists
- calcium antagonists can be used as monotherapy when contraindications to the use of beta-blockers and nitrates are present and can be added when optimum 2-drug (nitrates and beta-blockers) therapy is not adequate for symptom control (Am Heart J 1989;118:1093–1097)
- triple-drug therapy (maximum therapy) has not had advantages over optimized therapy with nitrates and beta-blockers and should be reserved for patients who are symptomatic while taking double-drug (nitrates and beta-blockers) therapy (J Am Coll Cardiol 1984;3:1051–1057)
- if there is concomitant hypertension, calcium channel blockers should be chosen in patients unable to take beta-blockers
- if concomitant diabetes or chronic obstructive pulmonary disease or asthma is present, calcium channel blockers should be chosen in patients who cannot tolerate nitrates or in whom nitrates are ineffective
- all calcium channel blockers are equally effective; however, diltiazem is usually the best tolerated calcium channel blocker and should be chosen instead of the other agents unless there are significant price differences
- calcium channel blocking agents are considered the drugs of choice for the management of Prinzmetal's variant angina

Chronic (noncrisis) hypertension

- use only in patients who do not tolerate, do not respond to, or have contraindications to thiazide diuretics and beta-blockers because thiazide diuretics and beta-blockers have proven long-term benefit and are generally less expensive than calcium channel blockers
- calcium channel blockers are useful for hypertension in patients with ischemic heart disease if beta-blockers are not effective or tolerated and in patients with asthma, diabetes, or moderate to severe hyperlipidemias, as they have no effect on these disease states
- all calcium channel blockers are equally effective; however, diltiazem is usually the best tolerated calcium channel blocker and should be chosen instead of other agents unless there are significant price differences
- choose verapamil rather than diltiazem if the patient has concomitant atrial fibrillation

Atrial fibrillation or flutter

- verapamil is used in patients who do not respond to digoxin and beta-blockers as long as the patient does not have poor left ventricular function
- verapamil should also be used after digoxin and beta-blockers to control ventricular rate in patients with paroxysmal atrial fibrillation or flutter, even though digoxin may not be effective (Br Heart J 1990;63:225–227)
- verapamil may be more effective than digoxin in controlling ventricular rate in atrial fibrillation or flutter associated with increases in the levels of circulating catecholamines (e.g., due to anxiety or exercise)
- has greater atrioventricular nodal blocking properties than other calcium channel blockers

Atrioventricular nodal reentrant tachycardia

Acute episodes

- is considered the drug of choice when adenosine does not work or when the arrhythmia returns after adenosine treatment (JAMA 1992;268:2199–2241)
- verapamil should not be used for the treatment of a wide QRS tachycardia unless it is known to be supraventricular in origin; administration of verapamil in patients with ventricular tachycardia may result in acceleration of the tachycardia and severe hemodynamic deterioration (Am J Cardiol 1987;59:1107–1110)

Long-term therapy

- there are no studies comparing the efficacy of agents in preventing atrioventricular nodal reentrant tachycardia, but most sources consider digoxin the drug of choice (Arch Intern Med 1987;147:1706–1716)

- because response to intravenous verapamil does not accurately predict long-term response to oral verapamil (Circulation 1980;62:996–1010), and because many of these patients have concomitant left ventricular dysfunction, digoxin is a reasonable choice as a first-line agent for long-term therapy
- verapamil can be used when digoxin is ineffective

Migraine prophylaxis

- verapamil should be tried if there are contraindications to the use of or failure of beta-blockers
- these agents are expensive but probably better tolerated than the antidepressants
- selection of preferred calcium channel blocker therapy should be based on efficacy, toxicity, and cost
- majority of the studies have been done with verapamil and flunarizine, and no comparative trials have been done
- flunarizine is more expensive than verapamil but can be given as a single daily dose; however, flunarizine does cause weight gain and somnolence in 40–50% of patients (Headache 1991;31: 388–391)
- flunarizine is investigational in the United States
- toxicity profile of flunarizine likely limits its availability and widespread use
- during long-term therapy, extrapyramidal reactions have been reported with flunarizine (Drugs 1989;38:481–499)
- nifedipine can cause headaches and studies have not confirmed its effectiveness (Neurology 1989;39:284–286)

▶ When Should I Not Use This Drug?

Post–myocardial infarction patients

- addition of a calcium antagonist is indicated only if optimum (beta-blocker and nitrate) therapy does not control anginal symptoms
- data for empirical use of calcium antagonists after myocardial infarction has not shown a decrease in mortality

Raynaud's syndrome

- verapamil does not appear to be effective (J Clin Pharmacol 1982;22:74–76)
- nifedipine has proven efficacy in the treatment of Raynaud's syndrome

Acute (crisis) hypertension

- no evidence of the use of diltiazem in this condition

▶ What Contraindications Are There to the Use of This Drug?

see Diltiazem

▶ What Drug Interactions Are Clinically Important?

Drugs that may increase the effect or toxicity of verapamil

BETA-ADRENERGIC BLOCKING AGENTS

- when used concomitantly with verapamil, this increases the incidence of congestive heart failure (CHF), arrhythmia, and severe hypotension
- these agents should be used together only when there is an ejection fraction greater than 30 and when anginal symptoms fail to be controlled by other drug therapy or either agent alone in maximum dosages

AMIODARONE

- when used concomitantly with verapamil, amiodarone increases the incidence of CHF, arrhythmia, and severe hypotension
- these drugs should not be used together

Drugs that may decrease the effect of verapamil

CALCIUM

- calcium therapy may result in antagonism of the beneficial effects and unwanted effects of calcium channel blocking agents, and therefore, concomitant use is not recommended
- calcium therapy for osteoporosis prophylaxis is not a contraindication

CAFFEINE, EPINEPHRINE, ISOPROTERENOL, THEOPHYLLINE

- drugs that increase cyclic adenosine monophosphate inhibit the calcium channel blocking activity and patients should be observed for an alteration in response
- if episodic hypertension is suspected because of these agents, an ambulatory blood pressure monitor may be useful

RIFAMPIN, PHENYTOIN

- may substantially reduce the oral bioavailability of verapamil by increasing first-pass metabolism via the induction of hepatic microsomal enzymes
- be aware of the effect and monitor within a few days for reduced clinical efficacy or for toxicity whenever these agents are initiated or discontinued, respectively (adjust the dosage of verapamil on the basis of changes in effect or toxicity)

Drugs that may have their effect or toxicity increased by verapamil

DIGOXIN

- digoxin concentrations may increase by 50–75% during the first week of verapamil therapy and may be more substantial in patients with underlying hepatic disease
- may raise digoxin levels (by inhibition of renal clearance and/or alterations at tissue-binding sites)
- decrease the digoxin dosage by 50% when adding verapamil and make further dosage changes on the basis of clinical response (efficacy and toxicity)

CARBAMAZEPINE

- hepatic metabolism is inhibited by verapamil via the cytochrome P-450 microsomal enzyme system, which may result in increased plasma carbamazepine concentrations and subsequent toxicity
- 40–50% reduction in carbamazepine dosage may be necessary during concomitant therapy
- use nifedipine in place of verapamil if possible
- if verapamil must be added for longer than 3 days, obtain a baseline serum carbamazepine concentration prior to adding inhibitor, recheck the concentration in 1 week, and reduce the dosage proportionally if the concentration is greater than 12 mg/L
- monitor for symptoms of toxicity, and if they occur, stop the drug administration, repeat serum concentration, and adjust the dosage accordingly
- if a concentration is not available within 24 hours, restart carbamazepine administration at 50% of the previous dosage as long as toxicity is not present
- if no toxicity occurs, measure concentrations weekly until a new steady state has been reached
- if verapamil administration is stopped, increase the dosage back to preinhibitor levels

CYCLOSPORINE

- inhibits hepatic metabolism of cyclosporine
- seen as early as 2 days after the start of therapy with these drugs
- use alternative if possible (e.g., nifedipine does not interact)
- monitor cyclosporine levels every other day until the full extent of interaction is seen and adjust the dosage accordingly
- may need to decrease the cyclosporine dosage by 30% or more

QUINIDINE

- quinidine clearance is decreased by verapamil and quinidine may attenuate the alpha-mediated reflex pressor response to verapamil-induced vasodilatation, leading to excessive hypotension
- these agents can be used together but be aware of the potential for an interaction

METOPROLOL

- bioavailability is increased 300% by verapamil therapy, decreasing metoprolol's hepatic clearance
- do not use this combination and choose a different beta-blocker

Drugs that may have their effect decreased by verapamil

- none

▶ *What Route and Dosage Should I Use?*

How to administer

Orally

- oral bioavailability of extended-release verapamil is not affected by halving the tablets
- extended-release verapamil should be taken with food

Parenterally

- verapamil is physically compatible with 5% dextrose injection or normal saline
- verapamil should be given slowly under continuous electrocardiographic and blood pressure monitoring, as a slow IV push, over a period of not less than 2 minutes or, in geriatric patients, of not less than 3 minutes

Chronic stable angina

- 120 mg of sustained-release verapamil (a once-daily product sometimes given twice daily when dosages exceed 240 mg/d) PO daily, increasing the dosage weekly by 120 mg daily until symptoms are controlled or a maximum dosage of 480 mg PO daily is reached
- sustained-release preparations are recommended, as they are more convenient and usually not much different in price from the regular-release products (unless generic regular-release is available)
- regular-release form is started at 80 mg PO Q8H, increasing the dosage weekly by 80 mg/d until symptoms are controlled or a maximum dose of 360 mg/d is reached

Chronic (noncrisis) hypertension

- 120 mg of sustained-release verapamil (a once-daily product sometimes given twice daily when dosages exceed 240 mg/d) PO daily increasing the dosage every 4 weeks by 120 mg/d until an effect is seen or a maximum dosage of 480 mg/d is reached
- sustained-release preparations are recommended, as they are more convenient and usually not much different in price from the regular-release products (unless generic regular-release is available)
- regular-release form is started at 80 mg PO Q8H, increasing the dosage every 4 weeks by 80 mg PO Q6H until an effect is seen or a maximum dosage of 360 mg/d is reached

Atrial fibrillation or flutter, atrioventricular nodal reentrant tachycardia

- 2.5 mg IV over 2–3 minutes
- if arrhythmia persists, additional doses of 2.5 mg every 5 minutes to a maximum of 10 mg or the development of hypotension should be administered
- pretreatment with calcium chloride 1 g IV over 10 minutes may prevent many of the hypotensive effects of verapamil without antagonizing the negative dromotropic effects (Am J Cardiol 1991;67:300–304)
- oral doses as above for chronic stable angina

Migraine prophylaxis

- 120 mg of sustained-release verapamil (a once-daily product sometimes given twice daily when dosages exceed 240 mg/d) PO daily, increasing the dosage weekly by 120 mg daily until headaches are controlled, toxicity develops, or a maximum dosage of 480 mg PO daily is reached
- regular-release form is started at 80 mg PO Q8H, increasing the dosage weekly by 80 mg daily until headaches are controlled, toxicity develops, or a maximum dosage of 360 mg/d is reached

Dosage adjustments for renal or hepatic dysfunction

- 70% of a dose of verapamil is excreted renally as metabolites
- specific verapamil dosage recommendations for patients with impaired renal or hepatic function are not available
- start with a low dose and titrate to effect

▶ *What Should I Monitor with Regard to Efficacy and Toxicity?*

see Diltiazem

▶ *How Long Do I Treat Patients with This Drug?*

see Diltiazem

How Do I Decrease or Stop the Administration of This Drug?

see Diltiazem

What Should I Tell My Patients About This Drug?

- extended-release verapamil should be taken with food to provide a more consistent serum concentration
- most common adverse effect of verapamil is constipation
- high-fiber diets are helpful in maintaining normal bowel habits
- excessive caffeine consumption (>5 cups per day) should be avoided, as this may inhibit the action of calcium channel blocking agents

Therapeutic Tips

- patients are usually more compliant with the use of extended-release products, and they are usually less expensive when the cost of daily therapy is considered.
- verapamil infusion can be helpful for rate control and arrythmia suppression for atrial fibrillation and multifocal tachycardia

Useful References

Follath F. The role of calcium antagonists in the treatment of myocardial ischemia. Am Heart J 1989;118:1093–1097

Tolins M, Weir EK, Chesler E, Pierpont GL. "Maximal" drug therapy is not necessarily optimal in chronic angina pectoris. J Am Coll Cardiol 1984;3:1051–1057

VITAMIN B12 (Cobalamin)

Eric Yoshida and Angela Kim-Sing

USA (Rubesol 1000, Sytobex, Crysti-12, Cyanoject, Cyomin, Kaybovite-1000, Cobex, Crystamine, Rubiamin PC, Berubigen, Betalin-12)
CANADA (Anacobin, Bedoz, Rubion, Rubramin)

When Should I Use This Drug?

Prevention of vitamin B12 depletion

- dietary vitamin B12 is abundant in dairy products, fish, meat, and liver
- because of its unique absorptive mechanism via gastric secreted binding protein (R protein), parietal cell-secreted intrinsic factor, and specific ileal receptor uptake, dietary deficiency rarely occurs
- exceptions to this are strict vegans, patients with gastric antral resection, diffuse atrophic gastritis, pancreatic insufficiency (impaired release of vitamin B12 from intrinsic factor), or diseases involving the distal ileum (e.g., Crohn's disease of the terminal ileum)
- requires a high index of suspicion during the care of patients with medical or dietary conditions mentioned above

Treatment of vitamin B12 deficiency

- body stores of vitamin B12 are such that 2–3 years are required to produce deficiency
- vitamin B12 deficiency can produce hematologic (macrocytic anemia with a high MCV) and neurologic (neuropsychiatric disturbance, peripheral neuropathy, and dorsal-lateral spinal cord degeneration) manifestations
- classically, vitamin B12 deficiency is a result of pernicious anemia, an autoimmune condition, but other conditions including those cited above as well as bacterial overgrowth/nematode infestation of the small bowel
- suspect deficiency when an increased MCV is reported with hematological profiles or when macrocytosis and hypersegmented neutrophils are seen on blood films
- if an increased MCV is reported, measure a serum vitamin B12 concentration to confirm the diagnosis
- a Schilling test should be done to detect vitamin B12 malabsorption

When Should I Not Use This Drug?

Enhancement of athletic performance

- there is no evidence that vitamin B12 injections enhance athletic performance or improve musculoskeletal injury

Treatment of lethargy or fatigue

- there is no evidence that vitamin B12 can improve lethargy or fatigue in a nondeficient patient

Alcoholism, psychological conditions

- although vitamin B12 is innocuous, the practice of injecting vitamin B12 as a placebo "treatment" for alcoholism and other psychological conditions is to be avoided

What Contraindications Are There to the Use of This Drug?

intolerance or allergic reaction to vitamin B12

What Drug Interactions Are Clinically Important?

What Route and Dosage Should I Use?

How to administer

- orally—take with food or milk or on an empty stomach
- parenterally—may be given IM or SQ

Prevention of vitamin B12 depletion

- in a patient without pernicious anemia or gastric or ileal disease, a normal diet should be sufficient
- in an absolute vegan, oral supplementation in the form of vitamin B12 tablets is recommended
- in those patients with partial or total surgical gastrectomy, diffuse gastritis, pancreatic insufficiency, or significantly diseased terminal ileum (Crohn's disease), parenteral vitamin B12, 100 μg IM monthly, may be advisable

Treatment of vitamin B12 deficiency

- 100 μg daily (IM or SQ) for 5 days, then a monthly 100 μg IM dose
- in patients without absorptive problems (e.g., absolute vegans), 1 mg PO daily may be used

What Should I Monitor with Regard to Efficacy and Toxicity?

Efficacy

Prevention of vitamin B12 depletion

- with adequate parenteral supplementation at recommended doses, no monitoring is required

Treatment of vitamin B12 deficiency • Hemoglobin and reticulocyte count

- reticulocytosis generally begins within 2–5 days following initiation of vitamin B12 therapy and the reticulocyte count should be checked 1 week after starting treatment
- if the reticulocyte response is inadequate, consider other coexisting deficiencies (e.g., folate, iron) or hematological conditions (e.g., myelodysplastic syndrome, hematological malignancy, etc.)
- check hemoglobin at 1 month following initiation of therapy to confirm rise toward normal concentration
- potassium shifts can occur during treatment; serum potassium should be checked within the first few days of treatment

Signs and symptoms of neurological manifestations of deficiency

- if deficiency is corrected early enough, reversal of neuropsychiatric abnormalities (e.g., dementia, psychosis, paranoia, depression), dorsal-lateral spinal cord degeneration (e.g., ataxia, loss of vibratory and proprioceptive sense), and peripheral neuropathy is possible
- improvement in the general condition of the patient may be seen in 24 hours
- vitamin B12 deficiency should always be considered in the investigation of dementia or confusion

Toxicity

- none, as excess vitamin B12 is excreted renally

▶ How Long Do I Treat Patients with This Drug?

Prevention of vitamin B12 depletion

- indefinitely as long as the medical condition that predisposes to deficiency exists

Treatment of vitamin B12 deficiency

- except in the rare case of dietary deficiency, treatment is lifelong

▶ How Do I Decrease or Stop the Administration of This Drug?

- may be stopped abruptly

▶ What Should I Tell My Patients About This Drug?

- patients should be made aware that the administration of vitamin B12 will require lifelong, monthly maintenance therapy

▶ Therapeutic Tips

- maintenance vitamin B12 injections need only be administered monthly

Useful References

McRae TD, Freedman ML. Why vitamin B12 deficiency should be managed aggressively. Geriatrics 1989;44(11):70–73,76,79

Clementz GL, Schade SG. The spectrum of vitamin B12 deficiency. Am Fam Physician 1990;41(1):150–162

National Academy of Sciences/National Research Council. Recommended Dietary Allowances, 10th ed. Washington, D.C., 1989

McEvoy G, ed. American Hospital Formulary Service Drug Information 91. Bethesda, MD: ASHP, Inc; 1991

VITAMIN K (Phytonadione)
Eric Yoshida and Angela Kim-Sing

USA (AquaMEPHYTON, Konakion)
CANADA (Konakion)

▶ When Should I Use This Drug?

Coagulopathy secondary to vitamin K deficiency

- indicated by an elevated INR
- deficiency may occur in malabsorption syndromes (celiac sprue, cholestatic liver disease, etc.), nutritional deficiency (''skid row'' alcoholics but also consider postsurgical patients with limited oral intake), and possibly in patients with marginal vitamin K intake, antibiotic use (diminished vitamin K3 from enteric flora)

Warfarin induced coagulopathy

- withdrawal of oral anticogulant usually corrects prolonged INR
- vitamin K administration should reverse the coagulopathy within 3–8 hours; however, if bleeding is present and urgent correction is needed, frozen plasma should be given

Prevention of vitamin K deficiency in patients receiving parenteral nutrition

- added to parenteral nutrition solution in patients with vitamin K malabsorption

Hypoprothrombinemia due to hepatocellular damage

- while vitamin K will not reverse coagulopathy secondary to severe liver damage, in cholestatic liver disease (e.g., primary biliary cirrhosis) or alcoholic liver disease there may be a component of vitamin K deficiency due to malabsorption or malnutrition
- in practice it is common to administer an empiric trial (3 days) of vitamin K

▶ When Should I Not Use This Drug?

Heparin anticoagulation

- vitamin K will not reverse effects of heparin (if rapid correction of heparin is required, consider reversal with protamine zinc or replace coagulation factors with frozen plasma)

Coagulopathy not secondary to vitamin K deficiency

- inappropriate to administer vitamin K in coagulopathy not secondary to vitamin K deficiency (e.g., disseminated intravascular coagulation [DIC], hemophilia)

▶ What Contraindications Are There to the Use of This Drug?

intolerance or allergic reaction to vitamin K

▶ What Drug Interactions Are Clinically Important?

Drugs that may increase the effect or toxicity of vitamin K

- none

Drugs that may decrease effect of vitamin K

- none

Drugs that may have their effect or toxicity increased by vitamin K

- none

Drugs that may have their effect decreased by vitamin K

COUMARIN AND DERIVATIVES (ANISINDIONE, DICUMAROL, WARFARIN)

- monitor patient's response with daily INR determinations for 3–5 days whenever vitamin K initiated, discontinued, or inadvertently given
- may need to use increased doses of the oral anticoagulant to overcome the temporary resistance
- if acute anticoagulation is required, administer heparin
- should advise patients not to take vitamin K supplements and/or a vitamin K-rich diet while on warfarin therapy

▶ What Route and Dosage Should I Use?

How to administer

- oral dosage form not commercially available in US or Canada
- parenterally—can be given IM, SQ, or IV
  SQ route preferred over IV or IM administration IM administration may result in intramuscular hematomas in presence of an elevated INR and should be avoided if possible if use via the IV route unavoidable, mix in D_5W or NS and administer at a rate not exceeding 1 mg/min

Coagulopathy secondary to vitamin K deficiency

- 10 mg SQ daily × 3 days
- in patients with syndromes limiting synthesis or absorption of vitamin K, give 10 mg SQ weekly

Warfarin induced coagulopathy

- if further anticoagulation is required and INR is <6 then simply holding the oral anticoagulant should correct the INR
- if the INR is between 6 and 10, give 0.5 mg and recheck INR in 24 hours
- if the INR is between 10 and 20, give 5 mg and recheck INR in 6–12 hours
- if reversal desired and further anticoagulation is not required, 10 mg SQ or IV as a single dose of vitamin K1 (not vitamin K3) may be administered
- if urgent reversal required (imminent or active bleeding), administer frozen plasma

Prevention of vitamin K deficiency in patients receiving parenteral nutrition

- 10 mg added to parenteral solution weekly

Hypoprothrombinemia due to hepatocellular damage

- 10 mg SQ daily for 3 days

Dosage adjustment for renal/hepatic dysfunction

- no adjustment needed in patients with renal or hepatic impairment

▶ What Should I Monitor with Regard to Efficacy and Toxicity?

Efficacy

Coagulopathy secondary to vitamin K deficiency, warfarin induced coagulopathy, hypoprothrombinemia due to hepatocellular damage

- measure INR daily until corrected

- if INR does not normalize within 3 days, consider other causes for coagulopathy (e.g., liver disease)

Prevention of vitamin K deficiency in patients receiving parenteral nutrition

- measure INR with pre-TPN bloodwork, then weekly

Toxicity
Rash, urticaria, pain
- inspect administration site for rash, urticaria, pain and swelling
- if allergic sensitivity or anaphylactoid reaction suspected, discontinue vitamin K

▶ *How Long Do I Treat Patients with This Drug?*
Coagulopathy secondary to vitamin K deficiency
- continue vitamin K therapy until underlying condition is reversed

Warfarin induced coagulopathy
- continue until INR is corrected

Hypoprothrombinemia due to hepatocellular damage
- if INR does not normalize within 3 days of giving vitamin K then the hypoprothrombinemia is due to liver disease and not an underlying vitamin K deficiency

Prevention of vitamin K deficiency in patients receiving parenteral nutrition
- continue vitamin K therapy for the duration of parenteral nutrition

Drug-induced hypoprothrombinemia
- continue until PT/INR is corrected

▶ *How Do I Decrease or Stop the Administration of This Drug?*
- may be stopped abruptly

▶ *What Should I Tell My Patients About This Drug?*
- vitamin K intake in the diet may be increased by including food sources such as leafy green vegetables, meat, cow's milk, vegetable oils, egg yolks, and tomatoes

▶ *Therapeutic Tips*
- it has been suggested that the parenteral formulation can be given orally; however, in the absence of pharmacokinetic data, it is recommended that vitamin K be given SQ in malabsorption syndromes

Useful References
Becker RC, Ansell J. Antithrombotic therapy. Arch Intern Med 1995; 155:149–161

Furie B. Disorders of the vitamin K dependent coagulation factors. In: Williams WJ, Beutler E, Erslev AJ, Lichtman MA, eds. Hematology. New York: McGraw-Hill, 1990:1510–1513

McEvoy, ed. American Hospital Formulary Service Drug Information 91. Bethesda, MD: American Society of Hospital Pharmacists, 1991: 2233–2236.

Vitamin K. In: Baumgartner TG, ed. Clinical Guide to Parenteral Nutrition. Melrose Park, IL: Educational Publications, 1984:229–239

American Medical Association Nutrition Advisory Group: Multivitamin preparations for parenteral use. [Statement]. J Parenteral Enteral Nutr 1979;3:258–262

WARFARIN
Frances Chow

USA (Coumadin, Panwarfin, Sofarin)
CANADA (Coumadin, Warfilone)

▶ *When Should I Use This Drug?*
Deep vein thrombosis or pulmonary embolism
- allows oral anticoagulation; however, warfarin takes 3–5 days to become effective and its administration must be overlapped with that of heparin

- initial treatment started in conjunction with heparin

Venous thromboembolism prevention
- for all patients undergoing hip surgery, warfarin has been shown to be more effective than heparin (Chest 1992;102:391S–407S)

Progressing stroke
- anticoagulation should be used only in cases of progressing stroke if hemorrhage has been ruled out by computed tomographic scan and there are major progressing neurological deficits; otherwise, do not anticoagulate

Prevention of cardiogenic cerebral embolism
Atrial fibrillation
- patients with paroxysmal or nonvalvular chronic atrial fibrillation should receive anticoagulation if other factors such as hypertension, coronary artery disease, and congestive heart failure are present (Arch Intern Med 1990;150:1598–1603)
- all other patients with atrial fibrillation should be anticoagulated to minimize the chance of systemic embolization from a cardiac source (Am J Cardiol 1990;65:24C–28C, N Engl J Med 1990; 323:1505–1511, N Engl J Med 1992;326:1264–1271) if patients do not have contraindications to anticoagulation
- in patients who will undergo pharmacological or electrical cardioversion for new-onset atrial fibrillation (not needed if atrial fibrillation < 3 days old) (Chest 1992;102:426S–433S)
- warfarin has been significantly more effective than aspirin for the prevention of stroke in atrial fibrillation (Lancet 1989;1: 175–179, N Engl J Med 1990;323:1505–1511, N Engl J Med 1990;322:863–868)

Mechanical prosthetic valves, bioprosthetic mitral valves
- warfarin is needed for long-term anticoagulation
- heparin need only be used if the patient cannot take warfarin

Myocardial infarction
- for many patients, the risks of warfarin therapy are high and prolonged anticoagulation after a myocardial infarction is not warranted
- consider warfarin therapy in patients with a prior embolus, left ventricular thrombus, large anterior infarcts, atrial fibrillation, or left ventricular aneurysm; patients who have or develop left ventricular dysfunction (failure); and patients who do not have contraindications and who are willing to undergo regular medical and laboratory follow-up
- start warfarin administration after arterial punctures are no longer required

▶ *When Should I Not Use This Drug?*
Transient ischemic attacks
- trials to date suggest that potential side effects are greater than benefit
- aspirin is the drug of choice

▶ *What Contraindications Are There to the Use of This Drug?*
Intolerance of or allergic reaction to warfarin
Pregnancy (first and third trimester are associated with congenital abnormalities)
Patients with recent eye, brain, or spinal cord surgery; head injury; or uncontrolled bleeding
- warfarin has the potential to make these conditions worse secondary to hemorrhage

▶ *What Drug Interactions Are Clinically Important?*
Drugs that may increase the effect of warfarin
NONSTEROIDAL ANTIINFLAMMATORY DRUGS, ASPIRIN
- these drugs affect platelet function and can increase the risk of hemorrhage

- use acetaminophen or narcotic analgesics
- in the case of post–myocardial infarction patients, low-dose aspirin therapy can be used in combination, as benefit outweighs risk
- in patients who require high-dose aspirin or nonsteroidal antiinflammatory drugs to adequately control a life-altering disease (e.g., rheumatoid arthritis), the combination can be used; however, keep INR at the lower end of desired values and make the patient aware of the potential for bleeding

CIMETIDINE

- inhibits warfarin metabolism and increases warfarin response
- switch to ranitidine or other H_2 antagonist if a combination must be used, as these agents have less of an effect on metabolism

AMIODARONE, TRIMETHOPRIM-SULFAMETHOXAZOLE, DISULFIRAM, METRONIDAZOLE

- interferes with warfarin metabolism and can increase INR
- use alternative agents if possible
- if not, monitor INR every 2 days until the full extent of the interaction is seen and adjust the dosage as for a warfarin dosage change
- on discontinuation of interacting drug, monitor INR every 2 days and adjust as for a warfarin dosage change

HIGHLY PROTEIN-BOUND DRUGS

- warfarin is highly protein bound and may be displaced by other highly protein-bound drugs
- the initial increase in free warfarin levels is followed by an increase in clearance, a fall in total warfarin concentrations, and the reestablishment of free warfarin concentrations, which are the same as they were before the interacting drug was added
- no special monitoring is required

Drugs that may decrease the effect of warfarin

BARBITURATES, RIFAMPIN

- induces hepatic enzymes and increases metabolism of warfarin
- if the patient is taking a barbiturate for epilepsy, there is no need to change if the barbiturate was started first and is continued after warfarin is discontinued
- if a barbiturate or rifampin is added after warfarin has been started, monitor INR every 2 days until the full extent of interaction is seen and adjust as for a warfarin dosage change

Drugs that may have their effect increased by warfarin

- none

Drugs that may have their effect decreased by warfarin

- none

▶ *What Route and Dosage Should I Use?*

How to administer

- orally—may be taken with food or on an empty stomach

Deep vein thrombosis of pulmonary embolism

- 10 mg PO daily starting at the same time as heparin
- adjust the dosage to achieve INR of 2–3 (a PT ratio of 1.3 to 1.5 times control values)
- during first 2–3 days of therapy, a desirable increase in PT is only 1–2 s/d and changes greater than this suggest that the dosage may be too high
- if PT increases greater than 1–2 s/d, reduce the daily dosage by 50%
- in general, titrate the daily dose by 0.5–2 mg on the basis of PT results
- changes in dosage after the initiation of therapy should not occur more frequently than every 4–5 days because of warfarin's long half-life

Venous thromboembolism prevention

- 5 mg PO daily starting 3–4 days prior to surgery
- PT should be approximately 2 seconds over baseline levels prior to surgery

- continue warfarin therapy after surgery, keeping an INR of 2–3 (a PT ratio of 1.3–1.5 times control values)

Progressing stroke

- 10 mg PO daily dosed to an INR of 2–3

Prevention of cardiogenic cerebral embolism

- 10 mg PO daily dosed to an INR of 2.5–3.5 for mechanical prosthetic values and 2–3 for bioprosthetic valves (Chest 1992;102[suppl]:445S–455S), myocardial infarction, and atrial fibrillation
- for atrial fibrillation, start 3 weeks prior to conversion and continue for 4 weeks after return to normal sinus rhythm

Dosage adjustments for renal or hepatic dysfunction

- hepatically metabolized
- no dosage adjustments for renal failure
- adjust the dosage on the basis of PT in patients with hepatic dysfunction

▶ *What Should I Monitor with Regard to Efficacy and Toxicity?*

Efficacy

Deep vein thrombosis

Limb circumference, swelling, tenderness, perfusion

- assess the patient daily

INR

- measure INR daily until INR is stable, then weekly for 2 weeks, and then every 2–3 weeks (Chest 1989;95:37S–51S)

Pulmonary embolism

Apprehension, cough, pleuritic chest pain, hemoptysis

- assess the patient daily

INR

- measure INR daily until INR is stable, then weekly for 2 weeks, and then every 2–3 weeks (Chest 1989;95:37S–51S)

Venous thromboembolism prevention

Clinical signs

- monitor daily for signs of venous thromboembolism

INR

- measure INR daily until INR is stable, then weekly for 2 weeks, and then every 2–3 weeks (Chest 1989;95:37S–51S)

Progressing stroke

Stroke stabilization

- assess whether the stroke is stabilizing

INR

- measure INR daily until INR is stable, then weekly for 2 weeks, and then every 2–3 weeks (Chest 1989;95:37S–51S)

Prevention of cardiogenic cerebral embolism

Evidence of cerebral embolism

- transient ischemic attacks or strokes

INR

- measure INR daily until INR is stable, then weekly for 2 weeks, then every 2–3 weeks (Chest 1989;95:37S–51S)

Toxicity

Symptoms of bleeding

- risk of minor bleeding episodes is 2–10%
- assess the patient for symptoms of bleeding with the same frequency as the PT is evaluated
- check for epistaxis, bleeding gums, hemoptysis, orthostatic hypotension, melena or bright red stools, blood in urine, increased bruising, local irritation, erythema, and hematomas
- if minor hemorrhage occurs, a lowering of the dosage should be done but not discontinuation of therapy because the hemorrhage

can be treated but the consequences of an embolism may not be easily treated

- for severe hemorrhage, stop warfarin therapy and give vitamin K_1 (phytonadione) 10 mg IV at a rate not exceeding 1 mg/min, plus fresh frozen plasma
- PT returns to normal values within 4–24 hours after vitamin K administration
- after vitamin K has been given, a relative resistance to warfarin therapy for 7–14 days occurs
- for surgical procedures, give 200–400 mL of fresh frozen plasma, which gives immediate reversal of anticoagulation for 4–6 hours

Local thrombosis, vasculitis

- occurs 2–10 days after the initiation of therapy
- if this occurs, stop warfarin administration, give vitamin K, and use heparin as the anticoagulant

"Purple toe" syndrome (blue-tinged discoloration of toes with pain but no necrosis)

- reversible if warfarin therapy is stopped; use heparin as the anticoagulant

▶ *How Long Do I Treat Patients with This Drug?*

Deep vein thrombosis or pulmonary embolism

- warfarin therapy should be continued for 3 months for a first episode, for 1 year for the second episode, and indefinitely for more than 2 episodes

Venous thromboembolism prevention

- should be continued until the patient is ambulatory (i.e., no longer confined to bed)

Progressing stroke

- continue anticoagulation either until stabilization or roughly 3–5 days
- if the stroke has not stabilized after 48 hours of therapy, stop anticoagulation and be sure that worsening of the clinical condition is not due to hemorrhagic stroke or another medical condition

Prevention of cardiogenic cerebral embolism

Atrial fibrillation

- continue anticoagulation for 4 weeks after successful cardioversion
- institute long-term anticoagulation for patients with chronic rheumatic or nonrheumatic atrial fibrillation (Am J Cardiol 1990;65: 24C–28C, N Engl J Med 1990;323:1505–1511), rheumatic paroxysmal atrial fibrillation (Am J Cardiol 1990;65:24C–28C), and nonvalvular chronic atrial fibrillation if cardiac disease such as hypertension, coronary artery disease, and congestive heart failure is present (Arch Intern Med 1990;150:1598–1603)

Mechanical prosthetic valves

- mechanical valves necessitate anticoagulation indefinitely (J Am Coll Cardiol 1986;8:41B)

Bioprosthetic mitral valves

- bioprosthetic mitral valves necessitate warfarin therapy for 3 months, followed by low-dose aspirin indefinitely; however, warfarin therapy should be continued indefinitely in patients with a history of systemic embolism

Myocardial infarction

- continue warfarin therapy for 3 months after myocardial infarction and continue aspirin administration indefinitely

▶ *How Do I Decrease or Stop The Administration of This Drug?*

- no need to taper the dosage after a decision to stop therapy
- may be stopped abruptly

▶ *What Should I Tell My Patients About This Drug?*

- women of childbearing age should be counseled about contraception because of the teratogenicity of warfarin

- American Academy of Pediatrics allows breast-feeding during warfarin therapy
- avoid over the counter products that contain aspirin or other nonsteroidal antiinflammatory drugs such as ibuprofen
- many cold or cough remedies and pain or headache medications contain aspirin; therefore, use acetaminophen for fever, headaches, and mild pain
- check with your pharmacist before purchasing any cold or cough preparations
- inform your dentist that you are taking warfarin prior to any dental extraction work or fillings
- many drugs interact with warfarin, ensure that any specialist is aware of possible interactions when prescribing new drugs
- take at same time each day
- if you miss a dose and remember on the same day, take the missed dose
- if you miss a dose and remember the next day, forget the missed dose and continue with the daily dosage
- do not double the dose
- get your refill several days before your supply runs out, and if you plan to go on holidays, ensure that you have an adequate supply to last the whole trip
- you tend to bleed a little longer on getting a cut, but applying pressure to the area should stop the bleeding, and if it does not and the cut is deep, go to the emergency department

▶ *Therapeutic Tips*

- start warfarin administration simultaneously with heparin to decrease the time required to get the patient anticoagulated with warfarin and to decrease the length of hospital stay
- initial response in PT on starting warfarin therapy reflects the rapid decrease in factor VII (half-life of 5 hours) only, and factor IX and X levels must be reduced for effective anticoagulation
- therefore, initially PT is not reflective of protection from thrombosis formation, and warfarin therapy must be overlapped with heparin administration for 4–5 days to ensure adequate anticoagulant effect
- avoid IM injections if possible to prevent the risk of hematomas while the patient is taking warfarin; however, if necessary, give IM injections to the upper extremities to allow easy access for compression and inspection of the site for bleeding

Useful References

Third ACCP Consensus Conference on Antithrombotic Therapy. Chest 1992;102:303S–550S
Hirsch J. Oral anticoagulant drugs. N Engl J Med 1991;324:1865–1875
Smith P, Arnesen H, Holme I. The effect of warfarin on mortality and reinfarction after myocardial infarction. N Engl J Med 1990;323:147–152

ZIDOVUDINE (AZT)

Ann Beardsell

USA (Retrovir)
CANADA (Retrovir)

▶ *When Should I Use This Drug?*

Human immunodeficiency virus infection

Asymptomatic patients

- if CD4 count is consistently less than 500/mm³ (N Engl J Med 1990;322:941–949)

Patients with acquired immunodeficiency syndrome (AIDS) or AIDS-related complex

- regardless of CD4 count (N Engl J Med 1987;317:185–191)

Patients with human immunodeficiency virus thrombocytopenia

- regardless of CD4 count (J AIDS 1990;3:565–570)

Prophylaxis

- for health care workers (physicians, nurses, dentists, laboratory workers, and so on) after a high-risk exposure to prevent possible infection and subsequent seroconversion
- high-risk exposures include transfusion of infected blood, injection of more than 1 mL of infected blood or body fluid, parenteral

exposure to laboratory materials or research specimens containing high viral titers, and exposure to blood or body fluids from a severely ill, HIV-positive person

▶ *When Should I Not Use This Drug?*

Human immunodeficiency virus infection only

- patients without evidence of immunological compromise should not be treated

▶ *What Contraindications Are There to the Use of This Drug?*

- intolerance of or allergic reaction to AZT

▶ *What Drug Interactions Are Clinically Important?*

Drugs that may increase the effect or toxicity of AZT

PNEUMOCYSTIS CARINII PNEUMONIA ANTIINFECTIVES (DAPSONE, PENTAMIDINE, TRIMETHOPRIM-SULFAMETHOXAZOLE)

- when treating acute *P. carinii* pneumonia (PCP), concurrent use with AZT may result in anemia and/or neutropenia
- monitor hemoglobin, reticulocyte, granulocyte, and white blood cell count (WBC) every 3–4 days
- withhold AZT if hemoglobin (HgB) dramatically decreased by 2 g or less than 8 g/dL, with reticulocyte count below the normal range and/or WBC of less than 1.5/mm³ and granulocyte count of less than 0.8/mm³
- resume AZT therapy after PCP treatment is completed and laboratory measures have recovered
- if HgB level and/or WBC improves but is still low compared with the levels before PCP, start AZT administration at a lower dosage and increase slowly only if counts improve
- if the HgB level and/or WBC declines but not to the lower limits, reduce the AZT dosage by 100–200 mg daily and continue to monitor closely and resume the regular dosage after treatment is completed and laboratory values return to pre-PCP levels
- if using as PCP prophylaxis in conjunction with AZT, anemia and/or neutropenia is infrequent but may necessitate AZT dosage reduction or a change of PCP prophylaxis medication

CYTOTOXICS (VINCRISTINE, VINBLASTINE, DOXORUBICIN, BLEOMYCIN)

- concomitant use of there agents with AZT may result in additive bone marrow suppression
- monitor WBC, granulocyte, and HgB counts every 3–4 days, and withhold AZT until chemotherapy is completed if WBC is less than 1.5/mm³, granulocytes is less than 0.8/mm³, and/or HgB count is less than 9 g/dL
- if the laboratory variables decline but are not as low as above, that reduce the AZT dosage by 100–200 mg daily and continue to monitor every 3–4 days

ANALGESICS (ACETAMINOPHEN, ASPIRIN, NONSTEROIDAL ANTIINFLAMMATORY DRUGS, MORPHINE)

- not a frequent problem with as needed use but high dosages for prolonged periods can be a problem, especially in patients with chronic active hepatitis
- may competitively inhibit glucuronidation and possibly decrease renal excretion of AZT, resulting in possible toxic effects
- monitor every 2 months for elevations in liver function test results (aspartate aminotransferase [AST], alkaline phosphatase, and lactate dehydrogenase [LDH]), greater than 5 times normal values and increases in nausea, headaches, and/or fatigue, and reduce the dosage of AZT or discontinue the analgesic and/or AZT therapy if they are severe

GANCICLOVIR

- neutropenia may occur with concurrent use of AZT
- monitor WBC and granulocyte count every 2 days during the induction period of ganciclovir and then weekly thereafter
- decrease the AZT dosage if the WBC and granulocyte count fall by 50%

- discontinue AZT therapy if the WBC is less than 1.5/mm³ or the granulocyte count is less than 0.5/mm³
- if AZT is believed necessary, then the ganciclovir therapy should be discontinued
- granulocyte-macrophage colony-stimulating factor has been used to prevent discontinuation of therapy with either drug, but if neutropenia persists, discontinue administration of one of the drugs

METRONIDAZOLE

- concurrent use frequently causes elevated liver enzyme levels and nausea, especially in patients with preexisting hepatic dysfunction
- monitor AST levels midtherapy and treat nausea symptomatically with antinauseants
- for AST levels less than 400, withhold AZT until therapy is completed or change to another antibiotic if appropriate

Drugs that may decrease the effect of AZT

RIBAVIRIN

- concurrent use antagonizes the antiviral activity of AZT; therefore, do not use together

Drugs that may have their effect or toxicity increased by AZT

- none

Drugs that may have their effect decreased by AZT

- none

▶ *What Route and Dosage Should I Use?*

How to administer

Orally

- take on an empty stomach

Parenterally

- intravenous form is available for use when oral therapy is contraindicated
- intravenous infusions should be run at a constant rate for 1 hour; avoid rapid infusion or bolus injection

Human Immunodeficiency virus infection

- 200 mg PO TID, although some clinicians recommend 100 mg PO Q4H while the patient is awake (the dosage regimen likely does not matter as long as the patient receives 500–600 mg PO daily)
- up to 400 mg PO TID in patients with nonresponding HIV-related thrombocytopenia, aggressive disease, or CNS involvement
- 100 mg PO QID if there is evidence of moderate bone marrow dysfunction or hepatic diseases
- give 100 mg PO Q8H if more significant bone marrow dysfunction is present
- if oral therapy is contraindicated, give 1 mg/kg IV Q4H or 2 mg/kg IV Q4H if there is neurological involvement

Dosage adjustments for renal or hepatic dysfunction

- renally eliminated
- for patients with renal dysfunction, start patients at 100 mg PO Q8H, and if the patient tolerates this dosage, increase to the above levels

▶ *What Should I Monitor with Regard to Efficacy and Toxicity?*

Efficacy

Human immunodeficiency virus infection

Clinical progression

- patients with low T4 counts but no other symptoms of HIV infection generally do not notice any difference with AZT therapy, except that their disease does not progress and infections do not develop as soon as expected without AZT
- patients with some constitutional symptoms (fever, night sweats, weight loss) generally notice an improvement within 2–8 weeks with, in some cases, resolution of symptoms and weight gain
- many patients respond with a transient increase in T4 counts

- patients with HIV-related dementia may show some improvement in cognitive function
- patients with HIV-related thrombocytopenia may show higher platelet counts for some time
- for the first 6 weeks of therapy, patients should be monitored every 1–2 weeks
- after they are stable, patients can be monitored every 4 to 8 weeks

CD4 counts

- every 3–6 months if initially greater than 300/mm^3 to guide the use of agents for PCP prophylaxis and every 3 months if less than 300/mm^3 to guide the use of alternative therapy

Toxicity

Many adverse effects are dose related and can be more severe in patients with advanced disease

Hematological effects

- anemia and neutropenia are the most common adverse effects of AZT
- monitor CBC and differential count every 2 weeks initially and then monthly
- if HgB level is less than 12 g/dL when starting AZT therapy or decreases by 2 g/dL or more and the reticulocyte count is low (<40), reduce the zidovudine dosage by 100–200 mg daily
- if the HgB level continues to drop and/or the patient becomes symptomatic (lightheadedness, racing heart, fatigue), withhold AZT for 1–2 weeks, then resume AZT therapy at a low dosage, and increase sowly if laboratory testing results improve
- in patients whose HgB level drops below 8 g/dL, transfusions of packed red blood cells to maintain HgB level while taking AZT or change of antiretroviral agent must be considered
- if HgB level is in the normal range when starting AZT therapy, decreases by 2–3 g/dL, and then stabilizes and the patient has no symptoms of anemia, the AZT dosage need not be reduced
- if the HgB level falls further and the reticulocyte count is below normal, reduce the AZT dosage by 200 mg daily
- if the WBC or granulocyte count decreases to less than 1.5/mm^3 or less than 0.8/mm^3 respectively, reduce the AZT dosage by 200 mg daily
- if the WBC or granulocyte count decreases to less than 1/mm^3 or less than 0.6/mm^3, respectively, stop AZT therapy for 1–2 weeks or until counts increase and then restart with a dosage that is 100–300 mg daily less than the previous dosage and monitor laboratory work weekly
- if WBC and granulocyte count continue to fall with AZT therapy, another antiretroviral agent should be considered

Gastrointestinal effects

- nausea, with some vomiting, is common (15%) in the first 2–4 weeks but generally slowly resolves
- if nausea and vomiting persists, antinauseants are helpful but a reduction in AZT dosage by 200 mg PO daily may be required, and as symptoms improve, slowly increase the dosage to a tolerable level (some patients resume the previous dosage without problems)
- metallic or bitter taste, loss of appetite, and abdominal bloating are also common and may resolve with time
- abdominal pain (less frequent) may resolve with administration of antacids or H$_2$ blockers or AZT dosage reduction
- if abdominal pain persists, discontinue AZT therapy and assess the patient for other problems that may be aggravated by AZT therapy

Neurological effects

- headaches are the most common problem and can usually be treated with analgesics
- if headaches are unresponsive to analgesics, reduce the AZT dosage by 200 mg PO daily and see if there is any improvement or discontinue therapy for several days and restart with 100 mg daily and slowly increase and monitor the recurrence of headaches
- myopathy is seen, primarily in the leg muscles, and may be accompanied by elevated creatine kinase (CK) activity

- if muscle pain and wasting occurs, check CK activity and reduce the dosage by 200 mg PO daily or discontinue AZT therapy and monitor CK for improvement every 2 weeks
- if improvement occurs, restart AZT therapy at 100 mg daily and slowly increase to a dosage lower than the patient was previously taking and watch for recurrences
- if the CK activity is not elevated and there is no response to discontinuing AZT therapy, myopathy due to HIV must be considered

Dermatological effects

- rash has been seen early in treatment in some patients
- AZT regimen should be stopped and the patient desensitized, starting with a small dose (25 mg/dose) and slowly increasing the dosage back into the normal range

Hepatic effects

- liver function test results (AST and LDH) can increase with AZT therapy, especially when alcohol is being consumed, the patient has a history of hepatitis or hepatic impairment, or certain medications are being concurrently administered
- monitor AST and LDH activity every 2 weeks initially, then monthly
- if values increase to 5 times the upper normal levels, reduce the AZT dosage by 100–200 mg daily
- if values increase to 8–10 times normal levels, withhold AZT therapy until levels are below 5 times normal, and then resume the AZT regimen at a dosage 200 mg PO daily less than the previous dosage and monitor AST and LDH levels every 2 weeks
- if the laboratory values return to the normal range or remain stable, the dosage can be slowly increased by 100 mg every 2–4 weeks with laboratory test results being monitored every 2 weeks
- patients with chronic active hepatitis are sensitive to AZT and most likely cannot tolerate more than 100–200 mg daily, if any at all

▶ How Long Do I Treat Patients with This Drug?

Human Immunodeficiency virus infection

- indefinitely, unless side effects are intolerable or disease progression indicates resistance
- it is generally estimated that the duration of efficacy is 18–24 months, but this is variable, depending on the stage of disease at the initiation of AZT therapy and the virulence of the virus, and can be as short as several months or as long as 3–5 years in some cases

▶ How Do I Decrease or Stop the Administration of This Drug?

- may be stopped abruptly

▶ What Should I Tell My Patients About This Drug?

- this drug does not provide a cure for HIV infection but controls the replication of the virus to preserve, or even improve, the present level of your immune system
- side effects of the drug were common with the higher dosages previously used but are much less frequent with the dosages now being used
- most patients notice either no difference or an improvement after starting AZT therapy
- some patients experience some tiredness, nausea, and headaches, and these generally last for 2–4 weeks and then disappear; however, if they persist or are severe, inform your physician
- other side effects that patients have noticed are a metallic taste, bloating, frequent urination, and ''spacy'' feeling, and these generally resolve with time
- small percentage of people feel drowsy at first with this medication; so do not drive a vehicle or operate machinery until you see how you are going to react
- it is recommended that AZT be taken on an empty stomach, and if you find that it upsets your stomach, take with low-protein meals
- because this medication has the potential to slow the production of your blood cells, it is important that you have routine labora-

tory work done as outlined by your physician; do not go more than 2 months without having it checked
- because this medication and alcohol can affect your liver, alcohol consumption should be limited until you see if AZT affects your liver
- social drinking is probably usually fine, but excessive ingestion should be avoided by all patients taking AZT
- most other prescription medications and over the counter products do not cause problems when taken in conjunction with AZT, but always let your physician and pharmacist know what you are taking

▶ *Therapeutic Tips*

- encourage the patient to establish a comfortable routine for taking this medication to ensure compliance
- monitor laboratory work on a regular basis and assess the dosage on the basis of laboratory values, specifically WBC and neutrophils
- as the absolute dosage for this drug is not really known, adjust the dosage on the basis of the patient's overall condition (i.e., physical, emotional, psychological, and laboratory states)
- AZT may not always be the cause of physiological and laboratory changes; consider other infections or disease processes and other medications
- 100 mg PO QID is the lowest dosage at which a clinical benefit has been demonstrated (Br Med J 1992;304:13–17)
- beneficial effect on surrogate markers has been demonstrated with dosages of AZT as low as 300 mg/d; however, the clinical impact of this dosage of AZT has not yet been demonstrated

ZOLPIDEM

Jonathan Fleming

USA (Ambien)
CANADA (not available)

▶ *When Should I Use This Drug?*

Transient and short-term insomnia

- newer hypnotic with fewer and less severe side effects than benzodiazepines that may be free from rebound phenomena (some studies show an absence of rebound but some reports show its presence) and is not augmented by low dosages of alcohol, although additive effects on psychomotor performance have been demonstrated
- should be used for short-term management of insomnia in patients who must avoid the amnestic effects of the benzodiazepines, such as students prior to an examination
- likely more expensive than the benzodiazepines
- may replace benzodiazepines but, because it has only recently been released, not as much data are available on safety and efficacy
- main difference between zolpidem and zopiclone is that zopiclone may cause a metallic taste

▶ *When Should I Not Use This Drug?*

Sleep disorders when the insomnia is part of a syndrome in which anxiety predominates

- benzodiazepine given at night has more anxiolytic effect and is less expensive than zopiclone

▶ *What Contraindications Are There to the Use of This Drug?*

see Zopiclone

▶ *What Drug Interactions Are Clinically Important?*

see Zopiclone

▶ *What Route and Dosage Should I Use?*

How to administer

- orally—40 minutes before retiring

Transient and short-term insomnia

- 5 mg PO 40 minutes prior to retiring
- increase to 10 mg only if the lower dose is clearly ineffective

Dosage adjustment for renal or hepatic dysfunction

- hepatically metabolized
- no dosage adjustment is required; just start with the lowest available dose and titrate to effect

▶ *What Should I Monitor with Regard to Efficacy and Toxicity?*

see Zopiclone

▶ *How Long Do I Treat Patients with This Drug?*

see Zopiclone

▶ *How Do I Decrease or Stop the Administration of This Drug?*

- studies show less rebound insomnia on withdrawal compared with the case with benzodiazepines, but if zolpidem used for longer than 3 weeks at the 10 mg dosage, taper by using the 5 mg dosage for 1 week before discontinuing

▶ *What Should I Tell My Patients About This Drug?*

- if you have previously used benzodiazepine hypnotics, you may notice a qualitative difference in sleep induction owing to the absence of marked anxiolytic effects
- rebound insomnia may occur and transitory sleep disturbance on withdrawal of therapy is expected and is not an indication to restart the medication
- report any adverse effects as soon as they occur
- increasing the dosage can lead to unwanted side effects, and if the dosage is not effective, consult your physician before increasing the dosage on your own
- therapy should be stopped if you are planning to become pregnant
- disturbances in memory may occur particularly for material learned just prior to the sleep period or during the sleep period (e.g., physicians may forget orders given during the night, students may forget information learned that night)
- sedative properties are additive if zolpidem is used with over the counter antihistamines, as increased sedation may occur
- note the improvements in your sleep performance and daytime functioning so that these can be evaluated at the follow-up visit

▶ *Therapeutic Tips*

- advantage over zopiclone is the lack of metallic taste
- efficacy may be maintained for as long as 6 months
- may not be as effective as benzodiazepines if anxiety (either as part of an anxiety disorder or about the sleep process) is prominent
- some long-term users of benzodiazepines who are used to the cognitive and mood effects of the benzodiazepines may prefer benzodiazepines
- may eventually be preferred to benzodiazepines

Useful References

Scharf MB, Mayleben DW, Kaffeman M, et al. Dose response effects of zolpidem in normal geriatric subjects. J Clin Psychiatry 1991;52:77–83
Langtry HD, Benfield P. Zolpidem. A review of its pharmacodynamic and pharmacokinetic properties and therapeutic potential. Drugs 1990;40:291–313

ZOPICLONE

Jonathan Fleming

USA (not available)
CANADA (Imovane)

▶ *When Should I Use This Drug?*

Transient and short-term insomnia

- newer hypnotic with fewer and less severe side effects than benzodiazepines that may be free from rebound phenomena (some studies show an absence of rebound but some reports show its presence) and is not augmented by low dosages of alcohol

- should be used for short-term management of insomnia in patients who must avoid the amnestic effects of the benzodiazepines, such as students prior to an examination
- more expensive than the benzodiazepines
- may replace benzodiazepines, but because it has only recently been released, not as much data are available on safety and efficacy

Long-term treatment of insomnia

- effective in the intermittent treatment of long-term insomnia if the use of alternative, behavioral techniques for controlling insomnia are ineffective
- although studies on the efficacy of long-term use of hypnotics are scant and many sleep laboratory studies show a loss of hypnotic effect (tolerance) by the fourth week of continuous use, about 10% of patients benefit from continuous or intermittent use of hypnotics and long-term users often report high satisfaction with their sleep and few adverse effects (Age Ageing 1984;13:335–343)
- continued, intermittent medication use (provided there is demonstrable benefit) may be the most sensible approach

▶ *When Should I Not Use This Drug?*

Sleep disorders when the insomnia is part of a syndrome in which anxiety predominates

- benzodiazepines given at night have more anxiolytic effect and are less expensive than zopiclone

▶ *What Contraindications Are There to the Use of This Drug?*

Intolerance of or allergic reaction to zopiclone

Patients with severe chronic obstructive pulmonary disease and sleep-related breathing disorders (particularly obstructive sleep apnea)

- these conditions are worsened by the use of zopiclone

Pregnant or lactating females

- because effects are unknown

▶ *What Drug Interactions Are Clinically Important?*

Drugs that may increase the effect or toxicity of zopiclone

ALCOHOL

- about 20% of insomniacs may take alcohol and sleeping pills concurrently to aid sleep (Confin Psychiatry 1977;15:151–172)
- at low alcohol dosages, there appears to be minimal or no interaction (Int Clin Psychopharmacol 1990;5[suppl 2]:105–113)

CENTRAL NERVOUS SYSTEM DEPRESSANTS

- additive, sedative effects are expected when central nervous system depressants are used
- avoid combination if possible or minimize by starting with low dosages

Drugs that may decrease the effect of zopiclone

- none

Drugs that may have their effect or toxicity increased by zopiclone

- none

Drugs that may have their effect decreased by zopiclone

- none

▶ *What Route and Dosage Should I Use?*

How to administer

- orally—40 minutes before retiring

Transient and short-term insomnia

- 7.5 mg (3.75 mg in the elderly) PO 40 minutes before retiring
- maximum dosage is 11.25 mg, and exceeding this dosage causes hangover and other side effects (Int Clin Psychopharmacol 1990;5[suppl 2]:1–10)

Dosage adjustments for renal or hepatic dysfunction

- renally eliminated

Normal Dosing Interval	C$_{cr}$ > 60 mL/min or 1 mL/s	C$_{cr}$ 30–60 mL/min or 0.5–1 mL/s	C$_{cr}$ < 30 mL/min or 0.5 mL/s
Q24H	no adjustment needed	decrease dosage by 50%	decrease dosage by 75%

▶ *What Should I Monitor with Regard to Efficacy and Toxicity?*

Efficacy

Transient situational insomnia, short-term insomnia, long-term insomnia

Shortening of the time taken to fall asleep and improved sleep efficiency

- quantify through the use of a sleep diary and compare with pretreatment sleep performance

Improved daytime functioning

- quantify by comparing changes in the symptoms (e.g., anxiety, tension, and fatigue) with treatment with baseline values

Toxicity

Psychomotor and memory effects

- are less than with the benzodiazepines; monitor for these changes

Morning carryover effects

- are minimal (Int Clin Psychopharmacol 1990;5[suppl 2]:79–83), but idiosyncratic reactions such as marked sedation can occur

▶ *How Long Do I Treat Patients with This Drug?*

Transient situational insomnia, short-term insomnia

- although sleep laboratory studies show no loss of efficacy when used continuously for as long as 6 months (Can J Psychiatry 1988;33:103–107), the general rule of using short courses of hypnotics should still be applied

Long-term insomnia

- although studies on the efficacy of long-term use hypnotics are scant and many sleep laboratory studies show a loss of hypnotic effect (tolerance) by the fourth week of continuous use, with the exception of flurazepam (Behav Med 1978;5:25–31) and zopiclone (Can J Psychiatry 1988;33:103–107), which have demonstrated continued, objective effectiveness beyond 3 months of continuous use, about 10% of patients benefit from continuous or intermittent use of hypnotics and long-term users often report high satisfaction with their sleep and few adverse effects (Age Ageing 1984;13:335–343)
- continued, intermittent medication use (provided there is demonstrable benefit) may be the most sensible approach

▶ *How Do I Decrease or Stop the Administration of This Drug?*

- studies show less rebound insomnia on withdrawal compared with the case with benzodiazepines, but if used longer than 3 weeks at the 7.5 mg dosage, taper by using the 3.75 dosage for 1 week before discontinuing

▶ *What Should I Tell My Patients About This Drug?*

- metallic taste, caused by secretion of active drug in the saliva, is the most common side effect
- if you have previously used benzodiazepine hypnotics, you may notice a qualitative difference in sleep induction owing to the absence of marked anxiolytic effects
- rebound insomnia may occur, and transitory sleep disturbance on withdrawal of therapy is expected and is not an indication to restart the medication
- report any adverse effects as soon as they occur
- increasing the dosage can lead to unwanted side effects, and if the dosage is not effective, consult your physician before increasing the dosage on your own

- best not to use with alcohol; however, low dosages of alcohol do not potentiate its effect
- therapy should be stopped if you are planning to become pregnant
- disturbances in memory may occur, particularly for material learned just prior to the sleep period or during the sleep period (e.g., physicians may forget orders given during the night, students may forget information learned that night)
- sedative properties are additive if the drug is used with over the counter antihistamines, as increased sedation may occur
- note the improvements in your sleep performance and daytime functioning so that these can be evaluated at the follow-up visit

▶ *Therapeutic Tips*

- efficacy may be maintained for as long as 6 months

- may not be as effective as benzodiazepines if anxiety (either as part of an anxiety disorder or about the sleep process) is prominent
- some long-term users of benzodiazepines who are used to the cognitive and mood effects of the benzodiazepines may prefer benzodiazepines
- may eventually be preferred over benzodiazepines

Useful References

Fleming JAE, Bourgouin J, Hamilton P. A sleep laboratory evaluation of the longterm efficacy of zopiclone. Can J Psychiatry 1988;33: 103–107

Hindmarch I, Musch B, eds. Zopiclone in clinical practice. Clin Psychopharmacol 1990;5[suppl 2]

ISBN 0-7216-4215-2

90038

9 780721 642154